Respiratory Disease in Children

Diagnosis and Management

Respiratory Disease in Children

Diagnosis and Management

Edited by

GERALD M. LOUGHLIN, M.D.

Associate Professor
Department of Pediatrics
The Johns Hopkins University School of Medicine
Director, Eudowood Division of Pediatric Respiratory Sciences
Baltimore, Maryland

HOWARD EIGEN, M.D.

Professor
Department of Pediatrics
Indiana University School of Medicine
Director, Section of Pulmonary and Intensive Care
Associate Chairman for Clinical Affairs
James Whitcomb Riley Hospital for Children
Indianapolis, Indiana

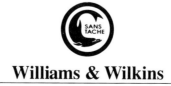

Williams & Wilkins

BALTIMORE • PHILADELPHIA • HONG KONG
LONDON • MUNICH • SYDNEY • TOKYO

A WAVERLY COMPANY

Editor: Jonathan C. Pine, Jr.
Managing Editor: Molly L. Mullen
Copy Editor: John M. Daniel
Designer: Norman W. Och
Illustration Planner: Ray Lowman
Production Coordinator: Kimberly M. Nawrozki

Copyright © 1994
Williams & Wilkins
428 East Preston Street
Baltimore, Maryland 21202, USA

EAST GLAMORGAN GENERAL HOSPITAL
CHURCH VILLAGE. near PONTYPRIDD

Accurate indications, adverse reactions, and dosage schedules for drugs are provided in this book, but it is possible that they may change. The reader is urged to review the package information data of the manufacturers of the medications mentioned.

Printed in the United States of America

Library of Congress Cataloging in Publication Data

Respiratory disease in children: diagnosis and management / edited by Gerald M. Loughlin and Howard Eigen.
    p.   cm.
    Includes index.
    ISBN 0-683-05190-3
    1. Pediatric respiratory diseases.   I. Loughlin, Gerald M.   II. Eigen, Howard.
    [DNLM: 1. Lung Diseases—in infancy & childhood. 2. Lung Diseases—diagnosis. 3. Lung Diseases—therapy.
WS 280 P3663 1994]
RJ431.P38   1994
618.92′2—dc20
DNLM/DLC
for Library of Congress   93-1902
          CIP

93   94   95   96   97
1   2   3   4   5   6   7   8   9   10

To my wife, Barbara, and my daughters, Ceila and Shaye, for their love, support, and patience during preparation of "the book," and to my parents, Mary and Joe, who without benefit of a medical education are superb role models for a physician.

—G.M.L.

To Linda, my wife, and my daughters, Sarah and Lauren, for their unwavering support and love.

—H.E.

Foreword

This textbook, *Respiratory Disease in Children: Diagnosis and Management*, comes as the field of pediatric pulmonology passes into the hands of a second generation of lung specialists. It is the first and only American textbook of substance that has been conceptualized and edited by formally trained pulmonologists. The pulmonary generation prior to theirs was for the most part necessarily sui generis, which says a great deal about the newness of the field.

Drs. Loughlin and Eigen now head their own broadly based divisions of pediatric pulmonology at the Johns Hopkins University and Indiana University, respectively. Both have made major contributions to the pulmonary field through clinical research and the development of innovative teaching methods. Through the years they have come to know the leaders in their field throughout the world. They have their own pulmonary fellows who, over a 3-year period, must digest an increasingly diverse body of knowledge, master skills that didn't exist a few years ago, and conduct basic and clinical research. These fellows will then be eligible to take examinations prepared by the American Board of Pediatrics' Subboard of Pediatric Pulmonology, which awarded its first certificates in 1981.

In addition, Drs. Loughlin and Eigen are in daily contact with medical students, pediatric house officers, and practitioners in the field who refer problem patients to them for diagnosis and management. Each of these groups presents its own challenge to the teacher, and each must be given information appropriate to its level of knowledge and expertise.

It is this background that positions Drs. Loughlin and Eigen ideally to (1) create a list of topics concerning pediatric pulmonology that practitioners should know about, (2) match those vital topics with experts, including themselves, and (3) edit the whole artfully, in a logical and apparently seamless way.

This is an unashamedly clinical text aimed pointblank at the practitioner facing the problems of children with lung problems that threaten lives or that at least won't go away. Carefully read and acted on, this book will lead to fewer such unsolvable challenges to pediatricians.

WILLIAM W. WARING, M.D.
Jane B. Aron Professor of Pediatrics
Department of Pediatrics
Section of Pulmonary Diseases
Tulane University School of Medicine
New Orleans, Louisiana

Preface

This book had its genesis in the problems faced in the clinical practice of pulmonology. Questions arise as to what to do, when to do it, and why. Clinical medicine is not neatly compartmentalized by sections and diseases. Patients come to us with a set of symptoms and complaints that are troublesome to them and confusing to us as physicians. Our job, based on our knowledge of the pathophysiology and the complaints brought to us, is to diagnose and treat the patient and family.

The book was thought of as one that would be practical and helpful to the practitioner while not forgetting the need to establish medical scientific underpinnings for decisions both diagnostic and therapeutic. We wanted a book that gave the reader perspective of what is done by a group of expert clinicians, and so the recommendations for diagnosis and management are modified by our clinical experience over the past 15–20 years. It represents how the contributors to this book practice pediatric pulmonology. We want to impart these clinical tips to the reader to use where the science of medicine must be combined with the art of medicine and common sense.

Since the process of development has important influences on the pathogenesis and natural history of lung disease in children, the first section is devoted to discussion of how growth and development affect the respiratory system. We then update applications of the diagnostic tools used in evaluating children with respiratory disease. The next three sections focus on clinical problems, first as unknowns (i.e., how the child presents to us as clinicians), then as specific respiratory diseases, and finally as respiratory aspects of non-pulmonary diseases. These sections represent our contributors' best knowledge on specific diseases and conditions so that once the diagnosis is made the reader can answer specific questions. The final section reviews the rationale behind modern respiratory care with an introductory chapter on how to evaluate the results of clinical trials.

We have tried to establish an even style that is useful, concise, and clear. We have intentionally omitted less common topics that could have been added for the sake of completeness and instead have focused on practicality.

The preparation of this book has involved many people. We thank the contributors for giving of their time, knowledge, and experience to help us make a useful book.

We acknowledge Lolita Goens, Kathie Bukowski and Mary Stainback for their great help in preparing the manuscripts of each chapter and coordinating this effort.

GERALD M. LOUGHLIN
HOWARD EIGEN

Contributors

Frank J. Accurso, M.D.
Associate Professor
Department of Pediatrics
University of Colorado School of Medicine
Denver, Colorado

Veda L. Ackerman, M.D.
Assistant Professor
Department of Pediatrics
Indiana University School of Medicine
James Whitcomb Riley Hospital for Children
Indianapolis, Indiana

Max M. April, M.D.
Assistant Professor
Department of Surgery and Pediatrics
State University of New York at Stony Brook
Stony Brook, New York

Steven T. Baldwin, M.D.
Fellow, Pediatric Critical Care Medicine
Department of Pediatrics
University of Alabama at Birmingham
Birmingham, Alabama

Diane L. Barsky, M.D., F.A.A.C.P., F.A.C.N.
Attending Physician
Divisions of General Pediatrics and
    Gastroenterology & Nutrition
Children's Hospital of Philadelphia
Philadelphia, Pennsylvania

C. Michael Bowman, Ph.D., M.D.
Associate Professor
Department of Pediatrics
University of Southern California
Los Angeles, California

John G. Brooks, M.D.
Professor
Department of Pediatrics
Chief, Pediatric Pulmonary Medicine
University of Rochester School of Medicine and
    Dentistry
Rochester, New York

Susan M. Brugman, M.D.
Assistant Professor
Department of Pediatrics
University of Colorado Health Sciences Center
Staff Physician
Department of Pediatrics & Pediatric Pulmonology
National Jewish Center for Immunology and
    Respiratory Medicine
Denver, Colorado

Preston W. Campbell III, M.D.
Assistant Professor
Department of Pediatrics
Vanderbilt University School of Medicine
Medical Director, Cystic Fibrosis Center
Nashville, Tennessee

Gerard J. Canny, M.D., B.C.H., F.R.C.P.(C), F.C.C.P.
Associate Professor
Department of Pediatrics
Faculty of Medicine
University of Toronto
Pediatric Pulmonologist
The Hospital for Sick Children
Toronto, Ontario
Canada

John L. Carroll, M.D.
Assistant Professor
Department of Pediatrics
The Johns Hopkins University School of Medicine
Director, Infant Apnea Program
Baltimore, Maryland

Michelle M. Cloutier, M.D.
Professor
Department of Pediatrics
University of Connecticut Health Center
Farmington, Connecticut

Allan L. Coates, M.D., C.M.
Professor
Department of Pediatric Respiratory Medicine
McGill University School of Medicine
Director, Respiratory Medicine
The Montreal Children's Hospital
Montreal, Quebec
Canada

Karen L. Daigle, M.D.
Assistant Professor
Department of Pediatrics
University of Connecticut Health Center
Farmington, Connecticut

Sally L. Davidson-Ward, M.D.
Associate Professor
Division of Neonatology and Pediatric
    Pulmonology
University of Southern California School of
    Medicine
Childrens Hospital Los Angeles
Los Angeles, California

G. Michael Davis, M.B., Ch.B.
Assistant Professor
Department of Pediatrics
McGill University School of Medicine
Montreal, Quebec
Canada

Henry L. Dorkin, M.D.
Associate Professor of Pediatrics
Tufts University School of Medicine
Chief, Pediatric Pulmonology & Allergy Division
Director, Cystic Fibrosis Center
New England Medical Center
Boston, Massachusetts

Howard Eigen, M.D.
Professor
Department of Pediatrics
Indiana University School of Medicine
Director, Section of Pulmonology and Intensive
    Care
Associate Chairman for Clinical Affairs
James Whitcomb Riley Hospital for Children
Indianapolis, Indiana

Leland L. Fan, M.D.
Professor
Department of Pediatrics
University of Colorado School of Medicine
National Jewish Center for Immunology and
    Respiratory Medicine
Denver, Colorado

Elizabeth Farrington, Pharm.D.
Assistant Professor of Clinical Pharmacy
Department of Pharmacy Practice
Purdue University
West Lafayette, Indiana

Alvin H. Felman, M.D.
Clinical Professor
Department of Radiology and Pediatrics
University of South Florida College of Medicine
Staff Radiologist
Tampa General Hospital
Tampa, Florida

J. Julio Perez Fontan, M.D.
Associate Professor
Department of Pediatrics
Washington University
Director, Division of Critical Care Medicine and
    Pediatric Intensive Care Unit
St. Louis, Missouri

Claude Gaultier, M.D., Ph.D.
Professor
Department of Physiology
Hopital Antoine Beclere
Clamart, France

Deborah C. Givan, M.D.
Associate Professor
Department of Pediatrics
Indiana University School of Medicine
Indianapolis, Indiana

J. Roger Hollister, M.D.
Professor
Department of Pediatrics
University of Colorado School of Medicine
The Children's Hospital
Denver, Colorado

Bonnie B. Hudak, M.D.
Assistant Professor
Department of Pediatrics
State University of New York at Buffalo
Buffalo, New York

J. Heyward Hull, Pharm.D., M.S.
Clinical Professor
Division of Pharmacy Practice
University of North Carolina School of Pharmacy
Chapel Hill, North Carolina
Director, Cardiovascular Medicine
Burroughs Wellcome Company
Research Triangle Park, North Carolina

Laura S. Inselman, M.D.
Associate Professor
Department of Pediatrics
Jefferson Medical College of Thomas Jefferson
    University
Philadelphia, Pennsylvania
Associate Pulmonologist
Medical Director
Respiratory Care Department and Pulmonary
    Function Laboratory
Attending Physician, A.I. du Pont Institute
Wilmington, Delaware

Richard F. Jacobs, M.D., F.A.A.P.
Horace C. Cabe Professor
Department of Pediatrics
University of Arkansas for Medical Sciences
Arkansas Children's Hospital
Little Rock, Arkansas

Meyer Kattan, M.D., C.M.
Professor
Department of Pediatrics
Mount Sinai School of Medicine
New York, New York

Thomas G. Keens, M.D.
Professor
Department of Pediatrics
University of Southern California School of
    Medicine
Associate Division Head for Pediatric Pulmonology
Division of Neonatology & Pediatric Pulmonology,
    Childrens Hospital of Los Angeles
Los Angeles, California

Louis I. Landau, M.D., F.R.A.C.P.
Professor
Department of Pediatrics
The University of Western Australia
Perth, Western Australia
Australia

Gary L. Larsen, M.D.
Professor
Department of Pediatrics
University of Colorado School of Medicine
Chief, Division of Pediatric Pulmonary Medicine
National Jewish Center for Immunology and
    Respiratory Medicine
Denver, Colorado

Beth L. Laube, Ph.D.
Assistant Professor
Environmental Health Sciences
The Johns Hopkins University School of Hygiene
    and Public Health
Baltimore, Maryland

Henry Levison, M.D., F.R.C.P.(C)
Professor
Department of Pediatrics
Faculty of Medicine
University of Toronto
Head, Chest Division
The Hospital for Sick Children
Toronto, Ontario
Canada

George Lister, M.D.
Professor
Department of Pediatrics and Anesthesiology
Yale University School of Medicine
New Haven, Connecticut

Gerald M. Loughlin, M.D.
Associate Professor
Department of Pediatrics
The Johns Hopkins University School of Medicine
Director, Eudowood Division of Pediatric
    Respiratory Sciences
Baltimore, Maryland

Jeffrey D. Macke, M.D.
Lecturer
Department of Pediatrics
Indiana University School of Medicine
Indianapolis, Indiana

Carole L. Marcus, M.B.B.Ch.
Assistant Professor
Department of Pediatrics
The Johns Hopkins University School of Medicine
Medical Director, Pediatric Sleep Laboratory
Baltimore, Maryland

Bernard R. Marsh, M.D.
Professor
Department of Otolaryngology, Head & Neck
    Surgery
The Johns Hopkins University School of Medicine
Baltimore, Maryland

Bruce H. Matt, M.D., M.S. (otol)
Assistant Professor
Department of Otolaryngology, Head & Neck
    Surgery
Indiana University School of Medicine
Indianapolis, Indiana

Maggie McIlwaine, M.C.S.P., P.T., C.P.A.
Clinical Coordinator
Medical Surgical & Orthopedics
Physiotherapy Department
British Columbia Children's Hospital
Vancouver, British Columbia
Canada

David F. Merten, M.D.
Professor
Department of Radiology and Pediatrics
University of North Carolina School of Medicine
Chapel Hill, North Carolina

Esther L. Moe, Ph.D.
Research Associate
Department of Pediatrics
Oregon Health Sciences University
Portland, Oregon

Ian Nathanson, M.D.
Chairman
Department of Pediatrics
Nemours Children's Clinic
Jacksonville, Florida

Christopher J.L. Newth, M.B., F.R.C.P.(C)
Professor
Department of Pediatrics
University of Southern California School of
    Medicine
Director
Division of Pediatric Intensive Care
Childrens Hospital of Los Angeles
Los Angeles, California

Bruce G. Nickerson, M.D.
Director, Respiratory Services
Pulmonary-Critical Care
Children's Hospital of Orange County
Orange, California

David M. Orenstein, M.D.
Professor
Department of Pediatrics
Department of Health, Physical & Recreational
    Education
School of Education
University of Pittsburgh School of Medicine
Pittsburgh, Pennsylvania

Susan R. Orenstein, M.D.
Associate Professor
Department of Pediatrics
University of Pittsburgh School of Medicine
Children's Hospital of Pittsburgh
Pittsburgh, Pennsylvania

Edward N. Pattishall, M.D., M.P.H.
Associate Director
Cardiopulmonary Medicine
Burroughs Wellcome Company
Research Triangle Park, North Carolina

Wayne R. Rackoff, M.D.
Assistant Professor
Department of Pediatrics
Indiana University School of Medicine
Indianapolis, Indiana

Gregory J. Redding, M.D.
Associate Professor
Department of Pediatrics
University of Washington School of Medicine
Head, Pulmonary Medicine Section
Children's Hospital and Medical Center
Seattle, Washington

Carolyn Lynn Rosen, M.D.
Assistant Professor
Department of Pediatrics
Yale University School of Medicine
New Haven, Connecticut

Beryl J. Rosenstein, M.D.
Professor
Department of Pediatrics
The Johns Hopkins University School of Medicine
Baltimore, Maryland

James A. Royall, M.D.
Assistant Professor
Department of Pediatrics
University of Alabama at Birmingham
Birmingham, Alabama

Paul S. Salva, M.D., Ph.D.
Fellow in Pediatric Pulmonology
Department of Pediatrics
Indiana University School of Medicine
Indianapolis, Indiana

Gordon E. Schutze, M.D.
Assistant Professor
Department of Pediatrics and Pathology
University of Arkansas for Medical Sciences
Arkansas Children's Hospital
Little Rock, Arkansas

Yakov Sivan, M.D.
Director
Pediatric Intensive Care Unit
Dana Children's Hospital
Tel-Aviv Medical Center
Tel-Aviv University
Sackler School of Medicine
Tel-Aviv, Israel

Mark Splaingard, M.D.
Associate Professor
Department of Physical Medicine and
    Rehabilitation/Pediatrics
Medical College of Wisconsin
Director, Pediatric Rehabilitation Cystic Fibrosis
    Clinic
Children's Hospital of Wisconsin
Milwaukee, Wisconsin

Virginia A. Stallings, M.D.
Associate Professor
Department of Pediatrics
University of Pennsylvania School of Medicine
Philadelphia, Pennsylvania

Arlene A. Stecenko, M.D.
Associate Professor
Department of Medicine
Vanderbilt University School of Medicine
Nashville, Tennessee

Paul C. Stillwell, M.D.
Director, Pediatric Pulmonology
Department of Pediatrics and Pulmonology
Cleveland Clinic Foundation
Cleveland, Ohio

Dennis C. Stokes, M.D.
Associate Professor
Department of Pediatrics
Division of Pediatric Pulmonary Medicine
Vanderbilt University School of Medicine
Clinical Director
Co-Director Cystic Fibrosis Center
Nashville, Tennessee

Derek A. Uchida, M.D.
Assistant Professor
Department of Pediatrics
University of South Alabama College of Medicine
Director, Division of Pediatric Pulmonary
    Medicine
Mobile, Alabama

Mary H. Wagner, M.D.
Assistant Professor
Department of Pediatrics
University of Florida School of Medicine
Gainesville, Florida

Michael A. Wall, M.D.
Professor
Department of Pediatrics
Oregon Health Sciences University
Chief, Pediatric Pulmonary and Critical Care
    Division
Portland, Oregon

Robert M. Weetman, M.D.
Professor
Department of Pediatrics
Indiana University School of Medicine
Indianapolis, Indiana

David F. Westenkirchner, M.D.
Clinical Associate Professor
Department of Pediatrics
Indiana University School of Medicine
Indianapolis, Indiana

Harry Wilson, M.D.
Staff Pathologist
The Children's Hospital
Denver, Colorado

Glenna B. Winnie, M.D.
Associate Professor
Department of Pediatrics
Albany Medical College
Head, Section of Pediatric Pulmonary
Albany, New York

Robert E. Wood, Ph.D., M.D.
Professor
Department of Pediatrics
University of North Carolina
Chapel Hill, North Carolina

Mervin C. Yoder, M.D.
Associate Professor
Department of Pediatrics
Indiana University School of Medicine
Indianapolis, Indiana

Jean H. Zander, R.N., M.S.N.
Pediatric Pulmonary Nurse Specialist
Staff Nurse, Pediatric Intensive Care Unit
James Whitcomb Riley Hospital for Children
Indianapolis, Indiana

Pamela L. Zeitlin, M.D., Ph.D.
Assistant Professor
Department of Pediatrics
The Johns Hopkins University School of Medicine
Baltimore, Maryland

Raezelle Zinman, M.D.C.M., F.R.C.P.(c)
Associate Professor
Department of Pediatrics
Dalhousie University Faculty of Medicine
Izzak Walton Killam Hospital for Children
Halifax, Nova Scotia
Canada

Contents

SECTION I

MATURATION OF THE RESPIRATORY SYSTEM: IMPLICATIONS FOR DISEASE

SECTION II

DIAGNOSTIC TECHNIQUES

SECTION III

APPROACH TO THE PATIENT WITH PULMONARY DISEASE

SECTION IV

COMMON PULMONARY DISEASES

SECTION VI
PRINCIPLES OF THERAPY

MATURATION OF THE RESPIRATORY SYSTEM: IMPLICATIONS FOR DISEASE

1

Maturation of Airway Mechanics

G. MICHAEL DAVIS AND ALLAN L. COATES

GROWTH OF THE LUNG

The mechanical function of the respiratory system is constantly undergoing maturational changes from infancy throughout childhood, and approximates that of the normal adult only after puberty. The embryologic development of the respiratory system begins from an outpouching of the primitive foregut at the 23 somite stage (approximately 26 days post conception). This blind pouch enlarges and bifurcates almost dichotomously to develop the asymmetric organization of the respiratory system. Weibel has demonstrated that symmetry or asymmetry in bifurcation of the lung structures does not materially alter the properties of the organ (1). Furthermore, replication of the airway structures continues throughout early fetal development, requiring amniotic fluid and, perhaps, the micro-pressure fluctuations produced by maternal blood pressure waves (2). At the same time there is caudal migration of all these structures, including the diaphragm, which itself originates as part of the third through fifth somites.

Following the completion of organogenesis at the thirteenth week of gestation, the development of the airways continues by extension of chords of cells into the loose parenchymal tissue. All 23 generations of the conducting airway precursors, both bronchi and bronchioles, are fully developed by 23-24 weeks of gestation. The canalization of these chords of epithelial cells occurs from about 18 weeks onwards and requires the presence of amniotic fluid (2). From this point in gestation there is progressive development of the future air-containing saccules, the precursors of alveoli, at the terminal end of the conducting airways. This process of alveolization is an integral constituent of the increase in surface area required for effective gas exchange. Alveolization begins with progressive flattening of the cuboidal epithelium, loss of the loose parenchymal tissue, and progressive approximation of blood vessels into more intimate contact with the epithelium. Finally, the basement membrane of the vascular endothelium fuses with that of the future alveolar epithelium. This relationship of the future gas-containing area to the vasculature is key to the subsequent extra utero viability of the fetus. As a generalization, this key developmental process of alveolization commences somewhere between 22 and 24 weeks of gestation.

The critical final step, starting around 30-34 weeks gestation, is the development and activation of the enzyme systems in the type II pneumocyte. These systems begin to produce and recirculate large amounts of a surface tension reducing substance, surfactant. The development of this system is enhanced by various hormones (corticosteroids, thyroixne) and may be delayed by certain maternal conditions such as diabetes (3). Surfactant has the unique property of reducing the surface tension in the alveolus, and sustains this ability over a wide range of surface areas. The practical implication of this is that, as the radius of an alveolus decreases, by Laplace's law, surface forces should increase; in the presence of surfactant, however, surface tension is reduced. The result is that large and small alveoli can coexist without the small collapsing into the large, which is what would be expected based on the Laplace relationship. This process of enzymatic maturation occurs in response to a paracrine secretion by the adjacent fibroblasts, *fibroblast-pneumocyte-factor* (FPF).

Throughout this process of canalization and alveolization of the lung, and most markedly in the last trimester of pregnancy (28-40 weeks gestation), the fetus makes rhythmic respiratory muscle efforts. These respiratory movements do not produce gas exchange in utero but, teleologically, they may represent training of respiratory muscles for postnatal function, along with the additive influence of the chest wall movement on lung growth. Animal studies would suggest that fetal respiratory movements may be present as much as 40% of the time. The reason for these bursts of respiratory movement is not clearly understood; nor are the factors that influence the frequency, depth, and periodicity of these bursts of central respiratory activity.

For the normal infant, birth should be considered a transient interruption of this maturational process. Following birth, the intrauterine stimulus to growth through micro-pressure fluctuations is replaced by the rhythmic stretching and relaxation of normal ventilatory movement in an air milieu, producing continued lung growth. A healthy, full-term infant has approximately 4×10^7 alveoli, a number that rapidly increases during the years of early growth to approximately 20×10^7 by 2 years. The adult number of alveoli, 40-80×10^7, is usually achieved by 8 years of age, with subsequent growth of the lung being mostly attributable to an increase in size of existing structures (4).

The growth of the central airways is not proportionally comparable to the growth of the rest of the lung (5). The trachea increases four times in diameter but only doubles in length, whereas the smaller airways increase less in diameter. More importantly, bronchial wall cartilage, which is present in small amounts at birth, increases over the first 4 years of life, adding to the structural rigidity of the airway.

TRANSITION TO AIR BREATHING

In utero, the fluid-filled lungs play no role in gas exchange and therefore neither require nor receive the full cardiac output. Oxygenated blood from the placenta bypasses the liver, via the ductus venous, to arrive at the right side of the heart. After partial mixing with systemic venous return, this blood will either pass through the foramen ovale into the left atrium, the left ventricle, and thus to the

aorta; or enter the right ventricle, to the pulmonary artery, through the ductus arteriosus, and into the descending aorta (Fig. 1.1). This results in an intrauterine milieu for the lungs that is very hypoxic, with a Po_2 in the range of 18 mm Hg. This degree of hypoxia results in vascular constriction and a very high pulmonary vascular resistance, effectively limiting pulmonary blood flow, since blood flow preferentially follows the path of least resistance through the ductus arteriosus. Furthermore, there is a very low resistance to flow within the systemic circulation, largely because of the extremely well vascularized placenta.

During the normal birth process, the lungs are compressed in the birth canal, helping to squeeze out the liquid in the airspaces, and the first breath brings air into the lungs with a Po_2 of approximately 150 mm Hg. Pulmonary vascular resistance falls and pulmonary blood flow increases, in part because of the abundance of oxygen, and in part because of mechanical factors. The foramen ovale (a flap valve) closes because the pressure in the left atrium exceeds that in the right as a result of

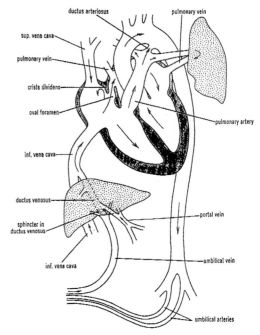

Figure 1.1. Plan of the human circulation before birth. Arrows indicate the direction of the blood flow. (From Langman J. *Medical embryology: Human development—normal and abnormal.* Baltimore, Williams & Wilkins, (1963.)

decreased venous return to the right atrium (the interruption of blood from the placenta) and the increased pulmonary blood flow within the lungs. At the same time, the systemic vascular resistance increases with removal of the placenta from the circuit. Pressures in the pulmonary and systemic circuits tend to remain balanced during the first several hours after birth; then pulmonary artery pressure progressively declines as the pulmonary vascular resistance falls.

The ductus arteriosus, under the influence of higher oxygen tensions, closes first by muscle spasm and then by fibrosis over the course of the next several weeks. This establishes the complete separation of the pulmonary and systemic vascular circuits, placing the lungs in the ideal position to eliminate CO_2 and oxygenate the systemic venous return. The fall of the pulmonary vascular resistance and hence right ventricular and pulmonary arterial pressures to the low levels found in adults takes place over the next several months. This normal progression can be interrupted or arrested by lung disease that results in alveolar hypoxia, or by congenital heart disease with large systemic-pulmonary shunts that give rise to greatly increased pulmonary blood flow.

Chest Wall

For the normal birth process the chest must be very compliant and relatively compressible so that it can pass through the birth canal without either obstructing labor or sustaining damage. This requires a soft chest wall in which much of each individual rib is composed of cartilage rather than bone. Thus, the chest of the newborn infant is susceptible to distortion by the application of forces generated by the muscles used for respiration (6). Chest wall distortion is promoted by both the compliant rib cage and the anterior insertion of the dome-shaped diaphragm into the lower ribs; this insertion is more horizontal than it is in older children. Contraction of the diaphragm during inspiration results in the downward displacement of the dome but, with muscle tension also acting horizontally, the lower ribs may be drawn inwards. This paradoxic inward movement of the chest wall during inspiration results in wasted work by the muscle, and can severely limit tidal volume (V_T).

The configuration of the rib cage changes with maturation, from an almost circular structure at birth to an ellipsoid one by 4 years of age. In concert with this, the angle of insertion of the diaphragm into the ribs changes from almost horizontal to the downward oblique insertion characteristic of the adult form. During the same period of maturation and growth, the cartilaginous rib ends undergo progressive ossification, giving rise to greater rigidity of the chest. The overall result is a more stable chest wall, a progressive increase in the role of the rib cage in ventilation, and the development of the "pump-handle" motion of displacement of the ribs during inspiration. This stability of the chest wall is important to ventilation.

The compliance of the chest wall in unanesthetized newborn infants under relaxed conditions (i.e., no respiratory muscle activity) has been measured as approximately three times that of the lung (7). Thus, for any effective ventilation to occur, the intercostal muscles must act to stiffen the rib cage and prevent paradoxic motion during inspiration. With maturation, and increasing ossification of the cartilage in the ribs and sternum, values of dynamic compliance become similar for both the chest wall and the lungs in both children and adults (Fig. 1.2). At birth, the majority of the muscle mass is type II "fast-twitch" fibers, but these fibers may differ from the adult type, in that they appear to be relatively "fatigue-resistant." Maturational changes in the respiratory musculature occur, with increased mass and a progressive increase in the fatigue-resistant type I muscle fibers, to approach adult values within the first year of life. The role of the intercostal and accessory muscles of respiration in stiffening the rib cage remains important throughout life. Even the relatively stiff rib cage of adults may exhibit paradoxic motion during inspiration if there is no intercostal activity, as may be seen in high cervical cord injuries (8). Inherent in this is the assumption that the lung is working on the steep part of its pressure-volume curve where small changes in pleural pressure give rise to a large V_T (Fig. 1.3). Furthermore, the resistance to airflow, which in health tends to be much less important than the elastic forces of the lung, is relatively small. The V_T resulting from the changes in the pleural pressure (Ppl) is sufficiently large that the wasted ventilation

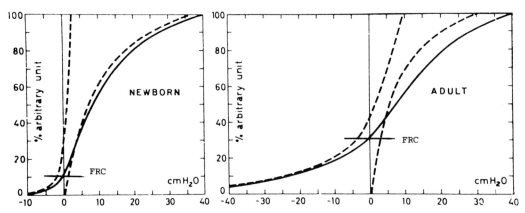

Figure 1.2. Schematic diagrams to illustrate the difference between the pressure-volume (P-V) curve of the respiratory systems in the newborn (within the 1st week of life) and the adult. The volume scale on the ordinate is expressed in arbitrary units, the lower limit at 0 pressure in the lung. In both diagrams the broken line to the left represents the thorax; the one to the right, the lung; and the solid line, the total respiratory system. Horizontal lines represent the FRC at which the elastic pressures of the thorax and the lung balance each other. (From Thibeault DW, Gregory GA, eds. *Neonatal pulmonary care,* ed 2. Norwalk, CT, Appleton-Century-Crofts, 1986.)

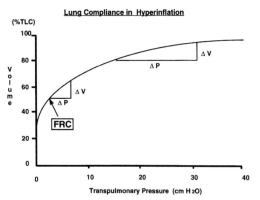

Figure 1.3. The pressure-volume (P-V) curve of the lung. At FRC, small changes in pleural pressure (ΔP) during inspiration give rise to relatively large changes in volume (ΔV), which represent tidal volume. During hyperinflation, the inspiration commences at a relatively flat part of the P-V curve, so large changes in pressure are required but the resulting tidal volume is low.

of the physiologic dead space (V_D) is relatively small, and therefore the breathing frequency (f_B) may be quite low.

MATURATION OF NORMAL BREATHING

The mechanisms responsible for the initial postnatal respiratory effort are not clear. It is apparent, however, that external stimuli are an important element of the first respiratory effort. A combination of chemical stimuli— the Pa_{O_2} and the Pa_{CO_2} tensions—along with external noxious stimuli such as temperature

and gravity result in a massive inspiratory effort. This initial effort has been documented to be in excess of -60 cm H_2O, resulting in a large pressure gradient between the airway and the alveolus. This overcomes the high surface forces of the fluid-filled alveoli, creating an air-liquid interface, and allowing for inspiratory gas flow. This initial distension of the lung results in the establishment of a residual volume of gas within the lung, optimizing the pressure-volume relationship.

LUNG VOLUMES

Functional Residual Capacity

Functional residual capacity (FRC) is that lung volume at which the inward recoil of the lung is balanced by the outward recoil of the chest wall (Fig. 1.4). At low lung volumes, near FRC and lower, the major contributor to elastic recoil of the lung is the surface tension at the air-liquid interface in the alveoli. At lung volumes above FRC, the elastic recoil is increasingly determined by the collagen matrix of the lungs. Elasticity happens in two ways: the first is the elastic recoil pressure or the pressure generated by the lungs or respiratory system when it is held at a volume different from the relaxed volume; the second is compliance, the volume change that results from a given change in the elastic recoil pressure.

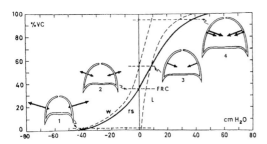

Figure 1.4. Static pressure-volume (P-V) curves of the lung (L), chest wall (W), and total respiratory system (rs). Static forces of the lung and chest wall are indicated by arrows (dimensions not in scale) in the side drawings. The volume at which pressures of the lung and chest wall balance each other is the FRC, indicated by the horizontal line corresponding to drawing 2. If lung compliance decreases, curve L becomes flatter, and the volume at which pressures are balanced (FRC) decreases. If lung compliance increases, curve L becomes steeper and FRC increases. (From Thibeault DW, Gregory GA, eds. *Neonatal pulmonary care,* ed 2. Norwalk, CT, Appleton-Century-Crofts, 1986.)

Although FRC is determined by the balance between these opposing forces in the healthy child and adult, the FRC (at the relaxation point) in the newborn is disproportionately small, on a per kilogram basis. (Fig. 1.2), and may be too small to allow for optimal gas exchange. What has been appreciated only relatively recently is the occurrence of modulation of passive expiration in infants to delay emptying of the lung (9). The newborn employs two different strategies to retard expiration, thus increasing the volume of gas in the lung at the end of expiration: laryngeal narrowing by partial vocal chord closure, and contraction of the inspiratory muscles before expiration is complete (i.e., before reaching the volume of relaxation). This creates an end expiratory volume that is greater than the "true" or relaxed FRC (10). Depending on the circumstances, both mechanisms come into play, but in the absence of lung diseases, the latter is the more important. The classic example of laryngeal modulation of expiration is the expiratory grunting of a premature baby with respiratory distress syndrome, but neither grunting nor laryngeal narrowing during expiration are unique to premature babies and, in one form or another, may be present throughout all ages. Older children and adults may also modulate expiration, usually by the persistence of inspiratory muscle activity during the first part of expiration. As in the neo-

nate, this increases the intrathoracic volume available for gas exchange during the expiratory phase of the respiratory cycle. This "dynamic establishment of FRC" is normal in neonates but, in older children, the end expiratory volume tends to be the relaxed FRC.

During normal quiet breathing, expiration is considered a passive event. This passive expiratory pressure gradient represents a combination of the static elastic recoil pressure of the lung and the recoil of the chest wall structures toward FRC. In response to stress and increased ventilatory needs, this expiratory pressure gradient may be augmented by active contraction of the expiratory muscles, especially the anterior abdominal wall muscles, to produce an increased expiratory airflow.

Ventilation

Ventilation, the movement of gas in and out of the respiratory system, depends on pressure gradients generated by the respiratory muscles acting on the chest wall and thus indirectly on the elastic recoil of the lung. The coordinated contraction of the inspiratory muscles—the diaphragm and the intercostal and accessory muscles—act to produce a negative pressure at the pleural border of the lung that is dispersed evenly over the pleural surface by the interdependence of the parietal and visceral pleura. This causes a pressure gradient between the alveolus (P_{alv}) and the airway opening (P_{ao}) at the mouth, resulting in gas flow down the pressure gradient and an increase in lung volume from FRC.

The walls of the intrapulmonary airways are tethered to the parenchyma of the lung. The negative intrapleural pressure on inspiration, because of this tethering, causes a pressure gradient across the airway wall, resulting in an increase in the diameter of the airways and facilitating airflow. This pressure gradient applies to the intrathoracic portion of the airway exposed to subatmospheric pressure. Conversely, the extrathoracic airway, which is exposed to a positive pressure from the surrounding tissues, narrows when the intraluminal pressures become subatmospheric. During passive expiration, the elastic recoil must generate a positive alveolar pressure to produce airflow. During forced expiration, when the expiratory driving pressure is the elastic recoil pressure (P_{el} + Ppl), there is dissipation of the driving pressure down the airway due to frictional losses. The Ppl may become positive relative to the pressure in the lumen of the airway, which promotes narrowing of malleable airways, particularly the small airways in the distal portion of the lung since they are without cartilaginous support. In the extrathoracic airway, where the intraluminal pressure is positive relative to the surrounding tissues, the diameter of the airway is enlarged. In pathologic conditions the extrathoracic airway may narrow during inspiration, leading to inspiratory stridor, and the intrathoracic airways may narrow during expiration, leading to expiratory rhonchi.

AIRWAY FLOW CHARACTERISTICS

Airflow is governed by a combination of pressure gradients and the physical characteristics of the conducting airways. The cross-sectional area is one of the major determining factors of the site of maximal airflow resistance within the respiratory tract. The branching network of the respiratory conducting airways results in a progressively greater number of smaller structures, arranged in parallel. This makes the total cross-sectional area of the airways multiply logarithmically in the periphery of the lung. Moreover, the smallest cross-sectional area of the airways, which represents the point of greatest resistance and airflow limitation, occurs at the laryngeal aperture. Since cross-sectional area increases as the site becomes more distal, large changes in the cross-sectional area of the peripheral airways must occur to make significant changes in the resistance to airflow. According to Poiseville's law, *resistance* (R) to laminar airflow through a vessel is defined as follows:

$$R = \frac{8\mu l}{\pi r^4}$$

where μ is the viscosity coefficient of the gas, l is the length of the tube, and r is the radius of the vessel. Because of the relationship between resistance and the fourth power of the radius, the small child is particularly susceptible to diseases that cause narrowing of the upper airway. For example, viral laryngitis gives rise mainly to hoarseness in the adult but to significant obstruction (stridor in infants).

The behavior of the moving column of gas within the conducting airway also varies with changes in velocity. It is evident that a given mass of gas passing through a region of airway constriction must have a greater velocity than that required in a larger diameter airway. Airflow occurs in three forms: laminar, turbulent, and transitional. Laminar airflow occurs principally in small airways where velocity is low and is more influenced by viscosity than by gas density. At the point of airway branching, where there is a rapid change in aperture, laminar flow may become turbulent. Turbulent airflow, which occurs principally in the central airways, is density-dependent, and may have a functional role in causing gas mixing. With laminar flow, only gas at the edge of the airway touches the airway wall, whereas turbulent patterns present the maximal mass of gas to the mucus blanket lining the large airways. The turbulent state facilitates filtration of inhaled particulate matter by leaving it trapped in mucus for subsequent clearance by the ciliary mechanism.

The relative size of the airways distal to the terminal bronchiole does not differ significantly between infancy and adulthood, the minimal size probably being limited by the effect of small radii on surface forces (Laplace's law). On the other hand, the size of the proximal airways varies greatly so that the transition from laminar to turbulent flow may happen in airways of very different generations in infants compared to adults.

RESPONSE TO STRESS

In the normal adult, the changes in Ppl during spontaneous ventilation are relatively small (approximately 8–10 cm H_2O, but are sufficient to generate adequate tidal volumes effortlessly and, coupled with a low breathing frequency, ensure adequate gas exchange at rest. Adequate gas exchange is defined as a minute ventilation ($\dot{V}_E$) sufficient to eliminate the mass of CO_2 produced by the metabolic activity of the body. In other words,

$$\dot{V}_{CO_2} = V_T \cdot f_B \cdot F_E{CO_2}$$

where $\dot{V}_{CO_2}$ is the production of CO_2 in liters per minute, f_B is the breathing frequency, and $F_E{CO_2}$ is the mixed expired concentration of CO_2. The $F_E{CO_2}$, or more properly the end-tidal carbon dioxide tension ($P_{et}CO_2$), can also be used as a reflection of the level of arterial partial pressure of CO_2 ($PaCO_2$).

In disease or during exercise, all of these parameters will change in an attempt to maintain a normal $PaCO_2$ and PaO_2. The greater sensitivity of the respiratory centers to PCO_2 means that PCO_2 rather than PO_2 tends to dominate the normal ventilatory response to exercise. During exercise at high altitude, however, hypoxia is the principal threat, and PO_2 dominates the response. The respiratory center's response to hypoxia is weak at birth but, as PO_2 increases with extrauterine life, it becomes progressively stronger during the first few months of life. If the PaO_2 does not increase significantly after birth (e.g., with cyanotic congenital heart disease), the hypoxic response remains blunted until corrective surgery raises the PaO_2.

The ventilatory response to increased respiratory drive occurs by two different mechanisms. Firstly, there is an increase in f_B, initially by decreasing the time of expiration (T_E) and subsequently by decreasing both T_E and inspiratory time (T_I). The V_T also increases, often very markedly because of an increase in inspiratory flow. The change in the CO_2 produced is linear with the change in f_B, but not with the change in V_T because of the changing fraction of tidal volume wasted in the V_D. Obviously, if the V_D is elevated because of disease, then the efficiency of this part of the response will be impaired proportionately.

Respiratory distress syndrome (RDS) of the newborn is an archetypical representation of lung disease associated with decreased compliance. To sustain gas exchange and to maintain the $PaCO_2$ in the normal range, there is an increased Ppl swing to produce an adequate V_T, along with an increase in f_B. Pardoxically, the increases in the Ppl swing are manifested as increased chest wall retractions and indrawing, thus limiting the efficiency of the respiratory pump. The more severe the disease, the greater the compensatory increases in Ppl that must occur to augment V_T and f_B. This increased respiratory drive must increase the energy expenditure of the respiratory muscles with a concomitant increase in $\dot{V}CO_2$. At some point the compensatory responses in V_T and f_B are insufficient to maintain adequate ventilation such that the $PaCO_2$ begins to rise, and acute respiratory failure supervenes.

Diseases associated with an increase in airway resistance—bronchiolitis being a classic example—are usually associated with a double compromise: an increased resistance and air trapping with hyperinflation of the lung. Under these conditions, larger swings in Ppl are necessary to overcome both the increased airway resistance and the lower compliance of the respiratory system at higher volumes. Increased upper airway resistance (the classic disease is croup) differs from increased lower airway resistance in that there is no associated hyperinflation. Under these conditions, the narrowed upper airway alone accounts for the increased swings in Ppl, such that there are marked retractions and indrawing, tachypnea, and inspiratory stridor.

The normal growth and maturation of the chest wall results in increased rigidity and hence resistance to deformation, undoubtadly offering the older child considerable protection against respiratory muscle fatigue and respiratory failure. Without this stabilizing action, children may have chest wall distortion even during normal quiet breathing (8). In children with neuromuscular diseases, the diaphragm is often relatively spared compared to the intercostal and accessory chest wall muscles, such that despite adequate function of the diaphragm, pradoxic chest wall motion may compromise the respiratory reserve of these children. The presence of pulmonary infection, to which these patients are prone because of poor cough and impaired mucus clearance mechanisms, can lead to early respiratory failure. The kyphoscoliosis that is often part of the disease further distorts the chest wall and impairs function.

PRINCIPLES OF ASSESSMENT OF LUNG FUNCTION

The basis of lung function testing in adults and older children is the ability to comprehend and follow specific commands. Pulmonary function testing is discussed in detail in chapter 8. The age at which testing can be performed varies with both the complexity of the test and the ability of the child to follow instructions without fear or anxiety. One extreme is neonates, who have no ability to cooperate; the other is enthusiastic, intelligent adolescents who are capable of performing very complicated respiratory maneuvers, with a vast range between the two extremes. Gas dilution FRC determinations have been made on children as young as 3 years, and most children 6 years of age or older can satisfactorily perform a forced vital capacity maneuver, allowing spirometric assessment of pulmonary "acceptable" function. Somewhere in between are children who manage to provide technically acceptable performances of peak expiratory flow assessments. Many children find the cooperation needed for plethysmographic assessment of lung volumes difficult. Part of this problem is difficulty in performing the panting maneuver, which can be overcome by measuring FRC from a single inspiratory effort (11). Nevertheless, it is unusual to have reproducible plethysmographic assessments of lung volumes in children less than 8 years of age.

The newborn infant spends a great deal of time asleep and, while interacting with other humans, does not yet discriminate his caregiver from the person attempting to do pulmonary function testing. This means that, provided the testing procedure is neither overly invasive nor uncomfortable, physiologic assessment of lung function in this age group may be accomplished with relative ease. This is in stark contrast to older infants, in whom the need for sedation for virtually any test is the rule rather than the exception. In part this is because of the natural fear of strangers, but also because the new stimuli to which the child is subjected leads to heightened awareness and activity that changes the respiratory pattern (e.g., crying). The newborn has two strong reflexes that in one instance may hinder, and in the other may facilitate, pulmonary function testing. The trigeminal area of the face is extremely sensitive to touch, and the presence of a face mask frequently results in an avoidance reaction with the infant often crying or turning his head. This makes obtaining a seal with the face mask quite difficult. The presence of respiratory disease and tachypnea appear to strengthen this reflex, thereby complicating the measurements in the very babies in whom it may be most useful. The Hering-Breuer reflex of the newborn is a vagally mediated reflex that is part of the control system of lung volume. It is likely responsible for the initiation of inspiratory activity to bring about the termination of expiration before lung volume reaches the true resting FRC. It also can be used to facilitate the assessment of lung physiology. The Hering-Breuer reflex also plays a role in the termination of inspiration.

The Hering-Breuer reflex tends to diminish with age as breathing becomes more modulated by other activities such as talking. In quiet sleep, however, when respiration tends to be completely automatic, it can be elicited in older children and adults, long after its convenience in respiratory physiologic measurements have disappeared.

Many physiologists consider esophageal pressure measurements invasive; if one uses a smooth-walled catheter, however—liquid-filled, open-ended, or with a balloon—esophageal pressure measurements tend to cause less disturbance to the neonate than the face mask. This is particularly true with the liquid-filled soft feeding tubes which, as well as causing minimal discomfort, tend to give rise to less esophageal spasm than the more irregular surfaces on the balloon catheter system (12). The use of a face mask connected to a pneumotachograph and an esophageal pressure measuring system allows the calculation of lung resistance and compliance. In those infants who are intubated, the difficulties with intolerance of a face mask is completely avoided, greatly facilitating physiologic measurements.

Many investigators have made use of the response of the normal newborn to an airway occlusion at end inspiration. In this situation the Hering-Breuer reflex causes relaxation against the occluded airway with the cessation of all inspiratory muscle activity (13). When the occlusion is released, the subsequent expiration is completely passive and approaches the relaxed FRC as opposed to the "dynamically determined" FRC. From the pressure generated during the relaxation against the occluded airway and the volume and flow characteristics of the subsequent expiration, the respiratory system resistance and compliance can be calculated, as will be described in the chapter on pulmonary function testing.

Spirometry has become so well established in the pulmonary literature because of its value in both prognosis and assessment of treatment of pulmonary disease that many investigators have tried to find some analogous way of evaluating lung function in children too young to cooperate. Although these techniques originally showed great promise, controversy continues concerning the effects of the measurement techniques on the parameters being measured. Since the basis of spirometry is the reproducible forced vital capacity maneuver, investigators generally employ some way of forcing expiration. Motoyama pioneered a technique in which anaesthetized and intubated infants have their lungs inflated to total lung capacity (TLC) by application of a standard positive pressure to the airway (14). Then, suddenly, the pressure is reversed, and a negative pressure is applied to the tube. The subsequent expiratory flow and volume characteristics are then analyzed to assess lung function over the volume range from TLC to residual volume.

A variation of this technique that requires sedation but not intubation has been to wrap the infant in an inflatable jacket and, at the end of a normal inspiration, apply a positive pressure to the jacket giving rise to a forced expiration from end inspiratory volume to a volume near or at residual volume ("baby hugging") (15).

Between the neonatal period, when newborns neither cooperate nor actively resist, and the age of 5 or 6 years, there is a period of life during which pulmonary function is rarely measured successfully. The liberal use of sedation to induce sleep may extend the period of relatively easy testing to 12 or 18 months of age, but toddlers frequently require so much sedation to stop them from actively fighting the procedures that they virtually require anesthesia. This results in a situation wherein the risk of the procedure may outweigh the potential benefits. Developing ways around these difficulties is one of the challenges to clinical respiratory research in the future.

REFERENCES

1. Weibel ER: *Morphometry of the Human Lung.* Heidelberg, Springer-Verlag, 1963.
2. Moessinger AC, Collin MH, Blanc WA, Rey HR, James LS: Oligohydramnios-induced lung hypoplasia: The influence of timing and duration of gestation. *Pediatr Res* 20:951–954, 1986.
3. Post M, VanGolde LMG: Metabolic and developmental aspect of the pulmonary surfactant system. *Biochem Biophys Acta* 947:249–286, 1988.
4. Thurlbeck WM: Postnatal human growth. *Thorax* 37:564–571, 1982.
5. Tepper RS, Morgan WJ, Cota K, et al: Physiologic growth and development of the lung during the first year of life. *Am Rev Respir Dis* 134:513–519, 1986.
6. Fleming PJ, Muller NL, Bryan MH, Bryan AC: The effects of abdominal loading on rib cage distortion in premature infants. *Pediatrics* 64:425–428, 1979.
7. Davis GM, Coates AL, Papageorgiou A, Bureau MA: Direct measurement of static chest wall compliance in animal and human neonates. *J Appl Physiol* 65:1093–1098, 1988.
8. De Troyer A, Heilporn A: Respiratory mechanics in quadriplegia. The respiratory function of the intercostal muscles. *Am Rev Respir Dis* 122:591–600, 1980.
9. Sherry JH, Megirian D: Respiratory EMG activity of the posterior cricoarytenoid cricothyroid and diaphragm muscles during sleep. *Respir Physiol* 39:355–365, 1980.
10. Mortola JP, Milic-Emili J, Noworaj A, Smith B, Fox G, Weeks S: Muscle pressure and flow during expiration of infants. *Am Rev Respir Dis* 129:49–53, 1984.
11. Desmond KJ, Demizio D, Allen P, Beaudry PH, Coates AL: An alternate method for the determination of functional residual capacity in a plethysmograph. *Am Rev Respir Dis* 137:273–276, 1988.
12. Coates AL, Stocks J: Esophageal pressure manometry in human infants. *Pediatr Pulmonol* 11:350–360, 1991.
13. Mortola JP, Saetta M: Measurement of respiratory mechanics in the newborn: A simple approach. *Pediatr Pulmonol* 3:123–130, 1987.
14. Motoyama EK: Pulmonary mechanics during early postnatal years. *Pediatr Res* 11:220–223, 1977.
15. Morgan WJ, Geller DE, Tepper RS, Taussig LM: Partial expiratory flow volume curves in infants and young children. *Pediatr Pulmonol* 5:232–243, 1988.

2

Maturation of Respiratory Control

CLAUDE GAULTIER

The respiratory control system matures functionally after birth. As it develops, this system is vulnerable and somewhat unstable, thus placing infants at risk for respiratory disturbances, especially during sleep. This chapter reviews our present knowledge of the maturation of respiratory control with advancing age. Recognition of these developmental changes is important to the clinician in dealing with a variety of clinical problems, such as apparent life-threatening events, sudden infant death syndrome (SIDS), and the response to respiratory disease. Current knowledge concerns mostly the first months of age and adolescence. There is a paucity of data concerning late infancy and early childhood. I shall review, in turn, data gathered during sleep on ventilatory mechanics including rib cage and upper airways, ventilation and apneas, gas exchange, chemical control of ventilation, and arousals.

VENTILATORY MECHANICS DURING SLEEP

Rib Cage and Abdomen

Changes in the rib cage during growth influence the evolution of respiration during sleep. At birth, the ribs extend almost at right angles from the vertebral column, making the thorax more circular than it is in the adult (1), and mechanically inefficient. In adults, the volume of the rib cage can be increased by elevating the ribs. In infants, the ribs are already elevated, which is why motion of the rib cage during room air breathing contributes little to tidal volume. The contribution of the rib cage to tidal breathing at 1 month of age has been estimated (using calibrated inductance plethysmography) to be 34% during quiet sleep (2). Between 1 and 2 years of age the round infantile form of the thorax changes to the more ovoid adult form. By age 1 year, the contribution of the rib cage to tidal breathing during quiet sleep resembles that seen in adolescents during non–rapid eye movement (NREM) sleep (i.e., approximatively 60% at 1 year) (3).

A high chest wall compliance (C_w) relative to lung compliance (C_L) is characteristic of the newborn mammal (4). In humans, C_w decreased relative to C_L with advancing postnatal age (5, 6). Given that each breath requires 5–10 cm H_2O pressure to expand the lung of a normal infant, chest wall muscles must augment the rigidity of the relatively compliant infant rib cage by tonic contraction. This stabilizes the chest wall, which would otherwise be pulled inwards by diaphragmatic contraction. The compliant rib cage of newborns and infants is easily deformed by a large diaphragmatic effort, or when the stabilizing effect of intercostal muscles is inhibited. This occurs during rapid eye movement (REM) sleep (7, 8) (Fig. 2.1), which accounts for more than 50% of total sleep time in full-term newborns, and is even more prominent in premature infants (9).

During REM sleep, with inhibition of the intercostal muscles, phasic inspiratory diaphragmatic contraction causes the rib cage to move inward rather than to expand (8). Associated with the rib cage distortion observed during REM sleep, general mechanical derangements have been reported: decrease in functional residual capacity (FRC) of variable magnitude compared to quiet sleep (10, 11), increase in the diaphragmatic work of breathing (12), and decrease in transcutaneous partial pressure of O_2 (13).

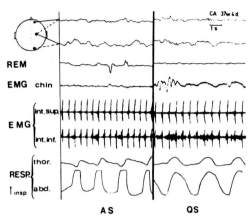

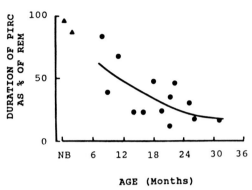

Figure 2.1. Recording in a newborn of 37.5 weeks. From top to bottom: EEG, EOG (REM), EMG chin, and EMG intercostal and diaphragmatic muscles obtained from surface electrodes in the 2nd (intercostal muscles) and 8th intercostal space (diaphragm); thoracic movements and abdominal movements obtained from strain gauges during REM and NREM sleep. In REM sleep, thoracic and abdominal movements are out of phase by 180°. EMG activity disappears at the level of the 2nd intercostal space. In NREM sleep, thoracic and abdominal movements are in phase, and inspiratory EMG activity is present at the 2nd and 8th intercostal spaces. (After Curzi-Dascalova L: Thoraco-abdominal respiratory correlations in infants: Constancy and variability in different sleep states. *Early Hum Dev* 2:25–38, 1978.)

Figure 2.2. PIRC: Pardoxic inspiratory rib cage (PIRC) movements. *Abcissa:* age in months (NB = newborns). *Ordinate*: duration of PIRC expressed as a percentage of REM time; *triangles* = previously published values of PIRC during REM sleep in neonates (7); *full circles*, individual values of PIRC in 13 healthy infants from 7 to 31 months of age. Duration of PIRC decreased significantly with age as a power function ($y = 339 \times {}^{0.84}$) ($r = -0.66$, $p < 0.002$). (After Gaultier CL, Praud JP, Canet E, Delaperche MF, D'Allest AM: Paradoxical inward rib cage motion during rapid eye movement sleep in infants and young children. *J Dev Physiol* 9:391–397, 1987)

The underlying mechanisms causing the fall in FRC during REM sleep in full-term newborns are not fully understood. In newborns there are compelling reasons to believe that because of a low outward recoil of the chest wall, dynamic and expiratory volume is substantially greater than the FRC determined by static passive balance of forces between the lung and chest wall. This is achieved by termination of expiration at substantial flow rates. Mechanisms that actively retard expiration include postinspiratory activity of the diaphragm and laryngeal narrowing. The disappearance of the active laryngeal braking observed in the newborn lamb during REM sleep (14) may partly explain the fall in FRC.

After 6 months of age, because of changes in rib cage geometry and chest wall compliance, the duration of paradoxic rib cage motion during inspiration seen in REM sleep decreases. It becomes rare or absent after 3 years of age (15) (Fig. 2.2). In adolescents no paradoxic movement of the rib cage is observed (3).

Reflexes originating from the lung and the rib cage play a role in respiratory adaptation during sleep. The Hering-Breuer reflex has been studied in human newborns. Its effect is greater during NREM than during REM sleep (16). With advancing age, the strength of the reflex decreases during NREM sleep (17). The rib cage distortion that occurs in newborns may elicit an intercostal phrenic inhibitory reflex that diminishes inspiratory time (T_I) (18). Continuous positive airway pressure diminishes rib cage distortion, and is associated with prolongation of T_I (18).

Lung mechanics have not been compared between states of alertness (awake, NREM sleep, and REM sleep) as has been done in adults (19). It is suggested that during periods of rib cage distortion, esophageal pressure swings do not reflect changes in pleural pressure (20). Tidal changes in esophageal pressure have been measured in healthy children of 2–4 years during both wakefulness and sleep. These changes increased during the course of sleep, particularly during REM sleep (21).

Upper Airways

The configuration of the upper airways changes with growth (22, 23). In the newborn, the upper airways is narrow. The epiglottis is large and can cover the soft palate, forming a low epiglottic sphincter and encouraging the obligatory "nasal breathing" of the newborn. This anatomic configuration is associated with a horizontal position of the tongue, and an elevated position of the hyoid bone and laryngeal cartilage. Over the course of the first 2 years of life, the upper airway anatomy changes, leading to a dynamic velolingual sphincter that permits buccal respiration and speech. The epiglottis, larynx, and hyoid bone move down the posterior portion of the tongue to take a vertical position during infancy. The facial skeleton enlarges vertically, and the mandible lengthens from front to back.

Although nasal breathing is considered obligatory in the newborn and infant, mouth breathing can occur if the nasal passages are obstructed (24–25). Responses vary according to sleep stage: during REM sleep, the response is slowest and weakest (24). As the infant grows older, the response is more rapid (25). Increased resistance of the upper airways secondary to blockage of one nasal orifice restricts ventilation more severely in REM than in NREM sleep (26).

Oropharyngeal dynamics have been studied in the baby during life and at postmortem examination (27–32). The relation between pharyngeal pressure and oropharyngeal patency has undergone postmortem analysis in infants up to 3 months of age (31). Closing pressure is, on average, 0.82 cm H_2O and is generally less than opening pressure. Position of the neck is a significant determinant of oropharynx dynamics (31, 32), and neck flexion is thought to play a role in the occurrence of obstructive apnea (28, 29). Oropharyngeal dynamics during sleep depend on the width of the airway and upper airway muscle function. During inspiration in normal children (33) and some normal premature infants (34), phasic activity of the genioglossus does not occur; when pharyngeal pressure increases, phasic genioglossus activity appears or is augmented (34).

Reflexes originating in the upper airways may elicit apnea in infants. Abnormal conditions (e.g., upper airway infection [35], anemia [36], or hypoxia [37, 38]) may increase the risk of apnea. In newborn animals, introduction of water or other liquids into the larynx leads to apnea (35, 39). In puppies, the duration of apnea elicited by water instillation into the larynx decreases with advancing age (39). In premature infants, reflex apnea has been reported after placing water or saline into the larynx during sleep (40–42). Prolonged apnea in preterm infants may be a pathologic extreme in the normal spectrum of airway protective responses to upper airway fluids (42). In newborn puppies, stimulation of other upper airway receptors, such as mechanoreceptors, by negative pressure causes apnea (43). This phenomenon disappears with age.

VENTILATION AND APNEAS

Studies of the patterns of breathing during sleep in full-term newborns and infants during the first year of life have assessed respiratory frequency, minute ventilation, sighs, apneas, and periodic breathing. Table 1.1 presents mean values of respiratory frequency in full-term newborns during the first 10 days of life (44–48). Total sleep time in these studies varied from 2 to 12 hours. Respiration was measured using thermistors, thoracic impedance, and barometric plethysmography. Ambient temperature varied from 22–24°C to 30°C. In general, respiratory frequency was higher during REM than during NREM sleep. Respiratory frequency decreases in both NREM and REM sleep with advancing postnatal age during the first year of life (44, 47, 49).

During sleep, minute ventilation (V_E) has been measured in full-term newborns during the first days of life using different techniques (Table 2.2) (16, 50–53). Measurements done using a face mask show the highest values because of the effects of stimulation of trigeminal afferents on breathing pattern (54).

Only two studies have reported extensive data on respiratory frequency and V_E in children and adolescents (3, 55). In children, respiratory frequency is lowest during stage 2 NREM sleep and the latter half of the night. Boys and girls have the same respiratory frequency, but girls breathe more regularly. In adolescents, respiratory frequency is highest and most variable during REM sleep and lowest in stage 3 and 4 NREM sleep (3). One study of adolescents has shown that V_E is sleep state dependent, decreasing by a mean of 8% from wakefulness to NREM sleep and increasing by 4% from NREM to REM sleep (3).

Table 2.1.
Mean Respiratory Frequency in Full-Term Newborns During the First 10 Days of Life

Reference	No. of Subjects	Sex	Time	TST (hours)	Method	Ambient Temperature (°C)	Respiratory Frequency REM	Respiratory Frequency NREM
44	4	9F/7M	Day	2	TH	22–24	47 ± 7	41 ± 4
45	22		AM	1–3	TH	25–26	47 ± 9	35 ± 8
46	15			2	Barpl	25	45	39
47	8		Night	12	I	23–25	46	38
48	120	60F	AM, PM	2	TH	30	57, 69	58, 72
		60M					62, 64	61,66

TH: thermistors; *I:* thoracic impedance; *Barpl:* barometric plethysmography.

Table 2.2.
Minute Ventilation and Tidal Volume in Full-Term Newborns and Infants

Reference	Newborns	No. of Subjects	Method		V_T (ml/kg)	V_E (ml/kg/min)
50	10 days of life	14	Barpl	REM	4.8	257[a]
				NREM	4.9	225
51	"	16	"	REM	5.6	299[a]
				NREM	6.3	243
52	"	10	PnN	REM	5	259 ± 19[a]
				NREM	4.9	204 ± 14
16	"	10	PnM	REM	5.2	352 ± 57[a]
				NREM	5.9	293 ± 43
53	Infants 3 months	16	PnN	REM	?	234 ± 85
				NREM	?	211 ± 11

V_T: tidal volume; V_E: minute ventilation; Barpl: barometric plethysmography; PnN: pneumotachograph connected to a nasal mask; PnM: pneumotachograph connected to a facial mask.
[a]Significantly different from NREM sleep.

These changes are caused by changes in respiratory rate, as tidal volume is unaffected by sleep state. The frequency of sighs, defined as respiratory cycles with an amplitude greater than 150% or 200% of the tidal volume of preceding breathing cycles, diminishes with postnatal age (56).

Numerous studies have looked at the frequency or the duration of apneas in newborns and infants. Apneas of short duration (< 10 sec) are common during the neonatal period, occurring more often during REM sleep than during NREM sleep (48, 57–60). During the first 6 months of life, frequency and duration of apneas, and especially of obstructive apneas, decrease (60) (Table 2.3).

The definition of periodic breathing is variable among studies. When periodic breathing is defined as three episodes of apnea lasting longer than 3 sec interrupted by respiration lasting 20 sec or less, the time spent in periodic breathing decreases during the first year of life, as shown in Table 2.4. These data were obtained from full-term infants examined during night sleep at home (61).

Many factors may increase the occurrence of apnea and/or periodic breathing in the neonatal period and during infancy: drug administration to the mother (62) or the infant (63), metabolic disorders (64), anemia (36), upper airway infection (35), hypoxia (65), viral infection (66), gastroesophageal reflux (67, 68), hyperthermia (69), sleep deprivation (70). The influence of three of these factors—administration of meperidine to the mother (62), hyperthermia (69), and sleep deprivation (70)—was significantly greater in active sleep than in quiet sleep.

Compared to the quantity of data gathered during the first months of life, there is little information concerning apneas in late infancy, childhood, and adolescence. Table 2.5 shows the available data for infants (7–54 months) (unpublished personal data), children, and adolescents during sleep (3, 55, 71, 72). Infants were studied during afternoon naps, and children and adolescents were studied during night sleep. In all studies but one (72) sleep states were scored using neurophysiologic criteria. During night sleep, mean total sleep

Table 2.3.
Apnea Index (Number of Apneas per Hour of Total Sleep Time) in Full-Term Infants from 6 wk to 6 mo of age.

Age	> 3–6 Seconds		> 6–10 Seconds		> 10 Seconds	
	C	M-O	C	M-O	C	M-O
3 wks (10)[b]	6.97 ± 2.44	0.31 ± 0.18	2.87 ± 0.45	0.24 ± 0.26	0.73 ± 0.72	0.07 ± 0.09
6 wks (10)	7.10 ± 1.57	0.66 ± 0.66	2.46 ± 1.15	0.38 ± 0.61	0.36 ± 0.66	0.10 ± 0.21
3 mo (9)	6.08 ± 2.28	0.28 ± 0.46	2.18 ± 1.49	0.13 ± 0.13	0.16 ± 0.19	0.02 ± 0.05
4.5 mo (10)	4.80 ± 1.53	0.15 ± 0.21	1.31 ± 0.93	0.07 ± 0.11	0.24 ± 0.32	0.00 ± 0.00
6 mo (9)	4.77 ± 1.35	0.17 ± 0.24	2.34 ± 0.93	0.03 ± 0.05	0.25 ± 0.30	0.00 ± 0.00

b: number of subjects; C: central apnea; M: mixed apnea; O: obstructive apnea.
Adapted from Guilleminault C, et al: Mixed and obstructive sleep apnea and near miss for sudden infant death syndrome.
2. Comparison of near miss and normal control infants by age. *Pediatrics* 64:882–891, 1979.

Table 2.4.
Time Spent in Periodic Breathing as a Percentage of Total Sleep Time

Age	0.0–0.2 wk	2–4 mo	5–6.5 mo	10–12 mo
PB% TST	0.7 ± 0.9 (3.5)[2]	0.4 ± 0.7 (2–4)	0.2 ± 0.2 (0.7)	0.2 ± 0.5 (1.7)

PB: periodic breathing (see text for definition); TST: total sleep time; wk: week; mo: month[a]
the numbers in parentheses indicate maximal values.
Adapted from Kelly DH, et al: Apnea and periodic breathing in normal full-term infants during the first 12 months. *Pediatr Pulmonol* 1:215–219, 1985.

Table 2.5.
Characteristics of Apneas in Healthy Infants after 6 mo of Age, in Children and Adolescents

Reference	No. of Subjects	Age	Duration (sec)	TST	AI	Duration (SEC) Mean	Max	% CA
[a]	14	7–54 mo	> 5	17.2 ± 18.8		6.5 ± 2.5	12	> 90
71	28	2–12 yr	> 5	25 ± 15		8.8 ± 1.3	< 30	100
72	50	1.1–17.4 yr	> 10		0.1 ± 0.5		26	100[b,c]
55	22	9–13 yr	> 5	F: 18.8 ± 8.5 M: 17.2 ± 11.4		< 10 "	25 "	100 "
			> 10	42%	0.4[d]			
3	9	13.5–16.5 yr	> 10	5.5	0.8[d]		24	100

TST: total sleep time; AI: apnea index, number of apneas per hour of TST; CA: central apnea.
[a]Unpublished personal data.
[b]Except in 9 children who had one or more obstructive apneas less than 10 sec.
[c]Central apneas following body movements were not counted.
[d]Estimated from available data.

time varied from 6 hours (72) to 9 hours (55). One study did not count central apneas following body movements (72). In children and adolescents, apneas longer than 5 sec (55, 71) or 10 sec (3) were always central. One study reported obstructive apneas lasting less than 10 sec in 9 children out of 50 (18%). When sleep states were scored, the greatest number of apneas occurred in stage 1 and 2 NREM sleep, followed by occurrence in REM sleep (3, 55, 71). From these data it can be seen that the apnea index (number of apneas per hour lasting longer than 10 sec) is less than 1 as a mean. Further investigations are necessary to define the expected normal apnea index according to age during childhood, however, episodes of periodic breathing are uncommon in children (55, 72).

GAS EXCHANGE

Although there are few reports on gas exchange during sleep in infancy, available data suggest that gas exchange improves during sleep with advancing age. Figure 2.3 shows oxygen saturation values (SaO_2) measured by pulse oximetry in healthy infants from 1 to

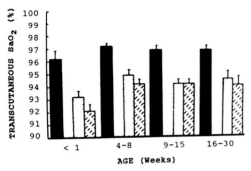

Figure 2.3. Transcutaneous oxygen saturation (SaO₂) measured by pulse oximetry. At different ages, from left to right, the columns refer to mean values ± 1 SEM during wakefulness, quiet sleep, and active sleep. (Adapted from Mok JYQ, McLaughlin J, Pintar M; Hak H, Amarao = Galvez R, Levison H: Transcutaneous monitoring of oxygenation. What is normal? *J Pediatr* 108:365–371, 1986.)

30 weeks during wakefulness, quiet (NREM), and active (REM) sleep (73). At 1 week, the difference between mean SaO₂ during wakefulness and active (REM) sleep amounted to 4%. With advancing postnatal age, the mean difference decreased to less than 3%, and the waking SaO₂ increased. Thus, during sleep, especially during active (REM) sleep, young infants are at risk for oxygen desaturation during apnea because of a relatively low oxygen tension, a high metabolic O_2 consumption (74), and a fall in O_2 stores (i.e., fall in FRC) (10, 11). In infants (7–40 months) studied during afternoon naps, the mean decrease in transcutaneous partial pressure of O_2 was 11 mm Hg (range 6–15) mm Hg (unpublished personal data). Table 2.6 shows SaO₂ measured by pulse oximetry after 2 years of age

during wakefulness and sleep (3, 72, 75, 76). Sleep states were scored in only one study (3).

Little information is available concerning partial pressure of CO_2 (Pco_2) during sleep. In newborns and infants, end-tidal Pco_2 (52, 77) or transcutaneous Pco_2 (78) is generally slightly greater in NREM sleep than in REM sleep. In infants from 7 to 54 months of age studied during afternoon naps, transcutaneous Pco_2 increased significantly from wakefulness to sleep without any difference among different sleep states (unpublished personal data). The difference between wakefulness and sleep never exceeds 10 mm Hg in these normal infants. During night sleep in 50 subjects aged from 1.1 to 17.4 years, maximal end-tidal Pco_2 during sleep was 46 ± 4 mm Hg (range 38–53 mm Hg) (72).

CHEMICAL CONTROL OF VENTILATION

In newborns, the increase in ventilation in response to hypoxia is transient, and is followed by a decrease in ventilation to control levels or below (79). The initial increase in ventilation has been attributed to peripheral chemoreceptor stimulation, whereas the origin of the second phase has been attributed to the central neural depressant effect of hypoxia. In premature infants studied approximatively 4 weeks after birth, the initial increase in ventilation to hypoxia during REM sleep was shown to be significantly lower than during wakefulness and NREM sleep (80). No such studies have been performed during infancy or childhood.

In contrast with the biphasic response to hypoxia, the newborn has sustained ventila-

Table 2.6.
Arterial Oxygen Saturation (SaO₂) Measured by Pulse Oximetry in Children and Adolescents

Reference	No. of Subjects and Age	Wake %	REM %	NREM %	Max Drop %	> 4% Dip /Hour	Lowest SaO₂
75	36 2–14 yr	97				1.13 (0.2–2.4)[a]	
72	50 9.9 yr ± 4.6					0.3 (0–4.4)	96(89–98)
76	9 13.8 yr ± 2.8	96.6 ± 1.5			2.2 ± 1.5	0	
3	9 15 yr ± 1.5	Max 97.5 ± 0.5 Min 97.2 ± 0.4	97.5 ± 0.5 96 ± 0.6	97.1 ± 0.3 96.1 ± 0.6	< 1.5	0	

[a]Mean and Range.

tory response to hypercapnia. Using the rebreathing method, three studies have reported a significantly lower response in active sleep than in quiet sleep (81–83) (Table 2.7). Thus in newborns as in adults (84), REM sleep is associated with a decrease in the ventilatory response to hypercapnia as compared to NREM sleep.

AROUSALS

Different types of arousals have been considered in the literature: behavioral, electroencephalograph (EEG), and movement arousals. Because of these differences and the ages of the subjects tested, there is no standard definition of arousal. This makes comparison between studies hazardous.

During sleep studies in which sleep states were not identified, behavioral arousals have been defined in infants from the first days of life to 3 months of age. However, the duration of behavioral events varied: longer than 5 sec (85) to 3 min (86, 87) (Table 2.8). Full-term and preterm infants have the same rate of spontaneous behavioral arousals lasting longer than 5 sec (85). In full-term newborns the rate of spontaneous behavioral arousals is close to the rate of EEG arousals lasting longer than 2 sec (88). Drugs such as phenothiazine can depress the arousal mechanisms in normal infants during sleep (63).

The arousal response from sleep is an important protective response that may prevent death during an apneic episode. Although apnea occurs to some extent in almost all preterm and full-term infants, little is known about the mechanisms that terminate an apneic episode. The occurrence of behavioral arousal has been studied in preterm apneic infants (84). Less than 10% of apneas ended by arousal. The frequency of arousal was significantly higher in long versus short, mixed versus central, and severe versus mild apnea (85). In children with obstructive sleep apnea syndrome, EEG and/or movement arousals have been studied at the end of obstructive apneas with (89) and without (90) identification of sleep states. During NREM sleep, 12% of obstructive apneas ended by an EEG arousal, and the remaining ended with a movement arousal. All obstructive apneas during REM sleep ended with a movement arousal. The lack of constant EEG arousal at the end of an obstructive apnea is in contrast to the typical apnea termination reported in adults with obstructive sleep apnea syndrome (91).

Behavioral arousal to hypercapnic stimuli has been studied in healthy infants and young

Table 2.7.
Ventilatory Response to CO$_2$

References	No. of Subjects	GA wk	PNA	Ventilatory Slope ml (min/kg/torr.P$_{ET}$CO$_2$)$^{-1}$	
				NREM	REM
80	6	36 ± 4	1–10 d	67.4 ± 17.4	35.7 ± 14.4[a]
81	14	40	3.3 d ± 0.9	67.3 ± 15.9	44.1 ± 23.7[a]
81	11	32 ± 0.4	9.9 d ± 1.6	50.5 ± 29.3	28.1 ± 14.2[a]
82	8	28-37	2-5 wk	40.8 ± 17.8	16.2 ± 9.3[a]

GA: gestational age; PNA: postnatal age; P$_{ET}$CO$_2$: end tidal partial pressure in CO$_2$.
[a]significantly lower than in NREM sleep.

Table 2.8.
Spontaneous Arousals in Healthy Preterm and Full-Term Infants

Reference	Subjects	PNA	Behavioral Arousal/min	EEG Arousal/min
84	Preterm infants (10)[a]	18 ± 13 d	0.24 ± 0.02	
84	Fullterm NB (7)	2 ± 0.7 d	0.23 ± 0.07	0.2
87	(13)	2 − 36h		
86	Infants (10)	7 wk	0.09	
85	(97)	10 wk	0.1	

[a]Number in brackets indicates the number of subjects.
PNA: postnatal age.

children during NREM sleep (92, 94). Hypercapnic challenge was accomplished by rapid change from room air to high inspired fraction of CO_2. All subjects were aroused from sleep at an end tidal partial pressure of CO_2 between 48 and 52 mm Hg. During a study of the ventilatory response to CO_2 using the rebreathing technique, one report showed that behavioral arousal occurred only in one third of tests during REM sleep in infants, but in 93% of the test in NREM sleep (83). Three studies have described behavioral arousals to hypoxic stimuli in NREM sleep, induced by rapid change from room air to low inspired partial pressure of O_2 (P_iO_2) (92, 93, 95). One study showed that all healthy infants (mean age 8.4 ± 3.2 months) were aroused at a mean P_iO_2 of 78 mm Hg (93). In another study, only 70% of the subjects (mean age 7.3 ± 0.7 weeks) were aroused at a mean transcutaneous PO_2 equal to 56 mm Hg (92). Finally, recent data show that the majority of infants younger than 7 months of age fail to arouse from NREM sleep in response to hypoxia (95).

Further investigations using standardized definitions of arousals, whether spontaneous or provoked by chemical stimulation, are of clinical relevance, since it has been suggested that some infants at risk for sudden death syndrome or apparent life-threatening events might have deficient arousal mechanisms (92, 93, 96).

REFERENCES

1. Openshaw P, Edwards S, Helm P. Changes in rib cage geometry during childhood. *Thorax* 1984; 39:624–627.
2. Hershenson MB, Colin AA, Wohl MEB, Stark AR. Change in contribution of the rib cage to total breathing during infancy. *Am Rev Respir Dis* 1990; 141:922–925.
3. Tabachnik E, Muller NL, Bryan AC, Levison H. Changes in ventilation and chest wall mechanics during sleep in normal adolescents. *J Appl Physiol* 1981; 51:557–564.
4. Agostoni E. Volume-pressure relationship to the thorax and lung in the newborn. *J Appl Physiol* 1959; 14:909–913.
5. Gerhart T, Bancalari E. Chest wall compliance in full-term and premature infants. *Acta Paediatr Scand* 1980; 69:359-364.
6. Sharp M, Druz W, Balgot R, Bandelin V, Damon J. Total respiratory compliance in infants and children. *J Appl Physiol* 1970; 2:775–779.
7. Curzi-Dascalova L. Thoraco-abdominal respiratory correlations in infants: Constancy and variability in different sleep states. *Early Hum Dev* 1978; 2:25–38.
8. Bryan AC, Gaultier C. Chest wall mechanics in the newborn. In Roussos C, Macklem PT (eds.): *The Thorax*. New York, Marcel Dekker, 1985, pp. 871–888.
9. Anders TF, Emde R, Parmelee A. A manual of standardized terminology. Techniques and criteria for scoring of states of sleep and wakefulness in newborn infants. UCLA Brain information service/BRI Publications office, Los Angeles, 1971.
10. Walti H, Moriette G, Radvanyi-Bouvet MF, Chaussain M, Morel-Kahn F, Pajot N, Relier JP. Influence of breathing pattern on functional residual capacity in sleeping newborn infants. *J Dev Physiol* 1986; 8:167–172.
11. Henderson-Smart DJ, Read DJC. Reduced lung volume during behavioral active sleep in the newborn. *J Appl Physiol* 1979; 46:1081–1085.
12. Guslits BG, Gaston SE, Bryan MH, England SJ, Bryan AC. Diaphragmatic work of breathing in premature human infants. *J Appl Physiol* 1987; 62:1410–1415.
13. Martin RJ, Okken A, Rubin D. Arterial oxygen tension during active and quiet sleep. *J Pediatr* 1979; 94:271–274.
14. Harding R, Johnson P, McClelland ME. Respiratory function of the larynx in developing sheep and the influence of sleep state. *Respir Physiol* 1980; 40:165–179.
15. Gaultier CI, Praud JP, Canet E, Delaperche MF, D'Allest AM. Paradoxical inward rib cage motion during rapid eye movement sleep in infants and young children. *J Dev Physiol* 1987; 9:391–397.
16. Finer NA, Abroms IF, Taeusch HW. Ventilation and sleeping states in newborn infants. *J Pediatr* 1976; 89:100–108.
17. Rabette PS, Costeloe KL, Stocks J. Persistence of the Hering-Breuer reflex beyond the neonatal period. *J Appl Physiol* 1991; 71:474–480.
18. Hagan R, Bryan AC, Bryan MH, Gulston G. Neonatal chest wall afferents and regulation of respiration. *J Appl Physiol* 1977; 42:362–367.
19. Hudgel DW, Martin RJ, Johnson B, Hill P. Mechanics of the respiratory system and breathing pattern during sleep in normal humans. *J Appl Physiol* 1984; 56:133–137.
20. Lesouef PN, Lopes JM, England SJ, Bryan MH, Bryan AC. Influence of chest wall distortion on esophageal pressure. *J Appl Physiol* 1983; 55:353–358.
21. Guilleminault C, Winkler R, Korobkin R, Simmons B. Children and nocturnal snoring: Evaluation of the effects of sleep related respiratory resistive load and daytime functioning. *Eur J Pediatr* 1982; 139:165–171.
22. Moss ML. The veloepiglottic sphincter and obligate nose breathing in the neonate. *J Pediatr* 1965; 67:330–331.
23. Bosma JF. Postnatal ontogeny of performances of the pharynx, larynx and mouth. *Am Rev Respir Dis* 1985; 131(Suppl):510–515.
24. Swift PG, Emery JL. Clinical observations on the responses to nasal occlusion in infancy. *Arch Dis Child* 1973; 48:947–951.
25. Rodenstein DO, Perlemuter N, Stanescu DC. Infants are not obligatory nasal breathers. *Am Rev Respir Dis* 1985; 131:343–347.
26. Purcell M. Response in the newborn to raised upper airway resistance. *Arch Dis Child* 1976; 51:602–607.

27. Tonkin SL, Partridge J, Beach D, Withey S. The pharyngeal effect of partial nasal obstruction. *Pediatrics* 1979; 63:261–271.
28. Thach BT, Stark AR. Spontaneous neck flexion and airway obstruction during apneic spells in preterm infants. *J Pediatr* 1979; 94:275–281.
29. Stark AR, Thach BT. Recovery of airway patency after obstruction in normal infants. *Am Rev Respir Dis* 1981; 123:691–693.
30. Roberts JL, Reed WT, Mathew OP, Menon AA, Thach BT. Assessment of pharyngeal airway stability in normal and micrognathic infants. *J Appl Physiol* 1985; 58:290–300.
31. Wilson SL, Thach BT, Brouillette RT, Abu-Osba YK. Upper airway patency in the human infant: Influence of airway pressure and posture. *J Appl Physiol* 1980; 48:500–504.
32. Reef WR, Roberts JL, Thach BT. Factors influencing regional patency and configuration of the human infant upper airway. *J Appl Physiol* 1985; 58:635–644.
33. Jeffery B, Brouillette RT, Hunt CE. Electromyographic study of some accessory muscles of respiration in children with obstructive sleep apnea. *Am Rev Respir Dis* 1984; 129:696–702.
34. Carlo WA, Miller MJ, Martin RJ. Differential response of respiratory muscles to airway occlusion in infants. *J Appl Physiol* 1985; 59:847–852.
35. Lucier GE, Story AT, Sessle BJ. Effects of upper respiratory tract stimuli on neonatal respiration: Reflex and single neuron analyses in kitten. *Biol Neonate* 1979; 35:82–89.
36. Lee JC, Dowing SE. Laryngeal reflex inhibition of breathing in piglets: Influences of anemia and catecholamine depletion. *Am J Physiol* 19:239 (Regulatory Integrative Comp Physiol, 8): R 25 6 R 30.
37. Lanier B, Richardson MA, Cummings C. Effect of hypoxia on laryngeal reflex apneas—Implications for sudden infant death. *Otolaryngol Head Neck Surg* 1983; 91:597–604.
38. Wennergren G, Hertzberg T, Milerad J, Bjure J, Lagercrantz H. Hypoxia reinforces laryngeal reflex bradycardia in infants. *Acta Paediatr Scand* 1989; 78:11–17.
39. Boggs DF, Bartlett D. Chemical specificity of a laryngeal apneic reflex in puppies. *J Appl Physiol* 1982; 53:455–462.
40. Perkett EA, Vaughan RL. Evidence for laryngeal chemoreflex in some human preterm infants. *Acta Paediatr Scand* 1982; 71:969–972.
41. Davies AM, Koenig JS, Thach BT. Upper airway chemoreflex responses to saline and water in preterm infants. *J Appl Physiol* 1988; 64:1412–1420.
42. Pickens DL, Schefft G, Thach BT. Prolonged apnea associated with upper airway protective reflexes in apnea of prematurity. *Am Rev Respir Dis* 1988; 137:113–118.
43. Fisher JT, San'Ambrogio G. Airways and lung receptors and their reflex effects in the newborn. *Pediatr Pulmonol* 1985; 1:112–126.
44. Adamson TM, Cranage S, Maloney JE, Wilkinson MH, Wilson FE, Yu VY. The maturation of respiratory patterns in normal full-term infants during the first six postnatal months. I. Sleep states and respiratory variability. *Aus Paediatr J* 1981; 17:250–256.
45. Curzi-Dascalova L, Lebrun F, Korn G. Respiratory frequency according to sleep states and age in normal premature infants: A comparison with full-term infants. *Pediatr Res* 1983; 17:152–156.
46. Haddad GG, Epstein RA, Epstein MA, Leistner HL, Marino PA, Mellins RB. Maturation of ventilation and ventilatory pattern in normal sleeping infants. *J Appl Physiol* 1979; 46:998–1002.
47. Hoppenbrouwers T, Harper RM, Hodgman JE, Sterman MN, McGinty DJ. Polygraphic studies of normal infants during the first six months of life. II. Respiratory rate and variability as a function of state. *Pediatr Res* 1978; 12:120–125.
48. Steinschneider A, Weinstein S. Sleep respiratory instability in term neonates under hyperthermic conditions: Age, sex, type of feeding, and rapid eye movements. *Pediatr Res* 1983; 17:35–41.
49. Katona PG, Egbert JR. Heart rate and respiratory rate differences between preterm and fullterm infants during quiet sleep: Possible implications for sudden infant death syndrome. *Pediatrics* 1978; 62:91–95.
50. Bolton DP, Hermans S. Ventilation and sleep state in the newborn. *J Physiol (Lond)* 1974; 340:66–67.
51. Hathorn MK. The rate and depth of breathing in newborn infants in different sleep states. *J Physiol (Lond)* 1974; 243:101–113.
52. Davi M, Sankaran K, MacCallum M, Cates D, Rigatto H. Effects of sleep state on chest distortion and on the ventilatory response to CO_2 in neonates. *Pediatr Res* 1979; 13:982–986.
53. Fagenholtz S, O'Connell SA, Shannon DC. Chemoreceptor function and sleep state in apnea. *Pediatrics* 1976; 58:31–36.
54. Dolfin T, Duffty P, Wilkes D, England S, Bryan MH. Effects of a face mask and pneumotachograph on breathing in sleeping infants. *Am Rev Respir Dis* 1983; 128:977–979.
55. Carskadon MA, Harvey K, Dement WC, Guilleminault C, Simmons FB, Anders TF. Respiration during sleep in children. *West J Med* 1978; 128:477–481.
56. Coup A, Coup D, Weathalls, Withy S. The development and abnormalities of breathing patterns. In Tiddon JT, Roeder LM, Steinschneider A (eds): *Sudden Infant Death Syndrome*. New York, Academic Press, 1983, pp. 423–449.
57. Hoppenbrouwers T, Hodgman JE, Harper RM, Hofmann E, Sterman MB, McGinty DY. Polygraphic studies of normal infants during the first six months of life. II. Incidence of apnea and periodic breathing. *Pediatrics* 1977; 60:418–425.
58. Hoppenbrouwers T, Hodgman JE, Arakawa K, Harper R, Sterman MB. Respiration during the first six months of life in normal infants. III. Computer identification of breathing pauses. *Pediatr Res* 1980; 14:1230–1233.
59. Curzi-Dascalova L, Christova-Guerguieva E. Respiratory pauses in normal prematurely born infants. A comparison with full-term newborns. *Biol Neonate* 1983; 44:325–332.
60. Guilleminault C, Ariagno R, Korobkin R, Nagel L, Baldwin R, Coons S, Owen M. Mixed and obstructive sleep apnea and near miss for sudden infant death syndrome. 2. Comparison of near miss and normal control infants by age. *Pediatrics* 1979; 64:882–891.
61. Kelly DH, Stellwagen LM, Kaitz E, Shannon DC. Apnea and periodic breathing in normal full-term infants during the first twelve months. *Pediatr Pulmonol* 1985; 1:215–219.

62. Hamza J, Benlabed M, Orhant E, Escourrou P, Curzi-Dascalova L, Gaultier CI. Neonatal pattern of breathing during active and quiet sleep after maternal administration of meperidine. *Pediatr Res* 1992, in press.

63. Kahn A, Hasaerts D, Blum D. Phenothiazine-induced sleep apneas in normal infants. *Pediatrics* 1985; 75:844–847.

64. Jansen AH, Chernick V. Development of respiratory control. *Physiol Rev* 1983; 63:437–483.

65. Manning DJ, Stothers JK. Sleep state, hypoxia and periodic breathing in the neonate. *Acta Paediatr Scand* 1991; 80:763–769.

66. Pickens DL, Schefft G, Thach BT. Characterization of prolonged apneic episodes associated with respiratory syncytial virus infection. *Pediatr Pulmonol* 1989; 6:195–201.

67. Herbst JJ, Minton SD, Book LS. Gastroesophageal reflux causing respiratory distress and apnea in newborn infants. *J Pediatr* 1979; 95:763–768.

68. Gaultier CL. Interference between gastroesophageal reflux and sleep in near miss SIDS. *Clin Rev Allergy* 1991; 8:395–401.

69. Berterottiere D, D'Allest AM, Dehan M, Gaultier C. Effects of increase in body temperature on the breathing pattern in premature infants. *J Dev Physiol* 1990; 13:303–308.

70. Canet E, Gaultier CL, D'Allest AM, Dehan M. Effects of sleep deprivation on respiratory events during sleep in healthy infants. *J Appl Physiol* 1989; 66:1158–1163.

71. Guilhaume A, Benoit O. Pauses respiratoires au cours du sommeil chez l'enfant normal. Observations de trois cas pathologiques. *Rev Electroencephalogr Neurophysiol Clin* 1976; 6:116–123.

72. Marcus CL, Omlin KJ, Basinski DJ, Bailey SL, Rachal AB, Von Pechmann WS, Keens TG, Davidson-Ward SL. Normal polysomnographic values for children and adolescents. *Am Rev Respir Dis* 1992; 146:1235–1239.

73. Mok JYQ, McLaughlin J, Pintar M, Hak H, Amaro-Galvez R, Levison H. Transcutaneous monitoring of oxygenation. What is normal? *J Pediatr* 1986; 108:365–371.

74. Stothers JK, Warner RM. Oxygen consumption and sleep state in the newborn. *J Physiol (Lond)* 1978; 278:435–440.

75. Stradling JR, Thomas G, Warley ARH, Williams P, Freeland A. Effect of adenotonsillectomy on nocturnal hypoxemia, sleep disturbances, and symptoms in snoring children. *Lancet* 1990; 335:249–253.

76. Chipps PE, Mak H, Schuberth KC, Talamo JH, Menkes HA. Nocturnal oxygen saturation in normal and asthmatic children. *Pediatrics* 1980; 65:1157–1160.

77. Anderson JV, Martin RJ, Abdoud EF, Zacharydyme I, Bruce E. Transient ventilatory response to CO_2 as a function of sleep state in full-term infants. *J Appl Physiol* 1983; 54:1482–1488.

78. Martin RJ, Herrel N, Pultusker M. Transcutaneous measurement of carbon dioxide tension. Effects of sleep state in term infants. *Pediatrics* 1981; 67:622–625.

79. Davis GM, Bureau MA. Pulmonary and chest wall mechanics in the control of respiration in the newborn. *Clin Perinatol* 1987; 14:551–579.

80. Rigatto H, Kalapesi Z, Leahy FN, Durand M, McCallum M, Cates D. Ventilatory response to 100% and 15% O_2 during wakefulness and sleep in preterm infants. *Early Hum Dev* 1982; 7:1–10.

81. Honma Y, Wilkes D, Bryan MH, Bryan AC. Rib cage and abdominal contributions to ventilatory response to CO_2 infants. *J Appl Physiol* 1984; 56:1211–1216.

82. Moriette G, Van Reempts P, Moore M, Cates D, Rigatto H. The effect of rebreathing CO_2 on ventilation and diaphragmatic electromyography in newborn infants. *Respir Physiol* 1985; 62:387–397.

83. Praud JP, Egreteau L, Benlabed M, Curzi-Dascalova L, Nedelcoux H, Gaultier CL. Abdominal muscle activity during CO_2 rebreathing in sleeping neonates. *J Appl Physiol* 1991; 70:1344–1350.

84. Douglas NJ, White DP, Weil JV, Pickett CK, Zwillich W. Hypercapnic ventilatory response in sleeping adults. *Am Rev Respir Dis* 1982; 126:758–762.

85. Thoppil CK, Belan MA, Cowen CP, Matthew OP. Behavioral arousal in newborn infants and its association with termination of apnea. *J Appl Physiol* 1991; 70:2479–2484.

86. Kahn A, Picard E, Blum D. Auditory arousal threshold of normal and near-miss SIDS infants. *Dev Med Child Neurol* 1986; 28:299–302.

87. Kahn A, Rebuffat E, Sottiaux M, Blum D, Yasik EA. Sleep apneas and acid esophageal reflux in control infants and in infants with an apparent life-threatening event. *Biol Neonate* 1990; 57:144–149.

88. Scher MS, Richardson GA, Coble PA, Day NL, Stoffer DS. The effects of prenatal alcohol and marijuana exposure: Disturbances in neonatal sleep cycling and arousal. *Pediatr Res* 1988; 24:101–105.

89. Praud JP, D'Allest AM, Nedelcoux H, Curzi-Dascalova L, Guilleminault C, Gaultier CL. Sleep-related abdominal muscle behavior during partial or complete obstructed breathing in prepubertal children. *Pediatr Res* 1989; 26:347–350.

90. McGrath-Morrow SA, McColley SA, Carroll JL, Pyzik P, Cybulski M, Loughlin GM. Termination of obstructive apnea in children is not associated with arousal. *Am Rev Respir Dis* 1990; 141:195.

91. Vincken W, Guilleminault C, Silvestri L, Cosio M, Grassino A. Inspiratory muscle activity as a trigger causing the airways to open in obstructive sleep apnea. *Am Rev Respir Dis* 1987; 135:372–377.

92. McCulloch K, Brouillette RT, Guzzetta AJ, Hunt CE. Arousal response in near-miss sudden infant death syndrome and normal infants. *J Pediatr* 1982; 101:911–917.

93. Van Derhal AL, Rodriguez AM, Sargent CW, Platzker ACG, Keens TG. Hypoxic and hypercapnic arousal responses and prediction of subsequent apnea in apnea of infancy. *Pediatrics* 1985; 75:848–854.

94. Marcus CL, Bautista DB, Amihyia A, Davidson-Ward SL, Keens TG. Hypercapneic arousal responses in children with congenital central hypoventilation syndrome. *Pediatrics* 1991; 88:993–998.

95. Davidson-Ward SL, Bautista DB, Keens TG. Hypoxic arousal responses in normal infants. *Pediatrics* 1992; 89:860–864, 908.

96. Coons S, Guilleminault C. Motility and arousal in near miss sudden infant death syndrome. *J Pediatr* 1985; 107:728–732.

3

Development of Increased Airway Responsiveness

ARLENE A. STECENKO

Increased airway responsiveness to a variety of chemical stimuli, such as histamine or carbachol, is thought to be the hallmark of asthma. For some, the sensitivity and the specificity of an increased airway responsiveness as a test for asthma approaches that of an elevated sweat chloride concentration as a test for cystic fibrosis. The suspicion that this may not be the case begins with the plethora of reports in children (many of whom are asymptomatic) of an association between increased airway responsiveness and a variety of lung injuries, some long-gone. An infection with respiratory syncytial virus (RSV) or Mycoplasma pneumoniae, premature birth without subsequent development of bronchopulmonary dysplasia (BPD), a hospital admission for croup, or a past history of croup or bronchiolitis by parental report are all associated with a significant increase in airway responsiveness (1–5). Although many of these children do develop asthma, particularly following an RSV infection severe enough to require hospitalization, a disturbing number of children with increased airway responsiveness have no respiratory symptoms and most certainly do not have asthma.

The complexity of the relationship between increased airway responsiveness and childhood asthma is underscored by the work of Pattemore and colleagues (6). They measured airway responsiveness to aerosol histamine in over 2000 New Zealand school children aged 7–10 years and correlated airway responsiveness with respiratory symptoms and with the presence of asthma. They found that only 52% of the 294 children diagnosed with asthma had increased airway responsiveness. Furthermore, half of the children with increased airway responsiveness had not been diagnosed as having asthma, and one-quarter reported no recent symptoms of cough or wheeze. This study is complemented by that of Stick et al., who found no increase in airway responsiveness to aerosol histamine in infants with recurrent wheeze (7). In contrast is the usually accepted notion that 100% of adult asthmatics demonstrate increased airway responsiveness during a symptomatic period. Thus, the development of asthma and the development of increased airway responsiveness from infancy to adulthood could be conceptualized as a Venn diagram (Fig. 3.1). During infancy, there may be little or no overlap between airway responsiveness and asthma. With progression through childhood, the overlap increases so that by adulthood, the two circles are superimposed. Therefore, consistently considering the phenomenon of increased airway responsiveness the sine qua non of childhood asthma may be overly simplistic.

In this chapter, the approach will be to describe events surrounding acute changes in airway caliber at a physiologic, cellular, and molecular level. The evidence for factors that enhance the development of increased airway responsiveness, and to a lesser extent the risk of developing asthma, will be presented at each step in the discussion.

PHYSIOLOGY OF AIRWAY RESPONSIVENESS

Classic bronchial provocation tests consist of challenging the lower airway with a stimulus, often applied in a graded, increasing fashion, then measuring the degree of airflow obstruction produced (8). The applied stimulus could be nonspecific,—that is, chemical, such as histamine or carbachol, or physical, such as cold

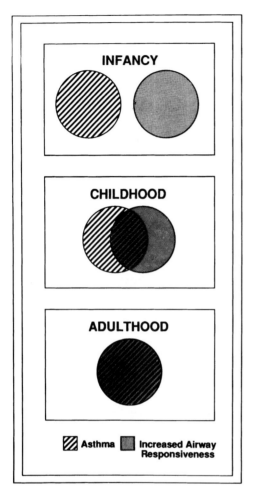

INFANCY

CHILDHOOD

ADULTHOOD

▨ Asthma ▉ Increased Airway Responsiveness

Figure 3.1. Hypothetical relationships between increased airway responsiveness and asthma at different levels of development.

whereby the percentage of change in lung function is plotted against the log of the concentration of aerosolized drug. The threshold dose (i.e., the concentration at which airflow obstruction begins) indicates the airway *sensitivity.* The slope of the dose-response curve, after the threshold dose is reached, indicates bronchial *reactivity.* Orehek and colleagues have found that adult asthmatic subjects differ from nonasthmatics in terms of reactivity but not necessarily in terms of sensitivity (9). Another difference between asthmatic dose-response curves and curves for normal controls may be the characteristics of the curve when the stimuli is increased once airflow obstruction has occurred. In normal subjects, a plateau in airway obstruction may occur. At this point, further increases in the concentration of aerosolized agent do not result in any increase in obstruction. This may not be the case with asthmatics (i.e., a plateau is not reached) (10).

In bronchial challenge tests in which a dose-response curve cannot be constructed, the percentage of change in lung function invoked by a constant stimulus (rather than a graded stimulus) can be used to quantitate the degree of responsiveness. For allergen challenge, the change in lung function is plotted against time, since the response may take over 8 hours for full expression (11). Usually, the maximal change in the first 2 hours following allergen challenge is used to describe the early asthma response (EAR), and the peak change in the second 4 or 6 hours is used to describe the late asthma response (LAR). Alternatively, the area under the curve for the EAR and the LAR can be calculated, thus including all data points (12).

Over the last several decades, efforts have been made to standardize these tests, resulting in reproducibility that one hopes is sufficient enough to permit comparisons of data from different centers. However, there are some inherent difficulties in bronchial challenge, particularly when addressing developmental issues such as comparisons between infants and adults or follow-up of an individual subject longitudinally over a long period, which are difficult to overcome. For example, the inability to document the dose delivered to the airway can pose a major problem when interpreting bronchial challenge data. Although careful control of the physical char-

air, an acid, or a hypotonic or hypertonic solution. Alternatively, the applied stimulus could be immunologic (i.e., a specific allergen). The response to the challenge is usually quantitated by measuring forced expired flows or airways resistance in a cooperative adult. In the infant or young child, who is unable to cooperate, tidal or partial forced maneuvers are used to quantitate the degree of airflow obstruction. The degree of airway responsiveness probably follows a unimodal distribution, with asthmatic subjects responding to much lower concentrations of the stimulus and nonasthmatics responding to much higher concentrations or not at all. For a quantitative description of these differences in responsiveness, a dose-response curve can be constructed acteristics of the output of the nebulization delivery system, such as particle size, and of breathing characteristics of the subject, such as flow rate and time of end-inspiratory breath hold, will help reduce variability in the amount of drug delivered (8), factors such as airway geometry, baseline airway caliber, and deposition can neither be controlled nor accurately quantitated. This translates to an inability to determine the *exact* amount of stimulus received by the lower airway. The difficulty this causes in interpreting data can be appreciated when comparing the degree of airway responsiveness between infants, children, and adults. In the past, several studies documented that airflow obstruction was induced by a much lower concentration of aerosol histamine or carbachol in infants and young children compared to adults or older children. One obvious problem was that the methods of measuring airflow obstruction in young children were quite different from the methods used in a cooperative subject. Nevertheless, it appeared that healthy, asymptomatic infants showed evidence of airflow obstruction at inspired concentrations of histamine that normally would only cause obstruction in adult asthmatics but not in asymptomatic controls. However, it appears that the problem may be one of aerosol delivery rather than true airway hyper-responsiveness. Infants normally have a much smaller minute ventilation than adults; therefore their minute ventilation is exceeded by the flow rate of a standard nebulizer. In contrast, the minute ventilation of adults exceeds the flow rate of the nebulizer. Thus, it is postulated that the inspired drug is "diluted" by room air through a Venturi effect in adults. This dilutional effect may not occur in the infant. Stick and colleagues showed that if the minute ventilation of the child is taken into account to estimate the potential dilutional effect, there is no increase in airway responsiveness to aerosol histamine in young children (13).

Despite these technical limitations, evaluating airway responsiveness in animals of different ages and in human population studies brings some clarity to the issue of how airway responsiveness develops. The first question is, how much does genetics contribute to the development of airway responsiveness (14)? Certainly there is evidence that the degree of nonspecific airway responsiveness to agents such as histamine and methacholine is determined, in part, by inheritance. Indeed, Longo has postulated that responsiveness to carbachol is inherited as an autosomal dominant trait in humans (15). This was based on the observation that 50% of nonasthmatic parents whose children had asthma demonstrated increased responsiveness. Hirshman and colleagues studied the inheritance of bronchial responsiveness in two breeds of dogs, both of which were allergic to Ascaris suum allergen as documented by positive skin test and bronchial challenge, but only one of which showed increased nonspecific airway responsiveness to citric acid and methacholine (16). All dogs and offspring were reared in the same environment. By evaluating airway responsiveness in these two breeds, these authors found that inheritance, rather than environmental factors, helped shape the degree of airway responsiveness in the offspring. Similarly, studies of parents of asthmatics or sons of patients with chronic obstructive pulmonary disease suggest a familial factor in determining the degree of responsiveness (15, 17). Unfortunately, these human studies could not control for the role of shared environmental exposure. Studies in twins provide some reasonable clues into the role of genetics in determining airway responsiveness in humans. Three separate studies on twins suggest that inheritance plays a much larger role in the ultimate expression of nonspecific airway responsiveness than in the clinical manifestations of asthma (15). Linkage analysis and gene mapping to determine the gene(s) responsible for shaping airway responsiveness certainly will be an important step in understanding the role of genetics in the development of airway responsiveness (18).

A reasonable assumption is that genetic factors will ultimately help shape the degree of airway responsiveness. However, this assumption does not address the issue of whether expression is complete at birth or whether baseline airway responsiveness develops postnatally. The dearth of intermittent airway obstruction, or "congenital asthma" if you will, in the newborn human infant would suggest that asthma is not present at birth. Is airway hyper-responsiveness also absent at birth? Sauder et al. measured nonspecific airway responsiveness to aerosol histamine, carbachol, and citric acid using the same techniques in sheep from age 1 month to adult-hood (19). They found significantly decreased responsiveness in young lambs that did not reach the adult range in responsiveness until 7 months of age. (Sheep reach sexual maturity by around 9 months of age.) Neither delivery to the airway nor amount of airway smooth muscle accounted for this decrease in airway responsiveness in the younger animals (20). In contrast, the contractile response of rabbit tracheal muscle strips to histamine decreased with age (21). In humans, the delineation of the effect of age on the development of non-specific airway responsiveness awaits appropriate techniques that permit a uniformly applied stimulus and a consistent measure of the outcome variable.

The physiology of the airway response to inhaled *allergens* provides insight into the development of asthma as well as the development of increased airway responsiveness. Aerosol challenge with an allergen in an asthmatic can produce an EAR only, a LAR only, or a dual phase response with both early and late obstruction. Approximately 50% of adult asthmatics who have an EAR will also have a LAR (11). This number is higher during childhood when 70–86% of children who have an EAR demonstrate a LAR (11, 22).

The presence of an airway response to inhaled allergen is thought to have significant clinical relevance because of several observations. First, the airflow obstruction following allergen exposure may last for hours and may be unresponsive to bronchodilator therapy. Second, there are multiple opportunities in today's environment for exposure to a host of allergens. Our energy-conscious society has built virtually air-tight houses that may have transformed homes into "exposure chambers" for its occupants. Finally, there is the interesting link between the response to a specific allergen and a subsequent increased nonspecific (i.e., nonimmunologic) airway responsiveness. For several days after allergen challenge (23), there is an increase in airway responsiveness to nonspecific agents, such as histamine and methacholine, which is first noted *prior* to the onset of the LAR. This increase in nonspecific airway responsiveness has also been found in several animal models of the dual-phase response (24). In asthmatics, the increase in nonspecific airway responsiveness to chemical stimuli may translate into a

heightened airway response to other, nonanti-genic stimuli such as exercise or viral infections. Additionally, the actual response to an inhaled allergen is accentuated if there already is heightened responsiveness to histamine (25). This has lead Cockcroft to postulate that a "vicious cycle" of exposure to natural allergens and heightened nonspecific airway responsiveness could lead to persistent, perennial asthma (26).

Considerable controversy exists as to the exact mechanism of the airway response to inhaled allergens because of the inaccessibility of the cellular and biochemical milieu of the human airway. A response to this problem has been either to study a more accessible human organ such as the skin (which does demonstrate a dual-phase response to antigen) or to study the airway of a more accessible animal such as the dog, sheep, guinea pig, horse, or monkey (24). Two types of animal models of the airway response to inhaled allergen are available. One is spontaneous or naturally occurring sensitization; the best examples of this model are found in adult sheep, dogs, horses, and monkeys. Animals are screened for cutaneous sensitivity to foreign protein, usually intestinal parasites. Skin test–positive animals are then challenged with the allergen and lung function measured to determine whether there is an airway response. This clearly can be tedious, since many animals may need to be screened before responders can be found. Sheep and monkeys, but not dogs, appear to be the species that most frequently have an LAR, with up to 50% of skin test–positive animals showing a dual phase response. The horse demonstrates some interesting reactions similar to those of asthma, but the horse's size precludes routine use in research protocols.

Other investigators have attempted to *induce* a dual-phase airway response. The key factors associated with success have been the sensitization schedule, the species, and the age of the animal at the initiation of sensitization. Successful induction of sensitization appears to require an adjuvant, usually aluminum hydroxide, to enhance the immune response, as well as frequent exposures to the allergen. Rabbits, sheep, and guinea pigs are the species that appear to be capable of an induction of a dual-airway response (24, 27–29). If the sensitization schedule is begun at birth, sensitization is optimal.

Perhaps the most elegant model of an inducible airway response is found in the rabbit (27, 28). Newborn rabbits are sensitized, beginning at birth, using multiple intraperitoneal injections of *Alternaria tenuis* extract and aluminum hydroxide. Sensitization requires 2–3 months. Sensitized animals have both an early and a late phase of airflow obstruction and positive passive cutaneous anaphylaxis (PCA). Transfusion of serum from a sensitized rabbit into a naive one results in a dual-phase airway response upon allergen challenge. The PCA response and the passive transfer experiment confirm the importance of specific immunoglobulin E (IgE) directed against the antigen in the pathophysiology of the dual-phase response. If the sensitization schedule is begun on the seventh day of life, the airway response is significantly diminished and these animals appear to have protective as well as reaginic serum antibodies.

Once asthma has developed, an increased airway response to inhaled protein is an important clinical event. An alternative approach, examining the role of frequent, repetitive exposures to inhaled protein on the development of asthma, provides some interesting speculation on the pathophysiology of asthma.

As discussed above, young animals given frequent, repetitive exposures to foreign protein can develop a dual-phase airway response to the allergen upon subsequent challenge. Interestingly, an RSV infection has also been used to achieve a reaginic response. Rodents infected with this virus produce serum IgE against concurrently inhaled nonviral antigen, whereas uninfected animals only produce IgG against the antigen (30).

As in these animal models, there are studies of humans that indicate that exposure to an antigen can eventually lead to airway sensitization. For example, infants with a high exposure to house dust mite antigen are twice as likely to have asthma at age 11 years than those with low exposure (31). Perhaps the best illustration that antigen exposure can result in airway sensitization in humans is occupational asthma. For example, workers in red cedar mills can eventually develop airway sensitization to the inhaled cedar dust as documented by a positive bronchial challenge test with pli-

catic acid (32). If the dust is removed from the work place, complete recovery occurs in 50% of subjects. However, if exposure continues, only 10% of patients improve, and none recover. Nonspecific airway responsiveness increases in those who remain exposed. Indeed, chronic asthma may develop, which is exacerbated by factors other than exposure to cedar dust. In this situation, it is unclear whether eventual removal from the workplace has any effect on asthma severity.

Thus, exposure to inhaled antigens may indeed promote the development of airway sensitization to that antigen and ultimately to asthma. Factors that may increase the risk of developing asthma could be the level of exposure; the age at the time of heightened exposure, with infancy and early childhood being the high-risk periods; and experience with acute respiratory tract injury, such as an RSV infection.

CELLULAR AND MOLECULAR BASIS OF AIRWAY RESPONSIVENESS

One of the major physiologic aberrations seen with bronchial challenge is airflow obstruction. It is reasonable to assume that the airway smooth muscle is an important component of the response at a cellular level. However, it has been rather difficult to correlate the in-vivo physiologic response of airflow obstruction with in-vitro characteristics of airway smooth muscle, such as quantity of muscle or the contractile response. For example, infants who wheeze, presumably because of asthma, do not respond well to bronchodilators. This was said to be because young children have less airway smooth muscle. This concept was supported by histologic data from autopsies of children and adults: children had less smooth muscle surrounding the small airways (but not major bronchi) than adults (33). However, examination of these data indicate that the number of lungs examined from subjects without pulmonary disease was very small (1 infant, 10 children, and 5 adults) and that there was considerable overlap between the quantity of smooth muscle in adults and in children. Thus, there may not be such a significant difference between adults and young children in terms of quantity of airway smooth muscle despite differences in bronchodilator response. Furthermore, studies in humans, dogs, and sheep have failed to find a correlation between in-vitro evaluation of the smooth muscle, such as the contractile response or the amount of airway smooth muscle, and the degree of nonspecific airway responsiveness found in the same subject on in-vivo testing (20, 34–36). In contrast, the responsiveness of tracheal smooth muscle from animals that have been sensitized to a foreign antigen is increased—that is, airway smooth muscle properties may be a determinant in the response to allergens (8, 37). Thus, it may well be that neither the quantity nor the inherent contractile properties of airway smooth muscle determine the degree of responsiveness to nonspecific bronchial challenge, but that these factors contribute to the responsiveness to specific antigens.

Other possible effector cells, besides airway smooth muscle, that may control the degree of airway responsiveness are inflammatory cells, particularly mast cells, alveolar macrophages, neutrophils, and T lymphocytes. Certainly, recruitment of inflammatory cells and release of mediators is an important component of the response to inhaled allergen. For the EAR, airflow obstruction begins within minutes of exposure, peaks in 10–30 minutes, and usually is resolved by 2 hours. The pathophysiology of the obstruction is thought to be due to IgE-mediated mast cell activation, release of mediators, and subsequent bronchoconstriction. Histamine appears to be released during the EAR as arterial histamine levels correlate; the degree of airflow obstruction and blocking histaminic action with antihistamines usually blocks the EAR (38, 39). The airflow obstruction is quickly *reversed* by inhaled beta sympathomimetics (11), suggesting that airway smooth muscle contraction is the final common pathway producing the airflow obstruction regardless of the mediators involved.

During the LAR, peribronchial edema and inflammation, rather than bronchoconstriction, are thought to produce the airflow obstruction (40). The initiating event causing the obstruction appears to be related to activation of mast cell–bound IgE during the EAR (11, 41). Several other cells appear to be recruited into the lung, such as the eosinophil, granulocyte, and T lymphocyte (11, 42). Release of mediators from these cells such as platelet activating factor (PAF), eosinophil-derived proteins, leukotrienes, interleukins, and products of the cyclo-oxygenase pathway

are important for the full expression of the response. It should be noted that one of the most potent inhibitors of the LAR is glucocorticosteroids.

Evaluation of the role of these mediators in the airway response to allergens provides insight into the development of airway responsiveness. PAF, in particular, has gained notoriety as a pivotal mediator in reversible airway disease (24, 43–45). PAF is an ether-linked phospholipid synthesized by a variety of inflammatory cells such as polymorphonuclear leukocytes (PMNs), platelets, eosinophils, mast cells, and macrophages. Through activation of phospholipase A_2 and a second cytosolic enzyme (which is the rate-limiting step), the inactive form of PAF is converted to the biologically active form. PAF is either released from the cell or remains in the cytoplasm. Plasma contains an enzyme, acetylhydrolase, which converts PAF to lyso-PAF, which has no biological activity. This conversion is very rapid, occurring within a few minutes. Interestingly, children with wheeze have a diminished plasma acetylhydrolase activity, implicating a role for PAF in asthma (46). Several of the biologic actions of PAF make it an excellent candidate, not only as a mediator of allergic disease, but as a key element in the development of such disease. For example, PAF is one of the most potent eosinophil chemotactic agents. As will be discussed later, recruitment of eosinophils to the lung and release of eosinophilic proteins that damage the airway epithelium is considered one of the first steps in the development of asthma. PAF is also one of the most potent bronchoconstrictors, recruits many other inflammatory cells to the lungs besides eosinophils, increases mucus secretion, and increases nonspecific airway responsiveness. This last action is unique among the inflammatory mediators. In man and in experimental animals, PAF is associated with increased airway responsiveness to inhaled histamine and methacholine that can last up to a few weeks. The exact mechanism of this increased nonspecific responsiveness is not clear, but it does not appear to be a direct effect on the airway smooth muscle. Thus, the biologic action of PAF would suggest that either excessive activity or delayed metabolism to the inactive form may play a critical role in the development of both nonspecific airway responsiveness and the response to inhaled allergens.

PMNs have been implicated as amplifiers of nonspecific airway responsiveness. Activation of PMNs in rabbits (47) or depletion in sheep (48) alters the degree of airway responsiveness to aerosol histamine: activation is associated with an increase in responsiveness, and depletion with a decrease. Surprisingly, baseline white cell count is correlated in a positive fashion with the degree of airway responsiveness to aerosol histamine in the sheep (48). In other words, the higher the peripheral white cell count, the more reactive the airways. Clinical correlates for this relationship between inflammatory cell activity and degree of airway reactivity are evident in children with asthma. Aggressive treatment of upper respiratory tract disease (allergic rhinitis or sinusitis) is associated with amelioration of lower airway symptoms. These clinical observations, coupled with the more invasive studies in animals, imply that an inflammatory load at a respiratory site somewhat distant from the predominant lower airway site of asthma may play a role in the cyclical variation in airway reactivity. This is of clinical relevance, since the variation in airway responsiveness seen in asthmatics correlates with the degree of symptoms (8, 49).

Another inflammatory cell, the eosinophil, is thought to play a key role in the pathogenesis of airway responsiveness to inhaled allergen and perhaps also in the development of nonspecific airway responsiveness (24, 44, 50). Eosinophils are derived from the bone marrow, but over 99% reside not in the bloodstream but in peripheral tissues. They are particularly prominent in epithelium that has contact with the external environment such as the gastrointestinal, genitourinary, or respiratory tract. The density of the eosinophil is often diminished in asthma. It is not clear whether these hypodense eosinophils are immature forms released from the bone marrow or are activated, mature eosinophils. At any rate, these eosinophils are considered activated, releasing preformed cationic proteins or newly synthesized proteins. The cationic proteins (major basic protein, eosinophilic cationic protein, and eosinophil-derived neurotoxin) and eosinophil peroxidase are highly basic proteins that are stored in granules in the eosinophil and are released upon stimulation.

The cationic proteins possess potent cytotoxic and helminthotoxic characteristics. Eosinophils also contain the appropriate intracellular machinery to synthesize and release newly generated mediators of inflammation such as leukotriene C_4, PAF, and monohydroxy and dihydroxy acids of arachidonic acid.

Several observations imply a critical role for the eosinophil in the development of airway hyper-responsiveness and/or asthma. For example, following antigen exposure in animal models or in asthmatic subjects, eosinophil recruitment to the airways is seen at the beginning of the late phase response and lasts for up to 4 days (24). Similarly, increased amounts of cationic eosinophilic proteins are found. These proteins have been shown to be toxic to respiratory epithelial cells causing ciliary dysfunction, alteration in chloride and water transport, and even desquamation of the epithelial cell (24, 50). Another interesting observation is that the degree of airway responsiveness to methacholine correlates with the number of eosinophils and the major basic protein content from bronchoalveolar lavage. Finally, transbronchial lung biopsies in asymptomatic asthmatics suggest an early role for the eosinophil in the pathogenesis of asthma. During an asymptomatic phase, asthmatics have extensive thickening of the basement membrane beneath the respiratory epithelium and an impressive number of what appear to be activated eosinophils, particularly immediately beneath the epithelial cells as well as in close proximity to endothelial cells in the postcapillary venules (50). It has long been recognized that patients dying with status asthmaticus can have a massive infiltration of the lungs with eosinophils. These relationships between the eosinophil and allergic airway disease has caused some to speculate that the eosinophil plays a pivotal role in the pathogenesis of asthma. Activation of inflammatory cells may cause complex interactions between the alveolar macrophage, mast cell, T lymphocyte, and neutrophil, ultimately resulting in migration of the eosinophil to the respiratory epithelium. The activated eosinophil releases preformed and/or newly synthesized mediators that damage the epithelium and continue the cascade of pathophysiologic events leading to asthma (44).

Dysfunction or disruption of the respiratory epithelium is associated with an increase in airway responsiveness. There are several possible mechanisms whereby damage to the epithelium could cause the development of airway hyper-responsiveness. For example, epithelial disruption could cause an increased permeability to inhaled antigens and subsequent access of these antigens to immunocompetent cells. This mechanism is hypothesized as the cause of the increased airway responsiveness seen in patients with severe bronchiectasis due to cystic fibrosis. Another consequence of epithelial desquamation would be exposure of sensory nerve endings in the submucosal area of the airway. This could result in an increase in local neuronal reflexes and subsequent increased reflex bronchoconstriction. Finally, the epithelial cells themselves could have a direct influence on airway smooth muscle. This latter possibility has recently gained substantial credibility. In dogs, cattle, guinea pigs, and humans, removal of the respiratory epithelium is associated with an increased responsiveness to a variety of bronchoconstricting agents (51, 52). Currently, the most plausible explanation of a series of experiments designed to evaluate the mechanism(s) of this observation is that respiratory epithelial cells secrete a substance that causes relaxation of airway smooth muscle. This substance has been called *epithelium-derived relaxing factor*. The exact nature of this factor or factors is somewhat elusive. There is considerable heterogeneity of activity depending on the species, the pharmacologic agent evaluated, or the location along the respiratory tree (53). Nevertheless, there is substantial evidence that the airway epithelium has a direct effect on the smooth muscle. It is a reasonable assumption that damage to the epithelium (whether through viral infections, through recurrent bacterial infections and ultimate bronchiectasis as in cystic fibrosis, or through the eosinophil in allergic disorders) could cause an increase in airway responsiveness via the absence of the bronchodilator effect of epithelial-derived relaxing factors.

A discussion on the development of airway responsiveness would not be complete without mentioning the lipoxygenase products of arachidonic acid (24, 50, 54). Lipids in the cell membrane are converted to arachidonic acid, which in turn is converted to a variety of monohydroxylated acids (hydroxyeicosatetraenoic acid, or HETE), dihydroyxlated acids

(leukotriene B_4 or LTB_4), trihydroxylated acids (lipoxins), or cysteinyl-leukotrienes (LTC_4 LTD_4 and LTE_4). The biologic properties of these lipoxygenase products are protean and indicate a clear potential as mediators in the pathogenesis of asthma and in the development of airway responsiveness. For example, the leukotrienes can cause bronchoconstriction, increased vascular permeability, increased sensitivity to histamine, and increased mucus production, as well as act as chemoattractants or activators for a variety of inflammatory cells. However, it is still unclear when these products are causing a direct affect, are acting as second messengers in the microenvironment of the lung, or are merely passive markers.

Clinical observations of patients with asthma suggest that a state of increased airway reactivity may be associated with leakiness of the bronchial endothelium and epithelium (44, 50). For example, the sputum from patients with asthma contain plasma proteins such as albumin, IgG, fibrin, and clotting factors. Even more interesting is the finding that ingestion of salt in asthmatics increases airway responsiveness to aerosol histamine (55). It is a difficult task to conceptualize, or organize into a cohesive framework, the effects of alterations in water and ion transport across the airway on airway responsiveness. However, some insight is available by reviewing the following information. Several of the mediators already mentioned as being involved in the pathogenesis of airway responsiveness have the capability to increase permeability of vascular endothelium. Because the airway, and not the alveolus, is the site of obstruction, bronchial vascular endothelial permeability is of interest. Many of the inflammatory mediators, such as the leukotrienes, cause bronchial vascular vasodilation and increased endothelial permeability. Also, release of substances from the sensory neurons in the airways (tachykinins, substance P, and neurokinin A) have been shown to increase airway microvascular permeability (50). Increased fluid in the interstitium surrounding the airway is thought to occur during the response to inhaled allergen. However, this does not explain the presence of plasma protein in the sputa of patients with asthma. Since the airway epithelium is approximately 10 times *less* permeable than the vascular endothelium, one must also hypothesize an increased permeability of the epithelial layer in order to explain this phenomenon. Disruption of the epithelium is thought to be an early lesion in asthma, but there also is evidence that epithelial permeability is increased. Several of the inflammatory mediators have the biologic property of increasing epithelial permeability. For example, prostaglandins and leukotrienes increase the flux of chloride ions into the lumen of the airway. Tachykinins also share this property. The possibility that excess Cl− secretion into the periciliary layer is important comes from several publications assessing the ability of diuretics to block airflow obstruction precipitated by exercise, ultrasonically nebulized distilled water, and allergen. Bianco et al. compared the effect of inhaled furosemide versus placebo on the EAR and the LAR to inhaled allergen in 11 adult asthmatics previously shown to have a dual-phase response to allergen (12). Furosemide markedly attenuated the early response in all 11 subjects and the late response in 10. Thus, abnormal movement of water and electrolytes may be intimately involved in the full expression of airway responsiveness.

The relationships between viral respiratory infections, exacerbations of asthma, and changes in airway responsiveness have attracted considerable study (56). Almost one-half of exacerbations of childhood asthma are associated with viral infections; RSV, parainfluenza, influenza, and rhinovirus are the more common pathogens. In contrast, exacerbations of wheeze in adult asthmatics are said to be infrequently due to viral infections. If this is true, it is difficult to explain the observation that experimental respiratory viral infections in adults with asthma are associated with increased nonspecific airway responsiveness. Even harder to understand is the British Thoracic Society retrospective study on factors associated with asthma mortality in adults (57). Almost one-half of adults dying during an asthma exacerbation were reported to have what was presumed to be a viral upper respiratory tract infection during the few days before their demise. Despite these conflicting observations in adult asthmatics, it appears that viral respiratory infections are associated with a period of increased airway responsiveness. There are several potential reasons for this association (56, 58). Respiratory viral infec-

tions may act as amplifiers of the inflammatory response since it has been demonstrated that IgE, histamine, and chemotactic factors are released with viral infections. Alternatively, viral infections may alter the neural control of airway smooth muscle. Besides the classic adrenergic and cholinergic systems, there is a nonadrenergic, noncholinergic (NANC) nervous system supplying the airway smooth muscle, mucous glands, and vasculature of the airways. There are both inhibitory (bronchodilating) and excitatory (bronchoconstricting) NANC nerves. Viral infections may alter airway responsiveness by decreasing adrenergic or NANC inhibitory activity and/or increasing cholinergic activity. Another possible mechanism is disruption of the epithelial layer and subsequent exposure of sensory receptors mediating reflex bronchoconstriction as well as loss of epithelial-derived relaxing factors.

CONCLUSIONS

Our genetic repertoire is the foundation upon which the architecture of our airway responsiveness is fashioned. A variety of external elements, such as exposure to inhaled protein and acute lung infections, alters the expression of the airway response. Of equal importance to the ultimate expression of the degree of airway responsiveness are inherent biologic factors such as the age of the individual, the exuberance of the inflammatory response, and the biochemical and neural milieu of the airway. Finally, the relationship between the degree of airway responsiveness and expression of disease is not straightforward.

REFERENCES

1. Gurwitz D, Mindorff C, Levison H. Increased incidence of bronchial reactivity in children with a history of bronchiolitis. *J Pediatr* 1981; 98:551–555.
2. Mok JYQ, Waugh PR, Simpson H. *Mycoplasma pneumoniae* infection: A follow-up study of 50 children with respiratory illness. *Arch Dis Child* 1979; 54:506–511.
3. MacLusky IB, Stringer D, Zarfen J, Smallhorn J, Levison H. Cardiorespiratory status in long-term survivors of prematurity, with and without hyaline membrane disease. *Pediatr Pulmonol* 1986; 2:94–102.
4. Gurwitz D, Corey M, Levison H. Pulmonary function and bronchial reactivity in children after croup. *Am Rev Respir Dis* 1980; 122:95–99.
5. Weiss ST, Tager IB, Munoz A, Speizer FE. The relationship of respiratory infections in early childhood to the occurrence of increased levels of bronchial responsiveness and atopy. *Am Rev Respir Dis* 1985; 131:573–578.

6. Pattemore PK, Asher MI, Harrison AC, Mitchell EA, Rea HH, Stewart AW. The interrelationship among bronchial hyperresponsiveness, the diagnosis of asthma, and asthma symptoms. *Am Rev Respir Dis* 1990; 142:549–554.

7. Stick SM, Arnott J, Turner DJ, Young S, Landau LI, LeSouef PN. Bronchial responsiveness and lung function in recurrently wheezy infants. *Am Rev Respir Dis* 1991; 144:1012–1015.

8. Hargreave FE. (ed) *Airway Reactivity.* Mississauga, Ontario, Canada, Astra Pharmaceuticals Canada Ltd, 1980.

9. Orehek J, Gayrard P, Smith AP, Grimaud C, Charpin J. Airway response to carbachol in normal and asthmatic subjects. Distinction between bronchial sensitivity and reactivity. *Am Rev Respir Dis* 1977; 115:937–943.

10. Woolcock AJ, Salome CM, Yan K. The shape of the dose-response curve to histamine in asthmatic and normal subjects. Am Rev Respir Dis 1984; 130:71–75.

11. O'Byrne PM, Dolovich J, Hargreave FE. State of art: Late asthmatic responses. *Am Rev Respir Dis* 1987; 136:740–751.

12. Bianco S, Pieroni MG, Refini RM, Rottoli L, Sestini P. Protective effect of inhaled furosemide on allergen-induced early and late asthmatic reactions. *N Engl J Med* 1989; 321:1069–1073.

13. Stick SM, Turnbull S, Chua HL, Landau LI, LeSouef PN. Bronchial responsiveness to histamine in infants and older children. *Am Rev Respir Dis* 1990; 142:1143–1146.

14. Levitt RC, Mitzner W, Kleeberger SR. A genetic approach to the study of lung physiology: Understanding biological variability in airway responsiveness. *Am J Physiol* 1990; 258:L157–L164.

15. Longo G, Strinati R, Poli F, Fumi F. Genetic factors in nonspecific bronchial hyperreactivity: An epidemiologic study. *Am J Dis Child* 1987; 141:331–334.

16. Hirshman CA, Downes H, Veith L. Airway responses in offspring of dogs with and without airway hyperreactivity. *J Appl Physiol* 1984; 56:1272–1277.

17. Britt EJ, Shelhamer J, Menkes H, Bleecker E, Permutt S, Rosenthal R, Norman P. Airways reactivity and functional deterioration in relatives of COPD patients. *Chest* 1980; 77(Suppl):260.

18. Levitt RC, Mitzner W. Expression of airway hyperreactivity to acetylcholine as a simple autosomal recessive trait in mice. *FASEB J* 1988; 2:2605–2608.

19. Sauder RA, McNicol KJ, Stecenko AA. Effect of age on lung mechanics and airway reactivity in lambs. *J Appl Physiol* 1986; 61:2074–2080.

20. Stecenko A, McNicol K, Polk S. Evaluation of the mechanism of decreased airway responsiveness in lambs. *J Appl Physiol* 1989; 66:727–731.

21. Hayashi S, Toda N. Age-related alterations in the response of rabbit tracheal smooth muscle to agents. *J Pharmacol Exp Ther* 1980; 214:675–681.

22. Warner JO. Significance of late reactions after bronchial challenge with house dust mite. *Arch Dis Child* 1976; 51:905–911.

23. Altounyan REC. Changes in histamine and atropine responsiveness as a guide to diagnosis and evaluation of therapy in obstructive airways disease. In Pepys J, Frankland AW. (eds) *Disodium Cromoglycate in Allergic Airways Disease.* London, Butterworth, 1970.

24. Dorsch W. (ed) *Late Phase Allergic Reactions.* Boca Raton, FL, CRC Press, 1990.

25. Cockcroft DW, Ruffin RE, Frith PA, Cartier A, Juniper EF, Dolovich J, Hargreave FE. Determinants of allergen-induced asthma: Dose of allergen, circulating IgE antibody concentration, and bronchial responsiveness to inhaled histamine. *Am Rev Respir Dis* 1979; 120:1053–1058.

26. Cockcroft DW. Mechanism of perennial allergic asthma. *Lancet* 1983; 2:253–256.

27. Shampain MP, Behrens BL, Larsen GL, Henson PM. An animal model of late pulmonary responses to *Alternaria* challenge. *Am Rev Respir Dis* 1982; 126:493–498.

28. Behrens BL, Clark RAF, Marsh WR, Larsen, GL. Modulation of the late asthmatic response by antigen-specific immunoglobulin G in an animal model. *Am Rev Respir Dis* 1984; 130:1134–1139.

29. Stecenko AA, McNicol KJ. Induction of a dual phase airway response in lambs [Abstract]. *Am Rev Respir Dis* 1991; 143:130.

30. Freihorst J, Piedra PA, Okamoto Y, Ogra PL. Effect of respiratory syncytial virus infection on the uptake of and immune response to other inhaled antigens. *Proc Soc Exp Biol Med* 1988; 188:191–197.

31. Sporik R, Holgate ST, Platts-Mills TAE, Cogswell JJ. Exposure to house-dust mite allergen (*Der p* I) and the development of asthma in childhood. *N Engl J Med* 1990; 323:502–507.

32. Cote J, Kennedy S, Chan-Yeung M. Outcome of patients with cedar asthma with continuous exposure. *Am Rev Respir Dis* 1990; 141:373–376.

33. Matsuba K, Thurlbeck WM. A morphometric study of bronchial and bronchiolar walls in children. *Am Rev Respir Dis* 1972; 105:908–913.

34. Yanta MA, Snapper JR, Ingram Jr RH, Drazen JM, Coles S, Reid L. Airway responsiveness to inhaled mediators: Relationship to epithelial thickness and secretory cell number. *Am Rev Respir Dis* 1981; 124:337–340.

35. De Jongste JC, Sterk PJ, Willems LNA, Mons H, Timmers MC, Kerrebijn KF. Comparison of maximal bronchoconstriction *in vivo* and airway smooth muscle responses *in vitro* in nonasthmatic humans. *Am Rev Respir Dis* 1988; 138:321–326.

36. Vincenc KS, Black JL, Yan K, Armour CL, Donnelly PD, Woolcock AJ. Comparison of *in vivo* and *in vitro* responses to histamine in human airways. *Am Rev Respir Dis* 1983; 128:875–879.

37. Souhrada M, Souhrada JF. Specific reaginic antibody IgG_1-induced changes of airway smooth muscle cells. *J Appl Physiol* 1988; 65:767–775.

38. Abraham WM, Oliver W, King MM, Yerger L, Wanner A. Effect of pharmacologic agents on antigen-induced decreases in specific lung conductance in sheep. *Am Rev Respir Dis* 1981; 124:554–558.

39. Wanner A, Mezey RJ, Reinhart ME, Eyre P. Antigen-induced bronchospasm in conscious sheep. *J Appl Physiol* 1979; 47:917–922.

40. Metzger WJ, Zavala D, Richerson HB, Moseley P, Iwamota P, Monick M, Sjoerdsma K, Hunninghake GW. Local allergen challenge and bronchoalveolar lavage of allergic asthmatic lungs. *Am Rev Respir Dis* 1987; 135:433–440.

41. Turner CR, Kolbe J, Spannhake EW. Rapid increase in mast cell numbers in canine central and peripheral airways. *J Appl Physiol* 1988; 65:445–451.

42. Blythe SA, Lemanske RF Jr. Pulmonary late-phase allergic reactions. *Pediatr Pulmonol* 1988; 4:173–180.

43. Townley RG, Hopp RJ, Agrawal DK, Bewtra AK. Platelet-activating factor and airway reactivity. *J Allergy Clin Immunol* 1989; 83:997–1010.

44. Barnes PJ. New concepts in the pathogenesis of bronchial hyperresponsiveness and asthma. *J Allergy Clin Immunol* 1989; 83:1013–1026.

45. Djukanovic R, Roche WR, Wilson JW, Beasley CRW, Twentyman OP, Howarth PH, Holgate ST. Mucosal inflammation in asthma. *Am Rev Respir Dis* 1990; 142:434–457.

46. Miwa M, Miyake T, Yamanaka T, Sugatani J, Suzuki Y, Sakata S, Araki Y, Matsumoto M. Characterization of serum platelet-activating factor (PAF) acetylhydrolase. *J Clin Invest* 1988; 82:1983–1991.

47. Murphy KR, Wilson MC, Irvin CG, Glezen LS, Marsh WR, Haslett C, Henson PM, Larsen GL. The requirement for polymorphonuclear leukocytes in the late asthmatic response and heightened airways reactivity in an animal model. *Am Rev Respir Dis* 1986; 134:62–68.

48. Hinson Jr JM, Hutchison AA, Brigham KL, Meyrick BO, Snapper JR. Effects of granulocyte depletion on pulmonary responsiveness to aerosol histamine. *J Appl Physiol* 1984; 56:411–417.

49. Woolcock AJ, Jenkins CR. Assessment of bronchial responsiveness as a guide to prognosis and therapy in asthma. *Med Clin North Am* 1990; 74:753–765.

50. International Symposium on Airway Hyperreactivity. *Am Rev Respir Dis* 1991; 143.

51. Vanhoutte PM. Epithelium-derived relaxing factor(s) and bronchial reactivity. *J Allergy Clin Immunol* 1989; 83:855–861.

52. Morrison KJ, Yuansheng G, Vanhoutte PM. Epithelial modulation of airway smooth muscle. *Am J Physiol* 1990; 258:L254–L262.

53. Stuart-Smith K. Heterogeneity in epithelium-dependent responses. *Lung Suppl* 1990; 168:43–48.

54. Raeburn D. Eicosanoids, epithelium and airway reactivity. *Gen Pharmacol* 1990; 21:11–16.

55. Javaid A, Cushley MJ, Bone MF. Effect of dietary salt on bronchial reactivity to histamine in asthma. *Br Med J* 1988; 297:454.

56. Busse WW. Respiratory infections: Their role in airway responsiveness and the pathogenesis of asthma. *J Allergy Clin Immunol* 1990; 85:671–683.

57. British Thoracic Society. Comparison of atopic and non-atopic patients dying of asthma: British Thoracic Society. *Br J Dis Chest* 1987; 81:30–34.

58. Barnes PJ, Baraniuk JN, Belvisi MG. Neuropeptides in the respiratory tract. *Am Rev Respir Dis* 1991; 144:1391–1399.

4

Development of Respiratory Defenses

MERVIN C. YODER

For the pulmonary system to function as a gas exchange organ, ambient air must be drawn continually into the lungs and delivered to the alveolar epithelial surface for oxygen and carbon dioxide diffusion into and from capillary blood. Unfortunately, the atmospheric gases we inhale are not pure, but a composite of gases and suspended particulates. Willingly or unknowingly, we breathe air contaminated with smoke, industrial and vehicle pollutants (sulfur dioxide, carbon monoxide, ozone, and hydrocarbons), products of natural disasters (dusts, ashes, and vapors from volcanic activity, forest fires, and hurricanes), and biologically active particles (viruses, bacteria, spores, and pollens). Because of well-developed local and recruitable systemic host defenses, the respiratory system is protected from potentially injurious inhaled material. This chapter provides an overview of the pulmonary components that recognize, filter, detoxify, and eliminate inhaled impurities. Since these protective mechanisms are not fully developed at birth, I will also review the process of maturation of pulmonary defenses.

OVERVIEW

Upper Airway Defenses

Pulmonary protective mechanisms begin at the level of the nostrils where nasal vibrissae filter out macroscopic contaminants of the inspired air. The high velocity of the inhaled air and the unique anatomy of the nasal chamber cause the airstream to flow turbulently through the nasal passages, and many of the largest inhaled particles collide into the mucus-coated epithelium of the nasal septum and turbinates. This mechanism of aerodynamic filtration is facilitated by the high humidity of the nasopharynx, which hydrates the aerosolized particles and alters their physical dimensions. As the airstream turns abruptly at the level of the nasopharynx, additional aerosolized contaminants collide into the posterior pharyngeal mucosa. So effective is this initial filtering mechanism that more than 90% of aerosolized particles greater than 10 μm and more than 75% of particles greater than 5 μm are captured (1). Beneath the pharyngeal mucosa lie the immunologically active adenoids and tonsils. These tissues contain lymphocytes and macrophages that participate in development of immunity against inhaled antigens. Particles trapped in the protective mucus overlying the nasopharyngeal epithelium may be bound and inactivated by macrophages, by antigen-specific lymphocytes originating from the tonsils and adenoids, or by enzymes, lipids, albumin, and antibodies (chiefly immunoglobulin A) present in the mucus. Nasopharyngeal mucus production is continually produced, with spent mucus being cleared continually from the nasopharyngeal surface by ciliary movement of the material toward the esophagus for eventual swallowing, or by rapid expulsion through sneezing (2).

Tracheobronchial Defenses

Aerosolized particles that elude upper airway filtration enter the trachea; many are filtered out at the level of the carina or within two bronchial divisions, the turbulent airflow of inspiration causing particles to collide into the walls of the branching airways (Fig. 4.1). Many foreign materials trapped in the mucus layer of the trachea and major bronchi are removed through coughing. Additional secretory and immunologic mechanisms of pulmonary defense are required for protection of more

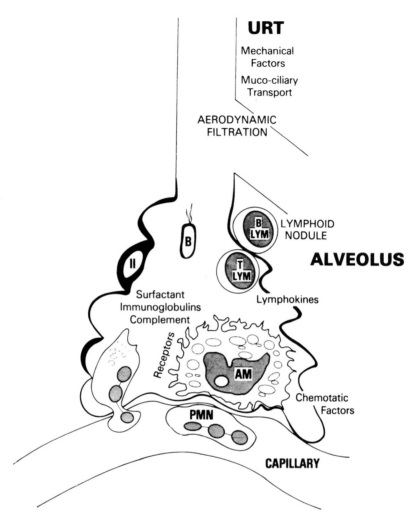

Figure 4.1. Factors responsible for clearance of bacteria *(B)* inhaled into the lungs are quite different in the upper respiratory tract *(URT)* and in the alveolus. A bacterium that is deposited in an alveolus may encounter surfactant (secreted by type II pneumocytes) and/or immunoglobulins (synthesized by B lymphocytes *[B lym])* and complement proteins that condition the organism for ingestion by alveolar macrophages *(AM)*. Additionally, the alveolar macrophages can liberate chemotactic factors that attract nearby neutrophils *(PMN* [polymorphonuclear neutrophil leukocyte]) marginated in the lung capillary adjacent to the alveolus, and thus initiate an inflammatory response. The microorganism may also trigger immune lymphocytes *(T lym)* to release lymphokines that activate and stimulate the alveolar macrophages' phagocytic and bactericidal capacity. (From Reynolds HY. Respiratory infections may reflect deficiencies in host defense mechanisms. *Dis Month* 1985; 31:13.)

distal smaller-diameter conducting airways. Numerous specialized secretory cells are present in the airway mucosa and submucosa. Secretory cells, interspersed with airway epithelium lining the airways or organized into submucosal glands, secrete mucin-type glycoproteins, glycosaminoglycans, lysozyme, phospholipids, and serum-derived proteins (1). These humoral (soluble) factors aid in preventing particle attachment to airway cells;

they also aid mucus entrapment, neutralization, and clearance of the inhaled contaminants by mucociliary transport. A few immunologically active cells (lymphocytes and macrophages) may be found on the surface of the airway epithelium, but a higher concentration of these cells is usually found in the submucosa. Antigen-specific lymphocytes and macrophages are capable of clearing pathogens deposited in the airway secretions independently, and also participate in initiating primary immune responses to new antigens and stimulation of airway epithelial secretory behavior. Collectively, tracheobronchial defenses efficiently remove most inhaled particulates, but some small (0.5–2 mm) particles, such as bacteria, viruses, spores, and toxic smoke and fumes, reach the respiratory bronchioles and alveoli (2).

Alveolar Defenses

Mechanisms of defense change significantly at the level of the respiratory bronchioles (2). Airflow velocity is nil in the respiratory bronchioles, and gases reach the alveolar epithelium through diffusion. Aerosolized particles no longer forcefully collide into the epithelial surface of the lung, as occurred in the upper and conducting airways. Specialized secretory glands and cells of the airways are not present in the alveoli; therefore, the secretory products of pneumocytes, macrophages, endothelial cells, and the diffusion of intravascular proteins into the alveolar fluid, play a prominent role in alveolar defense (3). Those biologically active particles which enter alveoli and are sequestered in the alveolar lining fluid are susceptible to opsonization by immunoglobulin (Ig) or other proteins present in the alveolar fluid (Fig. 4.1) and will be ingested more quickly by resident mobile macrophages (alveolar macrophages). Upon activation, complement proteins present in the fluid will opsonize the particles, serve as chemoattractants to recruit additional macrophages and intravascular neutrophils into the site of particle encounter, and in many instances lyse inhaled microbes directly (by inserting themselves into the cell membrane of the pathogen). Lymphocytes present in the area (Fig. 4.1) may be stimulated to secrete lymphokines (small peptide hormones) that activate the alveolar macrophages for a higher level of function, which results in microbial killing. Such activation may also lead to macrophage secretion of chemoattractants for mobilization of neutrophils and monocytes from the intravascular space into the alveolar space for added microbial elimination. The inflammatory response that ensues is a highly regulated sequence of humoral and cellular events (Fig. 4.2) that usually culminates in the removal of the offending pathogens and return of the alveolar epithelial surface to normal (4).

When appropriately directed, cellular mechanisms of pulmonary defense are highly protective. However, these same inflammatory mediators may result in structural damage to pulmonary epithelium and loss of gas exchange function in certain pathophysiologic states (5).

MATURATION OF PULMONARY DEFENSES

Upper Airway Defenses

Aerodynamic filtration of inhaled particulates in the nasopharynx is thought to be fully operative at birth. In the human newborn as in the adult, the nasal septum and turbinates contribute to the unique nasal chamber anatomy that imparts resistance to airflow and causes inspired air to flow turbulently into the nasopharynx; an important component of particle dispersion and aerodynamic filtration. Some researchers have speculated that preferential nasal breathing in the infant for the first 6 months of life serves to promote nasopharyngeal clearance of inhaled particulates, since oral breathing in any individual at any stage of life allows for larger inhaled particulates to penetrate to the level of the respiratory bronchioles (6).

Little is known of the mucus production rates in the nasopharynx of the human neonate or infant; nor is there information regarding nasal mucus composition in the infant at birth. Developmental differences in the concentration of nasal mucus Ig have been reported, however. Immunoglobulins G and A are detectable in nasal secretions as early as 10 days after term birth. IgG concentrations exceed IgA concentrations in nasal secretions of normal infants during the first 2 years of life, which is distinct from adults, in whom IgA far exceeds IgG. Acute respiratory infections in infants result in a shift to predominantly IgA and less IgG in the nasal secretions (7). Most (80–95%) of the IgA is locally synthesized, whereas only 5–10% of the IgG in nasal secretions is locally produced, most being derived from the serum. Finally, although the IgA concentration abruptly increases in the nasal secretions of infants during an acute respiratory infection, salivary and serum IgA concentrations are often unchanged from normal (7). This confirms the thought that local immune responses are

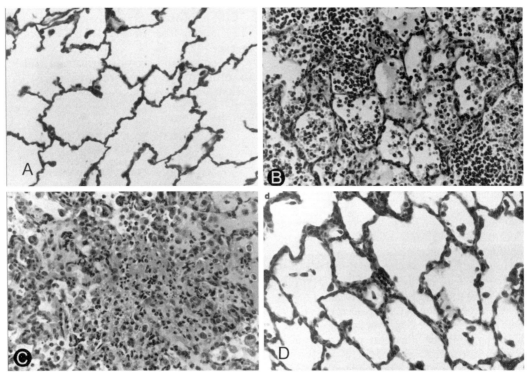

Figure 4.2. An acute inflammatory response induced by instillation of C5 complement fragments into the lungs of rabbits. *A,* Normal lung given saline. *B,* Early influx of neutrophils into alveoli filled with fluid in treated animals. *C,* At 48 hours neutrophils are declining and mononuclear cells are accumulating. *D,* Resolution complete at 5 days. (From Clark RAF, Henson P, eds. *The molecular and cellular biology of wound repair.* New York, Plenum, 1988, pp 188–189.)

present soon after birth and are highly responsive to the antigenic material directly presented to the mucosal surface.

Immunocompetent, differentiated B lymphocytes secreting antigen-specific antibody (plasma cells) appear in the tonsils of infants within 2 or 3 weeks of birth. The lymphocytes and antigen-presenting macrophages resident in adenoids and tonsils are exposed to a great variety of inhaled particulates and provide local immunity against this material throughout life. Peak lymphoid activity in these tissues occurs from ages 2 to 10 years and steadily declines with advancing age beyond the 18th birthday (8). IgG-synthesizing lymphocytes predominate in these tissues in normal children and adults, followed by cells producing IgA, IgM, and IgD. Virtually no IgE-synthesizing lymphocytes are detectable in the tonsils and adenoids of normal children. The proportion of plasma cells in the tonsils producing IgA increase, and cells producing IgG signifi-

cantly decrease, in children with recurrent tonsillitis (8).

It remains unclear how significant a role the humoral and cellular elements of the tonsils and adenoids play in pulmonary defense. Secretory IgA has been demonstrated to neutralize respiratory viruses in the nasopharynx and can neutralize certain microbes and exotoxins in vitro. Microbial and soluble antigenic material can be blocked effectively from mucosal attachment by secretory IgA (9). Unlike IgA, IgG can activate the complement system of proteins, and therefore is a powerful opsonin as well as an efficient agglutinator of particulates and neutralizer of exotoxins and viruses. Cell-mediated immunity to inhaled antigenic material or viral particles appears to afford greater defense to reinfection or challenge than if the initial exposure and primary immune response is to a systemic infection or challenge (10). This supports a role for the immunologic responsive tissues of the nasopharynx in augmenting pulmonary defenses.

Tracheobronchial Defenses

Important components of pulmonary defense in the conducting airways include (a) aerodynamic filtration, (b) mucus secretion, and (c) mucociliary clearance. As stated, aerodynamic filtration is operant in the newborn infant, although the capacity of the trachea and bronchi to "prevent" particulate penetration into the small airways is unknown. Maximal filtration would appear to be required since the gas exchange surface area of the lung has not fully developed and alveolar protective mechanisms are deficient at birth (see below).

Secretion of electrolytes and proteins by conducting airway epithelium in the fetus begins early in gestation (13–16 weeks). In utero, the lungs are filled with fluid, and the tracheobronchial mucosa functions in a more secretory than absorptive capacity (11). Just prior to birth, pulmonary fluid must be expelled from the conducting airways and gas exchange portions of the lung to prepare for normal respiration. The liquid layer that must remain to cover the conducting airway epithelium actually consists of an aqueous periciliary phase and a viscoelastic mucus superficial phase. This liquid is actively secreted in the distal airways and is gradually reabsorbed (primarily through sodium and chloride reabsorption) as it is moved by ciliary action toward the proximal airways. The high rate of fetal lung fluid production is driven by raising the electrolyte concentration in the fluid through active chloride secretion (sodium passively follows). Within 2 weeks of birth, the proximal airway epithelium fully develops the capacity to absorb sodium and chloride from the periciliary phase, and a decrease in chloride and fluid secretion by more distal airways is observed (11). Thus, adult-like secretory behavior of the proximal airways is achieved early in life.

Mucus-producing submucosal glands, goblet cells, and serous cells are present in the proximal airway of the developing human fetus by 12–16 weeks of gestation (12). Nearly 5000 mucus-producing glands are present in the trachea at birth (12); no further increase in the number occurs with postnatal growth and development. Airway mucus composition in the fetal lung changes slightly in the third trimester of human pregnancy, with increased content of some forms of glycosaminoglycans.

The content of mucus-type glycoproteins changes little from 26 weeks of gestation to 6 years of age. Unstimulated lysozyme secretion in the preterm infant is equivalent to that in the child, although cholinergic-stimulated lysozyme secretion is not apparent until 40 weeks of gestation (11). It is unclear if the lower concentration of the bacteriolytic enzyme, lysozyme, in the airways secretions diminishes pulmonary defense in the human preterm infant lung.

Although particle phagocytosis by airway alveolar macrophages and dendritic cells and direct-microbe cytotoxicity mediated by T lymphocytes may occur on the epithelial surface along the conducting airways, this is not a prominent mechanism for removal of trapped particles. Other specialized lymphoid tissues appear to participate in particle trapping and processing (13). Bronchus-associated lymphoid tissue (BALT) exists in aggregates or follicles throughout the lung and is covered by a specialized lymphoepithelium that is devoid of cilia and lacks specialized secretory cells. BALT is composed primarily of B lymphocytes (some mature antibody-secreting plasma cells), T lymphocytes, dendritic cells, and reticular cells. These lymphoid aggregates are most prominent along main bronchi, are found in higher concentration at bifurcations of the bronchi, and often lie between the bronchial epithelium and adjacent pulmonary arteries. The strategic location of BALT at branch points along the airways (where numerous particulates would impact by aerodynamic filtration) and the lack of cilia and goblet cells overlying the BALT aggregates (leading to slower mucociliary transport) seem adapted for most efficient particle capture. Indeed, antigen sampling and initiation of primary immune responses to inhaled material appears to be a primary function of BALT. Some of the antigenic material may be transported by macrophages present in BALT to more distant lymph nodes and augment the immune response. Furthermore, BALT belongs to a common mucosal immune system that includes gut-associated lymphoid tissue (GALT) and other mucosa-associated lymphoid tissues. The significance of this system is that antigen presentation to lymphocytes in one organ may result in redistribution of lymphocytes or plasma cells to other mucosal surfaces to provide a wider dissemination of anti-body protection (9).

Lymphoid aggregates representative of BALT are not present in the lungs of newborn human infants. Mononuclear cell aggregates present in the lamina propria of developing lung buds can be identified at 8–10 weeks of gestation. These cells are also present in the developing intestine and may represent the precursors of BALT and GALT. BALT first appears in the lungs of human newborn infants at 1 week of age. During the first year of life, BALT aggregates undergo a nearly tenfold increase in number and continue to develop through adolescence (13). The progressive development of BALT appears to be driven by the amount, type, and length of exposure to inhaled particulates.

Alveolar Defenses

Humoral and cellular elements present in the alveolar lining fluid are primary components of pulmonary defense at the level of the alveo-lus. Much of the information pertaining to the analysis of the protective factors is present in normal human alveolar lining fluid and has been obtained from human adult volunteers with the flexible fiberoptic bronchoscope (2). Our knowledge of the ontogeny of these alve-olar defense mechanisms in human infants and children is limited; therefore I will review data obtained from animal studies in those areas in which data on the ontogeny of human alveolar defenses are insufficient. I will focus on the role of Ig and complement as humoral factors, and alveolar macrophages and neutrophils as cellular factors, that function to protect the delicate alveolar epithelium from inhaled par-ticulate–induced injury.

IgG is the predominant Ig present in the alveolar fluid, accounting for nearly 9% of total protein recovered from bronchoalveolar lavage (BAL) fluid (14). IgA constitutes approximately 7%, and IgM 0.3%, of total BAL fluid protein (14). IgA concentrations slowly increase with age in the alveolar lining fluid of the normal human adult. Although IgG may be synthesized locally, most IgG in alveolar fluid is derived from serum. The large size of the IgM molecule probably accounts for the trace amount of this Ig that is able to traverse the alveolar-capillary barrier. The source of IgA in the alveolar fluid remains unclear; both upper airway secretion and aspi-

ration into the lower respiratory tract and local production have been proposed (2). Binding of IgG to inhaled particulate matter or formation of IgG complexes in alveolar fluid leads to particle ingestion by macro-phages and neutrophils and to activation of complement to generate several biologically active products (see below) that stimulate an inflammatory response. The role of IgA and IgM is less clear, though IgA is effective in preventing microbial attachment to epithelial cells and in neutralizing viruses.

The age at which mature (adult-like) Ig concentrations are achieved in alveolar fluid has not been defined in humans. IgG and secretory component (protein normally com-plexed with IgA) have been identified by immunohistologic techniques in the human fetus by 12 weeks of gestation. In one study, IgA and IgM were not detectable at the same gestational age, and no data regarding the presence of Ig in fetal lungs later than 22 weeks of gestation were reported (15). The ontogeny of B lymphocyte maturation and changes in serum Ig concentration during infant development have been studied, how-ever (16). This is relevant information since IgG and IgM in alveolar lining fluid are princi-pally derived from serum. Lymphocytes bear-ing surface Ig appear early in human gestation, and serum IgM is synthesized as early as 8 weeks of gestation. Serum IgG appears at 12 weeks, and IgA at nearly 30 weeks of gestation, but the endogenous synthesis of all classes of Ig remains very low until 6–8 weeks after birth (Fig. 4.3). Serum IgM concentrations are low at birth but reach adult values by 3–4 years of age (Table 4.1). Serum IgG concentrations are high (adult-like values) at birth, but only because of placental transfer of maternal IgG (Table 4.1). At 3–4 months of age, serum IgG concentrations have declined to the lowest point measured in infancy because maternal antibody has been continually catabolized and endogenous synthesis is only becoming engaged. A progressive increase then occurs to reach adult values by 4–6 years of age (Table 4.1). The importance of adequate Ig synthesis in pulmonary and host defense is demonstrated in infants and children with agammaglobulinemia or hypogammaglobuli-nemia who suffer recurrent upper and lower respiratory infections, as well as gastrointesti-nal and joint infections, early in life (17).

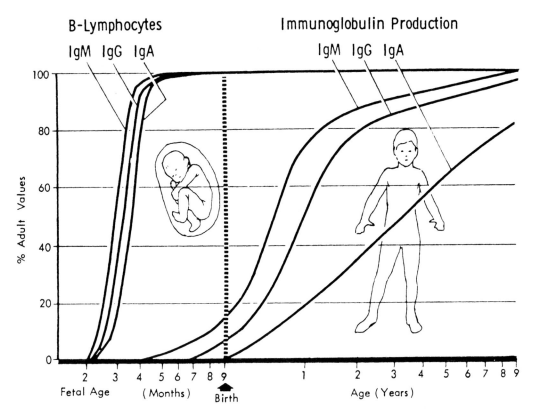

Figure 4.3. The development of B lymphocytes and age-dependant changes in serum immunoglobulins in the infant before and after birth. (From Goldman AS, Goldblum RM. Primary deficiencies in humoral immunity. *Pediatr Clin North Am* 1977; 24:281.)

Table 4.1.
Normal Values for Immunoglobulins at Various Ages

Age	IgG (mg/dl)	IgA (mg/dl)	IgM (mg/dl)
Newborn	600–1670	0–5	5–15
1–3 months	218–610	20–53	11–51
4–6 months	228–636	27–72	25–60
7–9 months	292–816	27–73	12–124
10–18 months	383–1070	27–169	28–113
2 years	423–1184	35–222	32–131
3 years	477–1334	40–251	28–113
4–5 years	540–1500	48–336	20–106
6–8 years	571–1700	52–535	28–112
14 years	570–1570	86–544	33–135
Adult	635–1775	106–668	37–154

From Fanaroff AA, Martin RJ, eds. *Neonatal-perinatal medicine: Diseases of the fetus and infant* (4th ed.) St. Louis, Mosby-Year Book, 1987, p 748.

The complement system plays an important role as one of the primary humoral effectors of the immune system. This group of proteins requires some form of activation to initiate the chain reaction in which one activated component serves as an enzyme to cleave and acti-vate the next component in the sequence (Fig. 4.4). Activation of the classic pathway requires immune complex formation with comple-ment-binding Ig (IgG and IgM), whereas the alternative pathway can be activated by a vari-ety of substances (IgA, bacterial or fungal cell

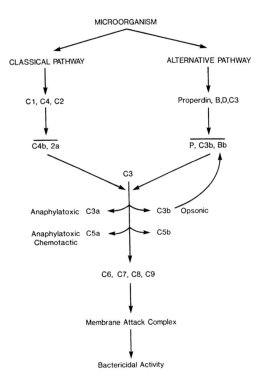

MICROORGANISM

CLASSICAL PATHWAY → C1, C4, C2 → C4b, 2a

ALTERNATIVE PATHWAY → Properdin, B,D,C3 → P, C3b, Bb

C3

Anaphylatoxic C3a ← → C3b Opsonic

Anaphylatoxic C5a ← → C5b
Chemotactic

C6, C7, C8, C9

Membrane Attack Complex

Bactericidal Activity

Figure 4.4. Activation of the classic pathway and/or alternative pathway results in generation of soluble factors that amplify phagocyte function and a membrane attack complex that damages cell membranes. (From McLean RH, Winkelstein JA. Genetically determined variation in the complement system. *J Pediatr* 1984; 105:180.)

sizing many complement components (2, 18). Even at low concentrations in the alveolar lining fluid, the biologically active fragments of activated complement may play an important role in amplifying the inflammatory response to aerosolized contaminants by serving as a chemoattractant for neutrophils and monocytes. Complement components have not been quantitated in alveolar lining fluid from normal human newborn infants and children.

Analysis of serum complement in the human fetus and newborn has been performed. Serum complement components are first detectable at 8 weeks of gestation in the human fetus (19). Classic complement components increase in concentration with increasing gestational age, but at term gestation the serum concentration of most classic pathway components are 50% of adult levels. Alternative pathway component concentrations are even lower (as a percentage of adult level) at term gestation and do not reach the adult serum concentration until nearly 1 year of age. It is unclear to what extent the lower serum complement concentrations in the human newborn infant diminish pulmonary and host defenses (16).

Alveolar macrophages serve as a first line of cellular defense for the epithelial surface of alveoli and conducting airways (20). Alveolar macrophages are members of the mononuclear phagocyte lineage and are derived from circulating monocytes, but may proliferate in situ to maintain adequate numbers of cells under normal conditions. These phagocytic cells are active in clearing and eliminating aerosolized pathogens that enter the lung, and they participate in several aspects of primary and secondary immune responses. Alveolar macrophages process and present antigen to T lymphocytes and secrete a wide variety of immunoregulatory cytokines including interleukins-1 and -6, tumor necrosis factor alpha, transforming growth factor beta, and several hematopoietic growth factors (21). Antigen-activated T lymphocytes, in turn, are capable of secreting a variety of cytokines that activate the alveolar macrophage for enhanced phagocytosis, production of toxic oxygen intermediates used for killing microbes, altered expression of cell surface receptors, and release of other cytokines that influence the behavior of resident fibroblasts and endothelial cells (16, 20, 21).

surfaces, and certain toxins). Generation of factor C3b from C3 is a critical point in the sequence (Fig 4.4), since further activation of components will result in release of C5a (which serves as a potent chemoattractant for leukocytes and alters capillary permeability) and formation of the membrane attack complex. Insertion of the complex into microbial or host cellular membranes causes disruption of cellular integrity. Alternatively, C3b may be cleaved into smaller fragments that are biologically active (opsonic) but do not result in C5 activation. Neutrophils, monocytes, and macrophages express cell surface receptors for C3b and C3bi and ingest particles bearing these complement components.

Low concentrations of complement proteins have been recovered from the BAL fluid of normal human adult volunteers. These proteins are probably derived from serum, but alveolar macrophages are capable of synthe-

Alveolar macrophages are not present in the developing human fetal lung prior to birth. Within 48 hours of birth, macrophages are present in the alveoli regardless of the gestational age of the newborn infant, but are particularly plentiful in those infants with pulmonary infections or respiratory distress (22). Similar kinetics of appearance have been reported for newborn rats, rabbits, and monkeys (23). The increase in alveolar surface-active material (surfactant and proteins) that occurs at birth may be a primary inducer of alveolar macrophage influx. Alveolar macrophage microbicidal activity, generation of reactive oxygen intermediates, chemotaxis, and synthetic capacity are impaired at birth but increase to near adult levels in the first weeks of life in newborn rats, rabbits, sheep, and monkeys (23, 24). Comparative data are not available for tests of alveolar macrophage function in normal newborn infants. Alveolar macrophages isolated by BAL from human premature and term infants who were intubated for respiratory distress were able to destroy Candida albicans in an in-vitro assay at a level equivalent to that of macrophages isolated by BAL from adult volunteers (24). The alveolar macrophages from the newborn infants did not restrict intracellular growth of the organisms to the same extent as did the "adult" macrophages, however, and it was postulated that in the face of a large intra-alveolar challenge, alveolar macrophage function may not provide adequate protection.

Under normal circumstances, the lung is able to remain sterile below the level of the carina. Normal pulmonary defenses may be overwhelmed on occasion, and additional defenses must be recruited. The stimuli that initiate an inflammatory response may come from the aerosolized particles directly or from activated humoral and cellular components of alveolar defense (Fig. 4.5). A normal host response to a localized infection involves release of chemical mediators of inflammation, vasodilatation, altered vessel permeability, and cellular infiltration (Fig. 4.5). Neutrophils accumulate at the site of infection because of a number of factors including changes in local blood flow, increased endothelial-neutrophil adhesion, presence of chemoattractants (alveolar macrophage, complement, or neutrophil derived), and extent of tissue damage (4). Usually, monocytes and

macrophages follow the influx of neutrophils by 48 hours and begin the process of resolution of inflammation and initiation of wound healing. A variety of factors determine at this point whether the acute inflammation resolves or persists and thus whether the area of infection heals or progresses to a chronic inflammatory condition (4).

Delivery of neutrophils and monocytes to localized areas of infection is blunted in the human preterm and term gestation infant (23). Some potential causes of limited neutrophil accumulation at infected sites are impairments in chemoattractant generation, neutrophil migration, and neutrophil production (25).

A striking histologic feature of the lungs of newborn infants dying of group B streptococcal pneumonia is the paucity of neutrophils present in alveoli filled with large numbers of bacteria. One explanation for the failure to elicit a more pronounced inflammatory response is that group B streptococci fail to generate significant activated complement components when incubated in vitro with newborn infant serum (25). This inability to activate complement is directly proportional to the low concentrations of complement components and type-specific IgG present in the newborn infant serum. Thus, impaired generation of complement-derived chemoattractants at sites of infection may account in part for the diminished inflammatory host response.

Impaired migration of neutrophils is a consistent finding in several studies of neutrophil function in newborn infants (26). A number of factors appear to be involved in causing this abnormality, including defective augmentation of adhesiveness and abnormal signal transduction following chemotactic stimulation, impaired redistribution of adhesion-promoting cell surface receptors following activation, diminished cell deformability, and perhaps heterogeneity in the maturational states of the circulating neutrophils. For all infants, neutrophil motility does not appear to reach adult levels of activity until 8 years of age (16).

Neutrophil production rates are limited in the fetus and newborn infant. Despite the fact that fetal and neonatal blood contains high concentrations of neutrophil progenitor cells, data from studies using fetal rats suggest that the bone marrow of these young animals has only one-tenth the number of progenitor cells

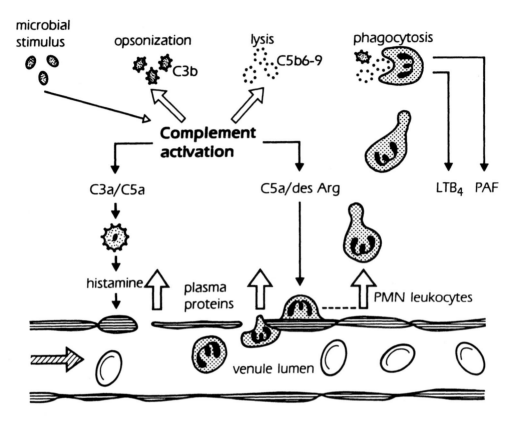

Figure 4.5. Depiction of some of the mediators and events of acute inflammation. Complement activation by microbial cell walls or antibody-coated microbes results in generation of additional opsonins (C3b) or the membrane attack complex (C5b6-9) that lyses some organisms. Other complement fragments, C3a and C5a, cause mast cell release of histamine and contribute to an early phase of vasodilatation and plasma protein leakage. An additional byproduct, C5a des Arg, serves as a chemoattractant for neutrophils *(PMN)*. PMN phagocytosis of opsonized material induces secretion of leukotriene B$_4$ (LTB$_4$) and platelet-activating factor (PAF), which promote continued PMN influx and plasma leakage. (From Clark RAF, Henson P, eds. *The molecular and cellular biology of wound repair.* New York, Plenum, 1988, p 138.)

compared to adult rat bone marrow (27). Studies of progenitor cell proliferation using human cord blood suggest that these progenitor cells are limited in their capacity to divide at greater rates when stimulated with a variety of hematopoietic growth factors, whereas progenitor cells from adult bone marrow are capable of fourfold or fivefold increases. Furthermore, the bone marrow storage pool of neutrophils is smaller and more rapidly depleted in the septic human newborn infant than in the adult. Thus, under the stress of delivering large numbers of neutrophils to sites of infection, the supply of neutrophils may irreversibly decline; neutropenia during sepsis is not uncommon and is a poor prognostic sign in human newborn infants (27). Phar-

macologic or immunotherapeutic correction of these developmental defects may enhance neutrophil contributions to local and systemic host defense in the newborn infant.

CONCLUSIONS

An extensive description of the maturation of pulmonary defenses is not currently possible because we know so little of the development of this system in the human newborn infant. At present it appears that most aspects of upper airway defenses are intact at birth. In the conducting airways, aerodynamic filtration is probably mature at birth, and changes in secretory behavior of the airway epithelium and in airway mucus composition are completed in the first few weeks of life. Significant maturation of the BALT system occurs throughout childhood and adolescence. Numerous aspects of pulmonary defense are deficient at the alveolar level in the newborn infant. Perhaps the most significant, deficit, sometimes life-threatening deficit is the impaired capacity of the immune system to generate inflammation at sites of microbial invasion. In spite of these apparent areas of pulmonary defense immaturity, most infants and children overcome the many exposures to injurious organisms and materials that are inhaled daily and lead full active lives.

REFERENCES

1. Newhouse MT, Bienenstock J. Respiratory tract defense mechanisms. In Baum GL, Wolinsky E, eds. *Textbook of pulmonary diseases.* Boston, Little Brown, 1989, pp 21–47.
2. Reynolds HY. Integrated host defense against infections. In Crystal RG, West JB, Barnes PJ, Cherniack NS, Weibel ER, eds. *The lung.* New York, Raven Press, 1991, pp 1899–1911.
3. Reynolds HY. Respiratory infections may reflect deficiencies in host defense mechanisms. *Dis Month* 1985; 31:1–98.
4. Larsen GL. Development of pulmonary defense mechanisms. In Chernick V, Mellins RB, eds. *Basic mechanisms of pediatric respiratory disease: Cellular and integrative.* Philadelphia, BC Decker, 1991, pp 347–360.
5. Hogg JC. Neutrophil kinetics and lung injury. *Physiol Rev* 1987; 67:1249–1295.
6. Mautone AJ, Cataletto MB. Mechanical defense mechanisms of the lung. In Scarpelli EM, ed. *Pulmonary physiology.* Philadelphia: Lea & Febiger, 1990, pp 192–214.
7. Cohen AB, Goldberg S, London RL. Immunoglobulins in nasal secretions of infants. *Clin Exp Immunol* 1970; 6:753–760.
8. Korsrud FR, Brandtzaeg P. Immune systems of human nasopharyngeal and palatine tonsils: histomorphometry of lymphoid components and quantification of immunoglobulin-producing cells in health and disease. *Clin Exp Immunol* 1980; 39:361–370.
9. Russel MW, Mestecky J. Induction of the mucosal immune response. *Rev Infect Dis* 1988: 10:S440–S446.
10. Ogra PL, Cumella JC, Welliver RC. Immune response to viruses. In Bienenstock J, ed. *Immunology of the lung and upper respiratory tract.* New York, McGraw-Hill, 1984, pp 242–263.
11. Wanner A, Phipps RJ, Kim CS. Mucus clearance: cilia and cough. In Chernick V, Mellins RB, eds. *Basic mechanisms of pediatric respiratory disease: Cellular and integrative.* Philadelphia, BC Decker, 1991, pp 361–382.
12. Thurlbeck WM, Benjamin B, Reid L. Development and distribution of mucous glands in the foetal human trachea. *J Dis Chest* 1961; 55:54–64.
13. Bienenstock J. Bronchus-associated lymphoid tissue. In Bienenstock J, ed. *Immunology of the lung and upper respiratory tract.* New York: McGraw-Hill, 1984, pp 96–118.
14. Banks DE, Bell DY, Davis GS, et al. Bronchoalveolar lavage constituents in healthy individuals, idiopathic pulmonary fibrosis, and selected comparison groups. *Am Rev Respir Dis* 1990; 141:S169–196.
15. Ogra SS, Ogra PL, Lippes J, Tomasi TB Jr. Immunohistologic localization of immunoglobulin, secretory component, and lactoferrin in the developing human fetus. *Proc Soc Exp Biol Med* 1972; 139:570–574.
16. Yoder MC, Polin RA. Developmental immunology. In Fanaroff AA, Martin RJ, eds. *Neonatal-perinatal medicine,* 5th ed. St. Louis, Mosby-Year Book, 1992, pp 587–618.
17. Goldman AS, Goldblum RM, Primary deficiencies in humoral immunity. *Pediatr Clin North Am* 1977: 24:277–291.
18. Johnson E, Hetland G. Mononuclear phagocytes have the potential to synthesize the complete functional complement system. *Scand J Immunol* 1988; 27:489–495.
19. Colten HR. Ontongeny of the human complement system: In vitro biosynthesis of individual complement components of fetal tissues. *J Clin Invest* 1972; 51:725–731.
20. Sibille Y, Reynolds HY. Macrophages and polymorphonuclear neutrophils in lung defense and injury. *Am Rev Respir Dis* 1990; 141:471–501.
21. Kelly J. Cytokines of the lung. *Am Rev Respir Dis* 1990; 141:765–788.
22. Alenghat E, Esterly JR. Alveolar macrophages in perinatal infants. *Pediatrics* 1984: 74:221–223.
23. Wilson CB. Lung antimicrobial defenses in the newborn. *Semin Resp Med* 1984: 6:149–155.
24. D'Ambola JB, Sherman MP, Tashkin DP, Gong H Jr. Human and rabbit newborn lung macrophages have reduced anti-candida activity. *Pediatr Res* 1988: 24:285–290.
25. Anderson DC. Neonatal neutrophil dysfunction. *Am J Pediatr Hematol Oncol* 1989: 11:224–226.
26. Hill HR. Biochemical, structural, and functional abnormalities of polymorphonuclear leukocytes in the neonate. *Pediatr Res* 1987: 22:375–382.
27. Christensen RD. Hematopoiesis in the fetus and neonate. *Pediatr Res* 1989: 26:531–535.

5

Origins of Chronic Lung Disease

LOUIS I. LANDAU

Chronic lung disease is a major cause of death and disability at most ages through life. There is increasing evidence that considerable morbidity from lung disease in later life is associated with prior lower respiratory illness in children. This association was originally proposed on the basis of both clinical and epidemiologic studies. Subsequently, physiologic studies have suggested pathogenetic mechanisms whereby the effects of childhood respiratory illness may result in chronic lung disease in later life. Colley and his colleagues (1) followed a group of children born in Great Britain in 1946 and found an increased prevalence of chronic cough and sputum at the ages of 20 and 25 years among those whose parents reported bronchitis or pneumonia in the first 2 years of life. Smoking compounded the effect. Burrows and colleagues in Tucson, Arizona (2) found a greater incidence of a history of childhood respiratory trouble in adults with chronic bronchitis. Holland et al. found that school children whose parents gave a history of previous bronchitis had significantly more respiratory symptoms and impaired airway function (3). Leeder et al. followed prospectively, from birth to age 5 years, a group of children in London and noted that those with bronchitis and pneumonia in the first year of life continued to have respiratory problems and reductions in peak expiratory flow rate (4).

The question arises as to whether the symptoms in early life identify those with a predisposition to chronic lung disease or whether the illnesses in early life cause lung damage that predisposes to further illness and progressive lung disease. An understanding of the association is further complicated by the spectrum of illness seen both in infancy and in later life. In infancy, there are no simple criteria

to differentiate viral bronchitis, asthma, and suppurative lung disease. Each may present with cough or wheeze. Particularly in the first year of life, any lower respiratory illness may produce wheeze that is not necessarily associated with asthma.

Similarly, in the older age group the separation of asthma and bronchitis is difficult because of the lack of specific diagnostic tests. Asthma may cause a spectrum of disease from nocturnal cough, to exercise-induced shortness of breath, to recurrent or chronic wheeze, to incorrectly diagnosed recurrent pneumonia related to atelectasis from mucus plugging (5). Most of the diseases in the first year of life that are associated with subsequent lung pathology have primary airway problems manifested as bronchitis and bronchiolitis. Pneumonia with alveolar destruction by organisms such as *staphylococcus* may have extensive radiologic changes yet do not appear to be associated with ongoing lung disease.

Some chronic lung diseases start at conception. A clear-cut genetic basis is present for diseases such as cystic fibrosis, alpha-1 antitrypsin deficiency, ciliary dyskinesia, some of the immune deficiency syndromes, and the rare familial types of fibrosing alveolitis. Genetic mechanisms are important in asthma and some of the variations in immunologic competence, although the genetic contribution is less clearly defined and environmental factors certainly contribute. Table 5.1 summarizes the genetic contribution to lung disease in these conditions.

Gender influences the expression of the genetic predisposition. Males are more prone to develop lower respiratory illness in the first 2 years of life. Lung function tests have suggested that boys have smaller airways relative

Table 5.1.
Genetic Basis for Conditions Associated with Chronic Lung Disease

Disease	Inheritance
Cystic fibrosis	Autosomal recessive
Alpha-1 antitrypsin deficiency	Autosomal recessive
Ciliary dyskinesia	
Kartagener syndrome	Autosomal recessive
Others	Uncertain
Asthma	Variously autosomal dominant/autosomal recessive/polygenic
Immunologic disorder	
Bruton agammaglobulinaemia	X-linked recessive
IgG subclass deficiency	Variable
IgA defiency	Variable
Mixed	Uncertain
Wiskott Aldrich syndrome	X-linked recessive
Ataxia telangiectasia	Autosomal recessive
Familial fibrosing alveolitis	Autosomal dominant

to lung size than girls, and this may be an important predisposing factor to an increased incidence of lower respiratory illness with infection (6). Similarly, males have more severe asthma during childhood. An interesting study has shown that the pattern of bronchial responsiveness to mediators in girls with Turner syndrome is very similar to that seen in boys, but the pattern changes to a female pattern once replacement estrogens are given (7). Pertussis is the one condition in which females are more prone to develop troublesome respiratory disease than males. The reason for this difference has not been elucidated.

In-utero experiences are very likely to contribute significantly to subsequent lung disease. Recent epidemiologic studies have implicated allergic influences during fetal life and around the time of birth. Associations have been documented between the month of birth and the development of asthma (8). Migration of populations from one environment to another show a change in asthma prevalence on migration. Those that migrate after birth tend to have the pattern of respiratory illness of the country from which they have come rather than that in which they subsequently live. Those born in the new environment have the prevalence of asthma most like others in that community (9).

Smoking during pregnancy is known to influence bronchial responsiveness after birth. Young and colleagues have demonstrated increased bronchial responsiveness in babies whose parents smoked during pregnancy (10). Martinez et al. have documented that boys whose mothers smoked during pregnancy had increased responsiveness to mediator in later childhood (11). Cord blood immunoglobulin E (IgE) levels have been found to be higher in those with a family history of asthma and those exposed to maternal smoking during pregnancy (12).

Influences that affect placental function and lead to preterm delivery indirectly result in a predisposition to chronic lung disease. Those born markedly preterm will develop respiratory distress syndrome in the newborn period and subsequently have an increased risk of chronic lung disease of prematurity with chronic airway dysfunction. Some have claimed that the preterm delivery and subsequent lung disease are related to an inherited tendency to hyper-responsiveness (13).

Airway function at birth has been measured in two major prospective studies, and abnormalities thought to be associated with differences in airway size or geometry have been described. Early evidence indicates that those infants with abnormal values have increased lower respiratory symptoms during the first year of life. Martinez and his colleagues recorded tidal breathing soon after birth and showed that those with a reduced ratio of the time to reach peak flow over the total time during a tidal breath had more lower respiratory symptoms in the first year of life (14). Similarly, Young and colleagues have shown that infants with lower maximum expiratory flows measured by forced expiration in the first month of life have increased symptoms through early infancy (15). These cohorts have not yet been followed beyond the early years of life.

There seems little doubt that differences in mucosal immunity and other host defense factors could explain some of the varying predisposition of particular infants to lower respiratory infections. However, the evidence for specific immune defects is lacking. It is most likely that subtle multiple dysfunctions of immune mechanisms are present.

There are many agents that may produce asthma or lower respiratory infection. With regard to asthma, it is necessary to separate those factors called inducers, which initiate the disease called asthma in a genetically predisposed host, from those called triggers, which produce acute asthma attacks (Fig. 5.1). Asthma inducers are thought to include viral infections, allergens, and irritants, and these agents may initiate a chronic inflammatory process likely to be seen in asthma. These agents also trigger attacks, but agents such as dry cold air, exercise, emotional factors, and gastroesophageal reflux may also trigger attacks without being able to induce the chronic asthma status. There may well be a critical period during which exposure to environmental agents is necessary to develop immunologic tolerance. Exposure at the wrong time or in the wrong dose may lead to sensitization and induction of the inflammation thought to be present in asthma in the predisposed individual.

Parental smoking increases the risk of respiratory illness in childhood. There is a definite dose relationship between maternal smoking and hospital admissions for bronchitis and pneumonia, increased lower respiratory illness, and abnormal lung function (16–18).

Respiratory syncytial virus (RSV) is responsible for considerable morbidity in young children. It contributes to at least 75% of episodes of bronchiolitis in infants admitted to the hospital. These infants have subsequently been found to have more frequent wheezing and persisting lung function abnormalities.

Although those with severe asthma may develop bronchiolitis as their first wheezing illness, most infants with bronchiolitis develop mild wheeze over the next few years and not continuous troublesome asthma. Increased airway resistance and lung over-inflation during acute viral bronchiolitis has been noted to persist for over 12 months (19). This airway obstruction does not appear responsive to bronchodilators (20). By mid-childhood, up to two-thirds of these infants have had further wheezing and continue to demonstrate reduced flow rates and increased airway responsiveness (21–23). By adolescence, bronchiolitis is no longer as strong a predictor of persisting wheeze, as passive smoking or family history of asthma has been (25).

It is not clear whether the RSV induces a wheezing status that is transient or if the RSV infection identifies those genetically predisposed to asthma and other lower respiratory illness. Clearly, those admitted to the hospital with RSV infection are different from those who acquire the infection in the community; the clinical syndromes seen later in childhood may be a combination of those whose asthma was induced by RSV, those who have smaller airways at birth and are predisposed to wheezing illnesses in early childhood, and those who have symptoms secondary to the damage caused by RSV.

Adenovirus, especially Types 3, 7, and 21, can cause bronchiolitis and be associated with severe residual abnormalities of the airways leading to bronchiolitis obliterans with chronic airflow limitation, hyper-inflation, and hyper-lucent lung or lungs on chest radiograph (26).

Measles can be complicated by severe pneumonia. In Western countries this usually occurs only in children with pre-existing disease or immunosuppression, but in disadvantaged children measles epidemics are associated with both a high mortality and secondary infection leading to chronic lung disease. Other viruses such as rhinovirus, influenza virus, and parainfluenza virus have all been associated with bronchiolitis and croup in infancy. It is not known whether these particular viruses cause long-term changes in the airways. Recurrent croup is also associated with an atopic predisposition and increased airway responsiveness to histamine (27).

Bordetella pertussis primarily causes bronchitis and bronchiolitis. It had been described as a predisposing infection to bronchiectasis since many adults with bronchiectasis gave a

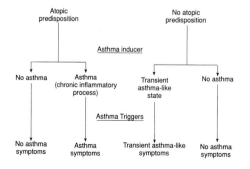

Figure 5.1. Algorithm of a model relating the genetic predisposition to asthma, with induction of the disease and triggering of attacks.

history of whooping cough in early childhood. However, more recent studies have suggested that this was an association related to socio-economic status and that pertussis per se does not predispose to bronchiectasis (28).

Haemophilus influenzae was considered an important organism causing bronchiolitis and pneumonia in infants. In developed countries it does not appear to be a significant organism responsible for infection in children or later chronic lung disease. It is a much more important pathogen in underdeveloped countries, where both acute and chronic infections are frequently related to the presence of *H. influenzae* (29). Chronic colonization appears to be associated with ongoing bronchial infection and airway obstruction in these populations.

Staphylococcus causes a severe destructive pneumonia in childhood. However, longitudinal studies have not shown the effects of *staphylococcus* to be associated with persisting lung function abnormalities (30). Infection of the pulmonary parenchyma with *Staphylococcos* has much less long-term detrimental effect than do agents like adenovirus, which predominantly affect the airways.

Mycoplasma pneumoniae can cause bronchiolitis in infants and bronchiolitis or pneumonia in older children. Chlamydia has also been shown to be a significant cause of bronchiolitis in infants. Both of these agents have been shown to be associated with chronic lung disease (31, 32). The airway function abnormalities in chlamydia tend to be very mild, and those usually seen in *Mycoplasma* are minor, although occasionally obliterative bronchiolitis producing McLeod syndrome or Swyer-James syndrome with unilateral hyperlucent lung has been reported.

Measles, tuberculosis, and adenovirus remain major pathogens for chronic lung disease in underprivileged racial groups in developing countries and in underprivileged groups within Western countries such as the Australian Aborigines, New Zealand Polynesians, and Native Americans. One difference between the consequences of acute respiratory illness in developing countries and those in developed countries is in the frequency of subsequent asthma. In many countries where the prevalence of lower respiratory illness in children is high because of poor social circumstances, asthma in childhood is uncommon.

In Western countries, the incidence of severe acute respiratory illness is lower but the prevalence of asthma is higher. The reason for these differences need further elucidation. Poor social circumstances may be associated with chronic colonization of the airway, recurrent lower respiratory infections, and chronic suppurative lung disease, but little asthma. The absence of lower respiratory illness in early childhood is associated with sensitization to common environmental allergens and subsequent asthma. The different inflammatory response with these two scenerios may contribute to the different patterns of lung disease in later life.

Infants born with cystic fibrosis have normal lungs at birth (33). Abnormalities in pulmonary function develop as a sequel to an initial insult, usually in early infancy. The underlying genetic abnormality in cystic fibrosis results in an abnormal amino acid content of the cystic fibrosis trans-membrane regulator. This abnormal protein prevents effective functioning of the chloride channel so that chloride and fluid are not excreted into secretions, which then become thick and viscous. Once the infant has an acute viral illness, the mucus produced is abnormal, and this leads to a predisposition for airway obstruction, secondary bacterial infection, airway damage, and further infection. Once the initial lung damage has occurred the infant is at risk for recurrent infections and progressive deterioration of lung function. This has led to the current approach of very aggressive therapy of every infection in cystic fibrosis with the aim of restoring airway function to as normal as possible (34).

Much adult chronic obstructive airway disease is clearly associated with previous pediatric respiratory illness. There is a more rapid deterioration in lung function through life in those who had childhood respiratory troubles (35). This is aggravated by cigarette smoking in adult life (Fig. 5.2). The question that remains to be answered is whether it is the predisposed host who developed early childhood respiratory troubles and subsequent lung disease or whether childhood injury in an otherwise normal host caused life long disease. The studies in infancy that demonstrate that the infant with small-caliber airways is the one who develops more lower respiratory symptoms may identify those who are predeter-

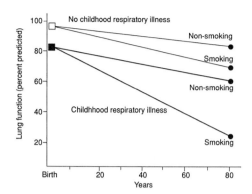

Figure 5.2. Summary curves demonstrating patterns of decline in lung function through adult life related to childhood respiratory illness and smoking.

mined to chronic obstructive airway disease through life.

There is increasing evidence that asthma is induced in early childhood.

Although up to 30% of children wheeze, many cease to have symptoms by early adult life, but they do not grow out of their asthma (36). Atopy, bronchial hyper-responsiveness, and small airway obstruction can be detected in those that have had anything more than mild, infrequent wheeze (37, 38). At 28 years they are frequently receiving less than adequate treatment for persisting symptoms, and a considerable proportion are smoking (39). Progressive age is associated with falling eosinophil counts but increased skin responsiveness to allergens. Atopy and airway hyper-responsiveness are both related to asthma but may not be directly associated with each other (40).

There is still some concern that asthma may become irreversible in later life and lead to chronic obstructive airway disease. If this is the case, can the natural history be changed by prevention of the initial induction of asthma or aggressive treatment of asthma through childhood?

There are many questions that need to be answered that will help reduce the morbidity and mortality from chronic obstructive airway disease. Establishment of the genetic library could lead to the identification of those at risk either because of their abnormal airway geometry or because of predisposition to asthma. More aggressive attempts to avoid insults in this group may lead to reduced prob-

lems in later life. In-utero exposures are important, and identification of the allergens and irritants that result in abnormal airway function at birth will help indicate those that should be avoided. Immunization or early anti-inflammatory agents may also prevent infection and the induction of asthma or the development of lower respiratory infections in infancy and may avoid the predisposition to chronic lung disease in adult life.

The interaction among determinants of host susceptibility, environmental factors, and infectious agents needs further definition to explain the association between childhood respiratory illness and chronic airway disease in adulthood. Standardized methods, accepted definitions of illnesses, large sample size, and very long follow-up are necessary to answer the questions raised. Prospective studies in progress may provide additional data that will improve our understanding about the origins of chronic lung disease (41).

REFERENCES

1. Colley JRT, Douglas JWB, Reid DD. Respiratory disease in young adults: Influence of early childhood respiratory tract illness, social class, air pollution and smoking. *Br Med J* 1973; 3:195–198.
2. Burrows B, Knudson RJ, Lebowitz MD. The relationship of childhood respiratory illness to adult obstructive airway disease. *Am Rev Respir Dis* 1977; 115:751–760.
3. Holland WW, Bailey P, Bland JM. Long term consequences of respiratory disease in infancy. *J Epidemiol Commun Hlth* 1978; 32:256–259.
4. Leeder SR, Cockhill RT, Irwig LM, Holland WW, Colley RJT. Influence of family factors on asthma and wheezing during the first 5 years of life. *Br J Prev Soc Med* 1976; 30:213–218, 219–224.
5. Eigen H, Laughlin J, Homrighausen J. Recurrent pneumonia in children and its relationship to bronchial hyper-reactivity. *Pediatrics* 1982; 70:698–704.
6. Taussig LM, Cota K, Kattenborn W. Different mechanical properties of the lung in boys and girls. *Am Rev Respir Dis* 1981; 123:640–643.
7. Villa MP, Bernardi F, Burnaccini M, Tura A, Martelli M, Mazzanti L, Bergamaschi R, Cacciari E. Bronchial reactivity and sex hormone: Study in a Turner's population. *Pediatr Pulmonol* 1990; 9:199–205.
8. Cole Johnson C, Ownby DR, McCullough J. Month of birth and risk of immediate hypersensitivity to seasonal and nonseasonal antigens. *Pediatr Asthma Allergy Immunol* 1989; 3:111–121.
9. Waite DA, Eyles EF, Tonkin SL, O'Donnell TV. Asthma prevalence in Tokelauan children in two environments. *Clin Allergy* 1980; 10:71–75.
10. Young S, LeSouef PN, Geelhoed G, Stick SM, Turner KJ, Landau LI. The influence of a family history of asthma and parental smoking on the level of airway responsiveness in early infancy. *N Engl J Med* 1991; 324:1168–1173.

11. Martinez FD, Antognoni G, Maeri F, Bonei E, Midulla F, DeCastro G, Ronchetti R. Parental smoking enhances bronchial responsiveness in 9 year old children. *Am Rev Respir Dis* 1988; 138:518–523.

12. Kjellman N-IM. Effect of parental smoking on IgE levels in children. *Lancet* 1981; 1:993–994.

13. Bertrand JM, Riley SP, Porkin J, Coates AL. Long term sequelae of prematurity: The role of familial airway hyper-reactivity and the respiratory distress syndrome. *N Engl J Med* 1985; 312:742–745.

14. Martinez FD, Morgan WJ, Wright AL, Holberg CJ, Taussig LM. Diminished lung function as a predisposing factor for wheezing respiratory disease in infants. *N Engl J Med* 1988; 319:1112–1117.

15. Young S, LeSouef PN, Arnott J, Geelhoed GC, Stick SM, Landau LI. Longitudinal evaluation of airway responsiveness and respiratory mechanics during the first 12 months of life in normal infants. *Am Rev Respir Dis* 1991:143:A23.

16. Harlap S, Davies AM. Infant admissions to hospital and maternal smoking. *Lancet* 1974: 1:529–532.

17. Wright AL, Holberg C, Martinez FD, Taussig LM and Group Health Medical Associates. Relationship of parental smoking to wheezing and non-wheezing lower respiratory tract illness in infancy. *J Pediatr* 1991; 118:207–214.

18. Tager IB, Weiss ST, Munoz A, Rosner B, Speizer FE. Longitudinal study of maternal smoking and pulmonary function in children. *N Engl J Med* 1983; 309:699–703.

19. Stokes EM, Milner ED, Hodges IG, Groggins RC. Lung function abnormalities after acute bronchiolitis. *J Pediatr* 1981; 98:871–874.

20. Sly PD, Lanteri CJ, Raven JM. Do wheezy infants recovering from bronchiolitis respond to inhaled salbutamol? *Pediatr Pulmonol* 1991; 10:36–39.

21. Pullan CR, Hey EH. Wheezing, asthma and pulmonary dysfunction 10 years after infection with respiratory syncitial virus in infancy. *B Med J* 1982; 284:1665–1669.

22. Kattan M, Keens TG, Lapierre LG, Levinson H, Bryan AC, Reilly BJ. Pulmonary function abnormalities in symptoms free children after bronchiolitis. *Pediatrics* 1977; 59:683–688.

23. Sly PD, Hibbert ME. Childhood asthma following hospitalization with acute viral bronchiolitis in infancy. *Pediatr Pulmonol* 1989; 7:153–158.

24. Welliver RC, Sun M, Rinaldo O, Ogra PL. Predictive value of respiratory syncitial virus specific IgE responses for recurrent wheezing following bronchiolitis. *J Pediatr* 1986; 109:776–780.

25. McConnochie KM, Roghmann KJ. Wheezing at 8 and 13 years: Changing importance of bronchiolitis and passive smoking. *Pediatr Pulmonol* 1989; 6:138–146.

26. James AG, Lang WR, Liant AY, et al. Adenovirus type 21 bronchopneumonia in infants and young children. *J Pediatr* 1979; 95:530–533.

27. Zach MS, Schnall RP, Landau LI. Upper and lower airway reactivity in recurrent croup. *Am Rev Respir Dis* 1980; 121:979–983.

28. Hughes DM, Newton-John H, Chay OM, Landau LI. Lung function after pertussis. *Aust Paediatr J* 1987; 23:277–282.

29. Jacobs NM, Harris VJ. Acute haemophilus pneumonia in childhood. *Am J Dis Child* 1979; 133:603–605.

30. Soto M, Demis T, Landau LI. Pulmonary function following staphylococcal pneumonia in children. *Aust Paediatr J* 1983; 19:172–174.

31. Harrison HR, Taussig LM. Fulginitti VA. Chlamydia trachomatis and chronic respiratory disease in childhood. *Pediatr Infect Dis* 1982; 1:29–33.

32. Stokes D, Sigler A, Khouri NJ, Talamo RC. Unilateral hyperlucent lung (Swyer-James Syndrome) after severe *Mycoplasma pneumonia* infection. *J Clin Pathol* 1968; 21(Suppl 2):93–97.

33. Chow CW, Landau LI, Taussig LM. Bronchial mucus glands in the newborn with cystic fibrosis. *Eur J Paediatr* 1982; 139:240–243.

34. Marks MI. The pathogensis and treatment of pulmonary infections in patients with cystic fibrosis. *J Pediatr* 1981; 98:173–179.

35. Burrows JM, Earle RH. Course and prognosis of chronic obstructive lung disease. *N Engl J Med* 1969; 280:397–404.

36. Martin AJ, McLennan LA, Landau LI, Phelan PD. The natural history of childhood asthma to adult life. *B Med J* 1980; 280:1397–1400.

37. Martin AJ, Landau LI, Phelan PD. Lung function in young adults who had asthma in childhood. *Am Rev Respir Dis* 1980; 122:609–616.

38. Martin AJ, Landau LI, Phelan PD. The natural history of allergy in asthmatic children followed to adult life. *Med J Aust* 1981; 2:470–474.

39. Kelly WJW, Hudson I, Phelan PD, Pain MCF, Olinsky A. Childhood asthma in adult life: a further study at 28 years of age. *B Med J* 1987; 294:1059–1062.

40. Kelly WJW, Hudson I, Phelan PD, Pain MCF, Olinksy A. Atopy in subjects with asthma followed to the age of 28 years. *J Clin Immunol* 1990; 85:548–557.

41. Samet JM, Tager IB, Spiezer FE. The relationship between respiratory illness in childhood and chronic airflow obstruction in adulthood. *Am Rev Respir Dis* 1983; 127:508–523.

6

Prevention of Lung Disease

MICHAEL A. WALL and ESTHER L. MOE

Acute and chronic lung diseases are the most frequent causes of pediatric outpatient visits and one of the most frequent reasons for hospital admissions. Disease prevention is often thought of in three broad categories: (a) primary prevention of disease, (b) secondary prevention of disease exacerbation, and (c) tertiary prevention of disease complications. A discussion of prevention can center around specific diseases such as bronchiolitis or on risk factors such as passive smoking and malnutrition. For organizational purposes this chapter is arranged around major disease categories, and the focus will be on primary and secondary prevention.

RESPIRATORY INFECTIONS

Scope of the Problem

Acute respiratory infections (ARIs) have become the leading worldwide cause of death in children. In developing countries about 50% of all deaths are in children under 5 years of age. Of the approximately 14 million child deaths in the world each year, one-fourth to one-third are caused by ARIs (1, 2). Mortality rates from ARIs in young infants are 10–30 times higher in the Third World than in industrialized nations, and the difference in mortality rates is even higher for children 1–4 years of age (1). Mortality rate differences between nondeveloped and industrialized nations have increased during this century as rates have declined in the industrialized world while they have remained virtually unchanged in much of the Third World. A decline in mortality rates from respiratory infections has been responsible for 25% of the overall mortality decline in developed countries and is the largest contributor to this decline (3). Most

studies have shown that ARI attack rates (three to eight per year) are similar in children around the world, so that mortality rate differences are due to theoretically preventable factors such as poverty, politics, nutrition, access to health care, and immunization rates. Respiratory deaths currently preventable by routine immunizations include those associated with measles, diphtheria, pertussis, tuberculosis, and *Haemophilus influenzae*. Measles causes about 2.5 million deaths per year, pertussis about 750,000, and tuberculosis another 30,000 (1).

In the United States ARIs are the leading cause of hospitalization in children 1–9 years of age, accounting for about one-third of all discharges (4). ARIs are the fourth leading cause of death in the immediate postnatal period. The United States is certainly not immune to major ARI risk factors, with 40% of the nation's poor being under age 18, over half of the pregnant teenagers in some locales being cigarette smokers, and many children being under- or un-immunized.

Causative Agents

There are no differences in the major causes of ARIs in developed versus nondeveloped areas of the world. Viral infections are the leading causes of ARIs in children (1–3, 5, 6). Respiratory syncytial virus (RSV) is the most common agent and is a particularly important cause of lower respiratory tract infection in young children. Other viruses frequently associated with ARIs include influenza, parainfluenza, adenovirus, and rhinoviruses. Measles virus infection is usually associated with clinically significant respiratory symptoms in non-immunized children.

Nonviral agents are also relatively common pathogens and mixed infections may be more frequent than is generally recognized (6). *Streptococcus pneumoniae* and *Haemophilus influenzae* are the most common bacterial infections of the lower respiratory tract beyond the first few weeks of life with infections caused by *Mycoplasma pneumoniae* becoming more frequent in children of school age. Nonimmunized children are susceptible to bacteria that cause diphtheria and pertussis, both of which are totally preventable. *Chlamydia trachomatis* is well recognized as a lower respiratory tract pathogen in inants, and in recent years evidence has arisen to implicate *Ureaplasma urealyticum* as a clinically relevant pathogen in premature infants (7). Tuberculosis is on the rise in the United States as a result of human immunodeficiency virus (HIV) infection, immigration patterns, and lack of funding for public health programs. In terms of preventable lung infections, one needs to consider the immunocompromised host, in whom at least some infections such as those due to *Pneumocystis carinii* and varicella zoster virus can be prevented.

Risk Factors And Prevention Strategies

SOCIOECONOMIC

It seems to be an unfortunate truism in today's world that the more effective a strategy is likely to be in preventing ARI–related morbidity and mortality, the less likely it is to be implemented. It is also interesting to note that there is an inverse correlation between the cost of prevention programs on an individual basis and their overall impact. The major risk factor for severe sequelae of ARIs is poverty and all that goes with it including malnutrition, lack of access to health care, lack of vaccines and medicine, high levels of indoor air pollution and overcrowding. Although ARI attack rates are similar in children throughout the world, ARIs are more severe in malnourished children (8). Maternal malnutrition leads to the delivery of low-birth-weight infants, and pneumonia is the leading cause of death in such infants in the Third World.

The World Health Organization and a small number of individual countries have set up demonstration projects in developing countries in an attempt to reduce ARI morbidity and mortality. A full description of these

laudable efforts is beyond the scope of this chapter. In general, the strategies that are being employed are "low tech" and include immunization, early recognition of serious ARIs by local health care workers, and early use of antibiotics. The early results of these trials are very encouraging, and it is to be hoped that their application will become more widespread.

PREVENTIVE STRATEGIES

Routine Immunizations

Respiratory diseases that are virtually completely eliminated by adherence to routine vaccination schedules include diphtheria, pertussis, and measles. Children with respiratory disease should receive routine immunizations, as is recommended by the American Academy of Pediatrics (9), regardless of the presence of chronic respiratory symptoms. The data with respect to respiratory disease caused by *H. influenzae* and the effectiveness of vaccination are not yet fully developed. The first influenza B (Hib) vaccine was unconjugated capsular polysaccharide and was approved for children 2–5 years of age (18 months in high-risk children). Unfortunately, at least half of the cases of serious *H. influenzae* disease occur before 18 months of age; furthermore, the protective efficacy achieved was quite variable. Since that time Hib conjugate vaccines have been developed, which consist of capsular polysaccharide covalently linked to a protein carrier that confers thymus-dependent properties. The vaccine has been approved for infants 2 months of age (10), but data are not yet available concerning protection from diseases such as pneumonia or epiglottitis.

Certain children at particularly high risk for developing severe respiratory infections should be protected with immunizations that are not routinely recommended in all children. (HIV infection is discussed separately.) Children with chronic lung disease, severe congenital heart disease, and sickle cell anemia, as well as those receiving immunosuppressive therapy, should receive influenza vaccine (9) (Tables 6.1 and 6.2). *Children with asthma who are steroid-dependent, have required frequent steroid bursts during the winter months, have had prior asthma episodes associated with respiratory failure, or have had frequent emergency room visits during the past year are candi-*

Table 6.1.
Recommendations for Influenza Immunization in Children

- Children with chronic pulmonary disease (BPD, cystic fibrosis, restrictive lung disease)
- Children with asthma who are steriod-dependent, have required frequent steroid bursts during the winter months, have had prior asthma episodes associated with respiratory failure, or have had frequent emergency room visits during the past year
- Children with complex congenital heart disease
- Children with sickle cell anemia
- Children who are HIV-positive
- Those receiving immunosuppressive therapy
- Residents of chronic care facilities
- Chronic medical conditions (e.g., diabetes mellitus, renal dysfunction)
- Those requiring chronic aspirin therapy
- Care providers (home and hospital) and siblings of the above high-risk patients, especially infants who cannot be immunized

Table 6.2.
Recommended Initial Dosage Schedule

Age	Type	Dosage	No. of Doses	Route
6–35 mo	Split virus	0.25 ml	2[a]	IM
3–8 yr	Split virus	0.5 ml	1 or 2[a]	IM
9–12 yr	Split virus	0.5 ml	1	IM
> 12 yr	Whole or split	0.5 ml	1	IM

[a]Repeat immunization may be administered as a single dose.

dates for influenza immunization. For patients who may be allergic to egg or who cannot receive the influenza immunization for other reasons or who would otherwise be candidates for immunization, the use of amantadine (11) or rimantadine (12) at the earliest signs of an influenza infection or as a prophylactic medication during the flu season has been recommended. Experience with these medications is limited in children, and concern has been raised about the emergence of resistant organisms (11, 12). Pneumococcal vaccine is not fully protective but should be administered to children with sickle cell anemia, asplenia, nephrotic syndrome, and selected immunosuppressed patients. There is no need to administer pneumococcal vaccine to children with asthma, bronchopulmonary dysplasia (BPD), cystic fibrosis (CF), or other chronic lung disease in children, since these children are capable of mounting an appropriate response to pneumococcal infection. Similarly, the efficacy of pseudomonas vaccine for patients with CF is unproven and thus is not recommended routinely. Varicella zoster immunoglobulin should be administered to immunosuppressed children who have had significant clinical exposure as well as to selected newborns and premature infants, depending on gestational age and history of maternal chicken pox (9).

Future directions in prevention of ARI should lie in the development of safe and effective immunizations against the common respiratory viruses, especially RSV.

Bacille Calmette-Guérin (BCG) vaccine is a live attenuated strain of *Mycobacterium bovis.* It is widely used in countries with a high incidence of tuberculosis but its level of protective efficacy is still debated (9) (see Chapter 29). In the United States, it is recommended in infants who are tuberculin skin test–negative and who live in a household where they are exposed to persons with sputum positive for *M. tuberculosis* who have not been adequately treated.

Tobacco Smoke

Of all the measures one might consider to reduce the burden of lung disease in the developed world, smoking prevention would without a doubt have the most impact. It is estimated that smoking is a causative factor in approximately 350,000 deaths each year in the United States. Cigarette smoking can be thought of as a "pediatric" problem in that 90% of adult smokers start as teenagers. Each day in the United States 3000 teenagers become regular smokers, with over 1 million starting annually. Adolescents in the United States purchase about 1 billion packs of cigarettes per year, and sales of tobacco products to teenagers currently total about $1.25 billion. Passive smoking also constitutes a major health hazard for children. Over the past 20 years numerous articles have been published concerning the health effects of passive smoking on children (13–15). Debate still exists concerning the exact extent of the health effects of passive smoking on children and the mechanisms involved, but there is strong consensus that passive smoking is a major preventable cause of respiratory morbidity and mortality.

The health effects of involuntary smoking on the developing fetus include low birth weight, an increased incidence of premature birth, and an increased incidence of spontaneous abortion (16). Animal studies (17) as well as epidemiologic data in humans (18) suggest that maternal smoking has an impact on lung development, and that part of what appears to be the postnatal effect of involuntary smoking on respiratory infections and lung function may be ascribed to in utero exposure.

The problem of involuntary smoke exposure is extremely widespread. Studies from North Carolina demonstrated that 60% of young infants had detectable cotinine (a metabolite of nicotine) in their urine as well as a correlation between home air nicotine levels and urinary cotinine levels (19, 20). The major impact of environmental tobacco smoke (ETS) is an increased incidence of respiratory infections, particularly in the first 2 years of life (21–24). In most studies, maternal smoking has the greatest impact, but paternal smoking also plays a role in increasing respiratory disease. ETS exposure has been reported to increase all types of respiratory infections from otitis media and tonsillitis to lower respiratory infections (LRIs) such as bronchiolitis and pneumonia.

Passive smoking is a risk factor for wheezing-associated respiratory illness in young children (25) and for recurrent wheezing later in childhood (26, 27). School age children who are exposed to ETS have greater degrees of airway hyper-responsiveness than those who are not (28, 29), and exposure to ETS may precipitate wheezing in children with pre-existing lung disease (30).

A number of studies have examined the effect of passive smoking on lung function in subjects 6–20 years of age (13, 15). The consensus from such studies is that ETS exposure is associated with small but statistically significant reductions in expiratory flow rates. Differences exist among the studies in terms of which measure of flow rate is reduced and whether the impact is greater on boys or on girls. Maternal smoking appears to be a greater risk factor than paternal smoking, and debate continues concerning whether this is related to in utero exposure, societal factors, or both. The clinical impact in later life of a small reduction in expiratory flow in adolescence remains to be seen. However, the data from the large study of adults and children with lung disease from Tucson suggests that active cigarette smoking is associated with a more rapid decline in lung function in those adults who had a history of respiratory problems in childhood (31).

Given the data concerning the adverse health effects of passive and active smoking it is sad to note that we have very little data concerning effective means of preventing childhood ETS exposure or the onset of smoking in teenagers. Smoking-related issues should be a part of the routine prevention advice that is given by pediatric health care providers along with subjects such as use of seat belts and nutrition. Such advice can be given in the context of routine well child care; it has been shown that brief, direct physician advice to quit smoking can be effective in motivating patients to quit (32–34).

A household smoking history should be obtained in all patients referred for evaluation of respiratory symptoms. Smokers should be made aware of the adverse health effects of passive smoking. Direct, unambiguous advice should be given concerning means of reducing infant smoke exposure. Parental cessation is the most effective means of ensuring smoke avoidance. To accomplish this goal, principles of a physician-based smoking intervention program for use in a pediatric setting have been developed (35). The essential points of the intervention are described in Table 6.3 and are based on a medical model of Ask, Advise, Treat, and Follow-Up. The entire intervention can take as little as 2 minutes

Table 6.3.
Suggestions for Pediatric Provider Office-Based Smoking Cessation

1. *The physician as a role model.*
   The physician should not smoke, especially in the office. Smoking should be completely banned from the office, including staff, parents, and patients.

2. *Look for a teachable moment.*
   Throughout a person's life there will be teachable moments when one may be particularly open to a nonsmoking message. For physicians who treat children, such moments include office visits for recurrent otitis media, wheezing, etc.

3. *Take a smoking history.*
   All parents should be queried concerning smoking. The history should include not only asking about smoking but also a few questions relating to amount so that the physician can get a rough idea of the extent of nicotine addiction. If a person smokes more than 20 cigarettes per day he or she is likely to be physically addicted and may benefit from referral to a group program and/or nicotine replacement therapy.

4. *Personalize the health risk.*
   Relate the child's recurrent otitis, cough, wheeze, etc. to parental smoking. Many parents are aware that smoking is "bad" but they may not be aware of the specifics. Make eye contact, be concise, be personal, and be prepared to hear a wide range of rationalizations.

5. *Emphasize the parent as role model.*
   This is another potential psychologic wedge, since the majority of smokers do not want their children to smoke.

6. *Engage the parent in a discussion about his or her smoking.*
   Smoking cessation is a long-term process. A "successful" clinical encounter is one wherein the physician and smoker discuss smoking and, it is hoped, another step is taken along the road to cessation. Three potential psychologic wedges one has with a smoking parent are (a) the health effects of passive smoking on the baby, (b) the health effects on the parent, and (c) the parent as a smoking role model. During the discussion it is useful to determine factors such as whether the parent is willing to try to quit, previous experience with quit attempts, and barriers to quitting. The physician and the smoker should be aware that relapse does not equal failure. In fact, the data show that the more times one has tried to quit the more likely one is to eventually succeed.

7. *Give direct advice to quit.*
   It is interesting that when surveyed most physicians state that they always advise smokers to quit. Other surveys, however, show that when smokers leave a physician's office they often claim not to have heard such advice. Advice to quit should be given in an unambiguous fashion. Be prepared for all sorts of rationalizations. Some of the most common are as follows:
   a. *Weight gain.* The average is 7 lbs. Give common sense advice such as sugarless sweets and increased exercise.
   b. *Life stress.* There will never be a perfect time to quit but cessation efforts are likely to be most successful when one's life is relatively stable.
   c. *"I only smoke outside."* Many parents claim this is true. Emphasize their own health and the role model effect (75% of smokers come from a household where there were one or more smokers).
   d. *Fear of withdrawal.* Nicotine withdrawal is real but manageable. Nicotine gum may be useful for 3–6 months while one is breaking the psychologic habit.

8. *Try to establish a behavioral commitment.*
   Smoking intervention is more likely to be successful if one can get the patient to make a specific behavioral commitment. One hopes that this will be to set a quit date in the near future. Give the parent a prescription with the quit date written on it. For some smokers a commitment to set a quit date may be too overwhelming. Other valid commitments can include setting a date for a family meeting, reading a self-help brochure, or enrolling in a group cessation program.

9. *Commit to follow-up.*
   Plan to follow-up on any behavioral commitment the parent may have made. Let the parent see you write down their commitment in the chart, and use this chart notation as a basis for discussion at the next office visit.

10. *Have local resources available.*
    These can include pamphlets, self-help materials, and telephone numbers for local cessation programs. Most physicians are aware of resources in their community for parents who might have health problems, and we believe that smoking intervention should be one of these resources. Addicted smokers can be helped to quit through the use of nicotine chewing gum. However, nicotine replacement therapy cannot be used in an unsupervised fashion; in fact many smokers will say they have tried nicotine gum and it has not helped them quit. A major reason for such failures is that the gum has not been used in conjunction with a comprehensive plan for smoking cessation including follow-up and a plan for weaning from the gum. Many physicians will not have the time, training, or office structure to provide the supervision required for the use of nicotine replacement therapy. As for other referral patterns, we believe that physicians who do not intend to become experts in the area of nicotine replacement should identify at least one health professional in their area who has such expertise to whom they can refer heavy smokers who are willing to try to quit.

and centers on the notion that an encounter between the parent of a young child and a physician is a "teachable moment."

In the Ask phase a brief smoking history is taken to assess household exposure levels, level of parental addiction, and problems with past attempts to quit smoking. This phase is crucial since it is clear that if smoking is not raised as an issue no advice will be given. A review of 12 studies concluded that less than one-third of health care providers report advising all patients to quit smoking (36). In the Advise step three psychologic "wedges" are employed to try to motivate the parent: (a) the health effects of passive smoking on the infant, (b) the health effects of active smoking on the parent, and (c) the role model effect of a smoking parent on the child. The majority of smoking parents will claim that they do not smoke around their children. Identifying their position as role models (75% of smokers are raised in smoking households) is often the most effective means of starting a fruitful interaction. In the Treat phase an attempt is made to elicit a behavioral commitment. For some parents this will be to set a quit date; for most it will be to have a family discussion or read a brochure. A chart notation about the sort of commitment elicited is made, and in the Follow-Up phase the status of compliance with this commitment is reviewed. In summary, advising parents not to smoke around their children should be advocated strongly, and cessation advice must be included as a legitimate part of such counseling.

The major factors influencing a child's decision about whether to become a smoker or not include the 3 P's: peer pressure, parental smoking habits, and psychosocial status. The major trend in smoking prevention programs at present is to try to assist teenagers in the areas of avoiding peer pressure and psychosocial influences while working with smoking parents to quit. Although it is easy for adults to tell teenagers to "just say no," peer pressure can be overwhelming. It should be emphasized to the teenager that smoking is not the norm, and that in fact most other teenagers do not want to smoke, date smokers, or be around other smokers. Teenagers appreciate being shown directly how attempts are being made to influence them to become smokers through the media and promotional events,

in essence to try to raise their indignation. There is certainly no perfect strategy that can be employed to ensure that teenagers do not become smokers, but when one considers that 90% of adult smokers start as teenagers, an aggressive program is warranted.

Other Environmental Pollutants

Many indoor and outdoor air pollutants other than cigarette smoke have been reported to cause respiratory symptoms such as cough, phlegm, and wheeze in adults and children (15, 37). Such agents include wood smoke, cooking gas, nitrogen dioxide, sulfur dioxide, carbon monoxide, and formaldehyde, among others. Home and industrial pollutants are major respiratory health risk factors, and primary prevention of pediatric lung disease arising from these exposures must be based on elimination of these pollutants from the local environment.

Child-Rearing Practices

The impact of selected child-rearing practices on respiratory infections in young children are of interest. It is often suggested that breast feeding is protective against such infections, but the data are inconclusive (38, 39).

Group day care attendance has also been suggested as a potential risk factor for increased respiratory illnesses. The data support the notion that for at least the first few years of life there is an increased incidence of respiratory infections in children who attend day care, even when potential confounders are taken into account (40, 41). One study showed increased odds ratios for infections caused by *H. influenzae* and *Neisseria meningitides*, but not other serious bacterial infections (42). Preventive measures that can be taken in a day care setting include requiring parents to follow immunization schedules, strict adherence to hand washing, and segregating febrile children or ideally keeping them at home. *There are no established guidelines for participation of children with chronic lung disease in day care.* Considering the risks of viral respiratory infections in this population, participation in a day care setting with large numbers of children should be discouraged until the child has had an opportunity to grow and demonstrate respiratory stability.

Nosocomial Infections

Outbreaks of infections in children in hospitals, day care, and long-term care facilities are well-documented. Infection is most commonly spread via fomite contact, although for some pathogens such as varicella virus, airborne spread occurs as well. Varicella and RSV tend to be the most common concerns in pediatric hospitals, and effective isolation and cohorting procedures are well described (9). The major prevention issue with nosocomial infections is not a lack of data about how to prevent spread but rather a lack of compliance among institutional staff and parents. Hand washing before and after touching infected children and/or objects in the room is the most effective single measure that can be taken, and staff members need to be encouraged and reminded repeatedly. House staff members, attending physicians, and sometimes nursing personnel are the chief offenders in hand washing noncompliance, and frequent reminders in the form of inservices, lectures, and written materials are required to maintain effective compliance levels.

Human Immunodeficiency Virus (HIV) Infection

Acquired immunodeficiency syndrome (AIDS) caused by HIV infection has become one of the major scourges of the 20th century and is becoming a major cause of death in infants and young children. A number of reviews have been published on the subject (42–45), and in this section we will cover only the highlights of strategies for prevention of infection. Clearly primary prevention of HIV infection in infants depends on primary prevention in their mothers. Unfortunately, the ravages of poverty and drug addiction make primary prevention, yet again, more a sociopolitical issue than a medical one. About 25–35% of HIV-infected pregnant women will transmit infection to their infants (45). Because of maternal transmission of antibody, early diagnosis of HIV infection in such children can be difficult and depends on a combination of clinical and laboratory findings. Diagnosis of AIDS usually depends on demonstration of antibody plus characteristic opportunistic infections, lymphadenopathy, hypergammaglobulinemia, and decreased CD4+ counts. Newer strategies that are being developed include detection of antigen using polymerase chain reaction technology and HIV culture (45).

Prevention of AIDS in HIV-infected babies will no doubt depend on early diagnosis and therapy. Immunization schedules for HIV-infected infants have been published (9) and are basically the same as for other children with the exception of the use of inactivated polio vaccine. In addition, influenza and pneumococcal vaccines are recommended.

At the time of this writing zidovudine (Retrovir, AZT) is available for children only under research protocol. However, the drug has been shown to be somewhat effective in the treatment of class P-2 symptomatic infection (46) and may soon be released for open treatment. Other preventive strategies that may soon be adopted include prophylactic use of trimethoprim-sulfamethoxazole and intravenous immunoglobulin (47).

CYSTIC FIBROSIS

Primary prevention of CF at present entails prenatal counseling to parents who already have a child with CF or carrier detection in relatives followed by prenatal counseling. The discovery of the CF gene in 1989 raised the possibility of widespread carrier testing. To date, however, over 200 mutations in the CF gene have been discovered, accounting for perhaps 85–90% of the CF mutations in the population. Routine carrier testing is not likely to be recommended until at least 95% of all mutations are identified, if then (48). Carrier testing raises many ethical issues, especially since CF is no longer uniformly fatal early in life and advanced therapies such as gene transfer appear to be coming within reach.

Much can be done in terms of secondary and tertiary prevention of CF. Data from screening programs using the immunoreactive trypsin assay technology indicate that nutritional status is significantly improved with early diagnosis and treatment, but the data for progression of lung disease are not yet available. The Cystic Fibrosis Foundation strongly encourages specialized care through its regionalized care centers, and guidelines for care in such centers have been published (49). The mainstay of CF treatment is early recognition and treatment of nutritional, pulmonary, endocrine, and intestinal complications.

Cystic fibrosis is a chronic, remitting, and relapsing disease, and patients are prone to an array of psychosocial and compliance problems. Part of an overall prevention strategy in CF is the recognition of compliance issues (50–53) with initiation of appropriate behavioral intervention. Research is currently being done to improve techniques of teaching coping and self-management skills to CF patients with the notion that life quality and perhaps quantity will increase.

ASTHMA

Scope of the Problem

Asthma is the most common chronic disease of childhood, and of all chronic diseases is the most common cause of school absenteeism. The prevalence of asthma varies among countries, regions within countries, socioeconomic status, race, age, and definition of the disease. In the United States about 3 million people under age 18 suffer from asthma. As children age, the point prevalence rate tends to decrease, ranging from about 7% at age 6 months to 2 years to about 5% in the adolescent years (54). Death from asthma in childhood is not common, with rates ranging from approximately 0.2 per 100,000 in Caucasians to 0.7 per 100,000 in African Americans. Morbidity, however, is quite common. Asthma accounts for 20–25% of grade school absences and well over 100,000 hospitalizations each year (54). Recent data suggest that morbidity and mortality from asthma, particularly in the pediatric age group, may be on the rise (55).

Primary Prevention

Although considerable epidemiologic data have been acquired relating potential risk factors to the development of asthma, no hard data exist that firmly support the notion that any manipulation of an infant's environment will totally prevent the disease. Numerous studies have confirmed an association between atopy and asthma. Atopy appears to result from a combination of hereditary and environmental factors, with heredity being the most important. For instance, in family studies heredity appears to be responsible for 40–60% of the observed variance in serum IgE levels (56, 57).

The possibilities for manipulating the environment to reduce atopic disease have been reviewed (58, 59). The data with regard to diet (formula versus breast milk) are inconclusive, and no recommendation based on firm evidence is possible (58). The possibility of reducing infant aeroallergen exposure in order to prevent subsequent asthma has been raised, but the data are by no means clear and the practical aspects of such an undertaking would be daunting at best. Reduction of respiratory infections in early infancy may be the most practical primary public health measure that can be taken. It is now well established that wheezing-associated lower respiratory tract infections in infancy are a risk factor for subsequent wheezing (60). Maternal smoking is associated with elevated umbilical cord IgE levels (61) and a higher prevalence of positive skin tests to common aeroallergens (29, 60) and, as noted previously, correlates with a higher incidence of infant respiratory infections.

Secondary and Tertiary Prevention

Although asthma itself may not be amenable to primary prevention, it is quite clear that much of the morbidity and mortality caused by asthma is avoidable. Strategies to reduce the burden of suffering from asthma include better recognition and avoidance of asthma triggers, immunotherapy, improvements in pharmacologic therapy, improvements in health care access, and the adoption of co-management strategies to improve self-efficacy and compliance. Review of potential triggers (viral infections, allergens, airway irritants) with parents in order to determine which may be operative is required in all patients with asthma. Many triggers may be unavoidable or may not be advisable to avoid (exercise, for instance, which almost all asthmatic children can do with planning). However, some household triggers such as pet dander and tobacco smoke are avoidable, and efforts should be made to curtail exposure. The role of immunotherapy after trigger avoidance and failure of reasonable pharmacologic therapy is controversial, with little long-term, well-controlled study data available.

The therapy of asthma is discussed in detail in Chapter 21. One strategy for preventing morbidity and perhaps mortality that is underused is early use of oral corticosteroids when an exacerbation is not being controlled with usual maintenance therapy. Such a strategy may prevent repeated emergency room visits or hospitalizations (62, 63). One of the frequent obstacles to effective pharmacologic therapy is the refusal of physicians to allow patients to start oral corticosteroids on their own.

In recent years home peak flow meters have been shown to be useful in predicting the onset of exacerbations and guiding pharmacologic therapy such as increasing the frequency of inhalation of β-2 sympathomimetics or starting oral corticosteroids (64–66). The peak flow data are only useful if recorded two or three times each day so that each patient's "best baseline" can be established. Although there is great interindividual variability, a decrease in peak flow rate from best baseline of 20% or more is often a warning sign of an impending exacerbation and can be used in an overall management plan to reduce clinically significant morbidity.

A number of educational programs have been devised to help improve the self-efficacy and behavioral skills of children with asthma (65, 67–70). Target populations, methods, and settings vary from one program to another. Some programs rely on a group dynamic whereas others focus on the individual patient. In general, all of the programs are designed to improve avoidance of triggers, recognition of exacerbations, use of medications, and access into the health care system. Most programs have shown significant improvement in some or all of the following parameters: school absenteeism, health care utilization, emergency room visits, hospitalizations, knowledge about asthma, medication compliance, and self-efficacy attitudes. Data on long-term follow-up are scanty, but at least one recent study showed a fall-off in efficacy 1 year after completion of an educational intervention (65), suggesting that educational and motivational efforts must be sustained.

Children with asthma may spend 6–8 hours a day in school but often find it difficult if not impossible to gain timely access to their medications. Most school districts have no uniform policy for administration of medications; often this responsibility is left to secretaries or teachers' aides. Data from Great Britain reveal that the vast majority of teachers have almost no knowledge about the patho-

physiology or treatment of asthma (71, 72). Responsible students with asthma should be permitted to keep physician-prescribed inhalers in their possession (73), but few school districts permit this policy. Much more needs to be done to educate teachers, administrators, and coaches so that students with asthma will not suffer needlessly.

REFERENCES

1. Pio A, Ten Dem HG. The magnitude of the problem of acute respiratory infections. In Douglas RM, Kerby–Eaton (eds): *Acute respiratory infections in children.* Adelaide, Australia: University of Adelaide, 1985, pp 3–16.
2. Berman S, McIntosh K. Selective primary health care: Strategies for control of disease in the developing world. XXI. Acute respiratory infections. *Rev Infect Dis* 1985; 7:674–691.
3. Riley I. The aetiology of acute respiratory infections in children in developing countries. In: Douglas RM, Kerby-Eaton, eds. *Acute respiratory infections in childhood.* Adelaide, Australia: University of Adelaide, 1985, pp 33–41.
4. U.S. Department of Health & Human Services, Office of Maternal and Child Health. *Child health USA '90.* Washington, DC: Public Health Service, 1990.
5. Denny FW, Clyde WA. Acute lower respiratory tract infections in nonhospitalized children. *J Pediatr* 1986; 108:635–646.
6. Paisley JW, Lauer BA, McIntosh K, Glode MP, Schachter J, Rumack C. Pathogens associated with acute lower respiratory tract infections in young children. *Pediatr Infect Dis* 1984; 3:14–19.
7. Stagno S, Brasfield DM, Brown MB, Cassell GH, Pifer LL, Whitley RJ, Tiller RE. Infant pheumonitis associated with cytomegalovirus, chlamydia, pneumocystis, and ureaplasma: A prospective study. *Pediatrics* 1981; 68:322–329.
8. Kendall PA, Leeder SR. Environmental factors relating to acute respiratory infections in childhood: Possibilities for prevention. In: Douglas RM, Kerby-Eaton, eds. *Acute respiratory infections in childhood.* Adelaide, Australia: University of Adelaide, 1985, pp 72–77.
9. Committee on Infectious Diseases American Academy of Pediatrics. Report of the Committee on Infectious Diseases, 1988.
10. Centers for Disease Control. Food and Drug Administration approval of use of a Haemophilus b conjugate vaccine for infants. *MMWR* 1990; 39:925–926.
11. Douglas RG Jr. Prophylaxis and treatment of influenza. *N Engl J Med* 1990; 322:443–450.
12. Hall CB, Dolin R, Gala CL, et al. Children with influenza A infection: Treatment with rimantidine. *Pediatrics* 1987; 80: 275–282.
13. Department of Health and Human Services. *The health consequences of involuntary smoking: A report of the Surgeon General* (Publication no. DHHS [CDC] 87-8398). Washington, DC: Government Printing Office, 1986.
14. Fielding JE, Phenow KJ. Health effects of involuntary smoking. *N Engl J Med* 1988; 319:1452–1460.

15. Samet JM, Marbury MC, Spengler JD. Health effects and sources of indoor air pollution. Parts I & II. *Am Rev Respir Dis* 1987; 136:1486–1508, 137:221–242.
16. Butler NR, Goldstein H, Ross EM. Cigarette smoking in pregnancy: Its influence on birth weight and perinatal mortality. *Br Med J* 1972; 2:127–130.
17. Collins MH, Moessinger AC, Kleinerman J, et al. Fetal lung hypoplasia associated with maternal smoking: A morphometric analysis. *Pediatr Res* 1985; 19:408–412.
18. Taylor B, Wadsworth J. Maternal smoking during pregnancy and lower respiratory tract illness in early life. *Arch Dis Child* 1987; 62:786–791.
19. Greenberg RA, Bauman KE, Glover LH, et al. Ecology of passive smoking by young infants. *J Pediatr* 1989; 114:774–780.
20. Henderson, FW, Reid HF, Morris R, et al. Home air nicotine levels and urinary cotinine excretion in preschool children. *Am Rev Respir Dis* 1989; 140:197–201.
21. Harlap S, Davies AM. Infant admissions to hospital and maternal smoking. *Lancet* 1974; 1:529–532.
22. Colley JRT, Holland WW, Corkhill RT. Influence of passive smoking and parental phlegm on pneumonia and bronchitis in early childhood. *Lancet* 1974; 2:1031–1034.
23. Fergusson DM, Horwood LJ, Shannon FT, Taylor B. Parental smoking and lower respiratory illness in the first three years of life. *J Epidemiol Community Health* 1981; 35:180–184.
24. Pedreira FA, Guandola VL, Feroli EJ, Mella GW, Weiss IP. Involuntary smoking and incidence of respiratory illness during the first year of life. *Pediatrics* 1985; 75:594–597.
25. Wright AL, Holberg C, Martinez FD, Taussig LM, Group Health Medical Associates. Relationship of parental smoking to wheezing and nonwheezing lower respiratory tract illnesses in infancy. *J Pediatr* 1991; 118:207–214.
26. Gortmaker SL, Walker DK, Jacobs FH, Ruch-Ross H. Parental smoking and the risk of childhood asthma. *Am J Public Health* 1982; 72:574–579.
27. Neuspiel DR, Rush D, Butler NR, et al. Parental smoking and post–infancy wheezing in children: A prospective cohort study. *Am J Public Health* 1989; 79:168–171.
28. O'Connor GT, Weiss ST, Tager IB, Speizer FE. The effect of passive smoking on pulmonary function and non specific bronchial responsiveness in a population-based sample of children and young adults. *Am Rev Respir Dis* 1987; 135:800–804.
29. Martinez FD, Antognoni G, Marci F, et al. Parental smoking enhances bronchial responsive in nine year old children. *Am Rev Respir Dis* 1988; 138:518–523.
30. Burrows B, Knudson RA, Lebowitz MD. The relationship of childhood respiratory illness to adult obstructive airways disease. *Am Rev Respir Dis* 1977; 155:751–760.
31. O'Connell E, Logan G. Parental smoking in childhood asthma. *Ann Allergy* 1974; 32:142–145.
32. Wilson DM, Taylor W, Gilbert JR, et al. A randomized trial of family physician intervention for smoking cessation. *JAMA* 1988; 260:1570–1574.
33. Bronson DL, Flynn BS, Solomon LJ, Vacek P, Secker-Walker RH. Smoking cessation counseling during periodic health examinations. *Arch Intern Med* 1989; 149:1653–1656.
34. Fisher EB, Kaire-Joshu D, Morgan GD, Rehberg H, Rost K. Smoking and smoking cessation. *Am Rev Respir Dis* 1990; 142:702–720.
35. Ockene JK. Physician-delivered interventions for smoking cessation: strategies for increasing effectiveness. *Prev Med* 1987; 16:723–737.
36. Samet J, et al. Environmental controls and lung disease: Report of the ATS workshop on environmental controls and lung disease. *Am Rev Resp Dis* 1990; 142:915–939.
37. Rubin DH, Leventhal JM, Krasilnikoff PA, et al. Relationship between infant feeding and infectious illness: A prospective study of infants during the first year of life. *Pediatrics* 1990; 85:464–471.
38. Wright AL, Holberg CJ, Martinez FD, Morgan WJ, Taussig LM. Breast feeding and lower respiratory tract illness in the first year of life. *Br Med J* 1989; 299:946–949.
39. Fleming DW, Cochi SL, Hightower AW, Broome CV. Childhood upper respiratory tract infections: To what degree is incidence affected by day–care attendance? *Pediatrics* 1987; 79:55–60.
40. Wald ER, Dashefsky B, Byers C, Guerra N, Taylor F. Frequency and severity of infections in day care. *J Pediatr* 1988; 112:540–546.
41. Berg AT, Shapiro ED, Capobianco LA. Group day care and the risk of serious infectious illnesses. *Am J Epidemiol* 1991; 133:154–163.
42. Falloon J, Eddy J, Wiener L, Pizzo PA. Human immunodeficiency virus infection in children. *Pediatrics* 1989; 114:1–30.
43. Novello AC, Wise PH, Willoughby A, Pizzo PA. Final report of the United States Department of Health and Human Services Secretary's work group on pediatric human immunodeficiency virus infection and disease: Content and implications. *Pediatrics* 1989; 84:547–555.
44. Nicholas SW, Sondheimer DL, Willoughby AD, Yaffe SJ, Katz SL. Human immunodeficiency virus infection in childhood, adolescence and pregnancy: A status report and national research agenda. *Pediatrics* 1989; 83:293–308.
45. Husson RN, Comeau AM, Hoff RH. Diagnosis of human immunodeficiency virus infection in infants and children. *Pediatrics* 1990; 86:1–10.
46. Butler KM, Husson RN, Balis FM, et al. Dideoxyinosine in children with symptomatic human immunodeficiency virus infection. *N Engl J Med* 1991; 324:137–144.
47. Hague RA, Yap PL, Mok JYQ, et al. Intravenous immunoglobulin in HIV infection: evidence for the efficacy of treatment. *Arch Dis Child* 1989; 64:1146–1150.
48. Caskey CT, Kaback MM, et al. The American Society of Human Genetics statement on cystic fibrosis screening. *Am J Hum Genet* 1990; 46:393.
49. The Cystic Fibrosis Foundation Center Committee and Guidelines Subcommittee. Cystic Fibrosis Foundation Guidelines for patient services, evaluation and monitoring in cystic fibrosis centers. *Am J Dis Child* 1990; 144:1311–1312.
50. Meyers A, Dolan TR, Mueller D. Compliance and self medication in cystic fibrosis. *Am J Dis Child* 1975; 129:1011–1013.

51. Passero MA, Ramor B, Salomon J. Patient reported compliance with cystic fibrosis therapy. *Clin Pediatr* 1981; 20:264–268.
52. Johnson MR, Gerhowitz M, Stabler B. Maternal compliance and children's self concept in cystic fibrosis. *Develop Behav Pediatr* 1981; 2:5–8.
53. Bell L, Durie P, Forstner G. What do children with cystic fibrosis eat? *J Pediatr Gastroenterol Nutr* 1984; 3:S137–46.
54. Evans R, Mullally DI, Wilson RW, et al. National trends in the morbidity and mortality of asthma in the US. Prevalence, hospitalization and death from asthma over two decades: 1965–1984. *Chest* 1987; 91(suppl 6):65–74.
55. Buist AS, Vollmer WM. Reflections on the rise in asthma morbidity and mortality. *JAMA* 1990; 264:1719–1720.
56. Meyers DA, Beaty TH, Friedhoff LF, Marsh DG. Inheritance of total serum IgE (basal level) in man. *Am J Hum Genet* 1987; 41:51–62.
57. Hasstedt SJ, Meyers DA, Marsh DG. Inheritance of immunoglobulin E: Genetic model fitting. *Am J Med Genet* 1983; 14:61–66.
58. Zeiger RS. Challenges in the prevention of allergic disease in infancy. *Clin Rev Allergy* 1987; 5:349–373.
59. Kjellman NI. Epidemiology and prevention of allergy. *Allergy* 1988; 43(suppl 8):39–40.
60. Weiss ST, Tager IB, Munoz A, Speizer FE. The relationship of respiratory infections in early childhood to the occurence of increased levels of bronchial responsiveness and atopy. *Am Rev Respir Dis* 1985; 131:573–578.
61. Magnusson CG. Maternal smoking influences cord serum IgE and IgD levels and increases the risk for subsequent infant allergy. *J Allergy Clin Immunol* 1986; 78:898–904.
62. Harris JB, Weinberger MM, Nassif E, Smith G, Milavetz G, Stillerman A. Early intervention with short courses of prednisone to prevent progression

63. Tal A, Levy N, Bearman JE. Methylprednisolone therapy for acute asthma in infants and toddlers: A controlled clinical trial. *Pediatrics* 1990; 86:350–356.
64. Taplin PS, Creer TL. A procedure for using peak expiratory flow rate data to increase the predictability of asthma episodes. *J Asthma* 1978; 16:15–19.
65. Hughes DM, McLeod M, Garner B, Goldbloom RB. Controlled trial of a home and ambulatory program for asthmatic children. *Pediatrics* 1991; 87:54–61.
66. Plaut TF. Peak flow: The key to success in asthma treatment. *Am J Asthma Allergy Pediatricians* 1988; 1:172–177.
67. Wigel JK, Creer TL, Kotses H, Lewis P. A critique of 19 self-management programs for childhood asthma: Part I. Development and evaluation of the programs. *Pediatr Asthma Allergy Immunol* 1990; 4:17–39.
68. Creer TL, Wigal JK, Kotses H, Lewis P. A critique of 19 self-management programs for childhood asthma: Part II. Comments regarding the scientific merit of the programs. *Pediatr Asthma Allergy Immunol* 1990; 4:41–55.
69. Howland J, Bauchner H, Adair R. The impact of pediatric asthma education on morbidity. *Chest* 1988; 94:964–969.
70. Fireman P, Friday GA, Gira C, Vierthaler WA, Michaels L. Teaching self-management skills to asthmatic children and their parents in an ambulatory care setting. *Pediatrics* 1981; 68:341–348.
71. Hill RA, Britton JR, Tattersfield AE. Management of asthma in schools. *Arch Dis Child* 1987; 62:414–415.
72. Bevis M, Taylor B. What do school teachers know about asthma? *Arch Dis Child* 1990; 65:622–625.
73. Committee on Drugs, American Academy of Allergy and Immunology. The use of inhaled medications in school by students with asthma. *J Allergy Clin Immunol* 1989; 84:400.

of asthma in ambulatory patients incompletely responsive to bronchodilators. *J Pediatr* 1987; 110:627–633.

DIAGNOSTIC TECHNIQUES

7

History and Physical Examination

FRANK J. ACCURSO, HOWARD EIGEN, and GERALD M. LOUGHLIN

HISTORY TAKING

History taking should be conducted to allow the patient and family to tell their story about the illness that brings them to you. This is a very personal process and depends on the personalities of both the physician and the family members. It is important to put the child and the family at ease and to reassure the family that you are carefully considering their previous experiences with the child's medical problem and that you are taking any and all symptoms seriously. In dealing with the older child and adolescent, it is also essential to direct attention to their individual questions and concerns and not to focus solely on the parents.

History taking is not an exercise in asking questions, but an exercise in listening carefully. It always helps to evaluate the family first. Is the father present or not present? The presence of the father often means that the disease is being taken much more seriously by the family than if the father does not come to the visit. Is there a grandmother present, and what is her role in the family? How old are the parents? What type of work do they do? The history taking approach you might take towards an engineer might be very different than one you would take to a farmer. It is not a matter of education or intelligence but rather of the family's experiences and outlook. It is also very valuable to listen to the interaction and comments made among family members, as well as the story they are giving to you directly.

When you begin the discussion, it is helpful to mention the referring physician by name and indicate that you have reviewed or will review all the information provided by the family's local physician. If you have spoken directly, either by phone or in person, to the referring physician, it is worthwhile to mention this to indicate that past information is valued and that the physicians caring for the child work well together. Families usually come with a story to tell, and we always find it useful to start the history session with an open-ended question using the child's name, such as "Tell me about the problems that Jane has been having." This allows the parent to begin talking in her own words and to feel comfortable talking with you. After several minutes you can then begin to focus the questions a little more (Table 7.1).

The formal history begins with the reason for the visit; document this as closely as possible in the patient's or parent's words. It is important not to accept diagnoses from parents. Parents will frequently use the term "bronchitis" to describe any illness with cough, and the term "croup" to describe any cough. This can be misleading and serve to confirm misdiagnoses. The parents should be asked to describe the child's symptoms in their own words. The history of the present illness should then be developed fully. It is usually helpful to start with a description of the first symptoms and then trace the problem chronologically to the present. It is also helpful to find out why they have been referred now and not previously. Has the illness gotten worse recently or have symptoms become more frequent? This leads to important questions about the direction of the disease, its duration, and whether it has been getting worse and over what length of time. Are symptoms continuous or intermittent? What activities or factors make the symptoms better and what makes them worse? What therapies have been

Table 7.1.
An Approach to the History and Physical Examination in a Child with Respiratory Disease

Chief complaint:

Description of symptoms—not a diagnosis

Onset, duration, associated symptoms

Factors that make symptoms worse or better, effects of feeding or sleep

Previous occurrence of similar symptoms

Response to therapy (was it adequate or appropriate?)

History of allergies, exposure, travel

Past history of respiratory illness, hospitalizations, emergency room visits

Effects on growth and development

Family history

Physical examination:

Vital signs

Ear, nose, and throat
 Thorough evaluation of ears, nose, and throat, checking for signs of obstruction, signs of infection, signs of allergy, status of nasal mucosa, and secretions

Chest
 Observation of breathing patterns, activity level, respiratory effort
 Inspection—chest wall (symmetry, pectus, size, deformities)
 Percussion—dullness, hyper-resonance
 Palpation—tracheal position, vibration with respiration
 Auscultation of the chest
 Breath sounds, adventitial sounds
 Timing, distribution, pitch, and quality of sounds
 Amount of airflow for the effort

Cardiac—murmurs, second heart sound

Miscellaneous
 Digital clubbing
 Abdominal organs
 Location, tenderness
 Signs of atopy
 Allergic shiners, dennie's line, nasal mucosa, eczema

used in the past, and what has been the response to previous therapy? It is important to determine if medications prescribed previously were used in the appropriate manner and for a duration sufficient to be able to tell whether the drug could have benefitted the child.

By this time in the history, it is likely that the physician has in mind one, two, or three diagnoses that seem most likely from the historical events. For each of these, the physician has in his mind the template of symptoms and responses that characterize the disease. For example, if the history signifies asthma, we would think that the child should have had difficulties with exercise, may have a nocturnal cough, and may wheeze in cold weather. Specific questions can then be asked, based on the internal template for the suspected disease. When something glaringly inconsistent with the template occurs in the history, that new avenue must be pursued. For example, if we were dealing with a child suspected of having asthma and the mother began to describe abnormal stools consistent with steatorrhea, we would recognize that this is out of the template for asthma and would pursue other avenues of questioning.

The environmental history may also be helpful in diagnosis (see Chapter 51). Irritants in the home, smoke from tobacco or wood stoves, or paint fumes may be associated with respiratory symptoms including cough and wheeze, especially in infants. All adult smokers with consistent contact with the child should be identified. In the environmental history it is important to be sure that all adults in the household are accounted for, not just the parents, and that exposures that commonly occur outside the home, such as at a babysitter's house, are pursued. Triggers to reactive airways disease may be present in the home environment. These would include exposures to pets such as cats, dogs, or even horses. The presence of birds raises the possibility of hypersensitivity pneumonitis as well as Psittacosis. Other environmental irritants may come from wood-burning stoves, paints and hobbies, or in-home businesses.

A history of *active* smoking should be sought in all older children and adolescents. This is best obtained with the parents out of the room; otherwise the answers are not likely to be reliable. A travel history may provide a clue to the diagnosis, especially with children with unusual infiltrates and illnesses.

The discussion period following the history and physical examination is of paramount importance in communicating with the family. It is crucial that the family and the patient feel that their concerns and questions have been understood and, if possible, answered by the physician, or that at least there is a plan to answer these questions. In discussing the illness, it is important to remember that even intelligent and well educated patients and parents may be medically unsophisticated, and to use language appropriate for the patient and the family.

Occasionally, a child's symptom occurs episodically, and the child may appear normal during the visit. This situation can be frustrating for the family. We have found that use of an audiotape or videotape of the event or symptom may be particularly helpful in these situations and will go a long way toward making the family feel that they are not losing their minds.

PHYSICAL EXAMINATION

The physical examination provides a window to the pathophysiology of the child's illness. It is very helpful to begin the physical examination during history taking by carefully observing the child and his or her respiratory patterns. With young children, we usually have the child partially undressed during the history taking so that these observations can be made without any threatening moves toward the child. Vital signs should be obtained in a nonthreatening fashion. Resting heart rate and respiratory rate, as well as blood pressure, should be measured in all patients before anything else is done to the child. Age-dependent normal values for respiratory rate

are presented in Tables 7.2 and 7.3 (1, 2). Height or length and weight should be measured and the results plotted on a standard growth grid. These values should be compared to historical data obtained from the referring physician.

The color of the lips, tongue, and extremities should be noted. Mild desaturation may impart a gray color to the skin. Cyanosis is an ominous finding and a late sign of lung dysfunction. Infants frequently develop acrocyanosis secondary to alterations in peripheral circulation despite adequate oxygen content centrally. Thus, it is important to assess the child's color from a central location such as the lips, tongue, or conjunctiva. In a child with a normal hemoglobin level, approximately 3 g/100 ml of reduced hemoglobin must be present to detect cyanosis. The oxygen saturation at which cyanosis can be detected varies with the hemoglobin level; an anemic child will have a considerably lower saturation before becoming clinically cyanotic.

Pulsus paradoxus, a decrease in the systolic blood pressure reading of more than 10 mm Hg during inspiration, has been shown to correlate with the degree of airway obstruction

Table 7.2.
Normal Mean Respiratory Rates per Minute in Full-Term and Preterm Infants between 2 and 50 Weeks of Age[a]

Age (weeks)	Preterm (x ± 1 SD)	Full-Term (x ± SD)
2	41 ± 11	36 ± 7
4	46 ± 11	35 ± 6
6	43 ± 11	37 ± 7
8	48 ± 20	36 ± 6
10	44 ± 12	31 ± 4
12	42 ± 12	30 ± 3
14	39 ± 11	30 ± 3
16	39 ± 11	31 ± 3
18	34 ± 8	29 ± 3
22	30 ± 5	28 ± 3
26	32 ± 6	28 ± 3
30	32 ± 8	28 ± 3
34	29 ± 6	27 ± 3
38	30 ± 5	29 ± 6
42	27 ± 2	27 ± 7
46	28 ± 5	27 ± 6
50	27 ± 6	25 ± 3
	35.9 ± 8.8	30.2 ± 4.5

Data from Katona DG, Egbert JR. Heart rate and respiratory rate differences between preterm and full term infants during quiet sleep: Possible implications for sudden infant death syndrome. *Peds* 1978; 3:89–99.
[a]All observations made during quiet sleep. Standard deviations calculated from authors' data.

Table 7.3.
Age-Dependent Mean Respiratory Rates ($\pm$ 1 SD per Minute for Boys and Girls

Age(y)	Boys	Girls	Age(y)	Boys	Girls
0–1	31 ± 8	30 ± 6	9–10	19 ± 2	19 ± 2
1–2	26 ± 4	27 ± 4	10–11	19 ± 2	19 ± 2
2–3	25 ± 4	25 ± 3	11–12	19 ± 3	19 ± 3
3–4	24 ± 3	24 ± 3	12–13	19 ± 3	19 ± 2
4–5	23 ± 2	22 ± 2	13–14	19 ± 2	18 ± 2
5–6	22 ± 2	21 ± 2	14–15	18 ± 2	18 ± 3
6–7	21 ± 3	21 ± 3	15–16	17 ± 3	18 ± 3
7–8	20 ± 3	20 ± 2	16–17	17 ± 2	17 ± 3
8–9	20 ± 2	20 ± 2	17–18	16 ± 3	17 ± 3

From Iliff A, Lee VA. Pulse rate, respiratory rate and body temperature of children between two months and eighteen years of age. *Child Dev* 1952; 23:237–245.

in asthma (3, 4). This measurement can be attempted in the older child or adolescent whose respiratory rate and level of cooperation make it feasible to obtain. However, we have not found this measurement to be of practical value since it is so difficult to obtain reliably in young children. In young children, one's chances of success may be improved by allowing the mother to hold the child on her lap while measurements are made.

Inspection

The order of physical examination of children must be flexible, depending on the age, anxiety level, and degree of cooperation. In the young child, it is usually best to start with the chest examination while the child is being held by one parent. This can start in a playful manner while the child feels the security of being in his parent's lap. A baseline observation period, whether done during the history or during the early part of the physical examination, is important to determine if the child is making respiratory noises at rest. During the baseline period evidence of stridor, upper airway noise, cough, wheezing or frequent clearing of the throat should be noted. It should be determined if any of these findings have also been noted by the parents and if they are the source of concern for the parent. For example, asking "Is that the cough that he typically has at night?" can be helpful. During this observation the child is normally active and should be observed for any changes in respiration that result from this activity. Observation should also focus on the breathing pattern: is the child struggling or working hard to breathe? Does he or she appear short of breath at rest? Is the child breathing rapidly? If the opportunity

arises the child should be observed during sleep and bottle feeding, since a number of respiratory conditions are exacerbated by either of these activities. If the child is asleep, is the respiratory rate regular or is there apnea or periodic breathing? Does the child have inspiratory or expiratory stridor? If a noise is present when the child is awake what effect does sleep have on this noise?

Inspection should also determine if nasal flaring, intercostal or substernal retractions, or paradoxical movement of the chest and abdomen on inspiration is present. With small children with acute disease, it is important to observe for any respiratory pauses that might indicate diaphragmatic fatigue. In young infants, the presence of head bob is an interesting sign of increased work of breathing. With the child sleeping in the mother's arms and the head only loosely supported, look to see if the head moves forward on inspiration. This indicates use of the accessory muscles of inspiration in a child who is not yet old enough to fix the extensor muscles of the neck.

Finally, what is the shape and size of the of the thoracic cavity? The chest wall should be inspected for evidence of deformities or unusual shape and to be sure that the thoracic cage is of appropriate size for the child's age and height. Concern about maldevelopment of the chest wall can be confirmed by actual measurements of the thoracic dimensions. Standards for width and depth have been published by Waring and co-workers (5). These measurements require the use of calipers and thus are not used routinely. Measurement of chest circumference obtained at the nipple line is easier to perform and is a more practical way to follow the growth of the chest cavity.

A set of standards based on a measurement obtained at mid-inspiration have been published (6). All of these measurements should be standardized to a particular phase of the respiratory cycle so that the measurement can be repeated at follow-up and the data can be plotted as with other growth parameters (Fig. 7.1). Changes in the chest size with respiration should be assessed, and notice should be taken of whether these changes are symmetric.

Auscultation of the Chest

Auscultation of the chest begins with the child in the parent's arms. Infants and toddlers should be approached cautiously and playfully in order to avoid upsetting them before a resting examination of the chest can be obtained. By this point, clothing covering the chest should have been removed so that the child does not need to be disturbed at the time of the examination. Warming the head of the stethoscope before placing it on the patient's skin is appreciated by the patient of any age. Using a careful and anatomically valid pattern of auscultation is important. A double-headed stethoscope is very helpful in comparing the sounds from anatomically homologous segments (7). If a single-headed stethoscope is used, the examiner should move back and forth between homologous segments. Findings should be recorded with reference to the general area in which any abnormalities are heard (Fig. 7.2). It is important to gauge the relationship of inspiratory and expiratory timing as well as the amount of airflow for the degree of effort involved in breathing. The finding of increased respiratory effort associated with diminished or absent breath sounds is an important clinical finding (8).

Evaluation of adventitious sounds, if present, should come next. A classification of adventitious breath sounds is presented in

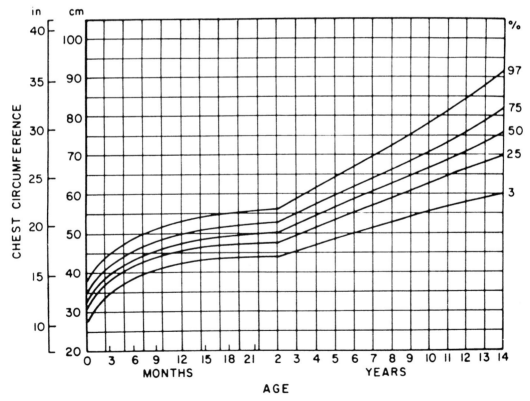

Figure 7.1. Graphic display of the growth of the chest circumference from birth through age 14. These measurements were obtained at mid-inspiration at the nipple line. A correction for gender differences between ages 2 and 12 can be made by adding 1 cm to the measured value for males and by subtracting 1 cm from the measured value for females. (From Feingold M, Bossert WH. Normal values for selected physical parameters. *Birth Defects* 1974; 10:14.)

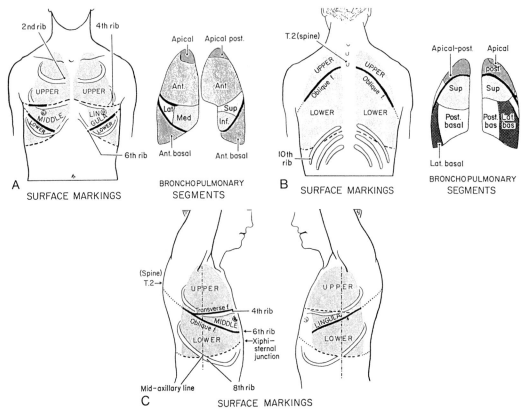

Figure 7.2. *A,* Surface markings of the lung from the anterior view with the appropriate bronchopulmonary segments displayed. *B,* Surface markings and underlying bronchopulmonary segments of the lung from the posterior view. *C,* Surface markings and underlying bronchopulmonary segments from the lateral view.(From Cherniack RM, Cherniack L, Naimark A. *Respiration in health and disease.* Philadelphia, WB Saunders, 1972, pp 236–238.)

Table 7.4 (9). The examiner should categorize the type of noise being made (stridor, wheeze, rhonchus, rale) and the timing of the noise in the respiratory cycle. Noisy breathing (wheeze, stridor, rhonchi) indicates the presence of airways obstruction. It is discussed in more detail in Chapter 14. *Crackles (rales)* are intermittent noises heard predominantly on inspiration. These sounds are produced by reopening of airways closed on the preceding expiration (3, 4). In healthy children and young adults, airway closure and thus rales should not occur; their presence suggests disease. In an attempt to link these sounds to a pathophysiologic process, researchers have given them a variety of qualifying labels such as sibilant or crepitant, wet or dry. However, we have found that from a practical standpoint, these labels are highly subjective and add little to the diagnostic approach. It is more useful to classify these sounds on the basis of

timing, inspiration versus expiration, and early versus late. Rales that occur late in inspiration or that are only detected with a deep inspiration are indicative of small airways disease. Expiratory rales indicate a marked discrepancy in the time constants of the small airways, with the more severely affected airways not opening (inspiring) until the bulk of the surrounding airways are in the expiratory phase. A differential diagnosis of crackles is presented in Table 7.5.

As auscultation proceeds, the examiner should note the following. Is the sound heard on inspiration, expiration, or both? Is the noise distributed symmetrically in both lung fields? Symmetry in the timing, quality, and distribution of adventitious sounds suggests that they are being generated above the tracheal bifurcation. Noises heard in inspiration should be judged for whether they occur early or late in the cycle. Although the examination

Table 7.4.
Classification of Adventitious Sounds

Acoustic Characteristics	Recommended ATS[a] Nomenclature	Terms in Some Textbooks	British Usage	Laennec's Original Term
Discontinuous, interrupted explosive sounds				
Loud, low-in-pitch sounds	Coarse crackle	Coarse rale	Crackle	*Rale muquex ou gouillement*
Softer than above and of shorter duration; higher in pitch than coarse rales or crackles	Fine crackle	Fine rale	Crackle	*Rale humide ou crepitation*
Continuous sounds				
Longer than 250 msec, high-pitched; dominant frequency of 400 Hz or more; a hissing sound	Wheeze[b]	Sibilant rhonchus	High-pitched wheeze	*Rale sibilant sec ou sifflement*
Longer than 250 msec, low-pitched; dominant frequency about 200 Hz or less; a snoring sound	Rhonchus	Sonorous rhonchus	Low-pitched wheeze	*Rale sec sonore ou ronflement*

Modified from Murphy LH. Lung sounds. *Basics of RD* 1980; 8(4).
[a]American Thoracic Society.
[b]Also describes inspiratory stridor—sound not modified by lung, which acts as a low-pass filter.

Table 7.5.
Common Causes of Crackles in Children

Pneumonia—viral, bacterial
Bronchiolitis
Asthma
Pulmonary edema
Interstitial pneumonitis or fibrosis
Bronchiectasis—cystic fibrosis, dyskinetic cilia, post-infectious

should begin with tidal volume breathing, it is often important to get the child to breathe deeply and rapidly during the examination. In older children, this can be done simply on request. In young children, tickling or playing with the child may increase both the speed and depth of respiration. Wheezes or stridor are sometimes heard only on forced or rapid exhalations, so it is important to have the patient perform some form of deep breathing maneuver during the physical examination. In older children, this can be done voluntarily, whereas in the infant and young child tickling or getting the child excited often produces the desired result.

Percussion of the Chest

Although it may be becoming a lost art, percussion of the chest wall can provide invaluable information on lung status and on the location of the edges of solid organs, and should be performed routinely over both hemithoraces in symmetric locations. The topical distribution of the various lung segments is depicted in Figure 7.2. Percussion is best performed by striking the distal phalanx of the middle finger, which is in contact with the chest wall. Other fingers should not be in contact with the chest wall. The percussion note is generated by a short, firm stroke. The information gathered from percussion is derived from both the sound and the feel of the vibration generated by the percussion note. A hyper-resonant percussion note indicates hyperinflation. It can be detected even in small infants. The presence of hyperinflation is also suggested by examination of the abdomen. Descent of the liver edge, spleen tip, or both below the costal margin confirms the finding of hyper-resonance. The span of the liver should always be evaluated to be sure that the liver edge is felt because of true enlargement. Atelectasis, consolidation, or pleural effusion can frequently be detected by the presence of a dull, flat percussion note in the chest.

Palpation of the Chest

Careful palpation of the chest is especially important in children complaining of chest pain, since it may elicit point tenderness. In the child with noisy breathing, palpation of the neck and supersternal area is important since it allows one to look for masses that might be impinging on the trachea. Position of the trachea should be determined, especially in children with breathing noises thought to originate from the large airways. Palpation of the upper abdominal muscles can be used to assess the presence of increased activity of these accessory muscles of expiration. Finally, gentle palpation of the chest wall will often detect the vibration produced by turbulent airflow through obstructed airways. This is what the parents describe as the child feeling rattly.

Upper Airway and Extremities

The respiratory examination does not end with examination of the chest. Examination of the nose should be carried out in all patients to evaluate for signs of nasal obstruction or rhinitis, either acute or chronic. In the newborn suspected of upper airway obstruction this should include passage of a No. 8 French feeding tube to rule out choanal atresia. The status of the nasal mucosa, the presence and nature of secretions, and the presence of nasal polyps should be commented on in the physical examination.

Examining the oropharynx is often quite difficult in young children, since they often have had a bad experience with a tongue blade and thus are orally defensive. Nonetheless, many times an adequate examination can be accomplished without the aid of a tongue blade if the examination is approached in a nonthreatening, almost casual manner with appropriate help from a parent. It is best not to force the issue unless examination of the oral pharynx is thought to be critical to establishing a diagnosis. Observation for any acute inflammation is part of the general physical examination. In the child with upper airway hypersecretion, looking for postnasal drip

with mucus dripping down from the nasopharynx into the oropharynx is very useful, as is the assessment of whether there is hypertrophic lymphoid tissue on the posterior wall of the oropharynx (cobble stoning). Tonsilar size and the ratio of their size to the oropharynx should be determined. It is important to note tonsilar tissue that extends posteriorly rather than medially. It is also quite important to examine the fingers to determine the presence or absence of digital clubbing (Fig. 7.3). This is done by holding the child's index finger so as to estimate the relative depth of the finger

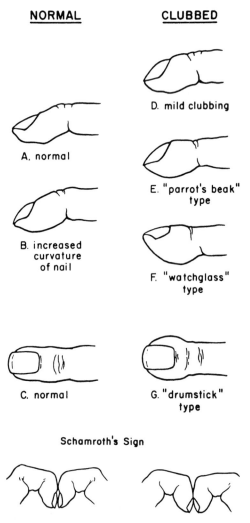

Figure 7.3. Normal variations and patterns of digital clubbing. (Modified from Hansen-Flaschen J and Nordberg J. Clubbing and hypertrophic osteoarthropathy. *Clin Chest Med* 1987; 8:287–298.)

at the base of the nail and the first interphalangeal joint (11, 12). If congenital heart disease and nonpulmonary causes of digital clubbing can be eliminated from consideration, the presence of digital clubbing indicates that there is significant destructive organic lung disease, either localized or generalized.

CONCLUSIONS

A thorough history and careful physical examination form the basis for care of patients with pediatric respiratory disease. The diagnosis is often apparent after the history and physical examination. When the diagnosis is not apparent after the history and physical examination, the information gained suggests the specifics of further diagnostic evaluation. The initial therapeutic plan is also greatly influenced by the history and physical examination. Follow-up histories and physical examinations pay a key role in longitudinal care.

REFERENCES

1. Iliff A, Lee VA. Pulse rate, respiratory rate and body temperature of children between two months and eighteen years of age. *Child Dev* 1952; 23:237–245.
2. Katona DG, Egbert JR. Heart rate and respiratory rate differences between preterm and full term infants during quiet sleep: Possible implications for sudden infant death syndrome. *Pediatrics* 1978; 3:89–99.
3. Wise RA, Summer WR. Pulsus paradoxus: Why it happens and how to treat it. *J Resp Med* 1982; 3:89–99.
4. Rebuck A, Pegelly LD. Development of pulsus paradoxus in the presence of airways obstruction. *N Engl J Med* 1973; 66–69.
5. Waring WW. Physical examination of children: Quantitative extensions. In Sackner MA, ed. *Diagnostic techniques in pulmonary disease*. New York: Marcel Dekker, 1980.
6. Feingold M, Bossert WH. Normal values for selected physical parameters. *Birth Defects* 1974; 10:14.
7. Forgacs P. The functional basis of pulmonary sounds. *Chest* 1978; 73:399–405.
8. Murphy RLD, Holford SK. Lung sounds. *Basics RD* 1980; 8(4).
9. Forgacs P. Crackles and wheezes. *Lancet* 1967; 2:203–209.
10. Forgacs P. *Lung sounds.* London, Casell & Coller, MacMillan Publishers, 1978.
11. Hansen-Flaschen J and Nordberg J. Clubbing and hypertrophic osteoarthropathy. *Clin Chest Med* 1987; 8:287–298.
12. Waring WW, Wilkinson RW, Wiebe RA, et al. Quantification of digital clubbing in children. Measurements of casts of the index finger. *Am Rev Resp Dis* 1977; 104:166–174.
13. Cherniack RM, Cherniack L, Naimark A. *Respiration in health and disease*. Philadelphia, WB Saunders, 1972, pp 236–238.

8

Lung Function Testing

HOWARD EIGEN

Pulmonary function testing is used to answer questions about the respiratory function of the child being evaluated. Specifically these fall into the following general questions:

Is the patient normal? or Is the previous clinical assessment of the patient's status by parents or medical personnel accurate?

Does the patient have restrictive or obstructive lung disease?

Is there bronchodilator responsiveness?

Does the patient have hyper-reactive airways?

Is the disease progressing or receding (prognosis)?

Has therapy or a change in therapy been beneficial?

The tests and testing conditions are then chosen to answer these particular questions depending on the clinical needs. To answer any of these questions, the laboratory must have equipment designed for testing children and a technician skilled in testing children and familiar with their special needs.

CHOICE OF EQUIPMENT

Most systems on the market are based on a pneumotachograph and use the signal from this to calculate flow and volume from which a flow-volume curve is plotted.

Choosing equipment entails a number of decisions that are particular to the laboratory making the purchase. Technical adequacy is of course essential. The equipment must meet the American Thoracic Society (ATS) standards for adults and other published standards for children (1, 2). The equipment must be easy to use for a child. Be sure to check that the arm holding the mouthpiece can be

Table 8.1.
Recommended Specifications for Pulmonary Equipment[a]

Flow	
Accuracy	±5% or ±.1 L/sec, whichever is greater
Response	±5% to 8 Hz
Volume	
Accuracy	±3% of reading or 30 ml, whichever is greater
Sensitivity	20–40 mm of chart equals 1 L
Response	±5% to 5 Hz
Time	
Discrimination	0.05 sec/mm
Timer threshold	50 ml/sec
Dynamic calibration	
Inertia	Low
Amplitude response	±5% to 15 Hz
Other considerations	
Ability to assess adequacy of inspiration effort (closed circuit or a pneumotachograph)	
Should produce a hard copy curve	

Data from Taussig LM, Chernick V, Wood R, et al. Standardization of lung function testing in children. *J Pediatr* 1980; 97:668.
[a]These recommendations from data generated in adults have been extrapolated for use in pediatric laboratories.

adjusted for the easy use of a child and/or that a hose can be attached to make use easy for small children. Many products do not provide proper adjustments for children, so this should be checked carefully. If a handheld pneumotachograph is part of the design be sure that the device can be held comfortably by a 5- or 6-year-old child and that it is not too large or too heavy. In using mechanical spirometers especially, check that the inertia of the system and the flow ranges and volumes that it can measure are appropriate for young or sick children. Often when testing children, the best technique to use is to allow them to put the mouthpiece in their mouth and let them breathe into the circuit before taking a deep breath for the forced maneuver. Systems that do not permit this technique should be avoided.

TESTING PROCEDURE

The room and environment should be free from distractions and especially from instruments associated with painful procedures. Most children entering a pulmonary function test laboratory for the first time will be curious, slightly timid, very willing to cooperate, and anxious to please the technician, physician, and parents by performing well. The laboratory and its staff should realize this and be careful not to alter this positive attitude by their actions.

Children are generally very responsive to explanations, even of technical material, and enjoy the chance to ask questions. Hospital personnel who do not deal with children daily tend to underestimate the child's ability to understand and his or her eagerness to do a good job. They often talk down to the child, or misinterpret tentative actions or genuine fear as lack of cooperation. Brough et al. (3) have shown that performance can be improved if children ages 5–7 are given 15 minutes of instruction that explain the test and how it works, are given a demonstration of the respiratory maneuvers, and are provided a chance to practice. A formal instruction period improved performance on forced vital capacity (FVC) and forced expiratory volume in 1 second (FEV_1) by 10% compared to a group given routine instruction just prior to testing. It is also helpful if a goal or element of competition is introduced to the test.

Obtaining an adequate expiratory curve may require a great deal of coaching. Children often cannot grasp the idea of blowing out with maximum force *and* for as long as possible. Children who blow a long time, obtaining a true vital capacity, will try to "save some air" and not blow out forcefully at the beginning of the effort.

All breathing maneuvers should be done wearing nose clips. Although the child may sit or stand for the test with no effect on its result, the technician should be certain that the trunk is held upright and the head is erect during the maneuver.

After the child has performed the test comes the problem of selecting the appropriate tracing for analysis. To obtain data representative of a child's actual lung function may require the performance and evaluation of many curves, since effort may vary greatly with each try. Although learning takes place in some cases, making later curves better than earlier ones, we have also experienced just the opposite, wherein the early efforts were the best, presumably because the test procedure exceeded the child's attention span or fatigue set in. In any case, a large set of curves must be generated and saved before a "best effort" can be chosen. This severely limits the usefulness of computer-based systems that store only three curves and those in which each effort must be rejected before the next attempt is made. The best-effort curve is selected as the one having the greatest sum of FEV_1 and FVC. Peak flow is usually measured separately as the best effort from three to five efforts using a peak flowmeter or from the best-effort flow-volume curve, which is reported as maximum forced expiratory flow (FEF_{max}). An incomplete effort is especially difficult to identify using a standard spirogram, yet in obtaining valuable data it is crucial to know that the effort is a true vital capacity maneuver. We find that it is easier to note an effort in which the child has stopped short of residual volume (RV) using a flow-volume plot rather than a volume-time tracing. More difficult still is judging whether the child has inspired to total lung capacity (TLC) as the start of the test, since curves blown from a lower lung volume will have the same shape as those blown from TLC using either graphic format.

PHYSIOLOGY

Testing lung function is based on the measurements of lung volumes and the rate of airflow from the lung. To make such measurements requires that the subject first inhale and then exhale naturally.

Normal respiration takes place with active inspiration caused by a contraction of the inspiratory muscles. The diaphragm accounts for two-thirds of the air movement achieved during quiet breathing. The intercostal muscles function to fix the chest wall. The accessory inspiratory muscles (scalenes, sternocleidomastoid) are inactive during tidal breathing and only become active at higher levels of respiration or with greater efforts. Exhalation is passive during quiet breathing.

The most basic maneuver in spirometry is the slow vital capacity maneuver. In a volume-time spirogram, the child first breathes quietly into the spirometer. Tidal inspiration is active and tidal exhalation is passive. The passive end expiratory resting point occurs when the forces of the elastic lung and the expansive chest wall are balanced and airflow ceases. The volume in the chest at this point is functional residual capacity (FRC), and by recording tidal breathing on a volume-time spirogram the level of FRC (but not its actual volume) is recorded. After recording quiet breathing a maximal volume effort is obtained. The child inhales slowly to TLC and then exhales steadily to RV. Recording this slow vital capacity maneuver on a volume-time spirogram defines the classic lung volumes (Fig. 8.1). The volume-time spirogram can be recorded from a *forced* maneuver in which the child maintains a maximum effort from TLC to RV. Both inspiration and expiration are active and maximal during a forced expiratory maneuver. This maximal maneuver is essential in order to define lung volumes and to reach flow limitation, which is the basis for interpreting an expiratory flow volume curve. By achieving flow resistive limitation we are testing the properties of the airways. In older children and adults, the larger airways, up to the 6th or 7th generation, account for the greatest portion (up to 80%) of airways resistance dur-

ing a maximal breathing effort. Thus, it is primarily the properties of these airways that we are testing during the forced expiratory maneuver. From the FVC effort, we can measure the volume exhaled at a specific time (e.g., FEV_1). Since flow is volume over time, the greater the volume exhaled over the first second the greater the average flow over that time. It is now more common to plot the forced spirogram as a flow-volume curve with 1-second time markers from the start of the effort. This gives an easy-to-read plot on which FVC, FEV_1, and FEF_{max} (peak flow) are easily identified.

FLOW-VOLUME RELATIONSHIPS

An assessment of the flow-resistive properties of the airways is obtained from the flow-volume curve. During the forced expiration, the rate of airflow rises quickly to a maximum value at or near TLC. As the lung volume decreases, intrathoracic airways narrow, airway resistance increases, and rate of airflow progressively falls.

A family of flow-volume curves is produced by repeating full expiratory maneuvers over the entire vital capacity at different levels of effort. At high lung volumes close to TLC, rate of airflow increases progressively with increasing effort. However, at intermediate and low lung volumes, expiratory flow reaches maximal levels after only moderate effort is exerted and thereafter increases no further despite increasing efforts.

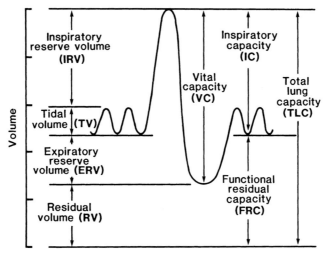

Figure 8.1. *Slow vital capacity maneuver.* The components of the TLC are identified.

The rate of airflow at any point during expiration is influenced both by lung volume and effort expended. The relationship between effort alone and expiratory airflow is illustrated by *isovolume pressure-flow curves* (Fig. 8.2). During repeated expiratory maneuvers performed with various degrees of effort, simultaneous measurements are made of airflow, pleural pressure, and lung volume. At given lung volumes, airflow is plotted against pleural pressure, providing a measure of effort.

At all lung volumes, pleural pressure becomes less subatmospheric and subsequently exceeds atmospheric pressure as the expiratory effort is progressively increased. Correspondingly, the rate of airflow increases. At lung volumes greater than 75% of vital capacity, airflow increases progressively with rising pleural pressure; airflow is thus considered to be effort-dependent. In contrast, at volumes below 75% of vital capacity, flow levels off as the pleural pressure exceeds atmospheric pressure and becomes fixed at a maxi-

mal level. Thereafter, further increases in effort and in pleural pressure effect no further rise in flow, and airflow is considered to be effort-independent. Since airflow remains constant despite an increasing driving pressure, resistance to airflow must also be increasing proportionally with pleural pressure, probably because of compression and narrowing of intrathoracic airways.

LUNG VOLUMES

The measurement of lung volumes may be helpful in following the course of chronic disease and occasionally in the diagnosis of some entities. For the purposes of volume measurement TLC can be divided into two parts: the vital capacity, which can be expelled into a spirometer, and RV, which cannot be exhaled and must be measured directly by the use of gas dilution or by plethysmography. In practice RV is not measured directly but is measured as part of FRC, which is a more reproducible lung volume and from which RV can be calculated. We use lung volume measure-

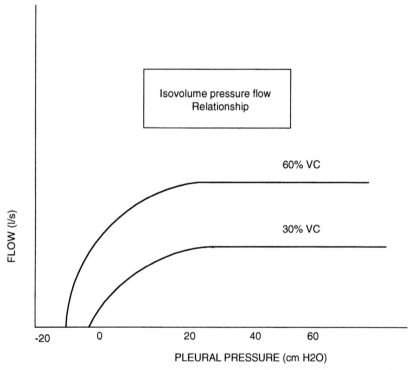

Figure 8.2. *Isovolume pressure flow curve.* This is the essence of the flow-volume curve relationship between flow and volume. The flow at any point is related to the lung volume, not to the pleural pressure. Even with increasing effort and increasing pleural pressure, there is not an increase in flow unless the volume of the lung is increased.

ments to follow the course of patients with cystic fibrosis by making serial comparisons of FRC over the years. Measuring lung volumes can also be helpful in those patients in whom the chest radiograph indicates hyperlucency but in whom spirometry is inconclusive. The finding of an elevated FRC or TLC would confirm the presence of obstructive lung disease.

MEASUREMENT OF GAS TRANSFER (DIFFUSING CAPACITY)

Gas transfer in the lung is measured as the diffusing capacity for carbon monoxide and is usually done as a single breath test (4). The patient inhales a low concentration of carbon monoxide mixed with a tracer gas such as helium. The dilution of the mixture can be calculated from the dilution of the helium; any further reduction in concentration of the carbon monoxide is related to its diffusion through the alveolar membrane and into the red cell. The uptake of CO is affected by any of the factors between the alveolus and the hemoglobin molecule in the red blood cell. Carbon monoxide is used as the test gas because it rapidly combines with hemoglobin, thus eliminating this reaction as a factor affecting the transfer factor measurement. Diffusing capacity for carbon monoxide ($D_{L}CO$) is primarily affected by ventilation perfusion relationships within the lung and the function of the pulmonary capillary bed, but it is affected by anemia and the lung volume at which it is measured. Because of this, $D_{L}CO$ is corrected for lung volume and for hemoglobin. A decrease in $D_{L}CO$ is most commonly seen in children with interstitial lung disease, sickle cell disease, and pulmonary vascular disease. It is very useful for monitoring the effects of chemotherapeutic agents and radiation on the lung in children being treated for malignancy. It is probably underused in this regard. We prefer to begin measuring $D_{L}CO$ at the beginning of a course of potentially pulmonary toxic drugs rather than waiting for clinical indication of toxicity.

INTERPRETATION

The first step is to have a technically adequate spirogram and to choose data from the best effort available. The recommendation of the ATS is to choose the best numeric values for FVC and FEV$_1$ from curves done at the same testing session, even if they come from different efforts.

Interpretation then depends on the reason testing is being done. If the question is whether the patient has "normal" function one must compare the results from the patient with those in an appropriate reference population (5). This is not as easy as it would seem, and the choice of reference population(s) is one that is both crucial and often not given sufficient thought. The reference population must match the patient being tested as closely as possible, especially in terms of the test equipment and techniques used, race, sex, and demographic data. The more differences that exist between the patient and the reference population the more likely it is that the patient will be misclassified as to whether he or she is normal or abnormal. The data of Hsu et al., obtained by testing a large group of children in the Houston public school system, provide a good reference group that has been stratified into separate equations for Caucasian, Mexican-American, and African-American children (6, 7). A normal value is generally described as one within 2 standard deviations (SDs) from the mean. In a normal distribution, 95.4% of observations fall within this interval and 2.3% fall outside on either side. In most clinical testing (FVC, FEV$_1$, peak expiratory flow rate [PEFR]) our interest is focused on the 2.3% of patients who have a value that is more than 2 SDs *below* the mean.

A reference population should be chosen that matches the group of children commonly tested in your laboratory; the laboratory director should be certain that the correct reference group is chosen by the computer for each patient group (1, 2). By all means do not allow the computer to choose the reference population by default. When establishing the laboratory, it is ideal to test a group of healthy children who match the reference population to be sure they fit in the normal range described for the reference group. There is general agreement that within the pediatric age range girls have smaller lungs than boys for the same standing height, so references should always be sex-specific. Because children of different races have different body proportion they will have different lung sizes for the same standing height. This must be corrected for when comparisons are made (8).

Adolescence presents another challenge. There is evidence that lung growth lags behind the increase in standing height associated with the pubertal growth spurt. For the same height, there may be differences in lung volumes depending on the degree of sexual maturity. This further complicates the process of judging a patient "normal" or not.

RESTRICTIVE DISEASE

If lung function is different from that expected in the referenced group, the patient can be placed in a physiologic class of restrictive disease or obstructive disease.

Restrictive disease is characterized on spirometry by a low FVC with a proportionate reduction in airflow. In this case, the FEV_1 will be low but will be reduced proportionately to the FVC such that the FEV_1/FVC ratio will be unchanged from normal (> 80%). Patients with pulmonary fibrosing processes and alveolar filling diseases will demonstrate a restrictive pattern.

OBSTRUCTIVE DISEASE

Obstructive disease is characterized by a reduction in airflow that is greater than any accompanying reduction in FVC. Thus the FEV_1 is reduced more than the FVC and the FEV_1/FVC ratio is low. Early in the course of obstructive disease there is a reduction in FEF_{25-75} and other measurements of flow in the middle portion of the vital capacity maneuver. When looking at a flow-volume plot this appears as a concavity or sag in the flow-volume envelope. The sag progresses with worsening disease, and the FEV_1 becomes reduced from normal (Fig. 8.3). As obstruction progresses, the air is trapped as RV encroaches on the vital capacity, which then begins to diminish. However, even when FVC is low, it is the low FEV_1/FVC ratio that distinguishes obstructive disease from restrictive disease.

LONGITUDINAL TESTING

In this case we are asking questions about how a patient is improving (or deteriorating) or whether a particular intervention has been successful.

The concept of normal or comparison with a reference population is not applicable when testing is done for this purpose. Instead, we are looking for a significant change (usually 1 SD) from the value obtained previously on the same patient. If no growth has taken place, absolute values can be compared. If the child has grown, it is best to compare patient data on the basis of changes in percentages of predicted values. It is important to differentiate a clinically significant change from one that is significant only by statistical analysis. In doing this, one must remember that the value of a significant change will vary with the test. Although there will be some differences for clinical purposes, one can use the same value for percentage of change in absolute value as for change in percentage predicted. Assessing change in lung function is often used to predict a need for change in therapy. Figure 8.4 shows a patient with cystic fibrosis (CF). In this case lung function as measured by FVC has been variable within a small range, one that is not significant. At point A, a significant reduction of FVC takes place and the patient is begun on therapy, which results in or is associated with an improvement in lung function. At this point, consideration is given to changing therapy back to baseline.

Is the Patient Bronchodilator Responsive?

This is an important clinical question and can be used to judge whether the patient would benefit from treatment with bronchodilators. This is obviously important therapeutically but may also be helpful diagnostically. The question arises when the patient is noted to have obstructive disease on initial testing. A bronchodilator is administered and the patient is retested to determine if a significant increase in airflow has taken place. Bronchodilator responsiveness is tested by administering an appropriate dose of an effective bronchodilator by aerosol and then retesting the patient. A significant response is one in which parameters of airflow increase by 1 SD. Usually this is taken to be 1 SD for the normal population, but it is better to use the SD of a previously tested sample of patients with the same disease. In CF, for example, the percentage of change required for significance for FEV_1 is 23%, whereas in most normal populations it is > 10–12% (5, 9). Ideally, each laboratory would establish its own normal values, but

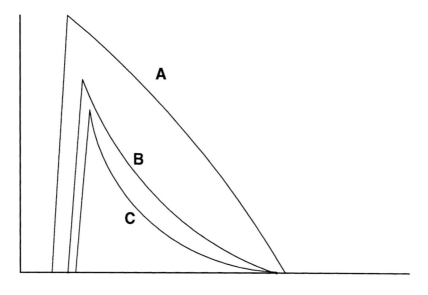

VOLUME

Figure 8.3. *Flow-volume curves with obstructive lung disease.* There is a progressive sag of the mid portion of the flow-volume curve as obstruction increases. Curve *A* is normal with a bowing-out of the cure (convexity) to the X-axis. In curve *B* we see the typical pattern of mild obstructive disease with the curve sagging toward the X-axis. This progresses in curve *C* as obstruction increases. This is a pattern seen in patients with cystic fibrosis as the disease progresses and in children with asthma who are having increasing airways obstruction. In asthma this can be corrected with a bronchodilator given in the laboratory by inhalation.

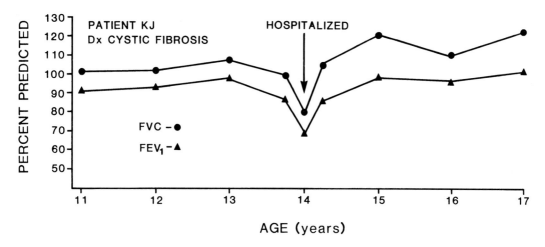

AGE (years)

Figure 8.4. Depiction of vital capacity measurement in a patient with CF over a 1-month interval. Point *A* indicates a significant reduction in FVC associated with a pulmonary exacerbation.

considering a response of 12% from baseline to be positive would seem reasonable.

The technique is simple but should be done with care. We give inhaled albuterol at a dose 0.5–1.0 ml to be certain that the patient has received an adequate dose. The patient is retested in 15 minutes. An increase in FEV_1 or FVC of 1 SD (12% of original value) or more indicates a positive response to the drug.

BRONCHOPROVOVATION TESTING

In a patient with a clinical history compatible with reactive airways disease, we may find normal lung function on the initial testing, which leads to the question: Does this patient have hyperactive airways? The question is answered by bronchoprovocation testing. Histamine, methacholine, cold air, and exercise are currently the most commonly used provocation agents. They all give the same information—that is, whether nonspecific hyper-reactivity is present in the patient. Each agent has its own advantages. Histamine and methacholine tests correlate well with each other and with exercise in the diagnosis of asthma. The chemical agents administered by inhalation are technically easier than exercise provocation. Two protocols are in general use for using methacholine and histamine. The patient can inhale increasing doses of methacholine from a nebulizer, inhaling five breathes of each concentration, from 0.0175 to 25 mg/ml; the number of breath units is then calculated. The response is positive at the cumulative dose that causes FEV_1 to drop 20% from baseline (the PD_{20}). In the second method, the patient breathes from a spirometer filled with aerosolized drug at the increasing concentrations. The concentration at which the patient responds with a reduction in FEV_1 of 20% from baseline (PC_{20}) is noted.

In either method, the lower the dose or concentration, the greater the nonspecific reactivity. The presence of hyper-reactive airways does not make a clinical diagnosis but adds information to the clinical picture already present.

During an exercise challenge, the normal airways dilate slightly and constrict slightly. Both of these responses are heightened in patients with airways hyper-reactivity. A positive response can be assessed by the fall in lung function or by using a lability index that accounts for the total response. We usually reserve exercise testing for children with specific exercise-induced symptoms, and even then will often use methacholine challenge as the first test to diagnose hyper-responsiveness of the airways. Although free running is most sensitive, most laboratories use treadmill running, which is only slightly less effective, but more practical, in inducing bronchospasm. Bicycle ergometry can also be used.

The next two questions—Is the disease process progressing, and has a change in therapy been beneficial?—are answered by sequential testing and comparison. The nature of how

these are approached is somewhat disease-specific.

In asthma, longitudinal testing is used to find early change in flows and lung volumes that would indicate deterioration in the child's condition but that has not yet become clinically apparent. Flows at low lung volumes (e.g., $FEF_{25-75\%VC}$) are particularly sensitive indicators. Reductions in these measurements occur earliest as the child's lung function deteriorates and so can be used as an early indicator of increasing disease. In clinical management, we use this measurement to follow a child closely as we reduce the level of medication. For example, we will discontinue a medication and then have the child return in 2–3 weeks for repeat testing. If the $FEF_{25-75\%VC}$ has fallen, we will reinstitute the medication prior to a more significant fall in lung function or the onset of clinical symptoms.

PEFR is an excellent way to use longitudinal testing at home to define the pattern of asthma in patients and as a guide for acute therapy (10). Interpretation is based on comparison with the patient's personal best effort or with his or her best effort as a percentage of predicted. The "personal best" approach takes into account that some patients may not have a "normal" PEFR even when well. The value is compared with the patient's best effort in order to classify the exacerbation as mild (> 70%), moderate (50–70%), or severe (< 50%). After an appropriate dose of an aerosolized beta agonist bronchodilator, PEFR is repeated and the response is classified as good (70–90%), incomplete (50–70%), or poor (< 50%). This approach as incorporated in the National Institutes of Health (NIH) report and used by others (11) gives objective criteria for action in a child with asthma. There is some question as to the best way of integrating PEFR and the role of this test in predicting clinical deterioration. It does not substitute for spirometry because it cannot detect small airways disease and so may be a relatively late indicator of pulmonary deterioration. It is probably equal to a carefully kept diary in its predictive function but is easier to perform. PEDF measurements do provide a practical and objective method for following a patient, especially those children who have a blunted dyspnea response. These children can develop severe airways obstruction without the perception of distress and become severely obstructed without becoming clinically distressed. In these children, we use PEFR to guide therapy instead of the patient's report of symptoms. It provides a good indicator of responsiveness to medication if the child is acutely ill. Use at home can give the physician objective data to deal with when the child's parents telephone. The PEFR can be measured, inhaled medication given, and the response measured by the parent. With this approach the physician can judge the need for evaluating the child in the emergency room or office and for starting additional medications.

Peak flow measurements are easy to make and can usually be performed satisfactorily by children older than 4 years. The child blows a short, sharp puff into the peak flow meter and stops. The measured flow (in liters per minute) is read off a dial or scale. The machine is reset and the maneuver is repeated. The maneuver should be done with nose clips and while standing. Peak flow obtained using a peak flow meter is similar to but not the same as the maximum flow (FEF_{max}) taken from a flow-volume curve, and so should be compared to different reference values.

In more chronic diseases such as CF the changes take place on a longer time scale. Longitudinal testing can establish a long-term baseline against which short-term changes in the child's lung function can be compared. In CF, changes in FEV_1 can occur acutely, but changes in FVC occur over longer periods (months) and may be more significant. A sharp reduction in FVC usually requires intervention on the part of the physician (either a change in medication or hospitalization). We usually use a decrease of 25% from the previously obtained value as an indication for the need for hospitalization. Once hospitalized, the patient with CF will be unlikely to have a significant increase in lung function for the first 5 days (12). Then lung function can be measured serially until it reaches a plateau, indicating that further therapy is not likely to be helpful in the next several days, and the child can be discharged. If the FVC continues to improve, continued hospitalization may be warranted.

In using serial testing one needs to reduce as much as possible the variation in results that might be due to other factors. Testing should be done at the same time of day, using the same equipment, and in the same position (sitting or standing). Medications should be discontinued for the same length of time prior to testing, and the patient should not consume foods or beverages that contain caffeine or related substances.

REFERENCES

1. Taussig LM, Chernick V, Wood R, et al. Standardization of lung function testing in children. Proceedings and recommendations of the GAP conference committee, Cystic Fibrosis Foundation. *J Pediatr* 1980; 97:668–676.
2. Gardner RM, Hankinson JL, Clausen JL, et al. Standardization of spirometry—1987 update. *Am Rev Respir Dis* 1987; 136:1285–1298.
3. Brough FK, Schmidt CD, Dickman M. Effect of two instructional procedures in the performances of the spirometry test in children 5 through 7 years of age. *Am Rev Respir Dis* 1972; 106:604–605.
4. Crapo RO, Gardner RM. Single breath carbon monoxide diffusing capacity (Transfer Factor). Official Statement of the American Thoracic Society. *Am Rev Resp Dis* 1987; 136:1299–1307.
5. Polgar G, Promadhat V. *Pulmonary function testing in children: Techniques and standards.* Philadelphia, WB Saunders, 1971.
6. Hsu KHK, Jenkins DE, Hsi BP, et al. Ventilatory functions of normal children and young adults, Mexican American, white and black: Spirometry. *J Pediatr,* 1979, 95: 14–23.
7. Hsu KHK, Jenkins DE, Hsi BP, et al Ventilatory functions of normal children and young adults, Mexican-American, white and black: Wright peak flow meter. *J Pediatr,* 1979, 95:192–196.
8. Taussig LM. Maximal expiratory flows at functional residual capacity: A test of lung function for young children. *Am Rev Resp Dis* 1977; 116:1031–1038.
9. Nickerson BG, Lemen RJ, Gerdes CB, et al. Within-subject variability and per cent change or significance of spirometry in normal subjects and in patients with cystic fibrosis. *Am Rev Resp Dis* 1980;122:859–866.
10. National Heart, Lung, and Blood Institute. Guidelines for the diagnosis and management of asthma. In *National Asthma Education Program: Expert panel report.* US Department of Health & Human Services, 1991.
11. Plaut TF. *Children with asthma—A manual for parents.* Amherst, MA, Pedipress, 1984.
12. Redding GJ, Restuccia R, Cotton EK, Brooks JG. Serial changes in pulmonary functions in children hospitalized with cystic fibrosis. *Am Rev Respir Dis* 1982; 126:31–36.

9

Imaging the Pediatric Chest

ALVIN H. FELMAN and DAVID F. MERTEN

Radiologic examination of the chest and lungs is an integral part of the diagnosis, treatment, and follow-up of patients with pulmonary disease. In addition to traditional radiographic film studies, cross-sectional imaging techniques have been developed, which include ultrasonography (1); computed tomography, or CT (conventional and high resolution) (1–3); and magnetic resonance imaging, or MRI (4, 5). Radionuclide scintigraphy (ventilation perfusion scan) and angiography are also applicable to the evaluation of chest diseases in childhood.

PRINCIPLES OF PEDIATRIC CHEST IMAGING
Conventional Radiographic Techniques

CHEST RADIOGRAPH

Plain chest films are the initial studies used in the work-up of children with respiratory symptoms. While frequently definitive, these studies may also serve to direct the selection of additional imaging modalities.

The respiratory phase of film exposure may vary considerably, especially in infants. Although inspiratory films are preferred, an expiratory film often indicates a normal chest (Fig. 9.1A). In expiration, the trachea buckles to the right with a normal left-sided aorta. In an adequately inspired chest film, the dome of the diaphragm usually lies at the level of the anterior 6th rib, and the trachea is straight from the subglottic area to the carina (Fig. 9.1B).

Standard Projections.
Frontal. In older children, the preferred position is erect, posterior-anterior (PA), if possible; anteroposterior (AP), if necessary. In

younger or less cooperative children (less than 3 years of age), AP supine is acceptable.

Lateral. As with the frontal projection, the preferred position is erect, but the lateral exposure may also be taken with the child supine (cross table lateral) or turned on the side with a vertical beam (turned up lateral).

Additional Projections.
Oblique. This view may improve rib detail (Fig. 9.2), visualize lung that is obscured on the frontal and lateral views, aid in cardiac contour analysis, and disclose mediastinal adenopathy.

Decubitus. This position is most often used for detecting free-flowing pleural fluid (Fig. 9.3). However, unilateral air trapping, as seen with a stem bronchus foreign body, may also be confirmed with decubitus views (Fig. 9.4) (6). On occasion, a subtle parenchymal process in the upper or nondependent lung may be more apparent on a decubitus film than on the frontal film.

Expiration. Exposing the film in expiration will sometimes disclose unilateral air trapping caused by partial stem bronchus occlusion (e.g., foreign body, tumor). In addition, the appearance of small pneumothoraces and/or effusions may be accentuated by expiratory films (Fig. 9.5). Firm epigastric pressure may be used to obtain an expiratory film.

Lordotic. Apical lordotic films may reveal lesions that are obscured by overlying ribs and clavicle. Sternal lordotic projections, centered lower on chest, may accentuate abnormalities in the right middle lobe and/or lingula (Fig. 9.6). Reverse lordotic projection will expose lesions in posterior costophrenic sulci that are occasionally obscured by the diaphragm.

High Kilovoltage, Filtered. This technique may also be used to facilitate visualization of

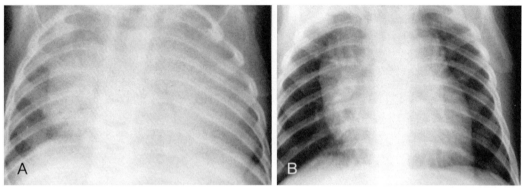

Figure 9.1.   Supine AP. *A,* Supine films tend to be exposed in an expiratory phase. This should not compromise interpretation, however, since infants who are able to empty their lungs usually are free of pulmonary infections. *B,* Film exposed several minutes later in improved inspiration shows normal heart and lungs.

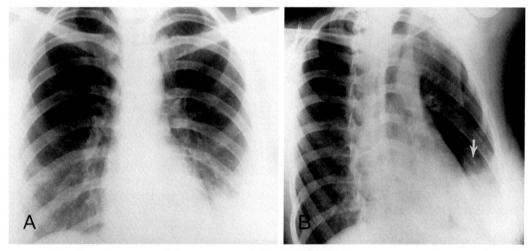

Figure 9.2.   Oblique exposure: Ewing sarcoma of rib. *A,* The frontal (PA) exposure reveals an opacity in the left lower hemithorax and costophrenic sulcus. The visible rib cage is normal although the left lower ribs are obscured. *B,* Right anterior oblique view shows the left lower thorax opacity to be quite peripheral and well defined against the adjacent lung. This view uncovers the destroyed left 7th rib.

the trachea and major bronchial airways (Fig. 9.7) (7).

Fluoroscopy (Video Tape). Fluoroscopy of the chest is helpful in assessing diaphragmatic excursion, mediastinal shift, thymic configuration, and upper airway and pharyngeal anatomy.

Contrast Esophagography. This procedure is used to evaluate esophageal anatomy, swallowing function, and gastroesophageal reflux. Vascular rings (Fig. 9.8), or mediastinal lesions that impinge on the trachea, are often detected with contrast esophagram.

Conventional Tomography The indications for conventional tomography include detection of calcification or cavitation, accurate localization of a lung opacity, delineation

of rib destruction, analysis of hilar and mediastinal shadows, and clarification of an indefinite pulmonary lesion. This technique, however, has largely been superseded by CT.

Cross-Sectional Imaging

ULTRASONOGRAPHY

Sonographic evaluation of the chest is limited by the air-filled lung and surrounding rib cage. Nevertheless, real-time ultrasonography, as well as Doppler techniques, can provide significant information regarding certain thoracic lesions.

Pleural Space. Ultrasonography can localize and help direct the drainage of intratho-

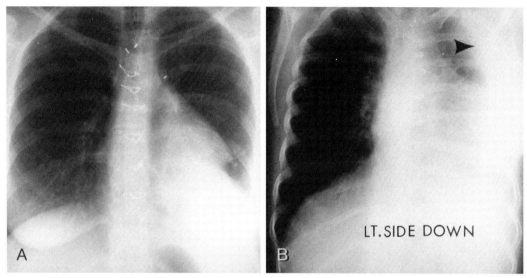

Figure 9.3. Subpulmonic pleural effusion. *A,* Erect frontal chest radiograph shows an apparent elevation of the left hemidiaphragm associated with a small lateral pleural effusion. *B,* Left decubitus view: large subpulmonic pleural effusion layers along the dependent left chest wall *(arrow).*

racic fluid collection(s) (Fig. 9.9). This is especially valuable when collections are loculated or subpulmonic.

Mediastinum. Mediastinal masses such as neuroblastoma, lymphoma, bronchogenic cysts, and others may be identified with ultrasonography.

Lungs. Sonographic evaluation of pulmonary abnormalities is limited to those processes adjacent to the chest wall, diaphragm, or mediastinum.

Diaphragm. Real-time sonography may provide significant information regarding diaphragmatic movement, as well as juxtadiaphragmatic abnormalities: diaphragmatic hernia/eventration (Fig. 9.10), neoplasms and cysts, subpulmonic pleural effusion, and subphrenic abscess.

COMPUTED TOMOGRAPHY (CT)

By using multiple projections and computer calculations of radiographic density, CT can record finer differences in absorption than can be achieved with conventional radiographs. CT is used to show abnormalities identified or suspected on plain chest radiograph, particularly in the mediastinum (Fig. 9.11). Outside the mediastinum, the major use of CT is to define the size, shape, and position of a pulmonary parenchymal abnormality that cannot be completely delineated on plain radiographs (2,

3). Thin-slice, high-resolution CT techniques can demonstrate interstitial (Fig. 9.12) and cystic processes (Fig. 9.13) not well-seen with conventional CT methods.

MAGNETIC RESONANCE IMAGING (MRI)

MRI is a major tool for evaluation of cardiovascular anomalies (Fig. 9.14) and for defining the position, morphologic characteristics, and extent of mediastinal and chest wall lesions (Fig. 9.15). Major advantages of MRI include the capability of multiplanar sectional imaging (axial, coronal, sagittal, and even oblique) without the use of ionizing radiation (Figs. 9.16, 9.17) (5). The additional expense, however, makes careful consideration of efficacy an important factor in determining MRI applications in pediatric chest imaging.

Lack of spatial resolution and decreased signal from surrounding air-filled lung obviates MRI in the evaluation of most small pulmonary parenchymal lesions.

Specialized Imaging

RADIONUCLIDE SCINTIGRAPHY

Ventilation-perfusion scans represent the primary application of nuclear medicine to chest imaging. Occasionally, bone scans define the presence and extent of skeletal lesions,

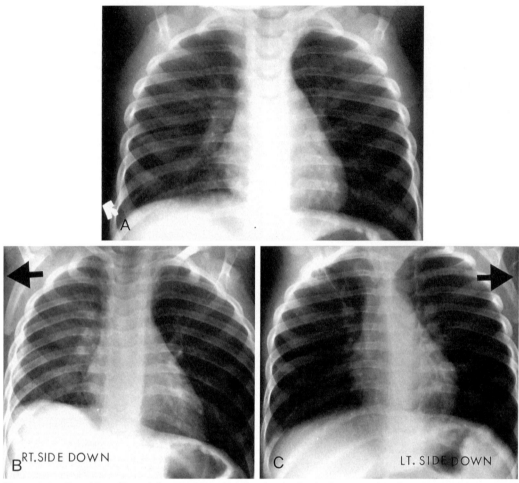

Figure 9.4. Decubitus films: left stem bronchus foreign body. A, Frontal upright film shows left lung hyper-aeration, consistent with partial obstruction to the left stem bronchus. B, On the right side down decubitus film, the dependent right lung contracts normally. C, Left side down decubitus confirms the inability of the dependent left lung to contract, thus suggesting a "ball-valve" obstruction of the left stem bronchus. *NOTE:* When expiratory films are difficult to obtain and fluoroscopy is not available, the use of decubitus films may help establish the presence of an obstructing foreign body in a stem bronchus.

although conventional radiography and CT will usually suffice. The role of gallium-67 in the evaluation of mediastinal lymphoma remains to be defined, although *single proton emission computed tomography (SPECT)* may provide additional diagnostic accuracy in defining the presence, extent, and recurrence of mediastinal lymphoma.

ANGIOGRAPHY

This technique has been of limited application in general pulmonary diagnostic imaging since the advent of ultrasonography and MRI. Current applications are limited to evaluation of suspected pulmonary arteriovenous malformations, major pulmonary anomalies requiring surgical removal, and patients with severe hemoptysis. Digital subtraction angiography has reduced both the radiation exposure and the necessity for more central vascular catheter access.

BRONCHOGRAPHY

Contrast examination of the airways is used less today than in the past but has some value in selected abnormalities, such as bronchiectasis (Fig. 9.18). Non-ionic contrast agents (metrizamide) are relatively safe and easy to use.

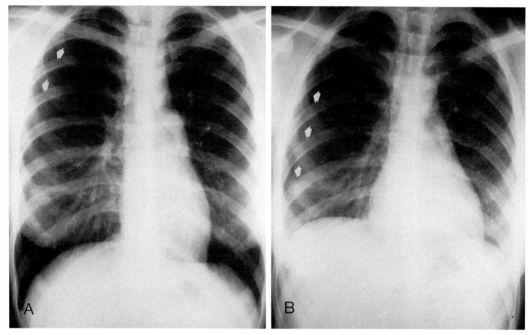

Figure 9.5. Pneumothorax. *A,* Inspiratory chest radiograph shows a small, subtle, apical, right-sided pneumothorax *(arrows)* B, Expiratory study accentuates the pneumothorax *(arrows).*

XERORADIOGRAPHY

This technique, with its high radiation dosage, has little role in the imaging of chest disease in children. Cross-sectional imaging (CT, MRI) has largely supplanted xeroradiography.

PRINCIPLES OF RADIOLOGIC INTERPRETATION AND PATTERN RECOGNITION

Radiographic Patterns

Pulmonary diseases frequently produce specific diagnostic patterns on chest radiographs. When a specific pattern can be recognized, the particular etiology or group (gamut) of etiologies may be suggested (8, 9). Although pattern recognition and gamut methods are often quite useful, certain pitfalls must be considered:

Radiographic patterns are not always typical
Similar diseases may produce different radiographic patterns
Similar radiographic patterns may be produced by different diseases

In spite of these reservations, four radiographic patterns seen in childhood lung disease will be considered in this chapter: (a) hyperinflation, (b) excess pulmonary fluid, (c) endobronchial obstruction/bronchial dilatation, and (d) major airway obstruction. These four patterns are reasonably consistent and recognizable, and may provide clues to the underlying pathologic process (10).

HYPER-INFLATION PATTERN

Terms such as diffuse hyper-aeration, hyper-inflation, over-aeration, over-expansion, and over-inflation are used interchangeably to describe enlarged lungs. Depending on the disease process at hand, the hyper-aeration may be generalized, asymmetrical, irregular, or focal. The salient radiographic features of generalized over-aeration are listed below. The first six are most useful, and the remaining three are less so:

Depressed diaphragm
Increased anteroposterior chest diameter
Narrow cardiothymic silhouette
"Elevated" or "elongated" heart
Clear retrosternal space
Present on sequential films (Fig. 9.19)
Horizontal, spread ribs
Separation of vessels
Disparity between lung size and chest size

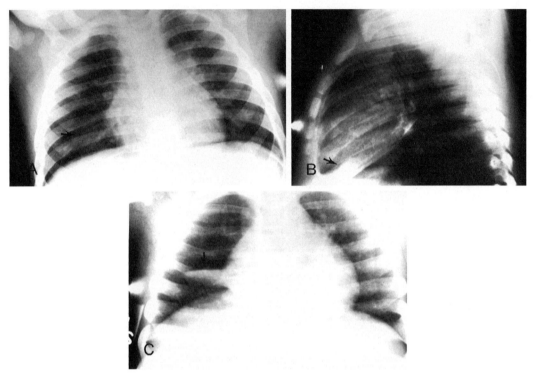

Figure 9.6.   Bronchiolitis with subtle right middle lobe atelectasis: lordotic projection *A,* Supine AP film shows a vague opacity in the right lung *(arrow),* and loss of right heart border silhouette. *B,* Lateral study reveals a radiodensity *(arrow)* in the region of the right middle lobe. *C,* Low centered lordotic projection clearly uncovers a wedge-shaped opacity *(arrow)* extending laterally from the right heart border, representing partial right middle lobe atelectasis.

In addition to the foregoing criteria, several additional factors should be considered in children with pulmonary over-aeration:

Age of patient—Radiographic over-aeration in infants and young children (under 18 months) is usually easier to identify and of greater clinical significance than in older patients

Position of patient—Infant supine chest films are often exposed in the expiratory phase because of upward pressure on the diaphragm; therefore, over-aeration on the supine chest study is a reliable indicator of air trapping and, as a corollary, an expiration film usually signifies absence of generalized lung disease (Figs. 9.1A, 9.19B) (11)

Generalized and/or Irregular Aeration (Scattered Atelectasis and Focal Over-Expansion). Such aeration is often produced by lower respiratory infections in children under 1 year of age. The following are conditions that frequently cause over-aeration:

Bronchiolitis and other diffuse peribronchial infections (Figs. 9.6, 9.20)
Aspiration (acute and chronic) (Fig. 9.21)
Asthma (Figs. 9.22, 9.23)
Cystic fibrosis (Figs. 9.13, 9.24)
Immune deficiency syndromes
Chronic infections (e.g., pertussis, chlamydia) (Figs. 9.25, 9.26)
Bronchopulmonary dysplasia (Fig. 9.27)
Others (acidosis, L-R intracardiac shunts, upper airway obstructions)

Asymmetrical Aeration. This condition may develop in the following conditions:

Unilateral "ball-valve" mechanisms (e.g., foreign body, tumor)
Focal or lobar atelectasis with compensatory emphysema
Congenital anomalies (hypoplastic lung [Fig. 9.28], lobar emphysema, adenomatoid malformation, bronchial atresia, abnormal vessels, vascular sling)

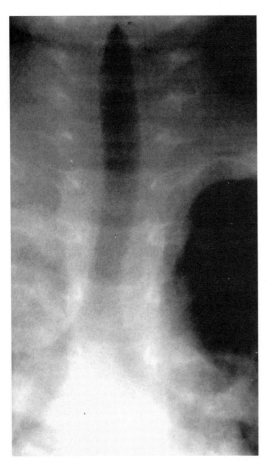

Figure 9.7. Airway—high kilovoltage—filtered. This technique allows for excellent visualization of the tracheal air column in the frontal projection.

Asymmetrical Density in Lung. This condition is caused by the following:

Absence of overlying soft tissue (e.g., Poland anomaly)
Vascular attenuation (e.g., bronchiolitis fibrosis obliterans/Swyer-James syndrome [Fig. 9.29], congenital vascular shunts)
Pleural fluid on supine chest
Intrapulmonary and extrapulmonary air (i.e., pulmonary interstitial emphysema, pneumothorax) (Fig. 9.30)

PULMONARY FLUID PATTERN

Normal lung tissue is radiolucent, except for branching, tapering vascular shadows, centrally located bronchi, and thin interlobar fissures. Excess fluid accumulation in the lung alters the appearance of these normal structures and produces a complex variety of radio-

graphic patterns (12). Several factors are responsible for these changes:

Type of fluid (transudate—edema; exudate—pus; blood; combinations)
Amount and rapidity of accumulation
Underlying etiology: cardiogenic, increased vascular permeability, overhydration, infection, trauma
Pre-existing pulmonary abnormalities: fibrosis, atelectasis, bullae
Gravitational force

In simplified anatomic terms, the lung may be divided into two compartments: (a) matrix or interstitium (vessels, lymphatics, connective tissue), and (b) air space or alveoli. Fluid may collect in these compartments and, in some cases, flow into a third compartment, the pleural space.

The radiographic pattern produced by excess fluid in any one of these three compartments rarely exists in pure form. Most frequently, rapidly changing densities are produced, which merge one into another. For the purpose of this discussion, however, the radiographic criteria of fluid in each of the three spaces (interstitial, alveolar, pleural) will be described and illustrated separately.

Interstitial Pattern. The interstitial pattern is produced when excess fluid accumulates in the lung matrix (Fig. 9.31). Interstitial fluid may produce any or all of the following changes:

Vascular unsharpness (13, 14)
swollen interlobular septa (Kerley A, B, C lines) (Fig. 9.32)
Thickened subpleural lymphatics/fissures (Fig. 9.32)
Peribronchial cuffing
Redistribution of pulmonary blood flow (14)

Comparison with previous film studies is often helpful in determining the changing nature of this fluid accumulation.

Alveolar/Air Space Pattern. The air space pattern is produced when fluid occupies the alveoli. Atelectasis or volume loss may produce a similar pattern but with some subtle differences. Alveolar/air space pattern is characterized by the following radiographic changes (8):

Fluffy, irregular margins (Figs. 9.31B, 9.33)
Coalescence (Fig. 9.34)

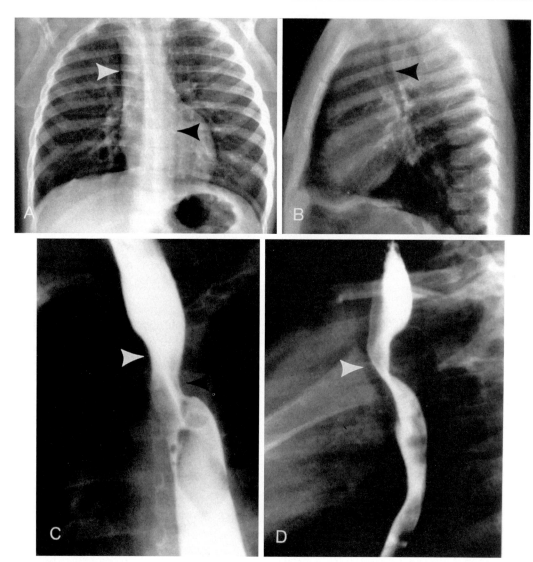

Figure 9.8. Vascular ring double aortic arch. *A,* Frontal film study shows a right-sided aortic arch *(white arrow),* but left-sided descending aorta *(black arrow). B,* Lateral view confirms anterior displacement of trachea *(arrow),* probably from a posterior aortic arch and suggestive of a vascular ring *C,* A-P projection of barium-filled esophagus confirms the presence of an indentation from a superiorly placed right arch *(white arrow)* but also shows a more caudally placed left arch indentation *(black arrow) D,* Lateral view shows large posterior indentation in the barium-filled esophagus. Note the narrowed tracheal air column *(arrow).*

Segmental and/or lobar distribution, often producing a sharply defined margin along a fissure (Fig. 9.35)

Occasional spherical or round configuration (Fig. 9.36)

Air bronchograms or alveolograms

Butterfly shadow; characteristic of pulmonary edema

Rapid timing

Two major categories of disease that cause the *alveolar* pattern are pulmonary edema and pneumonia. These two general disease processes will be considered independently, although they overlap considerably in their radiographic expressions.

Pulmonary Edema (PE). The excess lung fluid of PE may occupy the interstitium (lymphatics and perivascular space), the alveoli, and/or the pleural space. Thus, the radiographic features of PE will depend on the location of the fluid relative to these anatomic areas. Existing pathologic state of the lung,

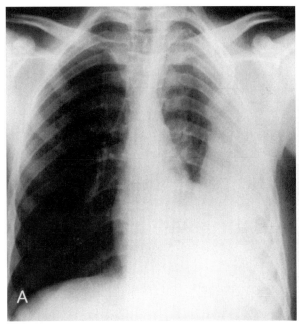
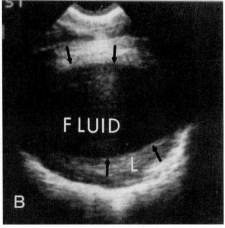

Figure 9.9. Pleural effusion—ultrasonography. *A,* Frontal chest study is strongly suggestive of a loculated left pleural collection. The homogeneous, left thoracic process has a well-defined convex border and obliterates the left hemidiaphragm and costophrenic sulcus. *B,* The ultrasound study over the left chest density confirms the presence of a loculated fluid collection *(arrows). The lung (L)* is compressed against the chest wall.

position in which the patient has been placed, and rapidity of accumulation are additional factors that may alter the radiographic appearance of PE.

By the very nature of the pathophysiologic process, pulmonary edema tends to be transient and evanescent. In addition, considerable overlap is to be expected in its clinicoradiologic presentation. Also, it is important to recognize at the outset that substances other than edema fluid (i.e., blood, purulence, and tumor) may, and often do, produce radiographic patterns indistinguishable from that of pulmonary edema.

There are two major groups of disease associated with pulmonary edema:

Cardiac—congestive failure (14)
Noncardiac—renal disease (chronic and acute), fluid overload, neurogenic, near drowning (Fig. 9.33), mechanical (croup [Fig. 9.37], epiglottitis, chronic airway obstruction), and drug ingestion

Pneumonia. Pneumonia is defined in pathologic terms as pulmonary inflammation. When the inflammatory reaction of pneumonia evokes the production of fluid (edema, pus,

blood), and this fluid occupies sufficient numbers of contiguous alveoli, the air space pattern is produced. Etiologic agent, patient age, host defense mechanisms, and other known and unknown factors all contribute to the radiographic manifestations of air space pneumonia. Some infections congregate into confluent segmental and/or lobar consolidations (Figs. 9.34, 9.35), whereas others disperse throughout the lungs, producing disseminated, patchy opacities (Fig. 9.31).

Rounded, separate, ill-defined opacities with rapid coalition and occasional cavitations, pleural effusions, and/or pneumothorax are characteristic of septic pulmonary emboli (Fig. 9.34). A spherical or round configuration proceeding in centrifugal fashion without relation to collateral air channels is yet another variation of pneumonic consolidation (Fig. 9.36).

In contrast to the over-aeration pattern of pneumonia, which usually results from viral infections (11) (see "Bronchiolitis"), consolidated or diffuse air space infections are generally, but not always, of bacterial origin. Pleural effusion, pneumothorax, and pneumatocele production suggest the presence of more

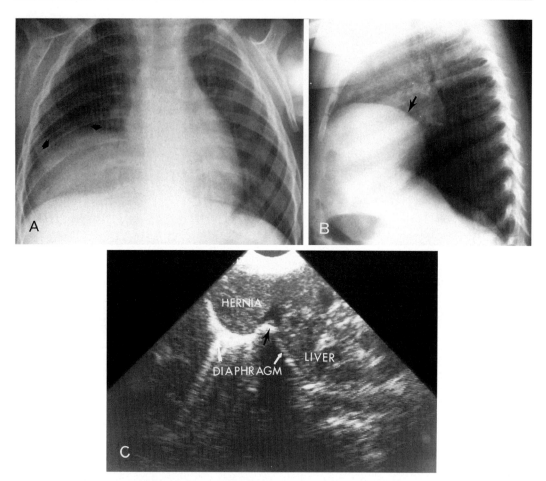

Figure 9.10. Anteromedial diaphragmatic defect *A,* A right cardiophrenic mass *(arrow)* displaces the heart to the left. *B,* The lateral view shows focal elevation of the diaphragm anteriorly *(arrow),* well above the posterior diaphragmatic margin. *C,* Longitudinal ultrasonography confirms focal herniation of the liver through an anterior medial diaphragmatic defect *(black arrow).*

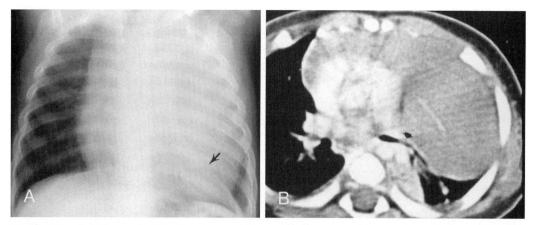

Figure 9.11. Anterior mediastinal lymphoma. *A,* The cardiomediastinal silhouette is enlarged to the left; there is left lower lobe atelectasis *(arrow). B,* Chest CT with intravenous contrast shows a large anterior mediastinal mass compressing the left bronchus *(arrow).*

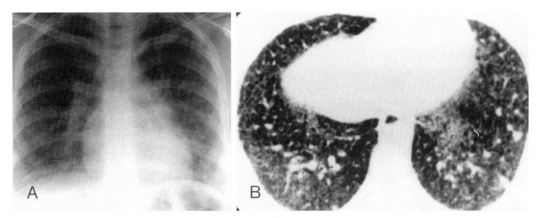

Figure 9.12. Fibrosing alveolitis/idiopathic pulmonary fibrosis. *A,* Chest radiograph shows a diffuse, fine reticular pattern, most prominent at the lung bases. *B,* High-resolution, thin slice chest CT discloses a generalized pattern of irregular linear opacities most evident in the subpleural lung regions with relative sparing of the central lung zones.

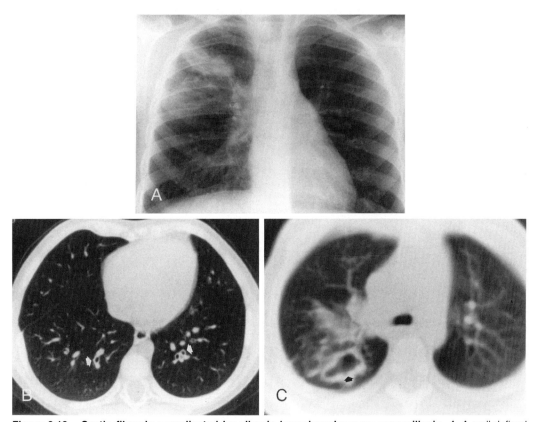

Figure 9.13. Cystic fibrosis complicated by allergic bronchopulmonary aspergillosis. *A,* A well-defined density with adjacent irregular cystic lucencies is present in the right upper lobe. The lower lobes appear normal. *B,* Chest CT of the right upper lobe contains a cavity *(arrow)* adjacent to focal consolidation. *C,* A scan centered lower in the chest shows mild bronchiectasis *(arrows).*

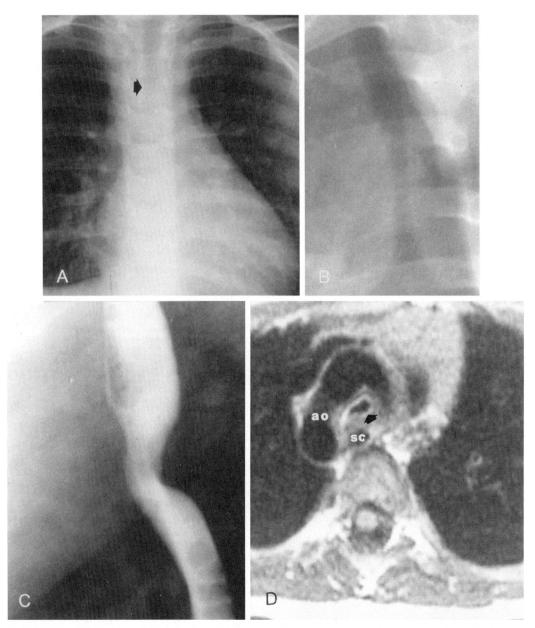

Figure 9.14. Vascular ring (right aortic arch, aberrant left subclavian artery). *A,* Chest radiograph shows a subtle impression on the trachea *(arrow)* by a right-sided aortic arch. The aorta descends on the right. *B,* On oblique fluoroscopic spot film, the tracheal impression is more obvious. *C,* Barium esophagram reveals an oblique posterior impression on the esophagus, caused by an aberrant left subclavian artery. *D,* T1-weighted axial MRI shows marked tracheal compression *(arrow)* between the right aortic arch *(ao)* and the aberrant left subclavian artery *(sc).*

virulent organisms. Less common, but of increasing importance in immunocompromised hosts, are infections and infiltrations caused by protozoa (Pneumocystis) (Fig. 9.38), rickettsia, fungi tuberculosis, and other less ubiquitous agents.

In selected patients, the characteristic radiographic pattern of pneumonia may be caused by other, non-infectious processes. Among these are hemorrhage (Fig. 9.39), contusion, atelectasis (Fig. 9.40), irritants, alveolar proteinosis, pulmonary vasculitides (e.g.,

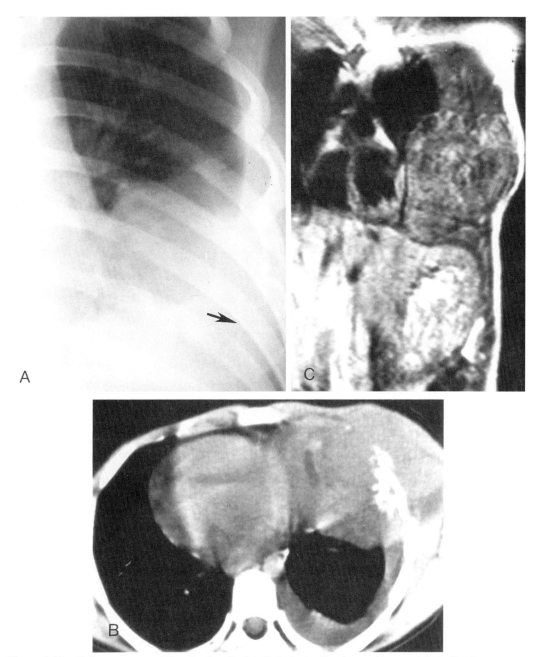

Figure 9.15. **Ewing sarcoma of the chest wall.** *A,* Left rib destruction *(arrows)* is associated with a large mass. *B,* Chest CT shows this to be a large intrathoracic and extrathoracic mass surrounding the expansile rib tumor. *C,* On coronal MRI, the bulky tumor abuts but does not invade the pericardial sac.

Wegener syndrome), sequestration, and many others.

Extrapulmonary lesions to be differentiated from pneumonia include tumors of the lung, chest wall, mediastinum, and paraspinal region (Fig. 9.17).

Pleural Fluid Pattern. Pleural fluid collections produce characteristic radiographic configurations (15). When subpulmonic, they may be difficult to identify or overlooked completely. Ultrasonography is a convenient tool for evaluation of pleural effusion, especially

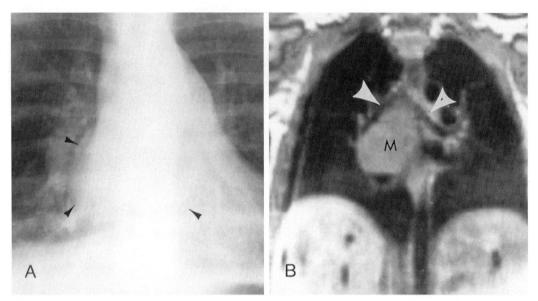

Figure 9.16.   Bronchogenic cyst. *A,* A round, soft tissue mass displaces and narrows the right lower lobe bronchus (arrow heads). *B,* T1-weighted MRI in coronal plane: a subcarinal soft tissue mass *(M)* displaces the right main and lower lobe bronchi *(arrowheads).* T2-weighted images confirmed the cystic nature of the lesion.

adjacent to the chest wall or in relation to the diaphragm (Fig. 9.9). CT may occasionally be useful in delineating the character and extent of pleural fluid collection (Fig. 9.41).

ENDOBRONCHIAL PATTERN (BRONCHIECTASIS)

In children, as in adults, certain pulmonary diseases produce pathologic processes that primarily affect the tracheobronchial tree. Inflammation and infection lead to mucosal edema, increased secretions, destruction of bronchial endothelium, dilation of bronchial lumina, and peribronchial inflammatory reaction.

Bronchiectasis may occur (a) following pulmonary inflammation (Figs. 9.18, 9.29), obstruction, edema, or other conditions, or (b) in association with immune deficiency syndrome, dysmotility cilia syndrome, cystic fibrosis, and related conditions (Fig. 9.24).

Pathologic alterations characterized by thickened and distorted bronchial walls, mucous-plugged lumina, and volume loss are responsible for the following radiographic pattern of bronchiectasis:

Ringlike densities with clear centers representing thick-walled bronchi seen on end

White, rounded, sometimes branching densities produced by mucopurulent material in the bronchial lumina

Parallel lines (railroad tracks) representing thick-walled bronchi seen from the side; these often branch and may contain plugs of mucous (gloved hand sign)

Irregular, ill-defined, distorted vascular markings adjacent to diseased bronchi

Unequal aeration with areas of focal atelectasis and/or emphysema resulting from either partial or complete bronchial obstruction

Well-exposed chest films usually demonstrate many of these features (16). If the films are taken at a time when bronchi are plugged with mucus, they appear as round, elongated, or sometimes branching (gloved hand) opacities. A study of sequential films will often show intermittent bronchial plugging; unplugged, thick-walled bronchi frequently simulate "railroad tracks." In many cases, old studies must be evaluated if subtle changes are to be appreciated. When only the most recent films are used for comparison, minor changes of bronchiectasis may be overlooked. Old film studies may also disclose an area of pre-existing pneumonia.

Although well-exposed plain films may arouse suspicion of the presence of bronchiec-

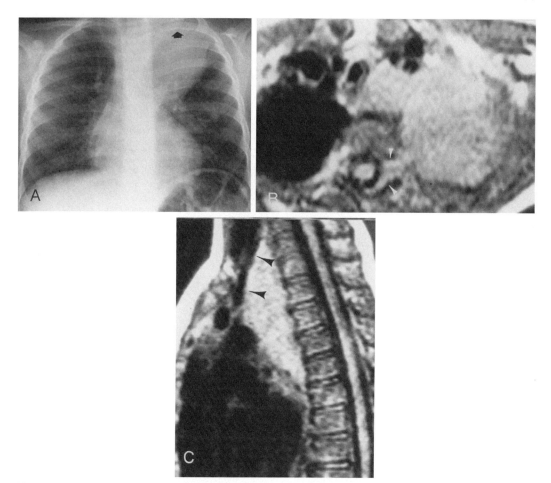

Figure 9.17.   Mediastinal ganglioneuroblastoma. *A,* Chest radiograph shows erosive scalloping of the inferior margin of the left third rib *(arrow)* with widening of the intercostal space. A soft tissue mass occupies much of the left upper hemithorax, and the trachea is deviated to the right. *B,* MRI, axial: the tumor extends into the spinal canal *(arrowheads). C,* On the sagittal view, the tumor also displaces the trachea anteriorly and causes minimal compression *(arrowheads).*

tasis, special imaging procedures are usually needed to confirm the diagnosis, delineate the extent of disease, and assess the condition of the remaining lungs. The following modalities are available:

1. Positive contrast bronchography (16)
2. Computed tomography (high-resolution CT): This method is most sensitive for the cystic type but is not as specific as bronchography (Fig. 9.13)
3. Radionuclide scintigraphy: Lung perfusion scintigraphy with ^{99m}Tc has been advocated in the evaluation of bronchiectasis, since bronchiectatic areas of lung will retain this radionuclide

MAJOR AIRWAY OBSTRUCTION

Radiographic evaluation will often define the nature and location of airway obstruction, but close clinicoradiologic correlation is of extreme importance in arriving at a proper plan of therapy. When radiographic evaluation is needed, care must be exercised during transport of these children to the radiographic department, and close monitoring is essential during the examinations. Portable studies may be obtained for critically ill children. A radiologist should be on hand to tailor and monitor all film studies (Fig. 9.42).

A large arsenal of imaging modalities is available and well-suited for evaluation of the

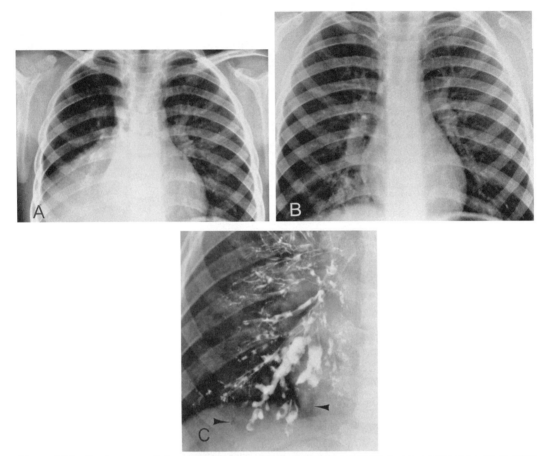

Figure 9.18.   Postpneumonic bronchiectasis. *A,* Right lower lobe consolidated pneumonia is present. *B,* After approximately 1 year, a persistent pattern of irregular alternating densities and lucencies is present in the medial segments of the right lower lobe. *C,* Contrast bronchography confirms the presence of irregularly dilated, tortuous bronchi containing excess secretions. Negative air bronchograms are visible beyond the filled bronchial lumina *(arrows).*

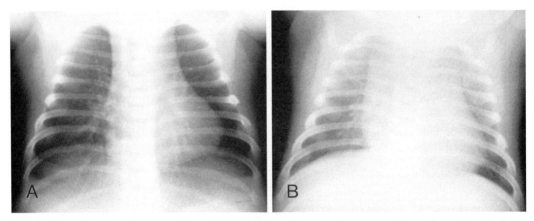

Figure 9.19.   Spurious hyper-aeration. *A,* This exposure demonstrates many of the radiographic criteria for hyper-aeration; depressed diaphragm, narrow cardiothymic silhouette, "elevated" heart, horizontal ribs. These changes, however, are the result of fortuitous exposure during deep inspiration. *B,* Film taken several minutes later is normally aerated.

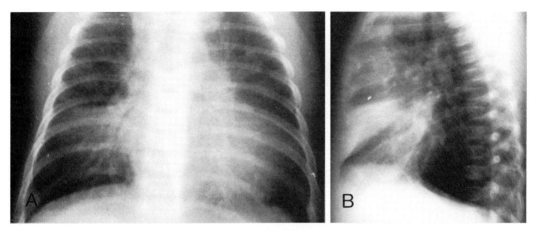

Figure 9.20. Bronchiolitis, *A, B,* Generalized over-aeration is apparent on the frontal and lateral film studies. Volume loss is evident in the right middle lobe and possibly the lingula.

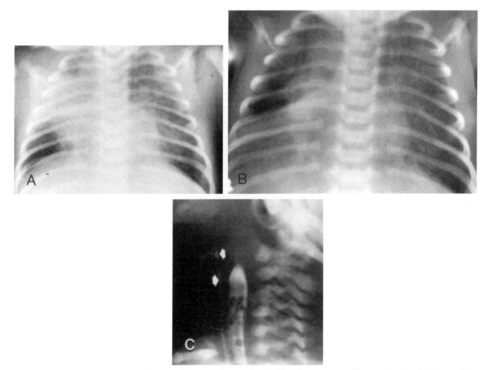

Figure 9.21. Chronic aspiration with shifting atelectasis. *A,* The lungs are diffusely involved with coalescent opacities in the right upper lobe and patchy infiltrates on the left. *B,* Five days later the right middle lobe and right lower lobe are consolidated and/or collapsed. *C,* Barium swallow shows aspiration of contrast into the trachea *(arrows).*

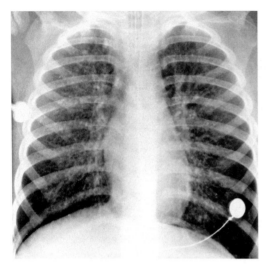

Figure 9.22. Asthma with diffuse lung disease. The lungs are generally over-aerated, although the patient is on a respirator. The normal vascular shadows are obliterated by diffuse, abnormal markings, some of which may represent thickened bronchial walls.

Fluoroscopy (Video Tape). Because of the marked malleability of the supporting soft tissues of the pediatric pharynx and hypopharynx, plain films may be confusing and inconclusive. Fluoroscopy in these circumstances is often definitive (Fig. 9.44). When airway obstruction occurs during sleep, sleeping video fluoroscopy is needed to show the nature of the obstruction process.

Contrast Swallow and Esophagram. These studies are readily available and often help define the anatomy and physiology of the pharynx and esophagus. Tracheal aspiration (Fig. 9.21C), congenital abnormalities, and fistulae, as well as vascular constrictions, are best evaluated by this method (Figs. 9.8, 9.14).

Computed Tomography. This study is not useful in most acute situations but is of value in the determination of (a) choanal atresia, (b) tracheal lumen and anatomy (Fig. 9.45) (17), and (c) mediastinal masses (18).

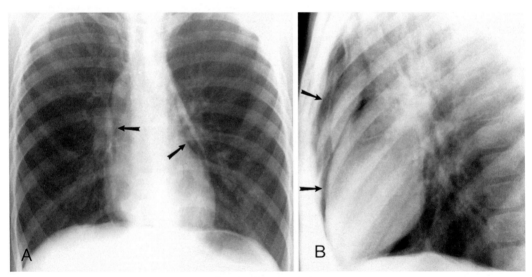

Figure 9.23. Asthma with pneumomediastinum. *A,* The frontal film shows over-aerated but clear lungs. Air *(arrows)* has dissected from lung into the mediastinum. *B,* The pneumomediastinum is represented by free air (arrows) in the retrosternal soft tissues.

nasopharynx and laryngotracheobronchial tree. The choice of methods and sequence of performance will depend on parochial expertise and the clinical circumstances.

AP and Lateral Plain Films of the Airway. Films of the airway should include the pharynx as well as the laryngotracheal air column. Except in rare instances, the frontal projection should be obtained, as well as lateral projection (Figs. 9.7, 9.42, 9.43) (7).

Magnetic Resonance Imaging. This technique is also useful for the delineation of masses and aberrant vascular structures that may impinge on the tracheobronchial air column (Figs 9.14, 9.17D) (5).

REFERENCES

1. Kirks DR, Fram EK, Vock P, Effman EL. Tracheal compression by mediastinal masses in children: CT evaluation. *AJR* 1983; 141:647–651.

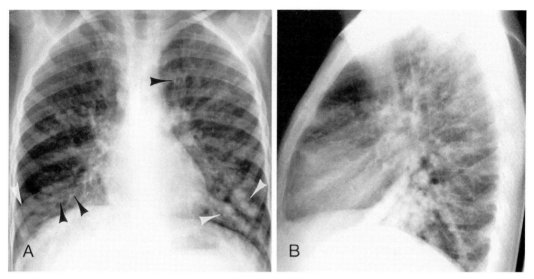

Figure 9.24. Cystic fibrosis—generalized bronchiectasis. *A,* The lungs are involved with a diffuse pattern representing abnormal bronchi. Some of these are air-bearing and thick-walled (black arrows), whereas others are mucous-plugged (white arrows). *B,* Similar changes are apparent on the lateral film. In spite of the extensive involvement, there is minimal over-aeration.

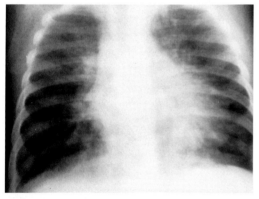

Figure 9.25. Pertussis. The lungs are over-aerated and contain diffuse, patchy, mostly paracardiac opacities. This appearance is also seen in many other lung diseases.

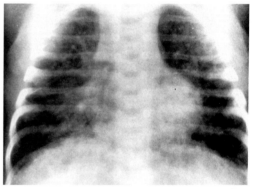

Figure 9.26. Chlamydia. This pattern of generalized over-aeration and scattered, mostly central, patchy opacities is characteristic of chlamydia pneumonia but is also produced by many other etiologic agents.

2. Muller NL, Miller RR. State of the art: Computed tomography of chronic diffuse infiltrative lung disease. Part 1. *Am Rev Respir Dis* 1990; 142:1206–1220.
3. Muller NL, Miller RR. State of the art: Computed tomography of chronic diffuse infiltrative lung disease. Part 2. *Am Rev Respir Dis* 1990; 142:1440–1450.
4. Bissett GS III. Pediatric thoracic applications of magnetic resonance imaging. *J Thorac Imaging* 1989; 4:51–57.
5. Siegel MJ, Molina PL. Respiratory system. In Cohen MD, Edwards MK, eds. *Magnetic resonance imaging of children.* Philadelphia, BC Decker 1990, pp 585–609.
6. Capitanio MA, Kirkpatrick JA Jr. The lateral decubitus film. An aid in determining air-trapping in children. *Radiology* 1972; 103:460–462.

7. Joseph DM, Berdon WE, Baker DH, Slovis TL, Haller JO. Airway obstruction in infants and children. *Radiology* 1976; 121:143–148.
8. Felson B. The roentgen diagnosis of disseminated pulmonary alveolar diseases. *Semin Roentgenol* 1967; 2:3–21.
9. Felson B. A new look at pattern recognition of diffuse pulmonary disease. *Am J Roentgenol* 1979; 133:183–189.
10. Felman AH. *Radiology of the pediatric chest; Clinical and pathological correlations* New York, McGraw Hill, 1987, p 201.
11. Griscom NT, Wohl MEB, Kirkpatrick JA Jr. Lower respiratory infections: How infants differ from adults. *Radiol Clin North Am* 1978; 16:367–387.

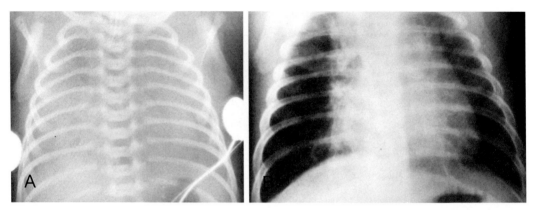

Figure 9.27. Hyaline membrane disease/bronchopulmonary dysplasia. *A,* A diffuse pulmonary opacity is produced by generalized atelectasis, characteristic of hyaline membrane disease. *B,* Three months later, generalized over-aeration and irregular diffuse parenchymal opacities represent chronic lung disease. *NOTE:* The appearance of *B* is remarkably similar to that of Figures 9.20, 9.21, 9.25, and 9.26, emphasizing the necessity for review of previous film studies.

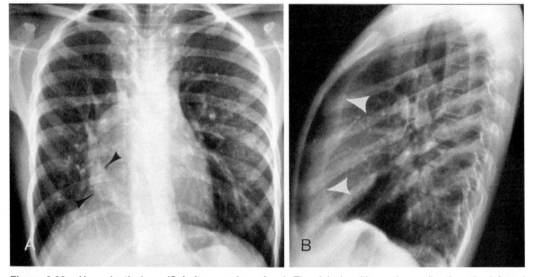

Figure 9.28. Hypoplastic lung (Scimitar syndrome). *A,* The right hemithorax is smaller than the left and contains a well-defined, curved shadow *(arrows)* in the lower medial sector. This shadow represents a pulmonary vein, resembling a "scimitar", that drains abnormally into the right atrium. *B,* The lateral study reveals an anterior chest opacity with well-defined, concave posterior border *(arrows).* This density probably represents areolar tissues interposed between the hypoplastic lung and anterior chest wall.

12. Milne ENC, Pistolesi M, Miniati M, Giuntini C. The radiologic distinction of cardiogenic and non-cardiogenic edema. *Am J Roentgenol* 1985; 144:879–894.

13. Johnson TH Jr, Gajaraj A, Feist JH. Vascular key to diagnosis of pulmonary interstitial disease. *Am J Roentgenol* 1971; 113:518–521.

14. Simon M. The pulmonary vessels: Their hemodynamic evaluation using routine radiographs. *Radiol Clin North Am* 1963; 1:363–376.

15. Fleischner FG. Atypical arrangement of free pleural effusion. *Radiol Clin North Am* 1963; 1:347–362.

16. Robinson AE, Campbell JB. Bronchography in childhood asthma. *Am J Roentgenol* 1972; 116:559–566.

17. Griscom NT. CT measurement of the tracheal lumen in children and adolescents. *AJR* 1991; 156:371–372.

18. Brown D, Magill HL, George P, Young LW. Tracheobronchial compression by thoracic neuroblastoma. *Am J Dis Child* 1986; 140:1171–1173.

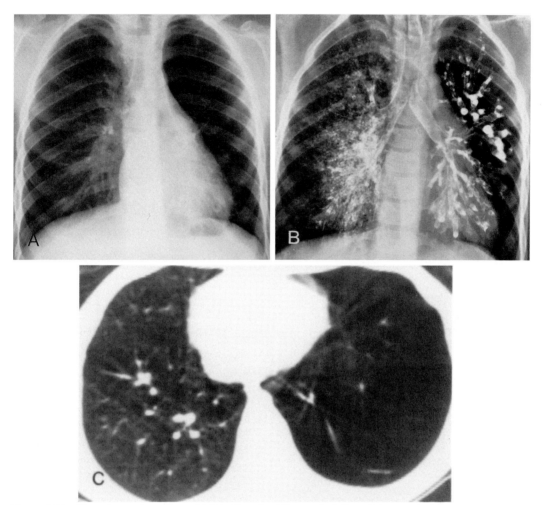

Figure 9.29. Hyperlucent lung (bronchiolitis fibrosis obliterans). *A,* Frontal chest study demonstrates hyperlucency of the left hemithorax resulting from attenuated vascular structures. *B,* Contrast bronchogram shows typical changes of bronchiolitis fibrosis obliterans on the left. The lumina are essentially obliterated at the bronchiolar level with secondary dilatation of the proximal radicals. Pulmonary vessels, adjacent to the bronchi, are similarly attenuated by this pathologic process. *C,* CT of different patient with same disease shows attenuated vascular supply to left lung compared to normal right pulmonary vessels.

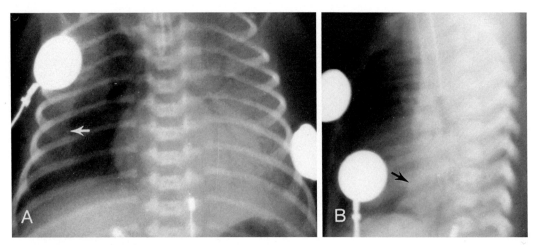

Figure 9.30.   Anterior-medial pneumothorax. *A,* Free air, located in the right hemithorax, produces a picture of increased lucency, defined by the anterior-medial lung edge *(arrow)* and sharply marginated right heart border. *B,* Lateral study in supine position confirms the anterior air collection and the posteriorly compressed lung *(arrow).*

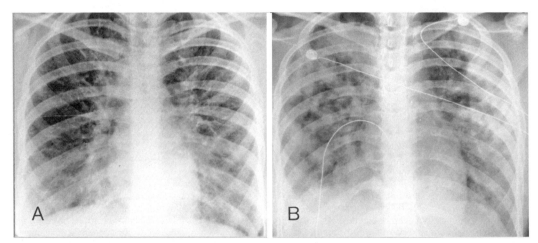

Figure 9.31.   Mycoplasma pneumonia. *A,* The initial film is characterized by diffuse, small, randomly placed linear densities. The normal, well-defined, vascular shadows are obliterated by interstitial pulmonary fluid. *B,* During the next 24 hours, the inflammatory process has extended to random air spaces and produced a disseminated alveolar pattern.

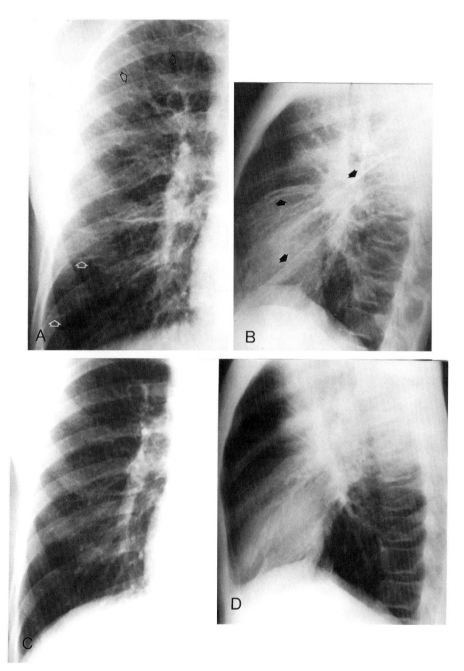

Figure 9.32. Interstitial edema. *A,* The diffuse, random, linear densities (Kerley lines) are produced by excess liquid filling the interlobular septa. Kerley B lines *(white arrows)* are located in the inferolateral segments of the lung. Kerley A lines *(black arrows)* are visible in the upper lungs. *B,* Lateral projection corresponding to *A* shows thickened fissures *(arrows)* as well as diffuse swollen interstitial septa. *C,* Several days later, the lungs have returned to normal. *D,* Follow-up lateral view, corresponding to *B,* continues to demonstrate indistinct hila, but the thickened fissure shadows are absent.

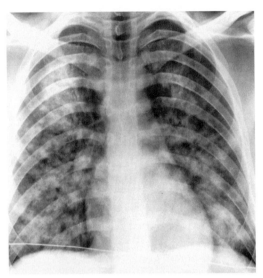

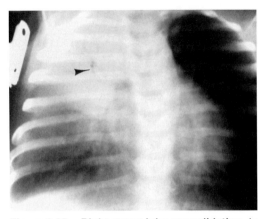

Figure 9.35.   Right upper lobe consolidation. In spite of the supine position, the lungs are over-aerated, a sign almost always associated with air trapping and diffuse pulmonary disease (see over-aeration pattern). In addition, there is a right upper lobe density that contains negative air bronchogram *(arrow),* thus identifying it as parenchymal rather than thymus (see air-space pattern).

Figure 9.33.   Near drowning. This film shows a typical disseminated alveolar (air-space) pattern. Patchy, fluffy, "cloud-like" opacities are scattered throughout the lung.

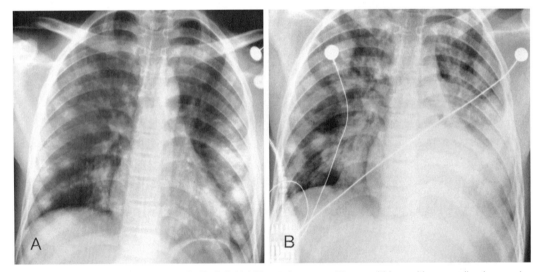

Figure 9.34.   Septic pulmonary emboli. *A,* Initial films taken on a 15-year-old boy with generalized muscular trauma shows multiple rounded, ill-defined opacities scattered throughout the lung, representing septic emboli. *B,* After 6 hours, these emboli have begun to coalesce into areas of consolidation, most evident in the left lower lobe. This child died after 1 week of intensive therapy.

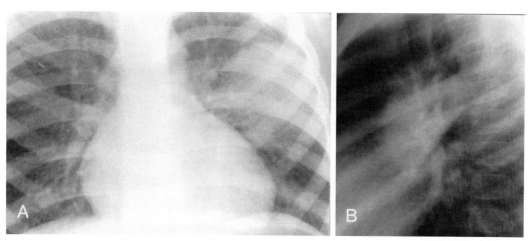

Figure 9.36.   Round pneumonia. *A,* A well-defined spherical opacity is present in the left mid-lung zone. *B,* On the lateral view, this consolidation abuts the major fissure and is hemispherical.

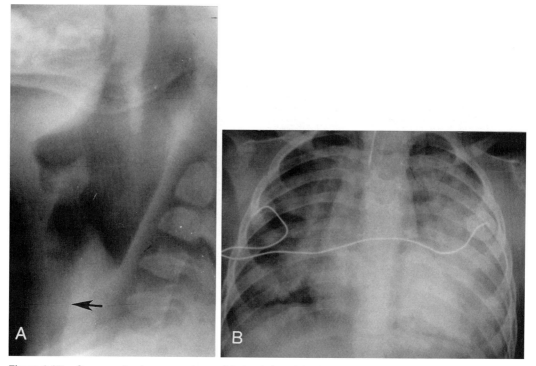

Figure 9.37.   Croup and pulmonary edema. *A,* Lateral view of the pharyngolaryngeal area shows typical changes of croup; dilated hypopharynx, edematous subglottis *(arrow),* and narrowed subglottic trachea. *B,* Generalized alveolar density represents pulmonary edema.

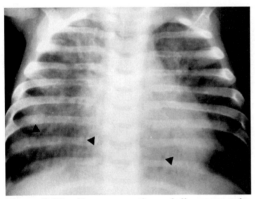

Figure 9.38.   Pneumocystis carinii pneumonia. Respiratory symptoms developed in this immunocompromised child. A chest film shows generalized confluence with numerous air bronchograms *(arrows)* and obscuration of the right heart border. Film 1 month before was normal.

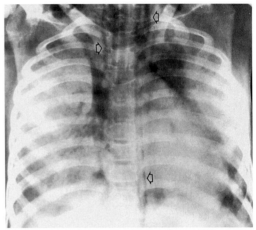

Figure 9.39.   Pulmonary hemorrhage. This patient has disseminated alveolar opacities secondary to chronic renal disease and pulmonary hemorrhage. The linear, central radiolucencies (arrows) represent extravasated mediastinal air associated with assisted respiration.

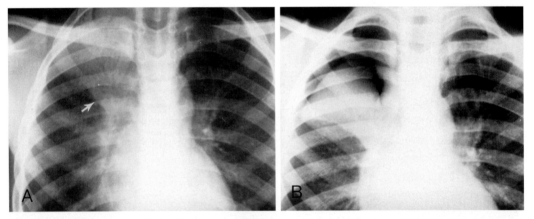

Figure 9.40.   Atelectasis with localized pneumothorax. *A,* Initial chest film in an asthmatic child shows right upper lobe volume loss characterized by air bronchograms and elevation of the horizontal fissure *(arrow). B,* As the lobe contracts, a localized pneumothorax has accumulated in the apical region. The pneumothorax disappeared several days later with re-expansion of the lung.

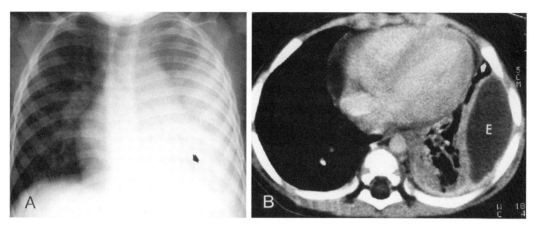

Figure 9.41. **Empyema.** *A,* Chest radiograph shows a large left-sided pleural effusion with opacification of the left lower lobe and scattered air bronchograms *(arrows). B,* Chest CT with intravenous contrast enhancement confirms the presence of a loculated pleural effusion *(E)* and adjacent left lower lobe atelectasis. There is also a small pericardial effusion *(arrow).*

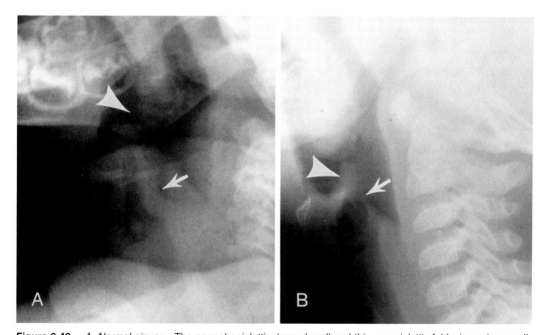

Figure 9.42. *A, Normal airway*—The normal epiglottis *(arrowhead)* and thin aryepiglottic folds *(arrow)* are well-visualized. The retropharyngeal soft tissue is of normal thickness and lies flat along the vertebral bodies. *B, Epiglottitis*—The epiglottis *(arrowhead)* is markedly enlarged and rounded; the aryepiglottic folds *(arrow)* are thickened. *NOTE:* This film is not well-exposed and must be "bright-lighted" for complete interpretation. Nevertheless, it is *diagnostic* of epiglottitis, and the patient's condition should not be compromised by having it repeated.

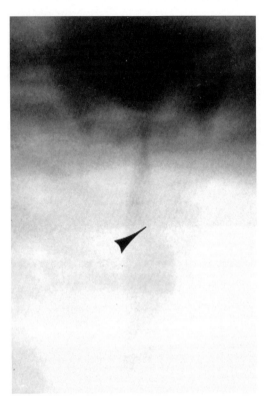

Figure 9.43.   Subglottic hemangioma. Frontal airway film shows an ovoid mass *(arrow)* protruding into the tracheal air column just below the larynx.

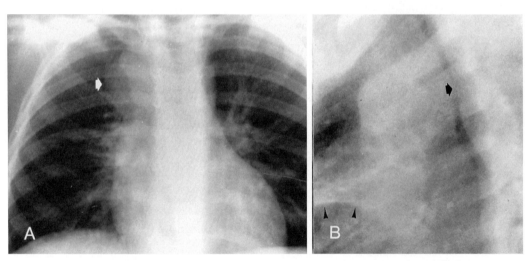

Figure 9.44.   Primary tuberculosis. *A,* Chest radiograph shows widening of the superior mediastinum to the right *(arrow). B,* Oblique fluoroscopic spot film reveals marked tracheal narrowing by enlarged paratracheal nodes *(arrows). A right upper lobe infiltrate extends anteriorly (arrowheads).*

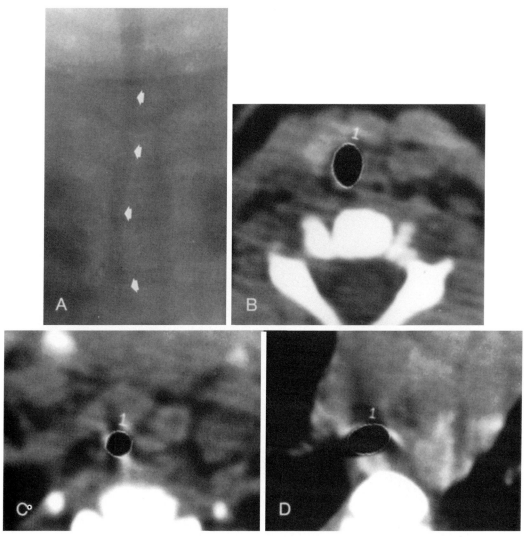

Figure 9.45. Congenital tracheal stenosis. *A,* A high-kilovoltage filtered chest radiograph shows tracheal stenosis extending from the thoracic inlet to just above the carina *(arrows)*. *B–D,* Tracheal CT at the cervical, upper thoracic, and carinal levels provides accurate definition and measurement of the degree and extent of tracheal stenosis.

10

Bronchoscopy

ROBERT E. WOOD

Bronchoscopy, the visual examination of the airways of a child from within, is an important diagnostic and therapeutic tool. A bronchoscope is used to visualize the airway structure and to study the dynamics of the larger airways. The appearance of the airway mucosa gives evidence of certain pathologic processes, whereas sampling of tissue (by biopsy or brushing) or secretions (by direct aspiration or washing) can lead to specific diagnosis. A bronchoscope can be used to restore airway patency by removing a foreign body, thick secretions, or tissue masses. In certain situations, the bronchoscope can be used to deliver therapeutic agents to the lower airways.

Bronchoscopy is not a simple procedure, and it must only be performed by physicians and assistants who are well trained and skilled in manipulating the bronchoscope and supporting the child. The necessary instruments and accessories must be readily available. Needless to say, bronchoscopy should only be performed when it is the best way to obtain the necessary information or clinical outcome.

INSTRUMENTATION

The original bronchoscopes were rigid metal tubes, passed through the mouth. During the past decade, flexible instruments suitable for use in infants and children have been developed.

Both types of instuments are necessary for full diagnostic and therapeutic capability. In general, for most therapeutic purposes, rigid bronchoscopy is the method of choice; for most diagnostic purposes, flexible bronchoscopy is preferred (Table 10.1). However, each instrument has advantages and disadvantages that influence its use (Table 10.2).

Rigid bronchoscopes have a much larger diameter than flexible instruments and can be used to view the orifices of the lobar and segmental bronchi. Visualization of more distal structures is limited in pediatric patients because of airway size and branching. Rigid bronchoscopes have some advantages in certain circumstances, such as the extraction of foreign bodies. The bronchoscope doubles as an endotracheal tube during the procedure, thus establishing and maintaining control of the airway and facilitating the delivery of oxygen and anesthetic gases. This fact, and the relatively large diameter that permits passage of ancillary instruments, are the major advantages of rigid bronchoscopes.

Rigid bronchoscopes are passed through the patient's mouth. This means that the bronchoscopist must be able to open the patient's mouth and extend the neck to provide a straight pathway. This has important implications in some patients, such as those with mandibular hypoplasia or cervical anklyosis, in whom rigid endoscopy may be difficult or impossible. Furthermore, certain mechanical forces must be applied to the airway and surrounding tissues. This may distort the anatomy somewhat, and care must be taken to ensure that the view obtained is correctly interpreted. In some circumstances, the instrument may be inserted through a tracheostomy incision. General anesthesia is required for rigid bronchoscopy.

The optics of a rigid bronchoscope make visualization of the airway anatomy beyond the tip of the bronchoscope very difficult. Fortunately, however, glass-rod telescopes can be used with rigid instruments, and these provide an image of extremely high quality. The telescopes do partially obstruct the airway, and

Table 10.1.
Indications for Bronchoscopy in Children

Indication	Preferred Technique	
	Flexible	Rigid
Stridor	X	May be needed
Persistent wheezing	X	
Chronic/recurrent infiltrates	X	
Abnormal airway radiographs	X	
Chronic/recurrent atelectasis	X	May be needed
Chronic cough	X	
Hemoptysis	X	May be needed
Foreign body aspiration:		
Suspected—no history	X	May be needed
High risk based on history, chest radiograph		X
Pulmonary TB with abnormal radiograph	X	
Vocal cord dysfunction	X	May be needed
Hospitalized patients		
Pulmonary toilet for debilitated patients	X	
Facilitate intubation	X	
Evaluate patient who fails extubation	X	
Pneumonia in immune-compromised host	X	
Management of artificial airway	X	
Endobronchial mass	May be useful	X
Bronchial stenosis	May be useful	X

must be removed temporarily in order to insert certain other instruments, and to ventilate very small children. In general, a rigid bronchoscope with a glass rod telescope provides the best possible view of the airways. Rigid instruments, inserted through the mouth, afford an excellent view of the posterior aspect of the glottis and trachea. In order to view the anterior aspect of the larynx and upper trachea, it may be necessary to employ an angulated telescope. Flexible instruments, inserted through the nose, approach the glottis from its posterior aspect, and the tip must be angulated forward to reach the glottis. Thus the view of the anterior portions of the glottis and upper trachea is excellent, although it may be more difficult to see the details of the posterior aspect of the glottis and trachea with a flexible bronchoscope. Need for a detailed examination of the posterior aspect of the larynx and upper trachea is a good indication for use of rigid instruments. Examples include the search for an "H-type" tracheoesophageal fistula or a laryngoesophageal cleft. Patients with bilateral vocal cord paralysis may also require examination with a rigid instrument, so that the cords can be passively abducted under direct vision.

Flexible instruments, although much smaller (the standard pediatric flexible bronchoscope is approximately 3.6 mm in diameter), are solid. The patient must breathe around them. Because they are flexible, they can be directed into airways that are inaccessible to rigid instruments, and their smaller diameter gives them greater peripheral range. Flexible instruments of appropriate size can be advanced under some circumstances into the 10th to 14th generation airways (although it is rarely important to do so in pediatric patients). Guidelines for the use of flexible bronchoscopy in children have been published by the American Thoracic Society (1).

Flexible bronchoscopes are almost always passed through the patient's nose (or through an endotracheal or tracheostomy tube). This means that the head and neck do not need to be extended; nor does the mouth need to be opened. The dynamics of the airway can thus be observed under relatively more physiologic conditions than with a rigid instrument. A major potential limitation, however, is that because the flexible instruments are solid, they must be sufficiently small to allow the patient to breathe around them. Furthermore, the patient must breathe spontaneously through-

Table 10.2.
Bronchoscopy Instrumentation

Rigid bronchoscope

Advantages:

Patient can be ventilated
Superior optics using telescope
Required for extraction of foreign bodies
Superior for evaluating posterior aspect of
subglottic space and upper trachea

Disadvantages:

Larger diameter
Requires general anesthesia and positive
pressure ventilation
Requires neck hyperextension and ability to
open mouth widely
Inadequate for evaluating dynamic airway
changes

Flexible bronchoscope

Advantages:

Smaller sizes
Improves visualization of upper lobes
Improves access to peripheral airways
Allows complete examination of both upper and
lower airways
Excellent for assessing dynamic airway changes
Usually requires only sedation and topical
anesthesia
Preferred method for bronchoalveolar lavage

Disadvantages:

Partially obstructs airway—patients must be able
to ventilate around scope
Limited visibility of posterior glottis and posterior
aspect of upper trachea
Limited suctioning capability

out the procedure (unless the instrument is inserted through an endotracheal or tracheostomy tube of sufficient diameter to allow ventilation around the bronchoscope). In the majority of circumstances, patients are quite able to breathe spontaneously, and the use of general anesthesia may be avoided. Nevertheless, the flexible bronchoscope always at least partially obstructs the airway, depending on the relative sizes of the instrument and the airway. Therefore, careful monitoring of the patient is essential throughout the procedure (2).

Transnasal passage of the flexible bronchoscope adds another dimension to the information gained with a flexible instrument since the examination includes the nasopharynx. In pediatric patients, a significant proportion of the pathologic findings are in this area, a fact that may not be adequately appreciated prior to the diagnostic procedure. Since the head

and neck may be kept in an anatomically neutral position (or even moved during the examination), and no distorting mechanical forces are applied to the airway, the usefulness of this instrument in evaluating the dynamics of the upper airway is increased. This may be especially important in infants with stridor.

Flexible endoscopes are often used for the primary purpose of examining the upper airway exclusively. However, a significant percentage of pediatric patients have more than one airway problem (3, 4), which is not always appreciated prior to the procedure. Therefore, it is important to examine the entire airway unless there is good reason not to do so. In some patients, the unexpected findings may be of much greater significance than the expected findings.

The image seen through a flexible instrument is composed of several thousand points of color and light intensity, and thus has a much lower optical resolution than the image from a glass rod telescope. On the other hand, the view is vastly superior to that obtained through a rigid bronchoscope without a telescope. For all but the most exacting requirements, the optical performance of contemporary flexible bronchoscopes is quite satisfactory.

Small, semi-disposable fiberoptic instruments are marketed as "aids to the management of endotracheal tubes," and sometimes are used as "bronchoscopes." These instruments have either no provision for distal angulation or only rudimentary distal control, and relatively poor optics. Although they may have some very limited utility in special circumstances (5), they are no substitute for a bronchoscope.

SPECIAL TECHNIQUES

Bronchoalveolar lavage (BAL) is used to obtain a representative sample of cells and secretions from the surfaces of small airways and alveolar spaces. The technique employed depends somewhat on the purpose of the procedure, but the primary principle is to obstruct an airway with a catheter and flood the airways and alveolar spaces distal to that site with saline. The airway must be occluded, or the instilled fluid will spill into adjacent airways, resulting in coughing, possible respiratory embarrassment, and loss of returned volume.

BAL may be performed with a rigid bronchoscope by advancing a catheter beyond the tip of the bronchoscope into the desired location. A flexible bronchoscope, however, is more ideally suited for BAL, since its tip can be easily directed to and wedged into the desired bronchus. The volume of lung lavaged will depend on the size of the catheter or bronchoscope in relation to the size of the airway. For example, the standard 3.5-mm pediatric flexible bronchoscope will wedge into a segmental airway in a newborn infant, and into a sub-sub-subsegmental airway in an 8-year old child.

The amount of fluid instilled during the course of BAL should be sufficient to reach the alveolar spaces, but there is little data in children on which to base an estimate of the required volume. In adults, BAL is typically performed with 3–5 aliquots of 50–100 ml of saline. There are no accepted standards for either the performance or the interpretation of BAL in pediatric patients. My approach involves the use of two 10-ml aliquots, with the flexible bronchoscope wedged into the same position (6). This will most likely obtain a representative sample of the airway and alveolar surface fluids distal to the tip of the bronchoscope, but it is difficult to prove this assertion. Since total lung capacity is in the range of only 100 ml/kg, however, it is apparent that very large volumes cannot be used in a single bolus. The volume typically returned with 1–3 aliquots is in the range of 40–60% of that infused, and increases with additional exchanges.

Transbronchial biopsy for sampling alveolar and small airways tissue is used frequently in adult patients, less frequently in adolescents (7, 8), and seldom in young children. As lung transplantation becomes more common in pediatric patients, this may change, but currently, for diagnostic purposes, if BAL cannot yield a satisfactory answer, open lung biopsy is probably the procedure of choice. Transbronchial biopsy yields very small tissue samples (~1 mm × 1 mm); for the diagnosis of many entities this may not be adequate. Currently, there are no biopsy forceps small enough to fit through the access port of the standard pediatric flexible bronchoscope.

Endoscope-guided nasotracheal intubation is an important technique (9) that may be life-saving. Patients with unstable cervical fractures, mandibular hypoplasia or ankylosis, cervical or pharyngeal mass lesions, and other conditions that make for very difficult intubation are ideal candidates for this relatively simple procedure. A flexible bronchoscope of appropriate size is passed through the selected endotracheal tube and then through the nose and into the trachea. The endotracheal tube is then advanced into the trachea, using the bronchoscope as a guide. This usually can be accomplished in about 30 seconds, and allows the visual examination of both the upper and lower airways at the same time.

Laser bronchoscopy for ablation of unresectable tumor or scar tissue is a well recognized procedure in adult patients. However, there are few indications for it in children. For upper airway lesions, such as subglottic hemangiomas, the carbon dioxide laser, used with an operating microscope, is the laser of choice. In selected patients with distal airway stenoses, the argon laser may be useful (10). The laser fiber may be passed through the suction channel of the flexible bronchoscope, and thus directed precisely to its target.

COMPLICATIONS

The risk of bronchoscopy is a function of many factors, involving the patient, the instrument, the operator, and the method used for anesthesia (3, 11–13). The sicker the patient, or the smaller the patient, the greater the potential risk. Although general anesthesia is much less risky than is commonly supposed, there is always some risk involved in the administration of any potent agent, including halothane and other general anesthetic agents, narcotics, benzodiazepines, and even topical anesthetics (14). On the other hand, the magnitude of this risk is generally quite low, but the risk of other complications is significantly increased if adequate sedation/anesthesia is not employed.

The relatively large diameter of the rigid bronchoscope (roughly equivalent to the appropriately sized endotracheal tube for the same patient) means that the subglottic space is potentially subjected to some trauma during the procedure. The cricoid ring in effect serves as a fulcrum about which the rigid bronchoscope is moved. For this reason, subglottic edema is a relatively common complication of rigid bronchoscopy, especially in prolonged or complicated procedures such as foreign body extraction. On the other hand, because of the small diameter of flexible bronchoscopes, sub-glottic edema is almost never seen after flexi-ble bronchoscopy (unless it was present before the procedure). Postbronchoscopy laryngeal edema does not necessarily mean that the pro-cedure was done improperly.

Other potential complications of bronchos-copy include epistaxis, laryngospasm, airway obstruction/hypoxia, cardiac arrhythmias, aspiration of oral or gastric contents, pneumo-thorax, hemoptysis, and pneumonia. The risk of each of these complications can be reduced by meticulous technique and choice of instru-ments, careful preparation of the patient, attention to detail, and the exercise of com-mon sense and good judgment. The highest rate of complications occurs in the extraction of foreign bodies; the patients are already compromised, and the manipulation of the foreign body may be very difficult. In a large published series of flexible bronchoscopies, the rate of minor complications such as epi-staxis or transient hypoxia or bradycardia was 2.5%, with 0.4% major complications (3). Many of these events should not really be considered complications, since very few had any effect on the patient or influenced the course or outcome of the procedure. Only one death has been reported as a complication of flexible bronchoscopy in a child (12).

Nosocomial infection from incompletely sterilized instruments, including broncho-scopes, has been reported many times (15, 16). In addition, contamination of the instrument may lead to misinterpretation of the results of cultures of specimens obtained from the patient (17). Finally, consideration must also be given to risk to the medical personnel per-forming procedures such as bronchoscopy. Physicians are often too casual in their approach to procedures in terms of their own protection, and are at risk of exposure to infec-tion with *Mycobacterium tuberculosis* after per-forming a bronchoscopy on a child in whom pulmonary tuberculosis was not thought likely (Wood, personal observation). Unsuspected human immunodeficiency virus (HIV) expo-sure is an increasing concern as well, and thus routine protection with gown, glove, mask, and eye protection is recommended. Good handwashing before and after the procedure is essential.

In view of the potential complications of bronchoscopy, it is clear that informed con-sent should be obtained from the parents for non-emergency procedures. In discussions prior to flexible bronchoscopy, it is very important for the child (if old enough) and his parents to understand all aspects of the procedure and that every attempt will be made to assure the comfort and safety of the child during the procedure. The risks of sedation and topical anesthesia, trauma to the airway (bleeding, pneumothorax), airway obstruc-tion, aspiration of stomach contents, and infection should be reviewed. The methods used to reduce risk and the fact that their child will be carefully monitored both electronically and by personnel trained and equipped to deal with any emergency should be stressed. The concept of risk versus benefit, the fact that in most instances the risk is small in relation to the potential benefit, and that alternative approaches either have greater risk or less potential for benefit should be presented to the family.

ANESTHESIA

Bronchoscopy, flexible or rigid, is not a proce-dure that most infants and young children willingly participate in. Therefore, some form of anesthesia/sedation is almost always neces-sary. Selected older patients may undergo flexible bronchoscopy with minimal sedation, or with hypnosis, but in any case, the child must be comfortable, yet not so deeply sedated as to impair spontaneous ventilation (unless, of course, the patient is intubated and mechanical ventilation is employed). It is also essential to anesthetize the nose and larynx completely. Topical application of lidocaine is usually sufficient but should be applied gently, with particular attention to the choanae and larynx.

General anesthesia is virtually mandatory for safe and effective rigid bronchoscopy. In some children, bronchoscopy (rigid or flexi-ble) is possible only with general anesthesia. This has some relative advantages. The child is totally unconscious, and thus more easily handled. With either a rigid bronchoscope or an endotracheal tube, the airway is controlled, and ventilation is reasonably ensured. How-ever, if the level of anesthesia is too deep, so that spontaneous respiration is inhibited, then airway dynamics and vocal cord movement

may not be apparent. Positive pressure ventilation can mask dynamic (expiratory) collapse
of the airways.

Children are usually anxious about impending procedures and separation from their parents. Therefore, some form of pre-sedation
can be very useful. In children up to age 5
years, oral chloral hydrate (75 mg/kg; maximum dose 1 g) given 30–45 minutes before
the scheduled procedure, or oral midazolam
(0.5–0.75 mg/kg) given 15–20 minutes before
the procedure, has been used successfully (18).
Rectal midazolam has also been used. A few
infants may require no further sedation, but
in the great majority of patients, after intravenous access is secured, additional sedation is
needed. The desired level of sedation is such
that the child will be comfortable (and cooperative) yet able to respond to command or stimulation and maintain patency of the airway
("conscious sedation" [19]). The child must
be carefully and constantly monitored; current
recommendations call for measurement of
oxygen saturation, pulse, and blood pressure,
in addition to observation. Hypnoanalgesic
techniques can add immeasurably to the comfort of the patient (as well as that of the parents
and staff), and reduce the dosages of chemical
agents required.

In my experience, general anesthesia has
been necessary in only 1% of patients undergoing flexible bronchoscopy. With proper
preparation and sedation, almost all flexible
procedures except those requiring a laser can
be done without general anesthesia (3). Occasionally, preprocedure anxiety in the older
child may interfere with sedation, and general
anesthesia is required in lieu of excessive doses
of sedatives. A wide variety of anesthetic
agents have been employed for sedation of
pediatric patients; the choice primarily
depends on the preferences and experience of
the individual physician as well the indication
for the bronchoscopy. For example, if the goal
of the examination is to evaluate vocal cord
function, caution must be observed in using
sedatives such as midazolam, which may transiently decrease vocal card movement (Loughlin, personal communication). Guidelines for
the safe use of sedation in pediatric patients
have been published (19, 20). Tables 10.3 and
10.4 outline a general approach to flexible
bronchoscopy and sedation in children. Several sedation protocols currently in use in cen-

ters with considerable experience in flexible
bronchoscopy are listed in Table 10.3. It is
important that the physician know and understand the agents being used, prepare the child
appropriately, monitor the child adequately,
and be prepared for all eventualities.

Topical anesthesia is readily achieved with
lidocaine, which should be placed on the nasal
mucosa (for transnasal passage of the bronchoscope) as well as the posterior pharynx and
larynx. Two-percent lidocaine can be used
above the glottis, and 1% below, since absorption is more rapid and complete below the
larynx. In very young infants, these concentrations should be reduced to 0.5%. Total lidocaine dosage should be kept below 7 mg/kg
(14), even though some fraction of what is
administered is suctioned away quickly. The
bronchoscopist must be familiar with the toxicity of lidocaine.

INDICATIONS

There is essentially only one indication for
diagnostic bronchoscopy: the need for specific
information from the airways that is most
safely, effectively, or definitively obtained by
bronchoscopy. If there is a better or safer way
to obtain the same information, then bronchoscopy is not indicated (1). For example,
bronchoscopy is sometimes employed to
obtain a specimen from the lower airways of
a young child to determine whether the lungs
are infected. This would not usually be indicated in an older patient who is able to produce
a sputum specimen (21). Radiographic or
magnetic resonance imaging (23, 24) should
at least be considered prior to bronchoscopy,
although these procedures have their own limitations. Bronchoscopy is expensive, relatively
difficult for patient and physician alike, and
involves some degree of risk. However, it is
often the most cost-effective technique, or it
may be the only technique that can yield the
necessary information.

Restoration of airway patency is essentially
the one indication for therapeutic bronchoscopy. Foreign body removal is the archetypal
indication, but removal of granulation tissue
or mucus plugs, and dilation of bronchial stenosis, are other good examples. A flexible
bronchoscope may be used to guide an endotracheal tube in a patient in whom traditional
methods for intubation are difficult or impossible, or to facilitate selective intubation of

Table 10.3.
Guidelines for Flexible Bronchoscopy[a]

- NPO—*solids:* 6 hours; *clears:* 2 hours
- Monitoring
- Person not performing procedure to monitor patient (pulse oximetry, EKG, BP, respiration), administer medications, maintain records, and help restrain patient
- Swaddling the small child is helpful in improving effectiveness of any sedative
- Supplemental oxygen and suction equipment available
- Crash cart immediately available
- Sedation—general principles

    All sedatives may effect vocal cord function

    If opioid is primary sedative, naloxone, a specific opioid antagonist, must be readily available (dose 0.01 mg/kg—can be given IV, IM, intratracheal, intra-osseous infusion)

    Monitoring requirements do not end when procedure is over; patient requires monitoring until consciousness returns to the level present before sedation was initated.

    Topical anesthesia:

    The key to successful bronchoscopy in a sedated patient is adequate topical anesthesia

    No amount of sedation will eliminate the risk of laryngospasm if there is inadequate topical anethesia; laryngeal reflexes may be operative even under general anesthesia

    A topical vasoconstrictor (penylephrine, oxymetazoline) may be helpful in the nose to reduce the risk of bleeding and to shrink swollen mucous membranes.

---

one mainstem bronchus; these applications can also be considered therapeutic.

Stridor

Stridor is one of the most common indications for endoscopic examination of the airway in infants and young children. The most frequent cause of acute stridor, infectious croup, should be readily diagnosed on clinical grounds alone and rarely warrants endoscopy. On the other hand, atypical or recurrent croup, especially if severe enough to require hospitalization, or croup occurring in the first 6 months of life, should make one suspicious of a chronic upper airway obstruction (see Chapter 27).

Persistent stridor following an acute upper respiratory infection (URI) in an infant less than a year of age is a strong indication for endoscopy. Croup that requires hospitalization for more than 10 days should be considered highly suspect. Endoscopic examination is indicated in such patients, many of whom will have anatomic lesions, such as subglottic stenosis, hemangiomas, cysts, vocal cord lesions or paralysis, and tracheal compression. It may be best especially with recurrent croup to wait until the acute symptoms have subsided to perform endoscopy, since the presence of acute edema may confuse the diagnostic picture. On the other hand, stridor is a visual diagnosis, and if the child is stridulous at the time of the examination, the source of the noise will always be visible.

Acute stridor, if not typical of infectious croup, may warrant endoscopic examination. Although visualization of the epiglottis and larynx is an important aspect of diagnosis and management of acute epiglotitis, a flexible bronchoscope should not be used to examine the larynx except perhaps in an operating room, by an expert bronchoscopist with full preparation for rigid laryngoscopy/bronchoscopy and even tracheostomy. Likewise, children in whom laryngeal foreign bodies are strongly suspected should undergo rigid laryngoscopy in the operating room.

Chronic stridor has a variety of causes, the most common of which is laryngomalacia (see also discussion in Chapters 27 and 40). In general, an infant with congenital stridor who has no respiratory distress, no evidence of vocal cord involvement (hoarseness, impaired glottic attack on coughing, or aspiration), and good growth and feeding patterns may be given a tentative diagnosis of laryngomalacia without visualization of the airway. Often, however, parental (or grandparental) anxiety may itself warrant further evaluation. Flexible endoscopy is ideal for this purpose, especially if the procedure is videotaped and the essential findings are reviewed with the family. Laryn-

Table 10.4.
Several Approaches to Sedation of Pediatric Patients Undergoing Bronchoscopy

University of North Carolina Protocol

Pre-procedure:

- Careful discussion with parents and patients—create the proper expectations of comfort and security; hypnoanalgesia begins well before the procedure begins
- Pre-procedure sedation:

  For children age 5 or younger:

  Oral chloral hydrate 75 mg/kg (maximal dose 1 g for children under 5) 30 minutes before the procedure

  For older, very anxious children (in pre-operative holding area or patient's room):
  IV midalzolam, 0.05 mg/kg over 2 minutes

- **If the child is pre-sedated, careful monitoring must be ensured from the time the drugs are given**

  In the bronchoscopy suite:

  - Initiate intravenous access if not done already
  - Re-establish monitoring (pulse oximetry, EKG, BP)
  - Hypnoanalgesic techniques—avoidance of loud noises, bright lights, inappropriate stimulation; positive suggestions of comfort, relaxation, displacement to another location and activity, etc.
  - Administer additional sedation if needed:

    IV midazolam 0.05-0.10 mg/Kg given over 2 minutes

    meperidine 0.5–2mg/kg given in increments of 0.5–1 mg/kg over 1–2 minutes (titrate to effect); it may be helpful to give part of the midazolam dose before and part after the narcotic; other narcotic agents may be used (e.g., fentanyl, morphine), since midazolam alone is unlikely to be sufficient.

  Topical vasoconstrictor (oxymetazoline, 0.05%), 0.25 ml, instilled into the nostril through which the bronchoscope will be passed

  Topical anesthetic (0.5–1 ml 2% lidocaine {1% should be used in infants}), instilled into the same nostril

  Before passing the bronchoscope, a scution catheter lubricated with lidocaine jelly is passed through the nose (and the stomach is aspirated in children less than 6 years old); this tests the level of sedation and topical anesthesia and also clears the nasal passage of secretions

  Maximum dose of lidocaine: 7 mg/kg

If additional sedation is needed:

- Titrate midazolam and/or meperidine to maximal dosage (0.2 mg/kg midazolam; 3 mg/kg meperidine); note that anxious, frightened children will require larger doses, and then will take longer to recover

                                                    or

- IV methohexital, 1 mg/kg, given rapidly—this produces near general anesthesia for about 60–90 seconds and usually induces a comfortable state of sedation upon arousal from the immediate effects of the methohexital; The dose may be repeated once or at most twice
- An occasional child simply cannot achieve satisfactory sedation with the above routines; general anesthesia is then required

Post-procedure

- Monitoring is continued until the child is awake and taking oral liquids well.
- Postprocedure hypnotic suggestions are given to facilitate comfort, a sense of hunger, and general well being; sedated children are very susceptible to suggestions (positive or negative) given to them

Riley Children's Hospital Protocol

- Initiate monitoring (EKG, oximetry) and start intravenous access
- Administer topical anesthetic (lidocaine—maximum dose 7mg/kg)
- Administer sedation as:

  Methohexital, 0.5–1 mg/kg, as the bronchoscope is about to be passed through the nose; this may be repeated to titrate level of consciousness

  For patients over 4 years—Midazolam; start with 0.05 mg/kg; increase in 0.05-mg/kg aliquots to maximum dose 0.2 mg/kg

- Post procedure, monitoring is continued until the patient has returned to preprocedure status

Johns Hopkins University—Pediatric Protocol

This protocol is based on the presence of an anesthesiologist to administer these medications

Pre-Procedure:

- Maintain calm, reassuring environment
- Midazolam, 0.5–1.0 mg/kg, per rectum 5–10 minutes before entering procedure room or oral midazolam, 0.5–1.0 mg/kg, 20 minutes before; oral midazolam can be made palatable by mixing it with liquid tylenol, coke syrup, or jello

In procedure room:

- Initiate monitoring (EKG, pulse oximetry, BP)
- Start intravenous line
- Administer additional medication as needed

Options available:

- Propofol, 2.0–3.0 mg/kg, IV bolus; give first 2–3 mg/kg of propofol as 0.5-mg/kg boluses until either sedation or general anesthesia is achieved; then 200 μg/kg/minute (propofol burns so it should be mixed with lidocaine and/or pretreat with IV fentanyl, 1–2 μg/kg

or

- Midazolam, 0.05 mg/kg (maximum dose 0.2 mg/kg)
- Fentanyl, 1–3 μg/kg (maximum dose 3 μg/kg) (titrate doses of these medications to appropriate level of sedation)

If additional sedation is needed:

- Ketamine, 0.25 mg/kg, IV; doses > 1–2 mg/kg will produce general anesthesia
- Alternatively, give 3–5 mg/kg IM, wait for nystagmus (approximately 3–5 minutes)
- If benzodiazepine has not been given, give with ketamine to decrease incidence of nightmares and "bum trips"
- Also administer atropine, 0.02 mg/kg (IV or IM)

Older children and adolescents:

- Depending on level of cooperation may need minimal sedation, especially if 3.6-mm OD pediatric bronchoscope is used
- Choices include:

    Propofol, 2–3.0 mg/kg, IV, in 0.5-mg/kg boluses

or

    Midazolam, 0.1–0.2 mg/kg, IV, in 0.05 mg/kg increments

Topical anesthesia:

- Lidocaine 1% (0.5% in infants)—1 ml in the nostril to be used for the procedure; this is followed by passing a cotton-tipped applicator saturated with viscous lidocaine jelly through the nostril that will be used; this permits the bronchoscopist to determine the anatomy and adequacy of the nasal passage and to assess the adequacy of the sedation.

Post-procedure:

- Patient is monitored in a recovery room until the child is returned to pre-procedure status and has tolerated oral feeding

[a]From Green et al.(1) and American Academy of Pediatrics (19).

gomalacia consists of either a floppy epiglottis or large, floppy arytenoids (or both). Care must be taken in the endoscopic diagnosis of laryngomalacia, since some part of the support of the epiglottis is muscular. Sedation can in some cases result in the appearance of a floppy epiglottis in a child with no history of stridor; this should not be over-interpreted. The examination should include visualization of the trachea and bronchi as well. At least 15% of children examined for stridor, in whom a plausible explanation for the stridor was found at or above the cricoid, also had a significant lesion in the lower airways (3, 4). In many cases, the lower airway lesions (such as complete tracheal rings or mass lesions) were far more important than the laryngeal lesion. However, the lower airways cannot always be safely examined, and the bronchoscope should not be passed through a very narrow opening unless one is prepared to deal with the consequences definitively.

Persistent Wheezing

Persistent wheezing that is poorly responsive (or unresponsive) to bronchodilators should be investigated by bronchoscopy. A significant proportion of children with such symptoms will have anatomic abnormalities such as tracheomalacia, bronchial or tracheal compression, and foreign bodies (3). Such abnormalities may be difficult to detect by non-endoscopic methods (22, 23). Although in many cases, such as in a child with bronchomalacia or tracheomalacia, there may be no effective treatment for the anatomic problem, definitive diagnosis may allow the physician to discontinue ineffective therapy. In other patients, the exclusion of anatomic causes may suggest more vigorous medical management. Persistent wheezing is the indication with the highest yield of detectable anatomic problems (3).

Pneumonia

Recurrent or persistent pneumonia may result from diverse etiologies, and may warrant bronchoscopic investigation. Patients in whom the pneumonia has been documented to recur in the same location are prime candidates for bronchoscopy, since localized abnormalities such as bronchial compression or stenosis, previously unsuspected foreign bodies, or congenital anomalies may be found. More often, even in patients with pneumonia localized to one area, the anatomy is normal and the most important information is derived from bronchoalveolar lavage. Cytologic and/or microbiologic analysis of BAL fluid (both of which should be performed) may reveal evidence of aspiration (24) or unusual infectious agents. In a few cases, what is thought on clinical and radiographic grounds to be pneumonia is in fact another disorder entirely, such as pulmonary hemosiderosis or alveolar proteinosis (25).

Persistent Cough

Persistent cough, if sufficiently severe, of long duration, or of unusual nature, warrants bronchoscopy, especially after more conventional approaches have proven nondiagnostic. Allergic or inflammatory (infectious) processes are the most common causes of cough, but anatomic factors must also be considered, espe-cially in younger children (see Chapter 15). Toddlers may aspirate a foreign body while out of sight of their caretakers, and thus there may be no history suggesting aspiration. Dynamic airway collapse (i.e., tracheomalacia or bronchomalacia) may also result in chronic cough (26). Culture and cytologic examination of bronchial washings may yield important clues to the inflammatory/infectious etiology of chronic cough.

Atelectasis

Atelectasis usually resolves without bronchoscopic intervention, but may warrant bronchoscopy if persistent or recurrent. In most pediatric patients with atelectasis, bronchoscopy will be done primarily for diagnostic purposes (culture, exclusion of foreign body or anatomic abnormality). However, in some situations, atelectasis may be of such magnitude as to produce respiratory distress or even respiratory failure. In such circumstances, bronchoscopy is clearly indicated, and may be therapeutic. With careful localized lavage and suctioning, most mucus plugs can be removed. It is probably useful in intubated patients to examine the lower airways with a flexible bronchoscope through the endotracheal tube prior to a decision to employ a rigid instrument. If a patient has many air bronchograms through the area of volume loss, it is relatively unlikely that bronchoscopy will yield immediate therapeutic results, since it is also unlikely that there are mucus plugs accessible to the bronchoscope. On the other hand, lavage for diagnostic purposes may be helpful even in this situation. Patients with large mucus plugs or foreign bodies may require rigid bronchoscopy (27).

Atelectasis in the premature infant may result from airway trauma produced by suction catheters or endotracheal tubes, and may be of massive proportions. Infants weighing as little as 700 g can successfully undergo bronchoscopy with a 3.5-mm flexible bronchoscope, and large central mucus plugs can be removed by suctioning (3). Since infants weighing less than about 2.5 kg will not be able to ventilate around the 3.5-mm instrument, however, great care must be taken to complete the procedure within 30–60 seconds. Multiple passes of the bronchoscope can be made if necessary. The small infant may require bag and mask ventilation between such passes with the bronchoscope, as well as reintubation at the end of the procedure. It is extremely helpful to examine the lower airways with an ultrathin instrument before attempting bronchoscopy with the larger instrument; infants as small as 540 g can breathe spontaneously around the ultrathin bronchoscope. This instrument can also be passed through endotracheal tubes as small as 2.5 mm inside diameter (ID). If a central mucus plug is discovered, then the infant can be extubated for bronchoscopy with a larger instrument, either flexible (3) or rigid (28).

Radiographic Abnormalities

Various radiographic abnormalities may warrant bronchoscopic evaluation. *Localized hyperinflation* may result from a foreign body, bronchial stenosis, bronchial compression, an endobronchial tumor, or localized bronchomalacia. In many children with localized hyperinflation, the bronchoscopic evaluation will be normal (the abnormality will be distal to the subsegmental bronchi), but bronchoscopy should be done to exclude treatable lesions in the central airways, especially if pulmonary resection is anticipated.

Bronchoscopy in pediatric patients with *hilar masses or adenopathy* is not a "high yield" process. One may see evidence of extrinsic bronchial compression, but it is usually very difficult to determine the cause of the compression. In older patients (adolescents or adults), transbronchial needle aspiration may be helpful, but this procedure is rarely warranted in children, and requires the use of an adult bronchoscope. High-resolution computed tomography or magnetic resonance image scanning may be more helpful in the majority of such patients. On the other hand, bronchoscopy may be very helpful if the etiology is inflammatory (e.g., tuberculosis) (28).

In adults with a *lung abscess*, bronchoscopy may be indicated to rule out the presence of a tumor (29), and occasionally to help establish intrabronchial drainage (30). In children with a lung abscess, a case can be made for diagnostic bronchoscopy. The probability of finding a foreign body is higher in children than in adults, and many children will be unable to produce a sputum specimen, so that bronchoscopic specimens may be quite useful for culture.

Hemoptysis is a relatively common indication for bronchoscopy in adults, but much less so in pediatric patients. On the other hand, bleeding from the respiratory tract in children, especially infants, may present primarily as hematemesis or melena, hiding the respiratory origin. Bronchoscopy and BAL may be very helpful in patients with bleeding in whom a gastrointestinal site cannot be found. BAL should be performed in any patient who undergoes bronchoscopy for suspected hemoptysis if blood is not seen in the airways; blood-tinged (or grossly bloody) BAL fluid is often obtained from such patients. The BAL fluid should also be stained for hemosiderin. Blood in the alveolar spaces will appear as hemosiderin in macrophages within about 48–72 hours (31).

When bronchoscopy is performed during active bleeding, the location of the bleeding may be clear, or may be obscured by the presence of blood in all areas. Bronchoscopy is not by any means always successful in localizing the site of a pulmonary bleed. In general, it is more likely to localize the site if done during active bleeding. Massive hemoptysis may require rigid endoscopy to handle the large volume of blood and to facilitate passage of bronchial packing or balloon catheters to tamponade the bleeding.

Tracheostomy

Children with tracheostomies often require endoscopic evaluation of their airways (3, 32). Development of granulation tissue masses above the stoma is common, and may progress to total obstruction; such masses should be removed in order to reduce the risk associated with dislodgement or occlusion of the tracheostomy tube. In other children, the tracheostomy tube may displace the anterior tracheal wall posteriorly, thus making decannulation more difficult. A flexible bronchoscope can be passed through the tracheostomy tube to evaluate such complications as improper length of the tube, bleeding, plugging of the tube, granulation tissue in the distal trachea or bronchi, and dynamic collapse of the trachea at the tip of the tube. In selected patients, retrograde laryngoscopy (through the tracheostomy stoma) may yield information not otherwise obtainable.

Bronchial or Tracheal Foreign Bodies

In patients with known bronchial or tracheal foreign bodies, rigid bronchoscopy is absolutely indicated, and should be performed as soon as appropriate equipment and facilities are available and the child is stabilized and ready for the procedure (33–35). Such patients may have a radiopaque foreign body, symptoms, or physical or radiographic findings supportive of the diagnosis, along with a history of aspiration (36, 37). In other children, however, the diagnosis may not be so readily apparent. There may be no history of choking or aspiration, physical or radiographic findings may be negative or misleading (38), or the child may present with recurrent pneumonia, atelectasis, recurrent wheezing, or other symptoms. In such patients, foreign body aspiration may be thought of only late in the course of the patient's management (or not at all). In over a thousand flexible bronchoscopies (3), a clinically unsuspected foreign body was found in 10. In a series of 52 children in whom foreign body was somewhere in the differential diagnosis, but with insufficient historical, radiographic, or physical evidence to warrant rigid bronchoscopy, a foreign body was found in 19% (39). It seems useful, therefore, to use flexible bronchoscopy for diagnostic purposes in children who might harbor a foreign body. However, in those who clearly have a foreign body or in whom the probability is high, the rigid instrument should be used.

Pulmonary Tuberculosis

The child with pulmonary tuberculosis may benefit from bronchoscopic evaluation. In children with a positive tuberculin test and abnormalities on chest radiograph, bronchoscopy and BAL may yield the organism (40), or may reveal significant endobronchial lesions warranting steroid therapy (28, 40). The recovery of organisms is lower in children who have been started on anti-tuberculous therapy. The prospect of finding significant endobronchial lesions and the relatively short time required for flexible bronchoscopy as an outpatient procedure makes this approach attractive in contrast to the more traditional 3-day collection of early morning gastric aspirates. Children with a positive tuberculin test and a normal chest film need not undergo bronchoscopy unless there is another indication for the procedure.

Vocal Cord Dysfunction

Vocal cord dysfunction can be evaluated by flexible laryngoscopy. In many cases, simple laryngoscopy (with clear visualization of the subglottic space) may be all that is needed, but occasionally bronchoscopy is also revealing. The left recurrent laryngeal nerve courses through the mediastinum to the level of the aortic arch, and is vulnerable to a variety of pathologic processes in this area, some of which may be diagnosed endoscopically. Vocal cord movement can be difficult to assess in some children. Videotape recordings of the endoscopic findings can be analyzed frame-by-frame, if necessary, to help evaluate the symmetry of cord motion. In some children, enlarged supraglottic structures (ventricular folds, aryepiglottic folds, arytenoids) may make direct visualization of the cords themselves very difficult; close attention should be given to the movement of the arytenoids. Rigid endoscopic instruments may have some special advantage in patients suspected of having bilateral vocal cord paralysis: not only can the posterior commissure be more easily examined than with a flexible instrument, but the cords can be passively manipulated under direct vision. Thus one can be certain that the putative paralysis is not due to interarytenoid fixation caused by (for example) scar tissue.

Additional Indications

In hospitalized patients there may be additional indications for bronchoscopy, including therapeutic removal of bronchial secretions ("bronchial toilet") and pneumonia in the compromised host (BAL and/or transbronchial biopsy, although the latter is rarely done in pre-adolescent patients). Bronchoscopy is very useful to aid in the difficult intubation (9, 41), in the evaluation of a child in whom extubation has failed, or to verify the position and/or patency of artificial airways. Flexible instruments, especially ultrathin instruments, may also facilitate visualization of areas not otherwise visible even with rigid instruments, thus allowing surgical procedures not possible by other methods (42).

Pneumonia in the compromised host may profitably be investigated by bronchoscopy if the patient does not produce sputum. Instead of relying on the clinical response to broad-based anti-infective therapy, examination and culture of BAL fluid can lead to more definitive (and hopefully effective) therapy (43–45). Whenever feasible, bronchoscopy/BAL should be undertaken very early in the clinical course of the patient's illness. Special care must be taken to reduce the problem of contamination of specimens by upper airway (mouth) flora. Once the larynx has been anesthetized, aspiration of oral contents may occur, thus confounding the diagnostic picture regardless of how the specimen is subsequently obtained. It may be useful to place the patient in a slight head-down position before applying topical anesthetic, to reduce the likelihood of aspiration. In adults and adolescents, protected brushes can be used to reduce the probability of contaminating the specimen with material from the bronchoscope suction channel, but this technique will not avoid the problem of aspirated oral secretions.

In the intensive care unit, bronchoscopy may be performed for virtually any of the indications cited above. One of the more specific applications, however, is the *management of the artificial airway*. The flexible bronchoscope can be passed through an endotracheal or tracheostomy tube, and the lower airways can be examined without removing the tube (42, 46, 47). The relationship of the end of the tube to the airway can be observed (for example, a tracheostomy tube may be partially occluded by the posterior tracheal membrane), and functional patency can be ascertained. In patients in whom intubation may be difficult or even impossible otherwise, a flexible bronchoscope can be used to guide the tube into the airway quickly and easily. Patients in whom extubation has failed may be examined with an endoscope at the time of an extubation trial to determine the cause of the failure. In this situation, the flexible bronchoscope is passed through one nostril and its tip is positioned just above the larynx. The patient is then extubated. A suitable endotracheal tube should be passed over the bronchoscope prior to starting the procedure, so that if reintubation is needed, it requires only a few seconds to do so. It is important in this situation to examine the subglottic space carefully, and to wait for at least 10 minutes before deciding that the patient will tolerate the extubation.

The presence of the endotracheal tube may prevent the formation of edema fluid in the subglottic space until the tube has been removed, and it is not uncommon to see an initially widely patent subglottis literally disappear before one's eyes over a 5-minute period as edema fluid accumulates.

Patients will benefit when bronchoscopy is used in a timely and appropriate fashion by a skilled bronchoscopist (48). Several cases are provided in the next section to illustrate this point.

ILLUSTRATIVE CASES

Case No. 1

An 18-month-old boy was referred for evaluation of stridor and wheezing since birth. He had been the 3.2-kg product of a full term, uneventful pregnancy, and had never been intubated. At 8 months of age he had undergone rigid bronchoscopy to evaluate his symptoms. At that time, a "slight anterior indentation of the trachea" was noted, but this was not felt to explain the child's symptoms.

Physical examination was remarkable for a harsh, low-pitched stridulous cough, inspiratory stridor, and an expiratory wheeze. A chest radiograph was unremarkable.

Flexible bronchoscopy revealed that the upper airway, including the larynx and subglottic space, was normal. At the thoracic inlet, the anterior tracheal wall was compressed by a pulsatile, extrinsic mass, so that nearly 90% of the lumen was obstructed. The membranous trachea could be seen to vibrate against the anterior wall at the site of the compression. This lesion was most consistent with tracheal compression by an anomalous innominate artery.

On examination of the remainder of the lower airways a kernel of popcorn, surrounded by granulation tissue, was found in the right mainstem bronchus.

This infant, with two lesions—a congenital anatomic anomaly, and an acquired airway obstruction due to an aspirated foreign body—illustrates a number of concepts: (a) Stridor is visible. If the patient is making noise at the time of the endoscopic examination, the vibrating structures should always be seen. (b) Rigid endoscopy can produce mechanical distortion of the airway, which can obscure the true nature of the pathology.

(c) Every child should be suspected of harboring a foreign body, even in the absence of historical or laboratory evidence of foreign body aspiration. (d) Many children have more than one lesion, whether congenital or acquired. Therefore, whenever airway endoscopy is performed, it is prudent to visualize the entire bronchial tree, at least to the level of the segmental bronchi, unless there is a very good reason not to do so.

Case No. 2

A 10-month-old girl was referred for evaluation of persistent pneumonia. At 6 months of age, she developed a respiratory illness characterized by fever, cough, and tachypnea; a chest radiograph revealed bilateral infiltrates. She was treated with antibiotics with slow improvement. Follow-up radiographs revealed persistence of the infiltrates, most prominently in the right middle lobe. Over the next 4 months, she had several episodes of similar respiratory symptoms; her chest film never cleared.

Her physical examination was completely unremarkable. A chest radiograph revealed bilateral infiltrates. Laboratory studies were notable only for a hematocrit of 28%.

Flexible bronchoscopy was performed to obtain bronchoalveolar washings for culture and cytology. The visual examination of the airways was normal, with no evidence of increased secretions. The right middle lobe was lavaged with sterile saline. The fluid that was returned was grossly and uniformly bloody, with no evidence of mucosal friability noted in the area into which the tip of the bronchoscope had been wedged for the lavage.

BAL bacterial cultures were sterile, but iron stains of the fluid revealed large amounts of hemosiderin in the alveolar macrophages, and a tentative diagnosis of pulmonary hemosiderosis was made. This was confirmed by open lung biopsy.

This patient illustrates an important concept: radiographic densities on a chest radiograph may not represent infection, even when there is a history consistent with infection. BAL fluid should be examined both by culture and also by microscopic techniques with appropriate staining.

Case No. 3

An 8-month-old boy was admitted to the hospital with a 3-week history of cough. He had received treatment with several antibiotics without improvement. Physical examination was remarkable only for tachypnea (respiratory rate = 44); he was afebrile. Chest film revealed a diffuse interstitial infiltrate.

Shortly after he was admitted, flexible bronchoscopy was done to obtain a BAL specimen for culture and cytology. The airway anatomy was normal; there were scant secretions. Examination of the BAL fluid with Wright stain (49) revealed numerous macrophages, a small percentage of neutrophils, an occasional eosinophil, and many areas of purple-staining debris containing many small dark dots surrounded by a lighter "halo." On this basis, a diagnosis of *Pneumocystis carinii* pneumonia was made, and later substantiated by a methenamine-silver stain. The child was started on appropriate chemotherapy, and evaluated for immunodeficiency. He was found to have very low serum IgG; HIV studies on the child and his mother were negative. This patient illustrates the concept that early diagnostic studies (i.e., bronchoscopy/BAL) can lead to early diagnosis and institution of specific therapy. The diagnosis of *Pneumocystis* pneumonia was established within 20 minutes of the time the bronchoscopy was performed, which in turn led to the search for an immunodeficiency.

Case No. 4

A 2.2-kg infant with severe mandibular hypoplasia had significant respiratory distress immediately after delivery, with retractions and poor air exchange. The larynx could not be visualized by direct laryngoscopy after multiple attempts by several experienced physicians. Barely adequate ventilation was maintained by bag and mask. A 2.2-mm flexible bronchoscope was passed through a 3.0-mm endotracheal tube and then advanced through one nostril.

Oxygen was insufflated into the posterior pharynx via a suction catheter passed through the opposite nostril; this provided the infant with some ventilation and also distended the pharynx to improve visualization with the bronchoscope. The larynx was noted to be normal, but the tongue was positioned very posteriorly, so that there was virtually no nasopharyngeal airway. The bronchoscope was passed into the trachea, the endotracheal tube advanced into the trachea, and the bronchoscope was then withdrawn. The bronchoscopic intubation required approximately 1 minute. The child later underwent a tracheostomy.

This patient illustrates the concept that a flexible bronchoscope can be a life-saving means of accomplishing an otherwise very difficult intubation.

Case No. 5

A 3-month-old infant was admitted to the hospital with croup. After 4 days he improved and was discharged. Three weeks later, he was readmitted with another episode of croup. On the second hospital day, he underwent nasopharyngoscopy with a flexible instrument; the findings were reported to be "normal." The symptoms continued, and the child was transferred from the outlying hospital. On physical examination, the child had significant suprasternal retractions with inspiratory stridor and a harsh, croupy cough. There were copious nasal secretions. A chest film showed normal results.

Despite the history of a previously normal endoscopic examination, the child was brought to the bronchoscopy suite for laryngoscopy/bronchoscopy. The supraglottic structures, including the vocal cords, were indeed normal. However, the subglottic space was nearly totally obstructed by a tissue mass arising from the lateral aspect of the subglottis; no airway could be visualized. The mass (almost certainly a hemangioma) was covered by normal-appearing epithelium. The bronchoscope was not advanced beyond the lesion, but the child was taken directly to the operating room and a tracheostomy was performed. The subglottic lesion was subjected to laser ablation in stages, and the tracheostomy was successfully removed after 8 months.

This case illustrates several concepts. Croup, when severe enough to require hospitalization, and especially when recurrent, is an indication for endoscopic evaluation. Although nasopharyngoscopy is an appropriate diagnostic approach, care must be taken to perform the examination with sufficient sedation and topical anesthesia so that the entire supraglottic and infraglottic airway can be carefully examined. Unless the airway can be seen to be widely patent, it cannot be safely assumed that there is no obstruction.

Case No. 6

A 7-year-old girl with cystic fibrosis developed increasing cough, and radiographic studies revealed an infiltrate in the right middle lobe. She was unable to produce sputum, but cultures obtained from the deep pharynx after vigorous coughing grew moderate amounts of *Pseudomonas aeruginosa*. She was treated with intravenous and aerosolized antibiotics, and more vigorous chest physiotherapy. There was slow but moderate improvement, and the radiographic findings did not improve. Repeated "gag sputum" cultures subsequently yielded only moderate amounts of "normal flora." Continued therapy with aerosolized aminoglycosides did not improve her condition, and bronchoscopy was therefore planned. At the time of the bronchoscopy, her chest was clear to auscultation, although she continued to have infiltrates in the region of the right middle lobe. Despite her nonproductive cough and unimpressive auscultatory findings, endoscopic examination of her airways revealed large quantities of extremely viscous secretions. Cultures of washings obtained from the right middle lobe yielded large numbers of *Mycobacterium avium* intracellulare; bacterial cultures were sterile (antibiotic therapy had been discontinued 2 weeks before the bronchoscopy).

This case illustrates two concepts: that bronchoscopy can be a useful and important technique for determining the lower respiratory tract flora in non–sputum-producing children with cystic fibrosis (or other chronic pulmonary diseases), and that there may be much more inflammatory airways disease than is apparent from clinical evaluation. Bronchoscopy is rarely warranted in patient who can produce adequate sputum specimens, but can be valuable in those who cannot.

REFERENCES

1. Green CG, Eisenberg J, Leong A, Nathanson I, Schnapf BM, Wood RE. Flexible endoscopy of the pediatric airway. *Am Rev Resp Dis* 1992; 145:233–235.
2. Schnapf BM. Oxygen desaturation during fiberoptic bronchoscopy in pediatric patients. *Chest* 1991; 99:591–594.
3. Wood RE. Spelunking in the pediatric airways: Explorations with the flexible fiberoptic bronchoscope. *Pediatr Clin North Am* 1984; 31:785–799.
4. Gonzalez C, Reilly JS, Bluestone CD. Synchronous airway lesions in infancy. *Ann Otol Rhinol Laryngol* 1987; 96:77–80.

5. Finkelhor BK, Healy GB. Disposable flexible fiber-optic mini-bronchoscope for evaluating the pediatric airway. *Otolaryngol Head Neck Surg* 1989; 101:511–512.

6. Wood RE. Bronchoalveolar lavage in infants and children. In Baughman RP, ed: *Bronchoalveolar lavage.* St. Louis, Mosby-Year Book, 1992, pp 26–28.

7. Fitzpatrick SB, Stokes DC, Marsh B, Wang KP. Transbronchial lung biopsy in pediatric and adolescent patients. *Am J Dis Child* 1985; 139:46–49.

8. Scott JP, Higenbottam TW, Smyth RL, Whitehead B, Helms P, Fradet G, De Leval M, Wallwork J. Transbronchial biopsies in children after heart-lung transplantation. *Pediatrics* 1990; 86:698–702.

9. Rucker RW, Silva WJ, Worcester CC. Fiberoptic bronchoscopic nasotracheal intubation in children. *Chest* 1979; 76:56–58.

10. Azizkhan RG, Lacey SR, Wood RE. Acquired symptomatic bronchial stenosis in infants: Successful management using an argon laser. *J Pediatr Surg* 1990; 25:19–24.

11. Lockhart CH, Elliot JL. Potential hazards of pediatric rigid bronchoscopy. *J Pediatr Surg* 1984; 19:239–242.

12. Wagener JS. Fatality following fiberoptic bronchoscopy in a two-year-old child. *Pediatr Pulmonol* 1987; 3:197–199.

13. Cohn RC, Kercsmar C, Dearborn D. Safety and efficacy of flexible endoscopy in children with bronchopulmonary dysplasia. *Am J Dis Child* 1988; 142:1225–1228.

14. Amitai Y, Zylber Katz E, Avital A, Zangen D, Noviski N. Serum lidocaine concentrations in children during bronchoscopy with topical anesthesia. *Chest* 1990; 98:1370–1373.

15. Nelson KE, Larson PA, Schraufnagel DE, Jackson J. Transmission of tuberculosis by flexible fiberbronchoscopes. *Am Rev Respir Dis* 1983; 127:97–100.

16. Pappas SA, Schaaff DM, Dicostanzo MB, King FW, Sharp JT. Contamination of flexible fiberoptic bronchoscopes. *Am Rev Respir Dis* 1983; 127:391–392.

17. Uttley AHC, Honeywell KM, Fitch LE, Yates MD, Simpson RA. Cross contamination of bronchial washings. *Br Med J* 1990; 301:1274.

18. Feld LH, Negus JB, White PF. Oral midazolam preanesthetic medication in pediatric outpatients. *Anesthesiology* 1990; 73:831–834.

19. American Academy of Pediatrics: Guidelines for monitoring and management of pediatric patients during and after sedation for diagnostic and therapeutic procedures. *Peds* 1992; 89:1110–1115.

20. Anderson JA, Vann WF Jr. Respiratory monitoring during pediatric sedation: Pulse oximetry and capnography. *Pediatr Dent* 1988; 10:94–101.

21. Ognibene FP, Gill VJ, Pizzo PA, Kovacs JA, Godwin C, Suffredini AF, Shelhamer JH, Parrillo JE, Masur H. Induced sputum to diagnose pneumocystis carinii pneumonia in immunosuppressed pediatric patients. *J Pediatr* 1989; 115:430–433.

22. Hernandez RJ, Tucker GF. Congenital tracheal stenosis: Role of CT and high kV films. *Pediatr Radiol* 1987; 17:192–196.

23. Myer CM III, Auringer ST, Wiatrak BJ, Bisset G. Magnetic resonance imaging in the diagnosis of innominate artery compression of the trachea. *Arch Otolaryngol Head Neck Surg* 1990; 116:314–316.

24. Colombo JL, Hallberg TK. Recurrent aspiration in children: Lipid-laden alveolar macrophage quantitation. *Pediatr Pulmonol* 1987; 3:86–89.

25. Martin RJ, Coalson JJ, Rogers RM, Horton FO, Manous LE. Pulmonary alveolar proteinosis: The diagnosis by segmental lavage. *Am Rev Respir Dis* 1980; 121:819–825.

26. Wood RE. Localized tracheomalacia or bronchomalacia in children with intractable cough. *J Pediatr* 1990; 116:404–406.

27. Muntz HR. Therapeutic rigid bronchoscopy in the neonatal intensive care unit. *Ann Otol Rhinol Laryngol* 1985; 94:462–465.

28. Toppet M, Malfroot A, Derde MP, Toppet V, Spehl M, Dab I. Corticosteroids in primary tuberculosis with bronchial obstruction. *Arch Dis Child* 1990; 65:1222–1226.

29. Sosenko A, Glassroth J. Fiberoptic bronchoscopy in the evaluation of lung abscesses. *Chest* 1985; 87:489–494.

30. Wanner A, Landa JF, Nieman RE Jr, Vevaina J, Delgado I. Bedside bronchofiberscopy for atelectasis and lung abscess. *JAMA* 1973; 224:1281–1283.

31. Sherman JM, Winnie G, Thomassen MJ, Abdul-Karim FW, Boat TF. Time course of hemosiderin production and clearance by human pulmonary macrophages. *Chest* 1984; 86:409–411.

32. Benjamin B, Curley JWA. Infant tracheotomy-endoscopy and decannulation. *Int J Pediatr Otorhinolaryngol* 1990; 20:113–121.

33. Puhakka H, Kero P, Valli P, Iisalo E, Erkinjuntti M. Pediatric bronchoscopy. A report of methodology and results. *Clin Pediatr* 1989; 28:253–257.

34. Friedman EM, Williams M, Healy GB, McGill TFI. Pediatric endoscopy: A review of 616 cases. *Ann Otol Rhinol Laryngol* 1984; 93:517–519.

35. Cohen SR, Herbert WI, Lewis GB, Geller KA. Foreign bodies in the airway: Five-year retrospective study with special reference to management. *Ann Otol Rhinol Laryngol* 1980; 89:437–442.

36. Wiseman NE. The diagnosis of foreign body aspiration in childhood. *J Pediatr Surg* 1984; 19:531–535.

37. Mantor PC, Tuggle DW, Tunell WP. An appropriate negative bronchoscopy rate in suspected foreign body aspiration. *Am J Surg* 1989; 158:622–624.

38. Svedstrom E, Puhakka H, Kero P. How accurate is chest radiography in the diagnosis of tracheobronchial foreign bodies in children? *Pediatr Radiol* 1989; 19:520–522.

39. Wood RE, Gauderer MW. Flexible fiberoptic bronchoscopy in the management of tracheobronchial foreign bodies in children: The value of a combined approach with open tube bronchoscopy. *J Pediatr Surg* 1984; 19:693–698.

40. deGracia J, Curull V, Riba A, Orriols R, Martin N, Morell F. Diagnostic value of bronchoalveolar lavage in suspected pulmonary tuberculosis. *Chest* 1988; 93:329–332.

41. Wood RE, Postma D. Endoscopy of the airway in infants and children. *J Pediatr* 1988; 112:1–6.

42. Wood RE, Azizkhan RG, Lacey SR, Sidman J, Drake A. Surgical applications of ultrathin flexible bronchoscopes in infants. *Ann Otol Rhinol Laryngol* 1991; 100:116–119.

43. deBlic J, Blanche S, Danel C, Le-Bourgeois M, Caniglia M, Scheinmann P. Bronchoalveolar lavage in

HIV infected patients with interstitial pneumonitis. *Arch Dis Child* 1989; 64:1246–1250.

44. Stokes DC, Shenep JL, Parham D, Bozeman PM, Marienchek W, Mackert PW. Role of flexible bronchoscopy in the diagnosis of pulmonary infiltrates in pediatric patients with cancer. *J Pediatr* 1989; 115:561–567.

45. Pattishall EN, Noyes BE, Orenstein DM. Use of bronchoalveolar lavage in immunocompromised children with pneumonia. *Pediatr Pulmonol* 1988; 5:1–5.

46. Schellhase DE, Graham LM, Fix EJ, Sparks LM, Fan LL. Diagnosis of tracheal injury in mechanically ventilated premature infants by flexible bronchoscopy. A pilot study. *Chest* 1990; 98:1219–1225.

47. Shinwell ES, Higgins RD, Auten RL, Shapiro DL. Fiberoptic bronchoscopy in the treatment of intubated neonates. *Am J Dis Child* 1989; 143:1064–1065.

48. Wood RE. Pitfalls in the use of the flexible bronchoscope in pediatric patients. *Chest* 1990; 97:199–203.

49. Bedrossian CWM, Mason MR, Gupta PK. Rapid cytologic diagnosis of Pneumocystis: A comparision of effective techniques. *Semin Diagn Pathol* 1989; 6:245–261.

11

Assessment of Respiratory Control

CAROL LYNN ROSEN

OVERVIEW

Respiratory control is an integrated process by which blood gas tensions and pH are kept in a narrow range despite changing metabolic and environmental conditions. It involves a complex interplay of chemical, neural, muscular, and bellows components to make ventilatory adjustments that meet a wide range of demands (Fig. 11.1) (1). Assessment of respiratory control requires evaluation of many complicated factors. Besides voluntary, psychologic, and behavioral influences, ventilation is modified by sensory information from the upper and lower airways, chest wall, and lungs that is sent to the medullary respiratory center. Respiration is stimulated by decreases in arterial pH and arterial P_{O_2} at the peripheral chemoreceptors (carotid and aortic bodies) and by a decrease in tissue pH in the medulla (as influenced by arterial P_{CO_2} and cerebrospinal fluid HCO_3^-). These afferent signals modify the central respiratory pattern generators that drive the upper airway, intercostal, and phrenic motor neurons. Thus, the rate, depth,

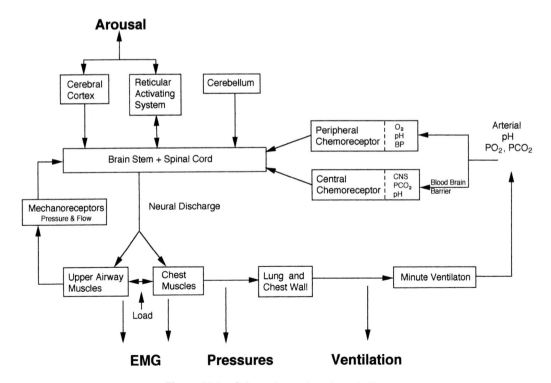

Figure 11.1. Schema for control of respiration.

and pattern of breathing reflect an elaborate interaction of neurohumoral and chemical regulatory mechanisms. Abnormalities anywhere along this control system can disrupt regulation of ventilation and impair arterial blood gas tensions and pH. With such diverse connections in the respiratory control system, the problem of determining mechanisms of abnormal ventilatory control is complex. This chapter provides an overview of pediatric respiratory control problems, a discussion of the methods to assess them, and a practical approach to their evaluation.

ABNORMALITIES OF RESPIRATORY CONTROL

Abnormalities of respiratory control are associated with a variety of pediatric problems (Table 11.1) (2–50). The clinical manifestations and therapy of these disorders are presented in Chapter 52. Except for congenital

Table 11.1.
Pediatric Conditions Associated with Abnormal Respiratory Control

Congenital central hypoventilation syndrome
(2–5, 7, 8)

Acquired central alveolar hypoventilation syndrome
  Asphyxia (9)
  Infarction (9)
  Infection (10–13)
  Trauma (14)
  Tumor (15, 16)

CNS malformations
  Chiari malformation (6, 17–22)
  Dandy-Walker malformation (23)
  Foramen magnum compression (24–26)
  Joubert syndrome (27)
  Moebius syndrome (28)
  Syringobulbomyelia (29)

Miscellaneous
  Autonomic nervous system dysfunction (30, 31)
  High altitude exposure (34)
  Hypothalamic dysfunction (32, 35, 36)
  Obesity-hypoventilation syndrome (38, 39)

Toxic—metabolic
  Inborn error of metabolism (40)
  Hypothyroidism (41)
  Leigh's disease (42)
  Metabolic alkalosis (43)
  Narcotic addiction (44)
  Pyruvate dehydrogenase deficiency (45, 46)

Reversible
  Severe upper airway obstruction (47)
  Congenital cyanotic heart disease (33, 48, 49)
  Chronic CO_2 retention (50)

central hypoventilation syndrome, most of these conditions have clear clinical evidence of underlying neurologic or other medical problems. Children with abnormal respiratory control are at risk for respiratory failure with minor stresses—infection, anesthesia, and sedation (2, 29, 37, 51). Problems with respiratory control should be suspected when hypercapnia or respiratory failure occurs without evidence of underlying lung disease, or is out of proportion to the severity of the lung disease, or when an abnormal respiratory pattern such as recurrent apnea is present.

Previously, clinical assessment of respiratory control was limited to arterial blood gases and pulmonary function tests. However, recently, several methods were developed to quantitate the output of the respiratory center. Unfortunately, the experience with the evaluation of respiratory control has been predominantly in adults (1, 52–61). Data in children other than newborns are limited, but since these responses seem to mature fairly rapidly, the data from adults will also be useful information to pediatricians.

ASSESSMENT METHODS

Assessment of respiratory control means measuring the outputs of central respiratory drive (Fig. 11.1). *Ventilation* was one of the earliest outputs to be measured. Since abnormal mechanical behavior of the lungs or chest wall can alter minute ventilation, other methods independent of these limitations were sought. Clearly, technical problems prohibit the direct measurement of the respiratory neuron activity in the brainstem. *Phrenic nerve activity* has been used to assess respiratory drive in spontaneously breathing laboratory animals, but is impractical for human investigation. Other measurable outputs from the respiratory control system appropriate for human studies include *integrated diaphragm electromyogram (EMG)* and *mouth occlusion pressure*. These techniques also have limitations (as discussed below) and are not generally useful for clinical testing. Finally, *arousal* is another measurable "output" of the respiratory control system that has important practical implications, particularly for sleep apnea patients (62).

Each of these respiratory center outputs must be "driven" by input stimuli such as hypercapnia, hypoxemia, and mechanical loading. The relevance of the test results from these unusual, unphysiologic stimuli to natural breathing is uncertain. Although measurement of these outputs is considered "noninvasive," the equipment used to make the measurement (nose clips, mouth pieces, or tight-fitting face masks) can alter respiratory patterns via trigeminal stimulation or increased dead space (63, 64). Finally, an "abnormal" response may not represent a primary respiratory control problem. Blunted responses can be secondary to underlying medical conditions (e.g., upper airway obstruction, chronic lung disease, or obesity) that expose the patient to chronic hypoxemia, hypercapnia, mechanical loads, or sleep disruption (65–69). The apparently "abnormal" response may disappear after treatment of the underlying problem, suggesting that these changes represent an adjustment of the respiratory control system to the stress of disease. At the present time, quantitative assessment of respiratory control is primarily a research tool, rather than a clinical tool. A brief discussion of the theory and methods will highlight the difficulties in performing and interpreting these tests.

Ventilatory Responses

Ventilatory responses to hypercapnia and hypoxia are commonly measured outputs of the respiratory system (70). Although these responses vary greatly even in normal patients, they have been used in the clinical evaluation of patients with unexplained respiratory depression, obesity, and sleep disorders.

Environmental influences such as anxiety about the testing, a recent meal, room noise, or a full bladder can alter breathing patterns and contribute to this variability (54).

VENTILATORY RESPONSE TO HYPERCAPNIA

The hypercapnic response is a measure of the change in ventilation associated with increased inspired CO_2 concentration when oxygenation is adequate. The normal ventilatory response is linear and increases as PaO_2 decreases (Fig. 11.2). In normal adults, the CO_2 response is highly variable and influenced by genetic and environmental factors (71). Twin studies of the ventilatory response to CO_2 have shown that tidal volume response is primarily genetically determined, whereas

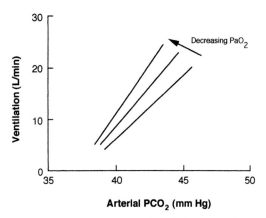

Figure 11.2. The linear relationship between minute ventilation (V_E) and arterial P_{CO_2}. The slope of the V_E versus arterial P_{CO_2} increases as P_{O_2} decreases.

the frequency response is acquired (72). Depressed ventilatory responses to CO_2 occur in endurance athletes, with aging, and in certain racial groups (73–75). Even within the same individual, these measures show significant variations when repeated on different days (76). Acid-base imbalances modify the ventilatory responses to CO_2. Low concentrations of bicarbonate in serum and in the brain enhance the response to CO_2; high concentrations of bicarbonate have the opposite effects (43). Drugs and hormones also alter the CO_2 response: aminophylline, salicylates, thyroxine, and progesterone increase responsiveness to CO_2, whereas narcotics, barbiturates, and other central nervous system (CNS) depressants decrease it (77). Behavioral state profoundly influences ventilatory responses to CO_2. The slope is greatest during wakefulness, falls during non–rapid eye movement (NREM) sleep to about one-half the waking value, and decreases even further during REM sleep (78).

In children, these techniques have been used to examine the maturation of respiratory control and to detect depression or absence of chemoreceptor responses in conditions such as central alveolar hypoventilation syndrome, cyanotic heart disease, morbid obesity, and asthma (2, 35, 38, 48, 79–81). Most of the experience with these methods has been in neonates. In this age group, rapid changes in behavioral state and rib cage distortion confounds the interpretation of CO_2 responses (82). The amount of ventilatory depression during wakefulness has not correlated with the severity of the hypoventilation during sleep in children with congenital central hypoventilation syndrome or in adults with obstructive sleep apnea (2, 69).

The ventilatory response to hypercapnia is measured with one of two methods: rebreathing and steady-state (54). The sensitivity or "gain" of the ventilatory response to CO_2 will be similar with these two methods. However, the threshold where ventilation increases in response to rising P_{CO_2} is higher in the rebreathing method (Fig. 11.3). This discrepancy is probably related to variable differences depending on the method used, between end-tidal CO_2 and tissue P_{CO_2} in the chemosensitive areas of the brain.

Steady-State Method

After a baseline period of breathing CO_2-free air through a mouthpiece, the patient breathes CO_2-enriched air for two or more periods. In adults, at least 10–20 minutes are required for a steady state to be reached in alveoli, arterial blood, cerebrospinal fluid, and the chemosensitive areas of the brain. The ventilatory response to CO_2 is determined from the ventilation (V_E)-Pa_{CO_2} plot. In patients free of lung disease, end-tidal CO_2 can be substituted for arterial P_{CO_2}. To eliminate the influence of variations in arterial PO_2 on the ventilatory response to CO_2, the inspired gas is enriched with O_2.

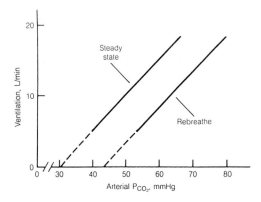

Figure 11.3. The relationship between ventilation and arterial P_{CO_2} as determined by the steady-state and rebreathing methods. Each method demonstrates the linear relationship between ventilation and P_{CO_2} and generates the same slope. However, the thresholds determined by the two methods are different, as discussed in the text.

Rebreathing Method

Because the steady state method is tedious and time consuming, it has largely been replaced by the rebreathing method. In this procedure, the patient rebreathes a CO_2-enriched gas mixture through a mouthpiece from a bag for approximately 4 minutes. The validity of this approach depends on the rapid equilibration of CO_2 between alveolar gas, arterial and mixed venous blood, and the chemosensitive areas of the brain. To promote this equilibration, the volume of the bag is adjusted to about 1 L greater than the patient's vital capacity and filled with a gas mixture that approximates the CO_2 in mixed venous blood. Oxygen is substituted for air in this mixture to avoid any hypoxic stimulus to the ventilatory drive. With these adjustments, equilibration generally occurs in 30–40 seconds. The test is stopped after 4 minutes, if the patient complains of dyspnea, or if the end-tidal CO_2 concentration exceeds 9%. The results are described using two terms: (a) the slope of the line relating ventilation to end-tidal P_{CO_2} (V_E/P_{CO_2}) and (b) the X-intercept of the relationship between V_E and end-tidal P_{CO_2}. The slope is the sensitivity of the control system and the X-intercept is the threshold (Fig. 11.3).

VENTILATORY RESPONSE TO HYPOXIA

The hypoxic response is a measure of the change in ventilation associated with reduced concentration of inspired oxygen. This response is determined by the peripheral arterial chemoreceptors when the level of hypoxia is mild to moderate. In severe hypoxia, the response may be attenuated because of depression of central respiratory drive. Unlike the linear response of V_E to progressive hypercapnia, the response to hypoxia is curvilinear. When oxygenation is expressed in terms of arterial saturation instead of Pa_{O_2}, the ventilatory response becomes linear (Fig. 11.4). The magnitude of the ventilatory response to a decrease in arterial PO_2 is influenced by the arterial P_{CO_2}, and the response increases as the concentration of CO_2 in the arterial blood rises. All other factors being equal, the rate of change in ventilation is greater over the lower range of oxygenation (i.e., when Pa_{O_2} falls below 60 mm Hg) than over the higher range (Fig. 11.5).

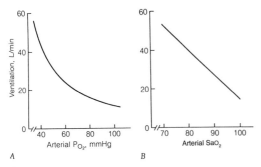

Figure 11.4. The ventilatory response to hypoxia. The relationship between ventilation and arterial P_{O_2} *(A)* is curvilinear, whereas that between ventilation and arterial saturation *(B)* is linear.

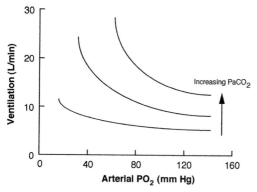

Figure 11.5. The curvilinear relationship between minute ventilation (V_E) and arterial P_{O_2}. The slope of the V_E versus arterial P_{O_2} increases as P_{CO_2} increases.

Many factors influence the ventilatory response to hypoxia and complicate the interpretation of these tests. First, even in normal individuals, the ventilatory response to acute hypoxia varies widely. This is probably on a genetic basis (70, 83, since higher ventilatory responses to CO_2 are linked with a high sensitivity to hypoxia. Second, the level of arterial P_{CO_2} is extraordinarily sensitive to the P_{O_2}. For example, when the O_2 tension falls to 40 mm Hg, ventilation in normal adult rises about 15 L/min. This response is abolished if the CO_2 tension is 5 mm Hg lower, and is double if the resting CO_2 tension is 5 mm Hg higher (84). The "normal" CO_2 tension for testing hypoxic responses is an open question, which becomes even more relevant when we consider what happens to the "baseline" CO_2 when a patient comes to a strange laboratory, anxiously awaiting this testing with nose clips, mouthpieces, and mysterious equipment.

Third, the duration of hypoxia before the test period influences sensitivity of the hypoxic response. Diminished chemosensitivity is observed after chronic hypoxia. For example, persons living at high altitude and persons with cyanotic congenital heart disease have blunted responses to acute hypoxia (33, 34), which can be reversed after successful surgery.

In pediatrics, the ventilatory response to hypoxia varies widely and differs from that of adults (82). In young infants, a transient increase in ventilation is followed by a decrease to baseline or even below. In older infants and adults, the response to hypoxia is sustained hyperventilation. In infants, environmental conditions, especially ambient temperature, profoundly affect ventilatory response to hypoxia because of the link between ventilation and metabolism. Oxygen response testing has also been used to study maturation of respiratory control. The same difficulties with rapidly changing behavioral state and rib cage distortion cloud the interpretation of ventilatory responses to hypoxia (82). Ventilatory responses to hypoxia have also been studied in severe asthmatics. Ventilatory responses were decreased, whereas occlusion pressure responses were not reduced (80, 81). These findings illustrate the limits of ventilatory response testing in the face of abnormal lung mechanics.

The methods for testing ventilatory responses to hypoxia, steady-state and non-steady-state, are less well standardized than those for CO_2 (54).

Steady-State Methods

The two approaches to steady state testing are based on different principles and have been used primarily as research tools. In the first method, the ventilatory response to hypoxia is expressed as the increase in ventilation produced by hypoxia from a series of increasingly more hypoxic gas mixtures. In the second method, the response is expressed as the increase in the ventilatory drive of central medullary CO_2 chemoreceptors caused by various levels of hypoxia. This method measures the effect of hypoxia on the slope of the line plotting V_E versus P_{CO_2} as P_{O_2} is lowered from hyperoxic (> 200 mm Hg) to hypoxic (< 40 mm Hg) levels. In both methods, the subject breathes each hypoxic gas mixture for 10 minutes. The P_{CO_2} is kept constant by adding CO_2 to the inspired gas mixture as the hypoxia-induced hyperventilation develops. Hypoxia dramatically increases the slope (i.e., the ventilatory response to hypercapnia). Because these steady-state methods require prolonged exposure to potentially dangerous levels of arterial hypoxia, clinical testing relies predominantly on non-steady-state methods.

Non-Steady-State Methods

Three non-steady-state techniques are currently in use: two are "rebreathing" and the other is a "few-breath" test. In the most popular rebreathing test, the subject rebreathes a hypoxic gas mixture containing 7% CO_2. As the hypoxia intensifies, causing ventilation and CO_2 elimination to increase, P_{CO_2} is held constant. The response to hypoxia is compared at two levels of hypercapnia. V_E is plotted against arterial P_{O_2} or arterial O_2 saturation. The advantage of using O_2 saturation instead of P_{O_2} is that the V_E-oxygenation relationship is linear when O_2 saturation is used. The slope of the line describing the relationship is increased by hypercapnia. An alternative rebreathing test uses progressive hypoxia by adding N_2 to the inspired gas mixture over a 20-minute period. In the original description of this method, ventilation was plotted as a function of a mathematical transformation of P_{O_2} that produced a linear relationship described by a slope. The greater the slope, the greater the sensitivity to hypoxia. Finally, in a simpler test, a transient drop in arterial P_{O_2} is induced by inhaling pure nitrogen for a few breaths (85). Minute ventilation is calculated from the two-breath period that coincides with the lowest oxygen saturation level (Sa_{O_2}). Hypercapnia augments the response to transient episodes of hypoxia. Because the duration of the hypoxia is brief, presumably only the peripheral chemoreceptors are stimulated.

Nonventilatory Measures of Respiratory Drive

The measurement of ventilatory responses to acute hypoxia or hypercapnia provides a useful index of respiratory output when the ventilatory apparatus (chest wall, diaphragm, abdominal muscles, lungs, and airway) is normal. When the mechanical behavior of the respiratory system is abnormal, minute ventilation fails to provide a reliable index of respiratory drive. Patients with severe asthma, kyphoscoliosis, muscular dystrophy, or obstructive airways disease are examples of conditions that may have intact chemosensitivity and respiratory drive, but abnormal ventilatory responses. Two newer methods measuring nonventilatory respiratory outputs have been used for the clinical assessment of respiratory control: (a) quantification of the diaphragmatic EMG (57) and (b) the measurement of the pressure generated by the inspiratory muscles during the first 0.1 seconds of an occluded inspiration ($P_{0.1}$) (56). Both methods need to be "driven" by input stimuli such as hypercapnia, hypoxia, or mechanical loading to make quantitative measurements.

DIAPHRAGM EMG

The electrical activity of the diaphragm is directly related to neural activity of the phrenic nerve, and thus should provide a measurement of efferent neural traffic to the diaphragm. Diaphragm EMG can be measured in two ways: (a) surface electrodes positioned over the anterior costal margin and (b) electrodes at the tip of an esophageal catheter positioned at the level of the diaphragm. These studies are technically difficult to perform. Since EMG signals depend on the conditions of the particular testing session, comparisons of absolute values of electrical activity between individuals are not useful. Lung volume and thoracoabdominal configuration also influence the responses and make standardization complicated. The esophageal method is invasive and difficult to standardize. With surface electrodes, intercostal activity can contaminate the diaphragm EMG, especially during hypercapnea resulting from the input stimuli. Although these studies have contributed greatly to our understanding of the maturation of chest wall mechanics in infants (86), the application of these techniques to clinical assessment of respiratory control in pediatrics is impractical.

$P_{0.1}$—MOUTH OCCLUSION PRESSURE

This method measures the negative pressure at the mouth generated by the inspiratory muscles during the first 0.1 seconds of an inspiratory effort made against an occluded airway. It is based on the principle that the force of an isometrically contracting skeletal muscle is directly related to the level of neural stimulation. Since there is no airflow during the occlusion, the test should be independent of mechanical problems in the respiratory system. This patient is connected to a two-way valve and a breathing circuit with separate inspiratory and expiratory lines by either a mouthpiece with nose clips or face mask. Airflow in the inspiratory line is randomly interrupted during the preceding expiration. The 0.1-second occlusion period has proved to be so brief as to be imperceptible to any conscious response. Occlusion pressures have been used to examine maturation of central chemosensitivity (87, 88). The equipment is inexpensive and the technique is quick and easy to perform, but the method still has limitations. Resting lung volume influences the measurement. The $P_{0.1}$ is reduced when functional residual capacity (FRC) is abnormally high.

AROUSAL RESPONSES

Arousal, an extremely important response in the termination of apnea, is defined as a change in state that can be induced by a variety of respiratory afferent stimuli (62). In humans, hypercapnia is a potent stimulus for arousal, whereas hypoxia appears to be less important. In addition to chemoreceptor inputs, stimuli to the larynx or tracheobronchial tree also produce arousal. Sleep state modifies arousal responses, and higher levels of stimuli are required to produce the same response in REM compared to NREM sleep. With repeated stimulation or sleep deprivation, adaptation and an increased threshold can develop. Abnormal arousal responses have been described in infants who have experienced apparent life-threatening episodes (89, 90). However, there was considerable overlap between study and control infants, precluding their usefulness in identifying respiratory control abnormalities. An abnormality in arousal responses has also been proposed as a factor contributing to the development of severe obstructive sleep apnea syndrome (91).

Limitations of Respiratory Control Measurements

The various methods for assessment of respiratory control—ventilatory responses, occlusion pressure, diaphragm EMG, and arousal—have made important contributions to our understanding of maturation of respiratory control and to the characterization of respiratory control problems in pediatrics. For example, patients with congenital central hypoventilation syndrome (CCHS) have abnormal ventilatory and arousal responses to CO_2 and O_2 during both sleep and wakefulness. Yet ventilation may be adequate during wakefulness and exercise in spite of the absence of these abnormal ventilatory responses (2). These children illustrate the powerful influence of behavioral state on respiratory control. Similar ventilatory control abnormalities can be found in patients with Arnold Chiari II or other CNS malformations. Depressed ventilatory responses are found in children with obesity-hypoventilation syndrome, Prader-Willi syndrome, hypothalamic dysfunction, and post encephalitis (11, 32, 37, 38, 48). Patients with poorly controlled asthma have decreased ventilatory responses to hypoxia, yet occlusion pressure responses are normal (80, 81), illustrating the difficulty in using ventilatory responses to assess respiratory drive in the face of lung disease.

Although the research contributions are substantial, several factors limit the clinical usefulness of these methods for assessment of respiratory control in pediatrics. First, these methods have not been standardized for children of different ages. Despite extensive experience with assessment of respiratory control in adults, the American Thoracic Society report on methods, standardization, and interpretation yielded more diversity than consensus (60). Even for the adult population, these methods have been primarily research tools that are not widely available. Since these tests are not standard care in pediatrics, research protocols with review by human investigation committees and informed consent procedures are required.

Prolonged exposure to severe hypoxia will be unacceptable for O_2 response testing in children. Since little ventilatory response to hypoxia occurs until Po_2 values fall below 60 mm Hg, changes at that end of the curvilinear response may be difficult to interpret. Second, these techniques, except arousal studies, require a connection to the airway. This means that the child must either be intubated, permit the application of a face or nasal mask (this usually means sleep or sedation), or be capable of cooperating in breathing through a mouthpiece with nose clips in place. Applying a mask to a child's face seriously distorts the normal respiratory pattern because of the added dead space and stimulation of the trigeminal nerve (63). "Non-invasive" techniques that require attachments such as nose clips, mouth pieces, tight-fitting face masks, or esophageal sensors become "invasive" in pediatrics. Barometric plethysmography is a non-invasive technique that avoids attachment to the airway. It has been used to assess ventilatory response to hypercapnia in infants, but the equipment is highly specialized (92). A child's anxiety and fear in a laboratory environment can cause hyperventilation and make the establishment of baseline ventilatory patterns difficult. These problems account for the paucity of data on respiratory control in children outside the neonatal period.

A PRACTICAL APPROACH

Since the methods for assessment of ventilatory control are primarily research tools, not readily available and difficult to perform in the pediatric age group, a practical clinical approach to patients with suspected abnormalities in respiratory control is recommended.

A variety of clinical signs and symptoms can be associated with defects in respiratory control (Table 11.2). Most children with respiratory control abnormalities will have other neurologic or other medical problems that are readily apparent on careful clinical assessment. When hypoventilation or apnea is discovered, a detailed history of respiratory behavior during sleep is needed. A history of stridor, loud snoring, struggling respiratory efforts, apnea, frequent arousals, or diaphoresis suggests serious impairment of gas exchange. Dyspnea associated with the supine position that is relieved in the upright position suggests diaphragm dysfunction. Craniofacial anomalies may be apparent on physical examination. A pectus excavatum deformity can develop in longstanding upper airway obstruction. Morbid obesity can mechanically load the chest wall and narrow the upper airway. Obesity hypoventilation syndrome may develop in obese children with pre-existing low chemosensitivity to O_2 or CO_2, or in children with hypothalamic dysfunction such as

Table 11.2.
Clinical Findings That May Be Associated with Abnormal Respiratory Control

History
Stridor
Loud continuous snoring
Struggling respiratory efforts during sleep
Observed apnea
Diaphoresis during sleep
Excessive daytime sleepiness
Severe breath-holding spells
Feeding or swallowing difficulties
Dyspnea in the supine position

Physical examination
Abnormal neurologic exam
  Cranial nerve dysfunction
  Weakness
  Hyper-reflexia
  Cerebellar abnormalities
  Loss of position or vibration sense
  Autonomic nervous system dysfunction
Adenotonsillar hypertrophy
Macroglossia
Micrognathia
Retrognathia
Pectus excavatum
Cor pulmonale unexplained by lung disease
Morbid obesity

Laboratory results
Unexplained hypercapnia $\pm$ metabolic alkalosis
Unexplained hypoxemia
Severe metabolic acidosis
Polycythemia
Hypothyroidism

Radiographic results
Cervical vertebral anomalies
Hindbrain abnormalities (Arnold-Chiari malformation; syringobulbomyelia)
Unexplained cardiomegaly $\pm$ pulmonary edema
Diminished diaphragm movement

Pulmonary function
Restrictive lung disease
Decreased inspiratory or expiratory pressures, or maximum voluntary ventilation
Inspiratory flow obstruction
Normal pulmonary function studies awake with hypoventilation asleep

Prader-Willi syndrome. A meticulous neurologic evaluation with particular attention to evidence of cranial nerve dysfunction, weakness and hyper-reflexia, loss of position and vibration sense, and cerebellar signs point to abnormalities in the cervicomedullary junction. Any specific neurologic signs require prompt evaluation with polysomnography and/or magnetic resonance imaging (MRI), focusing on the cervicomedullary junction and upper spinal cord and looking for evidence of cord compression or structural abnormalities.

The major laboratory finding in respiratory control problems is an elevated P_{CO_2} value out of proportion to the severity of the lung disease, suggesting alveolar hypoventilation. It is important from a diagnostic and therapeutic point of view to know (a) if this abnormality is present when the child is both awake and asleep or only during sleep and (b) the severity of the abnormality. Children with chronic hypoventilation can develop elevated serum bicarbonate as metabolic compensation for chronic respiratory acidosis. The severity of the problem can be determined by measurement of P_{CO_2}, but the sample must be obtained rapidly and painlessly to minimize the effects of crying or anxiety on the measurement of P_{CO_2}. Sampling from an indwelling arterial line avoids this problem, but is invasive and supplies only intermittent data. End-tidal CO_2 sampled from a nasal cannula or transcutaneous CO_2 values allow for continuous non-invasive measurement of this parameter in children. However, end-tidal recordings require maintenance of a cannula in the nostril for an extended period, and the accuracy of the reading is affected by the presence of underlying lung disease. Transcutaneous measurements may not accurately reflect arterial P_{CO_2} and are not responsive to rapid changes in CO_2. A capillary blood gas measurement can be quite helpful in infants in whom an arterial sample cannot be obtained in a timely fashion. If one chooses this approach, the extremity should be well warmed and the sample obtained quickly from a free-flowing stream of blood.

Measuring oxygen levels poses similar problems. Measurement of oxygen saturation (Sa_{O_2}) by pulse oximetry from a digital sensor provides easy, non-invasive monitoring for the presence of hypoxia. However, in children without chronic lung disease, changes in Sa_{O_2} can be subtle. Because of the shape of the oxyhemoglobin desaturation curve, a decrease in Pa_{O_2} from 100 to 60 mm Hg typically only changes the Sa_{O_2} from 99% to 90%. Recurrent hypoxia can stimulate erythropoietin and produce polycythemia.

Radiographic findings can provide important clues to the diagnosis of the cause of abnormal respiratory control. Most brainstem conditions have identifiable abnormalities on computed tomography (CT) or MRI. A notable exception is central hypoventilation syndrome (93). A cervical spine radiograph can detect an instability or congenital anomaly. Vertebral anomalies may be associated with major problems in neural tube development including hindbrain malformation and syringobulbomyelia. Serious disturbance of respiratory control including central alveolar hypoventilation, apnea, and vocal cord dysfunction has been associated with cervicomedullary abnormalities. These abnormalities are best characterized by MRI. Atlanto-axial instability or foramen magnum compression of the spinal cord can complicate skeletal abnormalities such as achondroplasia (26). Unexplained cardiomegaly and pulmonary edema can be the presenting symptom of alveolar hypoventilation. Diaphragm paralysis can be detected by carefully performed fluoroscopy.

If a child is old enough to cooperate for pulmonary function testing (≥ 6 years), certain findings may suggest respiratory control problems. In the presence of normal pulmonary function, the finding of hypoventilation strongly suggests the presence of a respiratory control abnormality. Spirometry can detect restrictive disease patterns in patients with neuromuscular weakness. Diminished maximal inspiratory and expiratory pressures can be further evidence of respiratory muscle weakness. Severe obstructive lung disease with chronic hypoxia and hypercapnia can lead to secondary blunting of the chemoreceptors. A flattening inspiratory portion of the flow-volume loop suggests fixed extrathoracic obstruction such as vocal cord dysfunction.

The clinical features and severity of most pediatric respiratory control problems can best be assessed by non-invasive continuous monitoring of multiple cardiorespiratory and neurophysiologic parameters (polysomnography). This testing uses changes in behavioral state as "input" stimuli to examine a variety of continuous outputs: respiratory frequency, Sa_{O_2}, airflow (end-tidal CO_2), respiratory effort, and heart rate. This information, with the clinical history, physical examination, and other ancillary tests should allow physicians to make appropriate patient care decisions. Consultation with an individual with expertise in the area respiratory control disorders is advised. For example, the diagnosis of congenital central hypoventilation syndrome is almost certain in the clinical context of an otherwise healthy infant who breathes normally during wakefulness, but who develops progressive hypercapnia and hypoxia during NREM sleep with REM sleep less impaired (2). In contrast, for respiratory dysfunction associated with upper airway dysfunction, gas exchange is most impaired in REM sleep, whereas it is better preserved in deep non-REM sleep. In a child without lung disease, hypercapnia with a normal or increased respiratory rate suggests hypoventilation secondary to either upper airway obstruction, neuromuscular weakness, or abnormal drive. If stridor, snoring, or paradoxical chest and abdominal movements are present, upper airway obstruction is most likely. Evidence of neuromuscular weakness should be apparent on clinical examination. In other recognizable neurologic conditions such as Arnold-Chiari malformation, polysomnography can characterize the respiratory dysfunction (obstructive vs. central hypoventilation) and its severity in terms of apnea, gas exchange impairment, associated arrhythmias, or sleep disruption. Hypothyroidism can be associated with both depressed chemosensitivity and obstructive sleep apnea. Profound metabolic acidosis and bizarre respiratory patterns can be seen in Leigh's encephalopathy.

REFERENCES

1. Lopata M, Lourenco RV. Evaluation of respiratory control. *Clin Chest Med* 1980; 1:33–45.
2. Weese-Mayer DE, Hunt CE, Brouillette RT. Alveolar hypoventilation syndromes. In: Hunt CE, Brouillette RT, Beckerman R, eds. *Respiratory control in infants and children.* Baltimore: Williams & Wilkins, 1991, pp 231–250.
3. Guilleminault C, McQuitty J, Ariagno RL, Challamel MJ, Korobkin R, McClead RE Jr. Congenital central alveolar hypoventilation syndrome in six infants. *Pediatrics* 1982; 70:684–694.
4. Haddad GG, Mazza NM, Defendi R, et al. Congenital failure of automatic control of ventilation, gastrointestinal motility and heart rate. *Medicine* 1978; 57:517–526.
5. Hunt CE, Matalon SV, Thompson TR, et al. Central hypoventilation syndrome. *Am Rev Resp Dis* 1978; 118:23–28.
6. Holinger PC, Holinger LD, Reichert TJ, Holinger PH. Respiratory obstruction and apnea in infants with bilateral abductor vocal cord paralysis, meningomyelocele, hydrocephalus, and Arnold-Chiari malformation. *J Pediatr* 1978; 92:368–373.
7. Shannon DC, Marsland DW, Gould JB, Callahan B, Todres ID, Dennis J. Central hypoventilation syndrome during quiet sleep in two infants. *Pediatrics* 1976; 57:342–346.
8. Mellins RB, Balfour HH, Turino GM, Winters RW. Failure of automatic control of ventilation (Ondine's curse). *Medicine* 1970; 49:487–504.
9. Brazy JE, Kinney HC, Oakes WJ. Central nervous system structural lesion causing apnea at birth. *J Pediatr* 1987; 111:163–175.
10. Jensen TH, Hansen PB, Brodersen P. Ondine's curse in listeria monocytogenes brain stem encephalitis. *Acta Neurol Scand* 1988; 77:505–506.
11. Brouillette RT, Hunt CE, Gallemore GE. Respiratory dysrhythmia: A new cause of central alveolar hypoventilation. *Am Rev Respir Dis* 1986; 134:609–611.
12. Liebhaber M, Robin ED, Lynn-Davies P, et al. Reye's syndrome complicated by Ondine's curse. *West J Med* 1977; 126:110–118.
13. Sarnoff SJ, Whittenberger JL, Affeldt JE. Hypoventilation syndrome with bulbar poliomyelitis. *JAMA* 1951; 147:30–34.
14. Quera-Salva MA, Guilleminault C. Post–traumatic central sleep apnea in a child. *J Pediatr* 1987; 110:906–909.
15. Kuna ST, Smickley JS, Murchison LS. Hypercarbic periodic breathing during sleep in a child with a central nervous system tumor. *Am Rev Resp Dis* 1990; 142:880–883.
16. Kelly DH, Krishnamoorthy KS, Shannon DC. Astrocytoma in an infant with prolonged apnea. *Pediatrics* 1980; 66:429–431.
17. Swaminathan S, Paton JY, Davidson Ward SL, Jacobs RA, Sargent CW, Keens TG. Abnormal control of ventilation in adolescents with myelodysplasia. *J Pediatr* 1989; 115:898–903.
18. Dure LS, Percy AK, Cheek WR, Laurent JP. Chiari type I malformation in children. *J Pediatr* 1989; 115:573–576.
19. Ruff ME, Oakes J, Fisher SR, Spock A. Sleep apnea and vocal cord paralysis secondary to type I Chiari malformation. *Pediatrics* 1987; 80:231–234.
20. Ward SL, Jacobs RA, Gaites EP, Hart LD, Keens TG. Abnormal ventilatory patterns during sleep in infants with myelomeningocele. *J Pediatr* 1986; 109:631–634.
21. Oren J, Kelly DH, Todres ID, Shannon DC. Respiratory complications in patients with myelodysplasia and Arnold-Chiari malformation. *Am J Dis Child* 1986; 140:221–224.
22. Papsozomenos S, Roessmann U. Respiratory distress and Arnold-Chiari malformation. *Neurology* 1981; 31:97–100.
23. Krieger AJ, Detwiler J, Trooskin BS. Respiration in an infant with the Dandy-Walker syndrome. *Neurology* 1974; 24:1064–1067.
24. Fremion AS, Garg BP, Kalsbeck J. Apnea as the sole manifestation of cord compression in achondroplasia. *J Pediatr* 1984; 104:398–401.
25. Pauli RM, Scott CI, Wassman ER, et al. Apnea and sudden unexpected death in infants with achondroplasia. *J Pediatr* 1984; 104:342–348.
26. Stokes DC, Phillips JA, Leonard CO, et al. Respiratory complications of achondroplasia. *J Pediatr* 1983; 102:534–541.
27. King MD, Dudgeon J, Stephenson JBP. Joubert's syndrome with retinal dysplasia: Neonatal tachypnea as the clue to a genetic brain–eye malformation. *Arch Dis Child* 1984; 59:709–718.

28. Sadarshan A, Goldie WD. The spectrum of congenital facial diplegia (Moebius syndrome). *Pediatr Neurol* 1985; 1:180–184.

29. Bokinsky GE, Hudson LD, Weil JV. Impaired peripheral chemosensitivity and acute respiratory failure in Arnold-Chiari malformation and syringomyelia. *N Engl J Med* 1973; 288:947–948.

30. Guilleminault C, Briskin JG, Greenfield MS, Silvestri R. The impact of autonomic nervous system dysfunction on breathing during sleep. *Sleep* 1981; 4:262–278.

31. Edelman NH, Cherniack NS, Lahiri S, Richard E, Fishman AP. The effects of abnormal sympathetic nervous system function on the ventilatory response to hypoxia. *J Clin Invest* 1970; 49:1153–1165.

32. DuRivage SK, Winter RJ, Brouillette RT, Hunt CE, Noah Z. Idiopathic hypothalamic dysfunction and impaired control of breathing. *Pediatrics* 1985; 75:896–898.

33. Edelman NH, Lahiri S, Braudo L, Cherniack NS, Fishman AP. The blunted ventilatory response to hypoxia in cyanotic congenital heart disease. *N Engl J Med* 1970; 282:405–411.

34. Severinghaus JW, Bainton CR, Carecelen A. Respiratory insensitivity to hypoxia in chronically hypoxic man. *Respir Physiol* 1966; 1:308–334.

35. Orenstein DM, Boat TF, Owens RP, et al. The obesity hypoventilation syndrome in children with the Prader-Willi syndrome: A possible role for familial decreased response to carbon dioxide. *J Pediatr* 1980; 97:765–767.

36. Moskowitz MA, Fisher JN, Simpser MD, Strieder DJ. Periodic apnea, exercise hypoventilation, and hypothalamic dysfunction. *Ann Intern Med* 1976; 84:171–173.

37. Moore GC, Zwillich CW, Battaglia JD, Cotton EK, Weil JV. Respiratory failure associated with familial depression of ventilatory response to hypoxia and hypercapnia. *N Engl J Med* 1976; 295:861–865.

38. Riley DJ, Santiago TV, Edelman NH. Complications of obesity-hypoventilation syndrome in childhood. *Am J Dis Child* 1976; 130:671–674.

39. Zwillich CW, Sutton FD, Pierson DJ, Creagh EM, Weil JV. Decreased hypoxic ventilatory drive in the obesity-hypoventilation syndrome. *Am J Med* 1975; 59:343–348.

40. Harpey J-P, Charpentier C, Couda M, Divry P, Paturneau-Jonas M. Sudden infant death syndrome and multiple acyl-coenzyme A dehydrogenase deficiency, ethylmalonic-adipic aciduria, or systemic carnitine deficiency. *J Pediatr* 1987; 110:881–884.

41. Zwillich CW, Pierson DJ, Hofeld FD, et al. Ventilatory control in myxedema and hypothyroidism. *N Engl J Med* 1975; 292:662–665.

42. Pincus JH. Subacute necrotizing encephalomyelopathy (Leigh's disease): A consideration of the clinical features and etiology. *Dev Med Child Neurol* 1972; 14:82–101.

43. Javaheri S, Kazemi H. Metabolic alkalosis and hypoventilation. *Am Rev Resp Dis* 1987; 136:1011–1016.

44. Olsen GD, Lees MH. Ventilatory response to carbon dioxide of infants following chronic prenatal methadone exposure. *J Pediatr* 1980; 96:983–989.

45. Johnston K, Newth CJL, Sheu KR, et al. Central hypoventilation syndrome in pyruvate dehydrogenase complex deficiency. *Pediatrics* 1984; 74:1034–1040.

46. Kretzschmar HA, DeArmond SJ, Koch TK, et al. Pyruvate dehydrogenase complex deficiency as a cause of subacute necrotizing encephalopathy (Leigh Disease). *Pediatrics* 1987; 79:370–373.

47. Hunt CE, Brouillette RT. Abnormalities of breathing control and airway maintenance in infants and children as a cause of cor pulmonale. *Pediatr Cardiol* 1982; 3:249–256.

48. Hunt CE. Reversible central apnea in an infant with cyanotic heart disease. *Chest* 1980; 77:565–567.

49. Blesa MI, Lahiri S, Rashkind W, Fishman AP. Normalization of the blunted ventilatory response to acute hypoxia in congenital cyanotic heart diases. *N Engl J Med* 1977; 296:237–241.

50. Mountain R, Zwillich CW, Weil JV. Hypoventilation in obstructive lung disease. *N Engl J Med* 1978; 289:521–525.

51. Plum F, Leigh RJ. Abnormalities of central control. In: Hornbein TF, ed. *Regulation of respiration.* New York, Marcel Dekker, 1981, pp 989–1067.

52. Milic-Emili J, Whitelaw WA, Grassino AE. Measurement and Testing of Respiratory Drive. In: Hornbein TF, ed. *Regulation of breathing.* New York, Marcel Dekker, 1981, pp 989–1067.

53. Lourenìo RV. Assessment of respiratory control in humans. *Am Rev Resp Dis* 1977; 115:1–5.

54. Cherniack NS, Dempsey J, Fencl V, et al. Workshop on assessment of respiratory control in humans: I. Methods of measurement of ventilatory responses to hypoxia and hypercapnia. *Am Rev Resp Dis* 1977; 115:177–181.

55. Milic-Emili J, Anthonisen N, Bryan AC, et al. Workshop on assessment of respiratory control in humans: II. Analyses of ventilatory responses. *Am Rev Resp Dis* 1977; 115:363.

56. Milic-Emili J, Anthonisen N, Campbell EJM, et al. Workshop on assessment of respiratory control in humans: III. Measurements of respiratory pressures in assessment of ventilatory drive. *Am Rev Resp Dis* 1977; 115:365.

57. Evanich MJ, Bruce E, Eldridge FL, et al. Workshop on assessment of respiratory control in humans: IV. Measurement of electrical activity in respiratory muscles. *Am Rev Resp Dis* 1977; 115:541–544.

58. Milic-Emili J, Anthonisen N, Bryan AC, et al. Workshop on assessment of respiratory control in humans: V. The use of loads to study ventilatory control. *Am Rev Resp Dis* 1977; 115:713.

59. Turino GM, Cugell DW, Goldring RM, Jones NL, Mellins RB. VI. The use of exercise to study ventilatory control. *Am Rev Resp Dis* 1977; 115:715–716.

60. Lourenco RV. Clinical methods for the study of regulation of ventilation. *Chest* 1976; 70(suppl 1):109–195.

61. Cherniack NS. The clinical assessment of the chemical regulation of ventilation. *Chest* 1976; 70:274–281.

62. Phillipson EA, Sullivan CE. Arousal: The forgotten response to respiratory stimuli. *Am Rev Resp Dis* 1978; 118:807–809.

63. Fleming PJ, Levine MR, Goncalves A. Changes in respiratory pattern resulting from the use of a face-mask to record respiration in newborn infants. *Pediatr Res* 1982; 16:1031–1034.

64. Gilbert R, Auchincloss JH, Baule G, Peppi D, Long D. Changes in tidal volume, frequency, and ventila-

tion induced by their measurement. *J Appl Physiol* 1972; 33:252–254.

65. Berthon–Jones M, Sullivan CE. Time course of change in ventilatory response to CO2 with long-term CPAP therapy for obstructive sleep apnea. *Am Rev Resp Dis* 1987; 132:144–147.

66. Leiter JC, Knuth SL, Bartlett Jr D. The effect of sleep deprivation on activity of the genioglossus muscle. *Am Rev Resp Dis* 1985; 132:1242–1245.

67. Lopata M, Onal E. Mass loading, sleep apnea, and the pathogenesis of obesity-hypoventilation. *Am Rev Resp Dis* 1982; 126:640–645.

68. Cooper KR, Phillips BA. Effect of short-term sleep loss on breathing. *J Appl Physiol* 1982; 53:855–858.

69. Garay SM, Rapoport D, Sorkin B, Epstein H, Feinberg I, Goldring R. Regulation of ventilation in the obstructive sleep apnea syndrome. *Am Rev Resp Dis* 1981; 124:451–457.

70. Rebuck AS, Woodley WE. Ventilatory effects of hypoxia and their dependence on PCO2. *J Appl Physiol* 1975; 38:16–19.

71. Irsigler GB. Carbon dioxide response lines in young adults: The limits of the normal response. *Am Rev Resp Dis* 1976; 114:529–536.

72. Arkinstall WW, Nirmel K, Klissovars V, Milic-Emili J. Genetic differences in the ventilatory response to inhaled CO2. *J Appl Physiol* 1974; 36:6–11.

73. Peterson DD, Pack AI, Silage DA, Fishman AP. Effects of aging on ventilatory and occlusion pressure responses to hypoxia and hypercapnia. *Am Res Resp Dis* 1981; 124:387–391.

74. Byrne–Quinn E, Weil JV, Sodal IE, Filley GF, Grover RF. Ventilatory control in the athlete. *J Appl Physiol* 1971; 30:91–98.

75. Beral V, Read DJC. Insensitivity of the respiratory centre to carbon dioxide in the Enga people of New Guinea. *Lancet* 1971; 2:1290–1294.

76. Sahn SA, Zwillich CW, Dick N, McCullough RE. Variability of ventilatory responses to hypoxia and hypercapnia. *J Appl Physiol* 1977; 43:1019–1025.

77. Robinson RW, Zwillich CW. The effect of drugs on breathing during sleep. *Clin Chest Med* 1985; 6:603–614.

78. Douglas NJ. Control of ventilation during sleep. *Clin Chest Med* 1985; 6:563–575.

79. Avery ME, Chernick V, Dutton RE, Permutt S. Ventilatory response to inspired carbon dioxide in infants and adults. *J Appl Physiol* 1963; 18:895–903.

80. Smith TF, Hudgel DW. Arterial oxygen desaturation during sleep in children with asthma and its relation to airway obstruction and ventilatory drive. *Pediatrics* 1980; 66:746–751.

81. Smith TF, Hudgel DW. Decreased ventilation response to hypoxia in children with asthma. *J Pediatr* 1980; 97:736–741.

82. Bryan AC, Bowes G, Maloney J. Control of breathing in the fetus and newborn. In: Cherniack NS, Widdicombe JG, eds. *The respiratory system.* Washington, DC, American Physiological Society, 1985, pp 621–647.

83. Hirschman CA, McCollough RE, Weil JV. Normal values for hypoxic and hypercapnic ventilatory responses in man. *J Appl Physiol* 1975; 38:1095–1098.

84. Severinghaus JW. Chemical regulation of ventilation: Who needs it? *N Engl J Med* 1976; 295:895–896.

85. Edelman NH, Epstein PE, Lahiri S, Cherniack NS. Ventilatory responses to transient hypoxia and hypercapnia in man. *Resp Physiol* 1973; 17:302–314.

86. Bryan AC, Gaultier C. Chest wall mechanics in the newborn. In: Roussos C, Macklem PT, eds. *The thorax.* New York, Marcel Dekker, 1985, pp 871–888.

87. Frantz ID, Adler SM, Thach BT, Tauesch HW. Maturational effects on respiratory responses to carbon dioxide in premature infants. *J Appl Physiol* 1976; 41:41–45.

88. Cosgrove JF, Neunburger N, Bryan MH, Bryan AC, Levison H. A new method of evaluating the chemosensitivity of the respiratory center in children. *Pediatrics* 1975; 56:972–980.

89. McCulloch K, Brouillette RT, Guzzetta AJ, Hunt CE. Arousal responses in near-miss sudden infant death syndrome and in normal infants. *J Pediatr* 1982; 101:911–917.

90. Van der Hal AL, Rodriguez AM, Sargent CW, Platzker AC, Keens TG. Hypoxic and hypercapneic arousal response and prediction of subsequent apnea in apnea of infancy. *Pediatrics* 1985; 75:848–854.

91. Phillipson EA. Arousal: The forgotten response to respiratory stimuli. *Am Rev Respir Dis* 1978; 118:807–809.

92. Haddad GG, Epstein RA, Epstein MAF, Leistner HL, Marino PA, Mellins RB. Maturation of ventilation and ventilatory pattern in normal sleeping infants. *J Appl Physiol* 1979; 46:998–1002.

93. Weese-Mayer DE, Brouillette RT, Naidich TP, McClone DG, Hunt CE. Magnetic resonance imaging and computerized tomography in central hypoventilation. *Am Rev Resp Dis* 1988; 137:393–398.

12

Exercise Testing

BRUCE G. NICKERSON

Exercise testing is an enormously helpful strategy for evaluating a child with pulmonary complaints. It can be used to elicit symptoms and physiologic findings that are not apparent to routine pulmonary function testing. A wide variety of methods of exercise testing are available. These range from a simple physical examination before, during, and after running down a hallway to sophisticated multichannel monitoring of precise exercise protocols. All these techniques have the goal of providing the clinician or researcher with a better understanding and a quantitative measure of the patient's physiologic response to exercise. Like other pulmonary function tests, exercise testing is a particularly valuable way of following the course of diseases such as interstitial pneumonitis and the response to therapy. Exercise testing allows the clinician to make or refute a number of diagnoses and to formulate a therapeutic program and/or conditioning prescription. Exercise testing provides a measurement of the patient's reserve above the resting state and can be used to explain symptoms, quantitate disability, and follow the progression of disease and the response to therapy.

The clinician should gain experience with different ages of children and severity of disease in order to develop judgement on choosing the type of exercise, the size of the increments of work, and interpretation of the physiologic response (1).

Assessing which organ system limits exercise is an important determination in exercise testing. Exercise is usually limited by cardiac and circulatory factors. In patients with lung disease, the mechanics of ventilation or gas exchange may limit exercise. In deconditioned patients the strength and endurance of the muscles involved may also limit exercise. Some patients may have pain or orthopedic and/or neurologic limitations that limit their exercise. Others may be poorly motivated or malingering. Symptoms such as bronchospasm induced by exercise may become apparent immediately after an exercise test. The clinician should carefully trace the patient's history and symptoms, design the exercise test, and pick workload increments and physiologic measurements in order to diagnose and quantitate the patient's response. The physician should select the equipment that is most suitable for the patient (treadmill vs. bicycle ergometer) and the specific question being asked. Attention should be given to safety and the ability to treat symptoms and handle untoward events, should they develop.

Prior to an exercise test, a complete medical history should be obtained that should include the patient's symptoms at rest and with exercise, as well as a history of underlying heart, lung, blood, orthopedic, neurologic, and muscle disease. A history of coronary artery disease, arrhythmia, or aortic or subaortic stenosis should be discussed with the patient's cardiologist to be sure that the proposed test would be safe. A history of cyanosis with exercise indicates the need for careful monitoring of oxygen saturation and immediate availability of supplemental oxygen. A history of cough, chest pain, tightness, or weakness associated with exercise suggests that spirometry before and after exercise should be done to look for the presence of exercise-induced bronchospasm. A history of stridor with exercise suggests that inspiratory flows and possibly fiberoptic laryngoscopy should be considered in order to look for subglottic stenosis or paradoxical vocal cord closure.

SELECTION OF THE EXERCISE TEST

Exercise testing equipment needed for a study depends on the purposes of the study and the resources available. If facilities for formal exercise testing are not available, measuring the distance a patient can run or walk around a measured track in 12 minutes is a well standardized test. Measurement of heart rate, respiratory rate, oxygen saturation, spirometry, and blood pressure before and after this simple test produces an objective physiologic record (2). In the laboratory, treadmill or bicycle tests are most commonly performed (3–5) (Table 12.1). It is best to become familiar with one of these tests in order to develop judgement of the most appropriate exercise load increments for individual patients. Useful tables are available (1). The bicycle ergometer tends to keep the chest and head more stable for easier measurement of gas exchange and EKG patterns. The workload on a bicycle ergometer can be set to compare different patients performing the same workload. Children are generally familiar with and enthusiastic about performing exercise on a bicycle ergometer. The workload can be easily adjusted in uniform steps. Calibrated bicycle ergometers are usually too large for children under the age of 7 years. They are difficult to use for individuals with cerebral palsy or orthopedic handicaps of the lower extremities. Usually a slightly lower maximum oxygen consumption is obtained with a bicycle ergometer than with a treadmill.

Treadmills are adjustable in speed and slope. Even small children quickly adapt to the treadmill. The problems of correcting workload for body size are avoided. Since conditioning is specific to muscle groups, the results of treadmill tests may be somewhat different from those obtained with a bicycle. Treadmills are somewhat larger and more expensive than bicycle ergometers.

Whichever form of exercise is used, usefulness is greatly enhanced by familiarity with it on the part of the physician and staff. This allows quick and appropriate adjustment of the workload to the capabilities of the patient.

There are numerous standardized exercise protocols. For children with lung disease I have found that a graded test with the workload increased each minute in uniform steps, with the patient's estimated maximum workload achieved in about 10 minutes, is most useful. This allows for demonstration of a fall in oxygen saturation with exercise, the anaerobic threshold (see the later section, "Ventilation"), maximum workload, and exercised-induced bronchospasm with reasonable accuracy and without the exercise exceeding the attention span or endurance of the child.

PHYSIOLOGY OF THE NORMAL RESPONSE TO EXERCISE

The following sections outline the normal pattern of response to a progressively increasing workload followed by a sudden stop with monitoring until recovery to baseline values.

Heart Rate

The heart rate increases very quickly at the onset of exercise and accelerates to match the degree of exercise. The heart rate correlates well with oxygen consumption and workload, and the heart rate response is quite reproduc-

Table 12.1.
Comparison of the Bicycle Ergometer and the Treadmill

	Advantages	Disadvantages
Bicycle ergometer	• Controlled work load • Easy to compare between subjects • Easier to monitor, less movement • Smaller and more portable • Easier to deliver and monitor respiratory gases (e.g., cold dry air)	• Unsuitable for small children • Slightly lower maximal work load • Subjects may faint with sudden stop
Treadmill	• No need to adjust for body size • Greater maximal work load • Suitable for all age groups • Patients with orthopedic handicaps may be able to use	• More difficult to monitor because of movement • Larger size and power requirements • Patients may fall off

ible for the same subject in different tests. Thus, the heart rate can be used to compare the intensity of exercise on different tests or between different laboratories or even different forms of exercise. The maximum heart rate expected for a healthy individual can be estimated as 210 minus the age in years. Most children reach a maximum heart rate of 170–190 with moderate coaxing. The heart rate usually becomes more regular with exercise as sinus arrhythmia and other rhythm disturbances disappear. After exercise, the heart rate gradually slows to baseline after several minutes. Premature ventricular contractions are sometimes seen during this recovery phase. In well-conditioned individuals the heart rate slows to baseline in 3 or 4 minutes, whereas those who are unaccustomed to vigorous exercise may take 5–10 minutes to recover fully.

Blood Pressure

The normal response of blood pressure to increasing exercise is an increase in systolic blood pressure, often closely matching the increase in heart rate. The maximum systolic blood pressure with exercise is usually 160–180. In children there is usually little change in diastolic pressure. Following exercise, there is a sudden drop in diastolic pressure because of venous pooling in the legs and a concomitant decrease in venous return to the heart. Some patients may faint if maximal exercise is suddenly stopped while they are in an upright position. This can be avoided by gradually decreasing the workload or free peddling to pump the calf muscles at the end of exercise.

Temperature

The body temperature stays stable with mild exercise and rises with moderate to severe exercise. In the typical exercise study described here, the subject's temperature will rise approximately 1°C. Obviously, the environmental temperature, humidity, and patient's clothing make a significant difference in the temperature response. Since most of the energy produced in an exercise test is heat, proper vasodilation of the skin and sweating to remove heat are crucial to an optimal exercise performance. Environmental temperature and humidity should be recorded, especially

in studies involving exercise-induced bronchospasm. In order to increase the likelihood of demonstrating exercise induced bronchospasm, the laboratory temperature should be less than 25°C, and the relative humidity should be less than 75%.

Ventilation

The response of minute ventilation to exercise occurs in three phases: With mild exercise ventilation increases in proportion to the increase in workload, heart rate, carbon dioxide production, and oxygen consumption. After the anaerobic threshold, minute ventilation increases with an even greater slope relative to workload, heart rate, and oxygen consumption and parallels carbon dioxide production. Finally, at maximum workload oxygen consumption and minute ventilation no longer increase with increasing workload.

Anaerobic Threshold

The anaerobic threshold is the level of exercise at which metabolism becomes anaerobic as marked by the appearance of lactic acid in the venous blood. The anaerobic threshold usually occurs at one-third to one-half of the maximum workload and is an important measurement to make. The anaerobic threshold as measured by gas exchange correlates well with the point at which lactic acid begins to accumulate in the blood stream. Thus, it represents the maximum level of exercise that can be sustained for long periods. Above the anaerobic threshold, the additional increase in minute ventilation above what is needed for oxygen consumption causes the Pa_{CO_2} to decrease and allows for respiratory compensation for the metabolic production of lactic acid.

The anaerobic threshold can be interpolated from a graph of minute ventilation, oxygen consumption, and CO_2 production versus workload (Fig. 12.1). It is the point at which the slope of the minute ventilation and CO_2 production increases more rapidly with respect to workload. The anaerobic threshold is more accurately defined by the ratios of minute ventilation to oxygen consumption (ventilatory equivalent for oxygen) and minute ventilation to carbon dioxide (ventilatory equivalent for carbon dioxide). The anaerobic threshold is the workload at which the ventila-

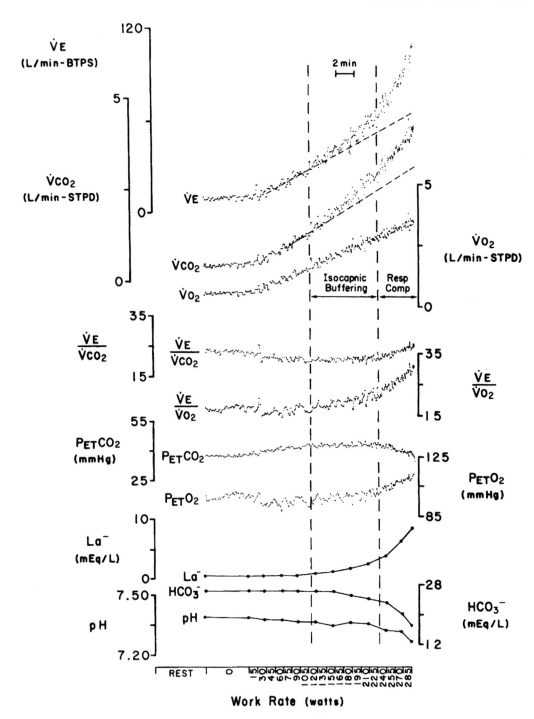

Figure 12.1. Breath-by-breath measurements of minute ventilation ($\dot{V}_E$), CO_2 output $\dot{V}_{CO_2}$), O_2 uptake $\dot{V}_{O_2}$), $\dot{V}_E/\dot{V}_{CO_2}$, $\dot{V}_E/\dot{V}_{O_2}$, $P_{ET}CO_2$, $P_{ET}O_2$, arterial lactate and bicarbonate, and pH for a 1-minute incremental work test on a cycle ergometer. The *AT* occurs when lactate increases. This is accompanied by a fall in HCO_3^- and generally an increase in $\dot{V}_E/\dot{V}_{CO_2}$. "Isocapnic buffering" refers to the period when $\dot{V}_E$ and $\dot{V}_{CO_2}$ increase curvilinearly at the same rate without an increase in $\dot{V}_E/\dot{V}_{CO_2}$, thus retaining a constant $P_{ET}CO_2$. After the period of isocapnic buffering, $P_{ET}CO_2$ decreases reflecting respiratory compensation for the metabolic acidosis of exercise. (From Wasserman K, Hansen JE, Sue DY, Whipp BJ. *Principles of exercise testing and interpretation.* Philadelphia, Lea & Febiger, 1986, p 12.)

tory equivalent for oxygen begins to increase while the ventilatory equivalent for carbon dioxide is still decreasing. The anaerobic threshold occurs simultaneously with the accumulation of lactic acidosis and is a consequence of respiratory compensation for this exercise-induced metabolic acidosis. The anaerobic threshold is a reproducible measurement and reflects the level of work that the patient can sustain for long periods. Exercise at workloads above this threshold are limited to relatively short periods by the accumulation of oxygen debt and lactic acidosis.

At maximum exercise, oxygen consumption actually plateaus with increasing workloads. This is the hallmark of a true maximum workload. Only subjects with substantial motivation are able to reach this level of work, and it can be sustained for only a minute or two, even in highly motivated patients. If this plateau is not observed, one cannot be entirely sure whether motivation or physiologic factors limited exercise. However, only about half of subjects, even under optimal circumstances, will be able to demonstrate this plateau.

Oxygen saturation or PaO_2 usually increases slightly with increased exercise. This reflects an increase in ventilation and blood flow with improved matching of ventilation to perfusion and a decrease in the alveolar arterial oxygen gradient. A fall in oxygen saturation with exercise is abnormal and indicates significant lung or cardiac disease or abnormal shunting. As exercise increases, normal subjects begin mouth breathing in order to decrease airways resistance. Normally, the tidal volume increases first with little change in exercise rate until tidal volume reaches one-half to two-thirds of the forced expiratory volume in 1 second (FEV_1). The tidal volume then plateaus at higher levels of exercise. Further increases in ventilation are achieved by increases in respiratory rate to a maximum of between 60 and 80 breaths per minute. The maximum ventilation with exercise often exceeds the predicted maximum voluntary ventilation of 35 times the FEV_1. The difference between maximum and resting ventilation defines the respiratory reserve. Following cessation of exercise, minute ventilation falls gradually to the baseline values, with reversal of the pattern in response to increasing exercise. Respiratory rate falls rapidly, and then tidal volume falls more gradually.

MONITORING

The goal of monitoring is to quantitate the physiologic and pathophysiologic response to exercise and to determine what system limits exercise. Monitoring depends somewhat on equipment available and questions being asked, but in general, the more parameters that are monitored, the more complete the understanding of the response to exercise.

The heart rate can be counted by taking a peripheral pulse. Electrocardiographic monitoring is enormously helpful. Subscapular or shoulder and precordial leads are most useful because there is less movement artifact than for limb leads. It is important to obtain a good tracing of both the P and QRS complexes. Careful skin preparation with 70% isopropyl alcohol or acetone to decrease skin resistance and securing the leads well with extra tape are very important steps, since the patient will sweat with exercise, and this may cause leads to loosen or fall off.

Pulse oximetry is the most important monitoring device for patients with lung disease. The pulse oximeter should be secured with tape and a tongue blade to reduce the amount of movement or artifact. With each recording it is important to compare the pulse rate from the pulse oximeter with electrocardiographic heart rate to be sure that rhythmic movement artifact is not causing a false reading of the pulse oximeter.

Work is the essence of exercise stress testing. For the treadmill, work is quantitated by the speed and slope of the treadmill. For an electronically braked bicycle ergometer, the work set on the dial determines the resistance to pedaling. The work set is based on a range of pedal speeds (usually between 40 and 80 rpm); the subject should be encouraged to pedal at a constant speed.

The blood pressure can be checked with an arm cuff with auscultation for Korotkoff sounds over the brachial artery. An automatic blood pressure plethysmograph is more convenient, can perform the blood pressure at regular intervals, and frees the observer. It is particularly important to check the blood pressure after exercise, since the diastolic pressures may fall and the patient may faint after suddenly stopping exercise.

Minute ventilation, tidal volume, and respiratory rate can be measured through a double-

4. Godfrey S, Silverman M, Anderson SD. The use of the treadmill for assessing exercise-induced asthma and the effect of varying the severity and duration of exercise. *Pediatrics* 1975; 56(Suppl):893–898.

5. Eggleston PA. The cycloergometer as a system for studying exercise-induced asthma. *Pediatrics* 1975; 56(Suppl):899–903.

6. Schonfeld T, Sargent CW, Bautista D, Walters MA, O'Neal MH, Platzker ACG, Keens TG. Transcutaneous oxygen monitoring during exercise stress testing. *Am Rev Respir Dis* 1980; 121:457–462.

7. Nickerson BG, Patterson C, McCrea R, Monaco F. In vivo response times for a heated skin surface CO_2 electrode during rest and exercise. *Pediatr Pulmonol* 1986; 2:135–140.

8. Monaco F, McQuitty JC, Nickerson BG. Calibration of a heated transcutaneous CO_2 electrode to reflect arterial CO_2. *Am Rev Respir Dis* 1983; 127:322–324.

9. Plaut TF. *Children with asthma—A manual for parents.* Amherst, MA, Pedipress, 1983.

10. Fitch KD, Morton AR. Specificity of exercise in exercise-induced asthma. *Br Med J* 1971; 4:577–581.

11. Anderson SD, Connolly NM, Godfrey S. Comparison of bronchoconstriction induced by cycling and running. *Thorax* 1971; 26:396–401.

12. Mellis CM, Kattan M, Keens TG, Levison H. Comparative study of histamine and exercise challenges in asthmatic children. *Am Rev Respir Dis* 1978; 117:911–915.

13. Kattan M, Keens TG, Mellis CM, Levison H. The response to exercise in normal and asthmatic children. *J Pediatr* 1978; 92:718–718

14. Green MA. Exercise-induced asthma. *N Engl J Med* 1980; 302:522.

15. Chen WY, Horton DJ. Heat and water loss from the airways and exercise-induced asthma. *Respiration* 1977; 34:305–313.

16. Strauss RH, McFadden ER, Ingram RH, Jaeger JJ. Enhancement of exercise-induced asthma by cold air. *N Engl J Med* 1977; 297:743–747.

17. Strauss RH, McFadden ER, Ingram RH, Deal EC, Jaeger JJ. Influence of heat and humidity on the airway obstruction induced by exercise in asthma. *J Clin Invest* 1978; 61:433–440.

18. Deal EC, McFadden ER, Ingram RH, Jaeger JJ. Hyperpnea and heat flux: Initial reaction sequence in exercise-induced asthma. *J Appl Physiol Respir Environ Exerc Physiol* 1979; 46:476–483.

19. Deal EC, McFadden ER, Ingram RH, Strauss RN, Jaeger JJ. Role of respiratory heat exchange in production of exercise-induced asthma. *J Appl Physiol Respir Environ Exerc Physiol* 1979; 46:467–475.

20. Deal EC, McFadden ER, Ingram RH, Jaeger JJ. Esophageal temperature during exercise in asthmatic and non-asthmatic subjects. *J Appl Physiol Respir Environ Exerc Physiol* 1979; 46:484–490.

21. O'Cain CF, Dowling NB, Slutsky AS, Hensley MJ, Strohl KP, McFadden ER, Ingram RH. Airway effects of respiratory heat loss in normal subjects. *J Appl Physiol Respir Environ Exerc Physiol* 1980; 49:875–880.

22. Haynes RL, Ingram RH, McFadden ER. An assessment of the pulmonary response to exercise in asthma and an analysis of the factors influencing it. *Am Rev Respir Dis* 1976; 114:739–752.

23. Hahn A, Anderson SD, Morton AR, Black JL, Fitch KD. A reinterpretation of the effect of temperature and water content of the inspired air in exercise-induced asthma. *Am Rev Respir Dis* 1984; 130:575–579.

24. Aitken ML, Marini JJ. Effect of heat delivery and extraction on airway conductance in normal and in asthmatic subjects. *Am Rev Respir Dis* 1985; 131:357–361.

25. Eschenbacher WL, Sheppard D. Respiratory heat loss is not the sole stimulus for bronchoconstriction induced by isocapnic hyperpnea with dry air. *Am Rev of Respir Dis* 1985; 131:894–901.

26. Edmunds AT, Tooley M, Godfrey S. The refractory period after exercise-induced asthma: Its duration and relation to the severity of exercise. *Am Rev Respir Dis* 1978; 117:247–253.

27. Morton AR, Fitch KD, Davis T. The effect of warm up on exercise-induced asthma. *Ann Allergy* 1979; 42:257–260.

28. Silverman M, Andrea T. Time course of effect of disodium cromoglycate on exercise-induced asthma. *Arch Dis Child* 1972; 47:419–422.

29. Sly RM. Effect of beta adrenoreceptor stimulants on exercise-induced asthma. *Pediatrics* 1975; 56(Suppl):910–915.

30. Shapiro GG, Pierson WO, Bierman W. The effect of cromolyn sodium on exercise-induced bronchospasm using a free-running system. *Pediatrics* 1975; 56(Suppl):923–926.

31. Godfrey S, Konig P. Suppression of exercise-induced asthma by salbutomol, theophylline, atropine, cromolyn and placebo in a group of asthmatic children. *Pediatrics* 1975; 56(Suppl):930–934.

32. Konig P, Jaffe P, Godfrey S. Effect of corticosteroids on exercise-induced asthma. *J Allergy Clin Immunol* 1974; 54:14–19.

33. Deal EC, McFadden ER, Ingram RH, Jaeger JJ. Effects of atropine on potentiation of exercise-induced bronchospasm by cold air. *J Appl Physiol Respir Environ Exerc Physiol* 1978; 45:238–243.

34. Schmidt-Nelsen K. Countercurrent systems in animals. *Scientific American* 1981; 244:118–128.

35. Cropp GA. Relative sensitivity of different pulmonary function tests in the evaluation of exercise-induced asthma. *Pediatrics*, 1975; 56:860–867.

36. Nickerson BG, Lemen RJ, Gerdes CG, Wegmann MJ, Robertson GR. Within subject variability and percent change for significance of spirometry in normal subjects or cystic fibrosis patients. *Am Rev Respir Dis* 1980; 122:859–866.

37. Petersen KH, McElhenney TR. Effects of a physical fitness program upon asthmatic boys. *Pediatrics* 1965; 35:215–299.

38. Hyde JS, Swats CL. Effect of an exercise program on the perennially asthmatic child. *Am J Dis Child* 1968; 116:383–395.

39. Keens TG. Exercise training programs for pediatric patients with chronic lung disease. *Pediatr Clin North Am* 1979; 26:517–526.

40. Nickerson BG, Bautista DB, Namey MA, Richards W, Keens TG. Distance running improves fitness in asthmatic children without pulmonary complications or changes in exercise-induced bronchospasm. *Pediatrics* 1983; 71:147–152.

41. Orenstein DM, Reed ME, Grogan FD, Crawford LV. Exercise conditioning in children with asthma. *J Pediatr* 1985; 106:556–560.
42. Wiens L, Sabath R, Ewing L, Gowdamarajan R, Portnoy J, Scagliotti D. Chest pain in otherwise healthy children and adolescents is frequently caused by exercise-induced asthma. *Pediatrics* 1992; 90:350–353.

13

Respiratory Monitoring

DAVID F. WESTENKIRCHNER

The goals of any respiratory monitoring system are to aid in diagnosis and prognosis, guide and assess therapy, alert caregivers to changes in status, and detect complications. In these ways respiratory monitoring may indicate (a) an acute need for therapy to treat or prevent respiratory failure, (b) progression of illness despite therapy, (c) improvement related to therapeutic intervention, (d) ability to maintain spontaneous ventilation, or (e) the unfortunate irreversible loss of respiratory function. Respiratory monitoring can serve as an indication of illness severity at one point in time as well as provide serial measure of changes.

Given that the major function of the respiratory system is gas exchange, two obvious categories of respiratory variables to be monitored are oxygenation and carbon dioxide removal via ventilation. Also, non–blood gas measures of respiratory system performance can be monitored. These include respiratory center function, respiratory muscle function, and respiratory mechanics. A last ill-defined category is estimation of work of breathing. These categories are outlined in Table 13.1. Some variables may be monitored easily in a clinical environment, whereas others are only research tools at this time. Technologic advances in the future may make bedside monitoring of more complex variables feasible. However, it is important to remember that a monitored variable should be used in conjunction with and cannot replace careful and repeated physical examination and bedside evaluation of the patient.

OXYGEN LEVEL

The ability of the respiratory system to contribute oxygen to the blood is of paramount

Table 13.1.
Respiratory Monitoring

Physical Examination
Oxygen level
ABG—PaO_2, SaO_2
Transcutaneous O_2
Pulse oximetry
CO_2 level
ABG—$PaCO_2$
Transcutaneous CO_2
Capnography
Respiratory drive
$P_{0.1}$
V_t/V_1
Respiratory muscle strength
P_IMax, P_EMax
NIF
Respiratory muscle endurance

importance in the maintenance of normal cellular respiration and organ function. Peripheral oxygen delivery is defined as the product of cardiac output and arterial oxygen content ($DO_2 = Q_t \times Cao_2$). Arterial oxygen content is determined by the saturation of hemoglobin and oxygen dissolved in plasma ($Cao_2 = [Hgb \times Sao_2 \times 1.34] + [Pao_2 \times 0.0003]$). The ability to monitor Pao_2 and Sao_2 is a reflection of cellular respiratory function.

Arterial Oxygen Tension

Arterial blood can be obtained by intermittent percutaneous collection or by intermittent withdrawal from an indwelling arterial catheter. Intravascular electrodes have been developed to allow continuous display of Pao_2; however, such devices have not gained wide acceptance because of technical problems (1).

Since Pa_{O_2} may not be a specific or sensitive indicator of efficiency of gas exchange because it is influenced by changes in ventilation, changes in the Fi_{O_2} and other nonpulmonary factors, various oxygenation indices have been developed to evaluate the Pa_{O_2} with respect to the Fi_{O_2}. One such index is the alveolar-arterial oxygen tension difference ($P[A-a]_{O_2}$), which is calculated as $Palv_{O_2}$ minus Pa_{O_2} when $Palv_{O_2} = [(P_B - P_{H_2O}) \times F_1O_2] - [Palv_{CO_2}/R]$ (P_B = barometric pressure, P_{H_2O} = 47 mm Hg, R = respiratory exchange ratio). The normal room air $P(A-a)_{O_2}$ of 5–10 mm Hg is not affected by changes in minute ventilation or $Palv_{CO_2}$, but this index changes unpredictability with Fi_{O_2} changes (2) and does not allow prediction of a change in Pa_{O_2} for a therapeutic change in Fi_{O_2}. However, increases in $P(A-a)_{O_2}$ occur with pulmonary dysfunction. A better index of oxygenation is the $Pa_{O_2}/Palv_{O_2}$ ratio. This ratio remains stable with changes in Fi_{O_2}. The lower limit of normal for the $Pa_{O_2}/Palv_{O_2}$ at any Fi_{O_2} is said to be 0.75 (4); lesser values signify pulmonary dysfunction. The $Pa_{O_2}/Palv_{O_2}$ ratio is more helpful for following a patient's status with serial changes in Fi_{O_2} can be used to predict the Fi_{O_2} required for a desired Pa_{O_2} (5).

Transcutaneous Oxygen Tension

Transcutaneous oxygen electrodes were developed in the early 1970s to measure oxygen values at the skin's surface. The device utilizes a small probe attached to the skin that includes a membrane-covered polarographic electrode, a heater, and a temperature-sensing thermistor. The arterialized Pa_{O_2} of the locally heated skin capillaries is measured and displayed. These devices have been used extensively in newborn intensive care units (NICUs) with good correlation between Ptc_{O_2} value and Pa_{O_2} value (6, 7). However, as skin thickness increases with age, the Ptc_{O_2} is proportionately lower than the Pa_{O_2} (8). One disadvantage of transcutaneous oxygen electrodes that has reduced their initial widespread use is a poor approximation of the transcutaneous value to the arterial value when there is poor perfusion and/or local skin hypoxia (9). They also require frequent calibration and site change to prevent local skin injury.

Arterial Oxygen Saturation

In an effort to have both an accurate and continuous monitor of oxygen, noninvasive pulse oximetry was developed in the middle to late 1970s (10). Pulse oximetry utilizes the principle of differential light absorption spectra for saturated oxyhemoglobin compared to reduce hemoglobin (11). The device consists of a probe, usually disposable, and a microprocessor/display unit. The probe is placed around a finger or toe tip, and contains a light source on one side that beams red and infrared light through the pulsating arteriovascular bed to a detector placed on the opposite side. The changing ratio of absorbed to transmitted light is measured and a microprocessor calculates Sa_{O_2}, which is continuously displayed. In some of the currently available pulse oximeters, the arterial pulse tracing may also be displayed. Under steady-state conditions, pulse oximeters measure Sa_{O_2} within 95% confidence limits of $+/- 4\%$ when the Sa_{O_2} is greater than 70%.

The reliability of pulse oximeters in pediatric patients has been demonstrated. They are able quickly to detect changes in Sa_{O_2} that may have otherwise gone unrecognized. One technical point of importance is that the pulse oximeter heart rate should be the same as an impedance-determined heart rate, or a false Sa_{O_2} value is likely to be displayed. Both technical and nontechnical factors may contribute to inaccuracy in the reading (12). In patients with very low cardiac output or peripheral perfusion the oximeter may not function correctly. Elevated carboxyhemoglobin levels, for example, in a patient with smoke inhalation, can cause the pulse oximeter reading to overestimate the true Sa_{O_2} since the oximeter cannot distinguish between oxyhemoglobin and carboxyhemoglobin (13). The same is true for the elevated methemoglobin levels (14). Skin pigmentation is known to effect the accuracy of pulse oximeters (15). Fluorescent lights may cause falsely low values, although ambient light can easily be excluded by covering the probed hand and foot with a sheet or diaper (16). A large source of error in the pediatric population is that of motion artifact causing poor pulse tracking and falsely low values. The utility of pulse oximetry in pediatrics has not been extensively investigated. Nonetheless, pulse oximeters are utilized routinely.

Beyond the technical uses, though, we find that too often medical personnel are falsely reassured by a satisfactory oxygen saturation and fail to consider the variable relationship between oxygen saturation and oxygenation at the tissue level. It is good to keep in mind that clinicians use oxygen saturation to reflect the status of oxygen content in blood. Oxygen content equals the percentage of oxygen saturation $\times$ 1.34 $\times$ Hgb gas/100 ml blood. Oxygen content can be markedly reduced by anemia although oxygen saturation remains normal. Oxygen delivery, regionally or generally, is not represented by oxygen saturation, and may be diminished in the face of a normal reading on pulse oximetry. On the other hand, pulse oximetry is not sensitive to hyperoxia because of the shape of the oxyhemoglobin desaturation curve, and should be supplemented with other measurements when high arterial pressures of oxygen are undesirable, as is the case with premature newborns.

CARBON DIOXIDE LEVEL

Arterial Carbon Dioxide Tension

The arterial carbon dioxide tension ($Paco_2$) is the best measure of ventilation. Increased $Paco_2$ is the hallmark of disorders of respiratory drive and one criterion of acute respiratory failure. Measurement of $Paco_2$ can be made from samples obtained by arterial puncture, a well-perfused capillary bed, or an indwelling arterial line. Intermittent sampling, although valuable, may miss sudden changes. Intravascular $Paco_2$ electrodes for continuous display have been developed but are even more problematic than Pao_2 electrodes (1).

Transcutaneous carbon dioxide tensions can be measured using a modified Severinghaus electrode (17). The underlying skin must be heated to 44° C to enhance carbon dioxide diffusion, but this can also cause local carbon dioxide production and thus transcutaneous carbon dioxide values higher than true arterial carbon dioxide values. Other disadvantages include technical problems, fragility of electrodes, difficult calibration procedures, and relatively sluggish response times (18).

Capnography

In healthy subjects, the end tidal carbon dioxide (Petco_2) value is normally 1 mm Hg <

$Paco_2$ and the measurement of $Petco_2$ provides a noninvasive means of monitoring arterial carbon dioxide tension (19). A capnometer measures and displays the breath-to-breath numeric values of carbon dioxide, while a capnograph also displays the wave forms of carbon dioxide during the respiratory cycle. This device operates on the principle that carbon dioxide absorbs infrared light within a narrow wavelength range. The absorption of the light is proportional to the carbon dioxide present. Monitors are of two types, side-stream or main-stream. Side-stream monitors aspirate a small sample of expired gas and transport it through a capillary tube to an infrared absorption chamber for measurement. A disadvantage of this sampling technique is the time delay for gas transport. False values may be obtained if the capillary tubing is occluded with water or secretions. Such devices are commonly used in sleep laboratories for noninvasive evaluation. Mainstream CO_2 monitors consist of a cuvette with a window in it onto which fits a small infrared CO_2 detector. Thus the analysis is performed on the main stream of gas and not on a sample drawn off into an analyzer. The problems with occlusion of a sample tube are avoided, but obviously this type of monitor is useful only if an artificial airway is in place. Its primary use is in the intensive care unit. The main-stream technique has other drawbacks in that the cuvette adds to the dead space of the breathing circuit. The weight of the device can be a problem when it is used in small infants, since it can kink the endotracheal tube. In patients requiring mechanical ventilation, $Petco_2$ may be helpful in monitoring changes in ventilatory status, guiding and assessing alterations in ventilatory status, or guiding and assessing alterations in ventilator settings, but main-stream capnometers are not used routinely outside the intensive care unit setting.

RESPIRATORY MUSCLE FUNCTION

The evaluation of respiratory muscle function can be divided into measurements of respiratory muscle strength and respiratory muscle endurance.

Inspiratory and expiratory muscle strength can be evaluated by monitoring maximum respiratory pressures. This is more commonly employed in adults and older pediatric patients. Respiratory muscle strength can be assessed by measures of maximum inspiratory pressure (Pi_{max}) and maximum expiratory pressure (Pe_{max}) obtained during inspiratory or expiratory maneuvers against an occluded mouth piece. These values depend on the lung volume at which the measurement is made, with Pi_{max} greatest following inspiration to total lung capacity. Proper performance of these tests requires patient cooperation and effort. In a child of appropriate age, the Pi_{max} or negative inspiratory force (NIF) is often employed as a criterion of ability to be weaned from mechanical ventilation. Values of NIF that are more negative than -30 cm H_2O are usually accepted as predictive of successful weaning.

The determination of respiratory pressure as NIF is helpful in evaluating patients with neuromuscular disease. We use it daily (or more often) in children with acute syndromes such as Guillain-Barré syndrome to evaluate them for impending respiratory failure. Children with weakness do not show the usual signs of respiratory distress that are based on muscle strength (retractions), and so a substitute and objective method is needed. With chronic disease, this method is helpful in long-term evaluation and can aid in making judgements regarding respiratory intervention.

Diaphragmatic muscle strength can be evaluated by measuring the pressure that can be generated across the diaphragm (Pdi). This has been measured invasively by manometric techniques utilizing transducer catheters that simultaneously measure lower esophageal (pleural) pressure and intragastric pressure. Such techniques have not been used clinically in children.

Routine spirometric measures such as lung volumes and flow rates may give practical information regarding respiratory muscle strength. Vital capacity is reduced in many forms of respiratory disease. Serial measurement of vital capacity may be used as a measure of chest wall weakness in disorders such as Guillain-Barré syndrome and myasthenia gravis. Decreases in vital capacity indicate deterioration of respiratory muscle function and can indicate the need for intubation and mechanical ventilation. In addition, measurement of vital capacity indicate the need for intubation and mechanical ventilation. In addition, measurement of vital capacity has often been used as a criterion to predict the ability to wean a patient from mechanical ventilation. It has been suggested that a vital capacity greater than 10–15 ml/kg may be used to predict successful weaning. Unfortunately, this value is an effort-dependent measurement and therefore less useful for younger pediatric patients or for those who are unable to cooperate with the measure, and its ability to predict successful weaning has been poor (22).

In addition to the measures of respiratory muscle strength, various techniques can measure respiratory muscle endurance and provide an assessment of the fatigability of the respiratory system. These include measures of transdiaphragmatic pressure response to phrenic nerve stimulation, electromyographic power spectral analysis of the diaphragm, relaxation rate of respiratory pressures, and maximum sustained ventilation (20, 21). However, these techniques have not proven useful for the clinical diagnosis of respiratory muscle fatigue because they depend greatly on patient cooperation and motivation. In addition, they are highly invasive techniques.

Although clinically attractive, the exact measure of respiratory muscle strength and fatigue remains elusive at the bedside.

PHYSICAL EXAMINATION

Despite the availability of various technologic respiratory monitors, their use is presently not widespread because of the lack of patient cooperation and motivation. Also, the predictive power of many of the monitors is low when considered individually. For these reasons, it is important to remember that monitoring is only an adjunct to careful bedside evaluation. The presence of cyanosis can be a bedside measure of arterial oxygenation. When present, cyanosis usually represents an arterial oxygen saturation of less than 80%. However, the utility of cyanosis is limited in that it can be a late finding in the assessment of respiratory failure, and there are differences between observers in their ability to detect cyanosis (12). Usually, examination of the chest is focused on auscultatory findings, but considerable information concerning the work of breathing and adequacy of respiratory muscle function can be obtained by careful observation and inspection of the breathing pattern. Simple measurement of the respiratory rate can be particularly helpful since tachypnea is an early sign of respiratory dysfunction and respiratory compromise. Another simple marker for the work of breathing is the degree of suprasternal and intercostal retractions. These can provide indirect evidence of increased pleural pressure swings (23). Patient effort can be estimated by determining the use of accessory muscles of respiration, particularly the sternomastoid muscles. Scalene and parasternal muscle recruitment during inspiration are increased as work of breathing is increased. Likewise, palpable tensing of the abdominal musculature during expiration is a marker for increased work of breathing (40). Paradoxical abdominal-ribcage movement with inward motion of the abdomen and outward motion of the ribcage during inspiration is a sign of increased work of breathing. The physical examination coupled with appropriate use of respiratory monitoring technology can provide valuable information regarding respiratory function.

REFERENCES

1. Ledingham FA, Macdonald AM, Douglas HS. Monitoring of ventilation. In Shoemaker WC, Thompson WL, Holbrook PR, eds. *Textbook of critical care*. Philadelphia, WB Saunders, 1984, pp 121–136.
2. Kanber GJ, King FW, Eshchar YR, et al. The alveolar-arterial oxygen gradient in young and elderly men during air and oxygen breathing. *Am Rev Resp Dis* 1968; 97:376–381.
3. Gilbert R, Auchincloss JH Jr, Kuppinger M, et al. Stability of the arterial/alveolar oxygen partial pressure ratio: The effects of low ventilation/perfusion regions. *Crit Care Med* 1979; 7:267–272.
4. Gilbert R, Keighley JF. The arterial/alveolar oxygen tension ratio. An index of gas exchange applicable to varying inspired oxygen concentrations. *Am Rev Resp Dis* 1974; 109:142–145.
5. Hess D, Maxwell C: Which is the best index of oxygenation—$P(A-a)o_2$, $Pao_2/Palvo_2$, or Pao_2/Fip_2? *Resp Care* 1985; 30:961–963.
6. Shoemaker WC, Vidyasagar D. Physiological and clinical significance of $Ptco_2$ and $Ptcco_2$ measurements. *Crit Care Med* 1981; 9:689–690.
7. Epstein MF, Cohen AR, Feldman HA, et al. Estimation of $Paco_2$ by two noninvasive methods in the critically ill newborn infant. *J. Pediatr* 1985; 106:282–286.
8. Tobin MJ: Respiratory monitoring. *JAMA* 1990; 264:244–251.
9. Tremper KK, Waxman KS: Transcutaneous monitoring of respiratory gases. In Nochomovitz ML, Cherniack NS, eds. *Non-invasive respiratory monitoring*. New York, Churchill-Livingstone, 1986:29–57.
10. Mauder RJ, Hudson LD: Respiratory monitoring in the intensive care unit. In Shoemaker WC, Abraham E, eds. *Diagnostic methods in critical care*. New York, Marcel Dekker, 1987, pp 33–45.
11. Wukitsch MW, Petterson MT, Tobler DR, et al. Pulse oximetry: Analysis of theory, technology, and practice. *J Clin Monit* 1988; 4:290–301.
12. Tobin MJ: Respiratory monitoring in the intensive care unit. *Am Rev Resp Dis* 1988; 138:1625–1642.
13. Barker SJ, Tremper KK. The effect of carbon monoxide inhalation on pulse oximetry and transcutaneous Po_2. *Anesthesiology* 1987; 66:677–679.
14. Eisenkraft JB. Pulse oximeter desaturation due to methemoglobinemia. *Anesthesiology* 1988; 68:279–282.
15. Ries AL, Farrow JT, Clausen JL. Accuracy of two ear oximeters at rest and during exercise in pulmonary patients. *Am Rev Respir Dis* 1985; 132:685–689.
16. Hanowell L, Eisele JH, Donns D. Ambient light affects pulse oximeters. *Anesthesiology* 1987; 67:864–865.
17. McLellan PA, Goldstein RS, Ramcharan V, et al. Transcutaneous carbon dioxide monitoring. *Am Rev Resp Dis* 1981; 124:199–201.
18. Leasa WJ, Sibbald WJ. Respiratory monitoring in a critical care unit. In Simmons DH, ed. *Current pulmonology*. Chicago, Year Book, 1988, pp 209–266.
19. Rebuck AS, Chapman KR. Measurement and monitoring of exhaled carbon dioxide. In Nochomovitz ML, Cherniack NS, eds. *Noninvasive respiratory monitoring*. New York, Churchill-Livingstone, 1986, pp 189–201.
20. Rochester DF. Tests of respiratory muscle function. *Clin Chest Med* 1988; 9:249–261.
21. Celli BR. Clinical and physiological evaluation of respiratory muscle function. *Clin Chest Med* 1989; 10:199–214.
22. Tahvanainen J, Salenpera M, Nikki P. Extubation criteria after weaning from intermittent mandatory ventilation and continuous positive airway pressure. *Crit Care Med* 1983; 11:702–707.
23. Heldt GP, Clements JA, McIlroy MB, et al. An intercostal retractometer for estimation of intrapleural pressure changes in infants. *J Appl Physiol* 1982; 52:1667–1671.
24. Pardee NE, Winterbauer RH, Allen JD. Bedside evaluation of respiratory disease. *Chest* 1984; 85:203–206.

APPROACH TO THE PATIENT WITH PULMONARY DISEASE

14

Noisy Breathing

HENRY L. DORKIN

For the most part breathing occurs quietly, so when it becomes audible, it is frequently a source of concern for parents and physicians alike. The common noises that initiate a pulmonary consultation include stridor, wheezing, snoring, and congestion. Another noise encountered in some patients with severe chronic bronchitis, asthma, or cystic fibrosis is a low pitched rumble during tidal volume breathing that can be heard several feet from the patient. This is in contrast to the patient with normal lung function, whose breathing typically can only be heard a few centimeters from the mouth. This sound most likely reflects increased turbulence at tidal volume flow rates (1). Its nondescript "white noise" quality frequently causes it to be overlooked by family members who have become accustomed to the noise. All of the other abnormal noises are of a magnitude and quality that they invariably attract attention of parents and concerned grandparents. Parents may seek consultation for their child with noisy breathing despite reassurance by the primary physician that nothing is seriously amiss. The role of the consultant is to rule out significant underlying pathology so that the family's fears can be allayed.

DEFINITIONS

Wheezing is a continuous, almost musical sound, typically heard on expiration. Wheezing arises from turbulence created by flow limitation through large and medium-sized intrathoracic airways (2, 3). Flow rates through small airways are generally insufficient to produce wheezing. The pitch of the noise depends on the flow rate and the degree of airway narrowing. Rhonchi, which are part of the wheeze continuum, are lower-pitched

sounds reflecting a lesser degree of obstruction and lower flow rates. Higher-pitched wheezes are best heard over the extrathoracic airways since the air-filled lung acts as a low-pass filter. Wheezing that originates from the trachea or major bronchi is usually monophonic, whereas that originating from lower airways will be polyphonic, reflecting the differing anatomic origins and degree of airway obstruction that contribute to the noise. This polyphonic quality is best appreciated with a stethoscope.

Stridor is a form of a wheeze, frequently a louder, harsher sound heard predominantly on inspiration. It also is generated by increased turbulent airflow secondary to obstruction in the extrathoracic trachea. The pitch of the stridor is also determined by the degree of obstruction and the velocity of airflow through the obstruction (1, 2).

Snoring is a sound produced by vibration of the pharyngeal soft tissue. It is usually a low-pitched, almost guttural sound heard on inspiration; except in extreme cases, it is heard only during sleep. In children with severe obstructive sleep apnea, this noise may take on a high-pitched, strident quality. Parents tolerate snoring perhaps more than they do any other respiratory noise.

Congestion is a catch-all term frequently used by parents. It means different things to different people and is used frequently to describe the nonspecific sound made by an infant who has increased secretions and mild narrowing of the major airways. Clinical experience allows us to correlate this noise with a variety of clinical problems. In some children, congestion is a wheeze equivalent. In others, it reflects nasopharyngitis or tracheobronchitis; if it follows a feeding or an episode of reflux, the sound is highly suggestive of aspiration. This noise is also frequently detected by feeling vibrations through the chest wall. Parents report that the child feels "rattly" when they have their hands resting lightly on the baby's chest.

When one is faced with a patient who presents with a complaint of noisy breathing, the primary goal of the evaluation is to determine if significant organic airway obstruction exists. A differential diagnosis based on the type of noise is presented in Table 14.1. As with the other chapters in this section, the material presented is heavily based on practical clinical experience.

APPROACH TO THE CHILD WITH NOISY BREATHING

One can organize the approach to this problem around the results of the history and physical examination. Frequently, the need for and type of laboratory studies will be evident at the completion of this process. The age of the patient, the acuity of onset, and the type of noise are the most helpful data (Table 14.2). The younger the patient, the more likely that a congenital lesion may underlie the problem. Was the noise present at birth or shortly thereafter? What preceded its onset? In some instances, a previously healthy infant will develop noisy breathing following a simple upper respiratory infection (URI), unmasking a previously undetected lesion such as subglottic stenosis or vascular ring. Is this a continuous or intermittent symptom? If the latter, what triggers the noise? Is this an acute problem? Is it associated with fever? If so, this suggests an infectious process (laryngotracheobronchitis, epiglottitis, tracheitis, abscess). In the adolescent, both acute and chronic recurrent stridor and wheezing have been reported as a functional (psychogenic) problem (3, 4). Typically, these patients present with very prominent noise that almost invariably disappears when the patient is asleep or thought to be unobserved. The intensity of this symptom may increase when the patient is stressed. C1 esterase inhibitor deficiency is a rare cause of acute and recurrent stridor. These patients usually manifest other symptoms, including abdominal pain and skin rash. Family history is often positive.

The quality of the noise, even as expressed in lay terms, can be very helpful in determin-

Table 14.1.
Differential Diagnosis of Noisy Breathing[a]

Stridor—acute onset

Laryngotracheobronchitis—viral croup
Epiglottitis
Spasmodic croup
Foreign body aspiration—tracheal or esophageal
Pharyngeal abscess
Trauma
Allergic reactions
Peritonsillar abscess
Angioneurotic edema
Psychogenic

Stridor—chronic

Laryngomalacia—infantile larynx
Subglottic stenosis—acquired or congenital
Laryngeal cysts, webs, hemangiomas
Vocal cord dysfunction
Laryngotrachealesophageal clefts
Retained foreign body
Epiglottic cysts—dermoid, aryepiglottic, thyroglossal duct
Laryngeal papilloma
Psychogenic

Wheezing—acute

Asthma
Viral bronchiolitis
Retained foreign body—often localized wheeze
Pulmonary hemosiderosis—associated with acute bleed

Wheezing—chronic

Asthma
Tracheomalacia
Retained foreign body
Chronic recurrent aspiration—dysfunctional swallowing, +/− GE reflux, tracheoesophageal fistula
Allergic bronchopulmonary aspergillosis
Vascular ring or sling
Tracheal stenosis

Snoring

Primary snoring—benign condition, no disruption of ventilation or sleep
Obstructive sleep apnea syndrome

Congestion

Nasal—choanal stenosis, nasopharyngitis (infection, irritant, allergic, dysfunctional swallow with nasopharyngeal reflux
Tracheobronchial—wheeze equivalent (asthma), tracheobronchitis (infectious, irritant, recurrent aspiration)

[a]These conditions are discussed in appropriate chapters.

ing the severity of the cause. Although many parents may not be able to determine if the sound occurs during inspiration, expiration, or both, it is still worth asking, especially in cases in which the sound is intermittent and not really apparent during the clinic visit. How

Table 14.2.
Differential Diagnosis of Noisy Breathing (Age, Noise, Acuity)

Stridor

Infancy—acute onset

Viral croup

Infancy—chronic

Laryngomalacia
Vocal cord dysfunction
Subglottic stenosis
Laryngeal cyst, hemangioma
Epiglottic cyst

Older child/adolescent—acute onset

Viral croup
Epiglottitis
Abscess—retropharyngeal (< 2 years), peritonsillar
Spasmodic croup
Allergic reaction
Trauma
Angioneurotic edema
Psychogenic—usually a teenager

Older child/adolescent—chronic

Subglottic stenosis
Retained foreign body
Papilloma
Laryngeal web
Psychogenic

Wheezing

Infancy—acute onset

Bronchiolitis
Asthma

Infancy—chronic

Asthma
Recurrent aspiration
Vascular ring/sling
Tracheal stenosis
Tracheomalacia
Cystic fibrosis
Environmental exposure—passive smoking

Older child/adolescent—acute

Asthma
Foreign body
Allergic reaction
Psychogenic

Older child/adolescent—chronic

Asthma
Retained foreign body
Cystic fibrosis
Vascular ring/sling
Tracheomalacia
Allergic bronchopulmonary aspergillosis
Pulmonary hemosiderosis
Psychogenic

Congestion

Infancy—acute onset

Viral nasopharyngitis

Infancy—chronic

Choanal stenosis
Recurrent NP reflux—dysfunctional swallow with aspiration
Asthma
Cystic fibrosis
Recurrent tracheobronchitis—immune deficiency, environmental pollution

Older child/adolscent

Congestion is usually not reported in the older child since symptoms are usually better defined by this age

---

loud is it? What makes it worse or better? Frequently, noise due to a dynamic obstruction (laryngomalacia, tracheomalacia) is lessened or even absent during sleep. Is the noise changed by feeding or exercise? Although snoring is heard almost exclusively during sleep, it is not the only noise that can occur during sleep. Wheezing and stridor may also occur. When the noise occurs exclusively during sleep or is dramatically affected by sleep, the physician should make every attempt to observe the sleeping child. If this cannot be accomplished during a clinic visit, the parents can be asked to obtain an audio or video tape of about 5 minutes of what they consider to be "the noise."

The next phase of the evaluation is designed to determine the clinical significance of the noise. Is this noise a social nuisance or does it compromise the child's respiratory status and well-being? In this context, increase in the work of breathing at rest associated with the noise should be assessed. Does the child retract at rest or only with exertion? For infants, this should include observation of feeding. Retractions and paradoxic respiratory movements at rest indicate more severe obstruction. What is the pitch of the noise? The higher the pitch, the more severe the obstruction. What is the child's growth and development status? Failure to grow is an important sign of clinically significant respiratory dysfunction. Is digital clubbing or evidence of pulmonary hypertension present? Does the child appear bothered by the noise? This is important in separating a benign condition such as laryngomalacia from a more significant lesion. Is there increased work of breathing? For noise that occurs during sleep, do the parents ever feel the need to intercede because they are concerned that the child is in significant danger? We have found that this correlates well with the severity of the obstructed breathing during sleep (5, 6).

Another important component of the history is the parents' perception of the significance of the problem. How concerned are they about the noise? Have other family members had similar problem and what was the outcome? It is also important to determine what other family members, especially grandparents, have said about the noise. Often, the mother of an infant with laryngomalacia is constantly harassed by concerned grandparents and other well-intentioned relatives that something must be wrong. If they listen to this harangue long enough, they begin to believe it. Consequently, parental concerns must be factored into the decision of how far to go with an evaluation, since a thorough work-up may be the only way to convince everyone that the infant will be fine.

The physical examination can be used to localize the source of the noise. From a physiologic standpoint, obstructing lesions of the upper airways (the region responsible for most of the noise) can be categorized by location (intrathoracic vs. extrathoracic) and by type (fixed vs. variable) (Table 14.3) (7, 8). *Fixed lesions* are those whose airway resistance does not change with phase of respiration. The resistance of *variable lesions*, on the other hand, changes with the location of the obstruction

(intrathoracic vs. extrathoracic) and on the phase of respiration. Noise that occurs on both inspiration and expiration suggests a fixed lesion that could be either intrathoracic or extrathoracic. However, the increased compliance of the airway of the child may help refine the diagnosis. If the infant or child can be made to breathe more forcefully, an additional dynamic obstruction may develop below an extrathoracic lesion and above an intrathoracic one. This will result in a worsening of the airflow on inspiration or expiration, depending on the location of the fixed obstruction. Variable lesions are easier to detect. A variable intrathoracic obstruction affects expiration primarily, since the variable lesion is dilated on inspiration by the negative intrathoracic pressure surrounding this airway. An extrathoracic variable obstruction is worse on inspiration and improves during expiration, since the positive intraluminal pressures distend this portion of the airway.

LABORATORY EVALUATION OF NOISY BREATHING

The options available to evaluate noisy breathing are fairly limited and are discussed in detail in the sections on diagnostic technology and under the specific conditions. In general terms, the choice of a particular diagnostic study is determined by the age of the patient, the acuity of onset of the noise, the degree of respiratory distress, and lastly the type of noise. This evaluation is summarized in Table 14.4. In most instances, the initial step in evaluating the child with noisy breathing is to obtain anteroposterior (AP) and lateral chest radiographs. If performed correctly, these can provide important screening information. On a routine chest radiograph, an air tracheobronchogram should be apparent in both the AP and lateral projections. Loss of this tracheal air column in the AP projection or a decrease in the AP diameter on the lateral view suggests tracheal narrowing (Fig. 14.1). Similarly, deviation of the tracheal air column from its usual position, leaning towards the right hemithorax, suggests the presence of extrinsic compression of the airway usually by vascular structures (10). This radiograph will also provide information on the presence of lower respiratory tract disease, including the possibility of a foreign body. Coupled with the findings of the history and physical exami-

Table 14.3.
Patterns of Upper Airway Obstruction

	Intrathoracic	Extrathoracic
Fixed	Noise occurs on both inspiration and expiration[a]	
Variable	Expiration: Wheeze dominates	Inspiration: Stridor dominates

[a]In young children, increased airway compliance may add a variable component to the findings of a fixed obstruction; for example, dynamic narrowing of the airway below a fixed extrathoracic obstruction will result in inspiration being affected more than expiration.

Table 14.4.
Diagnostic Evaluation of Noisy Breathing

Condition	Diagnostic Studies
Stridor—acute onset	
Laryngotracheobronchitis	AP neck radiograph
Epiglottitis	Lateral neck radiograph and/or direct visualization in a controlled setting
Spasmodic croup	History alone diagnostic
Foreign body aspiration	Inspiratory/expiratory radiograph, R and L lateral decubitus films, fluoroscopy, barium swallow for esophageal FB, rigid bronchoscopy
Pharyngeal abscess	Lateral neck radiograph
Trauma	History alone
Allergic reactions	History of exposure
Peritonsillar abscess	History and PE of pharynx
Angioneurotic edema	History, C_1 esterase inhibitor level
Stridor—chronic	
Laryngomalacia	History, fiberoptic laryngoscopy
Subglottic stenosis	History, PFT, bronchoscopy
Laryngeal cysts, webs, hemangiomas	Laryngoscopy
Vocal cord dysfunction	Laryngoscopy
Laryngotrachealesophageal clefts	Suspension laryngoscopy
Retained foreign body	Bronchoscopy
Epiglottic cysts	Laryngoscopy
Laryngeal papilloma	Laryngoscopy
Wheezing—acute	
Asthma	History PFT and bronchodilators
	Trial of bronchodilators in those too young to do PFT
Viral bronchiolitis	History, age, seasonal
Retained foreign body	Bronchoscopy
Pulmonary hemosiderosis	History, chest radiograph, CBC
Wheezing—chronic	
Asthma	As above for acute asthma
Tracheomalacia	Fluoroscopy, flexible bronchoscopy
Cystic fibrosis	Sweat chloride
Retained foreign body	Bronchoscopy
Aspiration—dysfunctional swallowing	Cine-swallowing study, bronchoscopy and lavage
GE reflux	Barium swallow, ph probe bronchoscopy and lavage
Allergic bronchopulmonary aspergillosis	Total and specific IgE
Vascular ring or sling	Barium swallow, MRI
Tracheal stenosis	High-resolution CT, bronchoscopy
Mediastinal nodes or mass	Chest radiograph, CT
Snoring	
Primary snoring	Polysomnography
Obstructive sleep apnea	Polysomnography
Congestion	
Nasal:	
Choanal stenosis	Pass 8-French catheter
Nasopharyngitis	H&P C&S, Gram stain secretions
Tracheobronchial:	
Wheeze equivalent (asthma)	PFT, bronchodilator
	Bronchoprovocation
Tracheobronchitis (infectious, allergic, aspiration)	Sputum C&S, Gram stain, flex bronchoscopy

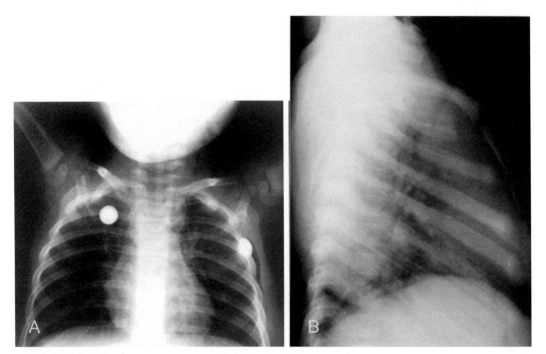

Figure 14.1. AP and lateral chest radiographs from a child with suspected tracheal obstruction. Note the loss of the air column above the carina in the AP projection *(A)* and the corresponding narrowing of the trachea seen on the lateral view *(B)*.

nation, this study will also determine the next best test. Chronic recurrent wheezing or biphasic noise with a dominant expiratory component is an indication for a barium swallow with airway fluoroscopy to rule out a vascular ring. In general, chronic noisy breathing, especially stridor, is best handled by proceeding to flexible fiberoptic bronchoscopy rather than performing other radiographic studies, which are not likely to yield a definitive diagnosis. In the older child (> 5 years), pulmonary function tests (inspiratory/expiratory

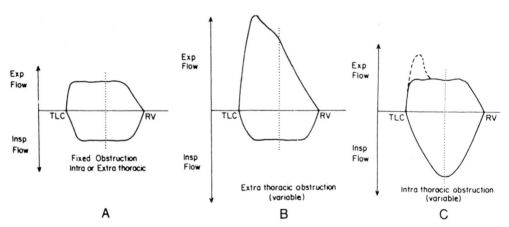

Figure 14.2. Flow-volume curve depicting the various types of upper airway obstruction. *A,* A fixed obstruction evidenced by flattening of both the inspiratory and expiratory flow volume curves. *B,* A variable extrathoracic obstruction evidenced by flattening of the inspiratory curve associated with a normal expiratory limb. *C,* A variable intrathoracic obstruction evidenced by flattening of the expiratory portion of flow-volume curve with a normal inspiratory limb. (From Kryger M, Bode F, Antic R, et al. Diagnosis of obstruction of the upper and central airways. *Am J Med* 1976; 61:85–93.)

flow volume curves) can assist in identifying the upper airway as the source of the noise (11) (Fig. 14.2). This information may also be available from tidal volume flow volume curves or partial flow/volume curves obtained in infants.

CONCLUSIONS

Noisy breathing is a common clinical problem in children, and as with the other respiratory symptoms presented in this section, may be either a benign process that will resolve with simply the tincture of time or the marker of a significant respiratory disorder. The pulmonary consultant's role is to make this determination as quickly and efficiently as possible so that therapy, if necessary, can be instituted, and the parent's concerns can be addressed.

REFERENCES

1. Forgacs P. The functional basis of pulmonary sounds. *Chest* 1978; 73:399–405.
2. Hollingsworth HM. Wheezing and stridor. *Clin Chest Med* 1987; 8:231–240.
3. Murphy RLH, Holford SK: Lung sounds. *ATS News* 1980; 8:24–29.
4. Rogers JH. Functional inspiratory stridor in children (case report). *J Laryngol Otol* 1980; 4:669–670.
5. Barnes SB, Grob CS, Lachman BS, Marsh BR, Loughlin GM. Psychogenic upper airway obstruction presenting as refractory wheezing. *J Pediatr* 1986;109:1067–1070.
6. Carroll JL, McColley SA, Marcus CL, Pyzik P, Curtis S, Loughlin GM. Can childhood obstructive sleep apnea syndrome be diagnosed by a clinical symptom score? *Am Rev Resp Dis* 1992; 145:A179.
7. Carroll JL, McColley SA, Marcus CL, Pyzik P, Curtis S, Loughlin GM. Reported symptoms of childhood obstructive sleep apnea syndrome (OSA) vs primary snoring. *Am Rev Resp Dis* 1992; 145:A177.
8. Loughlin GM and Taussig LM. Upper airway obstruction. *Semin Respir Med* 1979; 1:131–146.
9. Miller RD, Hyatt RE. Obstructing lesions of the larynx and trachea: Clinical and physiologic characteristics. *Mayo Clin Proc* 1969; 44:145–161.
10. Chang LWM, Lee FA, Gwinn JL, Normal lateral deviation of the trachea in infants and children. *Am J Roentgenol* 1970; 109:247–251.
11. Kryger M, Bode F, Antic R, et al. Diagnosis of obstruction of the upper and central airways. *Am J Med* 1976: 61:85–93.

debility, neuromuscular disease, or abdominal or chest surgery. Laryngeal disorders can be accompanied by ineffective glottic closure. As a result, a child with vocal cord paralysis or a nasotracheal or tracheostomy tube cannot cough as effectively as a child with a normal airway. And finally, because an effective cough requires high flow rates through stable airways, some children with bronchomalacia or tracheomalacia have ineffective coughs, as do children with widespread bronchopneumonia, severe asthma, or cystic fibrosis.

ACUTE VERSUS CHRONIC COUGH

The most common stimulus of cough is irritation or inflammation of the respiratory epithelium. At all ages viral upper respiratory tract infections (URIs) are responsible for most acute cough episodes. Cough due to a URI is most often nonproductive or minimally productive, lasts approximately 1 week, and is self-limited. As a general rule, a child with a cough of less than 3 weeks' duration, precipitated by a URI, in the absence of other symptoms, and with a normal physical examination does not need an extensive work-up. The parents of this child should be reassured; the protective and self-limited nature of cough should be explained; and the parents should be instructed to bring the child back if the cough persists.

A cough that lasts beyond 3 weeks is distinctly unusual for a simple URI and thus warrants an evaluation to identify the underlying condition so that specific therapy can be instituted.

A DIAGNOSTIC APPROACH TO THE CHILD WITH CHRONIC COUGH

History

The first step in the assessment of the child with a chronic cough is to determine the exact nature of the patient's and /or parent's major concern or complaint (Table 15.1). Important questions to ask include whether the cough is productive or dry and tight, single or paroxysmal. Expectoration is not the only criterion of a productive cough, since the young child usually swallows what he or she coughs up. Other questions include the following: When does the cough occur (time of day or year)? Does it persist during sleep? What does it

Table 15.1.
Evaluation of the Child with Chronic Cough

History
  Age of onset
  Nature (dry vs. productive), timing of the cough (day, night, during sleep, following exercise), associated symptoms (wheeze)
  Precipitating factors
  Characteristics of sputum
  Environmental or seasonal influences
  Response to previous therapy

Physical Examination
  Growth and development
  Nutritional status
  Digital clubbing
  Upper respiratory tract—signs of sinusitis, nasal polyps, allergic shiners
  Chest examination—crackles, rhonchi, wheeze, hyper-resonance

sound like? Are there any associated findings (fever, wheezing, shortness of breath)? Has it occurred before and, if so, how long does a typical illness last?

An important part of the history is to determine what makes the cough better or worse. Specifically, ask whether the common triggers of asthma (such as activity, laughing or crying, exposure to cold air or changes in the weather, exposure to irritants such as cigarette smoke, wood stove, or kerosene heater, or aeroallergens such as dog or cat dander, dust, or pollens) make the cough worse. Have previous therapies such as bronchodilators or antihistamines/decongestants improved the cough? What specific medications were used and what were the dosages and duration of therapy? Failure to respond to bronchodilator therapy is frequently seen, even in patients with cough asthma because of inadequate dosing and duration of therapy.

In addition to the cough, are other symptoms present? Has the child recently lost weight or had a difficult time gaining weight? Does the child appear chronically ill? Episodes of cough associated with high fever or infections in other parts of the body may suggest a child with immune dysfunction.

A good history will provide valuable clues to the diagnosis of cough. For example, a productive cough that begins after assuming a reclining position suggests postnasal drip or gastroesophageal reflux. A paroxysmal cough suggests pertussis, chlamydia, or a foreign body. Recurrent cough with wheezing may be due to tracheobronchial obstruction (e.g., asthma, foreign body, mediastinal tumor, or cystic fibrosis). A cough associated with swallowing or feeding suggests aspiration into the tracheobronchial tree, which may be due to gastroesophageal reflux, incoordination of swallowing due to neurologic impairment or, infrequently, a tracheoesophageal fistula (TEF). Cough with aphonia or dysphonia suggests a laryngeal foreign body, laryngeal papillomatosis, croup, or psychoneurosis. A ringing, brassy cough suggests tracheal irritation as seen in the tracheitis of rubeola. A croupy cough like the bark of a seal or a dog indicates glottic or subglottic disease. Hemoptysis may result from vigorous coughing of any cause, but foreign bodies, cystic fibrosis, bronchiectasis, pulmonary hemosiderosis, and tuberculosis should be considered. In a child with recurrent ear and sinus infections, immotile cilia syndrome and immune deficiency states (IgG, IgA, or IgG subclasses) should also be considered.

Physical Examination

Important elements of the physical examination of the child with chronic cough are presented in Table 15.1. Signs of atopy, when present, may include fluid or infection in the middle ear, allergic shiners, Dennie crease across the nasal bridge from allergic rhinitis, nasal discharge, or polyps (also seen in cystic fibrosis). In the child with asthma, the physical examination may be normal or reveal evidence of an increased anteroposterior diameter of the chest, retractions, wheezes, or crackles. Important physical findings in children with cough due to other etiologies include tracheal deviation suggestive of a collapsed lung or mediastinal mass, cobblestoning of the posterior pharynx suggestive of postnasal drip, a heart murmur suggestive of cardiac disease, and digital clubbing, which is most commonly seen in children with cystic fibrosis, bronchiectasis, and cyanotic congenital heart disease. A thorough examination of the ears looking for a foreign body is essential. Although it is unusual, stimulation of the external acoustic meatus, supplied by the auricular nerve (Arnold nerve), or stimulation of a branch of the vagus by a foreign body or excessive wax in the canal, can cause a cough.

The presence of crackles, wheezes, and rhonchi is not diagnostic in the child with cough but does indicate significant lower respiratory tract disease.

Laboratory Evaluation

The typical cough associated with an acute viral infection should not require any lab tests. However, in the child with a chronic cough, the laboratory evaluation can be divided into screening studies that should be obtained as part of the initial evaluation, and more specific tests that are guided by the results of the history and physical examination. This approach is outlined in the Table 15.2.

ETIOLOGY OF COUGH

In developing a differential diagnosis in a child with a cough, the age of the patient is particularly helpful. A differential diagnosis based on age is presented in Table 15.3. Certain conditions deserve further comment.

Cough in Infants

Cough in an infant is abnormal and should be investigated. Diagnostic considerations include congenital anomalies such as tracheoesophageal fistula and congenital heart disease with congestive heart failure, gastroesophageal reflux with aspiration, infection with *Bordetella pertussis* or *Chlamydia trachomatis*, cystic fibrosis, and perhaps the most common cause, involuntary exposure to cigarette smoke.

C. trachomatis infection has been recognized as a significant cause of pneumonia in young infants (8). Typically, these infants have tachypnea and a high-pitched, staccato, nonproductive cough that begins usually around 4 weeks of age; 50% of these infants have a history of conjunctivitis. Infants with chlamydia may cough for several weeks even after therapy with erythromycin.

Despite the availability of immunization, pertussis remains a serious health problem today. Immunization does not protect all children who receive it, and some parents neglect or fear having their children immunized. Moraxella catarrhalis can also produce cough and lower respiratory tract disease, especially in young children with lung disease or a tracheostomy (9).

Cough associated with feeding is typically seen in infants with dysfunctional swallowing

Table 15.2.
Laboratory Evaluation

Acute—in the absense of localized physical findings in the chest or upper airway, signs of sinusitis, or evidence of systemic infection, no lab tests are needed. These findings support obtaining a chest radiograph, CBC with differential, and/or sinus films.

Chronic—all patients should have a recent chest radiograph. If available, old films should be reviewed. Patients older than 5 years should have pulmonary function measured before and after use of bronchodilators. The following studies should be obtained based on the results of the history, physical examination, and the above findings and chest radiograph data.

Test	Indication
Sweat chloride	• Should at least be considered in all patients referred • Indicated in all patients with radiograph, failure to thrive, steatorrhea, productive cough + for *P. aeruginosa* or *S. aureus,* those whose cough is unresponsive to bronchodilators and routine antibiotics, and those with a positive family history.
Sinus radiographs	• Should be considered in child with purulent upper resipratory tract secretions, cough that is worse in the supine position, frontal headaches, and tenderness to percussion over the sinuses • Sinus computed tomography (CT) rather than plain radiography is the preferred mode of assessment, especially in the younger patient whose sinus cavities may be underdeveloped, making identification of an infection causing opacification very difficult
Barium studies (cine esophagram, swallowing study)	• Cough associated with feeding • Isolated coughing and/or choking after feeding • Cough associated with stridor or wheezing localized to a major airway
Immunology studies (IgG, A, M. & E) IgG subclasses	• Cough associated with chronic recurrent otitis • Bronchiectasis • Productive cough unresponsive to appropriate antibiotics
Cilia function studies	• Purulent otitis unresponsive to antibiotics • Above associated with sinusitis, bronchiectasis, or situs inversus

(Chapter 44) or with structural abnormalities such as a TEF or laryngeal tracheoesophageal cleft (Chapter 40). Similarly, sudden coughing episodes in an infant associated with gagging, choking, or chewing-like movements is suggestive of a diagnosis of gastroesophageal reflux (Chapter 44).

Passive Smoking

The incidence of chronic cough and pneumonia in infants in the first year of life is increased if one parent smokes, and is further increased if both parents smoke (10). Involuntary exposure to parental smoking is an independent risk factor for serious chest illness prior to 2 years of age (11). Passive smoking may also affect long-term pulmonary function as evidenced by decreased expiratory flow rates in teenage athletes exposed to parental smoke (12). Once children are removed from con-

stant exposure to cigarette smoke, parents often notice a rapid resolution of the cough.

Cystic Fibrosis

Cystic fibrosis (CF) is one of the most important causes of chronic cough in children (Chapter 22). It can present at any age, and chronic cough may be the only early manifestation of CF. Failure to thrive due to pancreatic insufficiency is not a prerequisite, since normal pancreatic function and normal growth are present in 10–20% of infants with CF during the first year of life (13). In a child of any age, the presence of digital clubbing should suggest CF.

Aspiration

Chronic cough secondary to aspiration is becoming increasingly common in young

Table 15.3.
Causes of Chronic Cough by Age

Infancy

Aspiration: Dysfunctional swallowing (developmental delay, CNS injury); gastroesophageal reflux; congenital malformations (Laryngotracheoesophageal cleft, H-type TEF)

Asthma: Wheezy bronchitis, asthmatic bronchitis

Congenital malformations: Laryngotracheomalacia or bronchomalacia; vascular compression (ring, sling innominate artery)

Cystic fibrosis

Infection: Viral: Parainfluenza, respiratory syncytial, adenovirus, cytomegalovirus influenza (uncommon in infants); pertussis; *Chlamydia, Pneumocystis, Ureaplasma,* maternally acquired *M. tuberculosis*

Miscellaneous: Passive smoking/environmental pollution; congenital heart disease with L-R shunt or pulmonary venous obstruction; idiopathic pulmonary hemosiderosis

Early Childhood

Aspiration: Retained foreign body

Asthma: Cough variant, asthmatic bronchitis

Bronchiectasis: Cystic fibrosis; postinfectious; immotile cilia syndrome; immunodeficiency syndrome (IgG, IgA, IgG subclasses, common variable immune deficiency, AIDS)

Chronic middle ear disease: Sinusitis infection: post viral infection especially influenza; Bacterial: *H. influenza, Moraxella catarrhalis, Mycoplasma, M. tuberculosis*

Pulmonary hemosiderosis

Late Childhood and Adolescence

Asthma

Brochiectasis: Postinfectious

Immotile cilia syndrome

Immunodeficiency syndrome

Cystic fibrosis

Infection: Viral; mycobacterial; mycoplasmal; fungal (histoplasmosis, coccidiomycosis)

Middle ear disease

Smoking (active, passive)

Occupational exposures

Psychogenic cough

Sinusitis/postnasal drip

Tumor

---

infants and those with neurologic impairment. Typically, symptoms are temporally related to feeding. Gastroesophageal reflux can cause cough either because of microaspiration of gastric contents into the lungs or reflex stimulation of the vagus nerve (14).

Sinusitis (Postnatal Drip)

Whether postnasal drip, with or without sinusitis, can cause chronic cough remains controversial (15). Typically the cough secondary to sinusitis is exacerbated in the supine position (Chapter 43). Adults with postnasal drip report a sensation of something dripping into the throat accompanied by frequent throat clearing. Although data in children are limited, clinical experience suggests that frequent throat clearing is also common in children with postnasal drip/sinusitis. On physical examination, mucoid or mucopurulent secretions are noted in the posterior pharynx, and the mucosa has a cobblestone appearance caused by chronic stimulation of submucosal lymphoid follicles.

In a study of adult patients with chronic cough, 30% were found to have postnasal drip as the sole cause of their cough (16). All of these adults responded to a combination of decongestants, antihistamines, nasal sprays, and antibiotics. In another study involving children with poorly controlled asthma and chronic cough, antibiotic therapy for sinus infection resulted in improved asthma control in 80% of the children (17).

Asthma: Wheezy Bronchitis, Asthmatic Bronchitis

The most common cause of chronic cough in children of all ages is asthma (18–20). Chronic cough can be the sole manifestation of asthma in children (Chapter 21). These children respond to bronchodilator and steroid therapy like other children with asthma. While cough has long been recognized as a symptom of bronchospasm in children known to have asthma, it has only recently been recognized as the only symptom of airway hyper-reactivity in children (18–20).

Cough in Adolescents

Since the Surgeon General's 1964 report on the hazards of smoking, the incidence of smoking among youths, especially adolescent girls, has risen dramatically (21). Mild conjunctivitis can sometimes be a telltale sign that an adolescent has been smoking in a closed room. Obtaining a history of smoking can be difficult, especially in the adolescent smoking against parental wishes. Thus, a history should be obtained with the parents excused. Confidentiality can be assured, increasing the chances of obtaining an accurate history.

Mycoplasma pneumoniae infection is common in this age group and may present with cough only (22). Positive cold agglutinins support the diagnosis, although a negative test does not exclude the diagnosis. Isolation of the organism from sputum is possible, and specific titers for mycoplasma (acute and convalescent) can be helpful in confirming clinical suspicion. However, in the appropriate clinical setting, an empiric trial of erythromycin is in order, since the results of these lab tests are not immediately available.

Psychogenic Cough

A psychogenic cough or cough tic should be considered in a child in whom no cause of cough can be detected after a thorough history, physical examination, and laboratory evaluation (23, 24). This is a diagnosis of exclusion, but is suggested when a cough dis-appears at night or when the child is distracted. There are two types of psychogenic cough. The most common is the perpetuation of a cough that was initially due to a viral infection. Airway irritation perpetuates the cough and parental anxiety and attention rewards the behavior. The other type of psychogenic cough usually has an explosive, barking, or crowing quality (like a Canadian wild goose) and is exacerbated when attention is drawn to it. A peculiar chin-on-chest posture with the hand held against the throat has been described in some patients while coughing; the cough is thought to be psychosomatic, due to emotional stress. The most common contributing cause of psychogenic cough in children is school phobia, which must be addressed with both child and parents. Cough suppressants are ineffective in relieving the psychogenic cough. Drinking water, sucking on a throat lozenge, or feedback coupled with an open discussion with the child and his family that addresses possible etiologic factors are effective measures in treating these children. However, before this is done, it is essential that a thorough work-up be performed. Sporadic testing can be misleading to the patient and can further heighten anxiety in the child. If the physician wants to make a diagnosis of a functional cough, he or she should be confident that there is no organic disease and stop ordering tests and new therapies.

Tumors

Mediastinal cysts and tumors may present as chronic cough and chest pain, as acute respiratory distress, or as an incidental finding on a chest radiograph. The most common causes of a widened mediastinum include malignant neurogenic tumors and bronchogenic cyst or esophageal duplication followed by teratoid cysts and tumors, lymphomas, thymic hyperplasia or cyst, and hemangioma or cystic hygroma.

TREATMENT OF CHRONIC COUGH

The treatment of chronic cough must be directed at the cause. In a study of adults with chronic cough, a specific diagnosis was made in 92% of patients; symptoms resolved with specific therapy in 98% (16). Such a goal also seems reasonable in children with chronic cough.

Reasonable standards of care in prescribing antitussive drugs have been proposed by the American Academy of Pediatrics Committee on Drugs (25). Since cough is a symptom of a disorder, the presence of cough is not always an indication for specific antitussive therapy. Cough associated with chronic pulmonary disease should not be suppressed but treated. Short-term symptomatic relief of a mild cough associated with the "common cold" or uncomplicated viral upper respiratory tract infection has not been proven to be either safe or harmful, or for that matter effective. These medications are discussed in more detail in Chapter 57. One study found no difference in clinical symptoms in children treated with brompheniramine, placebo, or no treatment for the common cold (26). That same study, however, pointed out that whether a treatment was successful or not depended more on whether the parent wanted medicine or not. Cough should be presented to patients and parents as a natural, protective, and beneficial mechanism and not "something to be stopped at all costs." Specific contraindications to centrally acting antitussives are the acute phase of pertussis and an acute asthma attack, since inspissated mucus plugs can lead to death.

Centrally active antitussive agents should rarely be prescribed for children less than 1 year old. Established safe doses for the use of antitussives in children are lacking. Symptomatic treatment of cough may mask serious underlying disease and delay its diagnosis. By suppressing cough, small airways may become plugged with thick mucus, thus increasing the morbidity and mortality of chronic pulmonary disease. The risk of overdosage in children, leading to respiratory depression, must be kept in mind when antitussive agents are prescribed. Single-ingredient preparations containing codeine or dextromethorphan should be used in place of combination preparations when antitussive therapy is considered, as when a nonproductive cough seriously disturbs sleep or school attendance.

Codeine and dextromethorphan are the two antitussives used most frequently in pediatrics. Codeine is a narcotic with addictive potential. Dextromethorphan is considered non-addictive, but abuse by teenagers ingesting huge doses has resulted in intoxication with bizarre behavior. Predictable dose-related manifestations of codeine toxicity are respiratory depression and narcosis. Other side effects of codeine include somnolence, ataxia, miosis, vomiting, rash, swelling, and itching of the skin. Doses of dextromethorphan equiantitussive to codeine may produce equivalent levels of central nervous system (CNS) depression, but no fatalities with the use of dextromethorphan have been reported. Arbitrary dosing guidelines for the antitussive effect of codeine are 0.2 mg/kg every 4–6 hours, not to exceed 1 mg/kg/day or 60 mg/day. Single oral doses of up to 5 mg/kg have produced no life-threatening effects. Doses of 1 mg/kg have been shown to cause respiratory depression in adults, however; therefore, the recommended pediatric dose offers only a fourfold margin of safety with regard to respiratory depression.

Other narcotic antitussives (e.g., hydrocodone bitartrate) are more potent than codeine and are classified as schedule II controlled drugs because of their dependency liability, and should be considered for use only in the instance of a severe, painful cough that is not suppressed by codeine.

CONCLUSIONS

The differential diagnosis of chronic cough in children is varied. The approach to chronic cough should be a carefully performed history and physical examination and consideration of specific disease entities given the child's age and clinical picture. A strong suspicion of asthma should be maintained as other possible diagnoses are ruled out.

REFERENCES

1. Widdicombe JM, Coleridge JCG. Reflexes from the upper respiratory tract, tracheobronchial tree, and lungs. In Fishman AP, Cherniack NS, Widdicombe JG, eds. *Handbook of physiology: The respiratory system.* American Physiological Society, 1986, pp 363–429.
2. Leith DE, Butler, JP, Sneddon SL, et al. Cough. In Fishman AP, Macklem PT, Mead J, eds. *Handbook of physiology: The respiratory system.* American Physiological Society, 1986, pp 315–319.
3. Wanner A. Clinical aspects of mucociliary transport. *Am Rev Respir Dis* 1977; 116:73–125.
4. Yanaura S, Nishimura T, Sakamoto M, et al. The role of bronchoconstriction in cough reflex. *Jpn J Pharmacol* 1975; 25:621–629.
5. Committee on Diagnostic Standards for Non-Tuberculous Respiratory Diseases, American Thoracic Society. Definition and classification of chronic bronchitis, asthma and pulmonary emphysema. *Am Rev Respir Dis* 1962; 85:762–766.
6. Taussig LM, Smith SM, Blumenfeld R. Chronic bronchitis in childhood: What is it? *Pediatrics* 1981; 67:1–5.

7. Umetsu DT, Ambrosino DM, Quinti I, et al. Recurrent sinopulmonary infection and impaired antibody response to bacterial capsular polysaccharide antigen in children with selective IgG-subclass deficiency. *N Engl J Med* 1985; 313:1247–1251.

8. Stagno S, Brasfield DM, Brown MB, et al. Infant pneumonitis associated with cytomegalovirus, pneumocystis and ureaplasma: A prospective study. *Pediatrics* 1981; 68:322–329.

9. Kasian GF, Shafran SD, Shyleyko EM. Branhamella catarrhalis broncho-pulmonary isolates in PICU patients. *Pediatr Pulmonol* 1989; 7:128–132.

10. Colley JR, Holland WW, Corkhill RT. Influence of passive smoking and parental phlegm on pneumonia and bronchitis in early childhood. *Lancet* 1974; 2:1031–1034.

11. American Academy of Pediatrics, Committee on Environmental Hazards. Involuntary smoking—A hazard to children. *Pediatrics* 1986; 77:755–757.

12. Tsimoyianis GV, Jacobsen MS, Feldman JG, Antonio-Santiago MT, Clutario BC, Nussbaum M, Shenker IR. Reduction in pulmonary function and increased frequency of cough associated with passive smoking in teenage athletes. *Pediatrics* 1987; 80:32–36.

13. MacLusky I, Levison H. Cystic fibrosis. In Chernick V, Kendig EL, eds. *Disorders of the respiratory tract in children*. Philadelphia, WB Saunders, 1990, pp 692–730.

14. Hoyoux CL, Forget P, Lambrechts L, et al. Chronic bronchopulmonary disease and gastroesophageal reflux in children. *Pediatr Pulmonol* 1985; 1:149–153.

15. Wald ER. Acute and chronic sinusitis: Diagnosis and management. *Pediatr Rev* 1985; 7:150–157.

16. Irwin RS, Corrao WM, Pratter MR. Chronic persistent cough in the adult: The spectrum and frequency of causes and successful outcome of specific therapy. *Am Rev Respir Dis* 1981; 123:413–417.

17. Rachelefsky GS, Katz RM, Siegel SC. Chronic sinus disease with associated reactive airway disease in children. *Pediatrics* 1984; 73:526–529.

18. Cloutier MM, Loughlin GM. Chronic cough in children: A manifestation of airway hyperreactivity. *Pediatrics* 1981; 73:526–529.

19. Konig P. Hidden asthma in children. *Am J Dis Child* 1981; 135:1053–1055.

20. Hannaway PJ, Hopper DK. Cough variant asthma in children. *JAMA* 1982; 247:206–208.

21. US Public Health Service. The health consequences of smoking. A report of the Surgeon General, 1964. Washington, DC, DHEW Publications, 1964.

22. Cassell GH, Cole BC. Mycoplasmas as agents of human disease. *N Engl J Med* 1981; 304:80–89.

23. Kravitz H, Gomberg RM, Burnstine RC, et al. Psychogenic cough tic in children and adolescents: Nine case histories illustrate the need for re-evaluation of this common but frequently unrecognized problem. *Clin Pediatr* 1969; 8:580–583.

24. Shuper A, Mukamel M, Mimouni M, et al. Psychogenic cough. *Arch Dis Child* 1983; 58:745–747.

25. American Academy of Pediatrics Committee on Drugs. Use of codeine and dextromethorphan-containing cough syrups in pediatrics. *Pediatrics* 1978; 62:118–122.

26. Hutton N, Wilson MH, Mellits ED, et al. Effectiveness of an antihistamine-decongestant combination for young children with the common cold: A randomized, controlled clinical trial. *J Pediatr* 1991; 118:125–130.

16

Apparent Life-Threatening Events

THOMAS G. KEENS and SALLY L. DAVIDSON-WARD

The respiratory system is immature at birth and develops rapidly during infancy. Stress on this unstable system from a variety of systemic disorders, including seizures, anemia, sepsis, metabolic disorders, pneumonia, lung disease, upper airway obstruction, pertussis, and heart disease (1, 2), may result in disruption of normal cardiorespiratory patterns. The clinical presentation of these disturbances may be perceived by the untrained observer as placing the infant at considerable risk. The current term for these episodes, apparent life-threatening events (ALTEs), is largely descriptive. *An ALTE is defined as event in which an infant has a convincing history of an episode of sudden onset characterized by color change (cyanosis or pallor), tone change (limpness, rarely stiffness), and apnea, which requires significant intervention (vigorous shaking, mouth to mouth breathing, or full cardiopulmonary resuscitation) to revive the infant and restore normal breathing* (1, 3). ALTEs are often frightening to the observer, who may believe that the infant is in the process of dying (3). The term should be reserved for severe ALTE episodes, not one in which a baby chokes on a feeding, turns red with crying, or is noted to have asymptomatic respiratory pauses while asleep. Mild episodes, which require little or no intervention, do not have the same prognostic significance, and in most instances do not require an aggressive diagnostic or therapeutic approach. The significance of a particular event is based largely on the history of the event, since there are currently no diagnostic tests that accurately and consistently confirm the presence or severity of ALTE (3–5). ALTE describes a clinical syndrome that may have many causes, some of which can be identified and some of which cannot. When no treatable cause for

an ALTE is found, there is concern that these infants may be at increased risk as compared to the general population of subsequently dying from the sudden infant death syndrome (SIDS) (1, 2, 5–14). Since the approach and SIDS risk may be slightly different for the various groups of infants who present with an ALTE, the presentation and management for each group will be reviewed separately.

APPARENT LIFE-THREATENING EVENTS IN OTHERWISE HEALTHY INFANTS

Previously healthy infants may present with an ALTE. Estimates for the incidence of ALTE in the general population range up to 3.0% (3). For infants with ALTE in whom no treatable cause for the ALTE can be identified, it has been estimated that the risk of subsequently dying from SIDS is more than 15 times that of the general population, depending on the severity of the event (6–10). As a group, these infants also have a high incidence of subsequent episodes of apnea (1, 2, 7, 11–14). Thus, diagnostic evaluation and management is required.

Diagnosis

As with making the diagnosis of a seizure disorder, the physician usually has not witnessed the event. Infants usually appear entirely normal by the time they reach medical attention following the ALTE. Optimal care of infants presenting with ALTE requires a thorough diagnostic evaluation to detect treatable causes of the event. The most important initial diagnostic step is to obtain a careful history from the person witnessing the event. One should specifically ask about the infant's color, gesting the presence or development of other clinical problems, such as a seizure disorder.

Discontinuing Home Apnea-Bradycardia Monitoring. Home apnea-bradycardia monitoring can be discontinued after 3 months of no apnea or bradycardia alarms that require intervention (3). An infant's tolerance of a physical stress (upper respiratory infection or other intercurrent illness) without apnea or bradycardia is reassuring, but is not required to discontinue home monitoring. Most infants with ALTE require 4–6 months of home monitoring, indicating that they had other events for 1–3 months after the initial ALTE. Some infants may continue to have lengthened breathing pauses, documented by polysomnogram or event recording, after these criteria for discontinuation have been met. However, if these episodes no longer require intervention, and are therefore not life-threatening, they do not necessarily require the continuation of home monitoring.

Outcome. It has been suggested that 40–60% of infants with an unexplained ALTE will have subsequent apnea during home monitoring (2, 7, 10–13, 24). From 30 to 40% of infants have subsequent apnea for which they receive at least vigorous stimulation for revival, and 5% receive mouth-to-mouth breathing or cardiopulmonary resuscitation (2). Most infants will have under 30 episodes total, but approximately 10% may have over 100 (2). Infants with ALTEs of unknown cause are more likely to have episodes when they are physically stressed, as with an upper respiratory infection (URI) or with fatigue. In most infants, episodes resolve before 1 year of age, but a few still have spells after their first birthday.

Even with the above diagnostic evaluation and home monitoring, infants with ALTEs of unknown etiology have twice the risk of dying from SIDS compared to the general population (9). Sleep studies are not predictive of subsequent apnea, SIDS, or death, and a normal sleep study does not eliminate the possibility that a child will die from SIDS (4, 9, 20). Following the initial ALTE, some infants have died when home monitor function and response to the alarms appeared to be appropriate (9, 10). Infants with ALTE who have received full CPR on more than one occasion are at high risk of dying (9, 10), and some of these infants have died even with appropriate

home monitoring. Some infants continue to die in temporal association with noncompliance or with errors in home monitoring technique (9). This reemphasizes the importance of parental teaching and reinforcement of monitoring skills.

MANAGEMENT OF OTHER CONDITIONS THAT CAN CAUSE ALTE

Inborn Errors of Beta-Oxidation of Fatty Acids. The rare association between inborn errors of fat oxidation and ALTE or SIDS-like deaths has been described (29, 30). An inborn error of metabolism is more likely to be associated with an ALTE if there is a family history of ALTE, consanguinity, seizure disorders, or SIDS. Inborn errors of fat oxidation may only be apparent during times of metabolic stress, such as fasting, when the infant is forced to utilize fatty acids rather than carbohydrates as substrates for energy production. The clinical presentation may include nonketotic-hypoglycemic attacks in a previously healthy infant, triggered by physical stress or a period of fasting. Progression of symptoms may mimic an ALTE. Medium-chain acyl-CoA dehydrogenase deficiency (MCADD) is the most common of these disorders, and the most likely to present as an ALTE. The frequency in the general population has been estimated to be between 1 in 10,000 and 1 in 25,000 (30).

A more extensive diagnostic evaluation is recommended in the following situations: an infant with an ALTE who has a positive family history for ALTE, seizure disorders, SIDS, or other sudden infant deaths; an infant who experiences an ALTE that occurs after an extended fast; or an infant with an ALTE who has a positive history of unexplained failure to thrive, developmental delay, or seizures. Laboratory evaluation should include assessment for hypoglycemia, hyperammonemia, metabolic acidosis, elevated liver enzymes, or abnormal hemostasis. This evaluation should also include blood and urine carnitine, urine nonvolatile organic acids, urine acylglycine, and urine acylcarnitine. The diagnosis of MCADD can be confirmed by DNA analysis. Treatment of MCADD involves the avoidance of fasting, L-carnitine supplementation, a low-fat/high-carbohydrate diet, and home apnea-bradycardia monitoring for infants who manifest this disorder with an ALTE (30).

Munchausen Syndrome by Proxy. Munchausen syndrome by proxy is a disorder of parenting and a form of child abuse, wherein the parent, usually the mother, creates a factitious illness in her child (31, 32). Because the diagnosis of ALTE is based on history, and there are no confirmatory laboratory tests available, it is particularly susceptible to the Munchausen syndrome by proxy. Most mothers afflicted with this syndrome do not harm their children, but rather the factitious illness is created by providing a fabricated history. However, Munchausen syndrome by proxy may involve inflicted physical injury to the child with suffocation used to induce "apneic spells" or even death.

There is a typical profile of the mother with Munchausen syndrome by proxy. She may have a background in the health care field, may be excessively involved with the clinic or hospital staff, may appear unconcerned about the severity of the child's illness, or may appear particularly brave or stoic in the face of tragedy. Fathers may be distant and not involved in caring for the child's illness, which has been described as "passive collusion" (32). Obviously, these traits are not diagnostic and may be present in the families of infants with a true illness, or conversely be absent in cases of proven Munchausen syndrome by proxy. Confirmation of this syndrome is often difficult. Physicians are trained to believe the parents' history and to treat illness, which makes recognizing factitious illness an uncomfortable task. Techniques that have been used include documenting induced "apneic spells" by hidden video camera or by separating the infant from the mother and documenting the resolution of the symptoms (31, 32). Treatment of Munchausen syndrome by proxy involves a team of specialists including psychiatric, social, and child protective services (32).

SUBSEQUENT SIBLINGS OF SUDDEN INFANT DEATH SYNDROME VICTIMS

Subsequent siblings of SIDS victims can present with ALTEs similar to those in otherwise healthy infants. SIDS siblings with ALTE should be evaluated and managed as any infant presenting with an ALTE would be. However, most subsequent siblings of SIDS victims are asymptomatic and survive without SIDS or apnea. Because of the devastating impact of a SIDS death in the family, parents of SIDS victims are usually anxious about their subsequent child's risk of dying from SIDS, and often seek diagnostic evaluation and management techniques to try and prevent a recurrence of SIDS.

SIDS is not thought to be hereditary. However, subsequent siblings of SIDS victims may be at increased risk of dying from SIDS (Table 16.4) (9, 33–40). After controlling for maternal age, birth order, and other important demographic characteristics, Peterson and coworkers found no greater SIDS risk for SIDS siblings than for infants born to non-SIDS parents (38). Conversely, Guntheroth and coworkers found that SIDS rates were elevated in SIDS siblings, but that the overall infant death rate was not elevated compared to controls (40). Thus, a family history of SIDS per se does not seem to confer a substantially increased risk of death as compared to infants born into *similar* non-SIDS families (38, 40). Because the recurrence risk is not markedly increased, current recommendations are that these SIDS siblings do not *require* laboratory evaluation or home apnea-bradycardia monitoring. However, some parents of SIDS victims may be sufficiently anxious that home apnea-bradycardia monitoring is indicated to reduce their anxiety. This is currently an acceptable indication for the use of home apnea-bradycardia monitoring (3).

There appear to be discrete groups of siblings of SIDS victims who have an increased risk of SIDS, above and beyond that of the group of siblings of one previous SIDS victim (35–37, 41). These include siblings of two or more previous SIDS victims, surviving twin siblings of SIDS victims, and SIDS siblings with an ALTE requiring cardiopulmonary resuscitation (35–37, 41–43). This suggests the possibility that the increased risk for SIDS attributed to SIDS siblings may be skewed by a small number of very-high-risk infants. Fortunately, some of these infants can be identified prospectively so that specific diagnostic and management techniques can be applied (35–37, 41).

Clinical management for asymptomatic siblings of a SIDS victim should include a review of the autopsy report of the SIDS victim to confirm the diagnosis of SIDS. The SIDS risk for siblings of one SIDS victim should be reviewed with the parents, and the option of using home apnea-bradycardia monitoring

3. National Institutes of Health Consensus Development Conference on Infantile Apnea and Home Monitoring. *Pediatrics* 1987; 79:292–299.
4. Wilson AJ, Stevens V, Franks CI, Alexander J, Southall DP. Respiratory and heart rate patterns in infants destined to be victims of sudden infant death syndrome: Average rates and their variability measured over 24 hours. *Br Med J* 1985; 290:497–501.
5. Keens TG, Sargent CW, Dennies PC, Bookout SM, Gates EP, Platzker ACG. Pneumograms do not predict subsequent apnea in near-miss sudden infant death syndrome infants [Abstract]. *Am Rev Respir Dis* 1982; 125:192.
6. Steinschneider A. Prolonged apnea and the sudden infant death syndrome: Clinical and laboratory observations. *Pediatrics* 1972; 50:646–654.
7. Kelly DH, Shannon DC, O'Connell K. Care of infants with near-miss sudden infant death syndrome. *Pediatrics* 1978; 61:511–514.
8. Steinschneider A, Weinstein SL, Diamond E. The sudden infant death syndrome and apnea/obstruction during neonatal sleep and feeding. Pediatrics, 1982; 70:858–863.
9. Davidson Ward SL, Keens TG, Chan LS, Chipps BE, Carson SH, Deming DD, Krishna D, MacDonald HM, Martin GI, Meredith KS, Merritt TA, Nickerson BG, Stoddard RA, van der Hal AL. Sudden infant death syndrome in infants evaluated by apnea programs in California. *Pediatrics* 1986; 77:451–455.
10. Oren J, Kelly D, Shannon DC. Identification of a high-risk group for sudden infant death syndrome among infants who were resuscitated for sleep apnea. *Pediatrics* 1986; 77:495–499.
11. Duffy P, Bryan MH. Home monitoring in "near-miss" sudden infant death syndrome (SIDS) and in siblings of SIDS victims. *Pediatrics* 1982; 70:69–74.
12. Ariagno RL, Guilleminault C, Korobkin R, Owen-Boeddiker M, Baldwin R. "Near-miss" for sudden infant death syndrome infants: A clinical problem. *Pediatrics* 1983; 71:726–730.
13. Rosen CL, Frost JD, Harrison GM. Infant apnea: Polygraphic studies and follow-up monitoring. *Pediatrics* 1983; 71:731–736.
14. Shannon DC, Kelly DH. SIDS and near-SIDS. *N Engl J Med* 1982; 306:959–965, 1022–1028.
15. Keens TG, Davidson Ward SL, Gates EP, Hart LD, Basile A, Tinajero LA, Lau AM, Chan CE. A comparison of pneumogram recordings performed in the hospital and at home. *Pediatric Pulmonology* 1986; 2:373–377.
16. Keens TG, Davidson Ward SL, Gates EP, Andree DI, Hart LD. Ventilatory pattern following DTP immunization in infants at risk for SIDS. *Am J Dis Child* 1985; 139:991–994.
17. Guilleminault C, Ariagno R, Souquet M, Dement WC. Abnormal polygraphic recordings in near-miss sudden infant death. *Lancet* 1976; 1:1326–1327.
18. Steinschneider A. Prolonged sleep apnea and respiratory instability: A discriminative study. *Pediatrics* 1977; 59(Suppl):962–970.
19. Kelly DH, Shannon DC. Periodic breathing in infants with near-miss sudden infant death syndrome. *Pediatrics* 1979; 63:355–360.
20. Southall DP, Richards JM, Rhoden KJ, Alexander JR, Shinebourne EA, Arrowsmith WA, Cree JE, Fleming PJ, Goncalves A, Orme RLE. Prolonged apnea and

cardiac arrhythmias in infants discharged from neonatal intensive care units: Failure to predict an increased risk for sudden infant death syndrome. *Pediatrics* 1982; 70:844–851.
21. Haddad GG, Leistner HL, Lai TL, Mellins RB. Ventilation and ventilatory pattern during sleep in aborted sudden infant death syndrome. *Pediatr Res* 1981; 15:879–883.
22. Hodgman JE, Hoppenbrouwers T, Geidel S, Hadeed A, Sterman MB, Harper R, McGinty D. Respiratory behavior in near-miss sudden infant death syndrome. *Pediatrics* 1982; 69:785–792.
23. Steinschneider A, Freed G, Rhetta-Smith A, Rice Santos V. Effect of diptheria-tetanus-pertussis immunization on prolonged apnea or bradycardia in siblings of sudden infant death syndrome victims. *J Pediatr* 1991; 119:411–414.
24. Weese-Mayer D, Brouillette RT, Morrow AS, Conway LP, L.M. Klemka-Waden LM, Hunt CE. Assessing validity of infant monitor alarms with event recording. *J Pediatr* 1988; 115:702–708.
25. Hunt CE, Hazinski TA, Gora P. Experimental effects of chloral hydrate on ventilatory responses to hypoxia and hypercapnia. *Pediatr Res* 1982; 16:79–812.
26. Shannon DC, Kelly DH, O'Connell K. Abnormal regulation of ventilation in infants at risk for sudden infant death syndrome. *N Engl J Med* 1977; 297:747–750.
27. Hunt CE, McCulloch K, Brouillette RT. Diminished hypoxic ventilatory responses in near-miss sudden infant death syndrome. *J Appl Physiol Resp Environ Exerc Physiol* 1981; 50:1313–1317.
28. Cain LP, Kelly DH, Shannon DC. Parents' perception of the psychological and social impact of home monitoring. *Pediatrics* 1980; 66:37–41.
29. Sinclair-Smith C, Dinsdale F, Emery J. Evidence of duration and type of illness in children found unexpectedly dead. *Arch Dis Child* 1976; 2:424–429.
30. Harpey JP, Charpentier C, Paturneau-Jouas M. Sudden infant death syndrome and inherited disorders of fatty acid beta-oxidation. *Biol Neonate* 1990; 58:70–80.
31. Rosen C, Frost JD, Bricker T, Tarnow JD, Gillette PC, Dunlavy S. Two siblings with recurrent cardiorespiratory arrest: Munchausen syndrome by proxy or child abuse? *Pediatrics* 1983; 71:715–720.
32. Meadow R. Suffocation, recurrent apnea, and sudden infant death. *J Pediatr* 1990; 117:351–357.
33. Adelson L, Kinney ER. Sudden and unexpected death in infancy and childhood. *Pediatrics* 1956; 17:663–697.
34. Froggatt P, Lynas M, MacKenzie G. Epidemiology of sudden unexpected deaths in infants ("cot death") in Northern Ireland. *Br J Prevent Soc Med* 1971; 25:119–134.
35. Peterson DR, Chinn NM, Fisher LD. The sudden infant death syndrome: Repetitions in families. *J Pediatr* 1980; 97:263–267.
36. Beal SM. Some epidemiological factors about sudden infant death syndrome (SIDS) in South Australia. In Tildon T, Roeder LM, Steinschneider A, eds. *Sudden infant death syndrome.* New York, Academic Press, 1983, pp 15–28.
37. Irgens LM, Skjaerven R, Peterson DR. Prospective assessment of recurrence risk in sudden infant death syndrome siblings. *J Pediatr* 1984; 104:349–351.

38. Peterson DR, Sabotta EE, Dalling JR. Infant mortality among subsequent siblings of infants who died of sudden infant death syndrome. *J Pediatr* 1986; 108:911–914.

39. Beal S. Recurrence incidence of sudden infant death syndrome. *Arch Dis Child* 1988; 63:924–930.

40. Guntheroth WG, Lohmann R, Spiers PS. Risk of sudden infant death syndrome in subsequent siblings. *J Pediatr* 1990; 116:520–524.

41. Oren J, Kelly DH, Shannon DC. Familial occurrence of sudden infant death syndrome and apnea of infancy. *Pediatrics* 1987; 80:355–358.

42. Spears PS. Estimated rates of concordancy for the sudden infant death syndrome in twins. *Am J Epidemiol* 1974; 100:1.

43. Beal SM. Simultaneous sudden death in infancy in identical twins. *Med J Aust* 1973; 1:1146.

44. Black L, David RJ, Brouillette RT, Hunt CE. Effects of birth weight and ethnicity on incidence of sudden infant death syndrome. *J Pediatr* 1986; 108:209–214.

45. Schwartz PJ, Southall DP, Valdes-Dapena M. *The sudden infant death syndrome: Cardiac and respiratory mechanisms and interventions.* New York, New York Academy of Sciences: *Ann N Y Acad Sci* 1988; 533:1–474.

46. Garg M, Kurzner SI, Bautista DB, Keens TG. Clinically unsuspected hypoxia during sleep and feeding in bronchopulmonary dysplasia. *Pediatrics* 1988; 81:635–642.

47. Davidson Ward SL, Bautista D, Chan L, Derry M, Lisbon A, Durfee M, Mills KSC, Keens TG. Sudden infant death syndrome in infants of substance abusing mothers. *J Pediatr* 1990; 117:876–881.

48. Chavez CJ, Ostrea EM, Stryker JC, Smialek Z. Sudden infant death syndrome among infants of drug-dependent mothers. *J Pediatr* 1979; 95:407–409.

49. Pierson PS, Howard P, Kleber HD. Sudden death in infants born to methadone-maintained addicts. *JAMA* 1972; 220:1733–1734.

50. Rajegowda BK, Kandall SR, Falciglia H. Sudden infant death (SIDS) in infants of narcotic-addicted mothers [Abstract]. *Pediatr Res* 1976; 10:334.

51. Finnegan LP, Reeser DS. The incidence of sudden death in infants born to women maintained on methadone [Abstract]. *Pediatr Res* 1978; 12:405.

52. Durand DJ, Espinoza AM, Nickerson BG. Association between prenatal cocaine exposure and sudden infant death syndrome. *J Pediatr* 1990; 117:909–911.

53. Davidson Ward SL, Schuetz S, Krishna V, Bean X, Wingert W, Wachsman L, Keens TG. Abnormal sleeping ventilatory pattern in infants of substance-abusing mothers. *Am J Dis Child* 1986; 140:1015–1020.

54. Chasnoff IJ, Hunt CE, Kletter R, Kaplan D. Prenatal cocaine exposure is associated with respiratory pattern abnormalities. *Am J Dis Child* 1989; 143:583–587.

55. Bauchner H, Zuckerman B, McClain M, Frank D, Fried LE, Kayne H. Risk of sudden infant death syndrome among infants with in utero exposure to cocaine. *J Pediatr* 1988; 112:831–834.

56. Deren S. Children of substance abusers: A review of the literature. *J Subst Abuse Treat* 1986; 3:77–94.

57. Suffet F, Brotmen R. A comprehensive care program for pregnant addicts: Obstetrical, neonatal, and child development outcome. *Int J Addict* 1988; 19:199–219.

17

Dyspnea

GERALD M. LOUGHLIN

Breathing, especially in children, is typically an effortless and almost imperceptible process. However, patients with acute and chronic cardiopulmonary and neuromuscular disease may experience difficulty in breathing (dyspnea) at rest and/or following exercise. Although there is no precise definition of dyspnea, especially in children, it can best be described as a sensation of difficult, labored, or uncomfortable breathing (1). It is a subjective symptom that involves not only a physiologic disturbance but also the patient's perception of the sensation as well as his or her reaction to it (2). Difficulty in identifying and understanding this symptom is more complicated in children, since it is more often the parents' perception that their child is either breathing too fast or appears to be laboring to breathe that causes them to seek medical attention. Thus the approach described in this chapter is based heavily on clinical experience and judgement.

In broad clinical terms, dyspnea arises from (a) an increase in respiratory drive or effort in response to an increase in the work of breathing (respiratory disease associated with increased resistance or decreased compliance), (b) an increased degree of muscle force required to maintain normal ventilation (neuromuscular disease or inefficient diaphragm position from over-inflation), and (c) increased ventilatory requirements (hypermetabolic states, anemia, hypoxemia, metabolic acidosis) (2). Although there has been limited attention to this problem in children, each of these situations is encountered commonly in children.

The mechanism or mechanisms responsible for dyspnea are not clearly established, even in adults. This is an extremely complicated subject, the study of which has been hampered by the lack of good experimental models, the difficulty in accurately reproducing the total symptom complex in experimental settings, and the extreme subjectivity of the symptom (2). These problems are magnified in children, thus severely restricting scientific investigation in children. However, for purposes of this discussion, an understanding of the basic mechanisms that account for the perception of dyspnea is not essential. The reader is referred to several reviews of the state of the art of studying dyspnea (3–5).

Dyspnea occurs in both acute and chronic forms. In children, without underlying lung or cardiac disease, acute onset of dyspnea is more often encountered by the general pediatrician. Some infants appear to be breathing fast but are in no distress and are not limited in their usual activities. These children may simply have adapted a strategy of breathing that is better suited to the mechanical properties of the lungs and chest wall. The differential diagnosis of acute dyspnea in a previously healthy child is listed in Table 17.1.

A more detail discussion of these causes of dyspnea is presented in the appropriate chapters. The cause of acute-onset dyspnea can usually identified by the associated clinical manifestations, the setting, and the age of the patient. For example, an infant who experiences acute onset of shortness of breath following an upper respiratory infection (URI) in the winter months most likely has bronchiolitis. Similarly, the most common cause of acute-onset dyspnea in older children is asthma. This may present as wheezing and/or shortness of breath with URIs or following exercise (6). The relationship between asthma and exertional dyspnea is underappreciated.

Table 17.1.
Causes of Acute-Onset Dyspnea/Tachypnea

Asthma

Foreign body aspiration (both airway and
    esophageal)
Bronchiolitis (primarily in infants)
Congestive heart failure (can be seen at rest but is
    more often seen with exertion; in infants this is
    usually seen with bottle feeding)

Pneumonia

Acute upper airway obstruction (croup, epiglottitis,
    allergic reaction)
Spontaneous pneumothorax (typically in the
    adolescent, frequently associated with chest pain)
Psychologic (anxiety, usually adolescents)
Exertional (asthma, poor conditioning, cardiac
    dysfunction)
Chest trauma (pulmonary contusion, rib fracture)
Recurrent aspiration (dysfunctional swallowing,
    gastroesphageal reflux; usually occur after bottle
    feedings)
Neuromuscular disease (Werdnig-Hoffman
    syndrome, diaphragmatic paralysis; usually seen in
    infants)
Chest syndrome (exacerbations of sickle cell
    disease)

In fact, as has been suggested for adults, no child should be labeled as having idiopathic or psychogenic dyspnea until the diagnosis of asthma has been excluded (7). Although it may occur as an isolated symptom in previously normal children, a spontaneous pneumothorax is more likely to occur in patients with underlying conditions such as asthma, cystic fibrosis, or Marfan syndrome. In most instances the onset of dyspnea is associated with chest pain. In fact, chest pain rather than dyspnea is more likely to initiate the referral. A chest radiograph is diagnostic. Acute onset of dyspnea in a toddler without evidence of infection should raise concern about the possibility of a retained foreign body. The degree of dyspnea associated with foreign body aspiration depends on the size and composition of the aspirated material as well as the anatomic location of the foreign body. Material that lodges in the upper airway or esophagus may cause significant dyspnea, whereas a more peripheral location typically produces more indolent symptoms. As with other respiratory symptoms such as cough or chest pain, dyspnea may be a manifestation of a functional or psychologic disorder. These patients are typically adolescents without evidence of cardiopulmonary disease. The symptoms usually arise when the child perceives a stressful situation and quickly abate when the stress is removed.

Dyspnea is also seen in children with underlying cardiopulmonary disease. In this clinical setting it reflects either worsening disease or an acute complication of the underlying condition. Table 17.2 summarizes the differential diagnosis of chronic dyspnea. (These conditions are discussed in the appropriate chapters.) In patients with underlying lung disease it is important to pay close attention to the patient's assessment of changes in disease status. By the same token, the physician caring for a patient with a chronic condition must be aware that dyspnea is a subjective symptom, and that patients may unwittingly under-represent the severity of their clinical condition and may not be very sensitive to physiologic changes in function. Table 17.3 presents complications of chronic conditions that may account for acute onset of dyspnea in a previously stable patient. Complications such as bronchospasm or pulmonary edema are common and thus thought of immediately when one encounters a patient who is experiencing an exacerbation of chronic dyspnea. Other causes, such as silent aspiration and pulmonary embolus, are frequently overlooked.

Table 17.2.
Conditions Associated with Chronic Dyspnea

Asthma (poorly controlled with chronic hyperinflation)
Bronchopulmonary dysplasia with and without
    pulmonary edema
Cystic fibrosis
Congenital heart disease with compromised cardiac
    function and pulmonary edema
Thoracic dystrophy (congenital asphyxiating thoracic
    dystrophy, kyphoscoliosis)
Extreme obesity
Pulmonary arteriovenous malformations
Interstitial lung disease (pneumonitis and fibrosis)
Chronic upper airway obstruction (subglottic or
    tracheal stenosis, vascular ring or sling)
Pulmonary hypoplasia (usually seen in infants)
Chronic recurrent aspiration (gastroesophageal reflux
    and dysfunctional swallowing)
Neuromuscular disease (Werdnig-Hoffman
    syndrome, polio, muscular dystrophy, myotonic
    dystrophy)
Congenital abnormalities of the airways, lung, and
    diaphragm
Chronic metabolic states (acidosis, anemia)
Deconditioning (usually a cause of exertional
    dyspnea)

Table 17.3.
Acute Exacerbations of Chronic Dyspnea

Congestive heart failure (congenital heart disease)
Pneumothorax (asthma, cystic fibrosis, Marfan
  syndrome, pulmonary fibrosis)
Pulmonary edema $+/-$ RV failure (superimposed on
  chronic lung disease, or following relief of upper
  airway obstruction or atelectasis)
Bronchospasm (superimposed on underlying
  conditions such as (cystic fibrosis or
  bronchopulmonary dysplasia)
Pulmonary embolus (debilitated chronically
  immobilized patient)
Infection (usually viral)
Aspiration

EVALUATION OF THE CHILD WITH DYSPNEA AND/OR TACHYPNEA

In the older child and adolescent who presents with dyspnea, the most important element of the history is the patient's report of the degree of shortness of breath. In the infant or young child, the physician must rely on the parents' interpretation that the child appears short of breath or has had trouble breathing. This is even more subjective than a patient's own report and is subject to the same sensitivity issues. Very observant or anxious parents are more likely to perceive an abnormality, whereas others are more tolerant of symptoms in their children and will only report them when they are extreme. Is dyspnea present at rest or only following exercise? If the latter, how much exertion is required to produce symptoms? The patient should be asked to quantify, if possible, the degree of dyspnea in terms of the activities of daily living. This will vary from patient to patient, and for some the dyspnea may only be seen with strenuous exercise. In the infant, exercise most often consists of bottle feeding. Does the infant fatigue or pull away to rest during feeding?

How long has the patient been dyspneic? What events or activities preceded the onset of dyspnea? Is it chronic or recurrent? Is there underlying cardiopulmonary or neuromuscular disease? What factors make it worse or better? Are there associated symptoms such as chest pain, cough, or wheezing? What has been the response to therapy?

In the infant or young child who cannot report dyspnea, the presence of shortness of breath must be inferred from the physical examination and from the parents' report of a change in the child's behavior or endurance

with normal infant or toddler activities. Evidence of respiratory distress, including an increased respiratory rate, inspiratory retractions, and nasal flaring and noisy breathing (stridor or wheeze), should be noted. Are breath sounds and the percussion note symmetric? Are rales present, and is there evidence of heart failure?

Laboratory evaluation of the patient who complains of dyspnea should at a minimum include a chest radiograph and a measure of gas exchange, preferably an arterial blood gas. If this is not easily obtainable, a capillary blood gas or end tidal CO_2 measurement coupled with pulse oximetry can provide a reasonable assessment of the underlying dysfunction accounting for the patient's complaint. A hematocrit and measure of serum electrolytes, including a bicarbonate level, should be obtained in all patients. Anemia may contribute to exertional dyspnea, whereas polycythemia indicates chronic hypoxemia. Total CO_2 level can be used to identify underlying metabolic acidosis or may suggest the presence of chronic hypoventilation. Avoid over-evaluation of the problem. If the above studies are normal, the subsequent evaluation can be approached conservatively. If the child is old enough, a bronchoprovocation test most likely will have the greatest yield, since asthma is such a frequent cause of dyspnea (6). In patients without evidence of cardiac dysfunction (murmur, signs of failure, or complaints about an irregular heart beat), a routine electrocardiogram (EKG) and echocardiogram are of limited value. Pulmonary function tests may provide an objective measure to correlate with the patient's reporting of shortness of breath. Similarly, an exercise stress test can be used in evaluating patients with exertional dyspnea. This study should include measures of the cardiac and ventilatory responses to exercise, as well as an assessment for exercise-induced bronchospasm.

TREATMENT

The treatment of dyspnea depends on the etiology not only of the acute cause but also of any underlying condition or exacerbating condition (Table 17.3) (2, 8). General therapy includes bronchodilators and steroids for relief of asthma symptoms. If hypoxia is present, supplemental oxygen is indicated. This may be particularly helpful for patients who complain of exertional dyspnea; however, formal testing to identify desaturation during exercise is needed in most patients. Although many patients report improvement, the benefits of supplemental oxygen in relieving dyspnea at rest are unclear. Work by Liss and Grant did not demonstrate any benefit of oxygen in patients with chronic obstructive pulmonary disease (COPD), leading them to postulate a placebo effect in wearing a nasal cannula as the responsible factor underlying the perceived benefit (9). Pulmonary edema can be managed with fluid restriction and diuretics. Furosemide is the most effective medication in managing acute pulmonary edema.

Attempts to treat dyspnea by reducing the increase in respiratory drive thought to be responsible for the sensation have largely been restricted to research studies. Benzodiazepines and opiates have both been tried. Although several studies report success in relieving symptoms of dyspnea and improving exercise performance, the side effects have been quite severe (2, 10, 11). At the present time, there does not appear to be any justification for routinely treating dyspnea in children with medications designed to reduce respiratory drive. However, in the terminally ill child these medications may have a role in keeping the patient more comfortable.

Other approaches to therapy that have been tried in adults include the use of breathing techniques, exercise training, alterations in nutritional intake, psychologic interventions, respiratory muscle training, and muscle rest (8). The results obtained have been quite variable. Many patients report feeling better without demonstrable change in function. Data on the application of these techniques to children is quite limited. Two of these techniques deserve mention for children. High-carbohydrate diets result in increased CO_2 production (12); for the child with chronic lung or neuromuscular disease, this may impose a greater respiratory burden and increase dyspnea. Since many young children are on high-caloric diets in order to facilitate growth, it is prudent to try to provide as many of these calories as possible through fat rather than carbohydrates (13). In adults with COPD, the benefits of intermittent rest of the respiratory muscles has been described by Braun and Marino (14). This approach is attractive for a wide range of children with chronic neuromuscular and pulmonary conditions who are prone to recurrent bouts of respiratory muscle failure. Perhaps the provision of a rest period, now possible noninvasively with the use of facemask ventilation, may improve the overall endurance of these patients. Additional studies are needed to determine the benefits of this approach in both children and adults.

CLINICAL IMPLICATIONS

Since this complaint has both a physiologic and psychologic or subjective component, it is not uncommon for there to be a discrepancy between a patient's or parent's reporting of dyspnea and the degree of pulmonary dysfunction. Some patients will experience acute dyspnea with minimal change in lung function, whereas others may experience a marked decrease in pulmonary function with little or no perception of difficulty in breathing. The perception of dyspnea may be linked to certain personality traits, with the more extroverted types typically possessing a heightened sense of dyspnea (15). Decreased perception of dyspnea may play a role in the increased morbidity and mortality associated with exacerbations of asthma (16). We have encountered a number of children with asthma who appear to have a decreased ability to perceive airflow obstruction and hypoxia. As a consequence, these children often develop severe airways obstruction and hypoxia before seeking additional medical attention for acute exacerbations because they simply don't recognize the severity of the obstruction. This group of patients can derived considerable benefit from the use of a peak flow meter to provide them with an objective measure of disease severity. They should be instructed to respond to a particular peak flow value, rather than to their perception of how dyspneic they are.

REFERENCES

1. Comroe JH. Some theories of the mechanism of dyspnea. In Howell JB, Campbell EJM, eds. *Breathlessness*. Boston, Blackwell Scientific, 1966, pp 1–7.
2. Tobin MJ. Dyspnea: Pathophysiologic basis, clinical presentation and management. *Arch Intern Med* 1990; 150:1604–1613.
3. Cherniack NS, Altose MD. Mechanisms of dyspnea. *Clin Chest Med* 1987; 8:207–214.
4. Burki NK, Tobin MJ, Guz A, et al. Dyspnea: Mechanisms, evaluation and treatment. *Am Rev Respir Dis* 1988; 1040–1041.
5. Altose MD. Assessment and management of breathlessness. *Chest* 1985; 88:77–82S.

6. Nudel DB, Diamant MD, Brady T, et al. Chest pain, dyspnea on exertion and exercise induced asthma in children and adolescents. *Clin Pediatr* 1987; 8:388–392.

7. Pratter MR, Bartter T. Dyspnea: Time to find the facts. *Chest* 1991; 100:1187.

8. Mahler DA. Dyspnea: Diagnosis and management. *Clin Chest Med* 1987; 8:215–230.

9. Liss HP, Grant BJB. The effect of nasal flow on breathlessness in patients with chronic obstructive pulmonary disease. *Clin Sci* 1987; 137:1285–1288.

10. Browning I, D'Alonzo GE, Tobin MJ. Effect of hydrocodone on dyspnea, respiratory drive and exercise performance in adult patients with cystic fibrosis. *Am Rev Resp Dis* 1988; 137:A305.

11. Rice KL, Kronenberg RS, Hedemark LL, et al. Effects of chronic administration of codeine and promethazine on breathlessness and exercise tolerence in patients with chronic airflow obstruction. *Br J Dis Chest* 1987; 81:287–292.

12. Gieseke T, Gurushanthaiah G, Glauser FL. Effects of carbohydrate on carbon dioxide excretion in patients with airway disease. *Chest* 1977; 71:55–58.

13. Angelillo VA, Sukhdarshan B, Durfee D, et al. Effects of low and high carbohydrate feedings in ambulatory patients with chronic obstructive pulmonary disease and chronic hyperpnea. *Ann Intern Med* 1985; 103:883–885.

14. Braun NMT, Marino WD. Effect of daily intermittent rest of respiratory muscles in patients with severe airflow limitation. *Chest* 1984; 85:59–60S.

15. Clark TJH, Cochrane GM. Effect of personality on alveolar ventilation in patients with chronic airways obstruction. *Br Med J* 1970; 1:273–275.

16. Rubinfeld AR, Pain MCF. Perception of asthma. *Lancet* 1976; 1:882–884.

18

Hemoptysis

C. MICHAEL BOWMAN

Hemoptysis is a relatively uncommon but potentially serious problem in children. Its profile has changed in recent years, becoming more prominent in patients with cystic fibrosis (CF) and less commonly associated with tuberculosis, bronchiectasis, or other infections in previously normal children. Its presentation is often so sudden and dramatic that it is important for the clinician to have a clear understanding of the problem and its treatment in advance so that key decisions can be made effectively.

Hemoptysis is "the spitting of blood derived from the lungs or bronchial tubes as a result of pulmonary or bronchial hemorrhage," according to *Stedman's Medical Dictionary* (1). The important consideration is that blood is coughed out. If pulmonary hemorrhage occurs in the parenchyma of the lung, slowly and without expectoration (particularly in young children), the severity may be underestimated. Conversely, bleeding from other sites, such as the oropharynx, esophagus, or stomach, may be mistakenly attributed to the lungs. In children, coughing and vomiting often occur together, obscuring the bleeding site. Since hemoptysis may be difficult to recognize in young children, who seldom expectorate sputum, the lungs should at least be considered a potential bleeding site for a young child who presents with melena or heme-positive stools associated with even mild respiratory symptoms.

The significance of true hemoptysis lies in the fact that it is seldom a "false positive" and usually indicates the presence of a significant problem. It is frightening to the patient and family, and although hemoptysis is not a disease in itself, it indicates the presence of another serious condition. The severity of the hemoptysis may or may not correlate with the severity of the underlying problem. The amount of bleeding can be difficult to quantitate, since blood is usually mixed in an unknown ratio with airway mucus, and the amount actually coughed out is often overestimated.

The pathophysiology of hemoptysis in children represents a dynamic balance between the forces keeping blood within blood vessels and the forces leading to extravasation. The forces that keep blood in pulmonary vessels and out of the airway are influenced by the physical integrity of the capillary walls and alveolar epithelium as well as by the hemostatic mechanisms in the blood and vessel walls. This is counterbalanced by the pressure and flow in the pulmonary (or bronchial) circulation. Pulmonary hemorrhage may occur from a discreet bleeding site, that is, an eroded or damaged blood vessel (artery, capillary, or vein), or it may result from diffuse bleeding. In the most severe form of pulmonary edema, which results from increased permeability of the pulmonary circulation, endothelial "pores" may be large enough to allow the passage of red blood cells. The resulting bloody pulmonary edema is usually sufficiently distinct from frank blood to be distinguished easily from hemoptysis. Infection, trauma, or inflammation, which damage the vasculature and often increase local blood flow, may lead to bleeding. Furthermore, shear forces, which are prominent in the patient with severe cough, may cause rupture of fragile pulmonary vessels. Since hemostatic mechanisms participate in maintaining the vascular barrier, dysfunction of hemostasis may lead to bleeding at any site in the body; given the large capillary network in the lung, the pulmonary parenchyma is commonly the site of bleeding. Bleeding that results purely from disordered hemostasis is a secondary type of hemoptysis but can still be severe. However, mild disorders in hemostasis may lead to significant hemoptysis when coupled with a minor breakdown in vascular integrity or an increase in pulmonary blood flow.

PATIENT PRESENTATION AND EVALUATION

The history of hemoptysis may be specific or vague, since it may be difficult for the family to identify the specific time of the bleeding or the cause of the hemorrhage. It may take careful questioning to elucidate whether the blood was produced in the gastrointestinal (GI) tract or in the lungs. Dyspnea and cough are common in patients with hemoptysis. Severe bleeding may be associated with pallor, although the patient who is in significant respiratory distress or who is frightened may appear pale anyway. It is important to inquire about the possibility of aspiration, since foreign bodies or caustic agents may lead to pulmonary or esophageal bleeding (2). Signs and symptoms of infection are also important, since pneumonia and other acute and chronic infectious processes can lead to pulmonary bleeding (3, 4). Any history of chest trauma is also important. The past medical history may reveal a previous bleeding diathesis or history of petechiae or easy bruising. Newborns may exhibit hemoptysis in association with sepsis or bleeding diatheses (5). Patients with chronic suppurative pulmonary disease such as CF or other forms of bronchiectasis may develop recurrent hemoptysis as their infection and inflammation worsens (3, 6). A patient with no significant history beyond intermittent respiratory symptoms may be a strong candidate for one of the pulmonary hemorrhage syndromes (7, 8) or for an unrecognized vascular malformation. Lastly, it is important to obtain complete documentation of any medication intake. Prescription medications are important, as are nonprescription medications, including those containing aspirin, other nonsteroidal anti-inflammatory agents, and other agents that may inhibit platelet function or lead to coagulopathies.

The physical examination and monitoring of the patient with hemoptysis are the keys to the assessment of the patient's status. Respiratory distress and circulatory stability are the primary indicators of the severity of the condition. Although the degree of distress may not correlate exactly with the severity of the bleed, it approximates the amount of lung affected by the bleed. Assessment of air exchange throughout both lung fields is important to help decide whether there is a discreet localized problem or a more generalized condition. Pulmonary hemorrhage may lead to altered air exchange and crackles (either coarse or fine), often with wheezing over the areas affected. As peripheral secretions and blood move proximally, the auscultatory findings may become more widespread. Blood loss may be large enough to cause pallor, tachycardia, and even blood pressure changes (orthostatic or sustained). The lung is capable of holding a relatively large volume of blood within the parenchyma and sequestering it from the circulation. Thus, circulatory support is an important early step in the care of patients with hemoptysis.

Laboratory studies to be pursued initially include measurement of oxygenation, because hypoxia indicates the extent of ventilation-perfusion (V/Q) mismatching. When present, anemia is of concern, but its absence is not reassuring. In the early stages of bleeding, the problem will be loss of whole blood with deficient circulation rather than preferential loss of red cells with resulting anemia. There may be leukocytosis, indicating bacterial infection.

A chest radiograph will indicate the extent of pulmonary infiltration and allow correlation with the physical examination. Radiographic findings may change suddenly or slowly; they may also indicate the presence of chronic changes. A chest computed tomography (CT) scan may define bronchiectasis or malformations more clearly than the plain chest film. Pulmonary function testing should not be performed at the time of an acute bleed, since forced expiratory maneuvers will often trigger coughing, which can lead to more severe hemorrhage. It is appropriate to do a culture of expectorated material to help guide antibiotic therapy, if any is necessary. Urinalyses and measurements of serum creatinine and blood urea nitrogen (BUN) are performed to look for signs of renal involvement.

TREATMENT
Stabilize the Patient

The immediate consideration for a patient with apparently massive hemoptysis is to maintain the circulation. This should be accomplished with fluids, transfusion, pressors, and other routine therapy to avoid shock and renal shutdown. The next treatment for all patients with hemoptysis is to maintain oxygenation. Oxygen can be given by nasal cannula, oxygen mask, non-rebreather mask, or head hood to maintain an oxygen saturation above 90% (preferably above 95% in most patients). Oxygenation may show marked fluctuations, depending on the condition and anxiety of the patient, and pulse oximetry may be difficult to use in the patient with impaired circulation. Although arterial blood gas determinations of PaO_2 are optimal, the agitation induced by an arterial puncture may outweigh the benefit of direct measurements of PaO_2. For this reason, in the severely ill patient consideration should be given to placement of an indwelling arterial catheter to allow repeated direct measurements of PaO_2 and $PaCO_2$ without inducing patient agitation and cough. Respiratory failure may ensue in the patient with severe hemoptysis, resulting from either impaired gas exchange due to massive involvement of many areas of the lung with hemorrhage or from increased respiratory work in the patient with limited reserve. In general, except in the terminal patient with CF or other destructive lung processes, the child with hemoptysis and respiratory failure should be intubated and supported with mechanical ventilation. Positive pressure ventilation with positive end-expiratory pressure (PEEP) may markedly improve gas exchange in the bleeding lung. The level of end expiratory pressure should be adjusted to keep the $FiO_2 < 0.60$, if possible. If the patient is an infant, the hemoptysis may represent part of a generalized infectious process. In this situation, the usual treatment for shock and disseminated intravascular coagulation (DIC) should be pursued. In the patient old enough to understand his or her surroundings and treatment, reassurance is an important part of patient care. Hemoptysis is frightening to patients far beyond its threat to life or the amount of respiratory embarrassment. Admission to an Intensive Care Unit with strange and frightening instruments may exacerbate this. Since sedatives may reduce respiratory drive and impair the patient's responses to further bleeding, their use should be restricted to patients monitored closely in an intensive care setting.

Patients with CF may know of previous patients with CF who have died after an episode of hemoptysis, so they too may overestimate the severity of their condition. Such patients will benefit from significant quiet reassurance when that is justified by their condition.

Quantitate the Severity and Treat the Hemorrhage

It is important to estimate the amount and rate of bleeding. This may be difficult if the patient has hemoptysis intermittently during an ongoing episode. For the patient old enough to cooperate, all of the products of hemoptysis should be expectorated into a large container kept at the bedside for the entire shift or day. It can then be measured and visualized by all caregivers. For the intubated patient, this type of assessment can be carried out by observation of the wall suction trap containing material removed from the airway. (One should realize that saline instilled into the airway will dilute and increase the volume of secretions removed). At times, measuring the hematocrit of the suctioned material or the expectorated blood may help quantify the actual amount of bleeding. Concomitant with the production of large amounts of hemoptysis material is an expected decrease in hemoglobin and hematocrit. In order for these indicators to decrease, there must be intake of free water, either enterally or parenterally. Thus, it may take several hours for a significant bleed to cause a drop in hemoglobin and hematocrit. The chest radiograph usually shows significant changes in patients who have experienced bleeding into the pulmonary parenchyma. However, these new infiltrates may be difficult to distinguish in a patient who has severe chronic abnormalities of their chest radiograph. Furthermore, it is difficult to distinguish a new infiltrate caused by infection from one caused by bleeding. Airway bleeding may produce more symptoms with less extensive radiographic changes.

Diagnose and Treat the Underlying Condition

Once the patient is stabilized and the severity of the bleeding is assessed, the next step is to diagnose and treat the underlying condition. Table 18.1 shows the more common condi-

Table 18.1.
Potential Primary Causes of Hemoptysis

Newborn (birth–30 days of age)	Infancy (1–12 months)
Hemorrhagic disorders	Pulmonary hemosiderosis
Sepsis	Pneumonia
Cardiopulmonary malformations	Cardiopulmonary malformations (e.g., bronchogenic
Bacterial pneumonia	cyst, AV malformation)
	Tumors

Childood (1–12 years)	Adolescence (12 + years)
Pulmonary hemosiderosis	Cystic fibrosis
Immune/collagen vascular disorders (I/CVD) (e.g.,	ICVD (e.g., Goodpasture syndrome, SLE, Wegener
systemic lupus erythematosis (SLE)	granulomatosis)
Foreign body aspiration	Bronchiectasis
Pneumonia	Foreign body aspiration
Lung abscess	Lung abscess
Cardiopulmonary malformations (e.g., sequestration,	Hemangioma
AV malformation, bronchogenic cyst)	Pulmonary hypertension
Hemangioma	

tions associated with hemoptysis with typical ages of presentation. It is intended primarily to expand rather than restrict the clinician's thinking about the range of possible causes of hemoptysis. The invasiveness and aggressiveness that are appropriate in a diagnostic workup, as well as its timing, are decided by the risk/benefit ratio for a particular patient at one time. Thoracotomy and open lung biopsy may be the only way to diagnose the cause of bleeding, but they may be appropriate only after stability has been obtained. Patients with hemoptysis and renal involvement often undergo renal biopsy rather than lung biopsy for most accurate diagnosis.

The treatment needed to limit hemoptysis depends on the specific pathophysiology. A patient with coagulopathy may benefit from infusion of fresh frozen plasma or other coagulation factors, as well as from vitamin K or other treatments aimed at remedying deficiencies. Patients who have insufficient numbers of active platelets may respond to infusion of platelets, preferably obtained from a single donor by platelet pheresis. Patients who have already lost significant amounts of red cell mass are likely to benefit from transfusion of packed red cells. Postural drainage treatments should be withheld during an acute bleed.

The underlying condition responsible for the hemoptysis must be treated appropriately. However, in the patient with suppurative lung disease (CF or bronchiectasis), aggressive intravenous antibiotic therapy is usually nec-

essary to limit an episode of hemoptysis. Patients who have an underlying immunologic cause for their pulmonary hemorrhage may need aggressive treatment with steroids and/ or other anti-inflammatory agents to limit hemoptysis (7–10). Patients with arterial venous malformation or other abnormality intrinsic to the lung may not terminate their hemoptysis until they have undergone surgical resection of the malformation.

MASSIVE HEMOPTYSIS IN THE PATIENT WITH CF

The treatment of a patient with CF who has hemoptysis is problematic and controversial. There are many reasons why a patient with CF might have hemoptysis; the treatment and the timing of such treatment, especially invasive treatment, is not the same in every CF center (6, 11, 12). As lung infection progresses in patients with CF, significant large bronchial arteries develop, feeding areas of infection and bronchiectasis. Because of exuberant flow, particularly at times of increased infection, increased cough or bronchial irritation may lead to significant episodes of bleeding. This abnormality of pulmonary circulation, especially when coupled with even mild platelet dysfunction or liver dysfunction, may exacerbate bleeding. Furthermore, the vigorous cough response of most patients with CF, as well as inhalation of irritating solutions such as tobramycin, may further increase their risk of hemoptysis. Patients with CF and severe hemoptysis previously underwent surgical removal of the presumed area of bleeding. With improved angiographic techniques now available, embolization of bronchial vessels is the technique of choice (11, 12). In general, the indications for embolization of bronchial arteries in a patient with CF are acute massive hemoptysis (a single life-threatening hemorrhage or hemoptysis of at least 300 ml of blood per day for 3 or more days), or recurrent moderate hemoptysis (100–200 ml/day for at least a week) (11).

Selective bronchial angiography with embolization of the affected vessels with alcohols, foam pellets, or metal coils may be chosen. Some angiographers feel that these invasive procedures should only be done when a patient is actively bleeding. Others feel that a history of several bleeds of > 100 ml make the patient a candidate for elective arterial embolization. Patients who are acutely bleeding are often agitated, unable to lie down comfortably, and recurrently coughing up blood. Such patients are much more difficult subjects for embolization. This is in contrast to the patient who has been adequately stabilized and is not currently bleeding massively. This patient is usually able to lie quietly and is more likely to be able to undergo the detailed (and at times prolonged) angiographic procedures necessary to selectively embolize the circuitous bronchial arteries with safety. Since there is not uniform agreement as to the single best treatment approach and material, this probably means that each modality has its benefits. Therefore, the skill and experience of the individual doing the treatment is more important than the treatment modality itself. For this reason, the pediatrician or the pediatric pulmonologist should discuss in advance with the available angiographers the approach that they would like to follow in dealing with the future patient with CF who has massive hemoptysis.

Aggressive therapy for hemoptysis may also include any of the following:

Flexible or rigid bronchoscopy to identify the site of bleeding

Ice saline bronchial lavage to constrict the bleeding vessels

IV Vasopressin and/or Desmopressin over a 24-hour to 36-hour period

Endobronchial balloon to apply direct pressure on the bleeding site or to limit the spread of the blood

Pulmonary resection (lobectomy or lobulectomy) may be necessary in patients with > 500–600 ml/hour of bleeding and in whom the bleeding site can be positively located and in whom embolization therapy has failed.

REFERENCES

1. *Stedman's Medical Dictionary*, 25th ed. Baltimore, Williams & Wilkins, 1990, p 701.
2. Case records of the Massachusetts General Hospital. *N Engl J Med* 1983; 309:1374–1381.
3. Firth JR, McGeady SJ, Smith DS. In Chernick V, ed. *Kendig's disorders of the respiratory tract in children*, 5th ed. Philadelphia, WB Saunders, 1990, pp 966–976.
4. Muthuswamy PP, Akbik F, Franklin C, Spigos D, Barker WL. Management of major or massive hemoptysis in active pulmonary tuberculosis by bronchial artery embolization. *Chest* 1987; 92:77–82.
5. Yeung CY. Massive pulmonary hemorrhage in neonatal infection. *Can Med Assoc J* 1976; 114:135–141.
6. Murphy S. Cystic fibrosis in adults: Diagnosis and management. *Clin Chest Med* 1987; 8:695–710.
7. Bradley JD. The pulmonary hemorrhage syndromes. *Clin Chest Med* 1982; 3:593–605.
8. Leatherman JW. Immune alveolar hemorrhage. *Chest* 1987; 91:891–897.
9. Heiner DC. Pulmonary hemosiderosis. In Chernick V, ed. *Kendig's disorders of the respiratory tract in children*, 5th ed. Philadelphia, WB Saunders, 1990, pp 496–509.
10. Leatherman JW, Davies SF, Hoidal JR. Alveolar hemorrhage syndromes: Diffuse microvascular lung hemorrhage in immune and idiopathic disorders. *Medicine* 1984; 63:343–361.
11. Sweezy NB, Fellows KE. Bronchial artery embolization for severe hemoptysis in cystic fibrosis. *Chest* 1990; 97:1322–1326.
12. Cohen AM, Doershuk CF, Stern RC. Bronchial artery embolization to control hemoptysis in cystic fibrosis. *Radiology* 1990; 175:401–405.

19

Chest Pain

GERALD M. LOUGHLIN

In contrast to its significance in adults, chest pain in children is infrequently associated with serious cardiopulmonary pathology. Nonetheless, it is a common problem in pediatrics, especially in adolescents, and one that is associated with increased anxiety in the patient and parent alike (1). The anxiety that surrounds this symptom stems largely from the incorrect notion that chest pain in a child means the same thing it does in adults (i.e., a heart attack or cancer). It is estimated that complaints about chest pain constitute approximately 2.5 per 1000 visits to a pediatrician in an outpatient setting (2, 3). It is unclear from the limited data available how often pediatric pulmonary consultants are asked to evaluate children with chest pain, since in most instances, this problem is handled by the general pediatrician (1). It would appear that the pulmonary consultant is more likely to encounter chest pain in children that is atypical, prolonged, associated with marked parental or patient anxiety, or associated with underlying conditions such as asthma or cystic fibrosis. Thus, it is important for those with a strong interest in pediatric pulmonary disease to recognize the spectrum of causes of chest pain in children and to know when diagnostic studies are needed.

EPIDEMIOLOGY

Chest pain is more often encountered in the older child and adolescent. The mean age of patients presenting to outpatient settings with chest pain is about 12 years (4–6). Girls tend to present at a slightly younger age, especially in the caucasian population (6). Approximately 650,000 visits per year come from children aged 10–18 (5). In inner-city black children, chest pain has been reported to be the seventh most common health concern (7, 8). Chest pain is reported fairly equally in males and females (2, 3, 5, 7).

ETIOLOGY

A differential diagnosis of chest pain based on the organ system responsible for the pain is presented in Table 19.1. Table 19.2 puts this into perspective by listing the common causes of chest pain in children presenting to pediatricians in the emergency department (5). The diagnostic criteria used to define these conditions are presented in Table 19.3.

The most common diagnosis in children without a pre-existing condition is idiopathic or unexplained (ranging from 20 to 67% of cases) (2, 5, 6, 9). In fact, the longer the duration of this symptom, the less likely one is to make a definitive diagnosis.

The most common organic cause of chest pain in children is musculoskeletal secondary either to injury (trauma or overexertion) or to costochondritis (1, 4). Typically, a history of excessive physical activity or trauma can be elicited. Costochondritis is diagnosed in approximately 20% of pediatric patients with chest pain. This is a sharp pain in the anterior chest wall that may radiate to the back or upper abdomen and that may last for several months. Onset of pain is often preceded by a viral respiratory illness or excessive exercise resulting in inflammation. The diagnosis is established by palpation of the anterior chest wall, which localizes the pain. This disorder should be distinguished from the far less common Tietze syndrome, a condition characterized by pain and localized swelling at the sternochondral junction (1, 4, 10).

Interestingly, cardiorespiratory causes of chest pain are uncommon, accounting for

Table 19.1.
Conditions Associated with Chest Pain in Children

Chest Wall

Muscoloskeletal—Usually associated with muscle strain or stress fracture of rib or costochondral cartilage secondary to over exertion from athletic activity or manual labor.

Inflammation.
- Costochondritis
- Tietze syndrome
- Myositis
- Herpes zoster (shingles)

Trauma.
- Major, direct blow to chest
- Minor, severity may not be appreciated
- Post tussive trauma

Miscellaneous.
- Precordial catch (Texidor twinge)
- Chest wall syndrome
- Slipping rib syndrome
- Hypersensitive xiphoid (xiphodynia)
- Bone tumors
- Connective tissue disorders (dermatomyositis and polymyositis)
- Breast development

Airways, Lungs, Pleura, and Diaphragm

Inflammation.
- Asthma–especially post exertion or associated with aggressive beta agonist therapy
- Tracheobronchitis (cystic fibrosis, smoking, viral infection
- Pneumonia
- Pleuritis with or without effusion
- Pleurodynia (coxsackie virus infection)
- Diaphragm irritation:
    Lower lobe pneumonia
    Intra-abdominal process, hepatic abscess, subphrenic abscess gonococcal infection (Fitz-Hugh-Curtis syndrome), splenic infarct
    stitch—strain on peritoneal ligaments attached to diaphragm

Miscellaneous.
- Pneumothorax:
    Spontaneous
    Obstructive lung disease (asthma, CF)
    Connective tissue disorders (Marfan syndrome)
    Chest syndrome (vaso-occlusive crisis—sickle cell disease)

Cardiovascular

Structural abnormalities.
- Mitral valve prolapse
- Coronary artery abnormalities
- LV outflow tract obstruction
- Aortic root dissection
- Aortic valve obstruction

Acquired lesions.
- Myocarditis, pericarditis
    Viral or bacterial
    Rheumatic
    Autoimmune
- Arteritis
    Kawasaki's syndrome
    Autoimmune
- Pulmonary embolism
- Ischemia–complication of hypoxemia and asthma therapy; may occur in sickle cell disease
- Pneumopericardium

Table 19.1.—continued

- Arrhythmia
  - Supraventricular tachycardia
  - Ventricular ectopy—ventricular tachycardia, premature ventricular contractions (rare)
  - Severe pulmonic stenosis

Gastrointestinal

Esophagus.
- Esophagitis—2° reflux
- Esophageal spasm
- Achalasia
- Foreign body

Stomach.
- Hiatal hernia

Referred Pain
- Peptic and duodenal ulcer
- Gastric distention
- Cholelithiasis—common in sickle disease

Miscellaneous

Hyperventilation—frequently complicates other causes
- Psychogenic:
  - Conversion reaction
  - Depression
  - Somatization disorder
- Drug use—Marijuana, cocaine

Table 19.2.
Common Causes of Chest Pain in Children Presenting to the Emergency Department

Diagnosis	% of Children
Idiopathic	21
Musculoskeletal	15
Cough	10
Costochondritis	9
Psychogenic	9
Asthma	7
Trauma	5
Pneumonia	4
Gastrointestinal	4
Cardiac	4
Sickle cell crisis	2
Miscellaneous	9

Modified from Selbst SM, et al. Pediatric chest pain: A prospective study. *Pediatrics* 1988; 82:319–323. Reprinted with permission.

about 10% of the cases (1, 2, 5). Asthma presenting as chest pain, especially following exertion, may be the most common etiology, especially considering the difficulty of diagnosing occult asthma in patients without frank wheezing or in those old enough to perform pulmonary function testing (11). This pain is typically retrosternal and may not be associated with wheezing. In fact, many younger children may misinterpret the uncomfortable

sensation of exertional dyspnea as chest pain. Pneumothorax as a cause of chest pain in children appears to be relatively uncommon, but must be considered, especially in those with asthma and advanced cystic fibrosis who present with acute onset of chest pain and dyspnea. Children and adolescents with Marfan syndrome are predisposed to pneumothorax secondary to rupture of cysts that develop in the lungs of these patients secondary to the underlying connective tissue disorder (12).

Cardiac disease is a very uncommon cause of chest pain (in most series it accounts for less than 5%), but it is perhaps the one group with the potential for significant morbidity and mortality if not recognized (Tables 19.2 and 19.3) (1, 3, 13, 14). Arrhythmias can result in chest pain at any age. Patients old enough to describe symptoms report a brief, sharp pain and may notice a fluttering or variation in the heart rate. Supraventricular tachycardia and premature ventricular contractions are the most common dysrhythmias. Myocardial ischemia caused by hypertrophic obstructive cardiomyopathy, aortic valve stenosis, or an anomalous coronary artery cause angina-like chest pain that usually occurs during exercise. Infection and inflammation of the pericar-

Table 19.3.
Clinical Criteria for Diagnostic Categories

1. *Referred pain from neck and shoulder:* movement or local palpation reproduces or aggravates pain.

2. *Referred pain from abdomen:* (a) tenderness or rebound of abdomen, (b) palpation reproduces or aggravates pain, (c) epigastric pain aggravated or alleviated with food, (d) colicky pain in epigastrium or right upper quadrant (RUQ) (radiation to scapula, nausea, and vomiting option features), (e) pain worse when lying flat or bending over, relieved by antacids or sitting upright, (f) associated with excess eructation or flatus.

3. *Dermatologic:* evidence of dermatologic change in area confined to area of pain.

4. *Breast-gynecomastia:* reproduction of pain on palpation of breast tissue.

5. *Pneumonia/pleurisy:* (a) clinical support: fever, tachypnea, rales, (b) radiographic documentation, (c) positive blood culture, (d) diffuse sharp pain aggravated by breathing in absence of radiographic evidence of tension pneumothorax, rib fracture, or point tenderness on clinical examination.

6. *Bronchitis:* (a) cough preceding symptom, (b) coarse rhonchi.

7. *Hyperventilation* (two of the following): (a) association of rapid breathing by history, (b) circumoral or acral paresthesias, (c) associated light-headedness or dizziness, (d) reproductive of symptoms (45-second timed hyperventilation).

8. *Musculoskeletal:* traumatic (includes rib fracture, tussive fracture) (a) trauma preceded/simultaneous with pain, (b) pain over bruised/traumatized area, (c) radiographic evidence swelling/fracture.

9. *Musculoskeletal:* chest wall syndrome, nontraumatic (includes xiphoidalgia, intercostal neuritis, myodynia, fibrositis, precordial catch, slipping rib, Tietze syndrome) (a) reproduction of pain by local application of pressure, (b) aggravated by isometric exercise of outstretched arm.

10. *Musculoskeletal:* costochondritis: reproduction of pain by local pressure directly over nonenlarged costochondral or chondrosternal junction.

11. *Isolated organic disease:* standard clinical criteria for (a) pericarditis, (b) pneumothorax, (c) asthma, (d) thoracic outlet syndrome, (e) pleurodynia, (f) pulmonary embolus (g) pain crisis of sickle cell anemia, (h) myocarditis.

12. *Idiopathic:* nonspecific description not classifiable into any of the above categories.

13. *Mixed:* clear indication of one or more etiologies. Example: historical evidence of hyperventilation during acute event but definite costosternal junction tenderness on examination reproducing chest pain.

Reprinted with permission from Pantell RH, Goodman BW Jr. Adolescent chest pain: A prospective study. *Pediatrics* 1983; 71:881–887.

dium, myocardium, or coronary arteries are also associated with chest pain; usually this pain is one component of a generalized illness, as with bacterial pericarditis or Kawasaki disease. Although frequently included in the differential diagnosis of chest pain, mitral valve prolapse is a relatively uncommon cause of chest pain in children (1, 2, 6, 12).

Approximately 4% of cases of pediatric chest pain are generally attributed to gastrointestinal (GI) disease (1–3,7). However, Berezin and co-workers reported that 78% of patients previously labeled as having idiopathic chest pain were found to have pain secondary to GI disease following a more intensive search for an underlying gastrointestinal cause (15). Diagnoses include esophagitis from gastroesophageal reflux, esophageal spasm, gastritis, and hiatal hernia. Chest pain that arises from a GI cause is characterized by a retrosternal location, occurrence at rest, and association with swallowing and with other gastrointestinal symptoms such as vomiting and dysphagia (16).

A psychogenic (functional) etiology for the pain must be pursued in all patients before the diagnosis of idiopathic chest pain can be applied. A functional cause is more common in girls, and the pain is more debilitating than one would imagine based on the physical examination. As with other functional respiratory symptoms such as cough, this chest pain, although not as intense as that from other organic causes, frequently results in considerable amounts of time lost from school and other activities of a teenager. Chest pain has also been reported as a manifestation of clinical depression in teenagers (17), as well as in association with use of marijuana and cocaine (18–20). It may also be the chief complaint of adolescent males and females concerned with excessive or unusual breast development at the early stages of puberty (1, 7).

Other rare but notable causes of chest pain in children include the slipping rib syndrome and the precordial catch, also known as Texidor twinge or "stitch in the side." The slipping rib syndrome has been reported following trauma to the 8th, 9th, or 10th rib, which are not attached to the sternum. The patient reports pain under these ribs or in the upper abdomen and a feeling that one of these lower ribs is moveable. Occasionally, the patient may report hearing a popping or clicking noise with lifting or truncal flexion (1, 21). A precordial catch is a brief, episodic, random left-sided chest pain usually triggered by sitting in a slouched position. This pain is relieved by standing up straight or by taking several shallow breaths. The etiology of this pain is unknown, but it may be due to pressure either on the parietal pleura or on an intercostal nerve (1, 22). Pleurodynia, also referred to as the "devil's grip" because of the severe thorax or upper abdominal pain secondary to infection with a coxsackie B virus, occurs in epidemics and fortunately is rare in children. In children with sickle cell disease, chest and abdominal pain can be seen as part of the typical vaso-occlusive crisis (1, 4).

APPROACH TO THE PATIENT WITH CHEST PAIN

History

As with the evaluation of other respiratory symptoms, the importance of a complete history cannot be understated. This is especially true in dealing with a child with chest pain since several series have demonstrated the limited value of laboratory studies in diagnosing the cause of the chest pain. Emphasis should be placed on the circumstances surrounding the onset of the pain, both initially and with recurrences. Does the pain occur spontaneously or is it associated with certain behaviors such as eating, sleep, or exercise? Are there other precipitating factors? Pain that awakens a child from sleep, or that is associated with fever or abnormal physical findings, is quite likely to be organic (3). Pain associated with exercise suggests a cardiopulmonary origin; the most likely diagnosis is exercise-induced asthma. Was there a history of trauma or of strenuous or unusual physical activity preceding the onset of pain? We have encountered several adolescents who developed severe chest wall pain localized to the costochondral junction following attempts at picking up lightweight but awkwardly shaped objects (such as a piece of pipe or a mattress). In both instances, the patient initially denied any trauma or strenuous activity. The pain was quite debilitating and was remarkable for eliciting exquisite point tenderness over the junction between the rib and the sternum. The pain originated from a fracture of the cartilage and eventually required surgery. Was the child short of breath? Has the patient experienced chest pain before? How has the pain altered the patients life? Does the child have any underlying cardiac or pulmonary disease? Asthma, cystic fibrosis, and Marfan syndrome all predispose a person to pneumothorax. In private, the adolescent and older child should be asked about smoking (23) and drug use (18–20). Has the patient experienced any recent emotional trauma? Is there a family history of cardiorespiratory disease or chest pain? What therapy has been tried and has it been effective?

Description of the pain in terms of sharp or dull has not been shown to correlate with a particular etiology (1, 2, 4). However, the localization of the pain is quite helpful (3). Diffuse pain and pain that radiates to the abdomen are rarely cardiac in origin. Substernal pain is infrequently cardiac (28%), whereas pain that radiates to the shoulder is frequently cardiac in nature (62% of the cases) (3).

It is also important to assess the patient and family's response to the pain. What significance does the family attach to the pain? Are they overly anxious about a possible heart attack or cancer? This knowledge will help guide the design of a therapeutic plan.

Physical Examination

The evaluation of the child with chest pain requires knowledge of the distribution of the thoracic dermatomes. The thorax from the clavicles to the xiphoid process is innervated by T1-T8. These thoracic dermatomes also include the anterior and medial portions of the upper arms. The diaphragm has dual innervation with input from both the thoracic spinal and cervical spinal nerves (3–5). Visceral pain in this region can arise from any of the organs contained within this zone (4) (Table 19.4). Pain originating from the upper dermatomes is typically most intense in the retrosternal and precordial regions, whereas that arising from the lower thoracic region

Table 19.4.
Distribution of Innervation of Thorax

T1-I4:

Myocardium
Pericardium
Aorta
Pulmonary arteries
Esophagus
Mediastinum

T5-I8:

Lower thoracic wall
Diaphragm (also fibers from C3, C4, C5)
Abdominal organs (gallbladder, liver, pancreas,
   stomach, duodenum, and peritoneum)

(T5-T8) tends to be maximal in the xiphoid region and may extend posteriorly and inferiorly to the region of the right scapula. Pain originating from the diaphragm has two distinct patterns depending on the portion of the diaphragm involved. Since the posterior and lateral parts are covered by the lower six thoracic dermatomes, pain arising from this region is sensed in the lower back, lower thorax, and upper abdominal regions. Pain arising from the anterior sections of the diaphragm is frequently sensed in the neck and shoulder since these areas are innervated by branches of the phrenic nerve (4).

Frequently, the examination of the chest is completely normal since most of time the source of the chest pain is not identified (idiopathic) or is psychogenic. Nonetheless, it is important to examine the chest carefully. Palpation of the chest wall to identify rib injury or costochondral inflammation should be performed in all patients regardless of the history. This examination should be focused over the area identified by the patient as being the source of the pain, but the entire thorax and upper abdomen should be examined. In patients who may have suffered a traumatic injury, the ribs should be compressed from opposite sides of the thorax to identify a rib fracture. Slipping rib syndrome can be diagnosed by hooking the rib in question with a finger and pulling gently. This should produce pain similar to that reported by the patient (1, 21). Diminished breath sounds, mediastinal shift, and a tympanic percussion note suggest the presence of a pneumothorax. Similarly, evidence of wheezing and hyperinflation may help identify a child with atypical presentation of asthma.

A thorough cardiac examination with the patient in a variety of positions helps to identify left ventricular outflow obstruction or mitral valve prolapse or other significant cardiac lesion (1, 12). A breast examination should be included for both males and females. Pubescent males may complain of chest pain when they are actually concerned about what may appear to them as unusual or excessive breast development.

Laboratory Studies

This is an area of some controversy. In the general pediatric practice office or pediatric emergency room, laboratory evaluation of the patient with isolated chest pain has been shown to be of limited value (2, 7). In fact, in most instances, few if any diagnostic tests are required as a part of the initial evaluation. A simple chest radiograph offers the greatest yield and should be obtained in the patient in whom a respiratory, cardiac, vertebral abnormality or traumatic injury is suspected as the etiology of the pain, or if there are associated symptoms such as dyspnea. However, the radiograph is frequently normal (5–7).

Routine electrocardiography (EKG) or echocardiography has not been shown to be helpful in identifying the cause of typical chest pain unless there is evidence of cardiac involvement on the physical examination (1, 7, 12).

Although a minimal work-up may be indicated initially when the child is seen in the emergency room or office setting, the situation is somewhat different in a referral practice. Since in most instances routine patients with chest pain who have no complications have been culled out by the pediatrician, the consultant is often faced with a patient whose pain is atypical, persistent, and debilitating or associated with signs and symptoms of underlying disease (1). Often there is be suspicion by the referring pediatrician that the pain is functional, but the pediatrician and family want to be sure. Although psychogenic pain is not totally a diagnosis of exclusion, it is important that the patient, parent, and physician be comfortable that the more common organic conditions have been ruled out. This is particularly important because chest pain causes considerable anxiety in all concerned. Any tests that are considered should be based on the presence of associated findings from the history, physical examination, or screening chest radiograph.

Other diagnostic studies that may be helpful in defining the etiology of chest pain include an echocardiogram in the patient with suspected cardiac disease, and esophagoscopy and a modified Bernstein test in the child with suspected esophagitis or gastritis (24). Pulmonary function tests are generally not needed except in the case of suspected asthma. These tests may detect reversible airways obstruction, but most likely some form of airway challenge study (exercise or methacholine) will be needed (11).

Treatment

Treatment of chest pain in children is largely symptomatic and dictated primarily by the underlying condition. Since most often chest pain turns out to be idiopathic, analgesia and reassurance that there is no significant problem underlying the pain is usually all that is needed. Anti-inflammatory agents are indicated in patients with costochondritis or following trauma. Pain secondary to post-exertional asthma is usually well controlled with bronchodilators before exercise. Treatment of pneumothorax is dictated by the size of the air leak, the nature of the underlying or predisposing condition, and the patient's degree of respiratory distress. A small air leak (e.g., < 15%) in an asymptomatic patient without a predisposing condition can be observed as the patient is given 100% oxygen to breathe to facilitate reabsorption. Occasionally, simple aspiration of the air is all that is needed. A larger pneumothorax in the same patient that is associated with respiratory distress and continued pain should be managed with a chest tube. Supplemental oxygen and analgesia should also be administered while the tube is in place. Patients with persistent leak or recurrent pneumothorax should undergo chest computed tomography (CT) to identify surface pleural blebs. These patients often require an open thoracotomy with pleurodesis in order to reduce the risk of recurrence. The management of pneumothorax in the patient with cystic fibrosis is discussed in Chapter 22.

Patients in whom a psychogenic origin is thought to be responsible for the pain should be referred for counseling. Management of chest pain in other conditions listed in Tables 19.1–19.4 should be directed at the underlying disease process (1, 4).

Prognosis

Follow-up data in children with chest pain have demonstrated that the pain will persist in 40–60% of the patients followed for up to 5 years (2, 6, 13, 25, 26). Interestingly, the initial diagnosis changed in 34%, but most importantly serious organic disease is rarely detected in the follow-up period. Nonetheless, close follow-up of the child with persistent pain is important, since this symptom is usually a continued source of concern to the patient and family and it is possible that what has been labeled as idiopathic pain may become definable at a latter date.

REFERENCES

1. Selbst SM. Evaluation of chest pain in children. *Pediatr Rev* 1986; 8:56–63.
2. Selbst SM. Chest pain in children. *Pediatrics* 1985; 75:1068–1070.
3. Zavaras-Angelidou KA, Weinhouse E, Nelson DB. Review of 180 episodes of chest pain in 134 children. *Pediatr Emerg Care* 1992; 8:189–193.
4. Coleman WL. Recurrent chest pain in children. *Pediatr Clin North Am* 1984; 31:1007–1026.
5. Selbst SM, Ruddy RM, et al. Pediatric chest pain: A prospective study. *Pediatrics* 1988; 82:319–323.
6. Driscoll DJ, Glicklich LB, Gallen WJ. Chest pain in children: A prospective study. *Pediatrics* 1976; 57:648–651.
7. Pantell RH, Goodman BW Jr. Adolescent chest pain: A prospective study. *Pediatrics* 1983; 71:881–887.
8. Bruswick AF, Boyle JM, Tarica C. Who sees the doctor? A study of urban black adolescents. *Soc Sci Med* 1979; 13A:45.
9. Fukushige J, Tsuchihashik, Harada T, et al. Chest pain in pediatric patients. *Acta Pediatr Jpn* 1988; 30:604–607.
10. Calabro J, Marchesano J. Tietze's syndrome: Report of a case with juvenile onset. *J Pediatr* 1968; 68:985.
11. Wiens L, Sabath R, Ewing L, et al. Chest pain in otherwise healthy children and adolescents is frequently caused by exercise induced asthma. *Pediatrics* 1992; 90:350–353.
12. Hall JR, Pyeritz RE, Dudgeon DL, et al. Pneumothorax in the Marfan syndrome: Prevalence and therapy. *Ann Thorac Surg* 1984; 37:500–504.
13. Brenner JI, Ringel RE, Berman MA. Cardiologic perspectives of chest pain in pediatric patients presenting to a cardiac clinic. *Pediatr Clin North Am* 1984; 31:1241–1258.
14. Fyfe DA, Moodie DS. Chest pain in pediatric patients presenting to a cardiac clinic. *Clin Pediatr* 1984; 23:321–340.
15. Berezin S, Medow MS, Glassman MS et al. Chest pain of gastrointestinal origin. *Arch Dis Child* 1988; 63:1457–1460.

16. Milov DE, Cynamon HA, Andres JM. Chest pain and dysphagia in adolescents caused by diffuse esophageal spasm. *J Pediatr Gastroenterol Nutr* 1989; 9:450–453.

17. Kashani JH, Lababidi Z, Jones RS. Depression in children and adolescents with cardiovascular symptomatology: The significance of chest pain. *J Am Acad Child Psychiatry* 1982; 21:187–189.

18. Lantner IL. Letter to the editor. *Pediatrics* 1983; 72:916.

19. Woodward GA, Selbst SM. Chest pain secondary to cocaine use. *Pediatr Emerg Care* 1987; 3:153–154.

20. Mofernson HC, Copland P. Caraccio TR. Cocaine and crack: The latest menace. *Contemp Pediatr* 1986; 3:44–50.

21. Porter GE. Slipping rib syndrome. An infrequently recognized entity in children: A report of three cases and review of the literature. *Pediatrics* 1985; 76:810–813.

22. Pickering D. Precordial catch syndrome. *Arch Dis Child* 1981; 56:401–403.

23. Friedman G, Sieglaub A, Dales L. Cigarette smoking and chest pain. *Ann Intern Med* 1975; 83:1–7.

24. Berezin S. Medow MS, Glassman MS, et al. Use of the intraesophageal acid perfusion test in provoking non-specific chest pain in children. J Pediatr 1989; 115:709–712.

25. Selbst SM, Ruddy R, Clark BJ. Chest pain in children. Follow-up of patients previously reported. *Clin Pediatr* 1990; 29:374–377.

26. Rowland TW, Richards MM. The natural history of idiopathic chest pain in children, a follow-up study. *Clin Pediatr* 1986; 25:612–614.

20

Chronic/Recurrent Pulmonary Infiltrates

HOWARD EIGEN

The child with recurrent pulmonary infiltrates or recurrent pneumonia presents what is an often difficult problem in diagnosis. The intent of this chapter, rather to be encyclopedic in the possible causes of recurrent infiltrates, is to present a clinical approach to such patients so that most often the most common diagnosis can be made quickly and with minimal testing and procedures.

Patients with recurrent or persistent respiratory infections can be categorized in many ways, but one useful device is to classify them into those with (a) persistent or recurrent radiologic findings with persistent or intermittent fever or other clinical signs of infection, (b) persistent radiologic findings without clinical evidence of infection, (c) recurrent pulmonary infiltrates with interval radiologic clearing. In the first group are patients with cystic fibrosis, immunodeficiencies such as hypogammaglobulinemia, pulmonary sequestration, bronchial obstruction (either intrinsic from foreign body or adenoma or extrinsic from nodes, tumor, or cyst), or bronchiectasis. In the second group anatomic lesions such as sequestrations, anatomic variants, granulomas, and pleural lesions would be considered. In the third group, asthma (and atelectasis) is probably the most common diagnosis, but aspiration syndromes (including tracheoesophageal fistula, gastroesophageal reflux, and dysfunctional swallowing disorders), mild immunodeficiency syndromes, hypersensitivity pneumonitis, and idiopathic pulmonary hemosiderosis could also be considered.

The first step in evaluating a child for recurrent infiltrates is to determine whether there truly has been a recurrent or persistent process in the lung. It is often the case that radiographs are over-read for minor abnormalities by persons unfamiliar with interpreting pediatric chest films. Expiratory chest films, those that are underpenetrated, and other such technical abnormalities can be misinterpreted as indicative of infiltrates or atelectasis. These "abnormalities" are then reread on subsequent films, creating the appearance of recurrent disease. Many times reports of pneumonia are passed along without the films being reread, or the diagnosis of recurrent pneumonia is made on clinical grounds alone without a confirming radiograph, which further confuses the picture.

To decide if a process is persistent or recurrent one must carefully define these terms. *Persistent pneumonia* is one that is prolonged past what would be expected from understanding the natural history of the illness. This definition requires knowing the infectious etiology of the original episode, which is often not possible. The radiologic course of specific viral pneumonia has been described by Osborne (1), who found surprisingly prolonged periods of radiographic abnormalities following viral pneumonia. Radiographic abnormalities seen in RSV pneumonia lasted 2–2½ weeks; those associated with adenovirus pneumonia lasted 2 weeks to 3 months; and those with parainfluenza lasted 2 ½ weeks to 3 months. Minor abnormalities could be seen as late as 1 year after the initial episode. In a study of adults, the normal course for chest radiographic abnormalities with pneumococcal pneumonia was 6 weeks (2). Without knowing the etiology of the pulmonary infiltrate, it is very difficult to make an assessment of what the course should be and what constitutes persistence. However, persistence of infiltrate on chest radiograph beyond 3 months is unusual and warrants follow-up

REFERENCES

1. Osborne D. Radiologic appearance of viral disease of the lower respiratory tract in infants and children. *Am J Roentgenol* 1978; 130:29–33.
2. Jay SJ, Johanson WG Jr, Pierce AK. The radiographic resolution of *Streptococcus pneumoniae* pneumonia. *N Engl J Med* 1975; 293:798–801.
3. Leonidas JC, Stuber JL, Rudavsky AZ, Abramson AL. Radionuclide lung scanning the diagnosis of endo-bronchial foreign bodies in Children. *J Pediatr* 1973; 83:628–631.
4. Eigen H, Laughlin JJ, Homrighausen. Recurrent pneumonia in children and its relationship to bronchial hyperreactivity. *J Pediatr* 1982; 70:698–704.
5. Kjellman B. Bronchial asthma and recurrent pneumonia in children. *Acta Pediatr Scand* 1967; 56:651–659.

COMMON PULMONARY DISEASES

21

Asthma

GERARD J. CANNY and HENRY LEVISON

Asthma is the most common chronic disease of childhood in industrialized countries. Although asthma is a rare cause of mortality among children (1), it remains a major cause of school absenteeism (2–5), restricted activity (2), and hospitalization (6), as well as a significant health care cost (7). Recent community surveys indicate that asthma morbidity is frequently due to underdiagnosis, undertreatment, poor education, and inadequate supervision of care (2–4, 8). Comprehensive treatment programs that address these issues have been shown to improve significantly the overall health of children with asthma (9, 10). Thus, the main objective of this chapter will be to provide a practical and flexible approach to the diagnosis and management of asthma of varying degrees of severity in children, and to focus on features that are unique to childhood asthma.

EPIDEMIOLOGIC CONSIDERATIONS

Prevalence

Epidemiologic studies indicate that asthma is strongly associated with a "Western" lifestyle. For example, the prevalence of asthma among children in developing countries is less than 1%, as compared to more than 20% in some industrialized countries (11). In addition, it has been shown that the prevalence of asthma in children who have emigrated to an industrialized country is more characteristic of the adoptive country than the society of origin (12). In developing countries, the prevalence of asthma is higher in urban than rural children, a difference that is likely due to environmental factors (13). In Western societies, estimates of the prevalence of childhood asthma vary widely (11). Unfortunately, these epidemiologic studies are difficult to interpret in view of differences in method, in the definition of asthma, and in the age of the children surveyed. In addition, some studies report point prevalence and others cumulative prevalence rates. On balance, the prevalence and severity of asthma in developed countries appears to be increasing, the cause of which is unclear (14).

A comprehensive picture of the prevalence of asthma among children in the United States is provided by the National Health and Nutrition Examination Survey (NHANES) (15, 16) and the National Health Interview Survey (NHIS) (17) (Table 21.1). These surveys found that asthma is more common in males (15–17), certain geographic locations (e.g., the South and West) (15), urban areas (15–17), and in blacks (15–17). The racial discrepancy in the prevalence of childhood asthma in the United States is at variance with reports from other multicultural societies (18), and appears to be due largely to social and environmental factors rather than to genetic differences (16, 17). The overall male-to-female ratio for asthma among children in the United States is 1.4:1, although this ratio declines with age (15). The cause of this male preponderance is unclear, but may be related to a greater degree of bronchial lability (19) and a higher occurrence of respiratory infections among boys.

Morbidity and Mortality

During the past two decades, a significant increase in hospital admission rates for childhood asthma has been noted in several Western countries, particularly in preschool children. In the United States, hospitalization rates for pediatric asthma have increased by 4.5% per annum (6), and by 12.5% in Canada (20). Likewise, asthma hospitalizations among

Table 21.1.
Estimates of Asthma Prevalence among US Children Related to Sex and Race

Survey and Asthma Definition[a]	Total	Sex		Race	
		Males	Female	White	Black
NHANES II, 1976–80 (children 3–17 years)					
Ever diagnosed by physician	7.0	8.3	5.5	6.4	10.1
Currently diagnosed by physician	3.6	4.3	2.9	3.3	5.6
Wheezing[b]	5.3	6.2	4.5	5.0	7.3
Ever diagnosed by physician or wheezing[b]	9.5	11.2	7.8	8.9	13.1
Currently diagnosed by physician or wheezing[b]	6.7	7.8	5.5	6.2	9.4
NHIS, 1981 (Children 0–17 years)					
Current asthma[c]	2.8	NA	NA	2.5	4.4

[a]*Abbreviations:* NHANES, National Health and Nutrition Examination Survey (15); NHIS, National Health Interview Survey (17); Data are mean percentages.
[b]Frequent trouble with wheezing (not counting colds or the flu) during the past 12 months.
[c]Based on parents' reports that their child had asthma at the time of interview, which had been present for longer than 3 months and had not been cured.

children have increased in Britain (14, 21), Australia (22), and New Zealand (23). The cause of these increased hospital admission rates is unclear, but could be the result of a combination of factors (Table 21.2) (6, 14, 20–24). The observation that the increase in hospitalization rates for asthma has occurred at a time of a decline in admissions for other pediatric respiratory conditions suggests that diagnostic transfer (recoding) is partly responsible (22). In addition, a change in medical practice has been noted in some countries, resulting in an increased use of hospital resources for the treatment of asthma (21, 25).

Although asthma is rarely fatal in children, an upward swing in death rates has been reported in children in several Western countries (1, 26). In the United States, mortality increased by 6.2% per annum among children and young adults in the 1980s, and is particu-

Table 21.2
Possible Explanations for Increased Hospitalization Rates for Asthma

- Diagnostic transfer (e.g., wheezy bronchitis to asthma)
- Asthma prevalence and/or severity may be increasing
- Changes in health care access, availability, utilization
- Change in the International Classification of Disease, from the 8th to 9th revisions in 1979
- Improved recognition and diagnosis of asthma
- Increasing levels of environmental pollution

larly high among blacks and in poor urban areas (1). The factors considered responsible for these rising mortality rates are similar to those put forward to explain the increasing morbidity rates (24). It has also been suggested that some deaths may be related to sympathomimetic and/or theophylline use (27). Several mechanisms have been postulated to explain this association, including (a) direct cardiotoxic effects of nonselective (28) and selective (29) beta agonists; (b) delivery of beta-2 agonists in high dosage by home nebulizers without supplementary oxygen (30); (c) synergistic cardiac toxicity from the concurrent use of beta-2 agonists and oral theophylline (31); and (d) paradoxical bronchoconstriction, induced by beta-2 agonists (32). However, the overwhelming evidence from epidemiologic studies is that deaths in asthma are usually preventable, and are often due to over-reliance on bronchodilators resulting in a delay in referral to hospital and treatment with systemic steroids, rather than to a direct toxic effect of beta-2 agonists (24, 33). These studies also provide a profile of children who are at higher risk of dying from asthma (Table 21.3), and these patients obviously require more intensive treatment and careful monitoring (33–35).

ETIOLOGIC ASPECTS

Airway inflammation has long been recognized as a characteristic pathologic feature in severe fatal asthma (36). The histologic find-

Table 21.3.
Characteristics of the High-Risk Child with Asthma

- Previous life-threatening episodes (e.g., ICU admission, hypoxic-related seizures)
- Recent hospitalizations or ER visits
- Dependency on multiple medications (particularly oral steroids)
- Discontinuous medical care
- Noncompliance/psychosocial problems (particularly in teenagers)
- Ethnic minority group—poor access to health care (e.g., Maoris/Polynesians in New Zealand; blacks in United States)

Data from references 34 and 35.

ings include subepithelial fibrosis and collagen deposition, epithelial shedding, goblet cell metaplasia, smooth muscle hypertrophy, and leukocytic (predominantly eosinophilic) infiltration of the submucosa (37). Other characteristic findings include mucosal edema due to microvascular leakage and hypersecretion of mucus from goblet cells, which results in mucus plugging of peripheral airways and focal atelectasis (37). More recently the presence of airway inflammation in some patients with relatively mild asthma has been recognized. Cutz et al. (38) found that the morphologic changes in open lung biopsy specimens from two children with well-controlled asthma were similar to the changes observed at autopsy in two children who had died from asthma, although a larger number of submucosal eosinophils and more extensive epithelial damage were noted in the latter patents. Likewise, transbronchial biopsies obtained from adult asthmatics have shown inflammation and epithelial damage (39, 40), although in some cases the bronchial epithelium may be normal (41).

Although the cause of asthma is not completely understood, its characteristic feature is bronchial hyperreactivity—up to 90% of children with frequent wheezing in the previous year demonstrate reactivity to methacholine/histamine, particularly when associated with atopy (42, 43). It is believed that the degree of bronchial reactivity is related to the extent of inflammation in the airways, although the role of various inflammatory cells and mediators in this link is still being debated (44). Bronchial hyper-responsiveness is detectable soon after birth (45), and it is postu-

lated that the expression of airway reactivity is determined by complex interactions between genetic, atopic, and environmental factors (45, 46) (Fig. 21.1) (see Chapter 3).

Genetic Influences

There is much evidence that asthma and other atopic disorders (e.g., eczema, allergic rhinitis) are partly hereditary in nature. There is an increased prevalence of asthma among first-degree relatives of index subjects (3, 47–50); likewise, the risk of having an asthmatic child is significantly greater when one or both parents have asthma than when neither parent is affected (51–53). Sibbald et al. showed that 17% of parents and 8% of the siblings of asthmatic children had asthma, as compared to 4% and 3% of the respective relatives of control children (47). Higgins and Keller found that the prevalence of asthma among boys increased from 7.4% when neither parent had asthma to 18.3% when one or both parent had asthma, and from 4.1% to 11.7% for girls (51). However, other studies have found that a history of parental atopy/asthma was associated with a higher prevalence of asthma in boys but not in girls (52, 53). A familial component is also thought to exist in the genesis of airway hyper-responsiveness to methacholine/histamine (54, 55) that may be independent of atopic status (56). A recent study found that airway responsiveness to histamine is present shortly after birth in normal, asymptomatic infants (57). The level of this airway responsiveness correlated with a family history of asthma and parental smoking, but not with atopic markers (e.g., IgE levels).

It could be argued that the tendency for asthma to cluster in families is due to the effect of a shared environment rather than to genetic

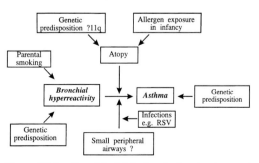

Figure 21.1. Possible risk factors for the development of asthma. *RSV* = respiratory syncytial virus.

influences. However, twin studies provide convincing evidence for a genetic component in asthma. A Scandinavian study of 7000 pairs of twins found a substantial concordance for asthma in monozygotic twins (19%) as compared to dizygotic twins (4.8%) (58). Likewise, Hopp and colleagues found greater concordance for asthma, atopy and methacholine sensitivity in monozygotic than for dizygotic twins (54). In a recent twin study from Australia, a common genetic influence on asthma and hay fever was reported, although 40% of the variation in the liability to these conditions was thought to be environmental in nature (59).

Atopy

Atopy, as an increased predisposition to form IgE antibodies on exposure to common environmental antigens, is present in the majority of patients with asthma (60). Family aggregation (48, 49, 52) and twin studies (54, 58, 59) indicate that atopy is at least partly hereditary, and recent data suggest an autosomal dominant pattern of inheritance (61), with the gene locus on chromosome 11 (62). Although atopy and airway hyper-reactivity may be inherited independently (64), exposure to high levels of inhaled allergens at an early age is an important determinant in the development of asthma. This is particularly true in the case of the house dust mite. In a recent prospective study of infants who were prone to allergic disease because of family history, Sporik et al. found a relation between the level of exposure to house dust mites in infancy and the age at which wheezing subsequently occurred (65). All but one of the children with diagnosed asthma at 11 years of age had been exposed to high levels (> 10 μg per gram of dust) of the house dust mite allergen (*Der p 1*) during infancy. In Papua, New Guinea, the increased prevalence of asthma has been related to greater exposure to aeroallergens, particularly house dust mites (66). It is also possible that exposure to other allergens (e.g., pollens and animal danders) in early life may influence the development of asthma (67). In recent years, several studies have shown a strong correlation between the degree of atopy and the prevalence of airway hyper-reactivity (42, 43, 68–71). Although the mechanism linking atopy and asthma is not entirely clear, it is possible that allergen-induced airway inflammation leads to increased airway responsiveness and is thus responsible for the development of asthma (71).

The role of food allergens in the pathogenesis of asthma is controversial. In general, pulmonary reactions to ingested foods are rare (72). In a study of young asthmatic children, it was found that 37 of 109 children were allergic to certain foods (e.g., milk, eggs, wheat) as defined by a high serum IgE antibody and a clinical history of a reaction to the food (73). Although eczema was more common in the food-allergic patients, the severity of asthma did not differ in the two groups. The question as to whether breast feeding prevents the subsequent development of asthma and other atopic conditions remains unresolved (74, 75). However, this should not detract from the many other benefits of breast feeding, including a protective effect against lower respiratory infections early in life (76).

Respiratory Infections

In children with asthma, respiratory viruses (e.g., rhinoviruses, respiratory syncytial virus [RSV], influenza, and parainfluenza viruses) are the most common precipitating cause of wheeze (77). Possible mechanisms of virus-induced wheeze include exposure of vagal receptors as a result of epithelial damage, a decreased beta adrenergic response, and IgE-related hypersensitivity (77). There is also evidence that respiratory illnesses in early childhood such as bronchiolitis (78–83), croup (84), chlamydia pneumonia (85), and pertussis (86, 87) contribute in a causal fashion to the development of airway reactivity and asthma. In this regard, the evidence is strongest for RSV-induced bronchiolitis. Moderately severe bronchiolitis in infancy is associated in about 50% of cases with the development of lung function abnormalities, enhanced airway reactivity, and an increased risk of asthma later in childhood, particularly in children with a family history of atopy. It is unclear whether RSV infections produce long-term abnormalities in airway function directly, or whether these infections are more likely to occur (and be more severe) in infants with a genetic predisposition to atopy or airway hyper-reactivity. In some infants with bronchiolitis, RSV-specific IgE antibodies and high histamine concentrations have been found in nasopharyngeal secretions (88), and these infants are more likely to develop subsequent episodes of wheezing than those with undetectable RSV IgE titers (89). The risk of wheezing during respiratory infections in the first few years of life is significantly higher in infants who have diminished lung function, possibly since birth (90, 91). This suggests that infants who are destined to wheeze with respiratory infections may have "critically narrower peripheral airways." On the other hand, citing the global distribution of asthma and respiratory infections, Burney and colleagues (92) have challenged the theory that there is a direct causal link between infection and asthma.

Parental Smoking

In children with asthma, maternal smoking increases the severity of symptoms, adversely affects lung function, and increases airway hyper-reactivity (93). This association is stronger for boys (94) and older children (93, 94) with asthma, and is affected by the duration of exposure and the number of cigarettes smoked by the mother each day (93). The relationship between passive smoking and the *acquisition* of asthma is less well defined (17, 95, 96). However, intrauterine exposure to cigarette smoke results in elevated cord IgE levels (97) and increased airway responsiveness at birth (57), and is a risk factor for the development of atopy (97) and asthma (98) in early childhood. Likewise, passive exposure to cigarette smoke is associated with wheezing and nonwheezing lower respiratory illness in infants, particularly in those who do not attend day care, whose mothers are heavy smokers (99). Children with atopic dermatitis are more likely to develop asthma if the mother is a smoker than if she is a nonsmoker (100). Finally, in older children, it has been suggested that parental smoking, by increasing the frequency of bronchial reactivity and atopy, may add to the risk and severity of asthma (101).

Air Pollution

Exposure to chemical (e.g., sulphur dioxide, ozone) and particulate pollution can induce symptoms in children with asthma. In the Harvard Six Cities Study, children with asthma were found to be particularly susceptible to respiratory symptoms when exposed to high particulate and SO_2 concentrations (102). Likewise, in a study from Utah (103), hospital admission rates for respiratory illnesses among children were found to relate to the level of ambient air particles arising from a local steel mill. In contrast, Vedal et al. failed to show an association between increased respiratory symptoms among children and SO_2 concentrations, although the levels were lower than the current air standards (104). The observation that the prevalence of asthma is low in certain highly polluted areas (105) does not support the view that atmospheric pollution contributes to the actual development of asthma.

Socioeconomic Factors

The racial discrepancy in the prevalence and morbidity from childhood asthma in the United States appears to be related to social and environmental factors associated with poverty and inner city living (16, 17). These risk factors for asthma include low family income, low birth weight, young maternal age, crowding in the home, and maternal smoking (16, 17). Likewise, the differences in the prevalence of asthma between Polynesian children and those of European descent in New Zealand appear to be related to socioeconomic status and home smoking rates (23). In contrast, no consistent relationship between social status and asthma prevalence has been found in other populations (53, 96).

ESTABLISHING A DIAGNOSIS OF ASTHMA

In the community, asthma is frequently underdiagnosed and inappropriately treated (2–4, 8, 68). This results from a reluctance on the part of physicians to apply the term "asthma" and from confusion over terminology. Although many definitions exist (Table 21.4), the diagnosis of asthma in childhood is essentially a clinical one, since pulmonary function measurements are not possible in

Table 21.4
Definitions of Asthma

Specialist	Definition
Clinician	Reversibility
Physiologist	Hyper-responsiveness
Pathologist	Inflammation

infants and young children (except in highly specialized laboratories). We suggest that any child, regardless of age, with recurrent (three or more) episodes of wheezing and/or dyspnea should be considered as having asthma until proven otherwise. The diagnosis of asthma is even more likely if these symptoms are episodic, aggravated by one or more of the factors listed in Table 21.5, and respond favorably to anti-asthmatic medications. The clinician should be aware that about 5% of children with asthma present with a persistent or recurrent cough as the sole symptom (106). The cough is usually nonproductive, mostly nocturnal, and often aggravated by exercise, allergen exposure, and viral infections. The study of Eigen et al. (107) indicates that some children are misdiagnosed as having persistent/recurrent pneumonia on chest radiographs, when in fact these infiltrates represent atelectasis from mucus plugging of peripheral airways in asthma. For a number of anatomic reasons, atelectasis in asthma affects the right middle lobe predominantly (108).

Clinical Evaluation

A careful history is the single most important element in the evaluation of a child suspected of having asthma. The key points to elicit in the history are listed in Table 21.6. It is also important in the course of the clinical evaluation to identify high-risk patients (Table 21.3) in order to provide them with the special attention they require (33–35). Physical examination should focus on overall growth and development and look for clinical evidence of airway obstruction, pulmonary hyperinflation, associated signs of allergy, and drug-related side effects. Finally, the clinical evaluation

Table 21.5.
Triggers of Asthma

- Respiratory infection (viral, mycoplasma)
- Exercise
- Allergens: Inhaled
             Ingested (rare)
- Irritants (cigarette smoke, air pollution)
- Weather changes
- Medications (ASA)
- Chemicals (tartrazine, sulfites, monosodium glutamate)
- Emotional stress
- Gastroesophageal reflux

Table 21.6.
Areas to Emphasize in Asthma History

- Nature of symptoms (wheeze, cough, dyspnea, chest tightness)
- Pattern of symptoms (severity, frequency, seasonal, and diurnal variation)
- Precipitating/aggravating factors
- Profile of typical acute episode (including ER visits, hospitalizations, ICU admissions)
- Previous and current drug therapy (response, dosage, delivery, side effects)
- Impact of disease on child and family (e.g., exercise tolerance, sleep disturbance, financial difficulties)
- Atopic history
- School performance and attendance
- Psychosocial evaluation of patient/family
- Environmental history (including active/passive smoking, housing conditions, pets)
- Family history
- General medical history of child

should be directed at excluding other potential causes of recurrent respiratory symptoms in infants and young children (Table 21.7). Clinical features suggestive of one of these alternative conditions are summarized in Table 21.8, and further investigations may then be necessary (e.g., chest radiograph, sweat chloride testing, barium swallow).

Diary Cards

A useful adjunct to the clinical history is to ask the parent and/or patient to record on a diary card the frequency and severity of symptoms over a period. In older children, peak expiratory flow rates (PEFRs) can be measured concurrently. Diary cards are invaluable in monitoring the response to treatment, particularly in preschool children who are unable to cooperate with pulmonary function testing.

Table 21.7.
Causes of Recurrent Wheeze/Cough in Infants and Children

Common	Uncommon	Rare
Asthma	Cystic Fibrosis	Left ventricular failure
	Foreign body	Vascular anomalies
Recurrent aspiration	Bronchopulmonary dysplasia	Mediastinal masses
		Tracheomalacia
		Bronchiolitis obliterans
		Immune deficiency states

Table 21.8.
Clinical Features Suggestive of an Alternative Diagnosis to Asthma

History

    Neonatal symptoms/ventilation
    Wheeze associated with feeding/vomiting
    Sudden onset of cough/choking
    Steatorrhea
    Stridor

Physical examination

    Failure to thrive
    Cardiac murmur
    Clubbing
    Unilateral signs

Investigations

    No reversibility of airflow obstruction with
      bronchodilator
    Focal or persistent chest radiographic findings

Lung Function Tests

Pulmonary function data can be used to support the diagnosis of asthma. Children from the age of 5–6 years onwards are usually able to perform simple lung function tests, such as PEFR and forced expiratory volume in 1 second (FEV_1). (Fig. 21.2) If airway obstruction is present at the time of evaluation, the diagnosis of asthma can be confirmed by demonstrating an improvement of at least 15% in FEV_1 after the inhalation of a beta-2 agonist from a metered dose inhaler (109). In a child with normal lung function at the time of examination and whose history is inconclusive, it may be possible to make a diagnosis of asthma by demonstrating a diurnal variability in peak flow rates, recorded twice daily on a diary card over a short period. In general, children have

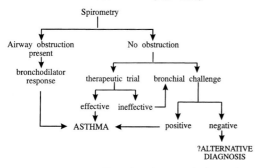

Figure 21.2. Role of lung function tests in the evaluation of asthma.

less diurnal lability in lung function than adult asthmatics do (110).

Bronchial Provocation Tests

Airway hyper-responsiveness is a characteristic feature of asthma, (42, 43, 68). It is arbitrarily defined as a ≥20% reduction in FEV_1 in response to stimuli such as histamine/methacholine, exercise, or cold air (111). However, these tests are of limited value in the diagnosis of asthma in children. In community surveys, significant overlap in bronchial responsiveness has been noted between children with asthma and symptom-free children (18, 112). In addition, bronchial hyper-reactivity may occur as a transient phenomenon after upper respiratory infections, and in a variety of other pulmonary disorders (e.g., cystic fibrosis) (111). Although the degree of airway hyper-reactivity has been found to correlate with asthma severity and treatment requirements in adult patients (113), this is not invariably the case (114), and we have been unable to reproduce these findings in children with asthma (115). Finally, the degree of bronchial responsiveness can change over time, depending on exposure to viruses, allergens, and other factors (111). While acknowledging these limitations, we find bronchial provocation tests useful in the evaluation of children with (a) normal spirometric results who have symptoms suggestive of asthma that do not respond to treatment, and (b) atypical symptoms (e.g., chronic cough) (116). It should be noted that some children with a chronic cough respond to anti-asthmatic therapy even in the absence of airway hyper-responsiveness (116).

Allergy Testing

The majority of asthmatic children over the age of 3 years are atopic (60, 65), and limited skin testing is a reasonable measure to determine sensitivity to environmental antigens after a comprehensive environmental history has been obtained. By identifying the offending allergens, the child's parents can be counseled with respect to appropriate avoidance measures. A skin prick is preferable to the intradermal technique, which is more likely to produce false-positive reactions (117). Although negative skin tests exclude clinical allergy with a high degree of reliability, positive results should be correlated with the clinical history (118). The extracts for skin testing should be selected on the basis of the history; the most important antigens to consider are dust mites (Dermatophagoides pteronyssinus, D. farinae), household pets, pollens, and molds (e.g., Alternaria). Saline (to exclude dermatographia) and histamine (to exclude recent antihistamine ingestion) controls should also be included. Radioallergosorbent tests (RASTs) are an alternative when skin tests are precluded because of skin disease or the risk of anaphylaxis (119). Finally, bronchial provocation testing with antigens remains essentially a research procedure.

MANAGEMENT

Once the diagnosis of asthma is established, a treatment plan must then be devised that is tailored to meet the needs of the individual child. The management of children with asthma should primarily take place in the community (9, 10). The long-term goals of asthma therapy are to abolish symptoms, maximize lung function, and allow children to lead normal lives with minimal interference from their illness (Table 21.9). In order to achieve these objectives, attention needs to be directed to three fundamental areas (120): (a) patient education and supervision, (b) preventative and environmental control measures, and (c) pharmacologic therapy. In addition, immunotherapy and behavior modification may be indicated for selected patients with asthma.

Patient Education and Supervision

Parents of children with asthma frequently have a poor understanding of the condition and its management (121), and this may contribute to the need for hospitalization (122). Health education programs, emphasizing self-management skills, can reduce morbidity and health-care costs and enhance the quality of life for children with asthma (123). The educational issues that need to be addressed are summarized in Table 21.10. As children with asthma approach adolescence, they should be encouraged to assume increasing responsibility for their own care. The control of asthma can be enhanced by having patients measure peak flow rates twice daily at home, thus allowing them to self-adjust therapy and make rational decisions about the need for emergency care (124). We recommend home monitoring of lung function particularly in children with (a) poor asthma control, (b) severe chronic asthma, and (c) a history of life-threatening asthma episodes. It should be pointed out that the accuracy of peak flow meters varies and can deteriorate over time (125).

Several self-management programs are now available for educating children with asthma and their parents (123), as are educational booklets (126). Some of this information needs to be transmitted to school personnel to ensure that school attendance and participation in recreational activities are disrupted as little as possible (127). A National Asthma Education Program has been initiated in the United States with the objectives of increasing public awareness of asthma as a serious disease, and of facilitating the education of physicians and parents about the management of the condition (120).

For optimal care of the child with asthma, regular follow-up by a consistent health care provider is essential. In this way, the child's progress, response to therapy, compliance, and inhalation technique can be reviewed, and lung function can be monitored. Unfortunately, the treatment of asthma is often crisis-orientated, at the expense of ongoing care and prophylactic measures (128, 129).

Table 21.9.
Specific Goals of Asthma Therapy

- Control symptoms
- No ER visits/hospitalizations
- No school absenteeism
- No exercise limitation
- No sleep disturbance
- Limit drug side effects
- Normal growth
- Normal pulmonary function

Table 21.10.
Parent/Patient Education

- Asthma—nature, aggravating factors, and prognosis
- Avoidance of trigger factors
- Medications—actions, administration, side effects
- Proper use of inhalation devices
- Acute exacerbations—recognition, treatment (written instructions), when and where to get medical help
- Monitoring—diary card, peak flow meters

Environmental Control

Specific allergic or irritant factors that aggravate the child's asthma should be eliminated or avoided if possible. Needless to say, family members should be urged not to smoke while in the house or car with their child. The observation that 20% of teenagers with asthma are cigarette smokers (15) highlights the importance of appropriate counseling in this age group. Exposure to wood-burning stoves and kerosene heaters should also be avoided.

HOUSE DUST MITES

The prevalence of house dust mite sensitivity in patients with asthma varies from 45–85%, as compared to 5–30% in control subjects (130). Dermatophagoides pteronyssinus and D. farinae are the most common dust mites, the major allergen (Der p 1) being found in mite fecal particles. A strong correlation was found between skin sensitivity to house dust mite and the presence of Der p 1 in air samples collected from the homes of asthmatic children (131). Mite sensitivity should be suspected if symptoms occur with sweeping, vacuuming, or dusting (132) and can be confirmed by skin (or RAST) testing. The efficacy of dust avoidance measures is supported by the observation that mite-sensitive asthmatics show reductions in airway reactivity following prolonged allergen avoidance (e.g., at high altitude [133] or in hospital rooms [134]). Although house mites cannot be eradicated from the home, dust avoidance measures applied to the bedroom are helpful in children with mite sensitivity, resulting in improved symptom control and lung function, and in reduced airway reactivity (135). Practical anti-dust measures are provided in Table 21.11. The measures instituted should be related both to the severity of the child's asthma and the financial circumstances of the family. If parents are unwilling to institute all of these measures, they should at least be encouraged to make the child's bed dust-free, as the highest dust mite levels are found in the mattress (65). House dust mites thrive when the relative humidity is over 50% (135). In humid climates, air conditioning during the summer can keep the relative humidity below this level, and significantly decrease the mite concentration in the home (136). Anti-mite chemicals (e.g., tannic acid, benylbenzoate) may also help to reduce dust mite concentrations in carpets and upholstered furniture (137), but these agents require further evaluation. On the other hand, electrostatic air cleaners appear to be of little help, unless high-efficiency particular air (HEPA) filters are used (138).

HOUSEHOLD PETS

Allergens from domestic pets, particularly cats (139), are a common trigger of symptoms in children with asthma. If there is clear evidence, based on history and positive skin (or RAST) tests, that the child is sensitive to pets, a trial separation is warranted or the pet should be kept outdoors (and certainly out of the child's bedroom). Parents should be aware that it may take up to 6 months after the removal of a pet before beneficial results are seen, since animal danders are cleared slowly from the environment (140). If parents are unwilling to remove the pet, the following recommendations from de Blay et al. (141) to reduce airborne cat allergen levels within the home can be instituted: (a) eliminate carpeting and maintain a polished flooring, (b) minimize upholstered furniture, (c) vacuum clean with a high-efficiency HEPA filter, (d) use an air filter in affected rooms, and (e) wash the cat weekly!

POLLEN AND MOLD SPORES

Mold spores and pollens are ubiquitous, and impossible to avoid completely. Exposure to the common mold, Alternaria alternata, has been identified recently as a risk factor for the development of life-threatening asthma (142). Indoor levels of pollens and spores can be reduced by closing windows and doors, avoiding the use of window fans, and installing window or central air conditioning (143, 144). The use of humidifiers in the home is to be discouraged, since they are a source of mold spores (135) and encourage the proliferation of dust mites.

FOOD ALLERGENS

Food allergens rarely trigger asthma symptoms; exclusion diets are, therefore, not warranted in the majority of children with asthma (72). An occasional child with asthma may be sensitive to aspirin or ingested chemicals such

Table 21.11.
How to Make a Bedroom Dust-Free

1. Move all the furniture, carpets, clothes, toys, and books out of the bedroom. The floor surface should be vinyl or hardwood.
2. Seal the hot air vent with tape. Heat the room with an electric baseboard radiator, or a hot water heater.
3. Clean the floor, window sills, and shelves with a damp mop or cloth, or one that has been treated with oil. Mop the floor once a week.
4. Encase the mattress and box spring in zippered vinyl covers.
5. Bedding is limited to synthetic fiber or foam chip pillows, and to a mattress pad, sheets, cotton thermal blankets or synthetic fiber blankets, and quilts. Launder these every 2–4 weeks (at a temperature of at least 140° F).
6. The room should ideally contain only the specially prepared bed, non-upholstered chairs, and a table. A chest of drawers is permitted, but should be cleaned out every few months. Laundered clothes that the child wears from day to day may be kept in these drawers and in the closet.
7. The room should contain no carpets, rugs, mats, stored blankets, books, stuffed toys, or other clutter. One toy, preferably a washable one, and one book may be taken to bed at night. Keep the bedroom door closed, if the child will allow it.

Other dust avoidance measures

1. Vacuum clean the carpets and furniture in other parts of the house once a week (but not when child is present).
2. Dust and animal danders accumulate in ducts leading from the furnace. Certain companies will clean out these ducts by powerful vacuum suction.

Adapted from Murray AB. Avoiding airborne allergens in the home. In *Treatment of Pediatric Asthma: A Canadian consensus (MEDICINE Publishing Foundation Symposium Series 29).* Toronto, MES Medical Education Services, 1991, pp. 33–38.

as tartrazine, sulfites, and monosodium glutamate and will need to be counseled accordingly.

Immunotherapy

Although immunotherapy is widely practiced, its role in the overall management of asthma remains uncertain in view of the variable results of clinical trials (135, 145–147). For example, in controlled trials of immunotherapy with dust mite extracts in asthma, symptomatic improvement has been shown to occur, but no significant difference in lung function between the mite- and placebo-treated groups has been demonstrated. In addition, the effect of dust mite immunotherapy on airway hyper-reactivity is extremely variable (148–151). One study found that mite immunotherapy increased bronchial responsiveness to histamine (151). Conflicting results have also been noted with immunotherapy to pollen, molds, and animal extracts (135, 145, 146, 152). Bacterial vaccines have no role in the management of asthma, since respiratory infections that induce wheezing in children are rarely bacterial in nature (77).

Immunotherapy, therefore, should be considered only in selected children with asthma that is triggered by one or more specific allergens and in whom allergen avoidance and pharmacologic therapy have been inadequate or associated with significant side effects (147). Accurate allergy diagnosis should precede treatment, and this should be based on a careful clinical history and skin (or RAST) testing. Immunotherapy should be used in conjunction with drug therapy and never as the sole form of treatment. Patients should be detained in the physician's office for 30 minutes after each injection to observe for possible adverse reactions (153). If a child does not show a favorable response after 12 months, immunotherapy should be discontinued (147).

Psychologic Management

It is generally agreed that psychosocial factors per se do not play a primary causal role in asthma, but they can profoundly affect the severity of the condition and the success of treatment (154). In some children, asthma symptoms can be related to emotional stimuli such as excitement, fear, or anger (154). Psychosocial problems (34) and depression (155) can lead to poor self-management, disregard of symptoms, and interpersonal conflict, factors that have been associated with asthma deaths in children. Some children can react to their asthma by using it to seek attention or avoid unpleasant activities (156). On a long-term basis, children with asthma (and their families) have to cope with stress factors such as uncertainty about future asthma episodes, the fear of emergency hospital admissions, and interference of the disease with school attendance, sleep, and physical and leisure activities. Inappropriate parental attitudes toward the condition, ranging from overprotectiveness to denial, can compound a child's problem (157). Theophylline therapy may also lead to psychological and behavioral problems in children with asthma (158). Finally, some children can mimic or aggravate asthmatic symptoms by inducing adduction of the vocal cords on inspiration (159).

Effective management of asthma should include close consideration of the psychosocial adjustments of the asthmatic child and the family. The primary physician can play a key role in correcting attitude and adjustment problems within a family by providing information concerning the etiologic, therapeutic, and prognostic aspects of asthma (156, 157). Intervention by a psychiatrist or social worker is indicated for selected children with asthma, and can lead to improvement in their clinical status (155, 160). Behavioral approaches have been used effectively to modify the reaction to situations that provoke episodes of asthma, to deal with manipulative behavior, and to improve compliance with medical regimens. The child's family should be included in such treatment programs, with the objective of bringing about a positive change in family relationships and perceptions. Finally, residential schooling with emphasis on family psychotherapy and self-management should be considered for children with severe asthma who fail to respond to outpatient medical and psychosocial care (161).

Pharmacologic Management

Pharmacotherapy remains the cornerstone of asthma management. Drug therapy of asthma must not only focus on relieving acute asthma episodes but should be used in a preventative fashion, particularly in children with frequent symptoms. For ease of discussion, the drugs currently available for the treatment of asthma can be divided (albeit somewhat artificially) into two main groups: bronchodilators and prophylactic (anti-inflammatory) agents. The

advantages, disadvantages, and delivery of these medications will be discussed as a background to an overview of their role in the management of asthma of different grades of severity.

BRONCHODILATORS

Beta-2 Agonists

Beta-2 agonists are the most potent bronchodilators available, and include albuterol (salbutamol), fenoterol, terbutaline, metaproterenol, bitolterol, pirbuterol, and procaterol (162). The usual doses of beta-2 agonists used at our institution are shown in Table 21.12 (these may differ from manufacturers' recommendations). Depending on the route of administration and product used these agents have a duration of action of 4–8 hours. Inhaled beta-2 agonists with a more sustained duration of action (up to 12 hours) are undergoing clinical trials (e.g., formoterol, salmeterol) (163). Other actions of beta-2 agonists pertinent to asthma therapy include inhibition of the release of inflammatory mediators and increased mucociliary clearance. The clinical importance of these effects remains unknown.

Beta-2 agonists should be administered by inhalation to ensure a rapid onset of action and to minimize adverse effects. They are the preferred initial treatment for acute exacerbations of asthma and for the prevention of exercise-induced asthma (162). On the other hand, several recent publications have questioned the role of beta-2 agonists in the maintenance treatment of asthma. In a study of adult asthmatics, it was found that in two-thirds of subjects, asthma was better controlled when an inhaled beta-2 agonist (fenoterol) was used only to control symptoms rather than taken regularly (164). In contrast, Shepherd et al. (165) reported that exacerbations of asthma were more common while patients received beta-2 agonists regularly rather than as required. Conflicting results have also been reported regarding the effect of beta-2 agonists on airway reactivity. Although some studies (164, 166–170) have shown that long-term treatment with beta-2 agonists has little effect or may even increase airway reactivity, other investigators (171, 172) have shown that albuterol has a transient protective effective against methacholine-induced bron-

Table 21.12.
Recommended Dosage Schedule for Bronchodilators[a]

B₂ Agonist	Oral Administration	Aerosol Administration	
		Formulations	Dose
Albuterol (salbutamol)	2 mg per 5 ml syrup; 2 mg or 4 mg tablets: 0.1 to 0.15 mg/kg/dose, 3–4 times daily	0.5% solution	0.01–0.03 ml/kg (maximum 1 ml) diluted with 3 ml saline, up to 4 times daily.
		Metered aerosol (100 μg/puff)	1–2 puffs, 4 times daily
		Dry powder (Rotohaler) (200 μg, 400 μg)	200–400 μg, 4 times daily
Fenoterol[b]	2.5 mg tablets; 0.1 mg/kg/dose, 3–4 times daily	0.1% solution	0.01–0.03 ml/kg (maximum 1 ml) diluted with 3 ml saline, up to 4 times daily
		Metered aerosol (200 μg/puff)	1 puff, 4 times daily
Metaproterenol (orciprenaline)	10 mg per 5 ml syrup; 20 mg tablets: 0.3–0.5 mg/kg/dose, 3–4 times daily	5% solution	0.01–0.02 ml/kg (maximum 1 ml) diluted with 3 ml saline, up to 4 times daily
		Metered aerosol (750 μg/puff)	1–2 puffs, 4 times daily
Terbutaline	300 mcg/ml syrup;[b] 2.5 or 5 mg tablets: 0.075 mg/kg dose, 3–4 times daily	1% solution	0.03 ml/kg (maximum 1 ml) diluted with 3 ml saline, up to 4 times daily
		Metered aerosol (250 μg/puff)	1 puff, 4 times daily
		Dry Powder (500 μg/actuation)	Inhalation, 4 times daily
Bitolterol	—	Metered aerosol (370 μg/puff)	1–2 puffs, 4 times daily
Proctaerol[b]	—	Metered aerosol (10 μg/puff)	1–2 puffs, 3 times daily
Anticholinergics Ipratropium bromide	—	Metered aerosol (20 mcg/puff)	2 puffs, 4 times daily
		0.025% solution[b]	0.5–1.0 ml, 4 times daily

[a]Doses given are those used in the author's unit and may differ from manufacturers' recommendations.
[b]Not available in United States.

choconstriction and that the longer-acting beta-2 agonists (e.g., formoterol) can provide protection for 12 hours. Twentyman et al. (173), studying a group of adult asthmatics, reported that salmeterol inhibited both the early and late asthmatic responses to allergen challenge and protected against nonspecific bronchial reactivity for up to 34 hours. In view of the aforementioned controversies, and the possible association between asthma deaths and chronic treatment with beta-2 agonists or theophylline (27–31, 33), it was recommended in the report of the National Heart, Lung, and Blood Institute (NHLBI) expert panel on Guidelines for the Diagnosis and Management of Asthma that it is preferred that beta

agonist aerosols be used on an as-needed basis and not as a regularly scheduled drug (not to exceed 1–2 doses daily) (174).

The principal side effects of beta-2 agonists are tremor, tachycardia, and hypokalemia (175), and are more common with the oral and systemic routes of administration. Although tolerance (tachyphylaxis) to the bronchodilator effects of beta-2 agonists may occur with chronic use, this does not appear to be of major clinical significance, and can be reversed by systemic steroids (176).

Anticholinergics

Ipratropium bromide, an atropine derivative, is currently available as a metered aerosol and as a nebulizing solution (Table 21.12). Although ipratropium has a slower onset of action and provides less maximal bronchodilation than beta-2 agonists, it has a more prolonged duration of action (up to 8 hours). In acute asthma, some (177–179), but not all (180, 181) reports indicate that additional bronchodilation can be achieved when ipratropium is used in combination with a beta-2 agonist. Ipratropium has a less clearly defined role in the maintenance treatment of asthma (182, 183) and does not appear to reduce airway reactivity (184). However, it can be used in combination with a beta-2 agonist in children with severe chronic asthma, and as an alternative to sympathomimetics or theophylline in children who experience intolerable side effects from these agents. The small subset of patients whose asthma is triggered by psychogenic factors appears to respond particularly well to ipratropium (185). Side effects are very uncommon, although paradoxical bronchoconstriction has been reported, possibly due to the hypotonicity or low pH of the nebulizing solution, or to additives such as benzalkonium chloride (32, 186).

Theophylline

The role of theophylline preparations in the maintenance treatment of asthma has become somewhat controversial in recent years (187–190). The trend is now towards introducing theophylline later in the therapeutic plan; several considerations account for this: (a) long-term treatment with theophylline does not appear to cause any sustained improvement in airway hyper-reactivity in asthma (191), although a recent study has challenged this contention (192); (b) theophylline preparations result in a high incidence of side effects, particularly in the presence of factors that reduce the metabolism of theophylline (e.g., viruses, erythromycin, liver disease) (193); (c) theophylline may cause cognitive, behavioral, and learning difficulties in some children (158) (one study indicates that these side effects are confined largely to children with pre-existing attentional and school achievement problems [194]); and (d) chronic use of theophylline has been associated with an increased risk of mortality from asthma (27, 31).

Theophylline, therefore, can no longer be regarded as "first line" therapy in pediatric asthma. It may have a role in selected children, specifically (a) patients with moderate to severe asthma, in whom therapy with beta-2 agonists and inhaled steroids is inadequate (196), (b) children who are unable to use or are noncompliant with inhaled medications, and (c) patients with nocturnal asthma (195). If theophylline is prescribed, a sustained-release preparation should be chosen, and dosage must be individualized and guided by serum theophylline assays. A suggested dosing regimen for various age groups is shown in Table 21.13 (196). This dosing regimen has been lowered from those previously recommended and is designed to achieve theophylline serum concentrations in the 12–15 mg/L range. These are recommended starting doses and should be adjusted according to symptoms, side effects, and pharmacokinetic information. Adverse side effects at the beginning of therapy can be minimized by commencing the patient on 50% of the calculated dose, followed by small increases at 3-day intervals until average doses for age are attained. The final adjustment in theophylline dosage and dosing interval should be based on peak and trough serum theophylline concentrations (196). After this initial individualization of dosing requirements, subsequent monitoring of theophylline concentrations at 6- to 12-month intervals is generally adequate. More frequent measurements may be necessary during periods of rapid growth, when control of asthma is suboptimal, or when situations that alter theophylline elimination develop. As a standard precaution, parents should be instructed to reduce the dose of theophylline by 50% if their child has a sustained fever and not to administer any other medication

Table 21.13.
Usual Dosage Requirements of Oral Theophylline to Maintain Serum Theophylline Concentration Within the Therapeutic Range

Age	Total Daily Dose (mg/kg)[a]
Infants 6–52 weeks	{0.3 × (age in weeks) + 8}
Children 1–9 years	18
Children 9–12 years	10–20
Adolescent 12–16 years	10
Adults	10 μg/kg or 600 mg/day (whichever is less)

[a]Use ideal body weight for age, sex, and height.
From Weinberger MM. Theophylline. *Immunol Allergy Clin North Am* 1990; 10:559–576.

without establishing the safety of the combination.

ANTI-INFLAMMATORY DRUGS

Cromolyn Sodium

Cromolyn sodium (CS) is exclusively a prophylactic agent, since it has no significant bronchodilator action (197). Although its mechanism of action is unclear, a single dose of CS prior to allergen challenge inhibits both the early and late asthmatic reactions (198). Pretreatment with CS has also been shown to attenuate bronchoconstriction in response to exercise (199) and methacholine (200). On the other hand, conflicting results have been reported regarding the long-term effect of cromolyn therapy on airway reactivity (201–204)—CS is certainly less effective than inhaled steroids in this respect (201–203).

Maintenance therapy with CS should be considered in children with moderate or severe asthma (204–206). The response to cromolyn therapy in the individual patient is unpredictable, but long-term studies have confirmed its efficacy in about two-thirds of children whose asthma is not adequately controlled by bronchodilators (205). On the other hand, cromolyn appears to be of little value in children who are steroid-dependent (207, 208). Cromolyn is available as a powder (spinhaler), a solution (for administration by nebulizer), and a metered dose inhaler. At the onset of treatment it is necessary to administer cromolyn four times daily, but with continued therapy many children can be managed with two to three doses per day. Table 21.14 provides dosage guidelines for the three formulations of cromolyn available.

In children with predictable seasonal asthma (e.g., grass pollen), best results are obtained if cromolyn is introduced several weeks before anticipated allergen exposure and continued throughout the entire season.

In the child with animal-sensitive asthma, cromolyn provides effective prophylaxis if taken 15–30 minutes prior to an anticipated encounter with animals. Similarly, exercise-induced asthma can be prevented by taking cromolyn, with or without a beta-2 agonist, 15–30 minutes before exercise (199).

Although relatively expensive, a major advantage of cromolyn is a virtual freedom from side effects. Some patients may experience airway irritation after inhaling the dry powder, but this can be alleviated by the prior inhalation of a beta-2 agonist. In view of this irritant property, cromolyn powder should be temporarily withdrawn during acute exacerbations of asthma.

Ketotifen

Ketotifen is an orally active agent with distinct anti-allergic and antihistaminic properties (209). In infants (210), children (211, 212), and adolescents (212) with mild to moderate asthma, ketotifen has been shown to diminish the severity of symptoms, bronchodilator requirements, and the frequency of acute episodes. In children with pollen-related asthma, its clinical efficacy appears to be equivalent to that of cromolyn (213). Conflicting results have been reported regarding the long-term effect of ketotifen on bronchial responsiveness (214, 215). Ketotifen does not inhibit exercise-induced asthma (216), and the addition of ketotifen to the drug regimen of children who require cromolyn does not confer any additional benefit (217, 218).

From the studies performed to date, it is clear that a minimum of 8–12 weeks is required before the beneficial effects of ketotifen are fully realized. The recommended dose is 1 mg twice daily in older children, and 0.5 mg twice daily in children less than 3 years of age (209). The drug appears to be remarkably safe, although weight gain and sedation are potential problems (219).

Table 21.14.
Prescription Guidelines for Cromolyn Therapy

Formulation	Dosage	Administration
Dry powder capsules	20 mg/capsule	1 capsule, 4 times daily
Solution (1%)	20 mg/2 ml ampoule	2 ml, 4 times daily
Metered aerosol[a]	1 mg/puff	2 puffs, 4 times daily

[a]A high dose inhaler (5 mg/puff) is available in some countries.

Nedocromil Sodium

Nedocromil is chemically unrelated to cromolyn but has a very similar clinical profile (220). It has been shown to be effective against antigen challenge and in preventing exercise-induced asthma. It is also effective in the long-term management of asthma (at a dose of 4 mg, four times per day), although no clear advantage over cromolyn has yet emerged (221). During the pollen season, nedocromil has some effect in reducing bronchial reactivity to histamine (222). Nedocromil may allow a reduction in the need for bronchodilators (223) and inhaled steroids (224), and this effect applies to some (225), but not all (226) patients who are dependent on oral steroids. Potential side effects include a bitter taste, headache, and nausea.

Corticosteroids

Inhaled corticosteroids, because of high topical anti-inflammatory activity but limited systemic absorption, have contributed greatly to the management of asthma. These preparations allow effective control of symptoms and improve lung function in the majority of children with asthma (227). The late asthmatic response and the subsequent increase in airway reactivity induced by allergen challenge can be inhibited by a single dose of an inhaled steroid preparation (198). Regular use of inhaled steroids reduces airway inflammation (228) and causes a gradual reduction in bronchial reactivity (166, 168–170, 191, 229–232), sometimes with full resolution (230, 231). A large variation in the rate of improvement in airway reactivity has been noted and appears to be related to dose and duration of therapy (229, 230). Although some investigators have shown that this reduction in reactivity may persist for 3 months after inhaled steroids have been discontinued (231), Vathenen et al. (232) have found that this effect is not maintained. Inhaled steroids do not provide any protection against bronchoconstriction when given immediately before exercise (233), although regular inhaled steroid therapy does reduce the severity of exercise-induced asthma (234).

Several inhaled steroid preparations are available (Table 21.15). Although flunisolide and triamcinolone have been in clinical use for several years, data regarding the efficacy and safety of inhaled steroids have been based largely on beclomethasone and budesonide. Although budesonide has a greater topical-to-systemic potency, both preparations appear to be equally effective clinically (227). Inhaled steroids are usually delivered by metered dose inhalers. A variety of dry powder delivery systems is now available. Nebulizing solutions of inhaled steroids are available in some countries, but data regarding the efficacy and safety of these preparations are limited.

For children, the generally recommended starting dose of inhaled steroids is 100 µg, four times daily. If a satisfactory clinical response occurs, conversion to a twice-daily dosing schedule may eventually be possible in some children, thus improving compliance (227). Patients with unstable asthma are, however, best advised to adhere to the standard four times daily regimen. Finally, in patients who respond poorly to conventional doses of inhaled corticosteroids, the use of high-dose inhaled steroids (up to 1600 µg/day) has been shown to improve asthma control and reduce systemic steroid requirements (235), although the risk of adrenal suppression is significantly increased. The introduction of "high-dose" inhalation devices in some countries has facilitated the delivery of inhaled steroids in children with severe asthma.

Studies that have examined the effect of inhaled steroids on adrenal function in children are difficult to interpret in view of the discrepancies in steroid dosage, the parameters of adrenal function examined, and the age of the children selected (236–239). It is reasonable to conclude that inhaled steroids can cause adrenal suppression in some children and that this effect is dose-dependent. One study indicates that biochemical evidence of suppressed adrenal function occurs when the dose exceeds 400 $\mu g/m^2/day$ (239). The clinical significance of this suppression is unclear at the present time. However, it may be advisable to measure adrenal function, particularly in children who require high-dose inhaled steroid therapy. Supplementary systemic steroids during prolonged periods of stress (e.g., trauma, surgery) should be considered in any child receiving chronic inhaled corticosteroid therapy. Likewise, linear growth should be monitored, although conflicting results have been noted regarding the effect of inhaled steroids on growth (240–242). Some investigators (243) have

Table 21.15.
Aerosol Corticosteroid Products

Trade Names	Active Ingredient	Dose Provided
Beclovent/Vanceril	Beclomethasone dipropionate	50 μg/puff 100 μg/rotacap[a] 200 μg/rotacap[a]
Beclodisk[a]	Beclomethasone dipropionate	100 μg/blister 200 μg/blister
Becloforte[a]	Beclomethasone dipropionate	250 μg/puff
AeroBid/Bronalide	Flunisolide	250 μg/puff
Pulmicort[a]	Budesonide	50 μg/puff 200 μg/puff 100, 200, 400 μg/actuation (Turbuhaler)
Azmacort	Triamcinalone	200 mcg/puff

[a]Not available in the United States.

found that the use of a spacer device may reduce the systemic effects of inhaled steroids, but this is not an invariable finding (244). Less common systemic effects of high-dose inhaled steroids include skin atrophy (245), cataracts (246), bone resorption, and demineralization (247).

Although oropharyngeal colonization with candida is common in children receiving inhaled steroids, overt infection is rare (248). The risk of infection can be reduced by rinsing the mouth with water after each inhalation, using a spacer device, and decreasing the frequency of inhalations to twice daily (244). Dysphonia caused by adductor vocal cord paralysis may occur (249), but responds to temporary withdrawal of corticosteroids. This problem can be avoided by inhaling the drug slowly, preferably through a spacer. Some patients experience airway irritation after inhaling corticosteroids, but this can be prevented by prior inhalation of a beta-2 agonist.

Fortunately, oral steroids are rarely necessary in the long-term treatment of pediatric asthma. If this situation does arise, the smallest dose of prednisone/prednisolone compatible with control of symptoms should be given as a single dose every other morning if possible. It should be noted that systemic side effects may occur even with alternate-day steroid therapy (250). Short courses of oral steroids (e.g., prednisone 1–2 mg/kg/day for 5–7 days) are extremely effective in treating acute exacerbations of asthma at home, and may reduce the need for hospitalization (251–253). Although short courses of oral steroids can cause adrenal suppression, rapid recovery in adrenal function occurs (254). However, children who are treated with more than four short bursts of oral steroids per year may develop more prolonged adrenal suppression (255).

Methods of Drug Delivery

Where possible, anti-asthmatic medications (particularly beta-2 agonists) should be delivered by inhalation (256). The rationale for using the inhaled route is that medication is deposited directly to the airways, allowing for a rapid onset of drug action, lower dosage requirements, and fewer systemic side effects as compared to oral therapy. Three inhalation systems are available at the present time for the delivery of aerosolized medications, and each of these will be considered briefly.

METERED DOSE INHALER (MDI)

Cromolyn, ipratropium bromide, and a variety of beta-2 agonists and inhaled steroid preparations can be delivered using inhalers. Metered dose inhalers are portable, inexpensive, and ideal for children over 7 years of age. However, even with optimal inhalation technique, only 10% of the drug released from an MDI reaches the airways: most of the aerosol spray impacts on the oropharynx. In view of this, children must be instructed carefully with respect to the correct use of an inhaler (Table 21.16), and their technique must be checked at subsequent visits. Unfortunately, inefficient use of MDIs is common and is a major cause of treatment failure (256). Some of the problems encountered include (a) lack

Table 21.16.
Suggested Inhalation Technique for Metered Dose Inhalers

- Shake the inhaler and remove the cap
- Hold the inhaler upright and breathe out fully
- Close lips around mouthpiece of inhaler

or

Hold mouthpiece 4 cm (2 finger widths) in front of open mouth

- Activate inhaler while inspiring slowly and deeply
- Hold breath for 10 seconds (or for as long as possible)
- If dose is to be repeated, wait a few minutes

of coordination of aerosol actuation with inspiration ("hand-lung dyscoordination"), (b) ceasing to inspire when the aerosol is released into the mouth ("cold freon" effect), (c) rapid inspiration, and (d) inhalation through the nose. Breath-activated inhalers have been introduced in some countries, and may prove useful in children with poor coordination.

In order to improve intrapulmonary drug deposition, various extension tubes (spacers) have been designed and marketed. Best results are obtained with large-volume (> 750 ml) spacers, but at the expense of portability (256). Spacers are indicated for patients with poor inhaler technique, particularly for young children (3–7 years) who are rarely able to use MDIs effectively. Spacers are also advisable when corticosteroid inhalers are used, in order to reduce the risk of oropharyngeal candidiasis. The addition of a face mask to the spacer may facilitate delivery of aerosolized medications to very young children (257). Maximal intrapulmonary deposition is achieved by loading one puff of aerosol into the spacer and having the patient take two slow vital capacity breaths, each followed by 10 seconds of breath holding (258). However, when multiple puffs of aerosol are required, a reasonable compromise is to load up to four puffs into the spacer at a time (258). In children who are unable to take vital capacity breaths, tidal breathing can be used and breath holding is not essential (259). The administration of multiple medications simultaneously by a spacer device is not advisable (260).

DRY POWDER INHALERS

Dry powder inhalers are available for the delivery of beta-2 agonists, cromolyn, and inhaled steroids. They require less coordination than MDIs and, hence, are particularly useful in 3- to 7-year-old children. Another advantage is that they do not contain freon. Recently, dry powder inhalers with a multi-dose facility (Diskhaler) and breath-activated inhalers (e.g., Turbuhaler) have become available. In order to achieve maximal effect from dry power inhalers, patients must be able to generate high inspiratory flow rates (>60 L/minute) (261). During acute exacerbations of asthma, when flow rates are reduced, powder inhalers may become less effective.

NEBULIZERS

Several beta-2 agonists, cromolyn, ipratropium bromide, and corticosteroids (in some countries) can be delivered by nebulizer. Nebulizers are used both in hospital and domiciliary practice with increasing frequency, although this trend is viewed with concern by some clinicians (30, 262). The main advantage of the nebulizer is that it requires little patient coordination, and therefore can be used to deliver medication to acutely ill or very young children; furthermore, their use in the home may reduce the need for hospitalization (263). On the other hand, nebulizers are expensive, not very portable, and an inefficient drug delivery system. Home nebulizers are of particular benefit in children with (a) severe, chronic asthma, (b) a history of life-threatening asthma episodes, and (c) a demonstrated inability to use MDIs or dry powder inhalers (e.g., very young children) or asthma that cannot be controlled with oral therapy alone (174). To ensure optimal lung deposition of drug particles, a gas flow rate of 6–8 L/minute and dilution of the drug solution in the nebulizer to a 3–4 ml volume is recommended (256). Parents should be carefully instructed in the use of nebulizers before home treatment is started, and must understand that failure on the part of the nebulizer to relieve their child's symptoms is an absolute indication to seek medical help (263)

Practical Aspects of Drug Use in Asthma

The maintenance drug therapy of asthma varies considerably, depending on the frequency and severity of the child's symptoms and the degree of airflow obstruction (264). Drug therapy should be considered in a stepwise fashion, with the child starting treatment at the level most appropriate for the severity of his or her asthma. For ease of discussion, it is useful to separate children with asthma into different groups according to disease severity (Table 21.17), and to consider the treatment of each group individually.

MILD INFREQUENT ASTHMA

About 60% of children with asthma have mild and infrequent episodes of coughing and wheezing in the course of the year, but in between have a normal quality of life (i.e., good exercise tolerance, uninterrupted sleep, regular school attendance) and normal lung function (264). (Fig. 21.3) The intermittent use of a beta-2 agonist may suffice in these children. If possible, beta-2 agonists should be delivered by inhalation, either by an MDI (with a spacer device if necessary) or a dry powder inhaler. Treatment can usually be discontinued after 5–7 days when symptoms have abated. For young children who are unable to use these inhalation devices, and whose asthma is not severe enough to warrant purchase of a home nebulizer, an oral beta-2 agonist may be adequate.

For children who experience symptoms mainly on a seasonal basis (e.g., on exposure to pollens), it may be necessary to introduce a prophylactic agent, such as cromolyn or ket-

Table 21.17.
NHLBI Classification of Asthma by Severity of Disease[a]

Characteristics	Mild	Moderate	Severe
Frequency of exacerbations	Exacerbations of cough and wheezing 1–2 times/week.	Exacerbation > than 2 times/week. Urgent care treatment in ER or office < 3/year.	Virtually daily wheezing. Exacerbations frequent, often severe. Tendency to have sudden severe exacerbations. Urgent visits to ER or office > 3/year. Hospitalization > 2/year.
Frequency of symptoms	Few clinical signs or symptoms between exacerbations.	Cough and low grade wheezing often present.	Continuous albeit low-grade cough and wheezing almost always present.
Exercise tolerance	Good exercise tolerance but may not tolerate vigorous exercise (e.g., running).	Exercise tolerance diminished.	Very poor exercise tolerance with marked limitation of activity.
Nocturnal asthma	Nocturnal asthma 1–2 times/month.	Nocturnal asthma 2–3 times/week.	Considerable, almost nightly sleep interruption. Chest tight in early A.M.
School or work attendance	Good school or work attendance.	School or work attendance may be affected.	Poor school or work attendance.
Pulmonary function			
• Peak Expiratory Flow Rate (PEFR)	PEFR > 80% predicted. Variability < 20%[b]	PEFR 60–80% predicted. Variability 20–30%.	PEFR < 60% predicted. Variability > 30%
• Spirometry	Minimal airway obstruction on spirometry. Usually a > 15% response to aerosol bronchodilator.	Airway obstruction on spirometry. Reduced flow at low lung volumes. Usually a > 15% response to aerosol bronchodilator.	Substantial airway obstruction on spirometry. F-V curve shows marked concavity. Incomplete reversibility to aerosol bronchodilator.
• Methacholine sensitivity	Methacholine PC_{20} > 20 mg/ml.[c]	Methacholine PC_{20} between 2 and 20 mg/ml.	Methacholine PC_{20} < 20 mg/ml.

[a]Characteristics are general: because asthma is highly variable, these characteristics may overlap. Furthermore, an individual may switch into different categories over time.
[b]Variability is the difference either between a morning and evening measure or among morning peak flow measurements each day of a week.
[c]Although the degree of methacholine/histamine sensitivity generally correlates with severity of symptoms and medication requirements, there are exceptions.
From Canadian consensus on the treatment of asthma in children. *Can Med Assoc J* 1991; 145:1449–1455.

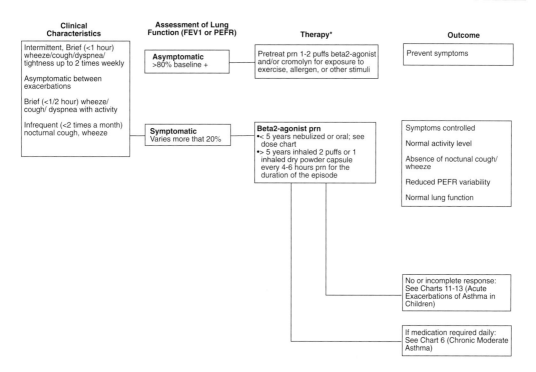

Clinical Characteristics	Assessment of Lung Function (FEV1 or PEFR)	Therapy*	Outcome
Intermittent, Brief (<1 hour) wheeze/cough/dyspnea/ tightness up to 2 times weekly	**Asymptomatic** >80% baseline +	Pretreat prn 1-2 puffs beta2-agonist and/or cromolyn for exposure to exercise, allergen, or other stimuli	Prevent symptoms
Asymptomatic between exacerbations			
Brief (<1/2 hour) wheeze/ cough/ dyspnea with activity			
Infrequent (<2 times a month) nocturnal cough, wheeze	**Symptomatic** Varies more that 20%	**Beta2-agonist prn** •< 5 years nebulized or oral; see dose chart •> 5 years inhaled 2 puffs or 1 inhaled dry powder capsule every 4-6 hours prn for the duration of the episode	Symptoms controlled Normal activity level Absence of noctunal cough/ wheeze Reduced PEFR variability Normal lung function

No or incomplete response: See Charts 11-13 (Acute Exacerbations of Asthma in Children)

If medication required daily: See Chart 6 (Chronic Moderate Asthma)

+PEFR % baseline refers to the norm or the individual, established by the clinician. This may be % predicted of standardized norms or % patient's personal best.

*All therapy must include patient education about prevention (including environmental control where appropriate) as well as control of symptoms.

Figure 21.3. Treatment algorithm for mild asthma. * = Unavailable in the United States. Modified from Canadian consensus on the treatment of asthma in children. *Can Med Assoc J* 1991; 145:1449–1455.

otifen, several weeks before anticipated allergen exposure, and to continue this treatment throughout the entire season (213). Similarly, in a child with animal-sensitive asthma, it may be possible to prevent symptoms by taking cromolyn 15–30 minutes before an anticipated encounter with animals.

FREQUENT EPISODIC ASTHMA

About 30% of children with asthma experience more frequent symptoms, and these children should be considered for daily prophylactic, anti-inflammatory therapy, used in conjunction with beta-2 agonists for symptom relief (Fig. 21.4). Suggested guidelines for the introduction of daily prophylactic therapy are listed in Table 21.18 (162).

In view of the potential for systemic effects with inhaled steroids (238, 239), we feel that a trial of a nonsteroidal prophylactic agent is warranted initially. Irrespective of which agent is chosen, certain rules need to be followed to ensure success with a preventative regimen: (a) prior to the introduction of a prophylactic medication, the child's asthma should be brought under control (and lung function optimized) by regular treatment with beta-2 agonists, and a short course of oral steroids, if necessary; (b) the patient and/or parent must understand the principles of a preventative drug regimen and the importance of compliance, and must appreciate that several weeks of therapy may be required before the full effects of the drug are realized; (c) during this time, a beta-2 agonist may need to be used concurrently, in order to maintain asthma control; and (d) while children are maintained on a prophylactic regimen, it is crucial that their parents have access to a beta-2 agonist (and appropriate delivery system) to treat acute exacerbations of asthma.

If no therapeutic effect is seen after a 6- to 8-week trial of cromolyn, or an 8- to 12-week trial of ketotifen, the child should be switched to low-dose inhaled steroid therapy (i.e., 100 μg four times daily). A beta-2 agonist can be used intermittently to manage acute symptoms. Once symptoms and lung function have

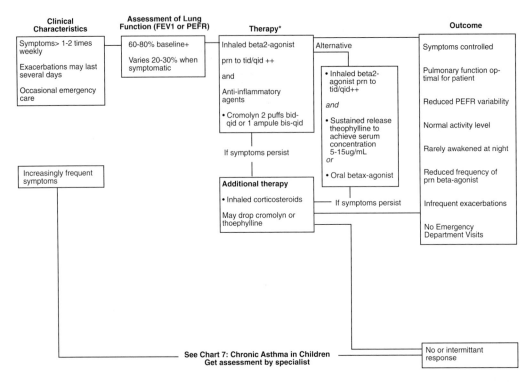

Clinical Characteristics	Assessment of Lung Function (FEV1 or PEFR)	Therapy*		Outcome

See Chart 7: Chronic Asthma in Children
Get assessment by specialist

+PEFR % baseline refers to the norm for the individual, established by the clinician. This may be % predicted based on standardized norms or % patient's personal best.
++If exceed 3-4 doses a day, consider additional therapy other than inhaled beta2-agonist.

*All therapy must include patient education about prevention (including environmental control where appropriate) as well as control of symptoms.

Figure 21.4. Treatment algorithm for moderate asthma. * = Unavailable in the United States. Modified from Canadian consensus on the treatment of asthma in children. *Can Med Assoc J* 1991; 145:1449–1455.

Table 21.18.
Criteria for Prophylactic Therapy in Childhood Asthma[a]

- Frequent acute episodes (> 6/year)
  (Acute episode = persistent wheeze/cough lasting > 24 hours)
- Frequent hospital admissions: > 2/year
- Bronchodilators used routinely twice a day or more
- Infrequent but severe asthma episodes (e.g., ICU admission)
- School absenteeism: > 4 days/month
- Sleep disturbance (e.g., 1–2 nights/week)
- Persistent airway obstruction (e.g., $FEV_1 < 70\%$)

[a]See also reference 162.

improved, the inhaled steroid (and beta-2 agonist) should be tapered to the lowest dose that maintains adequate control.

SEVERE, CHRONIC ASTHMA

Fortunately, less than 10% of children with asthma fall into this group (264), which is characterized by the presence of daily symptoms, frequent nocturnal coughing, limited exercise tolerance, and persistent airway obstruction. (Fig. 21.5) As an initial step in such patients, it may be worth adding a second bronchodilator (e.g., a sustained-release theophylline product or inhaled ipratropium bromide) to the pre-existing regimen of inhaled steroids in standard dosage plus regular therapy with a beta-2 agonist. Alternatively, the regular administration of bronchodilators (beta-2 agonists ± ipratropium) in higher doses by home nebulizer may be considered. If this approach is unsuccessful, high-dose inhaled steroid therapy (e.g., 800–1000 μg/day) should be attempted, preferably administered by a spacer device in three or four divided doses, in conjunction with bronchodilators. If necessary, the dose of inhaled steroids can be increased to a maximum of 1600 μg/day.

Maintenance treatment with oral prednisolone/prednisone should be instituted only if

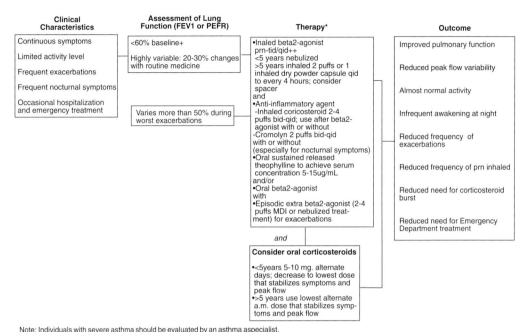

Clinical Characteristics	Assessment of Lung Function (FEV1 or PEFR)	Therapy*	Outcome
Continuous symptoms	<60% baseline+	•Inaled beta2-agonist prn-tid/qid++ <5 years nebulized >5 years inhaled 2 puffs or 1 inhaled dry powder capsule qid to every 4 hours; consider spacer and	Improved pulmonary function
Limited activity level	Highly variable: 20-30% changes with routine medicine		Reduced peak flow variability
Frequent exacerbations			Almost normal activity
Frequent nocturnal symptoms			
Occasional hospitalization and emergency treatment	Varies more than 50% during worst exacerbations	•Anti-inflammatory agent -Inhaled coricosteroid 2-4 puffs bid-qid; use after beta2-agonist with or without -Cromolyn 2 puffs bid-qid with or without (especially for nocturnal symptoms) •Oral sustained released theophylline to achieve serum concentration 5-15ug/mL and/or •Oral beta2-agonist with •Episodic extra beta2-agonist (2-4 puffs MDI or nebulized treatment) for exacerbations	Infrequent awakening at night
			Reduced frequency of exacerbations
			Reduced frequency of prn inhaled
			Reduced need for corticosteroid burst
			Reduced need for Emergency Department treatment

and

Consider oral corticosteroids

•<5years 5-10 mg. alternate days; decrease to lowest dose that stabilizes symptoms and peak flow
•>5 years use lowest alternate a.m. dose that stabilizes symptoms and peak flow

Note: Individuals with severe asthma should be evaluated by an asthma aspecialist.
+PEFR% baseline refers to the norm for the individual, established by the clinician. This may be % predicted of standardized norms or % patient's personal best.
++If exceed 3-4 doses a day, consider additional therapy other than inhaled beta2-agonist.

*All therapy must include patient education about prevention (including environmental control where appropriate) as well as control of symptoms.

Figure 21.5. Treatment algorithm for severe asthma. *TAO* = troleandomycin. * = Unavailable in the United States. Modified from Canadian consensus on the treatment of asthma in children. *Can Med Assoc J* 1991; 145:1449–1455.

adequate control cannot be achieved with maximal doses of inhaled steroid and bronchodilators. If possible, oral steroids should be administered on alternate days, and inhaled bronchodilator and high-dose inhaled steroid therapy used concurrently. The child's growth and blood pressure need to be monitored, a slit-lamp eye examination should be performed at 6- to 12-month intervals (to detect early cataract development), and urine samples should be checked regularly for glycosuria.

All patients with severe asthma should monitor lung function at home, their compliance and inhaler technique should be checked repeatedly, and close attention should be paid to their psychosocial status. A gradual reduction in steroid dosage should be attempted once the patient is stable.

In children with severe asthma who continue to be symptomatic despite the use of oral steroids, a trial of troleandomycin (TAO) has been recommended (265). When used concomitantly with methylprednisolone, this macrolide antibiotic has been shown to improve pulmonary function and symptom control in children with severe asthma, and to have a steroid-sparing effect. Potential side effects include elevation of hepatic enzymes, a cushingoid appearance, and abdominal pain, which generally resolve when the TAO dose is reduced. Because the elimination rate of theophylline is reduced by TAO, serum theophylline concentrations need to be monitored in patients who are on concomitant theophylline therapy. Whether TAO therapy is actually beneficial in terms of a true reduction in steroid dose is unclear. The dose may be reduced but the effects and side effects are equivalent to the higher dose of the effects of TAO on steroid activity (265).

Recent studies have shown that the use of low-dose weekly methotrexate in adults with steroid-dependent asthma allows a reduction in steroid dosage without associated clinical deterioration (266). Pending further investigation, the use of methotrexate in childhood asthma cannot be advocated at the present time. Likewise, gold therapy (267) cannot be recommended at present for the treatment of childhood asthma.

SPECIFIC PROBLEMS IN PEDIATRIC ASTHMA

Asthma in Infants and Young Children

A variety of physiologic and anatomic factors account for the increased vulnerability of infants and young children to the development of airway obstruction and respiratory failure (268) (Fig. 21.6). These include increased peripheral airway resistance, decreased elastic recoil of the lung, increased compliance of the rib cage, decreased collateral ventilation, and decreased fatigue-resistant diaphragmatic muscle fibers. It is not surprising, therefore, that the majority of children with asthma develop symptoms in the

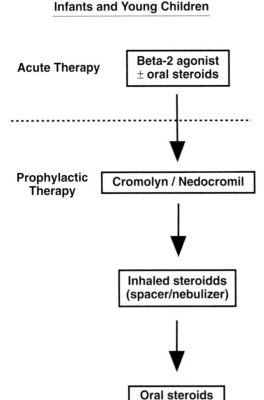

Figure 21.6. Treatment algorithm for asthma in infants and young children. * = Unavailable in the United States. Modified from Canadian consensus on the treatment of asthma in children. *Can Med Assoc J* 1991; 145:1449–1455.

first few years of life (15–17), and that emergency room (ER) visits (129) and hospitalizations (6, 20) for asthma are particularly high in this age group. In early life, asthma is typically aggravated by viral respiratory infections, whereas allergic triggers play a relatively unimportant role. Exposure to passive smoking in the prenatal and postnatal period increases the risk of atopic diseases, including asthma, in early childhood (98). Preterm delivery and neonatal ventilation are additional risk factors for the development of asthma in early life (269).

Unfortunately, clinicians remain reluctant to make a diagnosis of asthma in young children, and this frequently leads to inappropriate forms of treatment. The diagnosis of asthma in this age group must be made on clinical grounds, since tests of lung function and airway responsiveness are possible only in specialized laboratories (270). In babies with atypical symptoms (Table 21.8), additional investigations may be necessary to exclude other respiratory disorders that can mimic asthma. The diagnosis of asthma can be confirmed by demonstrating a favorable response to anti-asthmatic therapy.

Asthma in early life presents a major therapeutic challenge, largely because of the increased difficulty in administering medications, and the paucity of data concerning the value of many anti-asthmatic medications in this age group. In general, inhalation therapy in very young children is only possible with the use of nebulizers, although a spacer device with a facemask may be worth a trial (271). Although the efficacy of beta-2 agonists in children less than 18 months of age has been questioned (272), a beneficial clinical response to nebulized albuterol in young children with acute asthma has been shown (273, 274). For maintenance treatment of asthma in early childhood, therefore, a trial of a nebulized beta-2 agonist is warranted (oral beta-2 agonists may suffice for the treatment of very mild and infrequent symptoms). If this is not effective, the addition of nebulized ipratropium may be helpful (275), but this form is not available in the United States. Children with persistent symptoms should be treated prophylactically with nebulized cromolyn (276, 277) or oral ketotifen (210). Theophylline therapy may be beneficial in young children, but compliance is poor and side effects are common (277, 278). If the response to treatment is still inadequate, a trial of nebulized corticosteroids (if available) should be considered, although the efficacy of nebulized steroids in very young children seems quite variable (279–281). Preschool children may benefit from inhaled steroids delivered by MDI in conjunction with a spacer and a mask (282–284). The appropriate dose of inhaled steroids for young children is unknown—recent data indicate that adrenal suppression does not occur with doses in the range of 200–400 µg per day (285). As a last line of therapy, alternate-day oral steroids may be necessary, although the clinical response to oral steroid therapy in very young children may be disappointing (286).

Asthma During Adolescence

Although asthma symptoms frequently improve or disappear during adolescence, a deterioration may occur in some patients, and even new cases of asthma may arise in this age group. Specific issues in teenagers with asthma (287) include (a) denial of symptoms, (b) noncompliance, (c) psychosocial issues, (d) abuse of MDIs, (e) cigarette smoking, (f) poor relationship between the patient and the medical team, and (g) pregnancy (288).

Cough-Variant Asthma

Chronic cough may be the sole manifestation of asthma (106). Therapy should include a trial of therapy with bronchodilators, cromolyn, or inhaled steroids. Since cough-variant asthma may be related to hyper-responsiveness of cough receptors, antitussive therapy may have a role to play in such children (289).

Exercise-induced Asthma

Exercise-induced asthma (EIA) occurs in the majority of patients with asthma, and is particularly troublesome in children because of their high level of physical activity (290). In EIA, the bronchial obstruction reaches its peak 5–15 minutes after exertion, whereas a delayed asthmatic response after exercise is uncommon (291). EIA occurs after strenuous, continuous forms of exercise (e.g., running, skating), whereas sports not requiring sustained running and swimming are less likely to provoke symptoms (290). EIA is more marked with exercise in a cold, dry atmosphere. With adequate prophylaxis, the majority of children with asthma can participate in regular sporting and recreational activities—in fact, physical training programs have been shown to improve exercise tolerance and cardiorespiratory performance in patients with asthma (292, 293).

Warming-up before athletic events is helpful. EIA is prevented most effectively by inhalation of a selective beta-2 agonist from an MDI or dry-powder inhaler about 5 minutes before exercise (294). For children who are unable to use these inhalation devices, an appropriate dose of an oral beta-2 agonist 2 hours prior to exercise is a useful alternative (295). Premedication with cromolyn will prevent EIA in about 60% of children (199) and, if necessary, can be used in conjunction with a beta-2 agonist. Patients who take theophylline for prophylaxis of chronic asthma should be reasonably well protected against EIA, but inhalation of a beta-2 agonist may be necessary prior to strenuous exercise. Inhibition of EIA by theophylline occurs predominantly at serum theophylline concentrations greater than 10 mg/L (296).

Nocturnal Asthma

Children with asthma frequently complain of troublesome wheezing and coughing at night and in the early morning ("morning dippers"). In patients with asthma, the fall in lung function at night reflects an amplification of the normal circadian rhythm in airway caliber due to airway hyper-reactivity and inflammation (297). Since bronchial hyper-reactivity seems to be the underlying mechanism, the logical first step in treatment is to optimize daytime control of asthma with an inhaled steroid preparation (298). Control of nocturnal symptoms can be improved further by giving a single dose (10 mg/kg) of a slow-release theophylline preparation at bed-time (195). The use of an ultra-sustained theophylline preparation may be even more effective in this situation (299). Sustained-release oral beta-2 agonists are available and can help to control nocturnal symptoms (300). In the future, long-acting inhaled beta-2 agonists (e.g., salmeterol, formoterol) may prove particularly useful in treating nocturnal asthma (301). Environmental precautions may benefit patients with nocturnal symptoms who exhibit feather or dust mite allergy. Finally, a possible relationship between nocturnal wheezing and gastroesophageal reflux may need to be considered in selected patients (302).

"Impossible" Asthma

Some children with asthma continue to have symptoms despite apparent appropriate treatment. Several factors may be responsible for this (Table 21.19) (303). Compliance in particular is very important in the success of treatment, and this can be improved through education, providing consistent medical care, and keeping the therapeutic regimen as simple as possible.

Finally, small groups of children with asthma have been described who continue to have peripheral airway obstruction despite intensive bronchodilator and steroid therapy (304, 305).

ACUTE ASTHMA

Acute asthma is a common, potentially life-threatening medical emergency. At our institution, asthma accounts for 5.6% of patient visits to the ER (129) and for 11.2% of all medical admissions (306); even higher hospitalization rates for asthma have been reported from other pediatric centers (22, 307). It should be stressed that severe episodes of asthma can be prevented, or at least ameliorated, by early recognition and intensification of treatment. Unfortunately, deficiencies in both the assessment and treatment of children with acute asthma are common (129), and include (a) failure to measure lung function, (b) underuse of systemic steroids, and (c) inad-

---

Table 21.19.
Causes of Apparent Failure of Therapy[a]

- Incorrect inhaler technique
- Inappropriate drug dose or dosing interval
- Poor patient compliance
- Inadequate trial of preventative agents
- Failure to use medications in a systematic fashion
- Medical complications (e.g., gastroesophageal reflux, aspirin intolerance, allergic bronchopulmonary aspergillosis, sinusitis)
- Psychosocial factors and vocal cord paralysis
- Inappropriate treatment (e.g., antibiotics, antitussives)

[a]See also reference 303.

---

equate follow-up arrangements upon discharge from the ER.

Pathophysiology

The central event in acute asthma is widespread airway obstruction that results from bronchial smooth muscle spasm, inflammation, and mucus plugging (Fig. 21.7). Airway obstruction leads to increased airway resistance, reduced flow rates, gas trapping, and pulmonary overdistension. The potential benefit of pulmonary hyperinflation on respiration by helping to maintain patency of the airways is offset by a considerable increase in the work of the respiratory muscles resulting from increased airway resistance and decreased compliance.

The changes in airway resistance are not uniform throughout the bronchial tree: some lung units are overventilated, whereas others receive inadequate ventilation. This leads to ventilation-perfusion mismatching and, in turn, hypoxia. Although significant correlations have been found between the degree of airway obstruction (e.g., FEV_1) and both arterial oxygen tension (PaO_2) (308) and saturation (SaO_2) (309) in children with acute asthma, the scatter in individual values is high.

The changes in arterial carbon dioxide tension ($PaCO_2$) in acute asthma are more complex. As a result of hyperventilation, the majority of patients with acute asthma have respiratory alkalosis on presentation (308). However, in the presence of severe airway

Acute Asthma - Pathophysiology

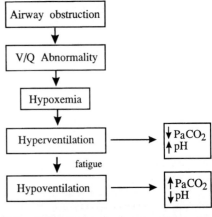

Figure 21.7. Pathophysiology of acute asthma. *V/Q* = ventilation/perfusion.

obstruction (FEV_1 >25% predicted), respiratory muscle fatigue and alveolar hypoventilation ensue, resulting in hypercapnia and respiratory acidosis. Thus, a rising $PaCO_2$, even into the "normal" range, must be regarded as a sign of fatigue and impending respiratory failure in acute asthma. Metabolic acidosis may also occur in severe acute asthma, and is due to lactic acidosis resulting from tissue hypoxia and lactate production by respiratory muscles (308, 310).

Assessment

The intensity of treatment in acute asthma is based on an accurate assessment of the severity of the event. This assessment should rely not only on history and physical examination, but should include simple laboratory measurements.

CLINICAL EVALUATION

Features in the history that indicate the potential for life-threatening asthma (34, 35) and the need for close monitoring and prompt care are listed in Table 21.3. In particular, children who have needed intubation and mechanical ventilation for asthma in the past should be treated very aggressively.

Clinical evaluation in the ER is the most important step in determining the severity of acute asthma and the need for hospitalization (311). Physical signs associated with severe acute asthma in children are listed in Table 21.20. Of these signs, accessory muscle use, dyspnea, and pulsus paradoxus of >15 mm Hg indicate that significant airway obstruction and arterial desaturation are likely to exist (309, 312). As a corollary, significant airflow

Table 21.20.
Clinical Manifestations of Severe Acute Asthma

Tachycardia > 120/minute
Tachypnea > 30/minute
Dyspnea
Inability to speak (or feeding difficulty)
Accessory muscle use
Pulsus paradoxus > 15 mm Hg

Life-threatening signs

Silent chest on auscultation
Cyanosis
Altered consciousness
Respiratory muscle fatigue (e.g., abdominal paradox)
Pneumothorax

obstruction and hypoxia can still be present in the absence of these signs. It should be emphasized that wheezing is an unreliable sign in severe asthma since, in the presence of severe obstruction, airflow is so reduced that wheezing may be eliminated. Cyanosis, confusion, and fatigue are ominous signs and indicate the need for immediate, intensive therapy and possibly intubation.

INVESTIGATIONS

In older children (>6 years), the assessment of acute asthma is incomplete without an objective measurement of the degree of airflow obstruction using a portable spirometer or a simple peak flow meter (129). Serial measurements should be made in order to determine the response to treatment; the results are expressed as a percentage of the predicted normal values for height and sex. A PEFR or FEV_1 value of less than 40% of the predicted norm indicates severe asthma.

Arterial blood gas analysis is rarely necessary prior to initiation of treatment. However, this procedure is mandatory in the presence of cyanosis, confusion, fatigue, or severe lung function impairment (e.g., FEV_1 >25% predicted), and in children who are not responding to treatment. Pulse oximetry is a non-invasive method of measuring systemic oxygenation, and can be used to determine the need for supplementary oxygen. Studies suggest that children with acute asthma who have SaO_2 values of 91% (in room air) before treatment should be hospitalized (311, 313).

Chest radiographs are not routinely necessary in acute asthma (129), but should be obtained in every episode of severe asthma or if physical findings suggest a complication (e.g., pneumothorax).

Treatment

Children with severe acute asthma require expeditious treatment, close observation, and serial measurements of physical signs and lung function (Fig. 21.8). The goals of treatment in acute asthma are to relieve hypoxia, reverse airway obstruction by the use of bronchodilators and systemic steroids, and prevent early relapse.

GENERAL MEASURES

Supplementary oxygen should be administered to hypoxic patients. Pulse oximetry is

Acute Asthma

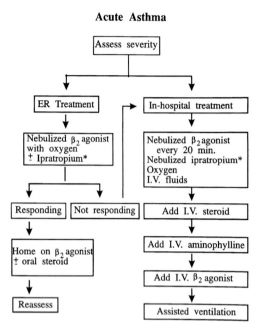

Figure 21.8. Treatment algorithm for acute asthma. * = Unavailable in the United States.

useful in titrating fractional inspired O_2 concentrations (FiO_2). An SaO_2 of 92% should be achieved (314). Nebulized medications should be delivered with oxygen, rather than air, since bronchodilators can occasionally cause transient oxygen desaturation (315).

Some children with acute asthma may be mildly dehydrated on presentation (316). Intravenous fluids may, therefore, be necessary to supplement oral intake and to provide access for the administration of medications. Care should be taken to avoid fluid overload, which can predispose to pulmonary edema in the presence of the abnormal swings in intrathoracic pressure found in acute asthma (317). Additional fluids above maintenance requirements are rarely necessary in acute asthma (316). A conventional hypotonic solution is recommended, and potassium supplementation may be necessary, since both bronchodilators and steroids can cause potassium wasting.

INHALED BRONCHODILATORS

A nebulized beta-2 agonist should be the first-line treatment for all patients with acute asthma (162). Two recent studies have demonstrated the efficacy and safety of frequent nebulizations of beta-2 agonists in severe, acute asthma (318, 319). Based on these data, our initial approach in severe acute asthma is to administer albuterol, 150 μg/kg (maximum 5 mg/dose), every 20 minutes until a clinical response is achieved. Oxygen should be used as the gas for the nebulizer. Possible side effects include tremor, (318, 319) tachycardia (319), and mild hypokalemia (319). In children who are less severely ill, hourly nebulizations of albuterol may suffice, and in this situation, a larger dose of nebulized albuterol, 300 μg/kg (maximum 10 mg/dose), can be used (320).

Recent data indicate that beta-2 agonists, administered by metered dose inhaler and spacer device, achieve bronchodilation equivalent to that effected by wet aerosol administration (321), but further studies are needed before this mode of delivery can be recommended in acute asthma, particularly in young, dyspneic children.

Although an aerosolized beta-2 stimulant is the first-line agent in acute asthma, residual airway obstruction may sometimes persist, even with 20-minute nebulizations (318, 319). Additional bronchodilation can be achieved by the administration of nebulized ipratropium every 4 hours (and hourly if necessary), in combination with albuterol (177–179). Based on the dose-response relationship for ipratropium, 125 μg/dose is recommended in children under the age of 4 years, and 250 μg/dose in older children (322). Unfortunately, ipratropium solution is not available in the United States.

CORTICOSTEROIDS

It should be emphasized that airway obstruction in asthma is caused not only by bronchial smooth muscle spasm, but also by edema of the airway mucosa, mucus plugging, and inflammation. Systemic steroids, therefore, are mandatory in children with severe acute asthma, and in those who respond poorly to nebulized bronchodilators (323). The factors listed in Table 21.1 are also indicative of the need for steroid therapy in acute asthma. It should be stressed that systemic steroids represent a supplement to, and not a substitute for, bronchodilator therapy.

The dose of systemic steroids in acute asthma is somewhat arbitrary. Depending on the clinical situation, steroids can be administered either orally (e.g., prednisone 1–2 mg/

kg/day) or intravenously (e.g., hydrocortisone 4–6 mg/kg or methylprednisolone 1–2 mg/kg, every 4–6 hours). Although recent data indicate that inhaled steroids may have a role in the treatment of acute asthmatic symptoms at home (324), this form of treatment cannot yet be recommended for the emergency care of acute asthma.

THEOPHYLLINE

Although it is relatively common practice to administer intravenous aminophylline to patients hospitalized with acute asthma, recent studies have questioned the value of this approach. Several trials in adult asthmatic subjects found that no additional bronchodilation was achieved when intravenous aminophylline was added to intensive sympathomimetic therapy, and that the addition of theophylline increased the risk of adverse effects (325). In contrast, Pierson et al. (326), in a double-blind, controlled pediatric study, found that intravenous aminophylline had a beneficial therapeutic effect when given in combination with nebulized sympathomimetics and systemic corticosteroids. We suggest that intravenous aminophylline be considered for use, in conjunction with nebulized beta-2 agonists, in all asthmatics who are seriously ill on hospital admission, and in those who fail to show a rapid response to adrenergic agents. In patients not taking theophylline, an initial loading dose of 6 mg/kg is administered intravenously over 20–30 minutes. For patients on maintenance oral theophylline, a serum theophylline concentration should be determined and the loading dose modified, as appropriate. Following the loading dose, the patient is started on maintenance intravenous aminophylline, which ideally should be given as a continuous infusion, rather than by intermittent bolus injections (327). Suggested maintenance doses of aminophylline are shown in Table 21.21, but the final decision on dosage will depend on the results of serum theophylline assays (196). There may be an advantage in maintaining serum theophylline concentrations close to the upper end of the therapeutic range in acute asthma (328).

ER Discharge

After treatment in the ER, up to 75% of children with acute asthma can be discharged

Table 21.21.
Continuous Theophylline[a] Dosage Following an Initial Loading Dose[b]

Patient Age/ Clinical Condition	Infusion Rate[c] (mg/kg/hr)
Infants 6–52 weeks	[(0.01 × age in weeks) + 0.03]
Children 1–9 years	1.0
Children 9–12 years	0.8
Children 12–16 years	0.7
> 16 years	0.6
Cardiac failure, cor pulmonale, and liver dysfunction	0.2

[a]Aminophylline is 80–85% theophylline.
[b]See also reference 196.
[c]Use ideal body weight.

home (129). The need for hospitalization can be reduced further if a holding room is available where children can be observed and treated for a prolonged period (329).

Follow-up studies in children recovering from acute exacerbations of asthma indicate that residual pulmonary function and blood gas abnormalities may persist for several weeks (305, 308). If a decision to discharge the child from the ER is made, it is essential that home therapy be adjusted. Inhaled bronchodilators should be continued at home, administered by an appropriate delivery system. A 5- to 7-day course of oral steroids is usually indicated. Prompt review of the child by the primary care physician is mandatory.

Criteria for Hospital Admission

One of the most difficult decisions in the emergency treatment of asthma is whether to admit the child to the hospital. Clearly all critically ill children with asthma should be admitted immediately. Children who continue to have persistent signs and symptoms and residual airflow obstruction (e.g., peak flow rate <60% predicted) after ER treatment should also be hospitalized (311), as should children with complications (e.g., pneumothorax, lobar atelectasis). Greater consideration for admission should be given to children who exhibit any of the features listed in Table 21.16. Finally, recent studies have intimated that children with acute asthma who have SaO_2 values of 91% (in room air) before treatment should be hospitalized (311, 313). Oxygen saturation measurements in the ER also appear to be more predictive of relapse than lung function measurements are (313, 330). Children who required aggressive bronchodilator therapy should be observed in the ER to make certain the improvement will be sustained on less aggressive therapy.

In-Hospital Management

Virtually all children admitted to hospital with acute asthma will have moderate to severe airway obstruction refractory to initial ER treatment (311). Careful ongoing assessment is, therefore, essential to determine the response to treatment and detect any deterioration. Lung function measurements, before and after bronchodilators, should be repeated several times each day, and SaO_2 should be monitored by oximetry. Serum potassium levels should be checked. Particular attention should be given to children with FEV_1 <25% predicted, or $PaCO_2 \geq 40$ mm Hg. In-hospital treatment should include hydration, oxygen, regular nebulizations of beta-2 agonists and ipratropium, intravenous steroids, and aminophylline (if necessary).

Treatment of Respiratory Failure

Despite optimal therapy, a small number of children with severe acute asthma develop respiratory failure with progressive hypoxia, hypercapnia, and fatigue, and require transfer to an intensive care facility. At this institution, approximately 20 children per year are admitted to the intensive care unit (ICU) with acute asthma, and about 33% of these children require intubation and mechanical ventilation (306). If possible, these children should be managed by an experienced critical care team, skilled in intubation techniques and ventilatory strategies.

The usual cause of death in asthma is severe asphyxia with acidosis (331), and correction of these abnormalities is of prime importance. On admission to the ICU (in children who do not require immediate intubation), children are placed on 100% oxygen until arterial blood gas results are available. Nebulized albuterol (150 μg/kg/dose) is administered continuously, a strategy that may avert the need for ventilation in some children with impending or actual respiratory failure (332). Intravenous steroids and aminophylline are given concurrently. Arterial blood gas tensions (obtained from an indwelling arterial catheter) are measured at 15- to 30-minute intervals, as demanded by the child's course. In the presence of severe acidosis (ph <7.2), the judicious use of sodium bicarbonate is a useful therapeutic adjunct in order to restore responsiveness to sympathomimetic agents (333). Supplementary potassium will be necessary if hypokalemia develops.

In children who fail to respond to the aforementioned measures, a continuous intravenous infusion of a beta-2 agonist is warranted, and may avert the need for intubation (332, 334). If albuterol is used, the infusion is commenced at a rate of 0.5 μg/kg/min and increased by 1 μg/kg every 15 minutes until the patient clinically improves and $PaCO_2$ falls, or intubation and ventilation become necessary. The maximum infusion rate of albuterol is 20 μg/kg/min, but patients generally respond to 4 μg/kg/min (334). The effect of albuterol is followed by cardiovascular and blood gas monitoring, and serum potassium levels should be checked regularly. In the United States, intravenous terbutaline is used as an alternative to albuterol.

If intubation becomes necessary, it should be done on an elective basis, prior to the development of cardiorespiratory arrest. The decision to intervene is based on an assessment of the child's clinical condition and response to therapy. Increasing fatigue and somnolence are particularly ominous signs. There is no absolute $PaCO_2$ value above which intubation is mandatory, since some children with very high $PaCO_2$ values respond rapidly to medical therapy. Intubation should be effected with the least systemic disturbance to the child. In order to achieve this, the use of intravenous thiopental or ketamine combined with a short-acting muscle relaxant (succinylcholine) is recommended. An orotracheal tube is inserted initially in order to secure the airway before changing to a nasotracheal tube. A tube with an internal diameter of 0.5 mm *greater* than that normally predicted for age is usually required to allow effective ventilation with a minimal air leak around the tube. Above the age of 9 years, a cuffed tube can be used. After placement of the endotracheal tube, neuromuscular blockade is maintained with a long-acting muscle relaxant (vecuronium or pancuronium) in order to keep airway pressures at a minimum.

The objectives of mechanical ventilation in severe asthma are the reversal of hypoxia, the relief of respiratory muscle fatigue, and partial compensation of respiratory acidosis, using the lowest peak airway pressures consistent with these objectives. It is not an objective to achieve a normal $PaCO_2$ in the first few hours of ventilatory support—any attempt to do so may result in pulmonary barotrauma. Arterial $PaCO_2$ values of 50–60 mm Hg are acceptable as long as they are accompanied by a pH of >7.3. This ventilatory strategy in asthma has been entitled "controlled hypoventilation" by Darioli and Perret (335). A volume-cycled ventilator is used, set at low ventilatory rates (8–12 per min), inspiratory/expiratory ratio of 1:4, and tidal volumes of 10–12 ml/kg. If possible, peak inspiratory pressures are maintained at less than 45 cm H_2O. The adequacy of the expiratory time can be gauged by auscultation of the chest or by scrutiny of the flow signal from the ventilator. Throughout the period of ventilation, beta-2 agonists are given by intravenous infusion or are nebulized into the inspiratory circuit of the ventilator. Bicarbonate is given to raise the pH above 7.25 if this cannot be achieved by mechanical ventilation. In order to maintain peak airway pressures at a minimum, muscle paralysis is continued and patients are sedated with a narcotic infusion.

The resolution of airway obstruction in the ventilated patient with severe asthma becomes evident when $PaCO_2$ values fall while the same or lower peak airway pressures are being used. Once the $PaCO_2$ is less than 45 mm Hg, peak airway pressure is less than 35 cm H_2O, and there is mild or no bronchospasm on auscultation, the muscle paralysis can be discontinued. As soon as respiratory muscle function has returned to normal, the patients can be placed on spontaneous ventilation. If a $PaCO_2$ of less than 45 mm Hg without assisted ventilation is maintained, rapid extubation is advisable. Most children who require ventilatory support for asthma can be weaned and extubated within 72 hours (306).

Using the above approach, the outcome for children with severe acute asthma who require ventilation is excellent, with low mortality and complication rates (306). However, follow-up studies of children who require ventilation for asthma show that they continue to be a high-risk group with ongoing morbidity and mortality (35, 336).

Management During Recovery in the Hospital

During the recovery phase of acute asthma, the frequency of inhalation therapy should be reduced gradually, and oral drugs should be substituted for intravenous medications. The child's inhalation technique should be checked, and re-education of the family may be indicated. Patients can be allowed home once symptoms have cleared and lung function has stabilized (e.g., PEFR >75% predicted). Children should be discharged on a course of oral steroids, inhaled bronchodilators, a prophylactic anti-inflammatory agent (usually an inhaled steroid), and possibly theophylline. Older children should be supplied with a peak flow meter on discharge. Early follow-up with the primary care physician is essential. It is hoped that by providing adequate supervision, education, and effective preventative treatment, future episodes of severe acute asthma will be avoided (337).

NATURAL HISTORY OF CHILDHOOD ASTHMA

The most comprehensive information on the natural history of asthma is provided by the Melbourne group, who followed children with asthma prospectively to the age of 28 years (338–341). At the age of 21, about 50% of the subjects who had mild, infrequent asthma as children had become symptom-free, whereas this was more the exception than the rule in those who had more severe asthma. Between 21 and 28 years, although some patients improved, others experienced a recurrence of symptoms (340). It was also found that some adults who had "outgrown" asthma continued to have occult pulmonary function abnormalities and increased airway reactivity—even greater pulmonary function abnormalities were found in symptomatic patients (341). The factors that may influence the long-term prognosis in childhood asthma are summarized in Table 21.22 (338–343). Although some children with asthma may experience some growth retardation around the time of puberty, normal stature is ultimately achieved in the majority of patients (240). Finally, the relationship between childhood asthma and

Table 21.22.
Factors Influencing the Outcome of Asthma

Sex	Variable pattern
Early age of onset	Possibly
Severity of asthma	Yes
Family history of atopy	Yes
Chronic eczema	Yes
Smoking (active/passive)	Yes
Level of lung function/ airway reactivity	Probably
Treatment	Not known

See also references 338–343 for more data on prognosis.

chronic obstructive lung disease in adult life remains unclear at this time (344).

Acknowledgement

The authors thank J. Chay for secretarial assistance.

REFERENCES

1. Weiss KB, Wagener DK. Changing patterns of asthma mortality: Identifying target populations at risk. *JAMA* 1990; 264:1683–1687.
2. Speight ANP, Lee DA, Hey EN. Underdiagnosis and undertreatment of asthma in childhood. *Br Med J* 1983; 286:1253–1256.
3. Clifford RD, Radford M, Howell JB, Holgate ST. Prevalence of respiratory symptoms among 7 and 11 year old schoolchildren and association with asthma. *Arch Dis Child* 1989; 64:1118–1125.
4. Hill RA, Standen PJ, Tattersfield AE. Asthma, wheezing and school absence in primary schools. *Arch Dis Child* 1989; 64:246–251.
5. Storr J, Barrell E, Lenney W. Asthma in primary schools. *Br Med J* 1987; 295:251–252.
6. Gergen PJ, Weiss KB. Changing patterns of asthma hospitalization among children: 1979 to 1987. *JAMA* 1990; 264:1688–1692.
7. Marion RJ, Creer TL, Reynolds RVC. Direct and indirect costs associated with the management of childhood asthma. *Ann Allergy* 1985; 54:31–34.
8. Editorial: Management of asthma in the community. *Lancet* 1989; 2:199–200.
9. Colver AF. Community campaign against asthma. *Arch Dis Child* 1984; 59:449–452.
10. Hughes DM, McLeod M, Garner B, Goldbloom RB. Controlled trial of a home and ambulatory program for asthmatic children. *Pediatrics* 1991; 87:54–61.
11. Sears MR. Epidemiology of asthma. In O'Byrne PM, ed. *Asthma as an inflammatory disease.* New York, Marcel Dekker, 1990, pp 15–48.
12. Waite DA, Eyles EF, Tonkin SL, O'Donnell TV. Asthma prevalence in Tokelauan children in two environments. *Clin Allergy* 1980; 10:71–75.
13. Keeley DJ, Neill P, Gallivan S. Comparison of the prevalence of reversible airways obstruction in rural and urban Zimbabwean children. *Thorax* 1991; 46:549–553.
14. Burney PGJ, Chinn S, Rona RJ. Has the prevalence of asthma increased in children? Evidence from a national study of health and growth 1973–86. *Br Med J* 1990; 300: 1306–1310.
15. Gergen PJ, Mullally DI, Evans R. National survey of prevalence of asthma among children in the United States, 1976–1980. *Pediatrics* 1988; 81:1–7.
16. Schwartz J, Gold D, Dockery DW, Weiss ST, Speizer FE. Predictors of asthma and persistent wheeze in a national sample of children in the United States. Association with social class, perinatal events and race. *Am Rev Respir Dis* 1990; 142:555–562.
17. Weitzman M, Gortmaker S, Sobol A. Racial, social and environmental risks for childhood asthma. *Am J Dis Child* 1990; 144:1189–1194.
18. Johnston IDA, Bland JM, Anderson HR. Ethnic variation in respiratory morbidity and lung function in childhood. *Thorax* 1987; 42:542–548.
19. Verity CM, Ven Heule B, Carswell F, Hughes AO. Bronchial lability and skin reactivity in siblings of asthmatic children. *Arch Dis Child* 1984; 59:871–76.
20. Mao Y. Canadian pediatric asthma: morbidity, mortality and hospitalization data. In *Treatment of pediatric asthma: A Canadian Consensus (MEDICINE) Publishing Foundation Symposium Series, 29.* Toronto, MES Medical Education Services 1991, pp 9–17.
21. Anderson HR. Increase in hospital admissions for childhood asthma: trends in referral, severity, and readmissions from 1970 to 1985 in a health region in the United Kingdom. *Thorax* 1989; 44:614–619.
22. Carman PG, Landau LI. Increased paediatric admissions with asthma in Western Australia—a problem of diagnosis? *Med J Aust* 1990; 152:23–26.
23. Dawson KP, Mitchell EA. Asthma in New Zealand children. *J Asthma* 1990; 27:291–297.
24. Buist AS, Vollmer WM. Reflections on the rise in asthma morbidity and mortality. *JAMA* 1990; 264:1719–1720.
25. Storr J, Barrell E, Lenney W. Rising asthma admissions and self referral. *Arch Dis Child* 1988; 63:774–779.
26. Burney P. Asthma deaths in England and Wales 1931–85: evidence for a true increase in asthma mortality. *J Epidemiol Community Health* 1988; 42:316–320.
27. Spitzer WO, Suissa S, Ernst P, et al. The use of beta agonist and the risk of death and near death from asthma. *N Engl J Med* 1992; 326:501–506.
28. Poynter D. Fatal Asthma—Is treatment incriminated? *J Allergy Clin Immunol* 1987; 80(Suppl): 423–427.
29. Grainger J, Woodman K, Pearce N et al. Prescribed fenoterol and death from asthma in New Zealand, 1981–7: A further case-control study. *Thorax* 1991; 46:105–111.
30. Sears MR, Rea HH, Fenwich J, et al. Seventy-five deaths in asthmatics prescribed home nebulizers. *Br Med J* 1987; 294:47–80.
31. Wilson JD, Sutherland DC, Thomas AC. Has the change to beta agonist combined with oral theophylline increased cases of fatal asthma? *Lancet* 1981; 1:1235–1237.
32. Snell NJC. Adverse reactions to inhaled drugs. *Resp Med* 1990; 84:345–348.

33. Sly MR. Mortality from asthma. *J Allergy Clin Immunol* 1989; 84:421–434.
34. Strunk RC. Workshop on the identification of the fatality-prone patient with asthma: Summary of workshop discussion. *J Allergy Clin Immunol* 1987; 80(Suppl):455–457.
35. Newcomb RW, Akhter J. Respiratory failure from asthma: A marker for children with high morbidity and mortality. *Am J Dis Child* 1988; 142:1041–1048.
36. Osler W. *The principles and practice of medicine*, 3rd ed. New York, Appleton, 1901, pp 628–632.
37. Djukanovic R, Roche WR, Wilson JW, et al. Mucosal inflammation in asthma. *Am Rev Respir Dis* 1990; 142:434–457.
38. Cutz E, Levison H, Cooper DM. Ultrastructure in airways in children with asthma. *Histopathology* 1978; 2:407–411.
39. Beasley R, Roche WR, Roberts JA, Holgate ST. Cellular events in the bronchi in mild asthma and after bronchial provocation. *Am Rev Respir Dis* 1989; 139:806–817.
40. Lozewicz S, Gomez E, Ferguson H, Davis RJ. Inflammatory cells in the airways in mild asthma. *Br Med J* 1988; 297:1515–1516.
41. Lozewicz S, Wells C, Gomez E, et al. Morphological integrity of the bronchial epithelium in mild asthma. *Thorax* 1990; 45:12–15.
42. Clough JB, Williams JD, Holgate ST. Effect of atopy on the natural history of symptoms, peak expiratory flow, and bronchial responsiveness in 7- and 8-year-old children with cough and wheeze. *Am Rev Respir Dis* 1991; 143:755–760.
43. Lee, DA, Winslow NR, Speight ANP, Hey EN. Prevalence and spectrum of asthma in childhood. *Br Med J* 1983; 286:1256–1258.
44. O'Bryne PM. Airway inflammation and asthma. In O'Byrne PM, ed. *Asthma as an inflammatory disease.* New York, Marcel Dekker, 1990, pp 143–158.
45. LeSouef PN, Geelhoed GC, Turner DJ, Morgan SEG, Landau LI. Response of normal infants to inhaled histamine. *Am Rev Respir Dis* 1989; 139:62–66.
46. Wilson NM. Wheezy bronchitis revisited. *Arch Dis Child* 1989; 64:1194–1199.
47. Sibbald B, Horn MEC, Brain EA, Gregg I. Genetic factors in childhood asthma. *Thorax* 1980; 35:671–674.
48. Sibbald B, Turner-Warwick M. Factors influencing the prevalence of asthma among first degree relatives of extrinsic and intrinsic asthmatics. *Thorax* 1979; 34:332–337.
49. Sibbald B, Horn MEC, Gregg I. A family study of the genetic basis of asthma and wheezy bronchitis. *Arch Dis Child* 1980; 55:354–357.
50. Zimmerman B, Feanny S, Reisman J, et al. The dose relationship of allergy to severity of childhood asthma. *J Allergy Clin Immunol* 1988; 81:63–70.
51. Higgins M, Keller J. Familial occurrence of chronic respiratory disease and familial resemblance in ventilatory capacity. *J Chronic Dis* 1975; 28:239–251.
52. Davis JB, Bulpitt CJ. Atopy and wheeze in children according to parental atopy and family size. *Thorax* 1981; 36:185–189.
53. Horwood LJ, Fergusson DM, Hons BA, Shannon FT. Social and familial factors in the development of early childhood asthma. *Pediatrics* 1985; 75:859–868.
54. Hopp RJ, Bewtra AK, Watt GD, Nair NM, Townley GD. Genetic analysis of allergic disease in twins. *J Allergy Clin Immunol* 1984; 73:265–270.
55. Townley RG, Bewtra A, Wilson AF, et al. Segregation analysis of bronchial response to methacholine inhalation challenge in families with and without asthma. *J Allergy Clin Immunol* 1986; 77:101–107.
56. Hopp RJ, Bewtra AK, Nair N, Townley R. Bronchial reactivity patterns in non-asthmatic parents of asthmatics. *Ann Allergy* 1988; 61:184–186.
57. Young S, LeSouef PN, Geelhoed G, et al. The influence of a family history of asthma and parental smoking on airway responsiveness in early infancy. *N Engl J Med* 1991; 324:1168–1173.
58. Edfors-Lub ML. Allergy in 7000 twin pairs. *Acta Allergol* 1971; 26:249–285.
59. Duffy DL, Martin NG, Buttistutta D, Hopper JL, Mathews JD. Genetics of asthma and hay fever in Australian twins. *Am Rev Respir Dis* 1990; 142:1351–1358.
60. Burrows B, Mortimer FD, Halonen M, Barbee RA, Cline MG. Association of asthma with serum IgE levels and skin-test reactivity to allergens. *N Engl J Med* 1989; 320:271–277.
61. Cookson WOCM, Hopkin JM. Dominant inheritance of atopic immunoglobulin–E responsiveness. *Lancet* 1988; 1:86–88.
62. Cookson WOCM, Sharp PA, Faux JA, Hopkin JM. Linkage between immunoglobulin E responses underlying asthma and rhinitis and chromosome 11q. *Lancet* 1989; 1:1292–1295.
63. Croner S, Kjellman NIM, Eriksson B, Roth A. IgE screening in 1701 newborn infants and the development of atopic disease during infancy. *Arch Dis Child* 1982; 57:364–368.
64. Longo G, Strinati R, Poli F, Fumi F. Genetic factors in non-specific bronchial hyperreactivity. *Am J Dis Child* 1989; 141:331–334.
65. Sporik R, Holgate SJ, Platts-Mills TAE, Cogswell JJ. Exposure to house-dust mite allergen (Der p 1) and the development of asthma in childhood: A prospective study. *N Engl J Med* 1990; 323:502–507.
66. Dowse G, Turner KJ, Steward GA, Alpers MP, Woolcock AJ. The association between Dermatophagoides mites and the increasing prevalence of asthma in village communities within the Papua New Guinea Highlands. *J Allergy Clin Immunol* 1985; 75:75–83.
67. Warner JA, Warner JO. Allergen avoidance in childhood asthma. *Resp Med* 1991; 85:101–105.
68. Clifford RD, Howell JB, Radford M, Holgate ST. Associations between respiratory symptoms, bronchial response to methacholine, and atopy in two age groups of children. *Arch Dis Child* 1989; 64:1133–1139.
69. Peat JK, Salome CM, Sedgwick CS, Kerrebijn J, Woolcock AJ. A prospective study of bronchial hyperresponsiveness and respiratory symptoms in a population of Australian school children. *Clin Exp Allergy* 1989; 19:299–306.
70. Witt C, Stuckey MS, Woolcock AJ, Dawkins RL. Positive allergy prick skin tests associated with bronchial histamine responsiveness in an unselected population. *J Allergy Clin Immunol* 1986; 77:698–702.

71. Cockcroft DW. Atopy and asthma. In O'Byrne PM, ed. *Asthma as an inflammatory disease.* New York, Marcel Dekker Inc, 1990, pp 103–125.
72. Bousquet J, Michel F-B. Food allergy and asthma. *Ann Allergy* 1988: 61(Suppl):70–74.
73. Zimmerman B, Chambers C, Forsyth S. The highly atopic infant and chronic asthma. *J Allergy Clin Immunol* 1988; 81:71–77.
74. Kramer MS. Does breast feeding help protect against atopic disease? Biology, methodology, and a golden jubilee of controversy. *J Pediatr* 1988; 112:181–190.
75. Wright AL, Holberg CJ, Martinez FD, Morgan WJ, Taussig LM. Breast feeding and lower respiratory tract illness in the first year of life. *Br Med J* 1989; 299:946–949.
76. Cunningham AS, Jelliffe DB, Jelliffe EFP. Breast-feeding and health in the 1980's: A global epidemiologic review. *J Pediatr* 1991; 118:659–666.
77. Busse WW. Respiratory infections: Their role in airway responsiveness and the pathogenesis of asthma. *J Allergy Clin Immunol* 1990; 85:671–683.
78. Kattan M, Keens TG, Lapierre J-G, Levison H, Bryan AC, Reilly BJ. Pulmonary function abnormalities in symptom-free children after bronchiolitis. *Pediatrics* 1977; 59:683–688.
79. Sims DG, Downham MAPS, Gardner PS, Webb JKG, Weighman D. Study of 8-year-old children with a history of respiratory syncytial virus bronchiolitis in infancy. *Br Med J* 1978; 1:11–14.
80. Gurwitz D, Mindorff C, Levison H. Increased incidence of bronchial reactivity in children with a history of bronchiolitis. *J Pediatr* 1981; 98:551–555.
81. Pullan CR, Hey EN. Wheezing, asthma, and pulmonary dysfunction 10 years after infection with respiratory syncytial virus in infancy. *Br Med J* 1982; 284:1665–1669.
82. Mok JYQ, Simpson H. Symptoms, atopy and bronchial reactivity after lower respiratory infection in infancy. *Arch Dis Child* 1984; 54:299–305.
83. Rooney JC, Williams HE. The relationship between proved viral bronchitis and subsequent wheezing. *J Pediatr* 1971; 79:744–747.
84. Gurwitz D, Corey M, Levison H. Pulmonary function and bronchial reactivity in children after croup. *Am Rev Respir Dis* 1980; 122:95–99.
85. Weiss SG, Newcomb RW, Beem MO. Pulmonary assessment of children after chlamydia pneumonia of infancy. *J Pediatr* 1986; 108:659–664.
86. Howenstine M, Eigen H, Tepper R. Pulmonary function in infants after pertussis. *J Pediatr* 1991; 118:563–566.
87. Johnston IDA, Bland JM, Ingram D, Anderson HR, Warner JO, Lambert HD. Effect of whooping cough in infancy on subsequent lung function and bronchial reactivity. *Am Rev Respir Dis* 1986; 134:270–275.
88. Welliver RC, Wong DT, Sun M, et al. The development of respiratory syncytial virus specific IgE and the release of histamine in nasopharyngeal secretions after infection. *N Engl J Med* 1981; 305:841–846.
89. Welliver RC, Sun M, Rinaldo D, Orga PL. Predictive value of respiratory syncytial virus–specific IgE responses for recurrent wheezing following bronchiolitis. *J Pediatr* 1986; 109:776–780.
90. Martinez FD, Morgan WJ, Wright AL, Holberg C, Taussig LM. Initial airway function is a risk factor for recurrent wheezing respiratory illnesses during the first three years of life. *Am Rev Respir Dis* 1991; 143:312–316.
91. Martinez F, Morgan W, Wright AL, Holberg C, Taussig L. Diminished lung function as a predisposing factor for wheezing respiratory illness in infants. *N Engl J Med* 1988; 319:1112–1117.
92. Burney PGJ, Anderson HR, Burrows B, Chan-Yeung M, Pride NB, Speizer PE. Epidemiology. In Holgate ST, ed. *The role of inflammatory processes in airway hyperresponsiveness.* Oxford, Blackwell Scientific, 1989, pp 222–250.
93. Murray AB, Morrison BJ. The effect of cigarette smoke from the mother on bronchial responsiveness and severity of symptoms in children with asthma. *J Allergy Clin Immunol* 1986; 76:575–581.
94. Murray AB, Morrison BJ. Passive smoking by asthmatics: Its greater effect on boys than on girls and on older than on younger children. *Pediatrics* 1989; 84:451–459.
95. Gortmaker SL, Walker DK, Jacobs FH, Ruch-Ross H. Parental smoking and the risk of childhood asthma. *Am J Public Health* 1982; 72:574–579.
96. Leeder SR, Corkhill RT, Irwig LM, Holland WM, Colley JRT. Influence of family factors on asthma and wheezing during the first five years of life. *Br J Prev Soc Med* 1976; 30:213–218.
97. Magnusson CG. Maternal smoking influences cord serum IgE and IgD levels and increases the risk for subsequent infant allergy. *J Allergy Clin Immunol* 1986; 78:898–904.
98. Weitzman M, Gortmaker S, Walker DK, Sobol A. Maternal smoking and childhood asthma. *Pediatrics* 1990; 85:505–511.
99. Wright AL, Holberg C, Martinez FD, Taussig LM. Relationship of parental smoking to wheezing and non-wheezing lower respiratory illnesses in infancy. *J Pediatr* 1991; 118:207–214.
100. Murray AB, Morrison BJ. It is children with atopic dermatitis who develop asthma more frequently if the mother smokes. *J Allergy Clin Immunol* 1990; 86:732–739.
101. Martinez FD, Antognoni G, Macri R, et al. Parental smoking enhances bronchial responsiveness in nine–year–old children. *Am Rev Respir Dis* 1988; 138:518–523.
102. Dockery DW, Speizer FE, Strom DO, Ware JH, Spengler JD, Ferris BG Jr. Effects of inhalable particles on respiratory health of children. *Am Rev Respir Dis* 1989; 139:587–594.
103. Pope CA. Respiratory disease associated with community air pollution and a steel mill, Utah valley. *Am J Public Health* 1989; 79:623–628.
104. Vedal S, Schenker MB, Munoz A, Samet JM, Batterman S, Speizer FE. Daily air pollution effects on children's respiratory symptoms and peak expiratory flow. *Am J Public Health* 1987; 77:694–698.
105. Anderson HR. Respiratory abnormalities in Papua New Guinea children: The effects of locality and domestic wood smoke pollution. *Int J Epidemiol* 1978; 7:63–72.
106. Reisman JJ, Canny GJ, Levison H. The approach to chronic cough in childhood. *Ann Allergy* 1988; 61:163–169.

107. Eigen H, Laughlin JJ, Homrighausen J. Recurrent pneumonia in children and its relationship to bronchial hyperreactivity. *Pediatrics* 1982; 70:698–704.

108. Altamirano HG, McGready SJ, Mansmann HC. Right middle lobe syndromes in asthmatic children. *Pediatr Asthma Allergy Immunol* 1991; 5:33–37.

109. Ries AL. Response to bronchodilators. In Clausen JL, ed. *Pulmonary function guidelines and controversies.* London, Grune & Stratton, 1984, pp 215–221.

110. Henderson AJW, Carswell F. Circadian rhythm of peak expiratory flow in asthmatic and normal children. *Thorax* 1989; 44:410–414.

111. Braman SS, Carro WM. Bronchoprovocation testing. *Clin Chest Med* 1989; 10:165–176.

112. Pattemore PK, Innes Asher M, Harrison AC, Mitchell EA, Rea HH, Stewart AW. The interrelationship among bronchial hyperresponsiveness, the diagnosis of asthma, and asthma symptoms. *Am Rev Respir Dis* 1990; 142:549–554.

113. Juniper EF, Frith PA, Hargreave FE. Airway responsiveness to histamine and methacholine and relationship to minimum treatment to control symptoms of asthma. *Thorax* 1981; 36:575–579.

114. Josephs LK, Gregg I, Mullee MA, Holgate ST. Nonspecific bronchial reactivity and its relationship to the clinical expression of asthma. *Am Rev Respir Dis* 1989; 140:350–357.

115. Amaro-Galvez R, McLaughlin FJ, Levison H, et al. Grading severity and treatment requirements to control symptoms in asthmatic children and their relationship with airway hyperreactivity to methacholine. *Ann Allergy* 1987; 59:298–302.

116. de Benedictis FM, Canny GJ, Levison H. Methacholine inhalation challenge in the evaluation of chronic cough in children. *J Asthma* 1986; 23:303–308.

117. Subcommittee of the Allergy Section, Canadian Pediatric Society. Skin testing for allergy in children. *Can Med Assoc J* 1983; 129:828–833.

118. Ferguson AC, Murray AB. Predictive value of skin prick tests and radioallergosorbent tests for clinical allergy to dogs and cats. *Can Med Assoc J* 1986; 134:1365–1370.

119. Allergy Section, Canadian Pediatric Society. Blood tests for allergy in children. *Can Med Assoc J* 1990; 142:1207–1208.

120. Sheffer AL. The National Asthma Education Program attacks asthma. *J Allergy Clin Immunol* 1991; 87:468–469.

121. Van Asperen P, Jandera E, De Neef J, Hill P, Law N. Education in childhood asthma: A preliminary study of need and efficacy. *Aust Pediatr J* 1986; 22:49–52.

122. Conway SP, Littlewood JM. Admission to hospital with asthma. *Arch Dis Child* 1985; 60:636–639.

123. Conboy K. Self-management skills for cooperative care in asthma. *J Pediatr* 1989; 115:863–866.

124. Cross D, Nelson HS. The role of the peak flow meter in the diagnosis and management of asthma. *J Allergy Clin Immunol* 1991; 87:120–128.

125. Shapiro SM, Hendler JM, Ogirala RG, Aldrich TK, Shapiro MB. The evaluation of the accuracy of Access and Mini Wright peak flow meter. *Chest* 1991; 99:358–362.

126. Canny GJ, Levison H. *Childhood asthma: A handbook for parents,* 4th ed. Boehringer Ingelheim (Canada) Ltd., 1993.

127. Hill RA, Britton JR, Tattersfield AE. Management of asthma in schools. *Arch Dis Child* 1987; 62:414–415.

128. Wissow LS, Warshaw MHS, Box J, Baker D. Case management and quality assurance to improve care of inner city children with asthma. *Am J Dis Child* 1988; 142:748–752.

129. Canny GJ, Reisman J, Healy R, et al. Acute asthma: Observations regarding the management of a pediatric emergency room. *Pediatrics* 1989; 83:507–512.

130. Report of international workshop. Dust mite allergens and asthma – a worldwide problem. *J Allergy Clin Immunol* 1989; 83:416–427.

131. Price JA, Pollock I, Little SA, Longbottom JL, Warner JO. Measurement of airborne mite antigen in the homes of asthmatic children. *Lancet* 1990; 336:895–897.

132. Murray AB, Ferguson AC, Morrison AJ. Diagnosis of house dust mite allergy in asthmatic children: What constitutes a positive history? *J Allergy Clin Immunol* 1983; 71:21–28.

133. Charpin D, Birnbaum J, Haddi E, et al. Altitude and allergy to house–dust mites. *Am Rev Respir Dis* 1991; 143:983–986.

134. Platts-Mills TAE, Tovey ER, Mitchell EB, et al. Reduction of bronchial hyperreactivity during prolonged allergen avoidance. *Lancet* 1982; 2:675–678.

135. Murray AB. Avoiding airborne allergens in the home. In *Treatment of pediatric asthma: A Canadian consensus (MEDICINE): Publishing Foundation Symposium Series, 29.* Toronto: MES Medical Education Services, 1991, pp 33–38.

136. Korsgaard J. Preventative measures in house-dust allergy. *Am Rev Respir Dis* 1982; 125:80–84.

137. Miller J, Miller A, Luczynksa E, et al. Effect of tannic acid spray on dust mite antigen levels in carpets [Abstract]. *J Allergy Clin Immunol* 1989; 83:262.

138. Georgitis JW, De Mais JM. A double-blind study of the effectiveness of a high-efficiency particular air (HEPA) filter in the treatment of allergic rhinitis and asthma. *J Allergy Clin Immunol* 1990; 85:1050–1057.

139. Murray AB, Ferguson AC, Morrison BJ. The frequency and severity of cat allergy compared with dog allergy in atopic children. *J Allergy Clin Immunol* 1983; 72:145–149.

140. Wood RA, Chapman MD, Adkinson NF, Eggleston PA. The effect of cat removal on allergen content in household-dust samples. *J Allergy Clin Immunol* 1989; 83:730–734.

141. de Blay F, Chapman MD, Platts-Mills TAE. Airborne cat allergen (Fel d 1): Environmental control with the cat in situ. *Am Rev Respir Dis* 1991; 143:1334–1339.

142. O'Halloran MT, Yunginger JW, Offord KP, et al. Exposure to an aeroallergen as a possible precipitating factor in respiratory arrest in young patients with asthma. *N Engl J Med* 1991; 324:359–363.

143. Solomon WR, Burge HA, Boise JR. Exclusion of particulate allergens by window air conditioners. *J Allergy Clin Immunol* 1980; 65:306–308.

144. Hirsch DJ, Hirsch SR, Kalbfleisch JH. Effect of central air conditioning and meteorologic factors

on indoor spore counts. *J Allergy Clin Immunol* 1978; 62:22–26.

145. Ohman JL. Allergen immunotherapy in asthma: Evidence for efficacy. *J Allergy Clin Immunol* 1989; 84:133–140.

146. Bousquet J, Hejjaoui A, Michel F-B. Specific immunotherapy in asthma. *J Allergy Clin Immunol* 1990; 86:292–305.

147. Eggleston PA. Immunotherapy for allergic respiratory disease. *Pediatr Clin North Am* 1988; 35:1103–1114.

148. Warner JO, Price JF, Soothill JF, et al. Controlled study of hypo-sensitization to Dermatophagoides pteronyssinus in children with asthma. *Lancet* 1978; 2:912–917.

149. Mosbech, H, Dreborg S, Frolund L, et al. Hyposensitization in asthmatics with mPEG modified and unmodified house dust mite extract. II. Effect evaluated by challenge with allergen and histamine. *Allergy* 1989; 44:499–509.

150. Van Bever HP, Stevens WJ. Evolution of the late asthmatic reaction during immunotherapy and after stopping immunotherapy. *J Allergy Clin Immunol* 1990; 86:141–146.

151. Murray AB, Ferguson AC, Morrison BJ. Non-allergic bronchial hyperreactivity in asthmatic children decreases with age and increases with mite immunotherapy. *Ann Allergy* 1985; 54:541–544.

152. Hill DJ, Hosking CS, Shelton MJ, Turner MW. Failure of hyposensitisation in treatment of children with grass-pollen asthma. *Br Med J* 1982; 284:306–309.

153. Norman PS, Van Metre TE. The safety of allergenic immunotherapy. *J Allergy Clin Immunol* 1990; 85:522–525.

154. Matus I. Assessing the nature and clinical significance of psychological contributions to childhood asthma. *Am J Orthopsychiatry* 1981; 51:327–341.

155. Miller BD. Depression and asthma: A potentially lethal mixture. *J Allergy Clin Immunol* 1987; 80(Suppl):481–486.

156. Quinn CM. Children's asthma: New approaches, new understandings. *Ann Allergy* 1988; 60:283–292.

157. Nacon A. Social and emotional impact of childhood asthma. *Arch Dis Child* 1991; 66:458–460.

158. Creer TL, Gustafson KE. Psychological problem associated with drug therapy in childhood asthma. *J Pediatr* 1989; 115:850–855.

159. Barnes SD, Grob CS, Lachman BSD, Marsh BR, Loughlin GM. Psychogenic upper airway obstruction presenting as refractory wheezing. *J Pediatr* 1986; 109:1067–1070.

160. Lask B, Matthew D. Childhood asthma – a controlled trial of family psychotherapy. *Arch Dis Child* 1979; 54:116–119.

161. Strunk RL, Fukuhara JT, LaBrecque JL, Mrazek DA. Outcome of long-term hospitalization for asthma in children. *J Allergy Clin Immunol* 1989; 83:17–25.

162. Canny GJ. The role of beta-2 agonists. In *Treatment of pediatric asthma: A Canadian consensus. (MEDICINE). Publishing Foundation Symposium Series, 29.* Toronto, MES Medical Education Services, 1991, pp 41–49.

163. Lofdahl CG, Chung KF. Long-acting beta₂-adrenoceptor agonists: A new perspective in the treatment of asthma. *Eur Respir J* 1991; 4:218–226.

164. Sears MR, Taylor DR, Print CG, et al. Regular inhaled beta–agonist treatment in bronchial asthma. *Lancet* 1990; 333:1391–1396.

165. Shepherd GL, Jenkins WJ, Alexander J. Asthma exacerbations in patients taking regular salmeterol, or salbutamol for symptoms [Letter]. *Lancet* 1991; 377:1424.

166. Kerrebijn KF, van Essen-Zandvlier EEM, Neijens HJ. Effect of long term treatment with inhaled corticosteroids and beta-agonists on the bronchial responsiveness in children with asthma. *J Allergy Clin Immunol* 1987; 79:653–659.

167. Vathenen AS, Knor AJ, Higgins BG, Britton JR, Tattersfield AE. Rebound increase in bronchial responsiveness after treatment with inhaled terbutaline. *Lancet* 1988; 1:554–558.

168. Kraan J, Koeter GH, Mark TW, Sluiter HJ, de Vries K. Changes in bronchial hyperreactivity induced by 4 weeks' treatment with antiasthmatic drugs in patients with allergic asthma: A comparison between budesonide and terbutaline. *J Allergy Clin Immunol* 1985; 76:628–636.

169. Haahtela T, Jarvinen M, Kava T. Comparison of a beta₂-agonist, terbutaline, with an inhaled corticosteroid, budesonide, in newly detected asthma. *N Engl J Med* 1991; 325:388–392.

170. Waalkens HJ, Gerritsen J, Koeter GH, et al. Budesonide and terbutaline or terbutaline alone in children with mild asthma: Effects on bronchial hyperresponsiveness and diurinal variation in peak flow. *Thorax* 1991; 46:499–503.

171. Becker AB, Simons FER. Formoterol, a new long-acting selective beta₂-adrenergic receptor agonist. Double-blind comparison with salbutamol and placebo in children with asthma. *J Allergy Clin Immunol* 1989; 84:891–895.

172. Ramsdale EH, Otis J, Kline PA, Gontovnick LS, Hargreave FE, O'Byrne PM. Prolonged protection against methacholine-induced bronchoconstriction by an inhaled beta₂-agonist formoterol. *Am Rev Respir Dis* 1991; 143:998–1001.

173. Twentyman OP, Finnerty JP, Harris A, Palmer J, Holgate SJ. Protection against allergen–induced asthma by salmeterol. *Lancet* 1990; 336:1338–1342.

174. Canadian consensus on the treatment of asthma in children. *Can Med Assoc J* 1991; 145:1449–1455.

175. Wong CS, Pavord ID, Williams J, Britton JR, Tattersfield AE. Bronchodilator, cardiovascular and hypokalaemic effects of fenoterol, salbutamol, and terbutaline in asthma. *Lancet* 1990; 336:1396–1399.

176. Ellul-Micallef R, Fenech FF. Effect of intravenous prednisolone in asthmatics with diminished adrenergic responsiveness. *Lancet* 1975; 2:1269–1270.

177. Beck R, Robertson C, Galdés-Sebaldt M, Levison H. Combined salbutamol and ipratropium bromide by inhalation in the treatment of severe acute asthma. *J Pediatr* 1985; 107:605–608.

178. Reisman J, Galdés-Sebaldt M, Kazim F, Canny G, Levison H. Frequent administration by inhalation of salbutamol and ipratropium bromide in the initial management of severe acute asthma in children. *J Allergy Clin Immunol* 1988; 81:16–20.

179. Watson WTA, Becker AB, Simoins FER. Comparison of ipratropium solution, fenoterol solution and their combination administered by nebulizer and face mask to children with acute asthma. *J Allergy Clin Immunol* 1988; 82:1012–1018.
180. Storr J, Lenney W: Nebulized ipratropium and salbutamol in asthma. *Arch Dis Child* 1986; 61:602–603.
181. Rayner RJ, Cartlidge PHJ, Upton CT. Salbutamol and ipratropium in acute asthma. *Arch Dis Child* 1987; 62:840–841.
182. Mann NP, Hiller EJ: Ipratropium bromide in children with asthma. *Thorax* 1982; 37:72–74.
183. Freeman J, Landau LI: The effects of ipratropium bromide and fenoterol nebulizer solutions in children with asthma. *Clin Pediatr* 1989; 28:556–560.
184. Raes M, Mulder P, Kerrebijn KF. Long-term effect of ipratropium bromide and fenoterol on bronchial responsiveness to histamine in children with asthma. *J Allergy Clin Immunol* 1989; 84:874–879.
185. Rebuck AS, Marcus HI: SCH 1000 in psychogenic asthma. *Scand J Resp Dis* 1979; 103(Suppl):186–191.
186. Rafferty P, Beasley R, Holgate ST. Comparison of the efficacy of preservative free ipratropium bromide and Atrovent nebulizer solution. *Thorax* 1988; 43:446–450.
187. Rooklin A. Theophylline: Is it obsolete for asthma? *J Pediatr* 1989; 115:841–845.
188. Marks MB. Theophylline: Primary or tertiary drug? A brief review. *Ann Allergy* 1987: 59:85–87.
189. Newhouse MT. Is theophylline obsolete? *Chest* 1990; 98:1–3.
190. Jenne JW. Theophylline is no more obsolete than "two puffs qid" of current beta-2 agonists. *Chest* 1990; 98:3–4.
191. Dutoit JI, Salone CM, Woolcock AJ. Inhaled corticosteroids reduce the severity of bronchial hyperresponsiveness in asthma but oral theophylline does not. *Am Rev Respir Dis* 1987; 136:1174–1178.
192. Pauwels RA. New aspects of the therapeutic potential of theophylline in asthma. *J Allergy Clin Immunol* 1989; 83:548–553.
193. Sessler CN. Theophylline toxicity: clinical features of 116 consecutive cases. *Am J Med* 1990; 88:567–576.
194. Schlieper A, Alcock D, Beaudry P, Feldman W, Leikin L. Effect of therapeutic plasma concentrations of theophylline on behavior, cognitive processing, and affect in children with asthma. *J Pediatr* 1991; 118:449–455.
195. Barnes PJ, Greening AP, Neville L, Timmers J, Poole GW. Single–dose slow-release aminophylline at night prevents nocturnal asthma. *Lancet* 1982; 1:299–301.
196. Weinberger MM. Theophylline. *Immunol Allergy Clin North Am* 1990; 10:559–576.
197. Altounyan REC. Review of clinical activity and mode of action of sodium cromoglycate. *Clin Allergy* 1980; 10(Suppl):481–489.
198. Cockcroft DW, Murdock KY. Comparative effects of inhaled salbutamol, sodium cromoglycate, and beclomethasone dipropionate on allergen–induced early asthmatic responses, late asthmatic responses and increased bronchial responsiveness to histamine. *J Allergy Clin Immunol* 1987; 79:734–740.
199. Corkey C, Mindorff C, Levison H, Newth C. Comparison of three different preparations of disodium cromoglycate in the prevention of exercise-induced bronchospasm. *Am Rev Respir Dis* 1982; 125:623–626.
200. Woenne R, Kattan M, Levison H. Sodium cromoglycate-induced changes in the dose–response curve of inhaled methacholine and histamine in bronchial asthma. *Am Rev Respir Dis* 1979; 119:927–932.
201. Molema J, van Herwaarden CLA, Folgering HThM. Effects of long-term treatment with inhaled cromoglycate and budesonide on bronchial hyperresponsiveness in patients with allergic asthma. *Eur Respir J* 1989; 2:308–316.
202. Jenkins CJ, Breslin ABX. Long–term study of the effect of sodium cromoglycate on non–specific bronchial hyperresponsiveness. *Thorax* 1987; 42:664–669.
203. Svendsen UG, Frolung L, Madson F, et al. A comparison of the effects of sodium cromoglycate and beclomethasone dipropionate on pulmonary function and bronchial hyperreactivity in subjects with asthma. *J Allergy Clin Immunol* 1987; 80:68–74.
204. Furukawa CT, Shapiro GG, Bierman CW, et al. A double-blind study comparing the effectiveness of cromolyn sodium and sustained-release theophylline in childhood asthma. *Pediatrics* 1984; 74:453–459.
205. Godfrey S, Balfour-Lynn L, Konig P. The place of cromolyn sodium in the long–term management of childhood asthma based on a 3–5 year follow-up. *J Pediatr* 1974; 87:465–473.
206. Eigen H, Reid JJ, Dahl R, et al. Evaluation of the addition of cromolyn sodium to bronchodilator maintenance therapy in the long-term management of asthma. *J Allergy Clin Immunol* 1987; 80:612–621.
207. Francis RS, McEnery G. Disodium cromoglycate compared with beclomethasone dipropionate in juvenile asthma. *Clin Allergy* 1984; 14:537–540.
208. Hiller EJ, Mann AD. Betamethasone 17 valerate aerosol and disodium cromoglycate in severe asthma. *Br J Dis Chest* 1975; 69:103–106.
209. Grant SM, Goa KL, Fitton A, Sorkin EM. Ketotifen: A review of its pharmacodynamic and pharmacokinetic properties and therapeutic use in asthma and allergic disorders. *Drugs* 1990; 40:412–448.
210. Neijens HJ, Knol R. Oral prophylactic therapy in wheezy infants. *Immunol Allergy Pract* 1988; 10:17–23.
211. Reid JJ. Double-blind trial of ketotifen in childhood chronic cough and wheeze. *Immunol Allergy Pract* 1989; 1:143–150.
212. Rackham A, Brown CA, Chandra RK, et al. A Canadian multicenter study with Zaditen (Ketotifen) in the treatment of bronchial asthma in children age 5–17 years. *J Allergy Clin Immunol* 1989; 84:286–296.
213. Graff-Lonnevig V, Kusoffsky E. Comparison of the clinical effect of ketotifen and DSCG in pollen-induced childhood asthma. *Allergy* 1980; 35:341–348.
214. Graff-Lonnevig V, Hedlin G. The effect of ketotifen on bronchial hyperreactivity in childhood asthma. *J Allergy Clin Immunol* 1985; 76:59–63.
215. Girard JP. Ketotifen and bronchial hyperreactivity in asthmatic patients. *Clin Allergy* 1981; 11:449–452.

216. Kennedy JD, Hasham F, Clay MJD, Jones RS. Comparison of action of disodium cromoglycate and ketotifen on exercise-induced bronchoconstriction in childhood asthma. *Br Med J* 1980; 281:1458.

217. Loftus BG, Price JF. Long-term, placebo-controlled trial of ketotifen in the management of preschool children with asthma. *J Allergy Clin Immunol* 1987; 79:350–355.

218. Dawson KP, Fergusson DM, Horwood LJ, Mogridge N. Ketotifen in asthma. *Aust Pediatr J* 1989; 25:89–92.

219. Maclay WP, Crowder D, Spiro S, Turner P. Post-marketing surveillance: Practical experience with ketotifen. *Br Med J* 1984; 288:911–914.

220. Thomson NC. Nedocromil sodium: An overview. *Respir Med* 1989; 83:269–276.

221. Geddes DM, Turner-Warwick M, Brewis RAL, Davies RJ. Nedocromil sodium workshop. *Respir Med* 1989; 83:265–267.

222. Dorward AJ, Roberts AJ, Thomson NC. Effect of nedocromil sodium on histamine airway responsiveness in grass-pollen sensitive asthmatics during the pollen season. *Clin Allergy* 1986; 16:309–315.

223. Rebuck AS, Kesten S, Boulet LP, et al. A 3-month evaluation of the efficacy of nedocromil sodium: A randomized, double-blind placebo–controlled trial of nedocromil sodium conducted by a Canadian multicenter study group. *J Allergy Clin Immunol* 1990; 85:612–617.

224. Bone MF, Kubik MM, Keaney NP, et al. Nedocromil sodium in adults with asthma dependent on inhaled corticosteroids: A double blind, placebo controlled study. *Thorax* 1989; 44:654–659.

225. Boulet L-P, Cartier A, Cockcroft DW, Gruber JM, Laberge F, et al. Tolerance to reduction of oral steroid dosage in severely asthmatic patients receiving nedocromil sodium. *Respir Med* 1990; 84:317–323.

226. Goldin JG, Bateman ED. Does nedocromil sodium have a steroid sparing effect in adult asthmatic patients requiring maintenance oral corticosteroids? *Thorax* 1988; 43:982–986.

227. Konig P. Inhaled corticosteroids—Their present and future role in the management of asthma. *J Allergy Clin Immunol* 1988; 82:297–306.

228. Lundgren R, Soderberg M, Horstedt P, Stenling R. Morphological studies of bronchial mucosal biopsies from asthmatics before and after ten years treatment with inhaled steroids. *Eur Respir J* 1988; 1:883–889.

229. Kraan J, Koeter GH, Van der Mark ThW, et al. Dosage and time effect of inhaled budesonide on bronchial hyperreactivity. *Am Rev Respir Dis* 1988; 137:44–48.

230. Juniper EF, Kline PA, Vanzieleghem MA, et al. Effect of long–term treatment with an inhaled corticosteroid (budesonide) on airway hyperresponsiveness and clinical asthma in nonsteroid–dependent asthmatics. *Am Rev Respir Dis* 1990; 142:832–836.

231. Juniper EF, Kline PA, Vanzieleghem MA, Hargreave FE. Reduction of budesonide after a year of increased use: A randomized controlled trial to evaluate whether improvements of airway responsiveness and clinical asthma are maintained. *J Allergy Clin Immunol* 1991; 87:483–489.

232. Vathenen AS, Knox AJ, Wisniewski A, Tattersfield AE. Time course of change in bronchial reactivity with an inhaled corticosteroid in asthma. *Am Rev Respir Dis* 1991; 143:1317–1321.

233. Konig P, Jaffe P, Godfrey S. Effects of corticosteroids on exercise–induced asthma. *J Allergy Clin Immunol* 1974; 54:14–19.

234. Henriksen JM, Dahl R. Effects of inhaled budesonide alone and in combination with low-dose terbutaline in children with exercise –induced asthma. *Am Rev Respir Dis* 1983; 128:993–997.

235. Smith MJ, Hodson ME. High-dose beclomethasone inhaler in the treatment of asthma. *Lancet* 1983; 1:265–269.

236. Springer C, Avital A, Maayan CH, Rosler A, Godfrey S. Comparison of budesonide and beclomethasone dipropionate for treatment of asthma. *Arch Dis Child* 1987; 62:815–819.

237. Goldstein D, Konig P. Effect of inhaled beclomethasone diproprionate on hypothalamo-pituitary–adrenal axis function in children with asthma. *Pediatrics* 1983; 72:60–64.

238. Tabachnik E, Zadik Z. Diurnal cortisol secretion during therapy with inhaled beclomethasone diprorionate in children with asthma. *J Pediatr* 1991; 118:294–297.

239. Priftis K, Milner AD, Conway E, Honour JW. Adrenal function in asthma. *Arch Dis Child* 1990; 65:838–840.

240. Balfour-Lynn L. Growth and childhood asthma. *Arch Dis Child* 1986; 61:1049–1055.

241. Littlewood JM, Johnson AW, Edwards PA, Littlewood AE. Growth retardation in asthmatic children treated with inhaled beclomethasone dipropionate [Letter]. *Lancet* 1988; 1:115–116.

242. Godfrey S, Balfour-Lynn L, Tooley M. A three- to five-year follow-up of the use of the aerosol steroid, beclomethasone dipropionate, in childhood asthma. *J Allergy Clin Immunol* 1978; 62:335–359.

243. Brown PH, Blundell G, Greening AP, Crompton GK. Do large volume spacer devices reduce the systemic effects of high dose inhaled corticosteroids? *Thorax* 1990; 45:736–739.

244. Toogood JH, Baskerville J, Jennings B, et al. Use of spacers to facilitate inhaled corticosteroid treatment of asthma. *Am Rev Respir Dis* 1984; 129:723–729.

245. Capewell S, Reynolds S, Shuttleworth D, Edwards C, Finlay AY. Purpura and dermal thinning associated with high dose inhaled corticosteroids. *Br Med J* 1990; 300:1548–1551.

246. Karim AKA, Thomson GM, Jacob TJL. Steroid aerosols and cataract formation. *Br Med J* 1989; 299:918.

247. Ali NJ, Capewell S, Ward MJ. Bone turnover during high dose inhaled corticosteroid therapy. *Thorax* 1991; 46:160–164.

248. Shaw NJ, Edmunds AT. Inhaled beclomethasone and oral candidiasis. *Arch Dis Child* 1986; 61:788–790.

249. Williams AJ, Baghat MS, Stableforth DE, et al. Dysphonia caused by inhaled steroids: Recognition of a characteristic laryngeal abnormality. *Thorax* 1983; 38:813–821.

250. Nassif E, Weinberger M, Sherman B, Brown K. Extrapulmonary effects of maintenance corticosteroid therapy with alternate-day prednisone and

inhaled beclomethasone in children with chronic asthma. *J Allergy Clin Immunol* 1987; 80:518–529.

251. Harris J, Weinberger M, Nasif E, et al. Early intervention with short courses of prednisone to prevent progression of asthma in ambulatory patients incompletely responsive to bronchodilators. *J Pediatr* 1987; 110:627–633.

252. Brunette MG, Lands L, Thibodeau L-P. Childhood asthma: Prevention of attacks with short-term corticosteroid treatment of upper respiratory tract infection. *Pediatrics* 1988; 81:624–629.

253. Deshpande A, McKenzie SA. Short course of steroids in home treatment of children with acute asthma. *Br Med J* 1986; 293:169–171.

254. Zora JA, Zimmerman D, Carey FL, et al. Hypothalamic-pituitary adrenal axis suppression after short-term, high-dose glucocorticoid therapy in children with asthma. *J Allergy Clin Immunol* 1986; 77:9–13.

255. Dolan LM, Kesarwala HH, Holroyde JC, et al. Short-term high-dose systemic steroids in children with asthma: The effect on the hypothalamic-pituitary-adrenal axis. *J Allergy Clin Immunol* 1987; 80:81–86.

256. Canny GJ, Levison H. Aerosols—Therapeutic use and delivery in childhood asthma. *Ann Allergy* 1988; 60:11–20.

257. O'Callaghan C, Milner AD, Swarbrick A. Spacer device with face mask attachment for giving bronchodilators to infants with asthma. *Br Med J* 1989; 298:160–161.

258. Newman SP, Millar AB, Lennard-Jones TR, Moran F, Clarke SW. Improvement of pressurized aerosol deposition with nebuhaler spacer device. *Thorax* 1984; 39:935–941.

259. Gleeson GJA, Green S, Price JF. Nebuhaler technique. *Br J Dis Chest* 1988; 82:172–174.

260. Clark AR, Rachelefsky G, Mason PL, Goldenhersh MJ. The use of reservoir devices for the simultaneous delivery of two metered-dose aerosols. *J Allergy Clin Immunol* 1990; 85:75–79.

261. Pederson S. How to use a Rotahaler. *Arch Dis Child* 1986; 61:11–14.

262. Editorial. The nebulizer epidemic. *Lancet* 1984; 2:789–790.

263. Bendefy IM. Home nebulizers in childhood asthma: Survey of hospital supervised use. *Br Med J* 1991; 302:1180–1181.

264. Zimmerman B, Stringer D, Feanny S, et al. Prevalence of abnormalities found by sinus x-rays in childhood asthma: Lack of relation to severity of asthma. *J Allergy Clin Immunol* 1987; 80:268–273.

265. Ball BO, Hill MR, Brenner M, Sanks A, Szefler SJ. Effect of low dose troleandomycin in glucocorticoid pharmacokinetics and airway hyperresponsiveness in severely asthmatic children. *Ann Allergy* 1990; 65:37–45.

266. Mullarkey MF, Lammert JK, Blumenstein BA. Long –term methotrexate treatment in corticosteroid-dependent asthma. *Ann Intern Med* 1990; 112:577–581.

267. Bernstein DI, Bernstein IL, Bodenheimer SS, Pietrusko RG. An open study of auroanofin in the treatment of steroid-dependent asthma. *J Allergy Clin Immunol* 1988; 81:6–16.

268. Muller NL, Bryan AC. Chest wall mechanics and respiratory muscles in infants. *Pediatr Clin North Am* 1979; 26:503–516.

269. Lucas A, Brooke OG, Cole TJ, Morley R, Bamford MF. Food and drug reactions, wheezing, and eczema in preterm infants. *Arch Dis Child* 1990; 65:411–415.

270. Milner AD. Lung function testing in infancy. *Arch Dis Child* 1990; 65:548–552.

271. O'Callaghan C, Milner AD, Swarbrick A. Spacer device with face mask attachment for giving bronchodilators to infants with asthma. *Br Med J* 1989; 198:160–161.

272. Silverman M. Bronchodilators for wheezy infants? *Arch Dis Child* 1984; 59:84–87.

273. Bentur L, Kerem E, Canny G, et al. Response of acute asthma to a beta-2 agonist in children less than two years of age. *Ann Allergy* 1990; 65:122–126.

274. Bentur L, Canny GJ, Shields MD, et al. A controlled trial of nebulized albuterol in children under the age of 2 years with acute asthma. *Pediatrics* 1992; 89:133–137.

275. Hodges IGC, Groggins RC, Milner AD, et al. Bronchodilator effect of inhaled ipratropium bromide in wheezy toddlers. *Arch Dis Child* 1981; 56:729–732.

276. Cogswell JJ, Simpkiss MJ. Nebulised sodium cromoglycate in recurrently wheezy preschool children. *Arch Dis Child* 1985; 60:736–738.

277. Newth CJ, Newth CV, Turner JAP. Comparison of nebulized sodium cromoglycate and oral theophylline in controlling symptoms of chronic asthma in preschool children—A double blind study. *Aust N Z Med* 1982; 12:232–238.

278. Loftus BG, Price JF. Treatment of asthma in preschool children with slow release theophylline. *Arch Dis Child* 1985; 60:770–772.

279. Storr J, Lenney CA, Lenney W. Nebulized beclomethasone diproprionate in preschool asthma. *Arch Dis Child* 1986; 61:270–273.

280. Webb MSC, Milner AD, Hiller EJ, Henry RL. Nebulized beclomethasone diproprionate suspension. *Arch Dis Child* 1986; 61:1108–1110.

281. Carlsen KH, Leegaard J, Larsen S, Orstravik I. Nebulized beclomethasone diproprionate in recurrent obstructive episodes after acute bronchiolitis. *Arch Dis Child* 1988; 63:1428–1433.

282. Gleeson JGA, Price JF. Controlled trial of budesonide given by the Nebuhaler in preschool children with asthma. *Br Med J* 1988; 297:163–166.

283. Freigang B. Adrenal cortical function after long-term beclomethasone aerosol therapy in early childhood. *Ann Allergy* 1990; 64:342–344.

284. Bisgaard H, Munck SL, Nielsen JP, Petersen W, Ohlsson SO. Inhaled budesonide for treatment of recurrent wheezing in early childhood. *Lancet* 1990; 336:649–651.

285. Varsano I, Volovitz B, Malik H, Amir Y. Safety of 1 year of treatment with budesonide in young children with asthma. *J Allergy Clin Immunol* 1990; 85:914–920.

286. Webb MSC, Henry RL, Milner AD. Oral corticosteroids for wheezing attacks under 18 months. *Arch Dis Child* 1986; 61:15–19.

287. de Benedictis, FM, Canny GJ, Levison H. The progressive nature of childhood asthma. *Lung* 1990; 168(Suppl):278–285.

288. Apter AJ, Greenberger PA, Patterson R. Outcomes of pregnancy in adolescents with severe asthma. *Arch Intern Med* 1989; 149:2571–2575.

289. Editorial: Cough and wheeze in asthma: Are they independent? *Lancet* 1988; 1:447–448.

290. Pierson WE. Exercise-induced bronchospasm in children and adolescents. *Pediatr Clin North Am* 1988; 35:1031–1040.

291. Rubinstein I, Levison H, Slutsky AS, et al. Immediate and delayed bronchoconstriction after exercise in patients with asthma. *N Engl J Med* 1987; 317:482–485.

292. Orenstein DM, Reed ME, Grogan FT, Crawford LV. Exercise conditioning in children with asthma. *J Pediatr* 1985; 106:556–560.

293. Cochrane LM, Clark CJ. Benefits and problems of a physical training programme for asthmatic patients. *Thorax* 1990; 45:345–351.

294. Editorial. Exercise and the asthmatic child. *Pediatrics* 1989; 84:392–393.

295. Francis PWJ, Krastins IRB, Levison H. Oral and inhaled salbutamol in the prevention of exercise induced asthma. *Pediatrics* 1980; 66:103–108.

296. Pollock J, Kiechel F, Cooper D, Weinberger M. Relationship of serum theophylline concentration to inhibition of exercised-induced bronchospasm and comparison with cromolyn. *Pediatrics* 1977; 60:840–844.

297. Martin RJ, Circutto LC, Smith HR, Ballard RD, Szefler SJ. Airways inflammation in nocturnal asthma. *Am Rev Respir Dis* 1991; 143:351–357.

298. Horn CR, Clark TJH, Cochrane GM. Inhaled therapy reduces morning dips in asthma. *Lancet* 1984; 1:1143–1145.

299. Arkinstall WW. Review of the North American experience with evening administration of Uniphyl tablets, a once-daily theophylline preparation, in the treatment of nocturnal asthma. *Am J Med* 1988; 85(Suppl)18:60–63.

300. Dahl R, Pedersen B, Hagglof B. Nocturnal asthma: Effects of treatment with oral sustained–release terbutaline, inhaled budesonide and the two in combination. *J Allergy Clin Immunol* 1989; 73:811–815.

301. Marsen FPV, Smeets JJ, Gubbelmans HLL, Zweers PG. Formoterol in the treatment of nocturnal asthma. *Chest* 1990; 98:866–870.

302. Orenstein SR, Orenstein DM. Gastroesophageal reflux and respiratory disease in children. *J Pediatr* 1988; 112:847–858.

303. Barnes PJ, Chung KF. Difficult asthma: Cause for concern. *Br Med J* 1989; 299:695–698.

304. Akhter J, Gasper MM, Newcomb RW. Persistent peripheral airway obstruction in children with severe asthma. *Ann Allergy* 1989; 63:53–58.

305. Canny GJ, Levison H. Pulmonary function abnormalities during apparent clinical remission in childhood asthma. *J Allergy Clin Immunol* 1988; 82:1–4.

306. Stein R, Canny GJ, Bohn DJ, Reisman JJ, Levison H. Severe acute asthma in a pediatric intensive care unit: six years' experience. *Pediatrics* 1989; 83:1023–1028.

307. Richards W. Hospitalization of children with status asthmaticus: a review. *Pediatrics* 1989; 84:111–118.

308. Weng TR, Langer HM, Featherby EA, Levison H. Arterial blood gas tensions and acid base balance in symptomatic and asymptomatic asthma in childhood. *Am Rev Respir Dis* 1970; 101:274–282.

309. Kerem E, Canny G, Tibshirani R, et al. Clinical-physiological correlations in acute asthma of childhood. *Pediatrics* 1991; 87:481–486.

310. Mountain RD, Heffner JE, Brackett NC, Sahn SA. Acid-base disturbances in acute asthma. *Chest* 1990; 98:651–655.

311. Kerem E, Tibshirani R, Canny G, et al: Predicting the need for hospitalization in children with acute asthma. *Chest* 1990; 98:1355–1366.

312. Rebuck AS, Tamarken JL. Pulsus paradoxus in asthmatic children. *Can Med Assoc J* 1975; 112:710–711.

313. Geelhoed GC, Landau LI, LeSouef PN. Predictive value of oxygen saturation in emergency evaluation of asthmatic children. *Br Med J* 1988; 297:395–396.

314. Jubran A, Tobin MJ. Reliability of pulse oximetry in titrating supplemental oxygen therapy in ventilator-dependent patients. *Chest* 1990; 97:1420–1425.

315. Seidenberg J, Mir Y, van der Hardt H. Hypoxaemia after nebulized salbutamol in wheezy infants: The importance of aerosol acidity. *Arch Dis Child* 1991; 66:672–675.

316. Potler PC, Klein M, Weinberg EG. Hydration in severe acute asthma. *Arch Dis Child* 1991; 66:216–219.

317. Stalcup SA, Mellins RB. Mechanical forces producing pulmonary edema in acute asthma. *N Engl J Med* 1977; 297:592–596.

318. Robertson CF, Smith F, Beck R, Levison H: Response to frequent low doses of nebulized salbutamol in acute asthma. *J Pediatr* 1985; 106:672–674.

319. Schuh S, Parkin P, Rajan A, et al. High– versus low–dose, frequently administered, nebulized albuterol in children with severe, acute asthma. *Pediatrics* 1989; 83:513–518.

320. Schuh S, Reider MJ, Canny G, et al. Nebulized albuterol in acute childhood asthma: Comparison of two doses. *Pediatrics* 1990; 86:509–513.

321. Noseda A, Yernault JC. Sympathomimetics in acute severe asthma: inhaled or parenteral, nebulized or spacer? *Eur Respir J* 1989; 2:377–382.

322. Davis A, Vickerson F, Worsley G, Mindorff C, Kazim F, Levison H. Clinical and laboratory observations: Determination of the dose-response relationship for nebulized ipratropium in asthmatic children *J Pediatr* 1984; 105:1002–1005.

323. Weinberger M. Corticosteroids for exacerbations of asthma: Current status of the controversy. *Pediatrics* 1988; 81:726–729.

324. Wilson NM, Silverman M. Treatment of acute, episodic asthma in preschool children using intermittent high dose inhaled steroids at home. *Arch Dis Child* 1990; 65:407–410.

325. Littenberg B. Aminophylline treatment in severe, acute asthma. *JAMA* 1988; 259:1678–1684.

326. Pierson WE, Bierman CW, Stamm SI, et al. Double-blind trial of aminophylline in status asthmaticus. *Pediatrics* 1971; 48:642–646.

327. Goldberg P, Leffert F, Gonzalez M, Gogenola L, Zerbe GO. Intravenous aminophylline therapy for asthma: A comparison of two methods of administration in children. *Am J Dis Child* 1980; 134:596–599.

328. Sakamoto Y, Kabe J, Horai Y. Effect of theophylline on improvement of the pulmonary function in the

treatment of acute episodes of asthma: The influence of the severity of acute asthma. *Ann Allergy* 1989; 63:21–27.

329. Willert C, Davis AT, Herman JJ, Holson BB, Zieserl E. Short-term holding room treatment of asthmatic children. *J Pediatr* 1985; 106:707–711.

330. Geelhoed GC, Landau LI, LeSouef PN. Oximetry and peak expiratory flow in assessment of acute childhood asthma. *J Pediatr* 1990; 117:907–909.

331. Molfino NA, Nannini LJ, Martelli AN, Slutsky AS. Respiratory arrest in near-fatal asthma. *N Engl J Med* 1991; 324:285–288.

332. Canny GJ, Bohn D, Levison H. Sympathomimetics in acute asthma—Inhaled or parenteral? *Am J Asthma Allergy Pediatr* 1989; 2:165–170.

333. Menitove SM, Goldring RM. Combined ventilator and bicarbonate strategy in the management of status asthmaticus. *Am J Med* 1983; 74:898–901.

334. Bohn DJ, Kalloghlian A, Jenkins J, Edmonds J, Barker GA. Intravenous salbutamol in the treatment of status asthmaticus in children. *Crit Care Med* 1984; 12:892–896.

335. Darioli R, Perret C. Mechanical controlled hypoventilation in status asthmaticus. *Am Rev Respir Dis* 1984; 129:385–387.

336. Seddon PC, Heaf DP. Long term outcome of ventilated asthmatics. *Arch Dis Child* 1990; 65:1324–1328.

337. Fletcher HJ, Ibrahim SA, Speight N. Survey of asthma deaths in the Northern region, 1970–85. *Arch Dis Child* 1990; 65:163–167.

338. McNicol KN, Williams HB. Spectrum of asthma in children. I. Clinical and physiological components. *Br Med J* 1973; 4:7–11.

339. Martin AJ, McLennan LA, Landau LI, Phelan PD. The natural history of childhood asthma to adult life. *Br Med J* 1980; 280:1397–1400.

340. Kelly WJW, Hudson I, Phelan PD, Pain MC, Olinsky A. Childhood asthma in adult life: A further study at 28 years of age. *Br Med J* 1987; 94:1059–1062.

341. Kelly WJW, Hudson I, Phelan PD, Pain MCF, Olinksy A. Childhood asthma and adult lung function. *Am Rev Respir Dis* 1988; 138:26–30.

342. Phelan PD. Hyperresponsiveness as a determinant of the outcome in childhood asthma. *Am Rev Respir Dis* 1991; 143:1463–1467.

343. Gerritsen J, Koeter GH, Postma DS, et al. Airway responsiveness in childhood as a predictor of the outcome of asthma in adulthood. *Am Rev Respir Dis* 1991; 143:468–469.

344. Strachan DP. Do chesty children become chesty adults? *Arch Dis Child* 1990; 65:161–162.

22

Cystic Fibrosis

BERYL J. ROSENSTEIN

Cystic fibrosis (CF) is the most common lethal or semi-lethal genetic disease affecting Caucasians (1). The triad of chronic obstructive pulmonary disease, pancreatic exocrine deficiency, and abnormally high sweat electrolyte concentration is present in most patients. It is the major cause of chronic debilitating pulmonary disease and pancreatic exocrine deficiency during the first three decades of life and accounts for a significant number of cases of neonatal intestinal obstruction. The name of the disease is derived from the characteristic histologic changes seen in the pancreas (2).

GENETICS

General

Estimates of the incidence of CF vary according to the population studied, but a reasonable figure for Caucasians is 1:2500 (1). The highest incidence is seen in persons of Anglo-Saxon ancestry. The incidence of CF in Afro-Americans is 1:17,000 (3). The CF gene is rare in African blacks and Asians (1). The disease is transmitted in an autosomal recessive manner. Based on incidence figures, it is estimated that 4% of Caucasians in the United States are carriers (heterozygotes) of the CF gene. A heterozygote advantage has been postulated but never documented (4). Heterozygotes have no recognizable clinical symptoms, although an increased incidence of airway reactivity has been reported in CF carriers, suggesting a subtle abnormality of autonomic function (5).

Gene Defect

The gene responsible for CF has been localized to 250,000 base pairs of genomic DNA located on the long arm of chromosome 7

(6–8). The gene encodes a protein of 1480 amino acids called the *cystic fibrosis transmembrane conductance regulator (CFTR)*. A three-base deletion removing a phenylalanine residue at position 508 of CFTR (F508 mutation) is present on approximately 70% of CF chromosomes (9). The remaining cases are accounted for by more than 300 different mutations, none of which accounts for more than 4% of cases (9). The ability to detect CF mutations by direct DNA analysis represents a major improvement in prenatal diagnosis and heterozygote detection, even in families wherein DNA is not available from an affected child. Unfortunately, the large number of mutations described in patients with CF limits the usefulness of DNA analysis as a screening test for CF (10). There is a correlation between genotype and pancreatic status (11), but there is no correlation between specific mutations and pulmonary phenotype (12).

PATHOPHYSIOLOGY

Initially CF was thought to involve the pancreas primarily, but it was soon realized that many of the clinical and pathologic findings might be explained by a generalized defect in mucous secretion (13). With the discovery of the sweat gland defect (14), it became apparent that there are abnormalities in all the exocrine glands. Most of the clinical manifestations can be related to the abnormal secretions that result in obstruction of organ passages, and abnormal function of the eccrine sweat glands (15). Involved glands are affected in varying distribution and degree of severity and fall into three types: (a) those which become obstructed by viscid or solid eosinophilic material in the lumen (pancreas, intestinal glands, intrahepatic bile ducts, gallbladder, submaxillary glands); (b) those which produce an excess of histologically normal secretions (tracheobronchial and Brunner glands); and (c) those which are histologically normal but secrete excessive electrolyte (sweat, parotid, and small salivary glands). The high concentration of electrolytes in the sweat is due to decreased transductal reabsorption of chloride and sodium (16).

Ion Transport Abnormality

The CFTR protein contains two nucleotide binding folds with adenosine triphosphate (ATP)-binding sites, a regulatory region that has many phosphorylation sites, and two hydrophobic regions that probably interact with cell membranes (17). It appears to be related to a family of membrane-bound glycoproteins involved in the transport of small molecules across cell membranes; there is evidence that CFTR itself is a cyclic adenosine monophosphate (cAMP)-activated chloride channel (18). Functional expression of the CF defect reduces the ability of epithelial cells in the airways and pancreas to secrete chloride in response to cAMP-mediated agonists (19). Enhanced absorption of sodium across the airway epithelium (20) and failure to secrete chloride (and thereby fluid) toward the airway lumen is thought to lead to dehydration of airway mucus and the abnormal mucociliary clearance and lung disease seen in patients with CF.

Pulmonary Manifestations

The respiratory tract is invariably involved, and pulmonary complications usually dominate the clinical picture (21). However, manifestations may not appear until weeks, months, or even years after birth (22). Autopsy studies suggest that the lungs are normal at birth. The initial pulmonary lesion is obstruction of the small airways by abnormally thick mucus secretions. Secondary to obstruction, there is bronchiolitis and mucopurulent plugging of the airways. Bronchial changes are more common than parenchymal changes (23). Bronchiectasis is present in almost all patients past the age of 18 months (23). It is progressive with age and is especially striking in older patients. Emphysema is not a common feature. A proposed mechanism for the pulmonary manifestations seen in patients with CF is shown in

Figure 22.1. Bacterial infection, first due to *Staphylococcus aureus* and later due to *Pseudomonas aeruginosa*, initiates a vicious cycle of chronic infection, tissue damage, and obstruction (21). With advanced disease, over 80% of patients consistently harbor strains of *P. aeruginosa*, the majority of which are heavy slime producers known as *mucoid variants* (24). These are rarely found in other diseases. The peculiar susceptibility of these patients to infection with mucoid *Pseudomonas* strains may be related to a defect in phagocytosis in the lung. Once established, *Pseudomonas* is virtually impossible to eradicate. Systemic defense mechanisms appear to be intact, and infection tends to remain localized to the respiratory tract. Septicemia and extrapulmonary infections are rare (25). Recently, the incidence of *P. cepacia* colonization among older CF patients has increased (26). Risk factors for colonization include increasing age

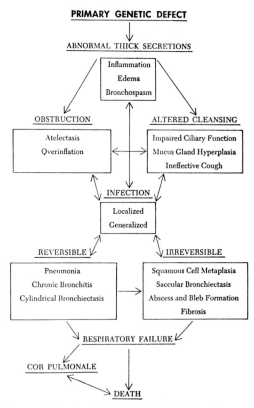

Figure 22.1. Proposed mechanism for the pulmonary manifestations seen in patients with cystic fibrosis. (From *Guide to diagnosis and management of cystic fibrosis.* Bethesda, MD, Cystic Fibrosis Foundation, 1979, p 8. Reproduced with permission.)

and severity of underlying disease, exposure to a sibling colonized with *P. cepacia*, and recent hospitalization (27). Person-to-person transmission has also been documented (28). Acquisition of this organism, especially by females with moderate or advanced pulmonary disease, may be followed by an unexpectedly rapid decline (29). The course of some of these patients is characterized by recurrent episodes of fever and bacteremia. In patients who do not show the expected response to antimicrobial therapy, one needs to consider infection with unusual organisms such as *Mycobacterium tuberculosis* and atypical mycobacteria (30).

There is evidence that immune-mediated inflammation contributes significantly to the lung damage present in patients with CF (31, 32). Recruitment and activation of neutrophils in the airways leads to a high level of elastolytic activity secondary to the release of proteases, such as granulocyte elastase and cathepsin G. This protease burden has been associated with both breakdown of the lung matrix and with cleavage and inactivation of a variety of opsonins, thereby contributing to the persistence of *Pseudomonas* in the lung. There is evidence of immune complex formation in 20–100% of patients with CF, which may also contribute to inflammatory lung damage (33). The presence of immune complexes correlates with disease severity and prognosis (34).

CLINICAL FEATURES

Fifty percent of patients come to diagnosis because of pulmonary manifestations, usually consisting of chronic cough and wheezing in association with recurrent or chronic infections (21). Young infants can present with atelectasis, often involving the right upper lobe, or a severe bronchiolitis syndrome (35). The most prominent and constant feature of pulmonary involvement is chronic cough (Table 22.1). At first the cough may be dry, but with disease progression it becomes paroxysmal and productive. Older patients expectorate mucopurulent sputum, particularly in association with pulmonary exacerbations. Physical findings include inspiratory rales and rhonchi and hyper-resonance to percussion. Wheezing is often a prominent feature, especially in association with pulmonary exacerbations, but it is unclear if this reflects inflammation and bronchial obstruction or coincidental atopy or

bronchial hyper-reactivity. Barrel-chest deformity, use of accessory muscles of respiration, growth retardation, digital clubbing, pulmonary hypertrophic osteoarthropathy, and cyanosis develop in association with disease progression.

The upper respiratory tract is usually affected secondary to hyperactive mucus-secreting glands and hyperplasia and edema of the mucous membranes. Chronic nasal congestion and rhinitis are common. Radiographic evidence of opacification of the paranasal sinuses is present in almost all patients and may be helpful diagnostically in patients with equivocal sweat test results (36). Clinically significant sinusitis is common and troublesome in some patients. Chronic sinusitis may contribute to infection of the lower respiratory tract (37). Computed tomography (CT) scans of the sinuses are useful in assessing the extent of sinus involvement and in the selection of patients who might benefit from a surgical procedure. Slowly progressive unilateral proptosis may occur secondary to formation of an inflammatory mucocele in the underlying maxillary and ethmoid sinuses (38).

Nasal polyps occur in 6–24% of patients (39) (Fig. 22.2). Clinical manifestations include obstruction to nasal airflow, mouth breathing, localized infection, epistaxis, rhinorrhea, and widening of the nasal bridge. Polyps occur at a much younger age in patients with CF as compared with those with underlying atopy, can be differentiated histologically (40), and tend to recur. The incidence of hearing problems in patients with CF is probably no higher than in the general population (41).

RADIOGRAPHIC CHANGES

The earliest chest radiographic findings include hyperinflation and bronchial wall thickening (43) (Fig. 22.3). Subsequent changes include areas of infiltrate, atelectasis, and hilar adenopathy. With advanced disease, segmental or lobar atelectasis, bleb formation, bronchiectasis, and pulmonary artery and right ventricular enlargement are seen. Branching, finger-like opacifications, representing mucoid impaction of dilated bronchi, are characteristic (43) (Fig. 22.4).

PULMONARY FUNCTION

Airway obstruction, air trapping, and ventilation-perfusion inequalities are the most

Table 22.1.
Summary of Clinical Manifestations

Upper Respiratory Tract	Hepatobiliary	Nutritional/Metabolic
Nasal Polyposis	Cholecystitis	Diabetes
Sinusitis	Cholelithiasis	Hypokalemic alkalosis
	Cholestasis	Hypoprothrombinemia
	Cirrhosis/portal hypertension	Iron deficiency anemia
		Salt depletion syndrome
		Protein-calorie malnutrition
		Vitamin A deficiency
		Vitamin E deficiency

Pulmonary	Gastrointestinal	Miscellaneous
Allergic bronchopulmonary aspergillosis	Gastroesophageal reflux	Arthritis/arthropathy
Atelectasis	Intussusception	Absent vas deferens
Bronchiectasis	Meconium ileus	Aspermia
Bronchiolitis	Meconium ileus equivalent	Decreased female fertility
Bronchitis	Meconium plug syndrome	Delayed puberty
Cor pulmonale	Pancreatic exocrine deficiency	Digital clubbing
Hemoptysis	Pancreatitis	Erythema nodosum
Pneumothorax	Peptic ulcer disease	Failure to thrive
Pneumonia	Rectal prolapse	Growth retardation
Reactive airway disease		Malnutrition
Respiratory failure		

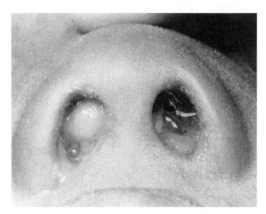

Figure 22.2. Nasal polyp obstructing nasal passage in a 10-year-old boy with cystic fibrosis.

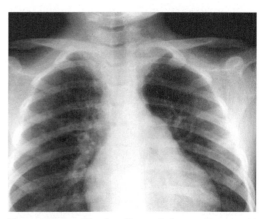

Figure 22.3. Chest radiograph from a 6-year-old patient showing increased lung markings and focal areas of peribronchial thickening.

important functional changes in CF (44). Ventilation-perfusion scans usually demonstrate focal areas of inequality (45). The earliest changes in pulmonary function are air trapping as evidenced by an increased residual volume to total lung capacity (RV/TLC) ratio and decreased expiratory flow rates at low lung volumes—decreased forced expiratory flow 50% (FEF_{50}) vital capacity (VC), FEF_{75} VC, and FEF_{25-75} VC. Forced vital capacity and the ratio of forced expiratory volume in 1 second to forced vital capacity (FEV_1/FVC ratio) decrease with advancing disease. Acute exacer-

bations are marked by a decline in vital capacity and flow rates. Recovery of lung function may be delayed following initiation of treatment of acute exacerbations, with improvement continuing during several weeks of inpatient therapy (46). Older patients with CF often develop a unique pattern of pulmonary function characterized by a mixture of both obstructive and restrictive lung disease (Fig. 22.5). This pattern arises as fibrosis reduces lung volume and counteracts the hyperinflation seen with earlier airway obstruction. Flow

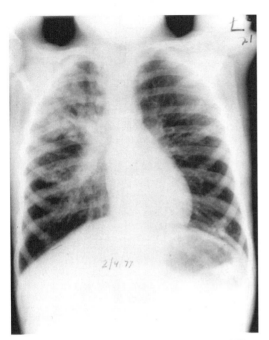

Figure 22.4. Chest radiograph from a 9-year-old boy with severe CF. Note the marked hyperinflation and finger-like mucus impactions of the right upper lobe bronchi.

volume curves demonstrate a characteristic "scooped out" appearance secondary to development of flow limitation at low lung volumes indicative of small airway disease. As disease progresses, the flow volume curve changes into a pattern seen almost exclusively in patients with CF (Fig. 22.6). The initial sharp peak is followed by severe flow limitation. The peak is thought to arise from flow transients from the trachea that empty early and contribute to the preservation of the peak flow rate (47) (Fig. 22.7).

Hypoxia develops as lung destruction occurs. Chronic severe hypoxia is a late occurrence. However, hypoxia is common in patients with advanced disease, especially during sleep (48).

Airway reactivity, based on broncho-provocative challenges, is present in 50% of patients and may be associated with more rapid progression of pulmonary disease (49). The response to bronchodilators is unpredictable and may vary over time and with changes in underlying pulmonary status (50). A paradoxical response to bronchodilators has been reported in patients with CF (51). Most likely, this results from the effects of decreasing

smooth muscle tone in an airway whose integrity has been compromised by airway infection and inflammation. The reduced tone of the airway wall increases the contribution of flow transients to flow rates that reflect large airway function (peak expiratory flow rate [PEFR] and FEV_1) and results in an apparent increase in flow. However, these highly compliant airways may collapse prematurely during forced expiratory maneuvers such as coughing and thus limit flow from the periphery (Fig. 22.7). Cough effectiveness is reduced despite the increased peak flow (52).

COMPLICATIONS

Pneumothorax

In patients with advanced lung disease, pneumothorax is a frequent complication occurring secondary to rupture of apical subpleural blebs. The overall incidence is 2–10%, and in adults may be as high as 16% (53, 54). Patients typically present with an acute onset of chest pain and shortness of breath. Following a pneumothorax on one side, there is a 50% incidence on the contralateral side within 6–12 months.

Hemoptysis

Patients often experience blood streaking of their sputum. This is most likely due to rupture of surface capillaries or small vessels secondary to vigorous coughing. More significant, even massive bleeding is due to erosion of bronchial arteries into a bronchus, often in association with an exacerbation of the underlying pulmonary infection. Massive hemoptysis is a serious complication associated with significant mortality, a high recurrence rate, and a poor prognosis (55). The site of bleeding is best localized by bronchoscopy.

Cor Pulmonale

Cor pulmonale, right ventricular wall hypertrophy with or without chamber enlargement, is seen in 70% of patients dying with CF and occurs in half the patients surviving past age 15 (56). Chronic alveolar hypoxia serves as a stimulus to reflex vasoconstriction and medial hypertrophy of the pulmonary arteries. Severe cor pulmonale has been consistently associated with Pa_{O_2} values of less than 50 mm Hg

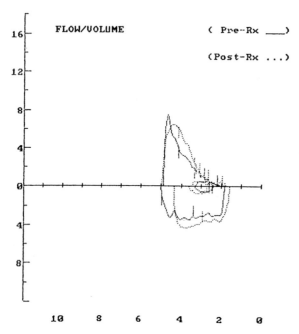

		PRED	PRE-RX BEST	%PRED	POST-RX BEST	%PRED	%CHG
SPIROMETRY	(BTPS)						
FVC	Liters	5.52	3.05 #	55*	3.38 #	61*	11
FEV1	Liters	4.68	2.06 #	44*	2.34 #	50*	14
FEV1/FVC	%	85	68 #	80*	69 #	81*	1
FEF25-75%	L/Sec	5.10	1.19 #	23*	1.31 #	26*	10
FEF25%	L/Sec		3.77		5.98		59
FEF50%	L/Sec		1.89		2.28		21
FEF75%	L/Sec		0.42		0.45		7
PEF	L/Sec		7.43		8.90		20
FIVC	Liters	5.52	3.27 #	59*	3.54 #	64*	8
PIF	L/Sec		4.60		4.28		-7

		PRED	PRE-RX AVG	%PRED	POST-RX AVG	%PRED	%CHG
LUNG VOLUMES	(BTPS)						
Vtg	Liters		2.91		2.88		-1
VC	Liters	5.52	3.47 #	63*	3.61 #	65*	4
TLC	Liters	6.65	5.31	80*	5.20	78*	-2
RV	Liters	1.28	1.84	144*	1.59	125	-14
RV/TLC	%	19	35 #	184	31 #	163	-11
FRC PL	Liters	3.13	2.83	91	2.77	89	-2

Figure 22.5. Spirometry and lung volume data from from a 29-year-old man with CF. Note the mixed picture of lung function—restriction as evidenced by a decreased TLC and FRC and obstruction evidenced by an increased RV/TLC, a decreased FEV$_1$/FVC ratio, and the concave appearence of the flow-volume curve.

(57). Clinically, cor pulmonale may be difficult to recognize. Peripheral edema is often a late manifestation and is present in only two-thirds of cases. Liver tenderness may be an early clue. The electrocardiogram does not consistently correlate with the presence of right ventricular hypertrophy. Echocardiography is probably the most practical and reliable way of documenting cor pulmonale and of following its course (58).

COURSE

The pulmonary course is characterized by chronic suppurative bronchitis with recurrent pulmonary exacerbations, often following viral respiratory infections (59). Infection with respiratory syncytial virus (RSV) may be an important cause of significant respiratory morbidity in young infants (60). By age 10, 90% of patients will have intermittent sputum production; by age 15, 90% of patients will

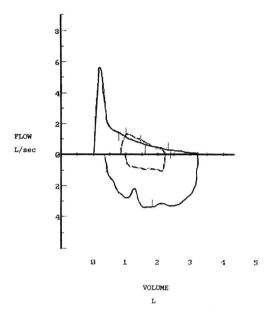

Figure 22.6. Flow-volume loop from a 23-year-old patient showing decreased flow at all lung volumes. There is a marked "scooped-out" appearance indicative of extensive medium and small airways disease. The sharp peak flow most likely results from the presence of flow transients (see Fig. 22.7).

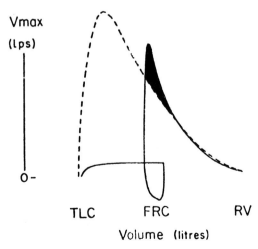

Figure 22.7. Maximal expiratory flow volume curve superimposed on a partial expiratory curve. The shaded area indicates the supramaximal flow transient arising from rapid compression of highly compliant conducting airways. These transients empty early and contribute to the preservation of peak flow seen in CF (see Fig. 22.6).

have daily sputum production. There is progressive shortness of breath and exercise intolerance. Pulmonary involvement advances at a variable rate, usually faster in females than in males (61), but eventually leads to respiratory or cardiac failure, or both.

Gastrointestinal Manifestations

PANCREATIC EXOCRINE DEFICIENCY

The most common gastrointestinal manifestations result from the loss of pancreatic enzyme activity and consequent intestinal malabsorption of fats and proteins and, to a lesser extent, carbohydrates. Complete loss of pancreatic activity is seen in 80–85% of patients (11). Loss of function may be progressive (62). Clinical manifestations include poor or absent weight gain; abdominal distention; lack of subcutaneous fat and muscle tissue; passage of frequent, pale, bulky, foul-smelling and often oily stools; and rectal prolapse. Steatorrhea and azotorrhea are pronounced. Secondary to pancreatic insufficiency, patients have low serum lipid levels and may be deficient in linoleic acid. Although infants may appear to have a voracious appetite, caloric intake is often deficient (63). In older patients there may be absence of a pubertal growth spurt and delayed maturation (64, 65). In general, however, growth retardation correlates more closely with the degree of pulmonary involvement. Adolescents and young adults with residual pancreatic function may have recurrent episodes of pancreatitis, sometimes as the presenting manifestation (66). Patients with residual pancreatic function tend to have lower sweat chloride values, less severe pulmonary involvement, and better survival (67).

Evaluation of Pancreatic Function

Tests of fat absorption, including 72-hour fecal fat excretion, provide indirect assessment of pancreatic exocrine function (68). The most direct measure involves analysis of duodenal fluid before and after the intravenous injection of pancreozymin and secretin (69). In patients with CF, volume and bicarbonate secretion (ductular activity) are grossly reduced, irrespective of the presence of steatorrhea. In those patients with steatorrhea, enzyme secretion (acinar activity) is virtually absent (69). Less invasive means of assessing pancreatic function include (a) measurement of stool trypsin and chymotrypsin (70), (b) measurement of urinary or serum levels of p-aminobenzoic acid after the oral administration of synthetic chymotrypsin substrates containing p-aminobenzoic acid (71), and (c) measurement of serum immunoreactive trypsin (ogen) (IRT) levels (72); with destruction of the pancreas there is progressive decline in IRT levels.

CARBOHYDRATE INTOLERANCE

In addition to pancreatic exocrine dysfunction, up to 40% of patients show carbohydrate intolerance, which progresses to frank diabetes in 2–5% of cases (73, 74). The incidence of carbohydrate intolerance increases with age, but diabetes has been seen as early as 6 months. Diabetes in patients with CF is characterized by insidious onset, mild clinical course, and virtual absence of ketoacidosis (74). Retinopathy, nephropathy, and vascular changes have been seen but are infrequent (75). There is evidence that CF-associated diabetes does not adversely affect the pulmonary course or shorten survival (73). The mild diabetic course in these patients may be due to preservation of some endogenous insulin output (76, 77), decreased glucagon secretion (76, 78), and compensatory enhancement of peripheral tissue sensitivity to insulin (79).

MECONIUM ILEUS

Meconium ileus, in which there is obstruction of the distal ileum by inspissated, tenacious meconium, occurs in 15–20% of newborn infants with CF (80). With rare exception (81), meconium ileus is always associated with CF. It is probably related to in-utero deficiency of proteolytic enzymes along with secretion of abnormal mucoproteins by the goblet cells of the small intestine. Clinically, infants present with evidence of intestinal obstruction (82). Abdominal films show distended bowel loops with a "bubbly" pattern of inspissated meconium in the terminal ileum, and contrast enema shows a microcolon from disuse secondary to intrauterine obstruction. Associated intestinal complications, including small-bowel atresia, volvulus, and perforation/peritonitis are present in 40–50% of cases (83). There is a tendency for meconium ileus to recur in the same family (84). A delay in the passage of meconium and distal colonic

obstruction secondary to the meconium plug syndrome may also be presenting manifestations of CF and are indications for a sweat test (85).

LATE INTESTINAL COMPLICATIONS

As a result of the abnormal behavior of the secretions of the intestinal glands, decreased chloride secretion across the colonic epithelium, deficiency of pancreatic enzymes, and prolonged intestinal transit time, the intestinal contents tend to be abnormally thick and putty-like. This may lead to a variety of late intestinal complications (86). There may be recurrent episodes of partial or complete obstruction of the small or large bowel, often preceded or accompanied by colicky abdominal pain and a palpable firm mass in the right lower quadrant. This symptom complex is referred to as *meconium ileus equivalent* or the *distal intestinal obstruction syndrome*, and occurs in up to 40% of patients (87). These episodes may be precipitated by decreased fluid intake, change in diet, or cessation of pancreatic enzyme supplements, and may be recurrent or associated with chronic symptoms. There may be episodes of small-bowel volvulus or intussusception. This latter complication occurs in 1% of older patients and may be the presenting manifestation (88).

The diagnosis of CF can be suggested by the histology of the appendix; goblet cells are increased in number and distended with mucous, and eosinophilic casts may fill the crypts and extend into the lumen (89). Mucoid impaction of the appendix may present as a right lower quadrant mass in the absence of other symptoms (90). Recurrent episodes of rectal prolapse occur in up to one-quarter of patients, most often between the ages of 1 and 2 years and usually before the diagnosis is established (91). They are probably related to the presence of frequent bulky stools, malnutrition, and raised intra-abdominal pressure secondary to paroxysmal cough. The diagnosis of CF should be considered in every patient with rectal prolapse.

UPPER GASTROINTESTINAL COMPLICATIONS

Patients with CF have an increased incidence of gastro-esophageal reflux, probably related to chest hyper-inflation along with increased

Table 22.2.
Indications for Sweat Testing

Pulmonary/Upper Respiratory	Gastrointestinal	Metabolic/Other
Atelectasis (especially right upper lobe)	Cirrhosis and portal hypertension	Acrodermatitis enteropathica
Bronchiectasis	Intestinal atresia	Aspermia/absent vas deferens
Chronic cough	Meconium ileus	Edema and hypoproteinemia
Digital clubbing	Meconium plug syndrome	Failure to thrive
Hemoptysis	Mucoid-impacted appendix	Hypoprothrombinemia
Mucoid *Pseudomonas* colonization	Prolonged neonatal jaundice	Metabolic alkalosis
Nasal polyps	Recurrent intussusception	Positive family history
Pansinusitis	Recurrent pancreatitis	Salt depletion syndrome
Recurrent/chronic pneumonia	Rectal prolapse	Salty taste/salt crystals
Tachypnea/retractions	Steatorrhea	Vitamin A deficiency (bulging fontanel)
Wheezing and hyper-inflation		

lected, and the electrolyte concentration is measured by accepted techniques (154). An acceptable alternative sweat testing procedure involves the collection of sweat with the MACRODUCT sweat collection system (Wescor—Logan, UT, 84321) and measurement of sweat electrolytes (155). With this system, weighing of samples and the manipulations involved in the elution of sweat from filter paper are avoided. The chloride concentration is usually measured, since it better discriminates between normal individuals and those with CF (156). A chloride concentration > 60 mEq/L is consistent with the diagnosis of CF. The sweat chloride concentration can also be measured by applying a chloride ion electrode directly to the sweating skin. However, this method has been associated with an unacceptably high rate of false-positive and false-negative results and should never be the basis of a definitive diagnosis (157). The sweat electrolyte abnormality is present from birth and persists throughout life. However, a volume of sweat sufficient for analysis may be difficult to obtain in the neonatal period.

It has been shown that patients with CF have an abnormality of transepithelial electrolyte transport manifested by increased sodium absorption across epithelium that is relatively impermeable to chloride (20). Abnormal electrolyte transport has been demonstrated in patients with CF shortly after birth; the measurement of nasal (158) or rectal (159) electrical potential differences may be a diagnostic adjunct to the sweat test in the early diagnosis of CF.

There is no correlation between the magnitude of the sweat gland abnormality and the severity of pulmonary manifestations. However, significantly lower but still abnormal sweat electrolyte concentrations have been reported in those CF patients with pancreatic sufficiency (67). Elevated concentrations of sweat electrolytes have been reported in other conditions (160) (Table 22.3). Most of these disorders can be easily differentiated on the basis of characteristic clinical features. Transient elevation of sweat electrolyte concentrations has been observed in children with evidence of abuse and neglect (161) and in adolescents with anorexia nervosa (162). In patients with a "confirmed" diagnosis of CF who do

Table 22.3.
Causes of a False-Positive Sweat Test

Adrenal insufficiency
Ectodermal dysplasia
Nephrogenic diabetes insipidus
Type I glycogen storage disease
Anorexia nervosa
Hypoparathyroidism
Mauriac syndrome
Familial cholestatic syndromes
Malnutrition
Hypothyroidism
Mucopolysaccharidoses
Fucosidosis

not follow a typical course, it is crucial to repeat the sweat test (163). Normal sweat electrolyte concentrations have been reported in some patients with CF in the presence of edema and hypoproteinemia (110). Values become abnormal with resolution of the edema. Most false-positive and false-negative results are due to technical errors, including inadequate sweat collection, sample contamination, and failure to interpret test results correctly (157). Physiologic variables such as sweating rate, salt intake, and acclimatization may affect the concentration of sweat electrolytes but do not usually interfere with the diagnostic value of the test. Although sweat electrolyte concentrations increase slightly with increasing age, they remain excellent discriminants for CF in older patients (164). The sweat test is not useful in diagnosing CF heterozygotes.

Intermediate sweat chloride concentrations in the range of 40–60 mEq/L have been reported in patients with chronic pulmonary disease and normal pancreatic function (*atypical cystic fibrosis*) (165). Borderline sweat electrolyte values are otherwise unusual. In such instances, CF mutation analysis may be helpful. Ancillary findings such as radiographic evidence of pansinusitis, aspermia, or the isolation of a mucoid *Pseudomonas* organism from the respiratory tract may also be helpful. Rarely, CF has been documented in patients with normal sweat electrolyte concentrations (166, 167). The diagnosis of CF should not be based solely on an elevated sweat electrolyte concentration but should be made only when it is associated with pancreatic exocrine deficiency, chronic pulmonary disease, meconium ileus, or a positive family history.

Newborn Screening

Screening of newborns for CF is now possible (168). It has been demonstrated that newborns with CF have elevated blood levels of IRT, presumably due to a secretory obstructive defect in the pancreas in utero. An alternative strategy for newborn screening involves direct mutation analysis of the blood spots of those infants with an elevated IRT value (169). Screening can be easily automated using the dried blood spots now routinely collected for metabolic screening, and is being carried out in many parts of the world. The potential benefits of screening include avoidance of diagnostic delays, decreased early morbidity, improved outcome, timely genetic counseling, and early and complete case detection for clinical and epidemiologic studies. Pending the results of cost-benefit analysis, however, mass newborn screening programs have not yet been recommended for the United States. The IRT test may also be helpful in evaluating neonates with a positive family history for CF. In such cases, it may yield useful information 2–3 weeks earlier than the age at which an adequate sweat sample can usually be obtained. In no case, however, should the IRT test be used as a substitute for the sweat test or as the basis of a definitive diagnosis. False-negative IRT results occur in up to 25% of newborns with intestinal obstruction (168).

MANAGEMENT

General

Because of the multisystem involvement, frequency of complications, psychosocial burden, and uncertain prognosis, a comprehensive and intensive therapy program is essential. Patients need to be followed at intervals of 2–3 months by an experienced and available physician, in conjunction with nursing, nutrition, physical-respiratory therapy, and counseling personnel (170). The Cystic Fibrosis Foundation in Bethesda, Maryland supports a nationwide network of centers that are involved in patient care, teaching, and clinical and basic research. Services provided by the centers include sweat testing and confirmation of the diagnosis; evaluation and provision of a therapeutic plan; continuity of outpatient and inpatient services; education of the patient and family; nutrition counseling; instruction in physical and respiratory therapy; psychosocial support, including individual counseling and education/support groups for patients, parents, and siblings; financial counseling; genetic counseling; subspecialty consultative services; and the opportunity to participate in clinical research projects. Vocational, educational, financial, and premarital counseling can help the increasing number of adult patients make a smooth transition to independent living. Optimal patient management involves coordination of services between the CF center and the primary care provider who is in a position to provide ongoing psychosocial support; to offer general medical care; to coordinate home, community, and educational services; and to interpret the significance of medical developments for the family (171). The goals of therapy include maintenance of adequate nutrition and normal growth, prevention or aggressive therapy of pulmonary complications, encouragement of a reasonable level of physical activity, and provision of psychosocial support.

Pulmonary

ANTIBIOTIC THERAPY

Treatment of the pulmonary manifestations of CF is directed at clearance of excess mucus from the tracheobronchial tree and aggressive antimicrobial therapy. Except in the case of acute respiratory illness, guidelines for the use of antibiotics in these patients are not well established (172–174). In some centers, patients are maintained continuously on one or more oral agents, usually directed against *Staphylococcus aureus, Hemophilus influenzae,* or both. In other centers, antimicrobial therapy is used only at times of respiratory exacerbations. Patients who do not respond to outpatient management are usually hospitalized for 10-day to 3-week courses of intensive antibiotic therapy, primarily directed against *Pseudomonas aeruginosa.* Combinations of an aminoglycoside (tobramycin, gentamicin) with an anti-*Pseudomonas* penicillin (carbenicillin, ticarcillin, piperacillin) are frequently used. A third-generation cephalosporin with anti-*Pseudomonas* activity (ceftazidime) as well as beta-lactams (aztreonam, imipenem) may be useful. Patients with CF may require high doses of aminoglycosides to achieve acceptable serum concentrations (175). Serum concentrations should be monitored and dosage adjusted to achieve a peak level of 8–10 μg/ml and a trough value of less than 2 μg/ml. Patients also show enhanced clearance of penicillins and may require large doses to achieve adequate serum levels (176). Quinolone derivatives such as ciprofloxacin are absorbed from the gastrointestinal tract and are the first oral agents shown to be effective against *Pseudomonas* pulmonary infections. In controlled trials in CF patients with pulmonary exacerbations, ciprofloxacin has been shown to be as effective as intravenous antibiotics (177). However, it is not approved for use in patients under 16

years. Its use is also limited by the rapid development of antibiotic resistance, and should be based on the results of sensitivity testing (178).

Improved methods for providing stable venous access have made home intravenous antibiotic therapy an attractive alternative to hospitalization (179). This type of therapy is cost-effective, associated with few complications, and does not interfere with normal activity. Long-term daily aerosol administration of anti-*Pseudomonas* agents such as tobramycin and gentamicin may be beneficial in patients with moderate-to-severe lung disease and chronic colonization with *P. aeruginosa* who require frequent hospital admission (180–182). Aerosol aminoglycoside therapy is well tolerated without significant side effects. There is very little systemic drug absorption, and there is no need to monitor serum drug levels. However, over time resistance may develop in a significant percentage of patients and should be monitored.

PHYSICAL AND RESPIRATORY THERAPY

Chest physiotherapy, consisting of postural drainage, manual or mechanical percussion, vibration, and assisted coughing, is used to enhance the removal of bronchial secretions and is usually recommended at the first indication of pulmonary involvement. Other useful methods of secretion removal include autogenic drainage and a variety of forced expiratory techniques (183). Treatments are carried out several times each day, depending on the degree of pulmonary disease. Although this is a cornerstone of CF therapy, objective assessments of its efficacy have yielded somewhat conflicting, but generally positive results (184, 185). In older patients, prolonged coughing in the absence of physiotherapy may yield similar results (186). Physical activity and exercise programs are useful adjuncts to physiotherapy and should be encouraged (187).

AEROSOL THERAPY

Although a variety of aerosolized agents have been used in CF, evidence to support their use is largely anecdotal. There are no data to document the efficacy of bland aerosols and N-acetylcysteine. In some patients, these agents may lead to reflex bronchoconstriction and worsening of pulmonary function. New approaches to mucolytic therapy include the nebulization of amiloride to normalize trans-epithelial electrolyte transport and increase sputum sodium and water content (188, 189), and human recombinant deoxyribonuclease (DNase) to enzymatically degrade the high concentration of DNA present in purulent sputum. In both short-term and long-term clinical trials, DNase has been shown to improve pulmonary function, decrease dyspnea, and decrease the need for parenteral antibiotics (190, 191). However, these agents are not yet approved for clinical use. Bronchodilators, administered either orally or by nebulization, may be useful in selected patients (192, 193). The response of CF patients to these agents is highly variable (51), and they should be used only after observing an obvious clinical response or documenting a beneficial response by pulmonary function testing. There are preliminary data that indicate that alpha-1 antitrypsin administered as an aerosol can neutralize the increased concentration of free proteases present in the airways of patients with CF (194).

IMMUNOTHERAPY

In patients with CF, the role for glucocorticoid therapy is controversial. In a double-blind study of alternate-day prednisone given to a small sample of patients with mild to moderate disease, at the end of 4 years the treatment group showed significant advantages in height, weight, pulmonary function, sedimentation rate, and serum immunoglobulin G values, and had fewer hospitalizations for CF-related pulmonary disease (195). However, in a much larger clinical trial, patients treated for 4 years with alternate-day prednisone, 1 mg/kg or 2 mg/kg, showed only modest short-term improvement in pulmonary function (Rosenstein BJ, Eigen H, personal communication) and had a high rate of complications, including carbohydrate abnormalities, cataracts, and growth retardation (196). The use of glucocorticoids in the treatment of CF should probably be limited to patients with severe bronchiolitic syndrome, significant airway obstruction that is not responsive to conventional bronchodilators, allergic bronchopulmonary aspergillosis, and evidence of hypersensitivity characterized by recurrent episodes of fever, rash, and joint pain (197). Patients on long-term glucocorticoid therapy need to be carefully monitored

for the development of carbohydrate abnormalities, cataracts, and growth retardation.

Infusion of intravenous immune globulin as an adjunct to antibiotic therapy has been shown to enhance short-term improvement in pulmonary function (198). Intravenous gamma globulin enriched with *P. aeruginosa* lipopolysaccharide antibodies has been associated with improvement in pulmonary function in patients infected with antibiotic-resistant phenotypes of *P. aeruginosa* (199). Routine use of these preparations awaits the results of further clinical trials.

MISCELLANEOUS THERAPIES

Tracheobronchial lavage has been used in an effort to remove impacted bronchial secretions, but there is no evidence that it is more effective than conventional therapy. Therapeutic bronchoscopy has been performed in patients with lobar and segmental atelectasis but the results are no better than those obtained with intensified medical therapy (200). Intermittent positive pressure breathing may worsen chest over-inflation and is usually contraindicated. There are no data to support the use of oral expectorants (201), and cough suppressants are contraindicated. Surgical treatment of pulmonary complications is infrequently undertaken since lung involvement is usually generalized, but lobectomy and segmental resection may be useful in selected cases of persistent atelectasis and localized bronchiectasis (202, 203).

UPPER AIRWAY PROBLEMS

Patients with symptomatic sinusitis should be treated with a 4- to 6-week course of antibiotics. For patients who do not respond and for those with chronic and/or recurrent symptoms, a surgical procedure to improve sinus drainage is indicated (204).

For patients with nasal polyps, intranasal glucocorticoids and oral antihistamines and decongestants may provide transient symptomatic relief but are rarely curative. Antibiotics and immunotherapy are not helpful. Patients with distressing symptoms are best treated by polypectomy. Associated sinusitis should be treated as outlined above.

PNEUMOTHORAX

Active intervention is indicated for pneumothorax greater than 10%. Conventional therapy consists of closed thoracostomy drainage via a chest tube followed by the intrapleural installation of sclerosing agents such as quinacrine and tetracycline. This form of therapy, however, has been associated with persistent air leak, prolonged hospitalization, and a high rate of recurrence (205). Because of these complications, an immediate open thoracotomy with pleural abrasion and resection of blebs has been recommended as an alternative form of therapy; it is associated with a recurrence rate of < 5% (206, 207). Intensive antibiotic therapy is usually used as an adjunct to these measures. The management of pneumothorax has been complicated by the availability of heart-lung and bilateral-lung transplantation. Prior sclerotherapy and pleural abrasion significantly increase chest wall bleeding at the time of transplantation; these procedures have been considered as relative contraindications to transplantation. An open thoracotomy with bleb resection and *localized* sclerotherapy may be an acceptable therapeutic option. This issue needs to be fully discussed with the patient and family prior to initiating therapy for pneumothorax.

HEMOPTYSIS

Heavy blood streaking of sputum and episodes of hemoptysis usually reflect increased pulmonary infection. The site of bleeding is best localized by bronchoscopy. In patients with heavy blood streaking, intensive antibiotic therapy alone may be sufficient. With massive hemoptysis (> 300 ml/24 hours) or with protracted or recurrent episodes of moderate bleeding, percutaneous catheter embolization of the involved bronchial arteries is the procedure of choice (208, 209). Immediate cessation of bleeding is achieved in over 80% of patients. Following the procedure, however, repeat bleeding is common, and one-third to half of patients will require repeat embolization (210).

COR PULMONALE

The management of right-sided failure includes therapy of the underlying pulmonary obstruction and infection along with diuretics, salt restriction, and oxygen (211). Digitalis is not generally useful. Overall, the results have not been favorable. In adults with chronic obstructive pulmonary disease, pulmonary

hypertension may be reversed by long-term continuous oxygen therapy (212). However, this has not been demonstrated in CF, and the role of oxygen therapy remains poorly defined. It is usually prescribed to relieve symptomatic hypoxia (i.e., headaches and dyspnea) and to improve exercise tolerance.

RESPIRATORY FAILURE

In general, assisted ventilation is not indicated for CF patients with progressive respiratory failure; such patients are rarely able to come off of ventilatory support (213). Its use should be restricted to the occasional patient with good baseline status in whom acute respiratory failure develops, patients awaiting transplantation, or in association with pulmonary surgery. Heart-lung and bilateral-lung transplants have been successfully performed in highly selected patients with chronic cardiorespiratory failure (214–217). The results are similar to those seen in non-CF patients with survival rates of 65–75% after 1 year and 50–60% after 2 years. Following successful transplantation, pulmonary function and exercise performance rapidly improve toward normal. The airways of the transplanted lungs maintain normal transepithelial ion transport (218). Early complications include rejection, bleeding, and infection, whereas infection and chronic rejection (bronchiolitis obliterans) are the leading late complications. Daily monitoring of lung function allows early detection of infection and rejection episodes with confirmation of the diagnosis by transbronchial biopsy. Wider application of heart-lung and bilateral-lung transplantation is limited by donor organ availability.

IMMUNOPROPHYLAXIS OF PULMONARY INFECTIONS

It is important to follow recommended vaccination schedules, especially for pertussis and measles. The *Hemophilus influenzae* type B vaccine should be given at the recommended age. Patients should be immunized against influenza starting at age 6 months, followed by a yearly booster. Household contacts should also be immunized. In patients who are exposed to influenza A and have not received vaccine, amantadine prophylaxis can be used until the risk of infection has passed. There has been no documented increase in susceptibility to or morbidity from pneumococcal infection, and routine use of pneumococcal vaccine is not recommended. *Pseudomonas* vaccines have been used investigationally (219, 220), but are not available for clinical use.

Gastrointestinal

PANCREATIC EXOCRINE DEFICIENCY

Pancreatic enzyme supplements, derived from hog pancreas, constitute the primary therapy of the pancreatic enzyme defect. The most effective preparations consist of capsules containing pancrelipase in pH-sensitive enteric-coated microspheres or microtablets (221–223). The enteric coating is designed to prevent gastric acid inactivation of the enzyme. Powdered preparations are usually used in infants. Enzyme supplements are given with all meals and snacks; the dosage is determined by the frequency and character of the stools along with the patient's growth pattern. The development of hard stools while a patient is taking enzymes is usually an indication for more, *not* less, enzyme. A misguided reduction in enzyme dosage in this situation may precipitate an episode of meconium ileus equivalent. It is rare to see an adverse reaction to an increased dose of enzyme.

Following the initiation of enzyme supplements, there is a reduction in the amount of both fat and nitrogen in the stools, although the values do not return to normal. Persistence of significant steatorrhea after enzyme therapy may be due to enzyme inactivation by gastric acid or to a low duodenal pH. In such cases, addition of bicarbonate or an H_2-receptor antagonist may be helpful (224). Complications of enzyme therapy are rare; skin and mucous membrane irritation may be seen in infants. Hypersensitivity reactions can occur in parents exposed to powdered extracts, but are rare in patients themselves (225).

NUTRITION

The goal of nutritional therapy is to promote normal growth. Contrary to earlier anecdotal reports of a voracious appetite in patients with CF, it is now known that most patients have a grossly deficient caloric intake (226). Because of incomplete correction of steatorrhea and increased metabolic demands, it is recommended that patients receive a diet that provides approximately 30% above recommended daily caloric allowances (227). This can usually be achieved by a well-balanced, high-protein diet with liberal fat. *Fat restriction is no longer recommended.* Infants can be breast-fed if they are receiving enzyme supplements, but weight gain must be closely monitored (228). For formula-fed infants, no advantage has been shown for predigested formulas containing medium chain triglycerides (MCTs) (229). However, these preparations are useful in infants with liver involvement or persistent steatorrhea, and following intestinal resection.

Older patients should be provided with a high-protein, high-calorie diet consistent with food preferences and lifestyle. Liberal fat should be allowed in the diet. Supplements with MCT oil and polycose can be used to boost caloric intake. In patients who have poor growth and inadequate caloric intake, in spite of nutritional counseling and attempts at oral supplementation, enteral supplementation may be useful (230–232). This is accomplished by the nightly infusion of high-calorie elemental formulas via a nasogastric, gastrostomy, or jejunostomy tube. There is evidence that this type of supplementation, when carried out over an extended period, may stabilize or even improve pulmonary function (233, 234). Parenteral hyperalimentation has been used but it is extremely costly and is associated with the complications of prolonged central line infusions. There is no evidence to strongly support the use of artificial elemental diets or supplements with essential fatty acids.

VITAMIN AND MINERAL SUPPLEMENTATION

Vitamin deficiencies can be prevented by the daily administration of a water-miscible vitamin preparation. Patients with achylia should receive a daily supplement of a water-miscible alpha-tocopherol preparation at a dose of 5–10 IU/kg, up to a maximum daily dose of 400 IU. Routine supplementation with vitamin K is not recommended, but may be indicated in patients with extensive liver involvement, at times of surgery, and in patients with demonstrated coagulation problems. Iron deficiency is frequently seen in CF patients. Iron status should be evaluated periodically, and appropriate supplementation should be provided in the face of anemia or low serum ferritin levels. The absorption of iron may be impaired in CF patients; response to therapy needs to be closely monitored (235). With pancreatic enzyme supplementation, there should be no need for supplementation with other trace metals. Additional dietary salt should be provided at times of thermal stress, including increased activity in hot weather. Supplementation with salt tablets is not usually indicated.

CARBOHYDRATE INTOLERANCE

Diabetes is usually easily managed by modest dietary changes along with low to moderate doses of insulin (74). Insulin requirements are based on the results of daily blood glucose monitoring and periodic glycosylated hemoglobin values. Oral hypoglycemic agents have not been useful. With improved survival, patients need to be closely monitored for retinal and renal vascular complications.

MECONIUM ILEUS

In uncomplicated cases of meconium ileus, the meconium can be removed nonoperatively by the use of hyperosmolar enemas administered under hydrostatic pressure (236, 237). In patients in whom this procedure is unsuccessful and in those with complications such as volvulus and perforation, it may be necessary to resect the involved segment of bowel. In some cases, mucolytics are used intraoperatively to liquify the inspissated meconium and may eliminate the need for intestinal resection (238). Patients who survive the newborn period have a prognosis similar to that for patients without meconium ileus (80, 84).

MECONIUM ILEUS EQUIVALENT

In cases of meconium ileus equivalent in which there is no evidence of intestinal obstruction, the oral administration of a cleansing electrolyte solution (Golytely—Braintree) is the treatment of choice (239, 240). If there is evidence of intestinal obstruction, enemas with hyperosmolar contrast material may be diagnostic as well as therapeutic. Large-volume saline and 2% N-acetylcysteine enemas have also been effective. Most episodes can be managed without surgical intervention. For patients with recurrent episodes, helpful measures include increased amounts of pancreatic enzyme, increased fluid intake, wetting agents,

high-fiber diet, oral N-acetylcysteine, lactulose, and mineral oil. In patients with intussusception, hydrostatic reduction should be attempted, although surgery may be necessary. Surgery is also indicated for episodes of volvulus.

MISCELLANEOUS COMPLICATIONS

Gastroesophageal reflux is treated by the administration of drugs such as metoclopramide and bethanechol to promote gastric emptying, and in infants by positioning and thickened feeds (241). Antacids and H_2-receptor antagonists are indicated in patients with esophagitis. The prokinetic agent cisapride may be helpful in reducing symptoms such as crampy abdominal pain, flatulence, and abdominal distention (242). Episodes of rectal prolapse are usually partial and easily treated by manual reduction. Surgical correction or injection of sclerosing agents is rarely necessary. In patients with recurrent episodes of prolapse, stool-wetting agents should be administered and the dosage of pancreatic enzymes should be increased.

Hepatobiliary

Although there is no specific therapy for liver complications, administration of the hydrophilic bile acid, ursodeoxycholic acid, has resulted in improvement in liver function (243, 243a) and dissolution of cholesterol gallstones (244) in patients with CF. In patients with bleeding secondary to portal hypertension and varices, portal-systemic shunting and splenectomy may be useful (244a). Post-shunt encephalopathy and hepatic failure are not usually a problem. However, a shunting procedure will decrease the patient's suitability for subsequent liver transplantation. The long-term results depend on the degree of underlying pulmonary disease. Endoscopic injection sclerotherapy can also be used to control acute or recurrent episodes of bleeding (245). In patients with severe liver disease and good pulmonary status, liver transplants have been carried out; early results indicate excellent 1- and 2-year survival rates (246). Although gallbladder abnormalities including cholelithiasis are common, patients are usually asymptomatic. Cholecystectomy should be reserved for the symptomatic patient in whom a trial of ursodeoxycholic acid has failed.

Psychosocial

Psychosocial support for the patient and other family members is especially important at the time of diagnosis, with exacerbations, and during the terminal phase of the disease. As with any chronic illness, consistency of medical care providers is essential. Members of the health care team should be willing to allow patients to develop close relationships with them and to provide ongoing support throughout life. It is important to know the entire family medically and psychosocially and to be sensitive to individual needs and coping mechanisms. Open communication is essential from the time of diagnosis. Questions should be answered honestly and directly but within a framework of guarded optimism.

Part of every visit should be devoted to a discussion of psychosocial issues. Parents should be encouraged to be open about CF rather than acting as though it did not exist. The involvement and support of extended family members should be encouraged. Parents constantly need to be encouraged to treat their child normally and to avoid overprotection. Special treatment and privileges should be discouraged. It is important to work with adolescents to promote independence and to encourage realistic academic and vocational goals. Families can be helped in a number of ways, including introduction to a CF family that is coping well, informational/support groups, respite care services, and individual counseling. It is the responsibility of the health care team to make appropriate referrals to and interface with mental health consultants, interact with the patient's teachers, ensure that the family is availing itself of all appropriate community and financial resources, arrange for vocational counseling, and in the case of adolescents to plan for a smooth transition to adult care. With appropriate support, most patients are able to make an age-appropriate adjustment at home and at school.

COURSE AND PROGNOSIS

The course of the disease is exceedingly variable from patient to patient, possibly related to genetic heterogeneity. Prognosis is largely determined by the degree of pulmonary involvement. Some patients retain near-normal lung function over a 5- to 7-year period (61); in general, however, there is an exponential decline in pulmonary function of approximately 2–3% per year. Early colonization with *Pseudomonas* may be associated with a more severe course (24, 247). Passive exposure to cigarette smoke has been associated with a more rapid decline in clinical status (248, 249) and should be avoided. Those patients with clinically intact pancreatic function have milder pulmonary disease and better survival (67). Improved prognosis has been related to early diagnosis and institution of a comprehensive treatment program prior to the establishment of irreversible pulmonary changes (250). There is evidence that survival may be correlated with intensity of the treatment regimen, particularly antibiotic use (251). Several clinical scoring systems are available for the longitudinal assessment of patients for prognosis counseling and for classifying patients for clinical studies (252, 253).

There has been steady improvement in prognosis over the past four decades. In 1950, survival past infancy was unusual. By 1991, the median age at time of death was 29.4 years (80) (Fig. 22.8). Approximately one-third of all patients under care at specialized CF centers are over 18 years of age (80). There is a trend toward poorer early survival, but better late survival among black patients (254, 255). For reasons that are not clear, the survival of male patients at every age appears better than that of female patients, but in recent years the gap has narrowed (80).

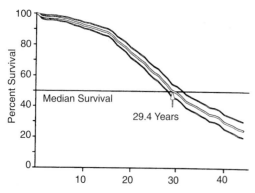

Figure 22.8. Survival curve for patients seen in CF centers in the United States in 1991. (Courtesy of the Cystic Fibrosis Foundation, Bethesda, MD.)

REFERENCES

1. Boat TF, Welsh MJ, Beaudet AL. Cystic fibrosis. In Scriver CL, Beaudet AL, Sly WS, Valle D, eds.

The metabolic basis of inherited disease, 6th ed. New York, McGraw-Hill, 1989, pp 2649–2680.

2. Andersen CH. Cystic fibrosis of the pancreas. *Am J Dis Child* 1938; 56:344–399.

3. Kulczycki LL, Guin GH, Mann N. Cystic fibrosis in Negro children: Results of a search. *Clin Ped* 1964; 3:692–705.

4. Danks DM, Allan J, Anderson CM. A genetic study of fibrocystic disease of the pancreas. *Ann Hum Genet* 1965; 28:323–356.

5. Davis PB. Autonomic and airway reactivity in obligate heterozygotes for cystic fibrosis. *Am Rev Respir Dis* 1984; 129:911–914.

6. Rommens JM, Iannuzzi MC, Kerem B, et al. Identification of the cystic fibrosis gene: Chromosome walking and jumping. *Science* 1989; 245:1059–1065.

7. Riordan JR, Rommens JM, Kerem B, et al. Identification of the cystic fibrosis gene: cloning and characterization of complementary DNA. *Science* 1989; 245:1066–1072.

8. Kerem B, Rommens JM, Buchanan JA. Identification of the cystic fibrosis gene: Genetic analysis. *Science* 1989; 245:1073–1080.

9. Cystic fibrosis genetic analysis consortium. Worldwide survey of the ΔF508 mutation—Report from the cystic fibrosis genetic analysis consortium. *Am J Hum Genet* 1990; 47:354–359.

10. Special report—Statement from the National Institutes of Health workshop on population screening for the cystic fibrosis gene. *N Engl J Med* 1990; 323:70–71.

11. Kerem E, Corey M, Kerem B, et al. The relation between genotype and phenotype in cystic fibrosis—Analysis of the most common mutation ΔF$_{508}$. *N Engl J Med* 1990; 323:1517–1522.

12. Santis G, Osborne L, Knight RA, Hudson ME. Independent genetic determinants of pancreatic and pulmonary status in cystic fibrosis. *Lancet* 1990; 336:1081–1084.

13. Farber S. Some organic digestive disturbances in early life. *J Michigan Med Soc* 1945; 44:587.

14. di Sant'Agnese PA, Darling RC, Perea GA, et al. Abnormal electrolyte composition of sweat in cystic fibrosis of the pancreas. Clinical significance and relationship to the disease. *Pediatrics* 1953; 12:549–563.

15. Bodian M. Fibrocystic disease of the pancreas. A congenital disorder of mucus production-mucosis. London, William Heinemann, 1952.

16. Quinton PM, Bijman J. Higher bioelectric potentials due to decreased chloride absorption in the sweat glands of patients with cystic fibrosis. *N Engl J Med* 1983; 308:1185–1189.

17. Bear CE, Li C, Kartner N, et al. Purification and functional reconstitution of the cystic fibrosis transmembrane conductance regulator (CFTR). *Cell* 1992; 68:809–818.

18. Anderson MP, Rich DP, Gregory RJ, et al. Generation of cAMP-activated chloride currents by expression of CFTR. *Science* 1991; 251:679–682.

19. Li M, McCann JD, Lieddtke CM, et al. Cyclic AMP–dependent protein kimase opens chloride channels in normal but not cystic fibrosis airway epithelium. *Nature* 1983; 331:358–360.

20. Boucher RC, Stutts MJ, Knowles MK, et al. Na$^+$ transport in cystic fibrosis respiratory epithelia: abnormal basal rate and response to adenylate cyclase activation. *J Clin Invest* 1986; 78:1245–1252.

21. Thomassen MJ, Demko CA, Doershuk CF. Cystic fibrosis: a review of pulmonary infections and interventions. *Pediatr Pulmonol* 1987; 3:334–351.

22. Esterly JR, Oppenheimer EH. Observations in cystic fibrosis of the pancreas. III. Pulmonary lesions. *Johns Hopkins Med J* 1968; 122:94.

23. Bedrossian CW, Greenberg SD, Singer DB, et al. The lung in cystic fibrosis: A quantitative study including prevalence of pathologic findings among different age groups. *Hum Pathol* 1976; 7:195–204.

24. Kerem E, Corey M, Gold R, et al. Pulmonary function and clinical course in patients with cystic fibrosis after pulmonary colonization with *Pseudomonas aeruginosa*. *J Pediatr* 1990; 116:714–719.

25. Fahy JV, Keoghan MT, Crummy EJ, et al. Bacteraemia and fungaemia in adults with cystic fibrosis. *J Infect* 1991; 22:241–245.

26. Thomassen MJ, Demko CA, Klinger JD, Stern RC. A new opportunist. Case reports—*Pseudomonas cepacia* colonization among patients with cystic fibrosis. *Am Rev Respir Dis* 1985; 131:791–796.

27. Tablan OC, Martone WJ, Doershuk CF, et al. Colonization of the respiratory tract with *Pseudomonas cepacia* in cystic fibrosis. *Chest* 1987; 91:527–532.

28. LiPuma JJ, Dasen SE, Nielson, et al. Person-to-person transmission of *Pseudomonas cepacia* between patients with cystic fibrosis. *Lancet* 1990; 336:1094–1096.

29. Lewin LO, Byard PJ, Davis PB. Effect of *Pseudomonas cepacia* colonization on survival and pulmonary function of cystic fibrosis patients. *J Clin Epideminol* 1990; 43:125–131.

30. Smith MJ, Efthimiou J, Hodson ME, et al. Mycobacterial isolations in young adults with cystic fibrosis. *Thorax* 1984; 39:369–375.

31. Berger M. Inflammation in the lung in cystic fibrosis: A vicious cycle that does more harm than good? *Clin Rev Allergy*, vol 9: *Cystic Fibrosis*. Gershwin E, ed. The Humana Press, 1991.

32. Suter S, Schaad UB, Roux L, et al. Granulocyte neutral proteases and pseudomonas elastase as possible causes of airway damage in patients with cystic fibrosis. *J Infect Dis* 1984; 149:523–531.

33. Dasgupta MK, Zuberbuhler P, Abbi A, et al. Combined evaluation of circulating immune complexes and antibodies to *Pseudomonas aeruginosa* as an immunologic profile in relation to pulmonary function in cystic fibrosis. *J Clin Immunol* 1987; 7:51–58.

34. Wisnieski JJ, Todd EW, Fuller RK, et al. Immune complexes and complement abnormalities in patients with cystic fibrosis. *Am Rev Respir Dis* 1985; 132:770–776.

35. Lloyd–Still JD, Khaw K, Shwachman H. Severe respiratory disease in infants with cystic fibrosis. *Pediatrics* 1974; 53:5.

36. Ledesma-Medina J, Osman MZ, Girdany BR. Abnormal paranasal sinuses in patients with cystic fibrosis of the pancreas. *Pediatr Radiol* 1980; 9:61–64.

37. Umetsu DT, Moss RB, King VV, et al. Sinus disease in patients with severe cystic fibrosis: relation to pulmonary exacerbation. *Lancet* 1990; 335:1077–1078.

38. Strauss RG, West PJ, Silverman FN. Unilateral proptosis in cystic fibrosis. *Pediatrics* 1969; 43:297–300.

39. Stern RC, Boat TF, Wood RE. Treatment and prognosis of nasal polyps in cystic fibrosis. *Am J Dis Child* 1982; 136:1067–1070.

40. Oppenheimer EH, Rosenstein BJ. Differential pathology of nasal polyps in cystic fibrosis and atopy. *Lab Invest* 1979; 40:445–449.

41. Forman–Franco B, Abramson AL, Gorvoy JD, et al. Cystic fibrosis and hearing loss. *Arch Otolaryngol* 1979; 105:338–342.

42. White H, Rowley WF. Cystic fibrosis of the pancreas. *Pediatr Clin North Am* 1964; 11:139–169.

43. Waring WW, Brunt CH, Hilman BC. Mucoid impaction of the bronchi in cystic fibrosis. *Pediatrics* 1967; 39:166–175.

44. Lamarre A, Reilly BJ, Bryan AC, et al. Early detection of pulmonary function abnormalities in cystic fibrosis. *Pediatrics* 1972; 50:291–298.

45. Alderson PO, Secker-Walker RH, Strominger DB, et al. Quantitative assessment of regional ventilation and perfusion in children with cystic fibrosis. *Radiology* 1974; 111:151–155.

46. Redding GJ, Restuccia R, Cotton EK, et al. Serial changes in pulmonary functions in children hospitalized with cystic fibrosis. *Am Rev Respir Dis* 1982; 126:31–36.

47. Loughlin GM, Cota K, Taussig LM. The relationship between flow transients and bronchial lability in cystic fibrosis. *Chest* 1981; 79:206–210.

48. Stokes DC, McBride JT, Wall MA, et al. Sleep hypoxemia in young adults with cystic fibrosis. *Am J Dis Child* 1980; 134:741–743.

49. Eggleston PA, Rosenstein BJ, Stackhouse CM, et al. Airway hyperreactivity in cystic fibrosis: Clinical correlates and possible effects on the course of the disease. *Chest* 1988; 94:360–365.

50. Hordvik NL, Koönig P, Morris D, et al. A longitudinal study of bronchodilator responsiveness in cystic fibrosis. *Am Rev Respir Dis* 1985; 131:889–893.

51. Landau LI, Phelan PD. The variable effect of a bronchodilating agent on pulmonary function in cystic fibrosis. *J Pediatr* 1973; 82:863–868.

52. Zach MS, Oberwaldner B, Forche G, et al. Bronchodilators increase airway instability in cystic fibrosis. *Am Rev Respir Dis* 1985; 131:537–543.

53. Lifschitz MI, Bowman FO, Denning CR, et al. Pneumothorax as a complication of cystic fibrosis: report of twenty cases. *Am J Dis Child* 1968; 116:633–640.

54. Luck SR, Raffensperger JG, Sullivan HJ, et al. Management of pneumothorax in children with chronic pulmonary disease. *J Thorac Cardiovasc Surg* 1977; 74:834–839.

55. Holsclaw DS, Grand RJ, Shwachman H. Massive hemoptysis in cystic fibrosis. *J Pediatr* 1970; 76:829–838.

56. Moss AJ. The cardiovascular system in cystic fibrosis. *Pediatrics* 1982; 70:728–741.

57. Siassi B, Moss A, Dooley RR. Clinical recognition of cor pulmonale in cystic fibrosis. *J Pediatr* 1971; 78:794–805.

58. Allen HD, Taussig LM, Gaines JA, et al. Echocardiographic profiles of the long-term cardiac changes in cystic fibrosis. *Chest* 1979; 75:428–433.

59. Wang EE, Prober CG, Manson B, et al. Association of respiratory viral infections with pulmonary deterioration in patients with cystic fibrosis. *N Engl J Med* 1984; 311:1653–1658.

60. Abman SH, Ogle JW, Butler-Simon N, et al. Role of respiratory syncytial virus in early hospitalizations for respiratory distress of young infants with cystic fibrosis. *J Pediatr* 1988; 113:826–830.

61. Corey M, Levison H, Crozier D. Five– to seven–year course of pulmonary function in cystic fibrosis. *Am Rev Respir Dis* 1976; 114:1085–1092.

62. Couper RTL, Corey M, Moore DJ, et al. Decline of exocrine pancreatic function in cystic fibrosis patients with pancreatic sufficiency. *Pediatr Res* 1992; 32:179–182.

63. Hubbard VS, Mangrum PJ. Energy intake and nutrition counseling in cystic fibrosis. *J Am Diet Assoc* 1982; 80:127–131.

64. Landon C, Rosenfeld RG. Short stature and pubertal delay in male adolescents with cystic fibrosis. Androgen treatment. *Am J Dis Child* 1984; 138:388–391.

65. Moshang T, Holsclaw DS. Menarchal determinants in cystic fibrosis. *Am J Dis Child* 1980; 134:1139–1142.

66. Shwachman H, Lebenthal E, Khaw K-T. Recurrent acute pancreatitis in patients with cystic fibrosis with normal pancreatic enzymes. *Pediatrics* 1975; 55:86.

67. Gaskin K, Gurwitz D, Corey M, et al. Improved respiratory prognosis in patients with cystic fibrosis with normal fat absorption. *J Pediatr* 1982; 100:857–862.

68. Durie PR, Gaskin KJ, Corey M, et al. Pancreatic function testing in cystic fibrosis. *J Pediatr Gastroenterol Nutr* 1984; 3:S89–S98.

69. Hadorn B, Zoppi G, Shmerling DH, et al. Quantitative assessment of exocrine pancreatic function in infants and children. *J Pediatr* 1968; 73:39–50.

70. Brown GA, Halliday RB, Turner PJ, et al. Faecal chymotrypsin concentrations in neonates with cystic fibrosis and healthy controls. *Arch Dis Child* 1988; 63:1229–1233.

71. Nousia-Arvanitakis S, Arvanitakis C, Greenberger NJ. Diagnosis of exocrine pancreatic insufficiency in cystic fibrosis by the synthetic peptide N-benzoyl-L-tyrosyl-p-aminobenzoic acid. *J Pediatr* 1978; 92:734–737.

72. Cleghorn G, Benjamin L, Corey M, et al. Serum immunoreactive pancreatic lipase and cationic trypsinogen for the assessment of exocrine pancreatic function in older patients with cystic fibrosis. *Pediatrics* 1986; 77:301–306.

73. Reisman J, Corey M, Canny G, et al. Diabetes mellitus in patients with cystic fibrosis: Effect on survival. *Pediatrics* 1990; 86:374–377.

74. Rodman HM, Doershuk CF, Rolano JM. The interaction of two diseases: diabetes mellitus and cystic fibrosis. *Medicine* 1986; 65:389–397.

75. Allen JL. Progressive nephropathy in a patient with cystic fibrosis and diabetes. *N Engl J Med* 1986; 315:764.

76. Milner AD. Blood glucose and serum insulin levels in children with cystic fibrosis. *Arch Dis Child* 1969; 44:351–355.

77. Wilmshurst EG, Soeldner JS, Holsclaw DS, et al. Endogenous and exogenous insulin responses in patients with cystic fibrosis. *Pediatrics* 1975; 55:75–82.

78. Stahl M, Girard J, Rutishauser M, et al. Endocrine function of the pancreas in cystic fibrosis: Evidence for an impaired glucagon and insulin response following arginine infusion. *J Pediatr* 1974; 84:821–824.

79. Lippe BM, Kaplan SA, Neufeld ND, et al. Insulin receptors in cystic fibrosis: Increased receptor number and altered affinity. *Pediatrics* 1980; 65: 1018–1022.

80. Cystic Fibrosis Foundation Registry. Bethesda, Maryland. 1991.

81. Dolan TF, Touloukian RJ. Familial meconium ileus not associated with cystic fibrosis. *J Pediatr Surg* 1974; 9:821–824.

82. Donnison AB, Shwachman H, Gross RE. A review of 164 children with meconium ileus seen at the Children's Hospital Medical Center, Boston. *Pediatrics* 1966; 37:833–850.

83. Oppenheimer EH, Esterly JR. Observations in cystic fibrosis of the pancreas: II. Neonatal intestinal obstruction. *Bull Johns Hopkins Hosp* 1962; III:1.

84. Kerem E, Corey M, Kerem B, et al. Clinical and genetic comparisons of patients with cystic fibrosis, with or without meconium ileus. *J Pediatr* 1989; 114:767–773.

85. Rosenstein BJ, Langbaum TS. Incidence of meconium abnormalities in newborn infants with cystic fibrosis. *Am J Dis Child* 1980; 134:72–73.

86. Rubinstein S, Moss R, Lewiston N, et al. Constipation and meconium ileus equivalent in patients with cystic fibrosis. *Pediatrics* 1986; 78:473–479.

87. Rosenstein BJ, Langbaum TS. Incidence of distal intestinal obstruction syndrome in cystic fibrosis. *J Pediatr Gastroenterol Nutr* 1983; 2:299–301.

88. Holsclaw DS, Rocmans C, Shwachman H. Intussusception in patients with cystic fibrosis. *Pediatrics* 1971; 48:51–58.

89. Shwachman H, Holsclaw D. Examination of the appendix at laparotomy as a diagnostic clue in cystic fibrosis. *N Engl J Med* 1972; 286:1300–1301.

90. Dolan TF, Meyers A. Mild cystic fibrosis presenting as an asymptomatic distended appendiceal mass: A case report. *Clin Pediatr* 1975; 14:862–863.

91. Kulczycki LL, Shwachman H. Studies in cystic fibrosis of the pancreas. *N Engl J Med* 1958; 259:409–412.

92. Scott RB, O'Loughlin EV, Gall DG. Gastroesophageal reflux in patients with cystic fibrosis. *J Pediatr* 1985; 106:223–227.

93. Rosenstein BJ, Perman JA, Kramer SS. Peptic ulcer disease in cystic fibrosis: an unusual occurrence in black adolescents. *Am J Dis Child* 1986; 140:966–967.

94. Taussig LM, Saldino RM, di Sant'Agnese PA. Radiographic abnormalities of the duodenum and small bowel in cystic fibrosis of the pancreas (mucoviscidosis). *Radiology* 1973; 106:369–376.

94a. Fiedorek SC, Shulman RJ, Klish WJ. Endoscopic detection of peptic ulcer disease in cystic fibrosis. *Clin Pediatr* 1986; 25:243–246.

95. Smith FR, Underwood BA, Denning CR, et al. Depressed plasma retinol-binding protein levels in cystic fibrosis. *J Lab Clin Med* 1972; 80:423.

96. Petersen RA, Petersen VS, Robb RM. Vitamin A deficiency with xerophthalmia and night blindness in cystic fibrosis. *Am J Dis Child* 1968; 116:662–665.

97. Abernathy RS. Bulging fontanelle as presenting sign in cystic fibrosis. *Am J Dis Child* 1976; 130:1360.

98. Hahn TJ, Squires AE, Halstead LR, et al. Reduced serum 25-hydroxyvitamin D concentration and disordered mineral metabolism in patients with cystic fibrosis. *J Pediatr* 1979; 94:38–42.

99. Mischler EH, Chesney PJ, Chesney RW, et al. Demineralization in cystic fibrosis. *Am J Dis Child* 1979; 133:632–635.

100. Walters TR, Koch HF. Hemorrhagic diathesis and cystic fibrosis in infancy. *Am J Dis Child* 1972; 124:641–642.

101. Farrell PM, Biere JG, Fratantoni JF, et al. The occurrence and effects of human vitamin E deficiency. *J Clin Invest* 1977; 60:233–241.

102. Oppenheimer EH. Focal necrosis of striated muscle in an infant with cystic fibrosis of the pancreas and evidence of lack of absorption of fat–soluble vitamins. *Bull Johns Hopkins Hosp* 1956; 98:353–359.

103. Willison HJ, Muller DPR, Matthews S, et al. A study of the relationship between neurological function and serum vitamin E concentrations in patients with cystic fibrosis. *J Neurol Neurosurg Psychiatry* 1985; 48:1097–1102.

104. Chase HP, Long MA, Lavin MH. Cystic fibrosis and malnutrition. *J Pediatr* 1979; 95:337–347.

105. Green CG, Doershuk CF, Stern RC. Symptomatic hypomagnesemia in cystic fibrosis. *J Pediatr* 1985; 107:425–428.

106. Godson C, Ryan MP, Brady HR, et al. Acute hypomagnesaemia complicating the treatment of meconium ileus equivalent in cystic fibrosis. *Scand J Gastroenterol* 1988; 143:148–150.

107. Ater JL, Herbst JJ, Landaw SA, et al. Relative anemia and iron deficiency in cystic fibrosis. *Pediatrics* 1983; 71:810–814.

108. Gunn T, Belmonte MM, Colle E, et al. Edema as the presenting symptom of cystic fibrosis: Difficulties in diagnosis. *Am J Dis Child* 1978; 132:317–318.

109. Lee PA, Roloff DW, Howatt WF. Hypoproteinemia and anemia in infants with cystic fibrosis. *JAMA* 1974; 228:585–588.

110. MacLean WC, Tripp RW. Cystic fibrosis with edema and falsely negative sweat test. *J Pediatr* 1973; 83:86–88.

111. Nussbaum E, Boat TF, Wood RE, et al. Cystic fibrosis with acute hypoelectrolytemia and metabolic alkalosis in infancy. *Am J Dis Child* 1979; 133:965–966.

112. Beckerman RC, Taussig LM. Hypoelectrolytemia and metabolic alkalosis in infants with cystic fibrosis. *Pediatrics* 1979; 63:580–583.

113. di Sant'Agnese PA, Blanc WA. A distinctive type of biliary cirrhosis of the liver associated with cystic fibrosis of the pancreas. *Pediatrics* 1956; 18:387–409.

114. Oppenheimer EH, Esterly JR. Hepatic changes in young infants with cystic fibrosis: possible relation to focal biliary cirrhosis. *J Pediatr* 1975; 86:683–689.

115. Valman HB, France NE, Wallis PG. Prolonged neonatal jaundice in cystic fibrosis. *Arch Dis Child* 1971; 46:805–809.

116. Craig JM, Haskell H, Shwachman H. The pathological changes in the liver in cystic fibrosis of the pancreas. *Am J Dis Child* 1957; 93:357–369.

117. Scott-Jupp R, Lama M, Tanner MS. Prevalence of liver disease in cystic fibrosis. Arch Dis Child 1991; 66:698–701.

118. Stern RC, Stevens DP, Boat TF, et al. Symptomatic hepatic disease in cystic fibrosis: Incidence, course, and outcome of portal systemic shunting. Gastroenterology 1976; 70:645–649.

119. Wilroy RS, Crawford SE, Johnson WW. Cystic fibrosis with extensive fat replacement of the liver. J Pediatr 1966; 68:67–73.

120. Schuster S, Shwachman H, Toyama W, et al. The management of portal hypertension in cystic fibrosis. J Pediatr Surg 1977; 12:201–206.

121. L'Heureux PR, Isenberg JN, Sharp HL, et al. Gallbladder disease in cystic fibrosis. Am J Roentgenol 1977; 128:953–956.

122. Kaplan E, Shwachman H, Perlmutter AD, et al. Reproductive failure in males with cystic fibrosis. N Engl J Med 1968; 279:65–69.

123. Oppenheimer EH, Esterly JR. Observations on cystic fibrosis of the pancreas. V. Developmental changes in the male genital system. J Pediatr 1969; 75:806–811.

124. Holsclaw DS, Perlmutter AD, Jockin H, et al. Genital abnormalities in male patients with cystic fibrosis. J Urology 1971; 106:568–574.

125. Anguiano A, Oates RD, Amos JA, et al. Congenital bilateral absence of the vas deferens. JAMA 1992; 267:1794–1797.

126. Cohen LF, di Sant'Agnese, Friedlander J. Cystic fibrosis and pregnancy: A national survey. Lancet 1980; 2:842–844.

127. Oppenheimer EH, Esterly JR. Observations on cystic fibrosis of the pancreas. VI. The uterine cervix. J Pediatr 1970; 77:991–995.

128. Kotloff RM, FitzSimmons SC, Fiel SB. Fertility and pregnancy in patients with cystic fibrosis. Clin Chest Medicine 1992; 13:623–635.

129. Palmer J, Dillon–Baker C, Tecklin JS, et al. Pregnancy in patients with cystic fibrosis. Ann Intern Med 1983; 99:596–600.

130. Fitzpatrick SB, Stokes DC, Rosenstein BJ, et al. Use of oral contraceptives in women with cystic fibrosis. Chest 1984; 86:863–867.

131. Cohen AM, Yulish BS, Wasser KB, et al. Evaluation of pulmonary hypertrophic osteoarthropathy in cystic fibrosis. Am J Dis Child 1986; 140:74–77.

132. Sagransky DM, Greenwald RA, Gorvoy JD. Seropositive rheumatoid arthritis in a patient with cystic fibrosis. Am J Dis Child 1980; 134:319–320.

133. Rose J, Gamble J, Schultz A, et al. Back pain and spinal deformity in cystic fibrosis. Am J Dis Child 1987; 141:1313–1316.

134. Newman AJ, Ansell BM. Episodic arthritis in children with cystic fibrosis. J Pediatr 1979; 94:594–596.

135. Schidlow DV, Goldsmith DP, Palmer J, et al. Arthritis in cystic fibrosis. Arch Dis Child 1984; 59:377–379.

136. Spaide RF, Diamond G, D'Amico RA, et al. Ocular findings in cystic fibrosis. Am J Ophthalmol 1987; 103:204–210.

137. Rimsza ME, Hernried LS, Kaplan AM. Hemorrhagic retinopathy in a patient with cystic fibrosis. Pediatrics 1978; 62:336–338.

138. Lietman PS, di Sant'Agnese, Wong W. Optic neuritis in cystic fibrosis of the pancreas: role of chloramphenicol therapy. JAMA 1964; 189:148–151.

138a. Katznelson D. Increased intracranial pressure in cystic fibrosis. Acta Paediatr Scand 1978; 67:607–609.

139. Roach ES, Sinal SH. Increased intracranial pressure following treatment of cystic fibrosis. Pediatrics 1980; 66:622–623.

140. Fischer EG, Shwachman H, Wepsie JG. Brain abscess and cystic fibrosis. Pediatrics 1979; 95:385–388.

141. Geller A, Gilles F, Shwachman H. Degeneration of fasciculus gracilis in cystic fibrosis. Neurology 1977; 27:185–187.

142. Borel DM, Reddy JK. Excessive lipofuscin accumulation in the thyroid gland in mucoviscidosis. Arch Pathol 1973; 96:269–271.

143. Azizi BF, Bentley D, Vagenakis A, et al. Abnormal thyroid function and response to iodides in patients with cystic fibrosis. Trans Assoc Am Phys 1974; 87:111–119.

144. Isolated growth hormone deficiency and cystic fibrosis: A report of two cases. Am J Dis Child 1980; 134:317–318.

145. Warwick WJ, Bernard B, Meskin LH. The involvement of the labial mucous salivary gland in patients with cystic fibrosis. Pediatrics 1964; 34:621–628.

146. Barbero GJ, Sibinga MS. Enlargement of the submaxillary salivary glands in cystic fibrosis. Pediatrics 1962; 29:788–792.

147. Lewiston NJ. Psychosocial impact of cystic fibrosis. Semin Respir Med 1985; 6:321–333.

148. Denning CR, Gluckson MM. Psychosocial aspects of cystic fibrosis. In Taussig LM, ed. Cystic fibrosis. New York, Thieme-Stratton, 1984, pp 461–492.

149. Walker LS, Ford MB, Donald WD. Cystic fibrosis and family stress: Effects of age and severity of illness. Pediatrics 1987; 79:239–246.

150. Gayton WF, Friedman SB, Tavormina JF, et al. Children with cystic fibrosis: I. Psychological test findings of patients, siblings, and parents. Pediatrics 1977; 59:888–894.

151. Spinetta J, Deasey-Spinetta P. Talking with children with a life-threatening illness. A handbook for health care professionals. Rockville, MD, Cystic Fibrosis Foundation, 1980.

152. Rosenstein BJ, Langbaum TS, Metz S. Cystic fibrosis: Diagnostic considerations. Johns Hopkins Med J 1982; 150:113–122.

153. Wood RE, Boat TF, Doershuk CF. State of the art: Cystic fibrosis. Am Rev Resp Dis 1976; 113:833–878.

154. Gibson LE, Cooke RE. A test for concentration of electrolytes in sweat in cystic fibrosis of the pancreas utilizing pilocarpine by iontophoresis. Pediatrics 1959; 23:545–549.

155. Barnes GL, Vaelioja L, McShane S. Sweat testing by capillary collection and osmometry: Suitability of the Wescor Macroduct System for screening suspected cystic fibrosis patients. Aust Paediatr J 1988; 24:191–193.

156. Kirk JM, Keston M, McIntosh I, et al. Variation of sweat sodium and chloride with age in cystic fibrosis and normal populations: Further investigations in equivocal cases. Ann Clin Biochem 1992; 29:145–152.

157. Rosenstein BJ, Langbaum TS, Gordes E, et al. Cystic fibrosis. Problems encountered with sweat testing. *JAMA* 1978; 240:1987–1988.

158. Gowen CW, Lawson EE, Gingras-Leatherman J, et al. Increased nasal potential difference and amiloride sensitivity in neonates with cystic fibrosis. *J Pediatr* 1986; 108:517–521.

159. Gowen CW, Gowen MA, Knowles MR. Colonic transepithelial potential difference in infants with cystic fibrosis. *J Pediatr* 1991; 118:412–415.

160. Ruddy RM, Scanlin TF. Abnormal sweat electrolytes in a case of celiac disease and a case of psychosocial failure to thrive. *Clin Pediatr* 1987; 26:83–89.

161. Christoffel KS, Lloyd-Still JD, Brown G, et al. Environmental deprivation and transient elevation of sweat electrolytes. *J Pediatr* 1985; 107:231–234.

162. Beck R, Goldberg E, Durie PR, et al. Elevated sweat chloride levels in anorexia nervosa. *J Pediatr* 1986; 108:260–262.

163. Rosenstein BJ, Langbaum TS. Misdiagnosis of cystic fibrosis. *Clin Pediatr* 1987; 26:78–82.

164. Davis PB, Del Rio S, Muntz JA, et al. Sweat chloride concentration in adults with pulmonary diseases. *Am Rev Respir Dis* 1983; 128:34–37.

165. Stern RC, Boat TF, Abramowsky CR, et al. Intermediate-range sweat chloride concentration and *Pseudomonas* bronchitis. *JAMA* 1978; 239:2676–2680.

166. Strong TV, Smit LS, Turpin SV, Cole JL, et al. Cystic fibrosis gene mutation in two sisters with mild disease and normal sweat electrolyte levels. *N Engl J Med* 1991; 325:1630–1634.

167. Davis PB, Hubbard VS, di Sant'Agnese PA. Low sweat electrolytes in a patient with cystic fibrosis. *Am J Med* 1980; 69:643–646.

168. Hammond KB, Abman SH, Sokol RJ, et al. Efficacy of statewide neonatal screening for cystic fibrosis by assay of trypsinogen concentrations. *N Engl J Med* 1991; 325:769–774.

169. Wilfond B, Gregg R, Laxova A. Mutation analysis for cystic fibrosis newborn screening: A two-tiered approach. *Pediatr Pulmonol* 1991; 56:238.

170. The Cystic Fibrosis Foundation Center Committee and Guidelines Subcommittee. Cystic fibrosis foundation guidelines for patient services, evaluation, and monitoring in cystic fibrosis centers. *Am J Dis Child* 1990; 144:1311–1312.

171. Stern RC. The primary care physician and the patient with cystic fibrosis. *J Pediatr* 1989; 114:31–36.

172. Marks MI. The pathogenesis and treatment of pulmonary infections in patients with cystic fibrosis. *J Pediatr* 1981; 98:173–179.

173. Govan JRW, Doherty C, Glass S. Rational parameters for antibiotic therapy in patients with cystic fibrosis. *Infection* 1987; 15:300–307.

174. Marks MI, Antibiotic therapy for bronchopulmonary infections in cystic fibrosis. In Hoiby N, Pedersen SS, Shand GH, Doring G, Holder IA, eds. *Pseudomonas aeruginosa infection. Antibiot Chemother:* Basel, Karger, 1989; 49:229–236.

175. Kelly HB, Menendez R, Fan L, et al. Brief clinical and laboratory observations —Pharmacokinetics of tobramycin in cystic fibrosis. *J Pediatr* 1982; 100:318–321.

176. Spino M, Chai RP, Isles AF, et al. Cloxacillin absorption and disposition in cystic fibrosis. *J Pediatr* 1984; 105:829–834.

177. Hodson ME, Roberts CM, Butland RJA, et al. Oral ciprofloxacin compared with conventional intravenous treatment for *Pseudomonas aeruginosa* infection in adults with cystic fibrosis. *Lancet* 1987; 1:235–237.

178. Jensen T, Pedersen SS, Nielsen CH, et al. The efficacy and safety of ciprofloxacin and ofloxacin in chronic *Pseudomonas aeruginosa* infection in cystic fibrosis. *J Antimicrob Chemother* 1987; 20:585–594.

179. Donati MA, Guenette G, Auerbach H. Prospective controlled study of home and hospital therapy of cystic fibrosis pulmonary disease. *J Pediatr* 1987; 111:28–33.

180. Hodson ME, Penketh ARL, Batten JC. Aerosol carbenicillin and gentamicin treatment of *Pseudomonas aeruginosa* infection in patients with cystic fibrosis. *Lancet* 1981; 2:1137–1139.

181. Gappa M, Steinkamp G, Tummler B, et al. Long-term tobramycin aerosol therapy of chronic *Pseudomonas aeruginosa* infection in patients with cystic fibrosis. *Scand J Gastroenterol* 1988; 23:74–76.

182. Ramsey BW, Dorkin HL, Eisenberg JD, et al. Efficacy of aerosolized tobramycin in patients with cystic fibrosis. *N Engl J Med* 1993; 328:1740–1746.

183. Schoni MH. Autogenic drainage: A modern approach to physiotherapy in cystic fibrosis. *J Royal Soc Med* 1989; 82:516.

184. Feldman J, Traver GA, Taussig LM. Maximal expiratory flows after postural drainage. *Am Rev Resp Dis* 1979; 119:239–245.

185. Reisman JJ, Rivington-Law B, Corey M, et al. Role of conventional physiotherapy in cystic fibrosis. *J Pediatr* 1988; 113:632–636.

186. Rossman CM, Waldes R, Sampson D, et al. Effect of chest physiotherapy on the removal of mucus in patients with cystic fibrosis. *Am Rev Respir Dis* 1982; 126:131–135.

187. Edlund LD, French RW, Herbst JJ, et al. Effects of a swimming program on children with cystic fibrosis. *Am J Dis Child* 1986; 140:80–83.

188. Knowles MR, Church NL, Waltner WE, et al. A pilot study of aerosolized amiloride for the treatment of lung disease in cystic fibrosis. *N Engl J Med* 1990; 322:1189–1194.

189. App EM, King M, Helfesrieder R, et al. Acute and long-term amiloride inhalation in cystic fibrosis lung disease. *Am Rev Respir Dis* 1990; 141:605–612.

190. Hubbard RC, McElvaney NG, Birrer P, et al. A preliminary study of aerosolized recombinant human deoxyribonuclease I in the treatment of cystic fibrosis. *N Engl J Med* 1992; 326:812–815.

191. Aitken ML, Burke W, McDonald G, et al. Recombinant human Dnase inhalation in normal subjects and patients with cystic fibrosis. A phase 1 study. *JAMA* 1992; 267:1947–1951.

192. Eggleston P, Rosenstein BJ, Stackhouse CM, et al. A controlled trial of long-term bronchodilator therapy in cystic fibrosis. *Chest* 1991; 99:1088–1092.

193. Tepper RS, Eigen H. Airway reactivity in cystic fibrosis. *Clin Rev Allergy*, vol 9: Cystic fibrosis. Gershwin E, ed. Humana Press, 1991.

194. McElvaney NG, Hubbard RC, Birrer P, et al. Aerosol α1-antitrypsin treatment for cystic fibrosis. 1991; 337:392–394.

195. Auerbach HS, Williams M, Kirkpatrick JA, et al. Alternate-day prednisone reduces morbidity and improves pulmonary function in cystic fibrosis. *Lancet* 1985; 2:686–688.

196. Rosenstein BJ, Eigen H. Risks of alternate-day prednisone in patients with cystic fibrosis. *Pediatrics* 1991; 87:245–246.

197. Lewiston NJ, Moss RB. Circulating immune complexes decrease during corticosteroid therapy in cystic fibrosis. *Pediatr Res* 1982; 16:354A.

198. Winnie GB, Cowan RG, Wade NA. Intravenous immune globulin treatment of pulmonary exacerbations in cystic fibrosis. *J Pediatr* 1989; 114:309–314.

199. Van Wye JE, Collins MS, Baylor M, et al. *Pseudomonas* hyperimmune globulin passive immunotherapy for pulmonary exacerbations in cystic fibrosis. *Pediatr Pulmonol* 1990; 9:7–18.

200. Stern RC, Boat TF, Orenstein DM, et al. Treatment and prognosis of lobar and segmental atelectasis in cystic fibrosis. *Am Rev Resp Dis* 1978; 118:821–826.

201. Ratjen F, Wönne R, Posselt HG, et al. A double-blind placebo controlled trial with oral ambroxol and N-acetylcysteine for mucolytic treatment in cystic fibrosis. *Eur J Pediatr* 1985; 144:374–378.

202. Marmon L, Schidlow D, Palmer J, et al. Pulmonary resection for complications of cystic fibrosis. *J Pediatr Surg* 1983; 18:811–815.

203. Mearns MB, Hodson CJ, Jackson ADM, et al. Pulmonary resection in cystic fibrosis. Results in 23 cases, 1957–1970. *Arch Dis Child* 1977; 47:499–508.

204. Cuyler JP. Follow-up of endoscopic sinus surgery on children with cystic fibrosis. *Otolaryngol Head Neck Surg* 1992; 118:505–506.

205. McLaughlin FJ, Matthews WJ, Strieder DJ, et al. Pneumothorax in cystic fibrosis: Management and outcome. *J Pediatr* 1982; 100:863–869.

206. Stowe SM, Boat TF, Mendelsohn H, et al. Open thoracotomy for pneumothorax in cystic fibrosis. *Am Rev Resp Dis* 1975; 111:611–617.

207. Rich RH, Warwick WJ, Leonard AS. Open thoracotomy and pleural abrasion in the treatment of spontaneous pneumothorax in cystic fibrosis. *J Pediatr Surg* 1978; 13:237–242.

208. Fellows KE, Khaw KT, Schuster S, et al. Bronchial artery embolization in cystic fibrosis: Technique and long-term results. J Pediatr 1979; 95:959–963.

209. Cohen AM, Doershuk CF, Stern RC. Bronchial artery embolization to control hemoptysis in cystic fibrosis. *Radiology* 1990; 175:401–405.

210. Sweezey NB, Fellows KE. Bronchial artery embolization for severe hemoptysis in cystic fibrosis. *Chest* 1990; 97:1322–1326.

211. Stern RC, Borkat G, Hirschfeld SS, et al. Heart failure in cystic fibrosis. *Am J Dis Child* 1980; 134:267–272.

212. Weitzenblum E, Sautegeau A, Ehrhart M, et al. Long-term oxygen therapy can reverse the progression of pulmonary hypertension in patients with chronic obstructive pulmonary disease. *Am Rev Respir Dis* 1985; 131:493–498.

213. Davis PB, di Sant'Agnese PA. Assisted ventilation for patients with cystic fibrosis. *JAMA* 1978; 239:1851–1854.

214. Higenbottam TW, Whitehead B. Heart-lung transplantation for cystic fibrosis. *J R Soc Med* 1991; 84:18–21.

215. Ramirez JC, Patterson GA, Winton TL, et al. Bilateral lung transplantation for cystic fibrosis. *J Thorac Cardiovasc Surg* 1992; 103:287–294.

216. Caine N, Sharples LD, Smyth R, et al. Survival and quality of life of cystic fibrosis patients before and after heart-lung transplantation. *Transplant Proc* 1991; 23:1203–1204.

217. Smyth RL, Scott JP, Higenbottam TW, et al. The use of heart-lung transplantation in management of terminal respiratory complications of cystic fibrosis. *Transplant Proc* 1990; 22:1472–1473.

218. Wood A, Higenbottam T, Jackson M, et al. Airway mucosal bioelectric potential difference in cystic fibrosis after lung transplantation. *Am Rev Respir Dis* 1989; 140:1645–1649.

219. Langford DT, Hiller J. Prospective, controlled study of a polyvalent pseudomonas vaccine in cystic fibrosis—Three year results. *Arch Dis Child* 1984; 59:1131–1134.

220. Pennington JE, Reynolds HY, Wood RE, et al. Use of a *Pseudomonas aeruginosa* vaccine in patients with acute leukemia and cystic fibrosis. *Am J Med* 1975; 58:628–636.

221. Beverley DW, Kelleher J, MacDonald A, et al. Comparison of four pancreatic extracts in cystic fibrosis. *Arch Dis Child* 1987; 62:564–568.

222. Stead RJ, Skypala I, Hodson ME, et al. Enteric coated microspheres with pancreatin in the treatment of cystic fibrosis: Comparison with a standard enteric–coated preparation. *Thorax* 1987; 42:533.

223. Constantini D, Padoan R, Curcio L, et al. The management of enzymatic therapy in cystic fibrosis patients by an individualized approach. *J Pediatr Gastroenterol Nutr* 1988; 7(Suppl 1)536–539.

224. Hubbard VS, Dunn GD, Lester LA. Effectiveness of cimetidine as an adjunct to supplemental pancreatic enzymes in patients with cystic fibrosis. *Am J Clin Nutr* 1980; 33:2281–2286.

225. Ganier M, Lieberman P. IgE mediated hypersensitivity to pancreatic extract (PE) in parents of cystic fibrosis (CF) children. *Clin Allergy* 1979; 9:125–132.

226. Daniels L, Davidson GP, Cooper DM. Assessment of nutrient intake of patients with cystic fibrosis compared with healthy children. *Hum Nutr Appl Nutr* 1987; 41A:151–159.

227. Roy CC, Darling P, Weber AM. A rational approach to meeting macro– and micronutrient needs in cystic fibrosis. *J Pediatr Gastroenterol* 1984; 3(Suppl 1)S154–S162.

228. Luder E, Kattan M, Tanzer-Torres G, et al. Current recommendations for breast-feeding in cystic fibrosis centers. *Am J Dis Child* 1990; 144:1153–1156.

229. Brennan J, Ellis L, Kalnins, et al. Do infants with cystic fibrosis and pancreatic insufficiency require a predigested formula? *Pediatr Pulmonol* 1991; 56:295–296.

230. Shepherd R, Cooksley WGE, Cooke WDD. Improved growth and clinical, nutritional, and respiratory changes in response to nutritional therapy in cystic fibrosis. *J Pediatr* 1980; 97:351–357.

231. Durie PR, Pencharz PB. A rational approach to the nutritional care of patients with cystic fibrosis. *J R Soc Med* 1989; 82(Suppl 16):11–20.

232. O'Loughlin E, Forbes D, Parsons H, et al. Nutritional rehabilitation of malnourished patients with cystic fibrosis. *Am J Clin Nutr* 1986; 43:732–737.

233. Levy LD, Durie PR, Pencharz PB, et al. Effects of long-term nutritional rehabilitation on body composition and clinical status in malnourished children and adolescents with cystic fibrosis. *J Pediatr* 1985; 107:225–230.

234. Shepherd RW, Holt TL, App B, et al. Nutritional rehabilitation in cystic fibrosis: Controlled studies of effects on nutritional growth retardation, body protein turnover, and course of pulmonary disease. *J Pediatr* 1986; 109:788–794.

235. Zempsky WT, Rosenstein BJ, Carroll JL, et al. Effect of pancreatic enzyme supplements on iron absorption. *Am J Dis Child* 1989; 143:969–972.

236. Noblett H. Treatment of uncomplicated meconium ileus by gastrografin enema: A preliminary report. *J Pediatr Surg* 1969; 4:190–197.

237. Wagget H, Bishop H, Koop E. Experience with gastrografin enema in the treatment of meconium ileus. *J Pediatr Surg* 1970; 5:649–654.

238. Meeker IA, Kincannon WN. Acetylcysteine used to liquefy inspissated meconium causing intestinal obstruction in the newborn. *Surgery* 1964; 56:419–425.

239. Cleghorn GJ, Stringer DA, Forstner GG, et al. Treatment of distal intestinal obstruction syndrome in cystic fibrosis with a balanced intestinal lavage solution. *Lancet* 1986; 1:8–11.

240. Koletzko S, Stringer DA, Cleghorn GJ, et al. Lavage treatment of distal intestinal obstruction syndrome in children with cystic fibrosis. *Pediatrics* 1989; 83:727–733.

241. Bendig DW, Seilheimer DK, Wagner ML, et al. Complications of gastroesophageal reflux in patients with cystic fibrosis. *J Pediatr* 1982; 100:536–540.

242. Koletzko S, Corey M, Ellis L, et al. Effects of cisapride in patients with cystic fibrosis and distal intestinal obstruction syndrome. *J Pediatr* 1990; 117:815–822.

243. Colombo C, Setchell KDR, Podda M, et al. Effects of ursodeoxycholic acid therapy for liver disease associated with cystic fibrosis. *J Pediatr* 1990; 117:482–489.

243a.Cotting J, Lentze MJ, Reichen J. Effects of ursodeoxycholic acid treatment on nutrition and liver function in patients with cystic fibrosis and long-standing cholestasis. *Gut* 1990; 31:918–921.

244. Salh B, Howat J, Webb K. Ursodeoxycholic acid dissolution of gallstones in cystic fibrosis. *Thorax* 1988; 43:490–491.

244a.Schuster SR, Shwachman H, Toyama WM, et al. The management of portal hypertension in cystic fibrosis. *J Pediatr Surg* 1977; 12:201–206.

245. Donovan TJ, Ward M, Sheperd RW. Evaluation of sclerotherapy of esophageal varices in children. *J Pediatr Gastroenterol Nutr* 1986; 5:696–700.

246. Mieles LA, Orenstein D, Teperman L, et al. Liver transplantation in cystic fibrosis. *Lancet* 1989; 1:1073.

247. Wilmott RW, Tyson SL, Matthew DJ. Cystic fibrosis survival rates. *Am J Dis Child* 1985; 139:669–671.

248. Campbell PW, Parker RA, Roberts BT, et al. Association of poor clinical status and heavy exposure to tobacco smoke in patients with cystic fibrosis who are homozygous for the (gd) F508 deletion. *Pediatrics* 1992; 120:261–264.

249. Rubin BK. Exposure of children with cystic fibrosis to environmental tobacco smoke. *N Engl J Med* 1990; 323:782–788.

250. Orenstein AM, Boat TF, Stern RC, et al. The effect of early diagnosis and treatment in cystic fibrosis: A seven-year study of 16 sibling pairs. *Am J Dis Child* 1977; 131:973–975.

251. Wood RE. Determinants of survival in cystic fibrosis. *Cystic Fibrosis Club Abstracts*, Rockville, MD, 1985; 26:69.

252. Shwachman H, Kulczyeki L. Long-term study of one hundred five patients with cystic fibrosis. *Am J Dis Child* 1958; 96:6–15.

253. Taussig LM, Kattwinkel J, Friedewald WT, et al. A new prognostic score and clinical evaluation system for cystic fibrosis. *J Pediatr* 1973; 82:380–390.

254. McColley SA, Rosenstein BJ, Cutting GR. Differences in expression of cystic fibrosis in blacks and whites. *Am J Dis Child* 1991; 145:94–97.

255. Stern RC, Doershuk CF, Boat TF. Course of cystic fibrosis in black patients. *J Pediatr* 1976; 89:412–417.

23

Bronchiolitis

VEDA L. ACKERMAN and PAUL S. SALVA

Bronchiolitis is an acute viral respiratory tract infection affecting the small airways of the young infant; it accounts for significant morbidity and mortality in this age group.

ETIOLOGY

The virus primarily responsible for bronchiolitis is respiratory syncytial virus (RSV), which is an RNA virus whose growth appears to be limited to the respiratory tract epithelium. Potency of RSV is increased by its ability to fuse cell membranes, thereby forming intracellular bridges that lead to the development of syncytia (multinucleated cells). These syncytia are particularly resistent to host defense mechanisms such as extracellular neutralizing antibodies. This negates the benefit of maternally acquired antibodies and allows reinfection to occur (1). Other viruses such as parainfluenza, adenovirus, rhinovirus, and influenza can produce a state that is clinically indistinguishable from that produced by RSV (2–4).

EPIDEMIOLOGY

Bronchiolitis occurs in annual epidemics, with the incidence peaking in mid-winter and early spring. Almost all children have been infected by age 3. The peak rate of hospitalization occurs in infants less than 6 months of age and in those who have underlying cardiorespiratory disease.

The severity of bronchiolitis is increased in infants with congenital heart disease or chronic pulmonary disease such as cystic fibrosis (CF) or bronchopulmonary dysplasia (BPD), with at least 50% of the mortality occurring in these infants. Other infants at risk include those with underlying immunodeficiency or suppression, neuromuscular disease, or inborn errors of metabolism (Table 23.1). Prematurity in itself is not a risk factor, but many prematurely born infants have chronic lung disease or immunosuppression, thus making them appear more at risk. Infants who live in crowded conditions, have multiple siblings, have not been breastfed, or have prenatal or postnatal exposure to tobacco smoke have a higher incidence of bronchiolitis. Though the rate of infection is the same in regard to gender, males experience a higher frequency of severe disease (5, 6).

Transmission of respiratory syncytial viral infections appears to occur primarily by direct contact with infected secretions. Attack rates are high, with 45% of family members becoming infected. Daycare transmission is thought to approach 98% in those infants previously uninfected (7). Hospitalized infants are at greatest risk, and nosocomial infection rates are directly related to the length of stay (8). It is important to remember that all persons infected with RSV become symptomatic, but that older children and adults tend to develop only upper respiratory symptoms, which are then misinterpreted as a simple "cold," thus promoting spread of the virus. Nosocomial transmission can be reduced by good hand

Table 23.1.
Risk Factors for Severe or Fatal RSV Infection

Congenital heart disease
Pulmonary disease
   Bronchopulmonary dysplasia
   Cystic fibrosis
Immunodeficiency
Immunosuppressive therapy
Inborn errors of metabolism
Neuromuscular disease or impairment

washing and cohorting of hospitalized infants. Viral shedding typically lasts 6–10 days, but may persist for several weeks in the very young or severely ill infant (9). Therefore contact isolation should continue for 30 days in the infant who remains hospitalized.

PATHOPHYSIOLOGY

The pathologic changes of bronchiolitis have been well characterized (10). Bronchiolitis is an infectious inflammation of bronchioles in the 75–300 μm diameter range. This invasion leads to necrosis of the respiratory epithelium and its sloughing into the airway lumen. A host inflammatory response ensues with migration and exudation of mononuclear cells consisting of lymphocytes, plasma cells, and macrophages. Tissue edema and mucus production occurs, resulting in thick plugs within the airway lumen. Pneumonia occurs when this process extends into the alveoli. Bronchiolitis has been associated with increased immunoglobulin E (IgE) levels in some but not all patients (11).

This process leads to a disruption of normal airflow. Some airways become partially occluded, leading to decreased airflow and air trapping; others become completely occluded, leading to atelectasis. These phenomena are quite characteristic of bronchiolitis and are accentuated because of the lack of collateral ventilation in the infant lung (12).

The findings on chest radiography are entirely consistent with the pathophysiology, and include bilateral perihilar and patchy parenchymal infiltrates, peribronchial cuffing, hyper-inflation with flattened diaphragms, atelectasis (commonly right middle lobe and right upper lobe subsegmental and segmental collapse), and emphysema (13).

The incidence of severe disease in otherwise normal infants correlates with size of the infant and the inoculum. In the younger infant, an inoculum of constant size could be expected to produce more significant illness because of the smaller lung volume and total number of alveoli. Also, infants living in crowded homes or with multiple siblings would be expected to receive a larger inoculum. The higher incidence of severe disease in males may be explained by the difference in lung growth reported between males and females, with females having proportionately larger airways relative to lung size (14) and therefore being less subject to obstruction of their small airways. Other possible explanations for an increased severity of disease in males may relate to differences in inherent immunity or host-defense responses in males versus females.

CLINICAL PRESENTATION

Bronchiolitis typically starts with a 1- to 3-day nonspecific viral upper respiratory infection (URI) prodrome consisting of rhinorrhea, congestion, cough, and at times a minor fever. For many children this is as far as the illness progresses. However, in a significant percentage of young toddlers and infants, the condition progresses to produce lower respiratory symptoms, giving the classic signs and symptoms of bronchiolitis (i.e., tachypnea, retractions, forced expiratory phase, rales, and high-pitched cough). Wheezing can occur but is a variable finding. Because bronchiolitis has multiple infectious etiologies, even during epidemics the physical findings are not homogeneous. The presence and severity of fever varies considerably, and otitis, conjunctivitis, and pharyngitis can also be present. Once lower respiratory symptoms appear they may worsen over 3–4 days, during which time tachypnea and dyspnea increase. Hypoxia is often present and commonly worse than the overall clinical appearance might suggest (15). Assessment of the infant with bronchiolitis should focus on the infant's chronologic and gestational age, the presence of underlying medical conditions, and the duration of illness. The physical examination will confirm the clinical history with abnormalities observed in the vital signs (particularly the respiratory rate) followed by signs of increased work of breathing (nasal flaring, retractions, use of accessory muscles). Altered mental status indicates hypoxia unless proven otherwise. Dehydration may develop in infants unable to feed because of respiratory distress (16).

The laboratory test that is easily available, noninvasive, and is the best predictor of severity of disease is the room air oxygen saturation test (17). In an otherwise normal infant, oxygen saturation of less than 95% on room air is a consistent predictor of severe disease. If the infant is sufficiently ill to be hospitalized, an arterial blood gas measurement is strongly recommended to assess the infant's ventilation and acid-base status.

In neonates and young infants the illness may present in a very atypical or rapidly evolving manner with minimal if any URI prodrome such that poor feeding, lethargy, and *apnea* may be the sole findings (18).

The incidence of apnea is inverse to age, with the youngest neonates at greatest risk. Apnea has been most closely correlated with RSV although other viruses (parainfluenza type 3, influenza A, rhinovirus, enteroviruses) have also been implicated. Patients with apnea tend to have higher cerebrospinal fluid (CSF) protein levels but it is not certain whether this is a cause or an effect. Bradycardia secondary to apnea or hyper-inflation may occur and is an ominous finding. Hyper-inflation triggers the Hering-Breuer reflex, resulting in vagally mediated bradycardia and increased respiratory rate due to stimulation of pulmonary stretch receptors. Because some infants less than 4 months old are obligate nose breathers, the usual nasal congestion and rhinorrhea seen in bronchiolitis can result in significant respiratory distress and fatigue. In addition, small infants have a more horizontally positioned, less efficient diaphragm, and a highly compliant chest wall. Thus, when hyper-inflation from air trapping occurs, they must generate increased respiratory effort to maintain effective alveolar ventilation. However, tidal volume may be decreased despite this effort because of collapse on inspiration of the highly compliant chest wall of the infant. Respiratory failure develops because of ineffective ventilation and evolving respiratory muscle fatigue.

DIAGNOSIS

Until recently, the diagnosis was based solely on clinical presentation because the identification of the specific virus responsible for a given case of bronchiolitis was limited to tertiary care centers with a large virology laboratory. The recent introduction of rapid viral diagnostic tests has made definitive testing more widely available.

Viral culture remains the gold standard, but is time-consuming and prone to error because of the lability of the RSV. Fluorescent antibody testing (RSV-FA) is rapid and has a high degree of sensitivity (61%) and specificity (89%) provided that an adequate specimen is obtained (19). Ideally, nasopharyngeal washings are used, and specimens that do not contain an adequate number of respiratory epithelial cells are rejected. An ELISA (enzyme-linked immunosorbent assay), which detects viral antigen, is reported to be as sensitive (69%) as tissue culture (72%) and highly specific (100%).

Clinical correlation remains crucial in making the diagnosis, although RSV-FA testing should be considered in all children who are hospitalized with bronchiolitis.

MANAGEMENT

Therapy for bronchiolitis remains primarily supportive, although for some selected individuals anti-viral therapy may be indicated. Specific management modalities to be considered include oxygen, fluid support, respiratory support, bronchodilators, steroids, and the antiviral agent ribavirin.

Oxygen Therapy

All patients with bronchiolitis have some impairment in oxygenation, and those who are ill enough to be hospitalized should be considered hypoxic until proven otherwise. Early studies have documented that oxygen therapy in bronchiolitis is helpful without inducing hypercarbia (20). Oxygen saturation can be determined by pulse oximetry and supplemental, humidified oxygen delivered to maintain O_2 saturations of at least 95%. It is important to remember that although oximetry is very helpful in assessing oxygenation, it does not assess ventilation, and thus a patient with an acceptable O_2 saturation may have a significant degree of hypercarbia and/or acidosis, which can only be documented by arterial blood gas analysis.

In addition, oxygen saturation does not measure actual oxygen delivery; thus, in an anemic infant, the oxygen saturation may be normal, despite an inadequate oxygen content.

Delivery of supplemental oxygen should use a humidified source, preferably a hood or a tent. Nasal cannulas should be used cautiously in small infants with URI symptoms, since nasal congestion may impede oxygen flow.

Fluid Support

Appropriate fluid balance is critical in infants with bronchiolitis. Infants may present with some degree of dehydration because of increased fluid losses from fever, tachypnea, and decreased oral intake. Dehydration can impair oxygenation by reducing perfusion to the lungs. However, overhydration of an infant with bronchiolitis may increase the risk of pulmonary edema from leakage through the injured alveolar capillary membranes, and further impair oxygenation by worsening ventilation perfusion mismatch. The rate of fluid administration should be based on the level of dehydration, with a goal of achieving isovolemia. Initially, oral feedings should be held in hospitalized infants who are tachypneic or exhibit increased work of breathing, in order to decrease the risk of aspiration. Once the respiratory status has stabilized, enteral feedings can be instituted in order to provide adequate caloric intake. Orogastric tubes may be required in the infant who remains too tachypneic to suck, but caution must be observed to prevent aspiration.

Respiratory Support

Infants with bronchiolitis are at significant risk of developing respiratory failure from fatigue and therefore require close monitoring of their ventilatory status. At particular risk are the very young, with a reported incidence of respiratory failure as high as 40% of infants less than 8 weeks of age who were hospitalized for bronchiolitis (17). Infants and children with underlying cardiac or pulmonary diseases are also at increased risk for respiratory failure, and may require early intervention with assisted ventilation. All hospitalized infants in the early stage of their disease should have continuous cardiac and apnea monitoring. Unless an infant has very mild disease, a baseline arterial blood sample is advisable to document P_{CO_2} and pH. Blood gas analysis should be repeated frequently as indicated by the clinical course. A change in status such as a sudden increase or decrease in respiratory rate, paradoxical breathing, or acute cyanosis, or if the infant has an oxygen requirement of 60% or greater, is an indication for repeated arterial blood gas analysis.

Interpretation of blood gas data requires close attention to the P_{CO_2} in relation to the degree of tachypnea, since an infant may not develop hypercarbia until immediately prior to respiratory arrest. Thus an infant breathing 90 times/minute with a P_{CO_2} of 45 is in respiratory failure, since the expected P_{CO_2} should

be in the low 30s. General guidelines are as follows:

P_{CO_2} less than 40 and respiratory rate less than 60: Monitor closely on ward.

P_{CO_2} 40–50: Monitor in pediatric intensive care unit or consider transfer to tertiary care center; place arterial line if possible for frequent blood gas analysis.

P_{CO_2} 50 or more: Consider intubation and assisted ventilation, especially if acidotic or extremely tachypneic (rate > 80).

It is important to establish an airway and assist ventilation before frank respiratory failure ensues, especially in the child with underlying cardiac disease, since these infants may not have adequate cardiac reserve to survive a respiratory arrest.

Infants who require mechanical ventilation for respiratory failure may be challenging to ventilate because of bronchospasm and air trapping. These infants generally require a short inspiratory time with a long expiratory time to allow for their prolonged expiratory phase, usually an inspiration/expiration ratio of at least 1:4. If this longer expiratory phase is not achieved, stacking of breaths can occur leading to increased air-trapping and CO_2 retention. Many infants require neuromuscular blockade and sedation to decrease ventilator-patient asynchrony and provide adequate oxygenation and ventilation. Barotrauma is fairly common, and any child with an acute deterioration should be considered to have a pneumothorax and appropriately evaluated and treated. Newer trends in ventilatory management of patients with air flow obstruction or acute lung injury suggest improvements in both mortality and morbidity through the use of controlled hypercarbia from relative hypoventilation (21). This lowering of tidal volume decreases mean airway pressure and may prevent iatrogenic deterioration of lung function (22). Although pediatric data are scarce (23), it seems reasonable to accept a P_{CO_2} in the 50–60 mm Hg range, provided that the pH is reasonably well compensated and the infant is hemodynamically stable.

Bronchodilator Therapy

The use of bronchodilators in acute bronchiolitis has long been controversial. Early studies failed to demonstrate an effect of beta agonists on pulmonary resistance in bronchiolitis (23, 25). These studies did not assess measurements of oxygenation or clinical work of breathing and thus may have failed to detect significant clinical improvement. Furthermore, since the clinical course of bronchiolitis is variable, the relative degree of bronchial hypersecretion versus bronchospasm versus inflammation may determine the response to bronchodilators in a specific patient. Recent data support the long-held clinical impression that bronchodilator therapy can be effective. Soto et al. demonstrated an improvement in specific conductance in 15 of 50 infants (30%) with RSV bronchiolitis. Potential responders could not be identified by sex, age, weight, family history of asthma or atopy, or passive smoke exposure (26). Severity of illness is not well documented except to show no difference in degree of illness between responders and nonresponders. In more severely afflicted infants who required mechanical ventilation, Mallory et al. were able to document airway reactivity that responded to bronchodilators in 13 of 14 infants as assessed by deflation flow-volume curves (27).

Schuh et al. describe a population of young infants (mean age 6 months) who clearly demonstrated improvement in accessory muscle use and oxygen saturation as compared to a placebo control group (28). Although Klassen et al. could not show improved oxygenation in the same age group, clinical scores were shown to be significantly improved (29). Klassen et al.'s group received a smaller dose of albuterol (0.10 mg/kg/dose versus 0.15 mg/kg/dose), which may explain this lack of improvement in oxygenation. A lack of demonstrable response may also be due to increased severity of bronchospasm and inflammation, as seen in status asthmaticus where continued administration of beta agonists will ultimately result in a good clinical response. Thus, initial failure to improve with bronchodilator therapy may not preclude a good clinical response if therapy is maintained.

Dosing of albuterol should be based on infant weight and clinical response. Nebulized albuterol, with oxygen as the source gas, should be given at 0.15 mg (0.03 ml)/kg/dose with a maximum dose of 5 mg (1 ml) as frequently as every hour with close observation for tachycardia. Frequency should be decreased as clinical improvement dictates. Oxygen saturation should be monitored continuously if aerosols are more frequent than every 3 hours because of the risk of inducing greater vasodilatation than bronchodilation, resulting in ventilation-perfusion mismatch and worsening of hypoxia (30). Frequent high dose use can also lead to an intracellular shift of potassium, producing hypokalemia.

Although the use of nebulized beta-2 agonists such as albuterol is now recommended, there are currently no well-controlled studies evaluating the use of theophylline in bronchiolitis. Given the narrow therapeutic range and the well-documented multiple adverse effects of theophylline, its use in bronchiolitis should be restricted to the critically ill infant who does not respond to frequent nebulized beta-2 agents such as albuterol. Theophylline should be discontinued if significant tachycardia or irritability develop or if there is not a clear and ongoing response.

If theophylline is used, it is critical to adjust the dosing for its highly variable half-life in the young infant. Additionally, infants with bronchiolitis are documented to have altered theophylline pharmacokinetics (31). An initial dose of a 5 mg/kg intravenous bolus, followed by an initial drip rate of 0.5 mg/kg/hour, may be used with appropriate adjustments as indicated by serum levels.

Corticosteroids

Since acute inflammation is a primary component of bronchiolitis, one would expect corticosteroid therapy to be helpful. Large, controlled studies have failed to document the efficacy of corticosteroids, but these studies were done prior to the development of pulse oximetry and infant pulmonary function techniques, and thus their outcome variables may not have been sensitive enough to detect a response (32). Tal et al. did show that infants treated with a combination of salbutamol and dexamethasone had a significantly greater improvement in clinical scores than infants treated with placebo, salbutamol alone, or dexamethasone alone. This may be due to the known potentiating effect of corticosteroids on the beta adrenergic receptors (33). A more recent study by Springer et al., employing measurements of pulmonary function, also failed to document any change in rate of improvement between the steroid-treated and control groups (34). In view of the multiple adverse effects of corticosteroids, it seems prudent to limit steroid use to a select group of patients who require prolonged ventilatory support or hospitalization secondary to copious airway secretions and bronchospasm. The use of steroids may also be beneficial in infants already known to have increased airway reactivity (35). It is particularly important to avoid steroids in the very young infant whose immature immune system is already compromised, thus increasing their risk of obtaining a potentially life-threatening nosocomial infection (36).

Ribavirin

Since its introduction to clinical use, therapy with ribavirin has been controversial. Ribavirin is a synthetic nucleotide that has in-vitro viricidal activity against RSV when delivered by small particle nebulization. The initial published studies documented improved severity scores, improved oxygenation (but not resolution of hypoxia), and reduced viral shedding (Table 23.2) (37–43). These studies have been criticized for errors in design and the small number of patients who received active drug. Guidelines for use of ribavirin were developed by the Academy of Pediatrics, which stated that "ribavirin therapy is recommended" in those patients at risk for severe or fatal disease (44) (Table 23.3). Unfortunately, the vast majority of the initial studies only evaluated previously normal infants, thus leaving efficacy for the child at high risk poorly documented. Additionally, because many of the infants at risk required mechanical ventilation, efficacy for this group of patients was unknown. A single small but well-designed, placebo-controlled study of the use of ribavirin in infants who required mechanical ventilation—both previously normal infants and infants with underlying cardiopulmonary disease—did document a reduction in the number of days requiring mechanical ventilation and in the number of days requiring supplemental oxygen (45). In addition, the previously normal infants, but not the infants with underlying diseases, had shorter hospital stays. All of the ribavirin studies used ultrasonically nebulized water as a placebo, which itself has been shown to induce bronchoconstriction in some individuals (46).

Other concerns regarding the use of ribavirin have centered on the potential teratogenic risk to the patient and to the health care provider. Studies of pregnant rodents fed large oral doses of ribavirin have documented fetal malformations and fetal loss, whereas studies of pregnant baboons exposed to aerosolized ribavirin did not reveal any fetal abnormalities (44). Risks to the health care provider are more difficult to quantitate. Studies of environmental exposure have revealed minimal to no absorption of active drug by providers. Rodriguez et al. found no adverse or toxic effects and no ribavirin in red cells, plasma, or urine from 19 nurses who cared for infants receiving ribavirin (47). A separate study by the Occupational Health group in California did document the presence of ribavirin in the red cells of a single caretaker out of 10 studied. The current recommendations regarding health care providers suggest that pregnant caretakers or those trying to become pregnant not provide direct care to patients receiving ribavirin and that aerosol administration be stopped whenever the hood is open (44). There is no evidence that further precautions are indicated at this time. The physical barriers imposed between patient and caregiver when ribavirin is used are considerable. The infant is already in respiratory isolation; the addition of a drug with potential adverse effects to the staff, and the isolation measures to combat this, further reduces the all-important human observation of the infant's clinical status.

Ribavirin should be reserved for use in the more severely ill child, in the child with an underlying disease increasing his or her risk for severe infection, and in those infants who require mechanical ventilation for respiratory failure. *Routine therapy for the previously healthy child with mild to moderate disease cannot be recommended at this time.* The documented decrease in viral shedding may also contribute to consideration of the use of ribavirin during severe epidemics with significant nosocomial spread.

Administration of ribavirin requires the use of a small particle aerosol generator (SPAG), which is supplied with the drug, through a hood or tent. The dose is constant at 6 g dissolved in 300 ml of sterile water nebulized over 12–18 hours for 3–7 days, based on the clinical response. Although administration of ribavirin through a ventilator circuit is not

Table 23.2.
Ribavirin Studies

Investigator	Patient Population	Results	Limitations
Hall	23 normal infants	Improved severity scores Improved oxygenation	Vague entry criteria Duration of therapy not well controlled Spontaneous improvement in placebo group before treatment Use of placebo that could potentially worsen bronchospasm
Taber	26 normal infants	Improved severity scores	No measure of severity at entry
Hall	13 infants with underlying illness	Increased rate of improvement	Statistical analysis questioned Same limitations as first study
Barry	26 normal infants	Increased rate of improvement (cough/rates)	Did stratify by severity Authors do not recommend routine use based on modest improvement
Rodriguez	30 normal infants	Improved severity scores	Modeled on Hall study with same limitations
Conrad	33 infants with underlying illness 97 untreated infants	Increased rate of improvement	Nonblinded, nonrandomized study
Groothius	47 infants with BPD or congenital heart disease	Improved analog score Improved oxygenation	Scoring again may be subjective with observer variability Placebo may induce bronchoconstriction
Smith	21 normal infants 7 with underlying disease (all required mechanical ventilation)	Decreased duration of mechanical ventilation Improved oxygenation Decreased hospital stay in normal infants only	Small sample size Placebo may not be benign

Table 23.3.
Indications for Ribavirin Therapy of Respiratory Syncytial Virus Infection

Infants at risk for severe or complicated disease

Congenital heart disease
Bronchopulmonary dysplasia
Cystic fibrosis
Immunodeficiency
Immunosuppression

Infants who are severely ill

Significant hypoxia
Hypercarbia

Infants at risk of progressing to severe disease

Multiple congenital anomalies
Neurologic disease
Metabolic disease

Infants who require mechanical ventilation for respiratory failure

recommended by the manufacturer, this can be safely accomplished provided that scrupulous attention is paid to cleansing of the filters and expiratory tubing. Ribavirin tends to crystalize, and thus can potentially plug off the filters, the tubing, or even the artificial airway, leading to life-threatening complications. Ventilator circuits and filters should be changed at least every 24 hours, and artificial airways should be watched closely for occlusion.

Although there are no reported major adverse effects associated with ribavirin administration, we and others have seen some infants, especially those with underlying lung disease such as bronchopulmonary dysplasia, develop severe, acute bronchospasm, presumably secondary to the aerosol delivery. The literature does report anemia with oral administration of ribavirin, but this has not been noted with aerosolized administration. Long-term effects of ribavirin are unknown at this time.

COMPLICATIONS

Complications of acute bronchiolitis include nosocomial or secondary infection, spontaneous pneumothorax, and the development or worsening of chronic lung disease. Secondary or co-infection occurs from other viruses and from bacterial pathogens, most commonly *Streptococcus pneumonia* and *Hemophilus influenzae* (48, 49). Infants who are younger at presentation or who present with significant fever and elevated white blood counts appear to be at increased risk. Infants who require intensive care also have a higher incidence of nosocomial infection that may be related to the need for invasive devices such as arterial catheters and endotracheal intubation. There is no evidence that pretreatment with antibiotics is beneficial. One study suggests a negative effect of antibiotic therapy (50). Antibiotic treatment should be limited to those infants with positive culture or for the critically ill infant with a high fever and elevated white blood count with immature neutrophils.

Spontaneous pneumothorax occurs in infants with bronchiolitis because of air-trapping and narrowed airways (51). The likelihood of air leaks in those infants requiring mechanical ventilation is similarly increased. Except for the very small, spontaneous, non-tension pneumothorax, most cases will require therapy with a chest tube.

The development or worsening of chronic lung disease can occur after any acute lung injury with a large inflammatory component. Infants who are very young or infants with mild BPD are at particular risk to have a protracted course requiring supplemental oxygen and other therapy for long periods.

PROGNOSIS AND LONG-TERM SEQUELAE

The long-term outcome for children who develop moderate to severe bronchiolitis in early childhood is far from normal. Although mortality is generally limited to infants with other concurrent disease processes, the morbidity is widespread and long-lasting. These children are predisposed to recurrent episodes of wheezing, especially if there is a family history of asthma, leading some clinicians to postulate that it was inherent airway hyper-reactivity that predisposed these infants to develop more severe disease, rather than acute lung injury from the infection itself (52, 53). The incidence of recurrent wheezing exceeds 50% in patients with bronchiolitis, and may reach 75% in infants with a family history of reactive airways.

Pulmonary function testing of older children who had documented bronchiolitis during infancy has demonstrated persistent airway hyper-reactivity and impairment of small airway function (54). More recent studies of infants have shown persistence of abnormalities in pulmonary function parameters and in the presence of hyper-inflation for at least 3–6 months after infection (55).

REFERENCES

1. Henderson FW, Collier AM, Clyde WA, Denny FW. Respiratory syncytial virus infections, reinfections and immunity. *N Engl J Med* 1979; 300:530–534.
2. Nohynek H, Eskola J, Laine E, Halonen P, Riwtu P, Saikku P, Kleemola M, Leinonen M. The causes of hospital treated acute lower respiratory tract infection in children. *Am J Dis Child* 1991; 145:618–622.
3. Schmidt HJ, Fink RJ. *Rhinovirus* as a lower respiratory tract pathogen in infants. *Pediatr Infect Dis J* 1991; 10:700–702.
4. Henderson FW, Clyde WA, Collier AM, Denny FW. The etiologic and epidemiologic spectrum of bronchiolitis in pediatric practice. *J Pediatr* 1979; 95:183–190.
5. Carlsen K, Larsen S, Bjerve O, Lecgaard J. Acute bronchiolitis: Predisposing factors and characterization of infants at risk. *Pediatr Pulmonol* 1987; 3:153–160.
6. Glezen WP, Paredes A, Allison JE, Taber AL. Risk of RSV infection for infants from low-income families in relationship to age, sex, ethnic group and maternal antibody level. *J Pediatr* 1981; 98:708–715.
7. Loda FA, Glezen WP, Clyde WA. Respiratory disease in group daycare. *Pediatrics* 1972; 49:428–437.
8. Avendano LF, Larranaga C, Palomino MA, Gaggero A, Montaldo G. Suarez M, Diaz A. Community and hospital-acquired respiratory syncytial virus infections in Chile. *Pediatr Infect Dis J* 1991; 10:564–568.
9. Hall CB, Douglas RG, Germon JM. Respiratory syncytial viral infection in infants. Quantitation 10 and duration of shedding. *J Pediatr* 1976; 89:11–15.
10. Aherne W, Bird T, Court SDM, Gardner PS, McQuillin J. Pathological changes in virus infections of the lower respiratory tract in children. *J Clin Pathol* 1970; 23:7–18.
11. Polmar SH, Robinson LD, Minnefor AB. Immunoglobulin E in bronchiolitis. *Pediatrics* 1972; 50:279–284.
12. Murray JF. *The normal lung.* Philadelphia, WB Saunders, 1986.
13. Simpson W, Hacking PM, Court SDM, Gardner PS. The radiological findings in respiratory syncytial

virus infection in children. II. The correlation of radiological categories with clinical and virological findings. *Pediatr Radiol* 1974; 2:155–160.

14. Tepper RS, Morgan WJ, Cota K, Wright A, Taussig LM, GHMA Pediatricians. Physiologic growth and development of the lung during the first year of life. *Am Rev Respir Dis* 1986; 134:513–519.

15. Hall CB, Hall WJ, Speers DM. Clinical and physiological manifestations of bronchiolitis and pneumonia. *Am J Dis Child* 1979; 133:798–802.

16. Shaw KN, Bell LM, Sherman NH. Outpatient assessment of infants with bronchiolitis. *Am J Dis Child* 1991; 145:151–155.

17. McMillan JA, Tristram DA, Weiner LB, Higgins AP, Sandstrom C, Brandon R. Prediction of the duration of hospitalization in patients with respiratory syncytial virus infection: Use of clinical parameters. *Pediatrics* 1988; 81:22–26.

18. Anas N, Boettrich C, Hall CB, Brooks JG. The association of apnea and respiratory syncytial virus infection in infants. *J Pediatr* 1982; 101:65–68.

19. Ahluwalia G, Embree J, McNicol P, Law B, Hammond GW. Comparison of nasopharyngeal aspirate and nasopharyngeal swab specimens for RSV diagnosis by cell culture, indirect immunofluorescence assay, and enzyme-linked immunosorbent assay. *J Clin Microb* 1987; 25:763–767.

20. Reynolds, EOR. The effect of breathing 40 percent oxygen on the arterial blood gas tensions of babies with bronchiolitis. *J Pediatr* 1963; 63:1135.

21. Hickling K, Henderson S, Jackson R. Low mortality associated with low volume pressure limited ventilation with permissive hypercapnia in severe adult respiratory distress syndrome. *Intensive Care Med* 1990; 16:372–377.

22. Marini J, Kelsen S. Re–targeting ventilatory objectives in adult respiratory distress syndrome. *Am Rev Respir Dis* 1992; 146:2–3.

23. Reynolds A, Ryan D, Doody D. Permissive hypercapnia and pressure–controlled ventilation as treatment of severe adult respiratory distress syndrome in a pediatric burn patient. *Crit Care Med* 1993; 21:468–471.

24. Phelan P, Williams H. Sympathomimetic drugs in acute viral bronchiolitis. *Pediatrics* 1969; 44:493–497.

25. Rutter N, Milner A, Hiller E. Effects of bronchodilators on respiratory resistance in infants and young children with bronchiolitis and wheezy bronchitis. *Arch Dis Child* 1975; 50:719–723.

26. Soto ME, Sly PD, Uren E, Taussig LM, Landau LI. Bronchodilator response during acute viral bronchiolitis in infancy. *Pediatr Pulmonol* 1985; 2:85–90.

27. Mallory G, Motoyama E, Koumbourilis A, Mutich R, Nakayama D. Bronchial reactivity in infants in acute respiratory failure with viral bronchiolitis. *Pediatr Pulmonol* 1989; 6:253–259.

28. Schuh S, Canny G, Reisman JJ, Kerem E, Bentur L, Petric M, Levison H. Nebulized albuterol in acute bronchiolitis. *J Pediatr* 1990; 117:633–637.

29. Klassen TP, Rowe PC, Sutcliffe T, Rapp LJ, McDowell IW, Li MM. Randomized trial of salbutamol in acute bronchiolitis. *J Pediatr* 1991; 118:807–811.

30. Prendiville A, Rose A, Maxwell DL, Silverman M. Hypoxaemia in wheezy infants after bronchodilator treatment. *Arch Dis Child* 1987; 62:997–1000.

31. Franko TG, Powell DA, Nahata MC. Pharmacokinetics of theophylline in infants with bronchiolitis. *Eur J Clin Pharmacol* 1982; 23:123–127.

32. Leer JA, Green JL, Heimlich EM, Hyde JS, Moffett HL, Young GA, Barron BA. Corticosteroid treatment in bronchiolitis: A controlled collaborative study in 297 infants and children. *Am J Dis Child* 1969; 117:495.

33. Tal A, Bavilski C, Yohai D, Bearman J, Gorodischer R, Moses S. Dexamethasone and salbutamol in the treatment of acute wheezing in infants. *Pediatrics* 1983; 71:13–18.

34. Springer C, Bar-Tishay E, Uwayyed K, Avital A, Vilogni D, Godrey S. Corticosteroids do not affect the clinical or physiological status of infants with bronchiolitis. *Pediatr Pulmonol* 1990; 9:181–185.

35. Driverman EJ, Neijens HJ, van Strik R, Affourtit MJ, Kerrebyn KF. Lung function and bronchial responsiveness in children who had infantile bronchiolitis. *Pediatr Pulmonol* 1987; 3:38–44.

36. Rizvi ZB, Halina AS, Myers TF, Zeller WP, Fisher SG, Anderson CL. Effects of dexamethasone on the hypothalamic-pituitary axis in preterm infants. *J Pediatr* 1992; 120:961–965.

37. Hall CB, McBride JT, Walsh EE, et al. Aerosolized ribavirin treatment of infants with respiratory syncytial viral infection. *N Engl J Med* 1983; 308:1443–1447.

38. Taber LH, Knight V, Gilbert BE, et al. Ribavirin aerosol treatment of bronchiolitis associated with respiratory syncytial virus infection in infants. *Pediatrics* 1983; 72:613–618.

39. Hall CB, McBride JT, Gala CL, et al. Ribavirin treatment of respiratory syncytial viral infection in infants with underlying cardiopulmonary disease. *JAMA* 1985; 254:3047–3051.

40. Barry W, Cockburn F, Cornall R, et al. Ribavirin aerosol for acute bronchiolitis. *Arch Dis Child* 1986; 61:593–597.

41. Rodriguez WJ, Kim WH, Brandt CD, et al. Aerosolized ribavirin in the treatment of patients with respiratory syncytial virus disease. *Pediatr Inf Dis J* 1987; 6:159–163.

42. Conrad DA, Christenson JC, Waner JL, Marks MI. Aerosolized ribavirin treatment of respiratory syncytial virus infection in infants hospitalized during an epidemic. *Pediatr Infect* Dis J 1987; 6:152–158.

43. Groothuis JR, Woodin KA, Katz R, Robertson AD, McBride JT, Hall CB, McWilliams BC, Lauer BA. Early ribavirin treatment of respiratory syncytial viral infection in high-risk children. *J Pediatr* 1990; 117:792–798.

44. Report of the Committee on Infectious Diseases. Use of ribavirin in the treatment of respiratory syncytial virus infection. *Pediatrics* 1993; 92:501–504.

45. Smith DW, Frankel LR, Mathers LH, Tang ATS, Ariagno RL, Prober CG, A controlled trial of aerosolized ribavirin in infants receiving mechanical ventilation for severe respiratory syncytial virus infection. *N Engl J Med* 1991; 325:24–29.

46. Sheppard D, Rizk NW, Boushey HA, Bethel RA. Mechanism of cough and bronchoconstriction induced by distilled water aerosol. *Am Rev Respir Dis* 1983; 127:691–694.

47. Rodriguez WJ, Dang Bui RH, Connor JD, Kim HW, Brandt CD, Parrott RH, Burch B, Mace J. Environ-

mental exposure of primary care personnel to ribavirin aerosol when supervising treatment of infants with respiratory syncytial virus infections. *Antimicrobr Agents Chemother* 1987; 31:1143–1146.

48. Tristram DA, Miller RW, McMillan JA, Weiner LB. Simultaneous infection with respiratory syncytial virus and other respiratory pathogens. *Am J Dis Child* 1988; 142:834–836.

49. Korppi M. Leinonen M, Koskela M, Makela PH, Launiala K. Bacterial coinfection in children hospitalized with respiratory syncytial virus infections. *Pediatr Infect Dis* J 1989; 8:687–692.

50. Hall CB, Powell KR, Schnabel KC, Gala CL, Pincus PH. Risk of secondary bacterial infection in infants hospitalized with respiratory syncytial viral infection. *J Pediatr* 1988; 113:266–271.

51. Pollack J. Spontaneous bilateral pneumothorax in an infant with bronchiolitis. *Pediatr Emergency Care* 1987; 3:33–35.

52. Young S, LeSouef PN, Geelhoed GC, Stick SM, Turner KJ, Landau LI. The influence of a family hisotry of asthma and parental smoking on airway responsiveness in early infancy. *N Engl J Med* 1991; 324:1168–1173.

53. Martinez FD, Morgan WJ, Wright AL, Holberg CJ, Taussig LM. Diminished lung function as a predisposing factor for wheezing respiratory illness in infants. *N Engl J Med* 1988; 319:1112–1117.

54. Pullan CR, Hey EN. Wheezing, asthma and pulmonary dysfunction 10 years after infection with respiratory syncytial virus in infancy. *Br Med J* 1982; 284:1665–1669.

55. Tepper RS, Rosenberg D, Eigen H. Airway responsiveness in infants following bronchiolitis. *Pediatr Pulmonol* 1992; 13:6–10.

24

Bronchitis

KAREN L. DAIGLE and MICHELLE M. CLOUTIER

ACUTE BRONCHITIS

Definition and Epidemiology

Acute tracheobronchitis (bronchitis) is defined as a transient inflammation of the lower airways from the distal trachea to the medium and large-sized bronchi. The pharynx and nasopharynx are also frequently involved but the laryngeal and subglottic regions are usually spared. In the immunocompetent pediatric host, this acute inflammatory process is usually caused by viral infection or by *Mycoplasma pneumoniae* (1). Primary bacterial infections are rare. The major symptom of acute bronchitis is cough, which usually resolves within 2 weeks. As with most respiratory viral infections, the peak incidence is winter and early spring. The attack rate is higher for males than for females, especially for children less than 9 years of age (1–4).

Etiology

The etiologic agents that most commonly cause acute bronchitis are listed in Table 24.1. The frequency with which these agents cause disease varies with age. In a study by Chapman and associates (1), parainfluenzae and respiratory syncytial virus were most often the cause

Table 24.1.
Etiologic Agents of Acute Bronchitis

Viral	Non-Viral
Adenovirus	Mycoplasma pneumoniae
Influenza A, B	Bordetella pertussis
Parainfluenza, type 3	Chlamydia trachomatis
Respiratory syncytial virus	Corynebacterium diphtheriae
Rhinovirus	

in children less than 6 years of age. For those less than 2 years of age, adenovirus was also frequently found. Influenza usually produced illness in older children (> 6 years). It is worth noting that rhinoviruses may cause a bronchitis-like illness, particularly in patients with airway hyper-responsiveness (2).

Mycoplasma pneumoniae is the most common nonviral etiology of acute bronchitis. The frequency of infection with *M. pneumoniae* is minimal in patients younger than 2 years, then steadily increases with age, reaching a peak in school-age children (1, 5, 6). Younger children are more likely to develop mild upper respiratory tract infections or tracheobronchitis, whereas pneumonia is much more common in older children.

Other nonviral etiologies of respiratory infection that cause or mimic acute bronchitis include *Bordetella pertussis*, *Corynebacterium diphtheriae*, and *Chlamydia trachomatis* (7, 8). Each is associated with a well-defined clinical syndrome in a specific host.

Pertussis is a disease of un-immunized children; the majority of cases occur by 12 months of age. The pathogenesis of this infection involves adherence of the bacteria to ciliated cells of the respiratory epithelium, causing abundant, tenacious secretions and impairment of mucociliary clearance. This gives rise to the three clinical stages of the disease (7). The initial or catarrhal stage is marked by mild upper respiratory symptoms and minimal cough. During the paroxysmal phase, secretions and airway edema increase, obstructing the airways. This obstruction results in cough paroxysms and the classic inspiratory "whoop." Apnea and cyanosis may occur, especially in young infants. The convalescent stage is characterized by chronic, nonparoxysmal cough that may persist for 4 weeks or longer.

Corynebacterium diphtheriae infects primarily unimmunized or partially immunized individuals. Like pertussis, diphtheria is also a disease characterized by damage to respiratory epithelium and elaboration of thick, organizing secretions. The most common clinical presentation is localized pseudomembranous tonsillopharyngitis. Occasionally, there is involvement of the larynx and trachea, which produces stridor and croup-like cough (7).

Infants less than 6 months of age are susceptible to infection with *Chlamydia trachomatis*, a perinatally acquired organism (3, 8). There is insidious onset of respiratory symptoms, usually a staccato cough and tachypnea in the absence of fever. Diffuse crackles are often found on chest examination, and wheezing is rare. Conjunctivitis may not be associated or may have already resolved. The presence of blood eosinophilia is helpful in making the diagnosis (3). The symptoms of a *Chlamydia* infection may be similar to those due to other infections (cytomegalovirus, *Pneumocystis carinii*, and *Ureaplasma urealyticum*) also encountered in young infants (9).

Pathology

Because of the low mortality associated with acute bronchitis, limited pathologic material is available for review. Findings consistent with the characteristic, nonspecific response of the airways to viral infection have been reported (10). This response includes desquamation of ciliated epithelium, mucosal congestion, increased mucus gland activity, and infiltration by neutrophils into the airway wall and lumen. These findings account for the production of sputum, which may appear purulent, even in the absence of bacterial infection. The loss of the ciliated epithelium disrupts mucociliary transport and contributes to secondary bacterial infection (11) and greater accessibility of cough receptors. Recovery of ciliated cells usually occurs within 5–7 days (11).

Clinical Manifestations

Cough is the primary symptom of acute bronchitis, and its characteristics change as the syndrome progresses. The initial phase of illness is marked by minimal cough but significant upper respiratory symptoms associated with rhinitis or nasopharyngitis. This typically lasts 3–5 days. Over the next week, symptoms of lower airway involvement and generalized illness appear. Cough in this phase is initially dry and brassy but eventually becomes loose and more productive. The patient usually has a low-grade fever. The cough may be so severe as to produce chest pain and/or post-tussive emesis. During the recovery phase of the next 7–10 days, fever resolves and the cough subsides as mucociliary clearance improves. However, the cough remains productive. A secondary bacterial infection should be considered when symptoms, especially fever, recur or persist beyond 2 weeks. Those bacteria implicated in secondary infection of viral bronchitis include *Hemophilus influenzae*, *Streptococcus pneumoniae*, and *Staphylococcus aureus* (12, 13).

Findings on physical examination vary with the phase of illness. Initially, involvement of the upper respiratory tract, particularly the nose, is predominant; the chest examination may be unremarkable. As the disease progresses, upper tract involvement decreases and lower tract signs are more prominent. Fever is frequently found and cough is always present. Auscultation reveals rhonchi and less frequently, coarse crackles. Wheezing may be evident, especially in patients with or predisposed to asthma.

A chest radiograph is usually normal but may show peribronchial thickening. In the later stages of more severe disease, atelectasis may result, which may be difficult to distinguish from pneumonia.

A specific etiologic diagnosis of acute bronchitis can be made by recovery of virus from nasopharyngeal secretions. *Mycoplasma pneumoniae* infection is suggested by the presence of cold agglutinins and confirmed by a positive throat culture or an increase in specific serum titers. Alternatively, the probable causative agent can be suspected based on the patient's age, season of the year (Table 24.2), and the presence of any concurrent epidemic infection in the community. If a secondary infection complicates the initial viral bronchitis, a specimen of airway secretions for culture can be obtained in several ways. Older, cooperative children may be able to produce a sputum sample. This should be checked to make certain that it is not contaminated by oral secre-

25

Bronchiectasis

PAUL C. STILLWELL

Bronchiectasis is defined as dilated bronchi, associated with varying degrees of acute and chronic inflammation as well as fibrosis (Fig. 25.1). Often the bronchioles are affected as well. With advanced disease, an increase in the bronchial vessels and microabscesses may develop in the peribronchial supporting structures (Fig. 25.2) (1). Bronchiectasis is becoming less common as treatment for acute lower respiratory tract infections improves and immunization programs decrease the frequency of pertussis and measles. Nevertheless, it remains a frequent problem in pediatrics as the final common pathway of several different lower respiratory tract insults (Table 25.1) (1–3).

PATHOGENESIS

With the exception of the congenital form, bronchiectasis begins after an acute airway injury such as infection or aspiration of gastric contents. In patients who have no existing impairment of the mucociliary escalator,

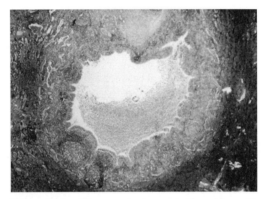

Figure 25.2. Microscopic demonstration of bronchiectasis following obstruction from a retained foreign body (resection specimen). The bronchial architecture and epithelium are disrupted and there is prominent inflammation of the bronchial walls.

either a single severe injury or multiple recurrent injuries may cause damage to the airway walls. Table 25.1 lists the causes of bronchiectasis; the common theme among these diverse diseases is a risk for recurrent and chronic airway damage, usually from recurrent infection. Once the bronchial architecture is sufficiently altered the local mucociliary transport becomes abnormal. Chronic bacterial colonization follows, usually with low-virulence pathogens. In diseases with impaired mucociliary clearance such as cystic fibrosis (CF) or ciliary dyskinesia, bacterial colonization becomes recurrent and chronic, independent of airway wall damage. In either case, this sets up a vicious cycle of inflammation, tissue destruction from the products of inflammation, and further impairment of mucociliary transport (4–6), contributing to the chronic inability to sterilize the airways (7, 8). The distended and floppy airway walls collapse

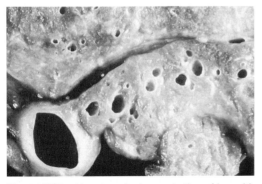

Figure 25.1. Macroscopic demonstration of bronchiectasis following a severe viral lower respiratory tract infection (autopsy specimen). The bronchi are markedly dilated both centrally and peripherally.

Table 25.1.
Etiology of Bronchiectasis

Idiopathic

Congenital

Deficient bronchial cartilage (Williams-Campbell
   syndrome)
Congenital tracheobronchomegaly (Mounier-Kuhn
   syndrome)
Yellow nail syndrome
Ectopic bronchus
Sequestration
Ehlers-Danlos syndrome
Marfan syndrome

Inflammatory

Cystic fibrosis
Ciliary dyskinesia
Immunodeficiency
Allergic bronchopulmonary aspergillosis
Chronic aspiration
   Swallowing incoordination
   Gastric contents from gastroesophageal reflex
(Alpha-1 antiprotease deficiency)

Post Infectious

Tuberculosis
Measles
Pertussis
Other viruses (adenovirus, influenza)
Necrotizing bacterial pneumonia (*Pseudomonas,
   klebsiella, Staphylococcus*)

Post Obstructive

Retained foreign body
Extrinsic Compression (i.e., RML syndrome)
Tumor

Miscellaneous

Bronchiectasis and azoospermia (Young syndrome)
Inhalation injury
Bronchiolitis obliterans and organizing pneumonia

during coughing, impairing the efficiency of cough as a mechanism of propelling mucus forward. Only if this cycle can be interrupted is there potential for healing and reversal of the bronchiectasis.

Clinical Aspects

The symptoms and signs of bronchiectasis depend on the severity of the architectural abnormality (Table 25.2). The hallmark symptom of bronchiectasis is a chronic productive cough (1, 2). It is often worse in the morning after rising and becomes less prominent as the day wears on. If the bronchiectasis is localized, morning cough may be the only symptom. Early on, abnormal auscultatory signs may be localized over the abnormal area, and inspiratory crackles may be heard only during deep inspiration. The crackles are typically coarse in nature. With generalized and advanced disease, dyspnea, chest pain, fever, and fatigue are present; widespread inspiratory crackles and wheezing become evident on examination.

Persistent crackles and wheeze after the period of acute lung injury suggests chronic lung damage. The intensity of breath sounds becomes diminished. This finding may be either localized and asymmetric or diffuse, depending on the degree of damage. The expiratory phase becomes prolonged. Although the abnormal auscultatory findings may change from moment to moment with deep breathing or coughing in moderate bronchiectasis, they become fixed with severe bronchiectasis.

Digital clubbing, which suggests considerable lung tissue destruction, is common in children with moderate to severe bronchiectasis, usually becoming evident in the school years. Hemoptysis occurs frequently with advanced bronchiectasis. Mild hemoptysis is due to bronchial wall inflammation, whereas major and life-threatening hemoptysis is due to erosion into the bronchial circulation or formation of arteriovenous malformations (9). Chronic hypoxia may develop, depending on the degree of lung damage and disturbance in gas exchange. If the hypoxia is untreated, cor pulmonale will ensue.

Diagnosis

Early on, minimal abnormalities are present on plain chest radiograph (CXR). As disease progresses and more severe bronchiectasis develops, findings suggestive of bronchiectasis on the CXR include increased peribronchial markings with tubular shadows and areas of atelectasis in the presence of generalized hyper-inflation (Fig. 25.3) (10). High-resolution computerized tomography (CT) of the chest has supplanted bronchography as the primary diagnostic tool (Fig. 25.4, 25.5). Findings similar to those found on CXR are evident on CT scan earlier in the course of disease. Since the CXR is not abnormal until moderate bronchiectasis is present, high-resolution CT scans should be performed in the patient who manifests the clinical features of bronchiectasis in order to establish the diagnosis early in the course of the disease. Bronchograms are occasionally performed to define the margins

Table 25.2.
Progression of Bronchiectasis

	Early (Mild)	Middle (Moderate)	Late (Severe)
Symptoms			
Cough	+	+ +	+ + +
Dyspnea	−	+	+ + +
Fever	−	+	+ + +
Hemoptysis	−	Mild	Major
Signs			
Localized crackles	+ +		
Localized wheeze	+ +		
Crackle/wheeze together		+ +	+ + +
Diffuse crackles/wheeze		+ +	+ + +
Prolonged expiratory phase		+	+ +
Increased AP diameter		+	+ + +
Clubbing		+	+ + +
Tests			
CT abnormal	+ +	+ + +	+ + +
CXR abnormal	−	+	+ +
Bronchogram abnormal	+	+ +	+ + +
Decreased FEV_1	−	+	+ + +
Decreased FEF_{50}	+	+ +	+ + +
Increased RV	+	+ +	+ + +
Decreased Pao_2	−	+	+ + +
Increased $Paco_2$	−	−	+ +

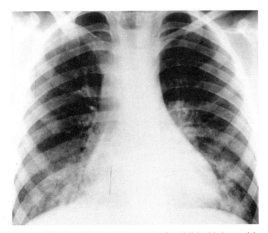

Figure 25.3. Chest radiograph of a child with bronchiectasis showing increased peribronchial markings, tubular shadows, and hyper-inflation.

of bronchiectasis if these are not clearly identified on CT (10, 11). The bronchogram demonstrates dilated bronchi with segmental volume losses and crowding of the airways (Fig. 25.4).

Pulmonary function tests only become abnormal after considerable disease progression and may remain relatively normal if the bronchiectasis is well localized. The earliest abnormalities are likely to be decreased flow at lower lung volume (i.e., decreased forced expiratory flow at 50% vital capacity [FEF_{50}]) (12). The shape of the expiratory flow-volume curve will become concave with the respect to the horizontal (volume) axis. With progression, the forced expiratory volume in 1 second (FEV_1) and FEV_1/forced vital capacity (FVC) ratio decrease; with severe obstruction, the FVC falls also. The corresponding plethysmographic abnormalities initially show an elevated residual volume (RV) and RV/total lung capacity (TLC) ratio; with progression the TLC increases and the specific airway conductance (SGaw) falls. Unless there is an accompanying reactive airways component, little improvement in flow rates occur post bronchodilator. Although measures of pulmonary functions are not diagnostic, they help determine and monitor the severity of the disease. Children with suspected bronchiectasis should undergo pulmonary function testing, and children with documented bronchiectasis should have pulmonary function followed routinely.

Once the diagnosis of bronchiectasis is established by CT scan, a vigorous attempt should be made to define the underlying

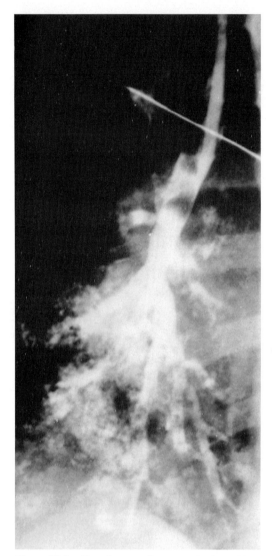

Figure 25.4. Bronchogram demonstrating bronchiectasis from chronic aspiration of gastric contents. The bronchi are dilated, irregular, and compressed.

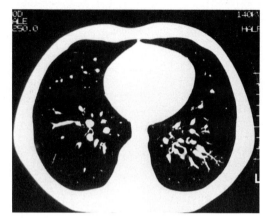

Figure 25.5. CT scan of the chest demonstrating bronchiectasis from chronic aspiration of gastric contents. The left lower lobe is most severely affected, showing dilated bronchi and thickened bronchial walls.

Table 25.3.
Evaluation of the Child with Suspected Bronchiectasis

Radiology
Chest radiograph
Chest CT scan (high-resolution, thin section)
Barium swallow
(Bronchogram)

Immunology
WBC and differential
Immunoglobulins
IgG, IgG subclasses
   Functional response to protein and polysaccharide
     antigen
  IgA, M, E
Cell functions
   Nitroblue tetrazolium test
   Chemotaxis
CH_{50}
T cell number and function
Skin test for tuberculosis (with positive control)
Skin test for *Aspergillus* if ABPA suspected

Other
Sweat test
Flexible bronchoscopy
  With bronchoalveolar lavage
  With transbronchial biopsy
Cilia evaluation
   Electron microscopy
   Beat frequency
   Wave form
(Mucociliary transport rate)
pH probe
Radionucleotide milk scan

cause, since therapy may be available that can control progression of the airway injury. Despite extensive evaluation, 30–50% of cases will remain "idiopathic" (13). Any evaluation of bronchiectasis should begin with a high-resolution CT scan or, if high-resolution CT is unavailable, a standard CT scan of the chest. Laboratory work should include at minimum a complete blood count (CBC) with differential count, immunoglobulins (IgG, A, M, and E), and a sweat test. Table 25.3 summarizes the gamut of diagnostic studies that may be needed to identify the etiology of the bronchiectasis. Additional studies will be dictated by factors such as age of onset of disease, distribution of bronchiectasis, and associated symptoms (Table 25.4). Specific conditions associated with bronchiectasis (CF, ciliary dyskinesia syndrome, immune deficiency, aspiration, and retained foreign body) are discussed in detail in other chapters.

Treatment

Therapy for moderate and severe bronchiectasis is focused on breaking the cycle that leads to progressive airways damage. If an underlying disease can be identified, it should be treated. Aerosolized bronchodilators, chest percussion, and postural drainage may facilitate mucociliary transport in some diseases causing bronchiectasis. Although these therapies have not been studied extensively in all diseases, a trial of bronchodilators and chest percussion should be considered for all children with bronchiectasis (14). High-dose antibiotics may decrease the bacterial colonization load, which may in turn minimize the host's inflammatory response. Chronic rotating antibiotic therapy (i.e., 3 weeks on, 1 week off, then change antibiotic for another cycle) has been recommended in patients with severe or moderate disease to provide relief of symptoms and perhaps reversal of bronchiectasis (15, 16). The prophylactic use of antibiotics in this fashion has not been critically evaluated

in children; nor have risks promoting colonization with resistant organisms.

Children with bronchiectasis often experience acute exacerbations characterized by increased cough and sputum production. The exacerbation is triggered by an upper respiratory tract infection (which is most certainly viral) in many cases. Antibiotics should be prescribed during an exacerbation if the patient is not already taking one. The antibiotics are usually given orally, but can be given intravenously or by inhalation, depending on the severity of the exacerbation and the response to previous therapy. The particular antibiotic can be selected based on sputum culture and sensitivity, if available; if culture results are not available, the choice of the antibiotic should be based on knowledge of the most likely pathogens. Choices for oral therapy include a cephalosporin (cefuroxime, cefpodoxime, cefprozil), trimethoprim-sulfamethoxazole, amoxicillin with clavulanic acid, or a macrolide antibiotic (erythromycin +/- sulfisoxazole, clarithromycin, azithromycin). Failure to respond to a course of antibiotics suggests the presence of a resistant pathogen and is an indication for more extensive evaluation and therapy (e.g., intravenous antibiotics). Choices for intravenous antibiotic therapy include ticarcillin plus clavulinic acid, ampicillin plus sulbactam, or cephalosporins (cefuroxime, cefoperazone, ceftriaxone, ceftazidime,

Table 25.4.
Findings That May Direct Clinical Evaluation of Bronchiectasis

Condition	Associated Findings	Additional Tests
CF	Steatorrhea, failure to thrive, sinusitis, + family history	Sweat chloride
Immotile cilia	Severe otitis media, infertility	Nasal turbinate biopsy
Immune deficiency	Recurrent infections	
Aspiration	Increased symptoms after feeding	Feeding/swallowing study
Foreign body	Localized findings, + history	Rigid bronchoscopy - ventilation - perfusion scan
Congenital bronchiectasis		
Mounier-Kuhn	Respiratory involvement of central airways	Flexible bronchoscopy
Williams-Campbell	Respiratory involvement of small and medium airways alone	
Ehlers Danlos	Skin involvement, skin ulceration	Skin biopsy
Marfan syndrome	Cardiac involvement, pectus, characteristic body habitus	Echocardiogram
Yellow nail syndrome	Discolored nails, lymphedema and pleural effusions	

ceftizoxime); aminoglycosides might be considered if *Pseudomonas aeruginosa* is present in the sputum. Bronchoscopy to obtain secretions for culture may be useful in order to direct subsequent antibiotic therapy; children who can tolerate the larger bronchoscopes should have the cultures done with a protected brush. Other treatments such as chest physical therapy (see Chapter 62) should be initiated or increased as well. Except for patients with CF, children with bronchiectasis do not often require hospitalization for treatment of these exacerbations.

The role for anti-inflammatory therapy, if any, remains to be defined. There is no definitive evidence that antihistamines, decongestants, or iodide preparations significantly alter the purulent secretions in bronchiectasis. New treatments directed at decreasing sputum viscosity and improving mucus clearance may prove valuable in decreasing the rate of progression of disease (17, 18).

Surgical therapy is rarely recommended for bronchiectasis due to generalized disease such as CF, ciliary dyskinesia, or immunodeficiency because of the certainty of progression of disease in the remaining airways. The spread and progression of bronchiectasis in these patients is most likely due to the primary disease process rather than "spread" of an endobronchial infection from an abnormal area to a normal area that would not otherwise be at risk. Resection of an area of localized bronchiectasis may be considered in selected patients, although it should be clear that the purpose of resection is relief of symptoms rather than prevention of spread of bronchiectasis (19). A favorable prognosis of the underlying disease process (such as IgG deficiency) makes a decision to proceed with surgery clearer, because subsequent bronchiectasis can be minimized by treatment. The presence of localized disease out of proportion to the status of the rest of the lung may warrant surgery even in patients with conditions with poorer prognosis, such as CF. For the patient with severe localized disease but no identifiable underlying etiology, resection should be considered since removal of the damaged lung unit generally results in complete resolution of symptoms, perhaps even for life.

Guidelines for considering surgical resection include severe symptoms that are unresponsive to aggressive medical management, recurrent episodes of pneumonia and atelectasis localized to one area, severe or recurrent hemoptysis, and interference with normal growth and development thought to be due to the consequences of chronic/recurrent infection. The extent of the disease should be established by high-resolution CT as a part of the preoperative evaluation. Timing of the surgery is also important. The patient should be as free from symptoms as possible. This may require an extended course of intravenous antibiotics, increased chest percussion, and bronchodilators prior to surgery. Once a diagnosis of severe, irreversible, localized bronchiectasis unresponsive to aggressive medical management has been established by CT, surgery should not be postponed. In the infant and toddler, this may allow the patient to capitalize on the potential for compensatory lung growth and minimize the theoretic risk of contamination of adjacent healthy lung units.

The prognosis for patients with bronchiectasis depends on the underlying disease or initiating events (13). The patient with ciliary dyskinesia may have a long life, whereas the patient with CF faces shortened survival. If there is a treatable underlying disease (i.e., immunodeficiency or chronic aspiration) there is a possibility that the bronchiectasis may be reversed if caught early in the disease progression.

REFERENCES

1. Barker AF, Bardana EJ. Bronchiectasis: Update on an orphan disease. *Am Rev Respir Dis* 1988; 173:969–978.
2. Murray JF. New presentations of bronchiectasis. *Hosp Pract* March 30, 1991.
3. Davis PB, Hubbard VS, McCoy K, Taussig LM. Familial bronchiectasis. *J Pediatr* 1983; 102:177–185.
4. Cole PJ. Inflammation: A two-edged sword—The model of bronchiectasis. *Eur J Respir Dis* 1986; 69(Suppl 147):6–15.
5. Lapa JR, Silva E, Jones JAH, Cole PJ, Poulter LW. The immunological component of the cellular inflammatory infiltrate in bronchiectasis. *Thorax* 1989; 44:668–673.
6. Currie DC, Peters AM, George P, et al. Indium-111–labelled granulocyte accumulation in respiratory tract of patients with bronchiectasis. *Lancet* Jan 13, 1987.
7. Wilson R, Sykes DA, Currie T, Cole PJ. Beat frequency of cilia from sites of purulent infections. *Thorax* 1986; 41:453–458.
8. Cochrane GM. Chronic bronchial sepsis and progressive lung damage. *Br Med J* 1985; 290:1026–1027.
9. Liebow AA, Hales MR, Lindskog GE. Enlargement of the bronchial arteries and their anastamoses with

the pulmonary arteries in bronchiectasis. *Am J Pathol* 1949; 25:211.

10. Stanford W, Galvin JR. The diagnosis of bronchiectasis. *Clin Chest Med* 1988; 9:691–699.

11. Munro NC, Cooke JC, Currie DC, Strickland B, Cole PJ. Comparison of thin section computed tomography with bronchography for identifying bronchiectatic segments in patients with chronic sputum production. *Thorax* 1990; 45:135–139.

12. Landau LI, Phelan PD, Williams HE. Ventilatory mechanics in patients with bronchiectasis starting in childhood. *Thorax* 1974; 29:304–312.

13. Ellis DA, Thornley PE, Wightman AJ, Walker M, Chalmers J, Crofton JW. Present outlook in bronchiectasis: Clinical and social study and review of factors influencing prognosis. *Thorax* 1981; 36:659–664.

14. Mazzocco MC, Owens GR, Kirilloff LH, Rogers RM. Chest percussion and postural drainage in patients with bronchiectasis. *Chest* 1985; 88:360–363.

15. Hill SL, Stockley RA. Effect of short and long term antibiotic response on lung function in bronchiectasis. *Thorax* 1986; 41:798–800.

16. Hill SL, Morrison HM, Burnett D, Stockley RA. Short term response of patients with bronchiectasis to treatment with amoxycillin given in standard or high doses orally or by inhalation. *Thorax* 1986; 41:559–565.

17. Aitken ML, Burke W, McDonald G, Shak S, Montgomery AB, and Smith A. Recombinant human DNase inhalation in normal subjects and patients with cystic fibrosis. *JAMA* 1992; 267:1947–1951.

18. Hubbard RC, McElvaney NG, Birrer P, Shak S, Robinson WW, Jolley C, Wu M, Chernick MS, Crystal RG. A preliminary study of aerosolized recombinant human deoxyribonuclease I in the treatment of cystic fibrosis. *N Engl J Med* 1992; 326:812–815.

19. Wilson JF, Decker AM. The surgical management of childhood bronchiectasis: A review of 96 consecutive pulmonary resections in children with nontuberculosus bronchiectasis. *Ann Surg* 1982; 195:354–363.

26

Acute Upper Airway Obstruction

YAKOV SIVAN and CHRISTOPHER J.L. NEWTH

Acute upper airway obstruction is a frequent problem in infants and children. Most cases are mild and short-lived, and can be managed adequately on an outpatient basis. The clinical importance of acute upper airway obstruction derives from the fact that some (often initially mild) cases can progress rapidly and result in severe and even complete airway obstruction. This situation is obviously a medical emergency that if not treated appropriately and quickly may cause severe hypoxia (with potential neurologic complications) and even lead to cardiorespiratory arrest. Some of the diseases causing acute upper airway obstruction should never be treated outside the hospital because the risk for complete airway obstruction is very high.

CAUSES

Chronic Upper Airway Obstruction Causing Acute Obstruction

Many situations that cause chronic partial upper airway obstruction may suddenly deteriorate to acute, severe obstruction if a mild respiratory infection is superimposed. Examples of lesions where this may occur are laryngomalacia, adenoidal and tonsilar hypertrophy, and mild subglottic stenosis (as in Down syndrome). These will also be discussed elsewhere.

Upper Airway Obstruction in the Newborn

Severe acute upper airway obstruction is infrequent in the newborn and is usually due to congenital anomalies or malformations. Relatively common examples are bilateral choanal atresia, Pierre Robin syndrome, vocal cord paralysis, subglottic stenosis/hemangioma, congenital laryngeal cysts and webs, laryngomalacia, and vascular ring. A different approach is required for these situations and is described elsewhere.

Upper Airway Obstruction in Children

The gross anatomy of the larynx is presented in Figure 26.1. The larynx is built of four major cartilages: thyroid, cricoid, arytenoid, and epiglottic; these are joined by muscles, ligaments, elastic tissue, and mucous membranes. The cricoid cartilage completely surrounds the lumen just inferior to the vocal cords. Infection or inflammation that involves the vocal cords and the area just below the cords is defined as *laryngitis*, or *laryngotracheobronchitis* when the disease progresses further down the trachea and bronchi. In fact, the airway of the child above the tracheal carina is narrowest at the cricoid level; thus the cricoid forms the border of a vulnerable airway orifice. The epiglottic cartilage is attached to the anterior surface of the thyroid cartilage. The aryepiglottic folds arise from the epiglottis and end posteriorly near the arytenoid cartilages on both sides. Infection of these structures is defined as *supraglottitis*. The space anterior to the epiglottis is the vallecula where saliva pools before deglutition. Thus, a disease involving these structures may impair swallowing, resulting in drooling of saliva.

Infection of the upper airways is the most common cause of severe acute upper airway obstruction, with laryngotracheobronchitis and spasmodic laryngitis being the two leading causes. Trauma to the larynx and accidents are also not uncommon as precursors of severe upper airway obstruction in children, but this

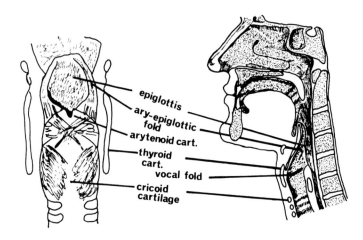

Figure 26.1.   Anatomy of the larynx. Posterior-anterior view (left) and saggital view (right).

chapter will focus on the more common infectious diseases (Table 26.1).

PATHOPHYSIOLOGY

When related to body size, the airways of a child are large in comparison with those of adults. However, the absolute diameter is small, causing higher resistance to airflow in the child. Since there is an inverse fourth-power relationship of the radius of an airway to its resistance to laminar airflow, a 1.0-mm

Table 26.1.
Causes of Upper Airway Obstruction in Children

Infections
  Acute laryngotracheobronchitis
  Epiglottitis
  Acute adenoidotonsillar enlargement (most
    common: infectious mononucleosis)
  Bacterial tracheitis
  Retropharyngeal abscess
  Diphtheria

Trauma, accidents
  Post-extubation subglottic edema
  Foreign bodies in larynx and upper esophagus
  Thermal injuries (burns) causing acute pharyngeal
    edema
  External trama to the neck
  Vocal cord paralysis secondary to trauma
    (including head injury)

Others
  Spasmodic croup
  Vocal cord paralysis secondary to neurologic
    lesions
  Angioneurotic edema
  Tumors of the anterior mediastinum

increase in the thickness of the mucosa at the subglottic level as a result of laryngotracheobronchitis, for example, will cause a 75% reduction of the cross-sectional area in the small infant (versus a 20% reduction in the adult). Hence, even a mild decrease in airway diameter in small children will increase the resistance significantly, and thus the work of breathing.

During forced inspiration against a fixed obstruction in the extrathoracic airways, large negative intratracheal pressures are generated below the obstruction by even small infants (1) with subsequent dynamic narrowing of the extrathoracic trachea (2) (Fig. 26.2). This results in increased turbulence and velocity of airflow, which causes the vocal cords and aryepiglottic folds to vibrate, resulting in inspiratory stridor. As a consequence of the increased negative pleural pressure during inspiration and the highly compliant chest wall in young children, much of the ventilatory effort during upper airway obstruction is wasted by "sucking in" ribs rather than air during forced inspiration. This results in asynchronous motion of the rib cage and abdominal compartments and is clinically manifested as chest retractions (3). During exhalation, the opposite occurs, with the extrathoracic trachea tending to "balloon" (Fig. 26.2). Thus, the obstruction to airflow is greater during inspiration than during expiration (Fig. 26.3).

Hypoxia is the earliest arterial blood gas abnormality and occurs out of proportion to carbon dioxide retention in croup as well as

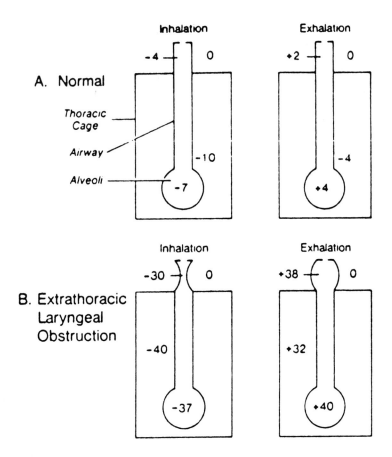

Figure 26.2. Each of the four diagrams represents the extra- and intra-thoracic airways, lung, and thoracic cage. The numbers represent average pressures developed during inhalation and exhalation in a normal child *(A)* and a child with acute upper airway obstruction *(B)*. Dynamic compression causing narrowing of the extrathoracic trachea results from the large negative pressures generated immediately below the obstruction and the increased airflow through the narrow segment (Venturi effect).

in epiglottitis (4–7). The hypoxia results from mismatching between ventilation and perfusion.

Several mechanisms may contribute to the ventilation-perfusion mismatch. Patients with croup and bacterial tracheitis have copious tracheobronchial secretions; in these situations and in epiglottitis, there is an impaired ability to produce an effective cough to clear the airways. Retention of these secretions can lead to subclinical plugging of small airways, resulting in ventilation-perfusion mismatching (7). Irritation of the larynx and trachea has been shown to produce reflex bronchoconstriction in animals (8), and this may also happen in croup, epiglottitis, and bacterial tracheitis. Patients with croup and epiglottitis sometimes present with frank pulmonary edema (9, 10). In less severe cases, a subclinical increase in lung water may flood some alveoli and cause ventilation-perfusion mismatching. The cause for this pulmonary edema is uncertain. It probably results from the increased negative intrapleural pressure that increases venous return to the right atrium of the heart, but at the same time also decreases the output of the left ventricle (net effect: an increase in intrathoracic pulmonary blood volume). The huge negative pressure that is applied also to the lung interstitium may increase fluid leakage out of the pulmonary vascular bed into the interstitium even further if the integrity of either the endothelial or epithelial linings is impaired by infection or endotoxin. The

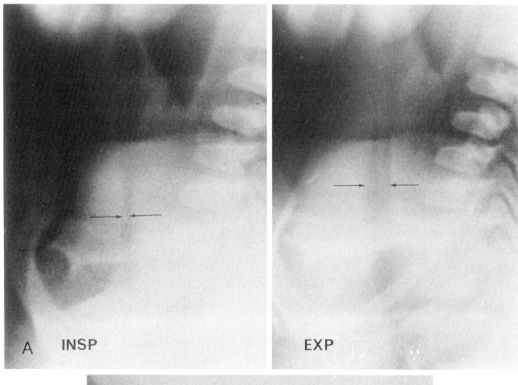

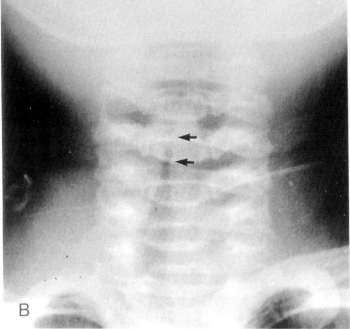

Figure 26.3.   A radiograph of the neck of a child with acute laryngotracheobronchitis showing the changes in the extrathoracic airway diameter during the respiratory cycle. *A,* Lateral view—the extrathoracic trachea is narrowed during inspiration *(arrows) (left),* and is relatively normal during expiration *(right). B,* An anterior-posterior view—subglottic narrowing and tapering of the upper trachea.

increased negative inspiratory pressure also impairs the ability of the interstitial lymphatic system to remove excessive fluid.

The exaggerated respiratory efforts are associated with pulsus paradoxus, which is sometimes difficult to measure in an agitated child. However, the degree of pulsus paradoxus has not been tested as a measure of the severity of upper airway obstruction, and its use as a clinical tool to follow the disease is thus limited.

Increased work of breathing, hypoxia, and lack of fluid and caloric intake cause respiratory fatigue, resulting in hypercapnia and respiratory acidosis. This situation of exhaustion may be misleading since the decreased air entry diminishes the intensity of the stridor and thus may erroneously be interpreted as clinical improvement, particularly if the listlessness of respiratory fatigue is mistaken for comfortable sleep.

EPIGLOTTITIS

Epiglottitis is an acute inflammation of the supraglottic structures involving the epiglottis and aryepiglottic folds. Classically, the disease does not involve the subglottic and tracheal regions. Its main importance stems from the fact that it is one of the true emergencies in pediatrics; when treatment is delayed it may rapidly progress to complete airway obstruction with cardiorespiratory arrest. Epiglottitis thus requires prompt diagnosis and management. When a well-organized approach is used, the outcome is excellent.

Epidemiology

Unlike croup, epiglottitis is a rare disease with a rate of only 1–10 per 10,000 pediatric admissions and 1.9–7.0% of pediatric admissions for upper airway infections (11–15). Epiglottitis occurs throughout the year. Peaks have been reported in all four seasons but mainly during the 6-month period from December to May (16–22) in both the Northern and Southern Hemispheres. Epiglottitis occurs almost equally in males and females (14, 23) with a slight male preponderance (24). It has been reported in all age groups from early infancy to old age. However, most of the cases occur between 2 and 6 years of age (14, 21, 23). Eighty percent of the cases occur before 5 years of age, 20% are children less than 2 years

of age, and up to 5% are less than 1 year old (22, 25).

Epiglottitis caused by *Haemophilus influenza* type B (HIB) is less common than meningitis caused by the same organism (25, 26). The yearly incidence and type of invasive HIB disease vary by country and by ethnic origin. Where the incidence is high, the median age of invasive HIB disease is low and epiglottitis is rare. For example, in Alaskan Eskimos, Navajo Indians, and Australian Aboriginals the incidence of HIB meningitis is extremely high: up to 400/100,000 in the age group 0–4 years (median age: 6 months), but epiglottitis is rare or nonexistent (25, 26). In Victoria, Australia the incidence of HIB diseases is low but the median age is higher (27 months), and 40% of the disease is epiglottitis.

There is some evidence that suggests genetic predisposition for epiglottitis. Increased frequency has been reported with certain M, N, and S erythrocytic antigens. Human leukocyte antigen A11 (HLA-A11) and HLA-B5 have been found more frequently in patients who had *H. influenza* type B epiglottitis than in patients who had meningitis from the same organism, and HLA-A28 and HLA-B17 were more common in infected patients than in those who never had epiglottitis (27, 28). These findings have not been confirmed by others (29).

Etiology

Epiglottitis results from infection of the supraglottic structures by HIB. Only a few cases caused by other organisms have been reported in children: *Streptococcus pneumoniae*, *Staphylococcus aureus*, beta-hemolytic *Streptococcus*, and *Haemophilus influenza* type A (12, 30–33). In most cases the infecting organism can be isolated from the upper airway as well as from the blood. This explains the systemic (toxic) nature of the disease, but not why distant organs (e.g., bones, meninges) rarely become secondarily infected. The rate of isolations from the blood is between 80% and 100% (21, 23, 31, 34–36). The rate of positive pharyngeal and laryngotracheal cultures is somewhat less.

Pathogenesis

Direct invasion by HIB causes inflammation of the supraglottic structures with subsequent bacteremia. This results in edematous swelling of these structures including the epiglottis (characteristically seen as cherry-red, aryepiglottic folds, and arytenoids with ensuing severe narrowing of the laryngeal orifice (Figs. 26.4–26.6). The subglottic area is not involved.

Clinical Picture

The onset of epiglottitis is usually abrupt. Minor upper respiratory infection may precede in some cases. The onset is characterized by high fever, toxic appearance, and sore throat, which progress over a few hours to dysphagia, drooling, and respiratory distress. The patient looks anxious and irritable. Breathing becomes noisy, and the voice and cry are muffled rather than hoarse. Cough is usually not a prominent feature, and stridor is a late finding.

On examination the patient looks sick, restless, and pale or cyanotic with marked tachycardia; he or she is sitting forward with hyperextension of the neck in order to increase airway patency (Table 26.2). Complete airway obstruction may occur at any time without any preceding deterioration in clinical signs—

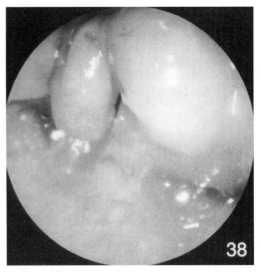

Figure 26.5. A view of the larynx in acute epiglottitis showing edema of the supraglottic structures obstructing the laryngeal orifice.

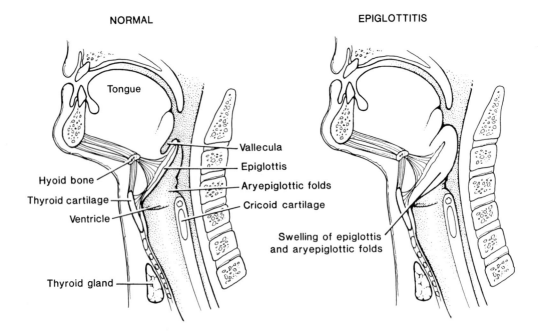

NORMAL   EPIGLOTTITIS

Tongue

Vallecula

Epiglottis

Hyoid bone   Aryepiglottic folds

Thyroid cartilage   Cricoid cartilage

Ventricle

Swelling of epiglottis
and aryepiglottic folds

Thyroid gland

Figure 26.4. Diagram of the the upper airway in the lateral projection showing the normal anatomy and the consequences of epiglottic swelling. The radiographic appearance is shown in Figure 26.7.

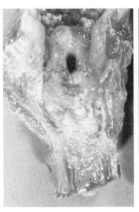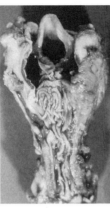

Figure 26.6. Post-mortem view of the larynx. Normal epiglottis *(right)* and the supraglottic inflammation and edema of acute epiglottitis *(left)*.

Table 26.2.
Epiglottitis—Symptoms and Signs

Symptoms	Signs
Dyspnea	Fever
Dysphagia	Toxic Appearance
	Aphonia/muffled voice
	Drooling
Sore throat	Respiratory distress
Irritability	Pallor/cyanosis
Lethargy	Sitting position
	Hyper-extended neck
	Stridor
	Tachycardia
	Decreased consciousness

thus the patient's consciousness may be already decreased by the time he or she reaches the hospital. Complete airway obstruction with respiratory arrest may be precipitated by inappropriate handling (such as attempts to visualize the epiglottis using a tongue depressor), by forcing the patient to lie flat for lateral radiographs of the neck, or by painful investigations such as venipuncture or the usually unnecessary procedure of obtaining arterial blood gases. The mechanism of this acute obstruction is not clear. Factors involved probably include vagal reflex, aspiration of saliva that accumulates in the supraglottic area, increased inspiratory efforts causing the epiglottis and aryepiglottic folds to be drawn onto the glottis, and laryngeal spasm.

The clinical presentation in children less than 2 years old is variable. Signs and symptoms not routinely described in children with epiglottitis but often observed in infants with epiglottitis include the absence of fever, the presence of only low-grade fever on a significant history of antecedent upper respiratory infection, and a prominent "croupy" barking cough (22). Occasionally, a child will present lying flat in a post-ictal state (secondary to fever rather than hypoxia); the presence of epiglottitis as the underlying and life-threatening problem may not be immediately appreciated.

In rare cases, extra-epiglottic infections may accompany the disease in the upper airway (e.g., meningitis, septic arthritis, pericarditis) (16). Other respiratory tract involvement is also rarely found (e.g., tonsillitis, otitis media, pneumonia).

Laboratory investigation reveals leukocytosis with neutrophilia and a left shift (12, 16, 37).

Diagnosis

The diagnosis of epiglottitis requires a high index of suspicion and should be considered in every child with acute upper airway obstruction who has a high fever and sore throat and who looks "toxic," especially when these signs have developed over only a few hours. The diagnosis is based primarily on the clinical signs. Infrequently, and more commonly in the younger age group, it may be difficult to differentiate epiglottitis from viral croup.

Because epiglottitis is an emergency, time should not be wasted on therapeutic trials such as inhalation of racemic epinephrine (see "Croup"). It is important to confirm the diagnosis as soon as possible. In cases that are clear-cut on clinical grounds, no further investigation is needed and the diagnosis is then confirmed by direct visualization of the swollen, erythematous, inflamed epiglottis and aryepiglottic folds at the time when airway control is established by intubation. However, many cases still require investigation, and two methods have been suggested: (a) Direct visualization of the epiglottis using a tongue depressor or laryngoscope will confirm the diagnosis, but we believe that this procedure is dangerous, since it may precipitate complete airway obstruction and respiratory arrest. This issue remains controversial only because some investigators still recommend (this unnecessary) inspection of the epiglottis by a pediatrician in the emergency room when the diagnosis of epiglottitis is in doubt (38). (b) A lateral neck radiograph is an excellent technique (23, 39, 40) when the diagnosis is in doubt, with very high sensitivity (23) while providing a good view of the epiglottitis and adjacent structures (Fig. 26.7). In supraglottitis, the appearance of a swollen epiglottis and aryepiglottic folds is characteristic. The best position to obtain the lateral neck film is with the patient upright, which also minimizes the risk for increased airway obstruction that accompanies the supine position. When a radiograph is needed, the patient must be accompanied to the radiology department by a physician who is skilled in intubation and carrying the appropriate resuscitation drugs and equipment.

Differential Diagnosis

Epiglottitis must be differentiated from the other causes of acute upper airway obstruction listed in Table 26.1. Traumatic and accidental causes are ruled out easily by history and absence of fever. The possibility that a foreign

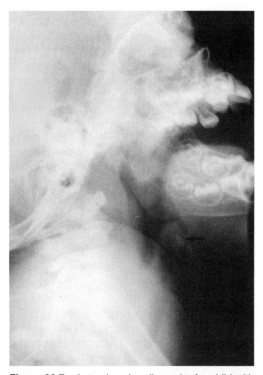

Figure 26.7. Lateral neck radiograph of a child with epiglottitis. Note the swollen epiglottis *(arrow)* and aryepiglottic folds.

body has been aspirated and lodged at the larynx or trachea should always be considered because it is also a true emergency that may cause complete obstruction within a short time. A history of choking while eating or of playing with small objects in the mouth, and the absence of fever, will make the diagnosis of foreign body aspiration very likely. Angioneurotic edema, which is a rare cause for acute upper airway obstruction, results from swelling of the tongue and supraglottic tissues. The diagnosis is often apparent because the lips, cheeks, and eyelids are usually involved, and urticaria may also be present.

In most cases viral croup, spasmodic laryngitis, and bacterial tracheitis can be easily differentiated from epiglottitis by history and clinical examination (Table 26.3).

Management

Most fatalities occur within the first few hours after the patient has arrived at the hospital. All deaths result from complete airway obstruction. Once the diagnosis of epiglottitis is made or even strongly suspected there should be no delay in therapy aimed at establishing an artificial airway. The child should be attended constantly by skilled personnel (usually a Pediatric Intensivist or Pediatric Emergency Room Physician) who can intubate the patient if respiratory arrest occurs. If the patient is stable and there is time, intubation should be performed in the operating room under general anesthesia. The personnel required for this procedure include at least an experienced anesthetist and a surgeon who can perform emergency tracheostomy in case intubation fails.

Several studies have reported that in up to 25% of the cases, acute epiglottitis can be managed by observation without "prophylactic" intubation (21, 41–44). Butt et al. recently reported 46 children with epiglottitis who did not receive prophylactic intubation (21). Only one of their patients subsequently required intubation. These 46 patients, however, represent only 13% of their series (349 children with epiglottitis over 8 years), and these patients were older and considered to have only mild airway obstruction. When all patients with epiglottitis are considered, the incidence of complete airway obstruction requiring emergency intubation under difficult conditions (which can lead to complica-

Table 26.3.
Comparison of Infections Causing Acute Upper Airway Obstruction

Factor	Epiglottitis	Viral Croup	Spasmodic Laryngitis	Bacterial Tracheitis
Age (years)	2–6	0.5–4	0.5–3	0–6
Organism	HIB	Parainfluenza 1,2,3 Influenza, adeno, RSV	?	HIB S. aureus
Season	All year	Late spring, late fall	All year	All year
Clinical presentation	Child sitting Toxic Drooling Dysphagia Muffled voice	Child lying down Nontoxic Barking cough Hoarseness	Nontoxic Barking cough Hoarseness	Toxic Barking cough Muffled voice
Onset (prodrome)	Rapid over a few hours	Variable; few hours to 4 days	Sudden	Variable: few hours to 5 days
Stridor	Less common	Common	Very common	Common
Fever	High	Low-grade	Afebrile	High
Chest retractions	Less common	Common	Common	Common
Lateral neck film	Swollen epiglottitis	Subglottic narrowing	No findings	Pseudomembrane
Progression	Rapid	Usually slow	Rapid	Usually slow
Recurrence	Rare	Fairly common	Very common	Rare

tions) is very high (24–50%) (23, 41–43). Mortality with conservative management has been reported as high as 6%, as opposed to less than 1% mortality when an artificial airway is used (45, 46). There is no way to predict which patient will do well without airway control. Thus, although a few patients may be managed conservatively with close observation, we advocate elective intubation in every patient with acute epiglottitis, and recommend intubation early regardless of the patient's respiratory status since delayed intubation may be dangerous.

SUGGESTED PROTOCOL FOR EPIGLOTTITIS

1. *Avoid disturbance.* Until the airway is secured, every effort should be made not to disturb the patient. The child should be placed in sitting position or allowed to lie face down. A venous line should be placed, but arterial blood gas sampling should be avoided, unless strongly indicated for other reasons.
2. *Oxygen.* Give humidified oxygen-enriched gas by face mask (at least 30% oxygen). A pulse oximeter should be used to obtain continuous information on arterial oxygen saturation.
3. *Radiographs.* If the clinical condition permits, a lateral x-ray film of the neck should be quickly obtained in the radiology department or in the emergency room with the patient

in the sitting position. If the radiograph confirms the diagnosis of epiglottitis, proceed with the next steps.
4. *Artificial airway.* Intubation should be performed in the operating room (unless the patient is too unstable to be transferred). Inspection of the larynx should be done at the same time. Anesthesia should be induced with halothane and oxygen, and oral intubation should be performed with a stilette in order to secure the airway. Bacterial cultures of the epiglottis can be taken with complete safety, and the endotracheal tube can be changed to a nasal one at leisure. Some particularly skilled intubationists prefer to use the nasal route initially and thus decrease the number of tube changes through the infected area. The recommended endotracheal tube sizes are given in Table 26.4 (11, 47).

Intubation has less morbidity and mortality than tracheostomy (19, 48–50), and only rarely is a skilled anesthetist unable to pass a

Table 26.4.
Sizes of Uncuffed Endotracheal Tubes for Acute Upper Airway Obstruction

Age of Child	Size of Tube (ID)
<6 months	3.0 mm
6 months–2 years	3.5 mm
2 years–6 years	4.0 mm
>5 years	4.5 mm

Never Xray neck

tube successfully, in which case tracheostomy should be performed.

5. *Sedation.* Sedate the patient in order to avoid the high risk of accidental extubation (which occurs in 28 of 294 cases) (5). Some investigators suggest that patients should be heavily sedated and electively ventilated, but we have had good experience with mild sedation (just enough to prevent agitation), combined with arm restraints to cover the elbows so the patient can move his arms but is not able to bend his elbows to reach the endotracheal tube (Fig. 26.8). The patient thus breathes spontaneously. Humidification is achieved by a headbox or a condenser humidifier (21). If the patient needs oxygen it is supplied by the headbox or through a T-tube. With this practice the risk of accidental extubation is minimized, and movement of the endotracheal tube through the inflamed area caused by "tethering" from ventilator circuits is eliminated.

6. *Antibiotics.* Cefuroxime, 100 mg/kg/day, or cefotaxime, 100 mg/kg/day, can be given intravenously after obtaining blood cultures. We prefer the second- or third-generation cephalosporins because of the increasing resistance to both ampicillin and chloramphenicol, which have traditionally been considered the drugs of choice. Treatment should last 7 days, but can be oral after the first 3–4 days of clinical progress with IV medication.

7. *Steroids.* There is no place for corticosteroids in the management of epiglottitis (43).

When to extubate remains controversial. In general, three criteria need to be met: (a) the fever and toxic appearance have resolved, (b) the supraglottic edema and pain have resolved to the extent that the patient can handle his own secretions, (c) there is a leak around the endotracheal tube (assessed daily), which signifies that airway narrowing from supraglottic edema has largely resolved.

Some investigators advocate that when repeated visualization at 24-hour intervals by direct pharyngoscopy reveals a reduction in the size of the epiglottitis, the patient is ready to be extubated (19, 34, 36, 51). Since this *always* occurs in association with resolution of fever and development of a leak, and the assessment is not quantitative, we do not recommend this procedure except for teaching purposes. A leak will be achieved usually in 24–48 hours. We recommend that if the child is otherwise well (even in the uncommon case of an inapparent leak), extubation should be performed after 48–72 hours (23).

Complications

Complete upper airway obstruction may be considered a part of the natural history of the disease rather than a complication. Otherwise, the main complications of epiglottitis are the rare extra-epiglottic infections (meningitis, arthritis, pneumonia) (16) and hypoxia. In one series, 17 of 22 children with epiglottitis had hypoxia and decreased arterial/alveolar oxygen ratios, even after their airways had been secured by a tube (7). One third of the patients had abnormalities on chest radiograph. The hypoxia could not be explained by alveolar hypoventilation (arterial carbon dioxide was normal) and may have been due to increased lung water causing mismatching of ventilation and perfusion. Pulmonary edema may rarely complicate the presence or relief of acute upper airway obstruction (9). This complication is usually treated with diuretics, positive pressure ventilation, and positive end-expiratory pressure (PEEP), and resolves within 1–4 days.

Prevention

HIB capsular polysaccharide vaccine has been recommended for use at 18 months of age (52, 53). It is expected to reduce the rate of epiglottitis by 48% (24). There are also promising trials of a conjugate vaccine given at 2 and 4 months of age (54).

In case of contact with epiglottitis, rifampin prophylaxis 20 mg/kg/day (maximum 600 mg) by mouth is recommended to all household

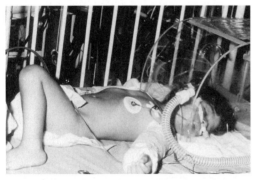

Figure 26.8. A child with epiglottitis breathing spontaneously through an endotracheal tube. Arms are restrained by plaster casts.

contacts if at least one contact is younger than 4 years, regardless of the immunization status of the child (55).

LARYNGOTRACHEOBRONCHITIS

Laryngotracheobronchitis (croup) is an infectious disease of the larynx causing upper airway obstruction in small children. In contrast to epiglottitis it is a common disease but rarely a medical emergency. The disease may be limited to the larynx (laryngitis) or the larynx and trachea (laryngotracheitis), or it may be spread all the way down to the medium and even small airways (laryngotracheobronchitis). The terms *laryngotracheobronchitis* or *croup* will be used here to describe any of these variants.

Epidemiology

Laryngotracheobronchitis occurs mainly in small children less than 5 years of age, with peak incidence between 6 months and 2 years (56). The disease occurs at all ages, but rarely causes symptomatic upper airway obstruction in older children and adults. Croup has been reported to occur at a rate of 4.7 cases per 100 children in the second year of life, but only 1.3% require admission to the hospital (56). However, wide regional variation exists. The attack rate during the first year of life in Tucson, Arizona was 107 cases in 961 children (11.1 per 100) (57). A survey at the Hospital for Sick Children in Toronto showed that croup accounted for about 3 cases per 1000 patients admitted and nearly 10.5 cases per 1000 patients admitted with a primary diagnosis of respiratory disease (11).

Laryngotracheobronchitis is more common in boys than in girls (the male/female ratio approximates 1.5:1). It occurs throughout the year but is especially common during the late autumn and winter months (56).

Etiology

Laryngotracheobronchitis is a viral disease. The most common infecting virus is parainfluenza type 1 followed by parainfluenza types 2 and 3, influenza A and B, adenovirus, respiratory syncytial virus, and rhinovirus. Some of the viruses are more associated with epidemic outbreaks (parainfluenza 1 and 2); others are responsible for outbreaks in closed populations (adenovirus 4 and 7); and others are responsible for sporadic instances (adenovirus, parainfluenza 3).

Pathogenesis

The primary site of the viral infection is usually the airways above the larynx; thus the involvement of the subglottic areas is preceded by nasal congestion and rhinorrhea. Once the virus has invaded the subglottic airway wall, it becomes edematous and red with fibrinous exudate. The vocal cords become edematous and their function is impaired. Histologic findings include edema and inflammation with infiltration of mononuclear and polymorphonuclear cells (58, 59). This narrows the airway, which then becomes clinically significant mainly in the more critical area of the subglottic cricoid cartilage, causing inspiratory stridor. When the narrowing is mild, the stridor is heard only when the child is agitated, cries, or hyperventilates. When the narrowing progresses, it is heard also during quiet breathing.

The disease may involve not only the trachea but also the lower (and smaller) airways, producing thick, viscid secretions and causing ventilation-perfusion mismatch (5). The combination of lower respiratory tract disease and narrowed subglottic region increases the work of breathing and hypoxia.

Clinical Picture

Typically the child has coryza for a few days before the larynx is involved. When this happens, the patient presents with a hoarse voice and harsh, barking cough. After a few hours, or even a day or two, inspiratory stridor develops. Agitation and crying worsen the stridor because the intrapleural pressure becomes more negative, resulting in further collapse of the already partially obstructed airway. When extreme narrowing takes place, the stridor may disappear, but one should not be mislead to believe that the upper airway obstruction has resolved. The opposite may also be true—the stridor disappears or becomes markedly diminished because little air is being inhaled. This may occur when the patient is exhausted; in this situation chest retractions also decrease. The patient is usually moderately febrile but the fever may sometimes be very high. The signs and symptoms of laryngotracheobronchitis tend to worsen at nights. The disease usually lasts 2–5 days in mild cases but may last a week or two in the more severe ones. Examination of the throat will reveal hyperemia and inflammation.

It is important to assess accurately the severity of the airway obstruction. If severe obstruction is not relieved, the patient will die of hypoxia. Fortunately, the vast majority of cases do not follow this pattern and resolve over a few days, although as many as 3% of patients admitted with acute laryngotracheobronchitis may require an artificial airway.

Several scoring systems have been suggested for the assessment of the severity of the upper airway obstruction; one example is shown in Table 26.5 (60). These scoring systems are based on assigning points to several clinical (and sometimes radiologic) parameters, and the severity of the upper airway obstruction is derived from their summation. However, scoring systems have been found to be somewhat unreliable and none has become standard (3, 60–62). The reason is that the clinical assessment relies on vague and subjective parameters. Respiratory rate and pulse rate, which are not informative in the awake child, are also unreliable as guidelines when the child is relaxed or asleep (3, 5) and are of much less value than the child's general appearance to an experienced observer. Warning signs for worsening upper airway obstruction are restlessness, fatigue, marked use of respiratory accessory muscles, increasing stridor, and marked chest retractions on inspiration. Asynchrony between the chest wall and abdominal compartments has been shown to be a sensitive and reliable measure of upper airway obstruction in children less than 4 years old (3). However, quantitative measurement of this asynchrony requires special equipment and, although easy to apply, is still experimental and not yet a bedside technique. Even objective measurements such as arterial blood gases do not correlate reliably with clinical findings because arterial hypoxia may occur very early, and hypercarbia occurs only late in the course of acute upper airway obstruction when urgent intervention is already needed (5, 61). Obtaining such measurements may agitate the child who is already in respiratory distress.

Laboratory investigation is usually not helpful except for ruling out other diseases. The blood count shows mild to moderate leukocytosis. Viral cultures do not contribute to diagnosis or management. Anterior-posterior and lateral neck radiographs demonstrate subglottic narrowing and tapering of the upper trachea (Fig. 26.3). The changes, however, do not correlate with the severity of the disease (62).

Differential Diagnosis

It is important to differentiate acute laryngotracheobronchitis from other causes of acute upper airway obstruction because the therapeutic protocols differ and some of the situations present an emergency. The differentiation is based mainly on clinical findings and a high index of suspicion, with the help of radiography in selected cases (Table 26.1). The most important differential diagnosis is epiglottitis (see Table 26.3 and the earlier section on epiglottitis). The two situations can usually be quickly differentiated by the rapid onset, toxic appearance, drooling, and sitting position that characterize epiglottitis. A lateral neck radiograph is helpful when the situation is not too urgent.

Management

There is no specific treatment for croup, and the rationale of therapy is to prevent an increase in airway obstruction and to secure the airway when obstruction is severe. The majority of children with croup can be treated

Table 26.5.
Croup Scoring System

Level of consciousness	
Normal	0
Disoriented	5
Cyanosis	
None	0
Cyanosis with agitation	4
Cyanosis at rest	5
Stridor	
None	0
When agitated	1
At rest	2
Air entry	
Normal	0
Decreased	1
Markedly decreased	2
Retractions	
None	0
Mild	1
Moderate	2
Severe	3

safely at home assuming that the parents are reliable. Indications for hospital admission include stridor at rest, chest retractions, cyanosis, pallor, and depressed sensorium.

TREATMENT AT HOME

Because agitation and crying may exacerbate the stridor, it is important to ensure minimal disturbance of the child.

The use of humidified mist is controversial. A mist vaporizer (either cool or warm) is helpful in increasing the humidity of the patient's environment. Mist may be helpful by moistening and decreasing the viscosity of the airway secretions and exudate, making it easier for the child to mobilize them and remove them by cough (63, 64). Dry air may cause the exudate to adhere to the airway wall. However, controlled studies have failed to show any beneficial effect of humidified air (relative humidity 87–95%) compared to room air (relative humidity 48–52%) on subglottic edema (the main cause of airway obstruction in croup) and respiratory resistance (65, 66). There is no advantage using cool as opposed to warm mist. However, cool mists are safer since they do not increase the temperature in the patient's environment, and burns have been reported when a warm mist vaporizer has been put too close to the patient.

We do not advocate the use of sedatives at home to treat agitation. Restlessness in a child with stridor should be presumed to be due to hypoxia until proven otherwise.

Antibiotics have no place in croup since this is a viral illness. However, when no improvement is observed within 3–4 days, or when fever or general appearance worsen, bacterial superinfection (see "Bacterial Tracheitis") should be suspected.

TREATMENT IN THE HOSPITAL

1. *Monitoring.* Clinical assessment by the physicians and nurses should be frequent. This is especially true when the patient is difficult to observe inside a mist tent and changes could be missed. Manipulations such as arterial punctures for blood gas analysis should be avoided unless there is reasonable doubt about the patient's clinical condition. Any such procedure will not only agitate the patient and thus worsen his stridor, but will not be reliable unless cleanly obtained on the first attempt before the child struggles and cries, rendering the results meaningless. In moderate to severe stridor oxygenation can be monitored easily and continuously by a pulse oximeter (67). In impending or actual respiratory failure (due to severe obstruction or to exhaustion), the patient should be transferred to a pediatric intensive care unit. Children with severe upper airway obstruction or in respiratory failure should be monitored with a cardiorespiratory monitor, and the carbon dioxide tension can also be continuously measured with clinical benefit by the non-invasive transcutaneous CO_2 monitor (68).

2. *Fever Control.* Stimulation that provokes anxiety will cause the child to hyperventilate, which leads to increased work of breathing and oxygen consumption. We recommend that fever control be achieved by drugs rather than by tepid sponging, which will further agitate a child.

3. *Feeding.* Hunger may agitate the child. On the other hand, feeding during dyspnea and tachypnea increases the risk for aspiration. We usually discontinue feeding during the first hours after admission to the hospital and make a decision about feeding a few hours later. If the patient is not agitated and does not have severe retractions, is not in respiratory failure or exhausted and can tolerate being out of oxygen therapy, then hydration and feeding can be accomplished orally. Otherwise, intravenous fluids should be started.

4. *Oxygen and humidification.* Children with moderate to severe croup require oxygen therapy. Although no controlled data exist for the efficacy of such treatment in a clinical setting, the demonstration of hypoxia in a significant proportion of children with croup who needed hospitalization (4, 5) is sufficient to convince a prudent clinician that oxygen should be used. Oxygen is best supplied using a headbox or tent with moist, nebulized oxygen. Face masks and nasal canulas are usually less tolerated in small children. An oxygen concentration of more than 30% is rarely required.

5. *Epinephrine.* Racemic epinephrine is believed to work via its topical alpha-adrenergic stimulation, which causes mucosal vasoconstriction, leading to decreased edema in the inflamed subglottic region (69). Several double-blind placebo-controlled studies that assessed the efficacy of racemic epinephrine using clinical scoring systems showed that the drug is effective (3, 60, 62, 70–72). Two stud-

ies (3, 62) also used an additional objective assessment to prove the efficacy of inhaled racemic epinephrine. Two of the studies (70, 72) demonstrated in addition that although a significant decrease in airway obstruction can be observed if measured within 30 minutes of administration of the drug, the degree of obstruction had returned to the pretreatment level when assessed 2 hours later. The initially progressive nature of croup ensures that the degree of obstruction resumes to an even greater degree compared to pretreatment as the drug effect wears off. This is often referred to as "the rebound phenomenon," a term for which there is no scientific or pharmacologic basis in this situation (73).

Two particular issues regarding the administration of epinephrine need to be addressed: (a) nebulized epinephrine administered via face mask and spontaneous breathing is as effective as delivery via intermittent positive pressure breathing (71) and is recommended; and (b) racemic epinephrine is not superior to a comparable dose of l-epinephrine. Racemic epinephrine is composed of equal parts of the d- and l-isomers of epinephrine. Since the l-isomer is the only active one, a 2.25% solution of racemic epinephrine will be virtually equipotent, volume for volume, with a 1% solution of l-epinephrine, which can be used instead. However, note that the commercial epinephrine preparation is only 1:1000 (i.e., 0.1%).

The dosage of racemic epinephrine is not critical, and lies between 0.5 and 2.0 ml of 2.25% solution diluted in distilled water to 4 ml. It can be given every hour (in ICU, even at closer intervals). However, if a patient is not improving after two to four treatments in 2–3 hours, an artificial airway should be considered.

6. *Corticosteroids.* The use of corticosteroids is controversial even after numerous investigations spanning almost 30 years, mainly because of methodologic problems (differences in definitions, dosage, and assessment). An analysis of the more critical studies reveals that dexamethasone at a dose of 0.6 mg/kg (up to 10 mg/dose) *may* shorten hospital stay, decrease the need for racemic epinephrine, decrease clinical scores, and reduce the need for endotracheal intubation (70, 74–79). A single dose of corticosteroids is unlikely to cause adverse effects, but nevertheless we do not routinely use corticosteroids in croup.

7. *Artificial airway.* Only a small proportion of children with croup need an artificial airway, in comparison to epiglottitis, where preventive intubation is the rule. The indications for intubation are respiratory failure resistant to conservative management, and exhaustion. Children with croup who need an artificial airway should be managed in a pediatric intensive care unit (PICU). Intubation should be performed in a controlled environment (i.e., the PICU or operating room). We advocate first oral, and later the nasal route with an endotracheal tube size as indicated in Table 26.4. Adequate humidification of inspired gas is needed. Patients may be allowed to awaken and breathe spontaneously without heavy tubing attachments, or may be kept immobile with heavy sedation and ventilated to prevent further irritation to the subglottic space by endotracheal tube movement (see "Management" under "Epiglottitis").

The duration of intubation is usually 3–7 days. The tube may be removed when (a) fever has subsided, and (b) tracheobronchial secretions have thinned and decreased. A "leak test" has been suggested as a reliable guideline for extubation. Theoretically, the occurrence of a leak signifies that airway obstruction has resolved to such a degree that the lumen is larger than the tube; hence it can be removed. However, this is not always the case (80). One reason is lack of standardization of the leak test with respect to the level of pressure needed to obtain the leak, head position, and the effect of muscle relaxants on the leak. Our approach is that if an air leak exists in combination with the other two conditions that imply that the patient is ready, the tube is removed. If there is no air leak after 7 days, direct laryngoscopy is performed and extubation is usually attempted. If the patient fails extubation, we re-intubate with a tube that is one size smaller than the previous tube (but never less than 3.0 mm ID unless this is the only tube that can be passed).

SPASMODIC LARYNGITIS

The term *spasmodic laryngitis* (spasmodic croup) refers to an entity of sudden onset consisting of stridor and acute upper airway obstruction of unknown etiology. Characteristically, the child goes to bed well, then awakens a few hours later with a classic cough, hoarseness, and stridor. The stridor is always reversible, usually within a few hours. The stridor may recur in the same patient on the next night or months later. Spasmodic croup rarely requires upper airway control.

Although respiratory viruses have been suggested as causative factors, the disease does not result from viral (or bacterial) inflammation of the upper airway. No prodromes of coryza or fever are associated with the clinical signs, and endoscopies have shown subglottic edema without inflammation (81). Other theories about causation include hyper-reactivity of the upper airway (82).

Treatment is the same as in acute viral laryngotracheobronchitis (see above).

BACTERIAL TRACHEITIS

Bacterial tracheitis (also referred to as membranous or pseudomembranous croup) is not a new disease. It was first reported in the earlier part of this century, but disappeared from the literature from the early 1940s until 1979 (83). Since 1979, the entity has been "rediscovered" and is now named *bacterial tracheitis*. It is a serious and potentially life-threatening disease through its complications and its ability to cause severe airway obstruction.

Etiology

As the term indicates, bacterial tracheitis is a bacterial disease. However, it usually follows a viral respiratory infection, most commonly due to parainfluenza 1 and 2 and less commonly influenza virus (84, 85). It is most common during increased seasonal activity of respiratory viruses (86). Thus, in many cases, bacterial tracheitis is a complication or superinfection of viral laryngotracheobronchitis (87, 88). It is believed that the virus predisposes the trachea to bacterial infection by initiating local mucosal damage, by facilitating bacterial adherence to the virus-infected cells, and by impairing the mucociliary clearance of the trachea (89, 90, 91). Pre-existing anatomic abnormalities in the trachea may predispose the child to tracheal bacterial infection (84, 85). Bacterial tracheitis can also begin as a primary bacterial disease.

The most common pathogen involved is *Staphylococcus aureus* followed by *Haemophilus influenza* type B. Cases due to beta-hemolytic streptococcus and a variety of other pathogens have been reported (85).

Clinical Picture

Bacterial tracheitis may occur at all ages; reports in children range from 3 weeks to 13 years of age (85), with most of the cases below 4 years of age.

When the disease follows a viral respiratory infection, a prodrome of 1–5 days precedes the bacterial phase. Classically, the child has "simple" viral laryngotracheitis that fails to resolve, and then becomes worse with high fever, toxicity, inspiratory stridor, barking cough, chest retractions, and leukocytosis with bandemia.

The primary bacterial disease is more rapidly progressive, and starts with only a few hours of prodromal illness or no prodrome at all (84, 92). The high fever lasts for several days. The tracheal secretions may be very copious, and necrotic mucosa forms pseudomembranes, which worsen the airway obstruction.

Bacterial tracheitis is diagnosed by the combination of the clinical picture and (after intubation) the presence of large amounts of thick, copious tracheal secretions. Visualization of the trachea and the secretions using endoscopy after intubation will confirm the diagnosis. Lateral neck radiographs may show irregularities of the tracheal walls from sloughing of the pseudomembranes and subglottic narrowing. However, a radiograph is often not helpful in the diagnosis and thus should not be done if it delays airway control of a patient at immediate risk of severe airway obstruction.

The most common complication is pneumonia due to extension of purulent material through the tracheobronchial tree (85). Other complications include sepsis, toxic shock syndrome, and pneumothorax (84).

Management

Monitoring, sedation, restraint, and handling of patients with bacterial tracheitis is no different from such procedures with patients with croup or epiglottitis. Specific measures include the following:

1. *Intubation.* Intubation is the rule. Death can result from thick secretions and the pseudomembranes obstructing the airways, so intubation is usually required to enable intensive toilet as well as airway control (92–94). Frequent suctioning is necessary.
2. *Humidification.* Humidification is essential and may help prevent inspissation of the tracheal secretions. Patients have suffered cardiopulmonary arrest, even after endotracheal

intubation, from tenacious secretions that were not adequately cleared (85).

3. *Antibiotics.* Because a variety of pathogens may be involved, it is essential to obtain tracheal aspirates early for both Gram stain and culture. Patients should initially receive broad-spectrum coverage, which includes coverage of *Staphylococcus aureus* and *Haemophilus influenza*. We recommend starting with a second-generation cephalosporin such as cefuroxime, 100 mg/kg/day IV, or other suitable coverage for *Staphylococcus* such as intravenous nafcillin, 150 mg/kg/day, which may be added in special circumstances (profound toxicity, extension of disease to other sites). Therapy is adjusted after receiving cultures results.

4. *Extubation.* Extubation can be attempted when fever has declined, secretions have thinned, and an air leak is present. Bacterial tracheitis usually resolves quickly (intermediate between epiglottitis and croup); it is unusual not to have a patient extubated after 4–5 days.

NOTE: Racemic epinephrine is not helpful in bacterial tracheitis.

ACUTE ADENOIDAL AND TONSILLAR ENLARGEMENT

One of the most alarming life-threatening complications of infectious mononucleosis is severe upper airway obstruction due to nasopharyngeal obstruction (95, 96). The obstruction can be severe enough to cause hypoxia and even death. The airway obstruction results from acute enlargement of the tonsils and the adenoids that obstruct the airway—a situation that should be looked for in every child with infectious mononucleosis. The clinical picture is that of a child with infectious mononucleosis who develops dyspnea a few days (mean 6–7 days) after the first symptom of infectious mononucleosis (97). The dyspnea is the ultimate symptom of the acute upper airway obstruction and is present in all patients with this complication. Other symptoms (which occur in 20–90% of the patients) include sore throat, dysphagia, and drooling. Physical examination reveals marked cervical adenopathy with swelling of the neck, fever, extremely enlarged tonsils covered with exudate, tonsillar membrane obstructing the pharynx, and nasal congestion and obstruction from viscous secretions (97). A lateral neck radiograph is usually not required but may be indicated when the physical examination does not reveal the site of obstruction (Fig. 26.9).

The diagnosis of infectious mononucleosis is based on clinical and laboratory work-up, the discussion of which is beyond the scope of this chapter.

Management

Once the diagnosis of impending upper airway obstruction is made, efforts to secure the airway should take priority. Two specific measures are important in this regard:

1. *Nasopharyngeal tube.* Passage of a nasopharyngeal tube into the hypopharynx can often be an effective initial treatment in the emergency department or during transport (the necessary

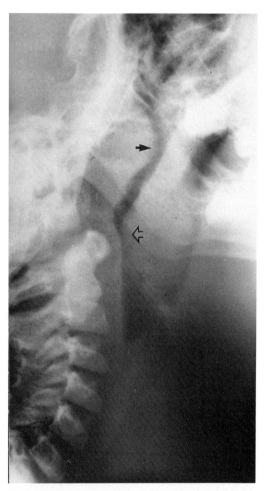

Figure 26.9. Lateral neck radiograph of a child with acute upper airway obstruction due to tonsillar *(arrowhead)* and adenoidal *(arrow)* enlargement secondary to infectious mononucleosis.

length of tube can be assessed by direct measurement on the patient prior to the procedure and on a lateral radiograph of the neck afterward). This procedure is relatively simple and quick, and can be accomplished by almost any caregiver. The nasopharyngeal tube will bypass the obstruction in most cases. In rare instances, endotracheal intubation is necessary because the glottic and subglottic regions are involved, being compressed by the enlarged cervical nodes.

2. *Corticosteroids.* It is well accepted today that acute upper airway obstruction due to infectious mononucleosis is an indication for steroid therapy (97–101). Most of the data comes from uncontrolled reports, but nevertheless, there are indications from the literature that the early administration of steroid therapy may result in the avoidance of endotracheal intubation. It is also possible that steroids shorten the time patients require an artificial airway (98, 101).

CONCLUSIONS

Acute upper airway obstruction is a syndrome dangerous only when physicians fail to suspect either the presence or the extent of the respiratory compromise when the child arrives at the hospital. There can be a further pitfall, in that having made the diagnosis of acute upper airway obstruction, time is wasted with various investigations that may not be helpful, are disturbing to the distressed child, and unnecessarily expose the patient to the risk of respiratory arrest from unrelieved airway obstruction. The management of epiglottitis, bacterial tracheitis, and laryngotracheobronchitis is straightforward once the specific diagnosis has been made. However, we lack objective, noninvasive techniques for assessing routinely the severity of upper airway obstruction and its response to various treatment modalities. The decision of when to intubate a child (in the cases requiring airway relief) depends entirely on good clinical judgement.

Despite the chest radiograph and arterial blood-gas data presented here, we do not advocate either investigation in the management of uncomplicated croup, bacterial tracheitis, or epiglottitis. We have reported these findings merely to emphasize that there is an underlying hypoxia irrespective of the relief of airway obstruction or the presence of normal chest radiographs. This hypoxia may be severe enough to be life-threatening, and these children should always be managed in humidified oxygen.

As indicated in Table 26.1, there are numerous other non-infectious causes of acute upper airway obstruction in children. Most are uncommon, but of these post-extubation subglottic edema (102) and intracranial pathology causing post-extubation vocal cord paralysis (103) seem relatively frequent. The former responds to epinephrine and other alpha-adrenoceptor agonists, and can be managed similarly to acute (viral) laryngotracheitis (see earlier). The latter occurs often in association with head injury and intracranial hypertension or hemiparesis and is suspected after the first attempts at extubation fail secondary to upper airway obstruction not related to subglottic edema. Management is usually re-intubation initially, and prognosis is related to the underlying neurologic problem. Ultimately, most of these children can be extubated.

REFERENCES

1. Newton-John H. Pulmonary edema in upper airway obstruction [Letter]. *Lancet* 1977; 2:510.
2. Wittenborg MH, Gyepes MT, Crocker D. Tracheal dynamics in infants with respiratory distress, stridor and collapsing trachea. *Radiology* 1967; 88:653–862.
3. Sivan Y, Deakers TW, Newth CJL. Thoracoabdominal asynchrony in acute upper airway obstruction in small children. *Am Rev Respir Dis* 1990; 142:540–544.
4. Wesley AG, Bruce R, Holloway R. Arterial blood gases as a guide to management of infective croup. *South Afr Med J* 1968; 42:1237–1239.
5. Newth CJL, Levison H, Bryan AC. The respiratory status of children with croup. *J Pediatr* 1972; 81:1068–1073.
6. Wesley AG. Indication for intubation in laryngotracheobronchitis in black children. *South Afr Med J* 1975; 49:1126–1128.
7. Costigan DC, Newth CJL. Respiratory status of children with epiglottitis with and without an artificial airway. *Am J Dis Child* 1983; 137:139–141.
8. Widdicomb JG, Sterling GM. The autonomic nervous system and breathing. *Arch Intern Med* 1977; 126:311
9. Travis KW, Todres ID, Shannon DC. Pulmonary edema associated with croup and epiglottitis. *Pediatrics* 1977; 59:695–698.
10. Soliman MG, Richer P. Epiglottitis and pulmonary edema in children. *Can Anaesth Soc J* 1978 ; 25:270–275
11. Levison H, Tabachnik E, Newth CJL. Wheezing in infancy, croup and epiglottitis. In Gluck L (ed): *Current problems in pediatrics.* Chicago, Year book, 1982, vol 12, pp 1–65.
12. Bass JW, Steele RW, Weiebe RA. Acute epiglottitis: A surgical emergency. *JAMA* 1974; 229:671–675.
13. Vetto RR. Epiglottitis: A report of thirty-seven cases. *JAMA* 1960; 173:990–994.

14. Baxter JD. Acute epiglottitis in children. *Laryngoscope* 1967; 77:1358–1367.
15. Fearon BW, Bell RD. Acute epiglottitis: A potential killer. *Can Med Assoc J* 1975; 112:760–766.
16. Molteni RA. Epiglottitis: Incidence of extraepiglottic infection. *Pediatrics* 1976; 58:526–531.
17. Baxter JD, Pashley NRT. Acute epiglottitis-25 years experience in management. *J Otolaryngol* 1977; 6:473–476.
18. Benjamin B, O'Reilly B. Acute epiglottitis in infants and children. *Ann Otolaryngol* 1976; 85:565–572.
19. Blanc VF, Weber ML, Leduc C, et al. Acute epiglottitis in children: Management of 27 consecutive cases with nasotracheal intubation with special emphasis on anesthetic considerations. *Can Anaesth Soc J* 1977; 24:1–11.
20. Cohen SR, Chai J. Epiglottitis-20 year study with tracheostomy. *Ann Otolaryngol* 1978; 87:461–467.
21. Butt W, Shann F, Walker C, Williams J, Duncan A, Phelan P. Acute epiglottitis: A different approach to management. *Crit Care Med* 1988; 16:43–47.
22. Brilli RJ, Benzing G 3rd, Cotcamp DH. Epiglottitis in infants less than two years of age. *Pediatr Emerg Care* 1989; 5:16–21.
23. Vernon DD, Sarnaik AP. Acute epiglottitis in children: A comprehensive approach to diagnosis and management. *Crit Care Med* 1986; 14:23–25.
24. Daum RS, Smith AL. Epiglottitis (supraglottitis). In Feigin RD, Cherry JD (eds): *Textbook of pediatric infectious diseases*, ed 2. Philadelphia, WB Saunders, 1987, vol 1, pp 224–237.
25. Clements DA, Gilbert GL. Immunization for the prevention of Haemophilus influenza type b infections: a review. *Aust N Z J Med* 1990; 20:828–834.
26. Trollfors B, Nylen O, Strangert K. Acute epiglottitis in children and adults in Sweden 1981–3. *Arch Dis Child* 1990; 65:491–494.
27. Gralnick MA et al. Host factors and antibody response in Haemophilus influenza type b meningitis and epiglottitis. *J Infect Dis* 1976; 133:448–455.
28. Tejani A, Mahadevan R, Dobias B Nangia B, Weiner M. Occurrence of HLA types in H. influenza type b disease. *Tissue Antigens* 1981; 17:205–211.
29. Granoff DM, Boies E, Squires JE, Pandey P, Suarez BK, Oldfather JW, Rodey GE. Histocompatibility leukocyte antigen and erythrocyte MNSs specificities in patients with meningitis or epiglottitis due to Hemophilus influenza type b. *J Infect Dis* 1984; 149:373–377.
30. Berenberg W, Kevy S. Acute epiglottitis in childhood: A serious emergency, readily recognized at the bedside. *N Engl J Med* 1958; 258:870–874.
31. Faden HS. Treatment of Hemophilus influenza type b epiglottitis. *Pediatrics* 1979; 63:402–407.
32. Lewis JK, Gartner JC, Galvis AG. A protocol for management of acute epiglottitis. *Clin Pediatr* 1978; 17:494–496.
33. Briggs WH, Altenau MM. Acute epiglottitis in children. *Otolaryngol Head Neck Surg* 1980; 88:665–669.
34. Schloss MD, Gold JA, Rosales JK, Baxter JD. Acute epiglottitis: Current management. *Laryngoscope* 1983; 93:489–493.
35. Bottenfield GW, Arcinue EL, Sarnaik A, Jewell MR. Diagnosis and management of acute epiglottitis—

Report of 90 consecutive cases. *Laryngoscope* 1980; 90:822–825.
36. Rothstein P, Lister G. Epiglottitis–duration of intubation and fever. *Anesth Analg* 1983; 62:785–787.
37. Ambrosino DM, Schiffman G. Gottschlich EC et al. Correlation between G2m(n) immunoglobulin allotype and human antibody response and suseptibility to polysaccharide encapsulated bacteria. *J Clin Invest* 1985; 75:1936–1942.
38. Mauro RD, Poole SR, Lockhart CH. Differentiation of epiglottitis from laryngotracheitis in the child with stridor. *Am J Dis Child* 1988; 142:679–682.
39. McCook TA, Kirks DR. Epiglottic enlargement in infants and children: Another radiologic look. *Pediatr Radiol* 1982; 12:227–234.
40. Rapkin RH. The diagnosis of epiglottitis: Simplicity and reliability of radiographs of the neck in the differential diagnosis of the croup syndrome. *Pediatrics* 1972; 80:96–98.
41. Glicklich M, Cohen RD, Rona JZ. Steroids and bag and mask ventilation in the treatment of acute epiglottitis. *J Pediatr Surg* 1979; 14:247–251.
42. Adair JC, Ring WH. Management of epiglottitis in children. *Anesth Analg* 1975; 54:622–624.
43. Storme M, Jaffe B. Epiglottitis—Individualized management with steroids. *Laryngoscope* 1974; 84:921–928.
44. Szold PD, Glicklich M. Children with epiglottitis can be bagged. *Clin Pediatr* 1976; 15:792–793.
45. Cantrell RW, Bell RA, Morioka WT. Acute epiglottitis: Intubation versus tracheostomy. *Laryngoscope* 1978; 88:994–1005.
46. Adair JC, Ring WH, Jordan WS, et al. Ten–year experience with IPPB in the treatment of acute laryngotracheobronchitis. *Anesth Analg* 1971; 50:649–655.
47. Shann FA, Phelan PD, Stocks JG, et al. Prolonged nasotracheal intubation or tracheostomy in acute laryngotracheobronchitis and epiglottitis? *Aust Pediatr J* 1975; 11:212–217.
48. Schultz RL, Morrison MV. Short-term intubation in children with acute epiglottitis. *South Med J* 1982; 75:158–160.
49. Breivik H, Klaastad O. Acute epiglottitis in children. *Br J Anaesth* 1978; 50:505–509.
50. Schuller DE, Brick HG. The safety of intubation in croup and epiglottitis: An eight-year follow-up. *Laryngoscope* 1975; 85:33–46.
51. Oh TH, Motoyama EK. Comparison of nasotracheal intubation and tracheostomy in the management of acute epiglottitis. *Anesthesiology* 1977; 46:214–216.
52. American Academy of Pediatrics. Committee in Infectious Diseases: Hemophilus influenzae type b conjugate vaccine. *Pediatrics* 1988; 81:908–911.
53. American Academy of Pediatrics. Committee on Infectious Diseases: Hemophilus influenzae type b conjugate vaccine: Update. *Pediatrics* 1989; 84:386–387.
54. Santosham M, Wolff M, Reid R, et al. The efficacy in Navaho infants of a conjugate vaccine consisting of Haemophilus influenzae type b polysaccharide and Neisseria meningitidis outer–membrane protein complex. *N Engl J Med* 1991; 324:1767–1772.
55. American Academy of Pediatrics. Committee in Infectious Diseases: Revision of recommendation

for use of rifampin prophylaxis of contacts of patients with Hemophilus influenzae infection. *Pediatrics* 1984; 74:301.

56. Denny FW, Murphy TF, Clyde WA Jr, Collier AM, Henderson FW. Croup: An 11-year study in a pediatric practice. *Pediatrics* 1983; 71:871–876.

57. Wright AL, Taussig LM, Ray CG, et al. The Tucson Children's respiratory study: II. Lower respiratory tract illnesses in the first year of life. *Am J Epidemiol* 1989; 129:1232.

58. Orton HB, Smith EL, Bell HO, et al. Acute laryngotracheobronchitis. Analysis of sixty-two cases with report of autopsies in eight cases. *Arch Otolaryngol Head Neck Surg* 1941; 33:926–960.

59. Richards LA. A further study of the pathology of acute laryngotracheobronchitis in children. *Ann Otol Rhinol Laryngol* 1938; 47:326–341.

60. Westley CR, Cotton EK, Brooks JG. Nebulized racemic epinephrine by IPPB for the treatment of croup. *Am J Dis Child* 1978; 132:484–7.

61. Kilham H, Gillis J, Benjamin B. Severe upper airway obstruction. *Pediatr Clin North Am* 1987; 34:1–14.

62. Corkey CWB, Barker GA, Edmonds JF, Mok PM, Newth CJL. Radiographic tracheal diameter measurements in acute infectious croup: An objective scoring system. *Crit Care Med* 1981; 9:587–90.

63. Parks CR. Mist therapy: Rationale and practice. *J Pediatr* 1970; 76:305–313.

64. Dulfano M, Adler K, Wooten O. Physical properties of sputum. IV. Effect of 100 per cent humidity and water mist. *Am Rev Respir Dis* 1972; 107:130–132.

65. Bourchier D, Dawson KP, Ferguson DM. Humidification in viral croup: A controlled trial. *Aust Paediatr J* 1984; 20:289–291.

66. Lenney W, Milner AD. Treatment of acute viral croup. *Arch Dis Child* 1978; 53:704–706.

67. Fanconi S, Doherty P, Edmonds JF, Barker GA, Bohn DJ. Pulse oximetry in pediatric intensive care: Comparison with measured saturations and trancutaneous oxygen tension. *J Pediatr* 1985; 107:362–366.

68. Fanconi S, Burger R, Maurer H, Uehlinger J, Ghelfi D, Muhlemann C. Transcutaneus carbon dioxide pressure for monitoring patients with severe croup. *J Pediatr* 1990; 117:701–705.

69. Baugh R, Gilmore BB. Infectious croup: a critical review. *Otolaryngol Head Neck Surg* 1986; 95:40–46.

70. Kuusela AL, Vesikari T. A randomized double-blind placebo-controlled trial of dexamethasone and racemic epinephrine in the treatment of croup. *Acta Paediatr Scand* 1988; 77:99–104.

71. Fogel LM, Berg LJ, Gerber MA, Sherter CB. Racemic epinephrine in the treatment of croup: Nebulization alone versus nebulization with positive pressure breathing. *J Pediatr* 1982; 25:1028–1031.

72. Taussig LM, Castro O, Beaudry PH, Rox WW, Bureau M. Treatment of laryngotracheobronchitis (croup). *Am J Dis Child* 1975; 129:790–793.

73. Morley J, Sanjar S, Newth C. Viewpoint: Untoward effects of beta-adrenoceptor agonists in asthma. *Eur Resp J* 1990; 3:228–233.

74. Koren G, Frand M, Barzilay Z, McLeod SM. Corticosteroid treatment of laryngotracheitis versus spasmodic croup in children. *Am J Dis Child* 1983; 137:941–944.

75. Muhlendahl KE, Kahn D, Spohr HL, Dressler F. Steroid treatment of pseudo-croup. *Helv Paediatr Acta* 1982; 37:431–436.

76. Skolnik NS. Treatment of croup. A critical review. *Am J Dis Child* 1989; 143:1045–1049.

77. Super M, Cartelli NA, Brooks LJ, Lembo RM, Kumar ML. A prospective randomized double-blind study to evaluate the effect of dexamethasone in acute laryngotracheitis. *J Pediatr* 1989; 115:323–329.

78. Kairys SW, Olmstead EM, O'Connor GT. Steroid treatment of laryngotracheobronchitis: A meta-analysis of the evidence from randomized trails. *Pediatrics* 1989; 83:683–693.

79. Smith DS. Corticosteroids in croup: A chink in the ivory tower? *J Pediatr* 1989; 115:256–257.

80. Adderley RJ, Mullins GC. When to extubate the croup patient: The "leak" test. *Can J Anaesth* 1987; 34:304–306.

81. Davison FW. Acute laryngeal obstruction in children. *JAMA* 1959; 171:1301–1305.

82. Zach MS. Airway reactivity in recurrent croup. *Eur Respir J* 1983; 128(Suppl):81–88.

83. Nelson WE. Bacterial croup: a historical perspective. *J Pediatr* 1984; 105:52–55.

84. Liston SL, Gehrz RC, Siegel LG, Tilelli J. Bacterial tracheitis. *Am J Dis Child* 1983; 137:764–767.

85. Donnelly BW, McMillan JA. Bacterial tracheitis: Report of eight new cases and review. *Rev Infect Dis* 1990; 12:729–735.

86. Chapman RS, Henderson FW, Clyde WA Jr, Collier AM, Denny FW. The epidemiology of tracheobronchitis in pediatric practice. *Am J Epidemiol* 1981; 114:786–797.

87. Edwards KM, Dundon MC, Altemeier WA. Bacterial tracheitis as a complication of viral croup. *Pediatr Infect Dis J* 1983; 2:390–391.

88. Naqvi SH, Dunkle LM. Bacterial tracheitis and viral croup. *Pediatr Infect Dis J* 1984; 3:282–283.

89. Fainstein V, Musher DM, Cate TR. Bacterial adherence to pharyngeal cells during viral infection. *J Infect Dis* 1980; 141:172–176.

90. Davison VE, Sanford BA. Factors influencing adherence of staphylococcus aureus to influenza A virus-infected cell cultures. *Infect Immunol* 1982; 37:946–955.

91. Loosli CG. Influenza and the interaction of viruses and bacteria in respiratory infections. *Medicine* 1973; 52:369–384.

92. Sofer S, Duncan P, Chernick V. Bacterial tracheitis—An old disease rediscovered. *Clin Pediatr* 1983; 22:407–411.

93. Han BK, Dunbar JS, Striker TW. Membranous laryngotracheobronchitis (membranous croup). *AJR* 1979; 133:53–58.

94. Liston SL, Gehrz RC, Jarvis C. Bacterial tracheitis. *Arch Otolaryngol Head Neck Surg* 1981; 107:561–564.

95. Snyderman NL. Otolaryngologic presentations of infectious mononucleosis. *Pediatr Clin North Am* 1981; 28:1011–1016.

96. Yeager H. Airway obstruction in infectious mononucleosis. *Arch Otolaryngol* 1964; 80:583–586.

97. Kaplan JM, Keller MS, Troy S. Nasopharyngeal obstruction in infectious mononucleosis. *Am J Fam Phys* 1987; 35:205–209.

98. Schumacher H, Jacobson W, Bemiller C. Treatment of infectious mononucleosis. *Ann Intern Med* 1963; 58:217–228.

99. Mandel W, Marilley R Jr, Gaines LM Jr. Corticotropin in severe anginose infectious mononucleosis. *JAMA* 1955; 158:1021–1022.

100. Bolden KJ. Corticosteroids in the treatment of infectious mononucleosis. An assessment using a double blind trial. *J R Coll Gen Pract* 1972; 22:87–95.

101. Doran J, Weisberger A. The use of ACTH in infectious mononucleosis. *Ann Intern Med* 1952; 38:1058–1062.

102. Tellez DW, Galvis AG, Storgion SA, Amer HN, Hoseyni M, Deakers TW. Dexamethasone in the prevention of postextubation stridor in children. *J Pediatr* 1991; 118:289–294.

103. Chaten FC, Lucking SE, Young ES, Mitchell JJ. Stridor: intracranial pathology causing postextubation vocal cord paralysis. *Pediatrics* 1991; 87:39–43.

27

Chronic Upper Airway Obstruction

MAX M. APRIL and BERNARD R. MARSH

Recurrent episodes of stridor or noisy breathing or persistence of stridor following an acute viral infection suggests the presence of an underlying obstructive lesion of the upper airway. The site of the obstruction can often be localized by a careful history, physical examination, and appropriate laboratory studies. Relevant history includes information on the age of onset, its duration, and previous airway injury or instrumentation. Feeding history and vocal performance may also provide useful information. The feeding process tends to be adversely affected by lesions involving oropharyngeal or supraglottic structures as well as by neurologic abnormalities. A harsh or breathy voice is usually caused by glottic lesions, whereas a muffled voice is more often secondary to supraglottic or oropharyngeal obstruction.

The timing and quality of the noise is quite helpful in localizing the site of obstruction. Inspiratory noise suggests an extrathoracic location, whereas expiratory noise places the obstruction within the thorax. Biphasic stridor or noise may be difficult to localize but suggests a fixed upper airway obstruction unaffected by the phase of respiration.

Details on the approach to evaluating suspected upper airway obstruction are contained in Chapter 26. High-kilovoltage airway radiographs (anteroposterior [AP] and lateral projections) and inspiratory-expiratory flow-volume curves can be used to confirm the location but not the nature of the obstructing lesion. A characteristic pattern of flattening of the flow-volume curve may be helpful in locating the obstruction and in distinguishing a fixed from a variable lesion. Although maximal inspiratory-expiratory flow-volume curve data is not available in children under 6 years of age, Abramson et al. have reported that the tidal volume flow-volume loop can provide similar information in infants and young children with marked upper airway obstruction (1). In infants with mild to moderate obstruction, partial flow-volume curves obtained by the rapid chest compression technique will demonstrate a pattern consistent with upper airway obstruction not detected by tidal curves since flow limitation may not be reached during spontaneous breathing in infants with less marked obstruction (2). Even though these techniques may confirm a clinical impression of obstruction of a central airway, bronchoscopy is required to establish a diagnosis and to determine the optimal therapeutic approach.

Although the management of clinically significant chronic upper airway obstruction frequently involves surgery, these problems are best approached as a joint effort between the pediatric pulmonologist and the otolaryngologist. The pulmonologist's role in this process involves organizing the initial diagnostic evaluation, providing the medical input into the timing and indications for surgical intervention, and consulting on the management of associated lower respiratory tract disease such as asthma.

The differential diagnosis of chronic upper airway obstruction is presented in Table 27.1. This chapter will focus on the surgical management of chronic upper airway obstruction in children with particular emphasis on conditions in which there have been recent advances in surgical treatment.

LARYNGOMALACIA

Laryngomalacia (congenital laryngeal stridor) is the most common cause of stridor in the infant. It accounts for approximately about

Table 27.1.
Site of Chronic Airway Obstruction

Nasal/Nasopharyngeal
Choanal atresia
Nasal mass
   Encephalocele
   Dermoid
   Glioma
Nasal polyposis
   Cystic fibrosis
Adenoid hypertrophy

Oropharyngeal
Tonsillar hypertrophy
Macroglossia
Glossoptosis (Pierre Robin sequence)
Vallecular cyst
Pharyngeal collapse

Supraglottic
Laryngomalacia
Laryngeal cyst (Saccular cyst/laryngocele)
Recurrent respiratory papillomatosis
Hemangioma
Lymphangioma

Glottic
Web
Laryngeal cleft
Recurrent respiratory papillomatosis
Vocal cord paralysis
   Bilateral
   Unilateral
Neoplastic
Neurofibroma
Hamartoma
Rhabdomyosarcoma

Subglottic larynx
Subglottic stenosis
   Acquired
   Congenital
Subglottic hemangioma
Subglottic cysts

Tracheobronchial
Tracheomalacia
Tracheal stenosis
Vascular ring/sling
Innominate artery compression
Tracheoesophageal fistula
Foreign body—airway or esophageal
External compression
Recurrent respiratory papillomatosis

60% of the cases of stridor in infants (3). Laryngomalacia is characterized by medial prolapse of the aryepiglottic folds, anterior collapse of the arytenoids, and/or posterior collapse of an omega-shaped epiglottis. This collapse causes inspiratory stridor that usually worsens with crying, exertion, or feeding and improves with the infant in the prone position or with neck extension. The diagnosis is established by fiberoptic laryngoscopy. This can be performed simply and safely with minimal or no sedation and is recommended in all children with stridor in order to diagnose other laryngeal anomalies such as laryngeal cyst or vocal cord dysfunction. Fiberoptic laryngoscopy will also allow the physician to reassure the parents about the diagnosis and natural history of the condition with confidence. It has been recommended by some that fiberoptic bronchoscopy be performed on children with laryngomalacia because of associated respiratory anomalies (4). Our experience suggests that one should consider the clinical and radiographic evidence in order to determine which infants may be at special risk for major anomalies of the tracheobronchial tree before proceeding with a full bronchoscopy.

Laryngomalacia is usually a benign, self-limited condition, typically presenting within the first month of life and resolving by 24 months of age. It does not require therapy other than parental reassurance that despite the noise, the infant will be fine and the condition will resolve on its own. Rarely, children exhibit severe airway obstruction associated with feeding problems, failure to thrive, cor pulmonale, apnea, and cyanosis (5). When indicated, a polysomnogram or continuous oximetry is helpful in determining the severity of the physiologic consequences of laryngomalacia. Since gastroesophageal reflux may contribute to the development of laryngomalacia, aggressive management of reflux followed by a period of observation to assess the effects on the severity of the malacia should be instituted prior to surgical intervention (6). Epiglottoplasty, the endoscopic resection of the obstructing supraglottic tissue, is advocated for these patients (5, 7, 8). Postoperative assessment, including polysomnography (8), has demonstrated dramatic resolution of airway obstruction with epiglottoplasty, thus reducing the need for tracheotomy.

SUBGLOTTIC STENOSIS

The subglottic space incorporates the region from the level of the vocal cords to the inferior margin of the cricoid cartilage and includes the only complete cartilaginous tracheal ring. In the normal term infant the subglottic space has a cross-sectional diameter of 5–6 mm. Subglottic stenosis is present when the cross-sectional diameter of airway in this region is less than 4 mm. It is labeled "congenital" if there is no history of endotracheal intubation or prior surgery (9). If the stenosis is severe (< 3 mm) the infant will present with stridor at birth or early in life and will require a tracheotomy.

More commonly, the child with congenital subglottic stenosis presents within the first year of life with recurrent episodes of croup or an episode of viral croup that results in persistent stridor. Airway radiographs (AP and lateral) may show a narrowed subglottic space, but the precise diagnosis is confirmed only by direct laryngoscopy under general anesthesia. Although flexible bronchoscopy may be useful to screen for subglottic abnormalities, general anesthesia is required to perform a suspension laryngoscopy with an operating microscope to evaluate the posterior aspect of the glottis and determine if fibrosis is present. In addition, precise measurements of the subglottic lumen should be made with rigid telescopes and/or ventilating bronchoscopes to guide therapy accurately. Direct laryngoscopy and rigid bronchoscopy have low complication rates and may reveal lesions in more than one anatomic site in the upper aerodigestive tract (10). Treatment of children with mild narrowing may consist of watchful waiting, allowing for enlargement of the subglottic lumen with growth. Children with more severe congenital stenosis should be considered for a cricoid split procedure (11) or tracheotomy if the stenosis is too severe to benefit from a cricoid split. Indications for surgery include the degree of respiratory distress under resting conditions, alterations in growth and development, evidence of cor pulmonale or CO_2 retention, and the response to common viral infections (i.e., a child who experiences life-threatening obstruction with an upper respiratory infection [URI] should be considered a candidate for intervention even if the infant has only mild to moderate obstruction at baseline). Other factors to be considered include the work of breathing at rest and the resultant airflow, as well as the pitch of the stridor; high-pitched stridor indicates a more severe stenosis. The cricoid split (laryngotracheal decompression) increases the lumen of the subglottic space by leaving a size-appropriate endotracheal tube in place after an incision in the cricoid, lower thyroid, and upper tracheal cartilages. The endotracheal tube is left in place for 7–14 days depending on the infants weight. Twenty-four hours prior to extubation, intravenous decadron is administered (12). If the cricoid split fails, a tracheotomy is performed. When the subglottic space remains severely stenotic, laryngotracheal reconstruction can be performed at about 2 years of age.

Over the past 25 years, as a consequence of long-term endotracheal intubation in premature neonates and their increased survival, acquired subglottic or laryngotracheal stenosis (LTS) has become more common than congenital stenosis. The incidence of LTS after intubation has been reported to be between 1% and 9%, but the true incidence, as well as the effect of endotracheal tube size, duration of intubation, and number of re-intubations is not known (11). With prolonged intubation, mucosal edema is followed by ulceration and infection, which may lead to perichondritis, loss of cartilage support, and circumferential scar formation. This condition usually presents with progressive or persistent airway obstruction after extubation (12).

Flexible nasolaryngoscopy should be performed to assess vocal cord motility and to search for other abnormalities. Direct laryngoscopy and examination with telescopes under general anesthesia is required. If there is a localized area of stenosis or a granuloma, microlaryngoscopy with CO_2 laser excision can be performed. If the stenosis is circumferential and the infant weighs more than 1500 g, does not require assisted ventilation, has oxygen requirements of less than 30%, and is free of upper or lower respiratory tract infection, then a cricoid split procedure can be considered (13). A tracheotomy is usually required if the cricoid split cannot be accomplished or if the split fails. A decision to perform surgery is based on the same criteria as for congenital stenosis. Tracheostomy in the pediatric patient can be associated with significant morbidity and mortality, especially in premature infants (14). These complications include those that occur in the immediate postoperative period (e.g., pneumothorax, accidental decannulation, and occlusion of the tube) and those that occur in the late postoperative period (e.g., granulation tissue, tube obstruction, infection, and accidental decannulation) (15). When providing care for children with tracheotomies, the physician must be aware of these potential problems and of the wide variety of types of tracheotomy tubes and their appropriate size selection for the growing child (Table 27.2) (16).

When endoscopic management of LTS has failed, surgical reconstruction is required to achieve decannulation. Prior to undertaking this procedure, assessment of pulmonary function, vocal cord motility, and the presence of gastroesophageal reflux must be made. If the child's lower respiratory tract disease would prevent decannulation even with an adequate airway, surgery should be postponed. Vocal cord motility must be determined by flexible laryngoscopy to select the appropriate surgical procedure. Acquired LTS refractory to laser excision or cricoid split is evaluated by laryngoscopy and tracheoscopy to establish an accurate diagnosis. If the subglottic/tracheal

lumen is less than 2.7 mm (Fig. 27.1), laryngotracheal reconstruction (LTR) with autogenous costal cartilage graft and placement of an internal Aboulker stent is performed (17). If there is posterior glottic fibrosis with limitation of vocal cord motility, or complete glottic and subglottic stenosis, division of the posterior cricoid cartilage is also performed. A costal cartilage graft may also be placed. The most commonly used internal stent is the Aboulker stent. The upper portion of this stent has a small opening that must be positioned carefully to lie just above the vocal cords (Fig. 27.2) in order to allow the supraglottic structures to cover this lumen adequately so that significant aspiration can be prevented. Aspiration of oral feedings is not uncommon following this procedure and underscores the need to control reflux. The stent is removed endoscopically 1–8 months later, depending on the severity of the stenosis. One month after stent removal, the child is examined under general anesthesia and any granuloma present is removed. After another month the airway is re-evaluated. If the airway is felt to be adequate, the child is admitted to the hospital for 24 hours of observation following decannulation.

If the subglottic lumen is greater than 2.7 mm (Fig. 27.3) and there is no posterior glottic

Table 27.2.
Common Tracheostomy Tube Sizes

Type	I.D. (mm)	O.D. (mm)	Length (mm)
Shiley			
00 NT	3.1	4.5	30
0 NT	3.4	5.0	32
1 NT	3.7	5.5	34
00	3.1	4.5	39
0	3.4	5.0	40
1	3.7	5.5	41
2	4.1	6.0	42
3	4.8	7.0	42
4	5.5	8.0	46
4 cuffed	5.0	8.5	67
5	5.0	7.0	58
Bivona			
60N025	2.5	4.0	30
60N030	3.0	4.7	32
60N035	3.5	5.3	34
60N040	4.0	6.0	36
60P025	2.5	4.0	38
60P030	3.0	4.7	39
60P035	3.5	5.3	40
60P040	4.0	6.0	41
60P045	4.5	6.7	42
60P050	5.0	7.3	44
60P055	5.5	8.0	46
Portex			
553025	2.5	4.5	30
553030	3.0	5.2	32
553035	3.5	5.8	34
555025	2.5	4.5	30
555030	3.0	5.2	36
555035	3.5	5.8	40
555040	4.0	6.5	44
555045	4.5	7.1	48
555050	5.0	7.7	50
555055	5.5	8.3	52

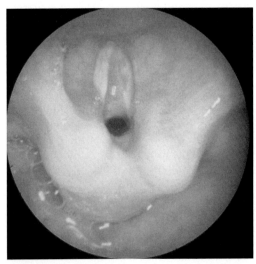

Figure 27.1. Suspension laryngoscopy showing an anteriorly based subglottic stenosis in a 2-month-old, formerly 25-week-premature infant, with tracheotomy since 3 months of life. Note right vocal cord abnormality. This child underwent LTR with anterior and posterior graft placement with an indwelling Aboulker stent.

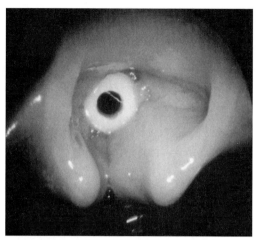

Figure 27.2. Indwelling Aboulker stent (at time of stent removal) with opening above false cords. Note small granulation of right vocal cord area.

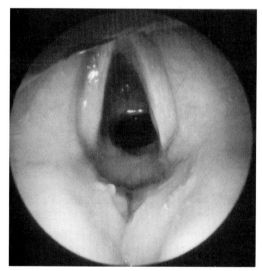

Figure 27.3. Eight-year-old child with intubation trauma after a motor vehicle accident. Note posterior glottic fibrosis. There was a marked decrease in vocal cord motility. He underwent an LTR with anterior and posterior cartilage grafts and placement of an indwelling stent.

involvement, a single-stage LTR can be considered (17). The tracheocutaneous fistula is excised with immediate reconstruction using an autogenous costal cartilage graft. Instead of an indwelling stent, an endotracheal tube is left in place until the pressure at which air leaks around the tube is less than 20 cm H_2O (18). This single-stage LTR allows definitive management in a single procedure.

Children who have been decannulated after LTR need close follow-up. The principal clinical factor in assessment of the upper airway is exercise tolerance. Direct laryngoscopy and bronchoscopy should rarely be required after decannulation. Pulmonary function studies have been used in cooperative older children in assessing the progression of the reconstructed area (19).

RECURRENT RESPIRATORY PAPILLOMATOSIS

The papillomas in recurrent respiratory papillomatosis (RRP) are the most common benign neoplasms of the larynx in children. They are exophytic pedunculated masses that can be single or multiple (Fig. 27.4), affecting the mucous membrane of the upper aerodigestive tract from the nasal cavity to the pulmonary parenchyma. The larynx is the most common site of involvement. The trachea and/or bronchi may become involved, especially if a tracheotomy is performed; therefore every effort is made to avoid tracheotomy (20).

RRP is caused by one or more of the human papilloma viruses (HPVs), a group of related DNA viruses that also cause cutaneous warts and genital condylomata. The most common types are HPV II and HPV G (21). Although spontaneous remission may occur, most cases have a tendency to progress, characterized by multiple recurrences requiring repeated ther-

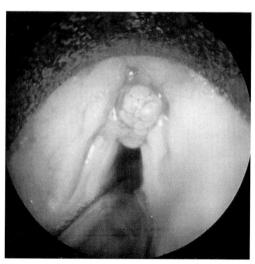

Figure 27.4. Recurrent respiratory papillomatosis at anterior commissure in a 2-year-old child after three previous laser procedures.

apeutic intervention, sometimes at very short intervals (22).

Over the years, a variety of adjuvants have been advocated, none with consistent success. The CO_2 laser delivered via microlaryngeal surgery or a bronchoscope has been the recommended treatment since the early 1970s (23). Kashima et al. reported that interferon alpha n-1 was an effective adjuvant to surgery in RRP management when given daily for 1 month and then three times per week (24). However, Healy et al. showed that while disease progression did slow with interferon in the first 6 months, this initial benefit was not sustained long-term (25). At present, RRP is best controlled by endoscopic microsurgical techniques, usually the CO_2 laser (26).

SUBGLOTTIC HEMANGIOMA

Another important cause of recurrent or a prolonged episodes of stridor is a subglottic hemangioma. Most patients (89%) present within the first 6 months of life. It appears to be more common in females (27). Approximately 50% of children with subglottic hemangiomas also have associated cutaneous hemangiomas. Airway radiographs prior to endoscopy show asymmetric subglottic narrowing. Endoscopy demonstrates a characteristic appearance of a smooth submucosal mass below the level of the vocal cords, usually in a posterolateral position (Fig. 27.5). If neces-

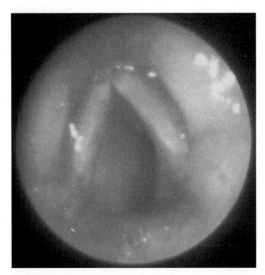

Figure 27.5. Large subglottic hemangioma in the left lateral position.

sary, biopsy can usually be performed without excessive bleeding (28). This should be done with a rigid endoscope under general anesthesia. Tracheotomy has traditionally been recommended for treatment for subglottic hemangioma, while waiting for resolution of the lesion at about 2 years of age. The decision to perform a tracheotomy is based on the criteria described for subglottic stenosis. The CO_2 laser delivered via a laryngoscope with operating microscope has been shown to be an effective alternative treatment for selected patients and carries a low complication rate (28). In many patients tracheotomy can be avoided.

REFERENCES

1. Abramson A, Goldstein M, Stenzler A, Steele A. The use of tidal breathing flow volume loop in laryngotracheal disease of neonates and infants. *Laryngoscope* 1982; 91:922–926.
2. Tepper RS, Eigen H, Brown J, Hurwitz R. Use of maximal expiratory flows to evaluate central airways obstruction in infants. *Pediatr Pulmon* 1989; 6:272–274.
3. Holinger LD. Etiology of stridor in the neonate, infant and child. *Ann Otol* 1980; 89:397–400.
4. Nussbaum E, Maggi JC. Laryngomalacia in children. *Chest* 1990; 98:942–944.
5. Zalzal GH, Anon JB, Cotton RT. Epiglottoplasty for the treatment of laryngomalacia. *Ann Otol Rhinol Laryngol* 1987; 96:72–76.
6. Belmont JR, Grundfast K. Congenital laryngeal stridor (laryngomalacia): Etiologic factors and associated disorders. *Ann Otol Rhinol Laryngol* 1984; 93:430–437.
7. Holinger LD, Konior RJ. Surgical management of severe laryngomalacia. *Laryngoscope* 1989; 99:136–142.
8. Marcus CL, Crockett DM, Ward SLD. Evaluation of epiglottoplasty as treatment for severe laryngomalacia. *J Pediatr* 1990; 117:706–710.
9. Cotton RT. Management and prevention of subglottic stenosis in infants and children. *Adv Otolaryngol Head Neck Surg* 1987; 1:241–260.
10. Friedman EM, Williams M, Healy GB, McGill TGI. Pediatric endoscopy: A review of 616 cases. *Ann Otol Rhinol Laryngol* 1984; 93:517–519.
11. Cotton RT, Gray SD, Miller RP. Update of the Cincinnati experience in pediatric laryngotracheal reconstruction. *Laryngoscope* 1989; 99:1111–1116.
12. Cotton RT, Myer CM, Bratcher GO, Fitton CM. Anterior cricoid split, 1977–1987: Evolution of a technique. *Arch Otolaryngol Head Neck Surg* 1988; 114:1300–1302.
13. Grundfast KM, Camilon FS, Pransky S, et al. Prospective study of subglottic stenosis in intubated neonates. *Ann Otol Rhinol Laryngol* 1990; 99:390–395.
14. Grundfast KM, Coffman AC, Milmoe G. Anterior cricoid split: A "simple" surgical procedure and a potentially complicated problem. *Ann Otol Rhinol Laryngol* 1985; 94:445–449.
15. Gianoli GJ, Miller RH, Guareisco JL. Tracheotomy in the first year of life. *Ann Otol Rhinol Laryngol* 1990; 99:896–901.

16. Irving RM, Jones NS, Bailey CM, Melville J. A guide to the selection of pediatric tracheostomy tubes. *J Laryngol Otol* 1991; 105:1046–1051.
17. April MM, Marsh BR. Laryngotracheal reconstruction for subglottic stenosis. The Johns Hopkins experience. *Ann Otol Rhinol Laryngol* 1993; 102:176–181.
18. Seid AB, Godin MS, Pransky SM, Kearns DB, Peterson BM. Prognostic value of endotracheal tube–air leak following trachael surgery in children. *Arch Otolaryngol Head Neck Surg* 1991; 117:880–882.
19. Zalzal GH, Thomsen JR, Chaney HR, Derkay C. Pulmonary parameters in children after laryngotracheal reconstruction. *Ann Otol Rhinol Laryngol* 1990; 99:386–389.
20. Weiss MD, Kashima HK. Tracheal involvement in laryngeal papillomatosis. *Laryngoscope* 1983; 93:45–48.
21. Abramson AL, Steinberg BM, Winkler B. Laryngeal papillomatosis: Clinical histopathologic and molecular studies. *Laryngoscope* 1987; 97:678–685.
22. Ossoff RH, Werkhaven JA, Dere H. Soft tissue complications of laser surgery for recurrent respiratory papillomatosis. *Laryngoscope* 1990; 101:1162–1166.
23. Strong MS, Vaughan CW, Healy GB, et al. Recurrent respiratory papillomatosis: Management with the CO₂ laser. *Ann Otol Rhinol Laryngol* 1976; 85:508–516.
24. Kashima H, Leventhal B, Clark K, et al. Interferon alfa-N1 in juvenile onset recurrent respiratory papillomatosis: Results of a randomized study in twelve collaborative institutions. *Laryngoscope* 1988; 98:334–340.
25. Healy GB, Gelber RD, Trowbridge AL, et al. Treatment of recurrent respiratory papillomatosis with human leukocyte interferon. *N Engl J Med* 1988; 319:401–407.
26. Robbins KT, Woodson GE. Current concepts in the management of laryngeal papillomatosis. *Head Neck Surg* 1984; 6:861–866.
27. Shikhani AH, Jones MM, Marsh BR, Holliday MJ. Infantile subglottic hemangiomas. An update. *Ann Otol Rhinol Laryngol* 1986; 95:336–347.
28. Healy G, McGill T, Friedman EM. Carbon dioxide laser in subglottic hemangioma: An update. *Ann Otol Rhino Laryngol* 1984; 93:370–373.

28

Foreign Body Aspiration

MARY H. WAGNER

Foreign body aspiration is an important cause of both morbidity and mortality in the pediatric age group. In 1987 aspiration of a foreign body was the fourth leading cause of accidental death in those under 5 years of age, accounting for approximately 8% of accidental deaths in this age group (1). Understanding the epidemiology, etiology, pathophysiology, treatment, and prevention of this problem is essential for the primary care provider as well as the pediatric pulmonary physician.

HISTORICAL PERSPECTIVE

As early as 1633 physicians recognized the importance of airway occlusion by foreign substances as a cause of death (2). The exact location of foreign materials and how they caused death was poorly understood, and patients often lingered for some time before succumbing. Muys described in 1690 a 7-year-old who died from "suffocation" 3 weeks after aspirating a bean (3). The first series of foreign body aspiration, the *Practical Treatise on Foreign Bodies in the Air Passages*, was reported in 1854 by S.D. Gross (3). This work included 200 case reports and demonstrated that foreign body aspiration was at least as common in children as in adults.

Therapies in these times were not very effective and included emetics and sternutatories (substances to stimulate sneezing) to promote expulsion of the foreign material. Bleeding, expectorants, purgatives and counter irritation were also used to counter the effects induced by the foreign substance. Surgical treatment of aspiration events was not widely accepted until the late 1800s. The initial surgical approach was a bronchotomy to open the airway to prevent suffocation as well as to allow for expulsion of the foreign object (3).

Although the idea was not new (Hippocrates had suggested placing a tube in the airway to prevent asphyxiation in cases of airway blockage), instrumentation of the airway with subsequent removal of foreign bodies was not attempted until the late 1800s. The development of esophagoscopy forged a path for airway endoscopy, and as early as 1825 physicians were "accidentally" passing tubes into airways. Killian has been credited with the early successful work in the area of bronchoscopy, and in 1897 he performed the first endoscopic removal of a foreign body (3). In 1898, the first successful bronchoscopy was performed in the United States at Massachusetts General Hospital using a urethroscope. Chevalier Jackson, in the early 1900s, advanced the practice of airway endoscopy by developing proper instruments (3, 4). Subsequent refinement of surgical instruments and techniques have made the treatment of airway foreign bodies much safer and more successful.

EPIDEMIOLOGY

Foreign body aspiration occurs most often in small children less than 5 years of age (5–8). Blazer reported on 200 cases of airway obstruction due to foreign bodies; 90% of their cases were in children less than 4 years of age (5). In the series reported by Svensson 65% of the 110 patients were under 4 years of age (8). Maximal frequency of aspiration occurs between ages 1 and 2 years (5, 8, 9). The high frequency of aspiration events in this age group can be attributed to their developmental activities of exploring their environment, often by putting objects in their mouths, and their expanding dietary repertoire. Boys

Laboratory Tests

At a minimum, oxygenation should be assessed by pulse oximetry or transcutaneous oxygen monitoring. In a group of 131 children suspected to have aspirated foreign bodies, Vane et al. noted evidence of impaired oxygenation in 62 prior to removal of the foreign body (11).

Radiologic Evaluation

The next step in the work-up of a child with a suspected foreign body should be lateral and anteroposterior chest radiographs. The chest radiograph is quite helpful if its results are abnormal. However, Svedstrom et al. found positive radiographic findings in 33% of children without foreign bodies at bronchoscopy (15).

A normal chest radiograph does not preclude the presence of a retained foreign body since various series have reported normal chest radiographs in 6–80% of children with foreign bodies in the respiratory tract (5–8, 14). Most foreign bodies are radiolucent, and therefore it is unlikely that a foreign body will be visualized on the chest radiograph. Changes on the chest radiograph may be related to the foreign body directly or due to secondary inflammatory changes from the foreign material. Abnormalities on chest radiographs include atelectasis (if there is complete airway obstruction), infiltrate, obstructive emphysema, mediastinal emphysema, and the presence of a radiopaque object (Fig. 28.1). The most common abnormality on plain chest radiograph is obstructive emphysema (7, 14, 15), which is more commonly seen with a bronchial foreign body (14) (Fig. 28.2). Abnormalities are less likely to be noted on the chest radiograph for foreign bodies located above the carina; Mu et al. noted that 80% of those with laryngotracheal foreign body had normal radiographic findings (14). Radiographic abnormalities are also more likely with longer diagnostic delay, with only 5% of cases having negative chest radiographs with a 30-day delay in the diagnosis of the foreign object (14). Blazer et al. found obstructive emphysema in 62% of children with bronchial foreign bodies and in 16% of those with laryngotracheal foreign bodies (5). Wiseman found that a delay in diagnosis was associated with more abnormalities noted on

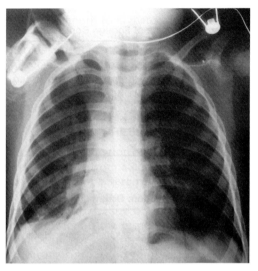

Figure 28.1. Chest radiograph demonstrating atelectasis involving the right middle and lower lobes in a 22-month-old child with a foreign body involving the right lower lobe bronchus. After removal of the foreign object, there was residual atelectasis for several weeks, which resolved with bronchodilator therapy and chest physiotherapy.

chest radiograph: 33% of those diagnosed early had normal study results, compared to only 9% of those diagnosed late (9).

Chest radiographs taken both on inspiration and on expiration may be helpful if the initial radiograph is normal. In the child with partial obstruction of the airway impairment of expiratory airflow will lead to differential lung deflation and air trapping on the affected side. The inspiratory film will demonstrate decreased inflation on the affected side if there is total occlusion of the airway. This technique is limited by patient cooperation.

An alternative approach involves the use of alternating right and left lateral decubitus views. In the normal situation, the lung in the dependent position should appear deflated. Finding a lung that does not deflate in the down position suggests the presence of a ball valve obstruction. This approach is particularly useful in younger uncooperative subjects, especially if fluoroscopy is not available.

Fluoroscopy of the chest can be used to make the diagnosis of a foreign body in the airway. This study may show obstructive emphysema, decreased diaphragmatic excursion, or mediastinal shift. Paradoxical mediastinal movement with an increase in size of mediastinal structures on inspiration was

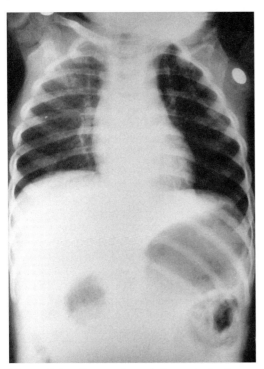

Figure 28.2. Chest radiograph demonstrating hyper-inflation involving the left lung in a 13-month-old child with a 1-week history of choking on a crayon and persistent wheeze. The initial chest radiograph was normal. At rigid bronchoscopy a small piece of orange crayon was removed from the left mainstem bronchus.

noted in 32% of patients with a laryngotracheal foreign body, and much less commonly in those with a bronchial foreign body (5, 16). Inspiratory shift of the mediastinal structures is a common finding (14), especially in those with a bronchial versus laryngotracheal foreign body (5, 14). Some children will have no demonstrable changes on chest fluoroscopy, particularly if the object is lodged in the laryngotracheal region of the respiratory tract or if a major airway is not involved.

Other radiologic modalities that have been used include computed tomography (CT) of the lung and pulmonary ventilation-perfusion scanning. Ventilation-perfusion scanning may demonstrate decreased or absent ventilation with a delay in washout of the involved region and a matched defect in perfusion (17). These modalities usually add little information to that obtained by careful history, examination, and inspiratory and expiratory chest radiographs or fluoroscopy, and are not necessary. Svensson found that the combination of plain chest radiography and fluoroscopy identified abnormalities in 76% of studied cases (8), and Wiseman found abnormalities in 84% of patients (9). Mu et al. found that these modalities identified abnormalities in 53% of their series of 400 (14).

TREATMENT

Children with a positive history of foreign body aspiration, such as a witnessed episode, should be evaluated by rigid endoscopy to facilitate removal of the foreign body as soon as possible. In the hands of an experienced pediatric bronchoscopist, this procedure is accomplished with minimal risk and few complications (10, 18). Unless the child is in respiratory distress the bronchoscopy should be scheduled to allow appropriate preoperative preparation including intravenous hydration, emptying of the stomach, and preoperative assessment of the child's respiratory status.

Rigid bronchoscopy allows the removal of the foreign body and any associated inflammatory material, as well as an assessment of the extent of airway damage. Most often the foreign body is removed using forceps and suctioning, although a balloon catheter has also been used by some bronchoscopists to aid in removing the object (8, 10, 11, 18). Secretions can also be obtained for microbiologic assessment. Wiseman reported increased bronchial inflammation at bronchoscopy in those diagnosed late when compared to those diagnosed early (9). Thus, early diagnosis and removal is important to prevent the possibility of airway occlusion from a dislodged foreign body, as well as prevention of inflammation that may further damage the tracheobronchial tree.

Flexible bronchoscopy should be considered in those children without a definitive history of foreign body aspiration who have unexplained respiratory tract pathology, including children with unexplained wheeze despite maximal medical management and children with localized wheeze, persistent infiltrates, atelectasis, or infiltrates that recur in the same lung segment.

Some children who have aspirated foreign bodies into the distal segments of the tracheobronchial tree may not be able to have their foreign body detected and removed by airway endoscopy. Persistent infiltrates/atelectasis associated with chronic cough, recurrent infection, or hemoptysis warrants a chest CT scan to identify and quantify bronchiectasis. In children with localized disease who are not responsive to intensive medical management and who develop persistent or recurrent symptoms, a thoracotomy should be considered. Timing of this surgery is variable and depends on the age of the patient, the severity of the patient's symptoms, and the frequency and severity of acute exacerbations localized to the damaged area. Examination of resected tissue may reveal a foreign body as the etiology of the persistent respiratory tract symptoms.

Antibiotics and steroids should not be routinely given except as indicated by bronchoscopic findings. Culture of bronchoscopic washings is important to determine if an infection secondary to the foreign body has further compromised the respiratory tract. Antibiotics should be instituted based on bronchoscopy findings including evidence of inflammation, purulent secretions, and positive cultures from bronchial lavage. Steroid therapy has been used occasionally to reduce airway inflammation and narrowing but there is little evidence that it helps. The use of antibiotics and steroids will not alleviate the underlying problem of a retained foreign body and should be considered for use on a case-by-case basis.

Chest physical therapy is contraindicated as primary therapy for a retained foreign body since there is increased risk of complete airway obstruction and respiratory arrest if the foreign body moves and lodges in the trachea or larynx (19, 20). Following removal of the foreign body, chest physical therapy may be helpful in clearing atelectatic lung segments and residual secretions. A follow-up chest radiograph is indicated in all patients whose initial radiograph was abnormal. In the asymptomatic patient, this study can be delayed for 6 weeks to assure sufficient time for resolution of the pneumonia/atelectasis. Conversely, it should be obtained sooner if symptoms persist or recur.

Persistent abnormalities may require repeat bronchoscopy to make certain that all of the foreign material has been removed from the lower respiratory tract and to assess residual airway damage. Follow-up studies in children several years after foreign body removal have demonstrated normal chest radiographs and pulmonary function, even in those patients

with evidence of marked airway inflammation on initial bronchoscopy (19).

COMPLICATIONS

Most of the complications related to foreign body aspiration events can be linked to a delay in the proper diagnosis. This delay can come in the form of unrecognized symptoms or recognized symptoms attributed to the incorrect disease process. This leads to a delay in the removal of the foreign object with the possibility of damage to the respiratory tract. Blazer et al. reported that only 54% of children in their series were referred to the hospital within 3 days of aspiration or onset of clinical signs (5). Often the delay in evaluation is prolonged, with 10–20% of patients experiencing a delay of more than 4 weeks (5, 8). Wiseman noted that children with peripheral foreign bodies that cause less bronchial obstruction, or objects lodged in the left side of the chest, were more likely to encounter a delay in diagnosis (9).

The misdiagnosis of foreign body aspiration as other disease entities can lead to ineffective therapies and persistent respiratory morbidity. Because the presenting respiratory symptoms are nonspecific and appropriate history may be lacking, many children with foreign body aspiration will be diagnosed as having a variety of other diseases. The differential diagnosis for the "acute" phase of foreign body aspiration includes laryngotracheitis, epiglottitis, laryngeal edema, pertussis, status asthmaticus, croup, and retropharyngeal abscess (6, 7). Conditions including asthma, recurrent pneumonia, bronchitis, tuberculosis, and bronchial stenosis are included in the spectrum of diseases that must be distinguished from a "chronically" retained foreign body (6, 7).

Retained foreign bodies can lead to a marked inflammatory response in the respiratory tract, particularly if organic material is involved. Materials such as nuts containing fats cause an intense inflammatory response. Recurrent infection from compromised airway defense mechanisms and secondary infection (Fig. 28.3) may also be linked to the inflammatory response. Often infiltrate will develop in the particular lung segment distal to the foreign body. However, foreign bodies can be dislodged by coughing leading to involvement of different lung segments.

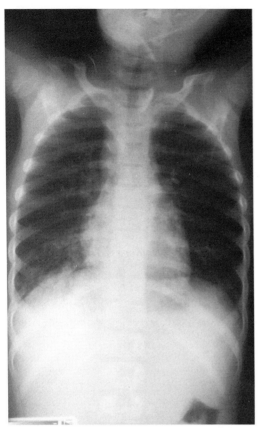

Figure 28.3. Chest radiograph demonstrating chronic changes involving the right middle and lower lobes in a 6-year-old girl with a 1-year history of recurrent pneumonias. There was no history of an aspiration event, although the child had decreased mental capacity. Because of persistent symptoms, a flexible bronchoscopy was performed, revealing a peanut in the bronchus intermedius. This was removed at rigid bronchoscopy performed immediately after the foreign body was discovered.

Other complications from delayed diagnosis include lung abscess, bronchiectasis, and infrequently bronchopleural fistula resulting from erosion through an airway wall either by the sharp edge of the aspirated material or secondary to the vigor of the inflammatory response. Improvement in the diagnosis of retained foreign bodies has lead to a decrease in serious late sequelae.

Postbronchoscopy complications include fever, atelectasis, infiltrate, bronchospasm, and pneumothorax (11, 20). Some children will require repeat bronchoscopy because of persistent respiratory symptoms related to incomplete removal of the object. Children

with laryngeal foreign bodies may also require tracheostomy if there is marked laryngeal damage or edema. Other complications include mediastinal and subcutaneous emphysema (5,7).

Asphyxiation and death can occur, particularly if the foreign body is lodged in larynx or trachea. Lima reported 11 cases with laryngeal foreign bodies (12). In this group, 45% of the children died as a result of their aspiration event, with another 27% suffering respiratory arrest and temporary anoxic encephalopathy. Asphyxiation can also result from an esophageal foreign body obstructing the airway by external pressure. Death has also resulted from dislodgement of a foreign body with subsequent obstruction of the trachea and contralateral bronchus after a prolonged asymptomatic interval.

PREVENTION

The most effective "therapy" for foreign body aspiration is prevention of the aspiration event. Risk factors that contribute to foreign body aspiration include the physical characteristics of potentially aspirated materials, the anatomy of the respiratory tract, the developmental status of the child, and environmental factors (2).

The physical characteristics of many objects may make them more likely to be aspirated if they are introduced into the mouth either inadvertently or during eating. The characteristics that facilitate foreign body aspiration include size, contour, shape, and consistency. Small size, smooth or slick surface, and round or cylindrical shape increase the risk of aspiration. These risk factors are found in foods such as hot dogs, grapes, peanuts, and small candies that are involved in the majority of foreign body aspiration events. Additional risk factors for foods include hard or tough foods (peanut, carrot) that resist chewing, viscous foods that may be difficult to clear from the oropharynx and airway, and pliable or compressible foods (hot dogs) that can plug the airway.

Developmental status also increases the risk of foreign body aspiration. Children in the age range 6 months–2 years commonly place objects in their mouth, increasing the risk of aspiration. Small children without molars are unable to chew foods such as nuts or hard candies in preparation for swallowing properly. When these children use their front teeth to chew these foods, fragments are created that may be propelled rapidly into the posterior pharynx, increasing the risk of aspiration. Thus, children less than 3–4 years of age should not be given nuts or hard candies to eat and must have other foods such as hot dogs and grapes appropriately prepared; furthermore, these children must be carefully supervised while eating such foods. Environmental factors such as the level of supervision and distractions can lead to aspiration episodes. Caregivers must be vigilant with small children to prevent them from putting objects into their mouths. During meals and snacks their foods must be appropriately prepared to minimize the physical characteristics of the food that predispose to aspiration. Distractions during eating must be minimized so that the child can concentrate on appropriately chewing and swallowing foods. Children must also be observed during play to prevent them from running or jumping with food or other objects in their mouths.

REFERENCES

1. *Accident facts.* Chicago, National Safety Council, 1990, p 12.
2. Harris CS, Baker SP, Smith GA, Harris RM. Child asphyxiation by food: A national analysis and overview. *JAMA* 1984; 251:2231–2235.
3. Clerf LH. Historical aspects of foreign bodies in the food and air passages. *S Med J* 1975; 68:1449–1454.
4. Witt WJ. The role of rigid endoscopy in foreign body management. *Ear Nose Throat J* 1985; 64:70–74.
5. Blazer S, Naveh Y, Friedman A. Foreign body in the airway: A review of 200 cases. *Am J Dis Child* 1980; 134:68–71.
6. Losek JD. Diagnostic difficulties of foreign body aspiration in children. *Am J Emerg Med* 1990; 8:348–350.
7. Steen KH, Zimmermann T. Tracheobronchial aspiration of foreign bodies in children: A study of 94 cases. *Laryngoscope* 1990; 100:525–530.
8. Svensson G. Foreign bodies in the tracheobronchial tree. Special reference to experience in 97 children. *Int J Pediatr Otorhinolaryngol* 1985; 8:243–251.
9. Wiseman NE. The diagnosis of foreign body aspiration in childhood. *J Pediatr Surg* 1984; 19:531–535.
10. Mantor PC, Tuggle DW, Tunell WP. An appropriate negative bronchoscopy rate in suspected foreign body aspiration. *Am J Surg* 1989; 158:622–624.
11. Vane DW, Pritchard J, Colville CW, West KW, Eigen H, Grosfeld JL. Bronchoscopy for aspirated foreign bodies in children. *Arch Surg* 1988; 123:885–888.
12. Lima JA. Laryngeal foreign bodies in children: A persistent, life-threatening problem. *Laryngoscope* 1989; 99:415–420.
13. Friedman EM. Caustic ingestions and foreign bodies in the aerodigestive tract of children. *Pediatr Clin North Am* 1989; 36:1403–1410.
14. Mu L, Sun D, He P. Radiological diagnosis of aspirated foreign bodies in children: Review of 343 cases. *J Laryngol Otol* 1990; 104:778–782.
15. Svedstrom E, Puhakka H, Kero P. How accurate is chest radiography in the diagnosis of tracheobronchial foreign bodies in children? *Pediatr Radiol* 1989; 19:520–522.
16. Grunebaum M, Adler S, Varsano I. The paradoxical movement of the mediastinum: A diagnostic sign of foreign-body aspiration during childhood. *Pediatr Radiol* 1979; 8:213–218.
17. Lull RJ, Tatum JL, Sugerman HJ, Hartshorne MF, Boll DA, Kaplan KA. Radionuclide evaluation of lung trauma. *Semin Nucl Med* 1983; 13:223–237.
18. Kosloske AM. Bronchoscopic extraction of aspirated foreign bodies in children. *Am J Dis Child* 1982; 136:924–927.
19. Law D, Kosloske AM. Management of tracheobronchial foreign bodies in children: A reevaluation of postural drainage and bronchoscopy. *Pediatrics* 1976; 58:362–367.
20. Cotton E, Yasuda K. Foreign body aspiration. *Pediatr Clin North Am* 1984; 31:937–941.

29

Pneumonia

PRESTON W. CAMPBELL III and DENNIS C. STOKES

Acute respiratory tract infections are the most common illnesses in the pediatric age group. Although pneumonia accounts for only 10–15% of all respiratory tract infections, it is a significant cause of morbidity and mortality in children. The United Nations Children's Fund (UNICEF) has estimated that worldwide approximately 3 million children die of pneumonia each year (1). Although most of these deaths occur in developing countries, pneumonia remains a major cause of acute morbidity in developed countries. In community-based studies, annual attack rates average 4 children per 100 preschool children, 2 per 100 children aged 5–9 years, and 1 per 100 children between the ages of 9 and 15 years (2, 3). Pneumonia, as defined by chest radiography, represented 7.5% of febrile illnesses in infants 3 months of age or younger (4) and 13% of infectious illnesses during the first 2 years of life (5).

Pneumonia is distinguished from the more common upper respiratory tract infection (URI) by the presence of lower tract signs and symptoms (cough, tachypnea, rales, and cyanosis) and an associated area of infiltration on chest radiograph. The challenge is not only to make the correct diagnosis, but also to rule out associated underlying conditions and begin rational treatment.

PATHOPHYSIOLOGY

A variety of mechanisms act to guard the lungs from infection. Inspired air is filtered by the nares. The lower respiratory tract is protected by the glottis and larynx, and material that manages to pass this barrier is usually expectorated by the cough reflex. Small particles impinging on the walls of the trachea and bronchi are trapped by the mucociliary blanket and carried by the cilia to the proximal airway, where they are then cleared. Particles reaching the alveolus are dealt with by the phagocytic activity of the alveolar macrophage and local immune defenses. Particles ingested by macrophages are then cleared by the lymphatic system. Any anatomic or physiologic derangement of these coordinated defenses renders the lung susceptible to infection (Table 29.1).

Viral agents are inoculated into the upper respiratory tract and spread distally. When infected, the respiratory epithelium loses its ciliary appendages, rounds up, and sloughs into the airway, resulting in stasis of mucus and accumulation of airway debris (6, 7). The associated inflammatory response is characterized by mononuclear infiltration into the submucosa and perivascular areas, further compromising the airway lumen. Smooth muscle contraction often occurs with this inflammatory process. These changes result in obstruction to airflow manifested clinically by the prolonged expiratory time, wheezes, radiographic hyper-expansion, and atelectasis (if complete obstruction has occurred) typical of viral bronchiolitis. Involvement of the alveolar type II cell and loss of its structural integrity results in diminished surfactant production, hyaline membrane formation, and pulmonary edema. Pneumonia results from viral proliferation and inflammation in the alveolar space. Collectively these changes diminish alveolar capillary gas exchange causing hypoxia from ventilation-perfusion mismatch.

Bacteria gain access to the lower airway primarily by aspiration of oropharyngeal organisms or inhalation of infectious respiratory droplets. Hematogenous spread occurs, rarely

Table 29.1.
Host Defense Disorders Leading to Pneumonia

Pulmonary Host Defense	Defective In:
Upper airway	
Turbinates	Intubation,
Epiglottis	Tracheostomy, aspiration syndromes
Mucociliary clearance	
Cilia	Ciliary dyskinesia syndrome, infections
Mucous blanket	CF, bronchitis
Cough	Muscle weakness, sedation
Immunoglobulin	
Secretory IgA	
IgA	IgA deficiency, IgG subclass deficiency
IgG, including subclasses	Agammaglobulinemia, hypogammaglobulinemia
IgE	Elevated in hyper-IgE with recurrent infections (Job syndrome)
Cellular	
Alveolar macrophage	Corticosteroids, chemotherapy, CGD
Polymorphonuclear leukocyte	
Numbers	Chemotherapy, congenital neutropenia
Mobility	Motility disorders
Function	Chronic Granulomatous disease
Lymphocytes	
Numbers	AIDS
Function	T-cell disorders, including CMC, SCID, others
Other	
Surfactant	?ARDS, edema
Fibronectin, lysozyme	
Complement	C3, C5 deficiency

arising from conditions such as staphylococcal skin abscesses and infected intravenous catheters. The alveolar involvement is more intense than that seen with viral pneumonias. Infection with pneumococci, for example, fills the alveoli with a proteinaceous fluid, followed by a brisk influx of red cells and polymorphonuclear cells. During resolution, alveolar macrophages fill the alveoli and remove the intra-alveolar debris, restoring normal lung morphology. In contrast, infection due to *Staphylococcus aureus* or *Klebsiella pneumonia* results in necrosis of intra-alveolar septa, making possible the formation of abscesses and destruction of underlying lung architecture.

ETIOLOGY

The causes of pneumonia in children vary with the season and the age and health status of the child (Table 29.2). It is important to understand which agent is most likely in a particular patient, since such knowledge will

guide both the diagnostic work-up and initial therapy.

Age and Season Considerations

NEONATE

Pathogens causing pneumonia in the newborn infant can be acquired by transplacental infection, aspiration of organisms present in the birth canal, and postnatal infection from human contacts or contaminated equipment. Organisms colonizing the maternal genital tract such as group B *Streptococcus* and gram-negative organisms (e.g., *Escherichia coli* and *Klebsiella pneumoniae*) are the most common causes of neonatal pneumonia.

Perinatally acquired infectious agents may cause illness later in infancy. For example, infants with perinatally acquired *Chlamydia trachomatis* develop an afebrile pneumonia with a staccato cough between 4 and 11 weeks of age (8). A similar syndrome can be caused by infection with *Ureaplasma urealyticum*,

Table 29.2.
Most Common Etiologic Agents of Pediatric Pneumonia

Ages	Causes
Community-Acquired Pneumonia	
Newborn	1. Group B *Streptococcus*
	2. Gram-negative bacilli
2–11 weeks	Afebrile pneumonitis syndrome
	Chlamydia trachomatous
	Ureaplasma urealyticum
	Mycoplasma hominus
	Cytomegalovirus
	Pneumocystis carinii
Preschool	1. Viruses
(1 month–5 years)	Respiratory syncytial virus (most common)
	Parainfluenza virus 1, 2, 3
	Influenza A and B
	Other—adenovirus, rhinoviruses
	2. Bacterial (less common)
	Streptococcus pneumoniae
	Hemophilus influenzae
	Other—*Staphylococcus aureus* other
	streptococci, *Moraxella catarrhalis*
School-aged	1. *Mycoplasma pneumoniae* (most common)
(6 years and older)	2. Viruses (parainfluenza, influenza)
	3. Bacteria (*Streptococcus pneumoniae, Haemophilus influenzae*)
Hospital-Acquired Pneumonia	
All ages	1. Enteric gram-negative bacilli
	2. *Pseudomonas aeruginosa*
	3. *Staphylococcus aureus*

Mycoplasma hominis, cytomegalovirus, and *Pneumocystis carinii,* and is now called the "afebrile pneumonitis syndrome of infancy" (9).

Community-acquired viral infections in the neonate usually occur in winter and are associated with illness in other family members (10). Respiratory syncytial virus (RSV) is the most commonly isolated virus, but enterovirus, rhinovirus, adenovirus, parainfluenza virus, and herpes simplex virus are also seen.

INFANT AND PRESCHOOL CHILD

After 1 month of age, viruses become the most common cause of pneumonia. Most of the viruses causing respiratory disease in children can produce a clinical spectrum ranging from rhinorrhea to pneumonia. Still, it is often possible to determine the most likely virus based on the age of the patient, season, clinical manifestations of the child, and other epidemiologic factors (Table 29.3).

RSV is the major cause of pneumonia and bronchiolitis in young children, with a peak incidence occurring between 2 and 5 months of age. It occurs in winter and early spring epidemics, with as many as 40% of children becoming infected during their first exposure. Most children have been infected at least once by one of the two subtypes by their second birthday. Next in importance are the parainfluenza viruses, of which there are three serotypes. Parainfluenza type 3 is most likely to affect younger infants and cause lower tract disease indistinguishable from RSV and occurs primarily in the spring. Parainfluenza types 1 and 2 occasionally cause pneumonia and are prevalent in the fall. Influenza A and B viruses can become the predominant isolates during winter epidemics. Influenza A is constantly changing its surface antigens (hemagglutinin and neuraminidase), which interferes with the development of lasting immunity and results in a renewable population of suscepti-

Table 29.3.
Respiratory Viruses Commonly Causing Pneumonia in Infants and Children

Virus	Age	Season	Associated Illness
Respiratory syncytial virus	Infants, young preschool	Winter	Bronchiolitis
Parainfluenza virus 1 and 2	Preschool	Fall	Croup
Parainfluenza virus 3	Infants and preschool	Spring	Bronchiolitis, croup pneumonitis
Influenza viruses A and B	Preschool, school aged	Winter	"Flu"
Adenoviruses	All ages	Year round	Pharyngitis, pneumonia bronchiolitis, tracheobronchitis

ble individuals. After a significant antigenic shift of the surface proteins, epidemics of influenza can occur with pneumonia as a complication. Adenovirus infections occur year-round, and are common causes of conjunctivitis and pharyngitis in young children. Of the 33 different adenovirus serotypes, types 3, 7, 11, and 21 can cause severe necrotizing pneumonia in young children and can result in obliterative bronchiolitis or death. Enteroviruses, rhinoviruses, coronaviruses, herpesviruses, and cytomegaloviruses have been less frequent isolates causing pneumonia in children.

Determining the true incidence of bacterial pneumonias in any age group is difficult because sampling the lower airway flora is difficult. Sputum samples are not easily obtained and invasive tests are not performed routinely. One study using bacterial antigen detection methods in an outpatient pediatric population determined the incidence of bacterial pneumonia to be 19% (11). Bacterial pneumonias occur throughout the year, but are most common during the winter months. *Streptococcus pneumoniae* and *Haemophilus influenzae* type b are the pathogens most likely to be isolated.

SCHOOL AGE AND ADOLESCENT

Once children are school aged, *Mycoplasma pneumoniae* becomes the most common etiologic agent. It accounts for up to 20% of all cases of pneumonia in the general population, 9–16% in early school aged children, 16–21% in older children, and 30–50% in college students and military recruits (12–16). Infections occur year round with sporadic epidemics in the fall or early winter, during which time the incidence of infection may increase three to five times. Older children and young adults are most commonly affected.

In this older age group the influenza viruses followed by parainfluenza virus and adenovi-

rus are the most common viral pathogens. *Streptococcus pneumoniae* remains the most common bacterial isolate; as children get older, *Haemophilus influenzae* becomes less common.

CLINICAL MANIFESTATIONS

Physical Examination

The signs and symptoms of pneumonia vary greatly and dependent on the pathogen, the age of the child, and the child's ability to mount an immunologic response. Although it may not be possible to differentiate between a viral and bacterial pneumonia in an individual case, it is helpful to understand the typical presentation of each.

Viral pneumonia typically begins with upper respiratory tract symptoms of several days' duration, including fever and rhinorrhea. The onset of respiratory distress and cough is usually gradual. Respiratory distress is usually manifested by tachypnea with or without tachycardia, nasal flaring, and retractions. Cyanosis and grunting respirations should alert the physician that the child requires prompt attention. Grunting results from partial closure of the vocal cords during expiration in an attempt to maintain a high alveolar pressure and prevent alveolar collapse.

Findings on physical examination are nonspecific. Percussion of the chest is less helpful in the smaller child than it is in the older child or adolescent. However, hyper-resonance may be detected if significant air trapping is present. Similarly, dullness to percussion may be present with consolidation of an entire lobe. Transmitted upper airway sounds may make interpretation of the lower airway findings on auscultation difficult. Coarse crackles are often heard and are secondary to partial obstruction of the larger airways by mucus and cellular debris. Wheezing is a variable finding and when present suggests associated bronchiolitis of viral etiology. Fine crackles may be heard focally, diffusely, or even intermittently.

Features suggestive of bacterial pneumonia include acute onset, toxic appearance, productive cough, and pleuritic pain. Lower lobe involvement with diaphragmatic irritation may cause severe referred abdominal pain. Often crackles will not be heard. Instead diminished breath sounds over the involved segment with dullness to percussion and tactile fremitus are appreciated. In some cases the only discernible findings will be fever and increased respiratory rate.

In all cases of pneumonia, extrapulmonary complications should be ruled out and clues that would suggest a particular pathogen should be searched for carefully. Poor oral intake and increased insensible losses from fever and tachypnea can lead to dehydration. The child with sepsis and early shock will have tachycardia, poor perfusion, and hypotension. A relative bradycardia in relation to fever should suggest *Legionella* pneumonia. Phlebitis or splinter hemorrhages indicate the possibility of a hematogenously spread pneumonia. Other cutaneous associations include a scarlatiniform rash in streptococcal disease and skin abscesses in staphylococcal infection. Meningitis and articular involvement are significant complications, and their identification may enable the identification of a specific pathogen and alter the duration and type of therapy chosen.

Radiographic Appearance

The classic radiographic appearance of viral pneumonia is that of a patchy bronchopneumonia. In infants, a perihilar pattern associated with hyper-expansion and atelectasis is often seen. Lobar pneumonia can be seen but is more often associated with a bacterial process. Consolidation, pleural effusion, pneumatoceles, or abscesses on the chest radiograph indicate that bacterial causes are likely.

Other Laboratory Studies

Peripheral white blood cell counts are usually elevated and not particularly helpful in diagnosis. A markedly elevated white blood cell count (greater than $30,000/mm^3$) with a predominance of neutrophils suggests a bacterial cause. The erythrocyte sedimentation rate is a nonspecific indicator of inflammation and therefore of little help.

SPECIFIC PATHOGENS

Streptococcus pneumoniae

Streptococcus pneumoniae is a gram-positive diplococcus having 84 different serotypes. Only a few serotypes (types 1, 3, 6, 7, 14, 18, 19, and 23) are responsible for the infections usually seen in children. *S. pneumoniae* is carried in the upper respiratory tract in 5–60% of asymptomatic individuals [17]. The prevalence is highest in infants (60%) and in families with children (25%) [18, 19]. The incidence of pneumonia from this organism is highest in infants under 2 years old, with a peak incidence between 3 and 5 months. It is more common in blacks and in males. Children with asplenia, functional asplenia, or immunosuppression are at special risk.

The onset of pneumococcal pneumonia is abrupt, with fever, chills, and dyspnea. Cough is an early manifestation and may produce blood-tinged sputum in the older child. The child usually appears acutely ill with shallow, rapid respirations. Crackles may be heard, but more commonly decreased breath sounds with dullness to percussion are noted. Chest radiographs typically show a lobar consolidation with air bronchograms (Fig. 29.1). Pleural inflammation is common and can result in small effusions or a pleural friction rub in some cases. Once appropriate antibiotic therapy is started dramatic clinical improvement is usually seen in 24–48 hours.

Haemophilus influenzae

Haemophilus influenzae is a small, pleomorphic gram-negative rod and is typed according to its polysaccharide capsule (a–f). Type b accounts for most cases of pneumonia. The spectrum of disease is wide, and those treated as outpatients may have minimal symptoms [20]. Children who require admission to the hospital tend to have a high rate of complications including pleural effusion, pneumothorax, pneumatoceles, associated meningitis, cellulitis, and pericarditis [21]. There was evidence suggesting that *H. influenzae* was

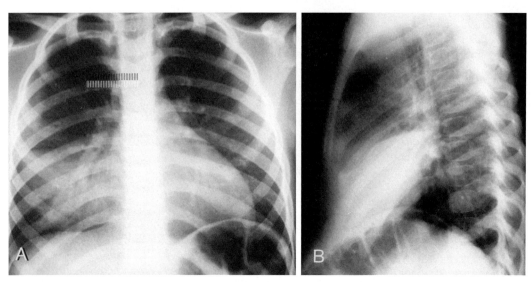

Figure 29.1. Pneumococcal pneumonia with lobar consolidation of right middle lobe. *A,* PA view: right heart border is obscured, illustrating silhouette sign. *B,* lateral view: wedge-shaped infiltrate in right middle lobe.

increasing in frequency (22–24), a trend that may be reversed with routine vaccination against *H. influenzae* type b.

Staphylococcus aureus

The incidence of staphylococcal pneumonia is greatest in the first 3 months of life. The prior use of antibiotics, altered host immunity, and an antecedent viral infection such as influenza are associated risk factors for staphylococcal pneumonia. In infants the onset is abrupt and rapidly progressive to severe disease with empyema, abscesses, and pneumatoceles. The presence of pneumatoceles is not diagnostic for *S. aureus* since they can also be seen in children with pneumonia caused by *S. pneumoniae, Haemophilus influenzae,* group A *Streptococcus,* and gram-negative enterics. In older children, staphylococcal pneumonia can be similar both clinically and radiographically to other bacterial pneumonias (Fig. 29.2).

Group B Streptococcus

Group B *Streptococcus* (GBS) serotypes I and II are associated with early-onset disease and pneumonia. When infected, neonates usually manifest clinical symptoms within the first 6–12 hours. It is a multi-system disease including fever, cardiovascular collapse, and pulmonary hypertension. The clinical and radiographic features of pneumonia due to GBS are similar to those of hyaline membrane disease except that apnea and shock are more common in group B streptococcal disease (25).

Chlamydia

The characteristics of chlamydial pneumonia are now well described (26). Affected infants are usually between 3 and 11 weeks of age and present with a persistent staccato cough, rales, and wheezing without fever. Laboratory findings include a mild peripheral eosinophilia and elevated immunoglobulin M (IgM) and IgG. The typical radiographic pattern is one of bilateral symmetrical interstitial infiltrates and hyper-expansion. Ureaplasma, cytomegalovirus, and *Pneumocystis carinii* can cause a similar illness (afebrile pneumonitis syndrome of infancy).

Mycoplasma

Mycoplasma pneumoniae pneumonia generally presents with the gradual onset of malaise, fever, and headache (27). A cough that begins 3–5 days after the onset of the illness, is initially nonproductive, and later becomes productive of white or blood-tinged sputum is typical (28). In Steven's review of 44 children with *M. pneumoniae* lower respiratory tract infection, cough was present in 93%, malaise in 86%, fever in 78%, nasal discharge or sore throat in 59%, vomiting in 39%, abdominal

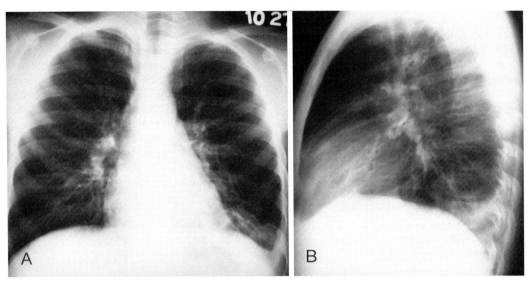

Figure 29.2. Staphylococcal pneumonia in an 11-year-old boy with cystic fibrosis. *A*, PA view: left lower lobe pneumonia with small effusion blunting left diaphragm. *B*, lateral view.

pain in 34%, and headache in 32% (29). Because of ciliostasis, cough is the most persistent symptom and can persist for weeks. Physical findings include crackles (78%), rhonchi (32%), and bronchial breath sounds (27%) (29). Levine noted that 40% of children wheeze (30). The radiographic appearance of *M. pneumoniae* is varied, but in a recent review 87% of patients had involvement of only one lung field, most frequently in the lower lobes (31). Early in infection the pattern is reticular and interstitial. Later patchy and segmental areas of consolidation are noted. Hilar adenopathy has been observed in 34% (31) of patients, and pleural effusion in 20% (32). Of the 7% of hospitalized patients who develop neurologic disease (33), most manifest meningoencephalitis, but transverse myelitis, cranial neuropathy, cerebellar ataxia, and Guillain-Barré syndrome are also seen. Approximately 10% of children develop an exanthem (27, 29, 41). Cardiac involvement occurs in 4.5% of patients, and as many as 36% have elevated hepatic transaminase enzymes.

Legionella pneumophila

In August of 1976, approximately 200 participants of an American Legion convention in Philadelphia developed an unusual form of pneumonia accompanied by encephalopathy, chills, myalgias, and liver dysfunction. Small pleomorphic rods were identified as the caus-

ative agent and designated *Legionella pneumophila*. Seroepidemiologic studies suggest that subclinical or mild infections occur in children (34, 35), but prospective studies of children with lower respiratory tract disease were able to identify only a few cases (36, 37). Features suggestive of *Legionella* pneumonia include high fever, nonproductive cough, slow pulse, and gastrointestinal problems. Most reports of *Legionella* pneumonia have occurred in immunocompromised children.

Anaerobic Bacteria

Children prone to aspirate oropharyngeal secretions may be infected with anaerobic bacteria including *Bacteroides melaninogenicus*, *Peptococcus*, *Peptostreptococcus*, *Fusobacterium nucleatum*, and *Veillonella*. Like gram-negative enterics and *Staphylococcus aureus*, these organisms cause tissue necrosis and abscesses. Sputum with a putrid smell strongly suggests an anaerobic pulmonary infection.

Tuberculosis

Recognition, prevention, and treatment of tuberculosis is covered in Chapter 30.

Fungal Pneumonias

The pulmonary mycoses are rare causes of pneumonia in non-immunocompromised hosts but are nevertheless important considerations in endemic regions, where they cause pneumonias in healthy individuals.

The dimorphic fungus, *Histoplasmosis capsulatum*, although distributed worldwide, is endemic to the Central United States. In Tennessee and Kentucky 90% of the population will have a positive histoplasmin skin test reaction by 20 years of age. The saprophytic form of the fungus grows in shady, acidic soil such as that seen in caves, in bird roosts, or beneath buildings. When the soil is disrupted, spores are inhaled, resulting in infection. When inhaled, the spores transform into small budding yeast within the alveoli. This infection spreads to adjacent lymph nodes and transiently to distal organs via the blood stream. In most cases infection with *H. capsulatum* is self-limited and mild. Most patients develop a flu-like illness with nonproductive cough. Eventually, the primary complex and adjacent nodes undergo caseous necrosis, fibrosis, and calcification that is similar in appearance to the Ghon complex of primary pulmonary tuberculosis. Secondary complications, including bronchial compression by enlarged nodes and mediastinal fibrosis, can also occur following histoplasmosis in children (38, 39) (Fig. 29.3). Severe and disseminated disease can occur and is usually seen in infants and immunosuppressed patients.

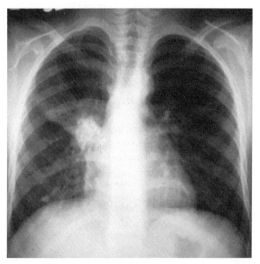

Figure 29.3. Histoplasmosis showing extensive mediastinal calcification and bronchial compression with partial atelectasis of the right upper lobe; a peripheral lung primary complex is also visible in the right lower lobe.

Coccidioidomycosis is an infection endemic to the arid regions of the Southwestern United States and is acquired by inhaling the minute arthrospores of the fungus *Coccidioides immitis*. Most infections are benign and self-limited. Sixty per cent of infections are believed to be asymptomatic, with the remainder causing influenza-like symptoms, night sweats, and possibly chest pain, arthritis, and skin rashes. Infrequently, a pulmonary cavity develops in an otherwise asymptomatic individual. Disseminated disease can occur in selected individuals.

NONINFECTIOUS CAUSES OF PNEUMONIA

Not all inflammation of the lung is infectious in origin. Pneumonitis can result from gastroesophageal reflux with aspiration, tracheoesophageal fistula with aspiration, smoke inhalation, hypersensitivity pneumonitis, and pulmonary hemosiderosis. Finally, a number of conditions can mimic pneumonia and need to be ruled out such as a prominent thymus, atelectasis, congenital structural anomalies, tumor, and congestive heart failure (Table 29.4).

SPECIAL CONSIDERATIONS

Children with recurrent (generally defined as more than one episode of pneumonia in a year or three or more in their lifetime), persistent, or atypical pneumonias are common diagnostic problems that deserve special emphasis (40). These patients often include those with underlying structural disorders as well as those with host defects in the lung defenses. Pleural effusions and empyema are the most frequent complications of pneumonia and are also considered briefly.

Recurrent or Persistent Pneumonias

Patients with recurrent or persistent respiratory infections can be categorized in many ways, but one useful way is to classify them into those with (a) persistent or recurrent radiologic findings with persistent or intermittent fever or other clinical signs of infection, (b) persistent radiologic findings without clinical evidence of infection, or (c) recurrent pulmonary infiltrates with interval radiologic clearing. In the first group are patients with

Table 29.4.
Non-Infectious Processes Complicating or Simulating Pneumonia

Process	Associated with:
Chemical pneumonitis	Aspiration syndromes, smoke inhalation
Immune-mediated	Hyper-sensitivity pneumonitis, collagen vascular disease
Atelectasis	Reactive airways disease
Hemorrhage	Hemosiderosis, thrombocytopenia, coagulopathy, *Aspergillus*
Pulmonary edema	CHF, fluid overload, poor myocardial function (anthracyline cardiotoxicity, sepsis, myocarditis), ARDS, pancreatitis
Drug-induced lung injury	Chemotherapy azathioprine
Radiation pneumonitis	Radiation 6–8 weeks previously
Leukostasis	Hyper-leukocytosis, amphotericin B, WBC transfusions
Leukemia, lymphoma	Active disease
Lymphocytic interstitial pneumonitis	HIV infection in children
"Idiopathic pneumonitis"	Allogeneic bone marrow transplantation
Other	Thymus, sequestration, tumor

cystic fibrosis, immunodeficiencies such as hypogammaglobulinemia, pulmonary sequestration, obstruction (either intrinsic due to foreign body, adenoma, or tuberculosis, or extrinsic due to nodes, tumor, or cyst), bronchial stenosis, and bronchiectasis. In the second group anatomic lesions such as sequestrations, anatomic variants, fibrosis, and pleural lesions would be considered. And in the third group, asthma (and atelectasis) is probably the most common diagnosis, but aspiration syndromes (including tracheo-esophageal fistula and gastro-esophageal reflux disorders), mild immunodeficiency syndromes, hypersensitivity pneumonitis, and idiopathic pulmonary hemosiderosis could also be considered. Whether the pneumonias are unilobar or are occurring in more than one lobe can also be a useful differential point in patients with recurrent pneumonia (Table 29.5) (40, 41). A number of early lung injury and repair syndromes are associated with repeated lung infections later in childhood, including bronchopulmonary dysplasia, tracheo-esophageal fistula repair, hydrocarbon pneumonitis, and severe viral infections such as adenovirus and measles pneumonias (42–44).

Unusually severe or prolonged pulmonary infections with common infectious agents can occur in compromised hosts. These include RSV infections in patients with immunodeficiencies, congenital heart disease, and bronchopulmonary dysplasia (45, 46). RSV commonly occurs as a nosocomial infection in hospitalized immunocompromised patients. Varicella-zoster, influenza, parainfluenza, and measles viruses are common childhood viral infections with generally mild respiratory symptoms that can be devastating in immuno-compromised children (47–49). *Mycoplasma* causes more severe pneumonias in patients with sickle cell disease (50). Although *Staphylococcus aureus* pneumonia also occurs in normal children, children with the hyper IgE and recurrent infection syndrome (Job syndrome) develop severe pulmonary damage from this organism, with chronic bullae and pneumatoceles (51). *S. aureus* is also a major cause of pneumonia in neutropenic patients.

Pneumonia in the Immunocompromised Host

The "opportunistic" infections are those infections typically not seen except in patients with altered immune status. The best example is *Pneumocystis carinii* pneumonia (PCP). PCP is also a common presenting manifestation of infants with hypogammaglobulinemia or agammaglobulinemia (52). The clinical course of opportunistic infections is varied and often depends on the degree of residual host immunity. Corticosteroid therapy may accelerate the resolution of *P. carinii* in AIDS patients, suggesting that residual host inflammatory response to this organism may be important in the pathogenesis of respiratory failure even in profoundly immunosuppressed patients (53, 54). Fungal pulmonary infections in patients with chemotherapy-induced neutropenia often result in mild clinical symptoms and radiographic findings until return of their neutrophil counts results in significant

Table 29.5.
Causes of Recurrent Pneumonia

Single Lobe	Multiple Lobes

I. Intraluminal obstruction
   A. Foreign body
   B. Bronchial adenoma
   C. Bronchial lipoma
   D. Broncholithiasis
	I. Aspiration syndromes
	   A. Gastroesophageal reflux
	   B. Tracheo-esophageal fistula
	   C. Laryngeal cleft
	   D. Altered consciousness (i.e., seizures)
	   E. Abnormal swallowing reflex

II. Extraluminal obstruction	II. Asthma

III. Structural abnormalities
   A. Tracheal bronchus
   B. Bronchial stenosis/atresia
   C. Bronchiectasis
      1. RML syndrome
   D. Sequestration
	III. Immunodeficiency syndromes
	   A. Acquired: AIDS, chemotherapy, malnutrition
	   B. Congenital: T-, B-cell, phagocytic disorders

	IV. Mucociliary dysfunction
	   A. CF
	   B. Ciliary dyskinesia

	V. Structural abnormalities
	   A. Lymph nodes
	   1. Infection
	      a. Tuberculosis
	      b. Histoplasmosis
	      c. Coccidiomycosis
	   2. Tumor

	VI. Congenital heart disease

	VII. Miscellaneous
	   A. AIAT
	   B. Hyper-sensitivity pneumonitis
	   C. Hemosiderosis

Adapted from Wald ER. Recurrent pneumonia in children. *Adv Pediatr Infect Dis* 1990; 5:183–203.

inflammation and clinical deterioration of their pulmonary status.

Development of pneumonia is a common occurrence in immunocompromised pediatric patients. Frequently this clinical situation is an emergency since the patient has rapidly progressive disease, significant respiratory distress, and hypoxia. We have used the term "pneumopathy X" to designate pulmonary processes in immunocompromised patients who cannot be diagnosed by non-invasive methods. Whether empiric antibiotic or antifungal therapy should be started or a diagnosis made by open lung biopsy or other invasive procedures is often a difficult clinical problem made more complex by the many non-infectious pulmonary processes that occur in this population (Table 29.4).

PNEUMONIAS BY "AT RISK" GROUPS

There are many ways to classify the types of pulmonary infections that can occur in immu-

nocompromised hosts. Table 29.6 shows the general classes of immunodeficiency disorders and the pulmonary pathogens most often associated with them.

Childhood Leukemia (ALL, Nonlymphocytic Leukemias). The major risk factor for pneumonia in patients with leukemia is chemotherapy-induced neutropenia. Because patients with nonlymphocytic leukemia undergo the most intensive chemotherapy, they are at greatest risk for developing pneumonia. Bacterial pneumonias are most common, but RSV, adenovirus, and enteroviruses are also significant causes of pneumonia in patients with leukemia. Fungal pneumonias occur in patients with prolonged neutropenia, hospitalization, and broad-spectrum antibiotic therapy. *Aspergillus* and *Zygomyces (Mucor, Rhizopus, Cunninghamella)* are the two most common fungal pulmonary pathogens (55). *Candida* spp are frequently causes of disseminated fungal infection, but their role in pulmonary disease is difficult to determine because

Table 29.6.
Typical Pulmonary Pathogens Associated with Immune Disorders

| Immune Disorder | Typical Pulmonary Pathogens | | | |
	Bacterial	Fungal	Viral	Protozoa/Other
Neutropenias:				
Chronic	H. influenzae, S. pneumoniae, S. aureus, Klebsiella,			
Acute	S. aureus			
Prolonged, hospitalized patients	Gram-negative, including Pseudomonas spp	Candida spp, Aspergillus spp, Mucor		
Agammaglobulinemia, Hypogammaglobulinemia	S. pneumoniae, H. influenzae, Pseudomonas spp	Aspergillus		PCP
Congenital T-Cell Disorders	Legionella, Nocardia, Listeria, M. tuberculosis, Salmonella	Candida, Cryptococcus	CMV VZV HSV	PCP
AIDS	M. tuberculosis, M. avium-intracellare	Cryptococcus	CMV	PCP Toxoplasmosis
Complement Deficiencies	Virulent encapsulated, (e.g., S. pneumoniae, H. influenzae)			
Immunosuppressive Therapy	S. aureus, Listeria, M. tuberculosis	Aspergillus, Mucor, Histoplasmosis, Cryptococcus	CMV VZV HSV	PCP Toxoplasmosis
Bone Marrow Transplant				
Early	Pseudomonas spp, other gram-negative organisms	Candida	HSV	
Late	S. aureus	Aspergillus	CMV, EBV, VZV	Toxoplasmosis PCP

they frequently contaminate sputum and bronchial washings of patients without *Candida* pneumonia (56). *Pneumocystis carinii* was a major cause of pneumonia in leukemia patients in the 1970s, but the use of trimethoprim-sulfamethoxazole prophylaxis has nearly eliminated it as a cause of pneumonitis in patients who receive prophylaxis (57). The incidence of varicella-zoster virus (VZV) pneumonia has also been reduced by effective prophylactic measurements, and early treatment with acyclovir has significantly reduced VZV pneumonia's impact (58).

Lymphomas (Hodgkin Disease, Non-Hodgkin Lymphoma). Patients with lymphoma are at risk for pneumonia because of neutropenia and from a variety of nonspecific immunologic defects, including anergy (59). Hodgkin disease patients are often infected with *T. gondii* and fungi such as *Cryptococcus neo-*

formans. The mediastinal adenopathy and lung nodules seen in these children require extensive evaluation to differentiate lymphoma from granulomatous diseases.

Bone Marrow Transplantation. The types of pneumonias seen in allogeneic bone marrow transplantation (BMT) vary with the time following transplantation (60, 61). Immediately following the BMT, patients are neutropenic and at risk for bacterial pneumonias with *Pseudomonas aeruginosa* and *Staphylococcus aureus.* As the transplant becomes established and neutrophils return, acute graft versus host pulmonary disease (GVHD) becomes a serious concern. Immunosuppressive therapy for GVHD with corticosteroids or cyclosporin A adds to the risk of pneumonia with viral pathogens (CMV, HSV, adenovirus) as well as *Pneumocystis carinii* and fungi. If engraftment fails and prolonged neutropenia occurs, the risk of fungal pneumonia rises significantly. Idiopathic interstitial pneumonias also occur during this later period, possibly related to radiation or chemotherapy. Late (> 4–6 months post transplant) causes of pneumonia include *Haemophilus influenzae* and *Streptococcus pneumoniae* and are associated with persistent immune deficits to these encapsulated organisms. A frequent cause of morbidity in the late transplant period is bronchiolitis obliterans, thought to be an immunologic disorder related to chronic GVHD. Infection may play a role in provoking or exacerbating chronic lung damage due to bronchiolitis obliterans (62–64).

Agammaglobulinemia, Hypogammaglobulinemia. In these patients, repeated bacterial pneumonias are most common, with *Pneumocystis carinii* seen in patients with hypogammaglobulinemia (65–67).

Chronic Granulomatous Disease. Fungi, primarily *Aspergillus* spp, and *Staphylococcus aureus* are the most common lung infections in children with chronic granulomatous disease (68). Extensive lung destruction and hilar adenopathy are common in these patents (69).

Chronic Mucocutaneous Candidiasis. Although persistent and recurrent *Candida albicans* infections of the mucous membranes and skin are associated with this T-cell disorder, 50% of patients have recurrent bacterial pneumonias, and they are at risk for other opportunistic pathogens, including *Pneumocystis carinii*, nocardia, and varicella-virus pneumonias. Pulmonary complications including bronchiectasis, empyema, and lung abscess frequently occur (70).

Acquired Immunodeficiency Syndrome (AIDS). The extensive list of pulmonary infections associated with AIDS includes *Pneumocystis carinii*, CMV, bacterial pneumonias, and atypical mycobacteria as major causes of pneumonia in this group (71).

Renal and Other Solid Organ Transplant. The development of pulmonary infections following transplant is attributable to chronic immunosuppression with cyclosporine A and corticosteroid therapy. CMV is the most significant pulmonary infection in all transplant patients and in heart and lung transplant patients; *Pneumocystis carinii* is also quite common (72).

RADIOGRAPHIC APPEARANCE

Pneumonias in this population can also be classified by their general radiologic appearance, including (a) diffuse alveolar and/or interstitial pneumonias, (b) localized alveolar lobar or lobular pneumonias (which may involve more than one lobe), and (c) nodular infiltrates, which may be cavitary or progress to frank lung abscess (73). The common causes of these general radiographic patterns are shown in Table 29.7, but it must be emphasized that radiographic appearances are often deceptive in immunocompromised hosts and usually not helpful in making a specific etiologic diagnosis.

Diffuse Interstitial and/or Alveolar Pneumonias. Pneumocystis carinii is the prototypical organism associated with this radiographic pattern (Fig. 29.4). As noted above the importance of *P. carinii* as a cause of diffuse pneumonia in pediatric oncology centers has declined significantly in patient populations receiving trimethoprim-sulfamethoxazole prophylaxis. However, *P. carinii* has emerged as the major pathogen associated with AIDS. Although this infection is usually a cause of diffuse pneumonia in patients with AIDS, atypical radiographic appearances of *P. carinii* pneumonia are common, including normal radiographs and cystic, unilateral, and granulomatous appearances (74–76). The use of aerosolized pentamidine for prophylaxis of *P. carinii* in AIDS may alter the radiographic presentation toward more upper lobe disease because of preferential distribution of the drug to the lower lobes (76). CMV is also associated with diffuse pneumonia in immunocompromised patients and is frequently seen with other infectious agents (77). Viral infections, including adenovirus, and influenza are also important causes of diffuse pneumonia.

Localized Alveolar Lobar or Lobular ("Bronchopneumonia") Pneumonias. Bronchopneumonias and lobar consolidation can occur in immunocompromised patients caused by the usual pathogens, such as *Streptococcus pneumoniae*, *Haemophilus influenzae*, and *Staphylococcus aureus*. However, since the radiographic pathology is a product of the host's response to the organism, patients with abnormal host defenses often show an altered initial radiographic pattern.

Nodular, Cavitary and Lung Abscess Lesions. Solitary pulmonary nodules, either

Table 29.7.
Radiographic Patterns of Pneumonia in Immunocompromised Hosts

Diffuse Interstitial/Alveolar Abscess	Lobar or Lobular ("Bronchopneumonia")	Nodules, Cavity, or Lung
Pneumocystis carinii	Bacteria, including *Streptococcus pneumoniae, Haemophilus influenzae, Staphylococcus aureus*	Bacteria (including *S. aureus*, anaerobes)
CMV	Nocardia	*Cryptococcus neoformans*
Crytococcus neoformans	*Aspergillus* spp	Nocardia
Aspergillus spp (unusual)	*Mucor*	*Aspergillus* spp
Candida albicans and other *Candida* spp (unusual)	*Mycobacterium tuberculosis* Viruses, including adenovirus	*Legionella pneumophilia*
	Legionella pneumophilia	

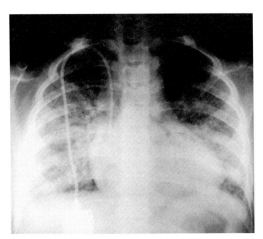

Figure 29.4. Staphylococcal empyema, same patient as in Figure 29.2; in the 2-day interval, a large left pleural effusion (empyema) has developed.

unilateral or bilateral, are a less common presentation of infection in most immunocompromised patients, but do occur frequently in pediatric oncology patients. Although most often these represent fungal pneumonias, other organisms including *Nocardia* can also present as pulmonary nodules.

Lung abscess is an uncommon occurrence in children. The development of a lung abscess generally indicates some degree of host immunity sufficient to localize an infection. The most common causes of cavitary lesions in pediatric cancer patients are fungi, especially *Aspergillus* spp.

Pleural Effusion

Pleural effusions are common in children with pneumonia, and thoracentesis is often necessary to establish a diagnosis and more rarely

to relieve respiratory distress caused by large fluid collections (see Chapter 37). Transudates occur commonly because of congestive heart failure, fluid overload, or hypoalbuminemia and must be considered in the differential diagnosis of an effusion. The presence of an exudate can by determined by a WBC of $> 1000/\text{mm}^3$, a pleural fluid/serum protein ratio of > 0.5, and lactate dehydrogenase (LDH) ratio of > 0.6 (or LDH $>$ two-thirds upper limit for serum) (78). Infection-related effusions may be parapneumonic or true empyema due to bacteria, tuberculosis, fungi, and (more rarely) viruses or mycoplasma (Fig. 29.5). Malignant effusions are also exudative and must be also considered in the differential diagnosis. Culture of pleural fluid is frequently negative in granulomatous disease, and pleural biopsy may be necessary. Patients with AIDS and pneumonia have been reported

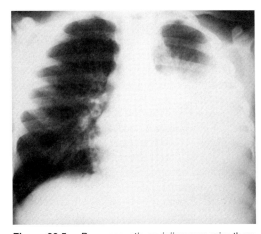

Figure 29.5. *Pneumocystis carinii* pneumonia; there is a ground-glass, opalescent appearance to both lung fields.

to have a variety of unusual pleural pathogens. Kaposi sarcoma or lymphoma commonly present with pleural involvement in adults with AIDS (79). In addition, *Pneumocystis carinii* extrapulmonary involvement has been reported to include the pleural space (80). Other opportunistic pathogens that can involve the pleural space in AIDS include the atypical mycobacteria, cryptococcus, histoplasmosis, and leishmania (81, 82).

DIAGNOSIS

The diagnostic evaluation of pneumonia is tailored to the age of the child, the season, the severity of the pneumonia, and whether the child has an underlying host immune disorder. The diagnosis of pneumonia in the normal child is usually made because of typical historical and physical findings. Although the presence of crackles is not necessarily correlated with consolidation on chest radiograph, a chest radiograph is essential when the diagnosis is uncertain or when the child is ill. It is required in the child seen for recurrent difficulties. Little or no evaluation may be necessary for the healthy child with a presumed viral illness. In contrast, the diagnostic workup may be complex and invasive in the child who has been treated with antibiotics and is deteriorating or in the child with an underlying immune disorder.

Diagnostic evaluation of the child with repeated or persistent pneumonias depends on a careful history and physical examination followed by initial screening laboratory studies directed toward excluding relatively common and significant causes of recurrent infection such as cystic fibrosis, asthma, tuberculosis, and foreign body aspiration (Table 29.8). Further studies become necessary only if this initial evaluation fails to provide an explanation for the repeated pneumonias. The presentation of a child with an opportunistic infection, such as *Pneumocystis carinii*, or recurrent pneumonia and sepsis with an encapsulated organism such as *Haemophilus influenzae*, should immediately focus the evaluation on the immune system.

In the abnormal host, consideration of specific types of pulmonary pathogens that occur in "at risk" groups (Table 29.5) and of general radiographic patterns (Table 29.7) may be useful. However, the list of potential pulmonary pathogens is much longer than summarized, their radiographic patterns overlap, and many non-infectious pulmonary processes may complicate the clinical evaluation. Nevertheless, an orderly diagnostic approach is possible in the immunocompromised patient with pneumonia, or "pneumopathy X" (Fig. 29.6). The ability to identify the pathogen responsible for pneumonia by non-invasive methods is improving. The challenge facing the physician is to know what tests are available and which tests are most appropriate. Understanding the advantages and limitations of each test will avoid over-interpreting their results or being falsely reassured by a negative test with low sensitivity. The proper selection and timing of invasive diagnostic methods is also important.

NON-INVASIVE TESTS

Sputum Culture and Gram Stain

Sputum samples are difficult to obtain in children under 10 years of age, and when obtained must be interpreted cautiously. Specimen collection may result in saliva alone and may not be representative of lower airway secretions. In addition, asymptomatic carriage of potential pathogens occurs. Therefore it is recommended that staining and culture be reserved for those specimens that have fewer than 10 squamous epithelial cells and more than 25 neutrophils per high-power field. If the sample is adequate, the presence of a single organism on Gram stain suggests the diagnosis. In adults, more than 10 gram-positive diplococci per oil immersion field has an 85% specificity and 65% sensitivity in the diagnosis of pneumococcal pneumonia. Sputum produced by cough induced with inhalation of hypertonic saline aerosols has also been useful in older children with AIDS and PCP (84). Gastric aspirates can be used in the younger child and are particularly helpful when the pathogen being considered is not a usual colonizing organism of the upper airway (e.g., tuberculosis).

Endotracheal Tube Aspirates

If the child requires endotracheal intubation for respiratory distress, endotracheal aspirates are easy to obtain. They seem to have their best predictive value in patients with community-acquired bacterial pneumonia in whom

Table 29.8.
Work-Up of the Child with Repeated or Persistent Pneumonia

Clinical

1. Review all previous radiographs, looking particularly at follow-up films for interval clearing of infiltrates, quality of films, unilobar versus multilobar disease, hyper-inflation; uncomplicated pneumonias may require 4–6 weeks to clear radiographically.

2. History of wheezing, chronic cough, otitis medias, skin infections, eczema, gastrointestinal disease (meconium ileus, steatorrhea, diarrhea, failure to thrive), TEF repair prematurity, previous ventilator therapy, history of transfusions, potential foreign body aspiration, household smoking history

3. Family history of CF, asthma, high-risk behavior for HIV infection (mother or child)

Physical

1. Lung: localization of auscultatory abnormalities, wheezing, clinical response to bronchodilator, clubbing.

2. Cardiac: murmurs, CHF, situs inversus.

3. Neurologic: cough effectiveness, muscle strength, swallowing disorders.

4. Skin: telangiectasia, abscesses, eczema

Laboratory

Primary (screening):

   1. Sweat test
   2. CBC with differential WBC
   3. Quantitative immunoglobulin, IgA, IgM, IgG, IgE
   4. Isohemagglutinins
   5. Barium swallow
   6. Sinus films
   7. PPD, histoplasmin skin tests
   8. Functional antibody titers if immunized (tetanus, diphtheria)
   9. Bronchoscopy, rigid and/or flexible (if FB suspected)

Secondary:

   1. IgG subclasses
   2. HIV antibody titer
   3. Pulmonary function testing, including response to BD, methacholine, or histamine
   4. Ciliary ultrastructure
   5. Screen for ciliary motility
   6. Allergy skin tests
   7. Response to polysaccharide vaccines (Hib, pneumococcus)
   8. T-cell studies (T4/T8 numbers, HA stimulation, etc.)
   9. pH probe study, other aspiration studies

an aspirate is obtained within 1 hour of intubation (85). After this time the lower airway is colonized with upper airway organisms and the irritation of the tube itself causes a low-grade inflammatory response. Endotracheal cultures obtained after 1 hour have a very low specificity and sensitivity.

Blood Culture

A blood culture should be obtained in all children suspected of having bacterial pneumonia. A positive result is highly specific, but in studies in which children with suspected bacterial pneumonias were studied, blood cultures were able to provide the diagnosis only about 10% of the time (5, 86). Therefore, blood cultures

are an accurate but insensitive method of diagnosis.

Bacterial Antigen Detection

The ability to detect capsular polysaccharide antigens of bacterial pathogens even after antibiotics have been administered is helpful in patients requiring hospital admission. A number of different tests are available, and most hospitals can routinely test for group B *Streptococcus*, *Neisseria meningitidis*, *Streptococcus pneumoniae*, and *Haemophilus influenzae*. Latex agglutination (LA) has replaced counter-immunoelectrophoresis (CIE) as the preferred technique because it is simpler and superior in sensitivity and specificity. Concen-

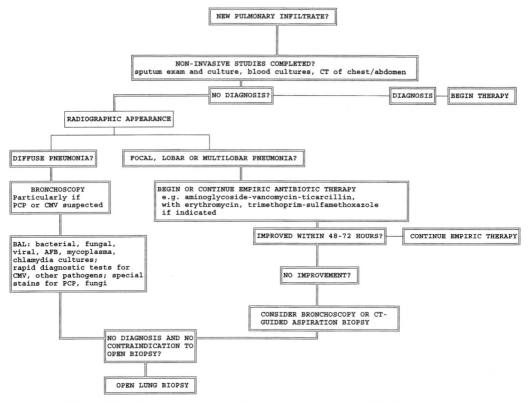

Figure 29.6. Diagnostic approach to the immunocompromised child with pneumonia.

trated urine samples are superior to serum samples. Antibiotic treatment does not affect the sensitivity of the test, which is between 30% and 45%, depending on the study. Specificity has been a concern because of the asymptomatic carriage of potential pathogens in normal children. In an outpatient population, Ramsey et al. found antigenuria in 24% of children aged 2 months to 18 years with acute lower respiratory tract infection (87). Antigenuria was found in 4% of asymptomatic children and in 16% of children with otitis media.

Direct immunofluorescence (IF) used to detect *Legionella* spp has a sensitivity of 50% and a specificity of 94% (88).

Direct Viral, *Mycoplasma,* and *Chlamydia* Detection

Rapid diagnosis of respiratory syncytial virus, influenza A virus, parainfluenza viruses, and *Chlamydia* infections by enzyme-linked immunosorbent assay (ELISA) and IF is now available. The sensitivities of these tests

depend partly on the adequacy of the sample provided to the laboratory. Viral cultures are generally available. Although *Mycoplasma pneumoniae* can be cultured on enriched media, this usually takes several weeks, and the diagnosis is usually based on serologic conversion. Genetic probes for detecting *Legionella, Mycobacterium,* and *Mycoplasma pneumoniae* are now commercially available. The ability of the polymerase chain reaction (PCR) to amplify specific regions of genomic DNA or RNA should allow a broader application of this approach.

Antibody Assays and Cold Agglutination Tests

Serologic tests demonstrating a fourfold or greater rise in antibody titer to an infectious agent are a sensitive and specific way to document an infection but usually are clinically impractical. Definitive diagnosis depends on a seroconversion on paired samples collected several weeks apart.

The cold agglutinin reaction measures an IgM autoantibody that agglutinates human erythrocytes at 4° C. Serum cold agglutinins are positive ($\geq$ 1:32) in 33–76% of patients with *M. pneumoniae* infection. In patients with pneumonia and positive cold agglutinins, specific antibody to *M. pneumoniae* will develop in 72–92%, suggesting that most cold agglutinin positive pneumonia is due to this organism. Usually cold agglutinins appear by the end of the first week of illness.

INVASIVE TECHNIQUES

Transtracheal Aspiration

Transtracheal aspiration to obtain sputum culture has been employed extensively in adults. Although transtracheal aspiration can be performed safely in children there does not appear to be justification for this procedure in most uncomplicated pneumonias; bronchoscopy is generally a better choice as a procedure to obtain cultures from the lower airway in pediatric patients.

Flexible Bronchoscopy

There is now extensive experience with the use of flexible bronchoscopy in children with pneumonia (83, 89–92). Bronchoscopy is safe in experienced hands and provides excellent culture material in the child with pneumonia. Indications for bronchoscopy in children with pneumonia include (a) failure of pneumonia or fever to clear with appropriate antibiotic therapy, (b) suspicion of foreign body or endobronchial obstruction, (c) recurrent pneumonia in a lobe or segment, and (d) suspicion of unusual organisms such as tuberculosis. Although the yield of gastric aspiration is probably superior to that of bronchoscopy for tuberculosis, bronchoscopy can also evaluate for endobronchial disease or bronchial compression.

The bronchoscope channel is usually contaminated by upper airway organisms, which makes simple washings through the bronchoscope channel generally useless. Several techniques have been developed to get around this problem; these include use of a double-sheathed, wax-protected sterile brush and quantitative culture of broncho-alveolar lavage (93). Brushings can also be obtained through the bronchoscope for cytologic examination and viral cultures.

Although bronchoscopy has limited application in normal children with uncomplicated pneumonia, it is the procedure of choice for most immunosuppressed children with pneumonia. Although the usefulness is well documented in this population, it is important to recognize the limitations of bronchoscopy (83). In patients on empiric broad-spectrum antibiotic therapy the yield of bacterial pathogens is likely to be low. *Pneumocystis carinii* is easily diagnosed by bronchoscopy, but in patients receiving prophylaxis for this infection the yield is likely to be low. CMV is another infection that can be diagnosed rapidly by bronchoscopy, but patients may have other complicating infections in addition to CMV that are missed by bronchoscopy. *Aspergillus* spp and other fungi are often difficult to diagnose by bronchoscopy, particularly early in the infection when therapy is most likely to be effective.

Transbronchial biopsies (TBBs) can also be taken through the bronchoscope. Although safe in adult patients, transbronchial lung biopsies may yield an unacceptable number of false negative results in immunosuppressed patients, and are most useful when organisms such as *Pneumocystis carinii* or granulomatous lesions are likely. Reported experience with TBB in pediatric patients is limited, but TBB has a significant role in monitoring rejection and infections in the pediatric lung transplant patient (94, 95).

Open Lung Biopsy

Open lung biopsy is the procedure of choice for obtaining definitive diagnostic information in immunosuppressed patients with pulmonary infiltrates. Timing of the biopsy is difficult. The clinician does not want to commit the patient too early, especially if empirical therapy appears to be working and the patient is in good condition. On the other hand the clinician does not want to wait so long in the face of marginally successful therapy that the patient deteriorates and the risk of biopsy is significantly elevated. We generally suggest relatively early biopsy in immunosuppressed patients with pneumonia. Any patient not clearly responding to therapy chosen on the basis of other culturing techniques or therapy chosen empirically would usually benefit from diagnosis by biopsy. In most medical centers this is a relatively safe procedure, especially when performed before the patient has the need for respiratory support. The risks only increase when the biopsy is delayed until the patient has become critically ill. When used for diagnosis of diffuse disease only a limited thoracotomy with a superficial subsegmental resection is necessary. In localized disease, typical of fungal infections, a more extensive procedure may be required to obtain an adequate specimen. In some cases lung biopsies can be performed using thorascopic techniques and a very limited incision (96).

Transthoracic Needle Aspiration Biopsy

Needle aspiration of the lung is useful for the diagnosis of PCP in pediatric cancer patients, and for the diagnosis of localized infections in other immunosuppressed patients (97, 98). In one study, pneumothoraces complicated 37% of the needle aspirates done for PCP (97), and this risk must be considered. Use of CT or fluoroscopic guidance greatly improves the yield and safety of this procedure, and it is the procedure of choice for many children with suspected fungal lesions that can safely be aspirated.

TREATMENT

The treatment of viral pneumonia is primarily supportive. With significant pneumonia close observation, monitoring of heart rate and oxygen saturation, oxygen supplementation, high humidity, bronchodilators, and chest physiotherapy are used as needed. In the vast majority of cases antibiotics are given because secondary bacterial involvement cannot be ruled out. This approach is both practical and reasonable although it may not alter the course. Specific antiviral therapy is available for respiratory syncytial virus (ribavirin) and influenza A (amantadine) and should be considered for infants and children with chronic lung disease, congenital heart disease, or immunodeficiency.

In infants antibiotic treatment should provide broad coverage and should follow the guidelines for presumed sepsis using ampicillin and an aminoglycoside. If staphylococcal disease is suspected methicillin or vancomycin should be initiated.

After age 3 months and until 5 years in a child with serious or life-threatening illness we would recommend cefuroxime or nafcillin and gentamicin given intravenously. For less severe illness where oral antibiotic therapy is thought sufficient, cefaclor or amoxicillin-clavulanic acid is a good initial choice.

Pneumonia not associated with fever in patients aged 4–11 weeks should be treated with erythromycin. After 5 years of age when *Haemophilus* is less likely and *Mycoplasma* becomes the most likely agent, the drug of choice is also erythromycin. If intravenous antibiotics are needed they should adequately cover the most likely organisms. A second-generation cephalosporin such as cefuroxime provides excellent coverage in most cases. When an organism is identified, therapy is guided by the sensitivity pattern of that organism. Intravenous therapy is continued until the patient's fever defervesces and sensitivity information is available. Oral antibiotic therapy can then be continued to complete the 14- to 21-day course.

The decision to hospitalize depends on the severity of the illness, the age of the child, the suspected organism, and the adequacy of the home environment. The majority of older children can be treated at home, but there should be a low threshold for admitting the young infant. Moderately severe respiratory distress, hypoxia, apnea, poor feeding, deterioration of clinical status on therapy, or an associated complication such as empyema should prompt immediate hospitalization.

Children with pneumonia should be reevaluated after 2 or 3 weeks. The child who has returned to his baseline status needs no further interventions. Repeat chest radiographs are indicated in children who have persistent respiratory difficulties, have had previous pulmonary disease, or have had complicated courses. Persistent radiographic abnormalities may simply reflect the inherently slow resolution of radiographic findings, and thus they should be compared to previous films and interpreted in the context of the clinical course. In the asymptomatic patient, a follow-up chest radiograph should be delayed at least 6–8 weeks to allow sufficient time for complete recovery. Early treatment is necessary for the immunocompromised patient with pneumonia, and empiric antibiotic therapy must generally be started at the first sign of clinical pneumonia. In many patients (e.g., the febrile, neutropenic patient), empiric antibiotic therapy may already have started before the pneumonia becomes clinically or radiographically apparent. Antibiotic therapy is typically broad-spectrum, aimed at both gram-positive and gram-negative bacterial infections (e.g., vancomycin-aminoglycoside/semisynthetic penicillin). If a patient presents with a new diffuse, bilateral pneumonia with respiratory distress and hypoxia, a rapid decision has to be made as to whether to proceed to open lung biopsy before the patient progresses to respiratory failure and open biopsy becomes more hazardous. Empiric therapy is usually guided by the underlying disorder and the radiographic and clinical features of the pneumonia. It might include trimethoprim-sulfamethoxazole for PCP as well as erythromycin for *Mycoplasma* and *Legionella*. Amphotericin B is often started in the febrile neutropenic patient who develops a new pulmonary infiltrate while on antibiotics. Empiric viral therapy with acyclovir for herpes simplex virus may sometimes be necessary, but the treatment of CMV pneumonitis with ganciclovir usually requires a histologic diagnosis of CMV pneumonitis. Because of its low morbidity, flexible bronchoscopy should be considered early in the course of the pneumonia. If bronchoscopy is negative, the risks and benefits of open lung biopsy must be weighed in each patient, particularly if the pneumonia progresses despite appropriate antimicrobial therapy. If the patient shows a good response to empiric antibiotic therapy it should be continued for a minimum of 2 weeks, and in the case of antifungal therapy may be required for much longer periods.

PROGNOSIS

The complications of bacterial pneumonia include empyema and lung abscess. Long-term alteration of pulmonary function is rare even when these complications are seen. Death occurs almost exclusively in patients with underlying conditions. The incidence of long-term complications after viral or *Mycoplasma* disease is unknown. Significant sequelae have been noted after adenoviral, influenza, and measles pneumonias. These include bronchiectasis, chronic pulmonary fibrosis, and desquamative interstitial pneumonitis. Evidence is accumulating to indicate that recurrent viral pulmonary infections in childhood in association with environmental irritants (e.g., passive smoking) can lead to chronic lung disease in adults.

REFERENCES

1. Grant JP. *The state of the world's children*. Oxford University Press, 1983, p 15.
2. Denny FW, Clyde WA Jr. Acute lower respiratory tract infections in nonhospitalized children. *J Pediatr* 1986; 108:635–646.
3. Foy HM, Cooney MK, Maletzky AJ, et al. Incidence and etiology of pneumonia, croup and bronchiolitis in preschool children belonging to a pre-paid medical care group over a four-year period. *Am J Epidemiol* 1973; 97:88–92.
4. Klein J, Schlesinger PC, Karasic RB. Management of the febrile infant three months of age or younger. *Pediatr Infect Dis* 1984; 3:75–79.
5. Fosarelli PD, Deangelis C, Winkelstein J. Infectious illnesses in the first two years of life. *Pediatr Infect Dis* 1985; 4:153–159.
6. Aherne W, Birch T, Court SDM, et al. Pathological changes in virus infections of the lower respiratory tract in children. *J Clin Pathol* 1970; 23:7–18.
7. Carson JL, Collier AM, Hu SS. Acquired ciliary defects in nasal epithelium of children with acute viral upper respiratory infections. *N Engl J Med* 1985; 312:463–468.
8. Tipple MA, Beem MO, Saxon EM. Clinical characteristics of the afebrile pneumonia associated with *Chlamydia trachomatis* infection in infants less than 6 months of age. *Pediatrics* 1978; 63:192–197.
9. Stagno S, Brasfield DM, Brown MB, et al. Infant pneumonitis associated with cytomegalovirus, Chlamydia, Pneumocystis and Ureaplasma: A prospective study. *Pediatrics* 1981; 68:322–329.
10. Abzug MJ, Ardene CB, Gyorkos EA, et al. Viral pneumonia in the first month of life. *Pediatr Infect Dis* 1990; 9:881–885.
11. Turner RB, Lande AE, Chase P, et al. Pneumonia in pediatric outpatients: Cause and clinical manifestations. *J Pediatr* 111:194–200.
12. Denny FW, Clyde WA, Glezen WP. *Mycoplasma pneumoniae* disease: Clinical spectrum, pathophysiology, epidemiology, and control. *J Infect Dis* 1971; 123:74–92.
13. Foy HM, Kenny GE, McMahan R, et al. *Mycoplasma pneumoniae* in the community. *Am J Epidemiol* 1970; 93:55–67.
14. Foy HM, Kenny GE, McMahan R, et al. *Mycoplasma pneumoniae* in an urban area. *JAMA* 1970; 214:1666–1672.
15. Stanfield S. Acute respiratory infections in the developing world: Strategies for prevention, treatment and control. *Pediatr Infect Dis* 1987; 6:622–629.
16. Mogabgab WJ. *Mycoplasma pneumoniae* and adenovirus respiratory illnesses in military and university personnel, 1959–1966. *Am Rev Respir Dis* 1968; 97:345–358.
17. Austrian R: Pneumococcal infections. In Thorn GW, Adams RD, Braunwald E, Isselbacher KJ, Petersdorf RG, eds. *Harrison's principles and practices of internal medicine*, 8th ed. New York, McGraw-Hill, vol 7, pp 802–808.
18. Gray BM, Converse GM III, Dillon HC. Epidemiologic studies of *Streptococcus pneumoniae* in infants: Acquisition, carriage and infection during the first 24 months of life. *J Infect Dis* 1980; 142:923–933.

19. Hendley JO, Sande MA, Stewart PM, Gwaltney JM Jr Spread of *Streptococcus pneumoniae* in families. Carriage rates and distribution of types. *J Infect Dis* 1975; 132:55–61.

20. Ginsburg CM, Howard JB, Nelson JD. Report of 65 cases of *Haemophilus influenzae* b pneumonia. *Pediatrics* 1979; 64:283–286.

21. Marshall R, Teele DW, Klein JO. Unsuspected bacteremia due to *Haemophilus influenzae:* Outcome in children not initially admitted to hospital. *J Pediatr* 1979; 95:690–695.

22. Nohynek H, Eskola J, Laine E, et al. The causes of hospital-treated acute lower respiratory tract infection in children. *Am J Dis Child* 1991; 145:618–622.

23. Jacobs NM, Harris VJ. Acute *Haemophilus* pneumonia in childhood. *Am J Dis Child* 1979; 133:603–605.

24. Potter AR, Fisher GW. *Haemophilus influenzae*, the predominant cause of bacteria in Hawaii. *Pediatr Res* 1977; 11:504.

25. Albow RC, Dirscoll SG, Effman EL, et al. A comparison of early onset group B Streptococcal neonatal infection and the respiratory distress syndrome of the newborn. *N Engl J Med* 1976; 294:65–70.

26. Shann F. Etiology of severe pneumonia in children in developing countries. *Pediatr Infect Dis* 1986; 5:247–252.

27. Copps SC, Allen VD, Sueltmann S, et al. A community outbreak of mycoplasma pneumonia. *JAMA* 1968; 204:123–128.

28. Cherry JD, Welliver RC. *Mycoplasma pneumoniae* infections of adults and children. *West J Med* 1976; 125:47–55.

29. Stevens D, Swift PGF, Johnston PGB, et al. *Mycoplasma pneumoniae* infections in children. *Arch Dis Child* 1978; 53:38–42.

30. Sabato AR, Martin AJ, Marmion BP, et al. *Mycoplasma pneumoniae:* Acute illness, antibiotics, and subsequent pulmonary function. *Arch Dis Child* 1984; 59: 1034–1037.

31. Niitu Y: *M. pneumoniae* respiratory disease: Clinical features—Children. *Yale J Biol Med* 1983; 56:493–503.

32. Fine NL, Smith LR, Sheedy PF. Frequency of pleural effusions in Mycoplasma and viral pneumonias. *N Engl J Med* 1970; 283:790–793.

33. Sterner G, Biberfeld G. Central nervous system complications of *M. pneumoniae* infection. *Scand J Infect Dis* 1969; 1:203–208.

34. Muldoon RL, Jaecker DL, Kiefer HK. Legionnaires' disease in children. *Pediatrics* 1981; 67:329–332.

35. Renner ED, Helms CM, Hierholzer WJ Jr, et al. Legionnaires' disease in pneumonia patients in Iowa. A retrospective seroepidemilogic study, 1972–1977. *Ann Intern Med* 1979; 90:603–606.

36. Anderson RD, Lauer BA, Fraser DW, et al. Infections with *Legionella pneumophila* in children. *J Infect Dis* 1981; 13:386–390.

37. Orenstein WA, Overturf GD, Leedom JM, et al. The frequency of Legionella infection prospectively determined in children hospitalized with pneumonia. *J Pediatr* 1981; 99:403–406.

38. Riggs W, Nelson P. The roentgenographic findings in infantile and childhood histoplasmosis. *Am J Roentgenol* 1966; 97:181–185.

39. Mathisen DJ, Grillo HC. Clinical manifestations of mediastinal fibrosis and histoplasmosis. *Ann Thorac Surg* 1992; 54:1053–58.

40. Wald ER. Recurrent pneumonia in children. *Adv Pediatr Infect Dis* 1990; 5:183–203.

41. Rubin BK. The evaluation of the child with recurrent chest infections, *Pediatr Infect Dis* 1985; 4:88–98.

42. Shermeta DW, Whitington PF, Seto DS, Haller JA. Lower esophageal sphincter dysfunction in esophageal atresia: Nocturnal regurgitation and aspiration pneumonia. *J Pediatr Surg* 1977; 12:871–876.

43. Nickerson BG. Bronchopulmonary dysplasia. Chronic pulmonary disease following neonatal respiratory failure. *Chest* 1985; 87:528–535.

44. Sly PD, Soto-Quiros ME, Landau LI, et al. Factors predisposing to abnormal pulmonary function after adenovirus type 7 pneumonia. *Arch Dis Child* 1984; 59:935–959.

45. Hall CB, Powell KR, MacDonald NE, Gala CL, et al. Respiratory syncytial virus infection in children with compromised immune function. *N Engl J Med* 1986; 315:77–81.

46. Committee on Infectious Diseases: Ribavirin therapy of respiratory syncytial virus. *Pediatrics* 1993; 92:501–503.

47. Feldman S, Stokes DC. Varicella zoster and herpes simplex virus pneumonias. *Semin Respir Infect* 1987; 2:84–94.

48. Feldman PS, Cohan MA, Hierholzer WJ Jr. Fatal Hong Kong influenza: A clinical, microbiological, and pathological analysis of nine cases. *Yale J Biol Med* 1972; 45:49–63.

49. Patriorca PA, Kendal AP, Zakowski PC. Lack of significant person-to-person spread of swine influenza-like virus following fatal infection in an immunosuppressed child. *Am J Epidemiol* 1984; 119:152–158.

50. Shulman SJ, Bartlett J, Clyde WA Jr. The unusual severity of mycoplasmal pneumonia in children with SS disease. *N Engl J Med* 1972; 287:164–167.

51. Merten DF, Buckley RH, Pratt PC, et al. Hyperimmunoglobulinemia E syndrome: Radiographic observations. *Radiology* 1979; 132:71–78.

52. Leggiadro RJ, Winkelstein JA, Hughes WT. Prevalence of *Pneumocystis carinii* pneumonitis in severe combined immunodeficiency. *J Pediatr* 1981; 99:96–98.

53. Rankin JA Pella JA. Radiographic resolution of *Pneumocystis carinii* pneumonia in response to corticosteroid therapy. *Am Rev Resp Dis* 1987; 136:182–183.

54. Gallacher BP, Gallacher WN, MacFadden DK. Treatment of acute *Pneumocystis carinii* pneumonia with corticosteroids in a patient with acquired immunodeficiency syndrome. *Crit Care Med* 1989; 17:104–105.

55. Gold JWM. Opportunistic fungal infections in patients with neoplastic disease. *Am J Med* 1984; 76:458–463.

56. Hughes WT. Systemic candidiasis: A study of 109 fatal cases. *Pediatr Infect Dis* 1982; 1:11–18.

57. Hughes WT. Five year absence of *Pneumocystic carinii* pneumonitis in a pediatric oncology center. *J Infect Dis* 1984; 150:305.

58. Feldman S, Hughes WT, Daniel CB. Varicella in children with cancer: Seventy seven cases. *Pediatrics* 1985; 56:388–397.

59. Young RC, Corder NP, Haynes HA, et al. Delayed hypersensitivity in Hodgkin's disease: A study of 103 untreated patients. *Am J Med* 1972; 52:63–72.

60. Johnson FL, Schofer O. Pulmonary complications of bone marrow transplantation. In Laray-Cuasay LR, Hughes, WT, eds. *Interstitial lung diseases in children*, vol 2. Boca Raton, FL, CRC Press, 1988.

61. Zaia JA, Forman SI. Management of the bone marrow transplant recipient. In Parillo JE, Mason H, eds. In *The critically ill immunosuppressed patient: Diagnosis and management*. Aspen, Rockville, 1987.

62. Johnson FL, Stokes DC, Ruggiero M, Dalla-Pozza L. Chronic obstructive airways disease after bone marrow transplantation. *J Pediatr* 1984; 105:370–376.

63. Chan CK, Hyland RH, Hucheon MA, et al. Small-airways disease in recipients of allogenic bone marrow transplants. *Medicine* 1987; 66:327–340.

64. Hamilton PJ, Pearson ADJ. Bone marrow transplantation and the lung. *Thorax* 1986; 47:497–502.

65. Conley ME, Park CL, Douglas SD. Childhood common variable immunodeficiency with autoimmune disease. *J Pediatr* 1986; 108:915–922.

66. Dukes RJ, Rosenow EC III, Hermans PE. Pulmonary manifestations of hypogammaglobulinemia. *Thorax* 1978; 33:603–607.

67. Saulsbury FT, Bernstein MT, Winkelstein JA. *Pneumocystis carinii* pneumonia as the presenting infection in congenital hypogammaglobulinemia. *J Pediatr* 1979; 95:559–561.

68. Park BH. Chronic granulomations disease of childhood. In Chernick V, ed. *Kendig's disorders of the respiratory tract in children*. Philadelphia, WB Saunders, 1990.

69. Caldicott WJH, Baehner RL. Chronic granulomations disease of childhood. *Am J Roentgenol* 1968; 103:133–139.

70. Chipps BE, Saulsbury FT, Hsu SH, et al. Non-Candidal infections in children with chronic mucocutaneous candidiasis. *Johns Hopkins Med J* 1979; 144:175–179.

71. Rubenstein A, Morechi R, Silverman B, et al. Pulmonary disease in children with acquired immune deficiency syndrome and AIDS-related complex. *J Pediatr* 1986; 108:498–503.

72. Gryzan S, Paradis IL, Zeevi A, et al. Unexpectedly high incidence of *Pneumocystis carinii* infection after lung-heart transplantation: Implications for lung defense and allograft survival. *Am Rev Resp Dis* 1988; 137:1268–1274.

73. Infectious disease of the lungs. In Fraser RG, Pare JAP, Pare PD, Fraser RS, Genereux GP, eds. *Diagnosis of diseases of the chest*, vol 2. Philadelphia, WB Saunders, 1989.

74. Chechani V, Zaman MK, Finch PJP. Chronic cavitary *Pneumocystis carinii* pneumonia in a patient with AIDS. *Chest* 1989; 95:1347–1348.

75. Klein JS, Warnock M, Webb WR, Gamsu G. Cavitating and noncavitating granulomas in AIDS patients with *Pneumocystis* pneumonitis, *AJR* 1989; 152:753–754.

76. Scannell KA. Atypical presentation of *Pneumocystis carinii* in a patient receiving inhalational pentamidine. *Am J Med* 1988; 85:881–884.

77. Stokes DC, Shenep JL, Horowitz ME, Hughes WT. Presentation of *Pneumocystis carinii* pneumonia as unilateral hyperlucent lung. *Chest* 1988; 94:201–202.

78. Light RW, MacGregor MI, Luchsinger PC, et al. Pleural effusions: The diagnostic separation of transudates and exudates. *Ann Intern Med* 1972; 77:507–513.

79. O'Brien RF, Cohn DL. Serosanguineous pleural effusions in AIDS-associated Kaposi's sarcoma. *Chest* 1989; 96:460–466.

80. Lubat E, Megibow AJ, Balthazar EJ, et al. Extrapulmonary *Pneumocystis carinii* infection in AIDS: CT findings. *Radiology* 1990; 174:157–160.

81. Katz AS, Niesenbaum L, Mass B. Pleural effusion as the initial manifestation of disseminated cryptococcosis in acquired immune deficiency syndrome. Diagnosis by pleural biopsy. *Chest* 1989; 96:440–41.

82. Newman TG, Soni A, Acaron S, Huang CT. Pleural cryptococcosis in the acquired immune deficiency syndrome. *Chest* 1987; 91:459–461.

83. Stokes DC, Shenep JL, Parham D, et al. Role of flexible bronchoscopy in the diagnosis of pulmonary infiltrates in pediatric patients with cancer. *J Pediatr* 1989; 115:561–567.

84. Kirsch CM, Jensen WA, Kagawa FT, Azzi RL. Analysis of induced sputum for the diagnosis of recurrent *Pneumocystis* pneumonia, 1992; 102:1152–1154.

85. Golden SE, Ziad MS, Bjelland JC, et al. Microbiology of endotracheal aspirates in intubated pediatric intensive care unit patients: Correlations with radiographic findings. *Pediatr Infect Dis* 1987; 6:665–669.

86. Teele DW, Pelton SI, Grant MJA, et al. Bacteremia in febrile children under 2 years of age: Results of cultures of blood of 600 consecutive febrile children seen in a "walk-in" clinic. *J Pediatr* 1975; 87:227–230.

87. Ramsey BW, Marcuse EK, Roy HM, et al. Use of bacterial antigen detection in the diagnosis of pediatric lower respiratory tract infections. *Pediatrics* 1986; 78:1–9.

88. Edelstein PH. The laboratory diagnosis of Legionnaire's disease. *Semin Respir Infect* 1987; 2:235–41.

89. Wood RE. The diagnostic effectiveness of the flexible bronchoscope in children. *Pediatr Pulmonol* 1985; 1:188–192.

90. Pattishall EN, Noyes BE, Orenstein DM. Use of bronchoalveolar lavage in immunocompromised children with pneumonia. *Pediatr Pulmonol* 1988; 5:1–5.

91. Bozeman PM, Stokes DC. Diagnostic methods in pulmonary infections of immunocompromised children: Bronchoscopy, needle aspiration, and open biopsy. In Patrick CC, ed. *Infections in immunocompromised infants and children*. New York, Churchill Livingstone, 1992.

92. deBlic J, McKelvie P, leBourgeois M, Blanche S, Benoist MR, Scheinmann P. Value of bronchoalveolar lavage in the management of severe acute pneumonia and interstitial pneumonias in the immunocompromised child. *Thorax* 1987; 42:759–765.

93. Rigal E, Roze JC, Villers D, Derriennic M, et al. Prospective evaluation of the protected specimen brush for the diagnosis of pulmonary infections in ventilated newborns. *Pediatr Pulmonol* 1990, 8:268–272.

94. Stokes DC. Is there room for another bronchoscope? *Pediatr Pulmonol* 1992; 12:201.

95. Whitehead B, Scott JP, Helms P, Malone M, Macrae D, Higenbottam TW, Smyth RL, Wallwork J, Elliott M, deLeval M. Technique and use of transbronchial lung biopsy in children and adolescents. *Pediatr Pulmonol* 1992; 12:240–246.

96. Daniel TM, Kern JA, Tribble CG, Kron IL, Spotnitz WB, Rodgers BM. Thoracoscopic surgery for diseases of the lung and pleura. Effectiveness, changing indications, and limitations. *Ann Surg* 1993; 217:566–574.

97. Chaudhary S, Hughes WT, Feldman S, et al. Percutaneous transthoracic needle aspiration of the lung. Diagnosing *Pneumocystic carinii* pneumonitis. *Am J Dis Child* 1977; 131:902–907.

98. Sokolowski JW Jr, Burgher LW, Jones FL Jr, et al. Guidelines for percutaneous transthoracic needle biopsy. *Am Rev Respir Dis* 1989; 140:255–256.

30

Tuberculosis

LAURA S. INSELMAN

Tuberculosis is an ancient disease that affects individuals from all socioeconomic strata and that still poses diagnostic and therapeutic challenges. The incidence and prevalence of tuberculosis declined during this century, but, since the late 1970s, has appeared to be on the rise (1–3). Since tuberculosis is highly contagious and children usually acquire tuberculosis from an adult with active infection, this resurgence includes both children and adults. The prevalence of tuberculosis in children reflects the prevalence of tuberculous infection in adults in the community (2–3). The total number of cases of tuberculosis in the United States reported to the Centers for Disease Control (CDC) in 1992 increased by 13.5%, representing 3178 new cases, when compared with 1989 (4, 4a, 5). In children younger than age 15 years, the number of cases increased by 21% between 1989 and 1990 (4, 5). Elevations of the case rate of tuberculosis during 1990 were particularly notable in New York, California, Texas, Florida, Mississippi, Hawaii, and Washington, D.C., with case rates considerably higher than the national rate of 10.3 cases per 100,000 population (4, 6). Several cities had markedly elevated case rates of tuberculosis during 1990: Newark (68.3), Miami (66.1), Atlanta (51.5), San Francisco (46.1), and New York (48.1) (6). Tuberculosis results in more than 7 million new cases and 3 million deaths yearly in developing countries (7, 8).

Factors contributing to this rise of tuberculosis in the United States include the increasing presence of a foreign-born population, particularly from Southeast Asia and the Caribbean, where the disease is widespread; multiple-drug resistant tubercle bacilli; poverty; overcrowding; homelessness; inadequate medical care; prisons; the elderly, who may now have tuberculosis as a result of reactivation of disease acquired when younger; and human immunodeficiency virus (HIV) infection (2, 9–13). The mortality from tuberculosis is 50% without chemotherapy (7).

PATHOGENESIS

Tuberculosis is caused by the acid-fast tubercle bacilli, *Mycobacterium tuberculosis (M. tb)* and *M. bovis* (2, 3, 14). In developed countries, inhalation of droplets containing *M. tb* is the usual mode of spread of the disease, whereas tuberculosis resulting from ingestion of milk containing *M. bovis* is more likely to occur in developing countries where control of tuberculosis in cattle and pasteurization of milk are not accomplished (2, 3, 14, 15). Disease with *M. bovis* has not been identified to a large extent in immigrants entering the United States from undeveloped countries. Other modes of infection with *M. tb*, which occasionally occur in the United States, include contamination of an open wound, such as could occur from an insect bite, a circumcision, or an abrasion of the skin; inoculation with a syringe containing tubercle bacilli; and congenital transmission, either transplacentally with infected blood or by inhalation of infected amniotic fluid at the time of delivery (2, 3, 14). *M. bovis* infection can also occur through these routes, and the clinical picture is similar with infection with either organism (15).

M. tb Disease

If inhalation of M. tb occurs, only those particles measuring 1–5 μm and composed of small clusters of one to three bacilli pass through the mucociliary defense mechanisms of the nasopharynx and large airways, reach the alveoli, and cause infection (2, 16–18). Larger clusters of inhaled organisms usually become trapped in large airways and do not cause disease. The tubercle bacilli that reach the alveoli multiply and initiate an acute inflammatory reaction with an influx of polymorphonuclear granulocytes and resultant vasodilatation, edema, and exudate formation (16, 19). Pulmonary alveolar macrophages (PAMs) are subsequently attracted to this area, ingest the bacilli, destroy most of them, and prevent spread of the tuberculous infection (2, 17). However, replication of virulent bacilli within PAMs can occur, with killing of the PAMs by the bacilli and release of the bacilli into the surrounding lung (2, 17). Lymphocytes then migrate to this area and liberate lymphokines (chemotactic factor, migration inhibitory factor, mitogenic factor, macrophage activating factor), which then attract hematogenous monocytes, or macrophages (16, 17). These macrophages, or histiocytes, ingest the bacilli and form epithelioid cells of a tubercle (2, 14, 16, 17). The tubercle functions to destroy the bacilli that were not killed by the PAMs (17). A primary complex results, which consists of the tubercles in the primary parenchymal focus (where the initial infection and inflammatory response occurred), the regional lymph nodes that drain this area, and the resulting lymphangitis (2, 14–16). A primary complex forms with every primary infection, irrespective of the initial portal of entry of the tubercle bacilli.

Tubercles resolve (3), may calcify and form a Ghon complex, or, in approximately 10% of cases, develop central caseation (18). The caseous lesion has large numbers of replicating bacilli, which travel from this primary focus through the draining lymphatics to the regional lymph nodes. As the organisms spread, they cause further inflammatory and secondary lung lesions, which may later resolve, calcify, or caseate. The bacilli can also spread hematogenously to infect other organs (2, 3, 14–17).

The time from when the tubercle bacilli enter the body until cutaneous delayed hypersensitivity to the organism develops is the incubation period, and is usually 6–8 weeks, with a range of 2–10 weeks (2, 3, 14, 16). At this time, the individual has a positive tuberculin skin test reaction, which indicates acquired immunity and coincides with macrophage activation (17, 18). Lesions heal and symptoms do not occur. The acquired immunity protects against future inhalation of additional tubercle bacilli. However, viable organisms in tissues can survive from the hematogenous spread of the initial infection, and these foci can eventually act as a source of subsequent disease (2, 3, 14–16).

When small quantities of bacillary antigen are present, the hyper-sensitivity reaction of acquired immunity benefits the host by causing bacillary death (17). However, large amounts of antigen can overwhelm the immunologic system, and the resultant hypersensitivity reaction is then destructive to cells and tissues. Caseation and liquefaction occur through release of hydrolytic enzymes, oxygen-derived free radicals, and cytotoxic lymphokines (16, 17). When liquefaction does occur, tubercle bacilli replicate extracellularly at a very high rate and further increase the antigenic load (17). The presence of liquefaction is an important marker of the occurrence of disease (16, 17). Healing ensues only when growth of tubercle bacilli is inhibited. With caseous, liquefied cavities, this is often accomplished by fibrosis, which isolates the diseased area (17).

The type and quantity of tubercle bacilli in a lesion correlate with the nature of the lesion that occurs. For example, extracellular cavities in the lung harbor rapidly multiplying organisms, whereas intracellular tubercle bacilli lie dormant for many years (2, 20). In addition, the number of bacilli in different lesions varies, with 10^7–10^9 organisms in aerobic cavities, 10^5 in vertebral lodes (Potts disease), and 10^2–10^5 in caseous lesions and nodules (16, 21). Bacilli that spread throughout the body replicate at sites of highest oxygen tension (i.e., the apices of the lung, which have an elevated ventilation/perfusion ratio; the kidneys; and the highly vascularized growing ends of long bones) (16). In contrast, primary pulmonary tuberculous lesions usually occur in the middle or lower lobes of the lung, which have a larger ventilation per unit lung volume than do the apices and are more likely to be sites for deposition of airborne organisms (15, 16).

CLINICAL MANIFESTATIONS

Tuberculous infection differs from tuberculous disease. When infection is present, the individual has a positive tuberculin skin test, indicating exposure to tubercle bacilli, but lacks clinical, radiographic, or laboratory evidence that reflects the occurrence of organ involvement (2, 3, 14). When such evidence does occur, the individual has tuberculous disease, and a positive tuberculin skin test is usually present. Approximately 5% of individuals develop pulmonary tuberculous disease within 5 years of the initial infection, whereas another 5% develop disease later on, with a risk of 0.01% per year in those with normal chest radiographs (18, 22). Although the likelihood of developing disease decreases after the first 5 years, an individual continues to remain at risk for developing disease, particularly if immunocompetence is lost (2, 3, 14). Development of disease in other organs appears to follow the "timetable of tuberculosis," with tuberculous meningitis usually occurring in 3–6 months, pleuritis in 3–9 months, bone and joint disease in 1–3 years, and renal disease in 5–25 years following the primary infection (14, 18). Factors influencing the development of tuberculosis include the age at acquisition of the infection, with the young and elderly more likely to develop severe disease; the amount of bacilli entering the body; the occurrence of lymphohematogenous spread; and the immunocompetence of the host at the time of the initial infection (2, 14–16, 22).

With few notable exceptions, the pulmonary manifestations of tuberculosis in children are similar to those in adults (Table 30.1). Unlike adults, children are more likely to have primary pulmonary tuberculosis with mediastinal adenopathy and without a primary parenchymal lesion (1–3). Regional lymphadenopathy, lymphohematogenous dissemination, and calcified lesions occur more frequently in children than in immunocompetent adults (2). Chronic pulmonary tuberculosis is a "reactivated" lesion and, therefore, does not occur in the young child. Unless endobronchial tuberculosis is present, children under 6 years of age usually do not have a cough deep enough to produce sputum for culture of tubercle bacilli (2, 15). Children with primary pulmonary tuberculosis, unlike adults, are often asymptomatic (2, 3, 14, 15).

The child with tuberculosis may also have systemic manifestations of illness, such as fever (particularly at night), fatigue, malaise, anorexia, and weight loss. Extrapulmonary disease may also be present, with manifestations suggestive of tuberculosis in other organs, including the skeletal system, central nervous system, gastrointestinal tract, genitourinary system, eyes, ears, heart, and skin (1–3, 14, 16). In fact, children are more likely to develop extrapulmonary disease than are immunocompetent adults (2, 3, 23).

Tuberculosis occurs with increased frequency with HIV infection, and its development may precede or follow the occurrence of HIV infection (13, 16, 22, 24). In children, tuberculosis is more likely to follow the onset of HIV infection, which is usually acquired prenatally, whereas in adults, tuberculosis frequently precedes the acquisition of HIV infection. Although its presence in HIV infection is believed to be reactivation of latent tuberculosis (25) and, therefore, not likely to be identified in young children, tuberculosis has been diagnosed in children with HIV (26). Atypical clinical, radiographic, and histologic manifestations of tuberculosis frequently occur in both children and adults with HIV (13, 24, 26). When compared with non-HIV infection, tuberculosis in adults with HIV is more likely to be associated with radiographic findings of mediastinal or hilar adenopathy, middle or lower lobe infiltrates, miliary disease, atelectasis, pleural effusion, and even a normal chest radiograph, and with histologic findings of granulomas that are both well-formed and atypical (i.e., lacking caseation necrosis, epithelioid cells, and acid-fast bacilli) (13, 24). In addition, extrapulmonary tuberculosis, particularly miliary and lymphatic disease, appears with increased frequency with HIV, unlike non-HIV infection (13, 24, 25).

DIAGNOSIS

The diagnosis of tuberculosis in children is made by a history of exposure; physical, laboratory, and/or radiographic abnormalities; and a positive tuberculin skin test (1–3, 14). The most accurate, definitive, and reliable skin test is the Mantoux tuberculin skin test, which uses 0.1 ml of 5 tuberculin units (TU), or intermediate-strength, purified protein derivative (PPD). The material is injected intracutaneously into the volar surface of the

Table 30.1.
Pulmonary Manifestations of Tuberculosis in Children

Pulmonary Tuberculosis	Signs and Symptoms	Radiographic Findings
Primary pulmonary tuberculosis	None, cough	Mediastinal adenopathy, may have primary complex and/or calcification
Tuberculous pneumonia	Cough, crackles, rhonchi, wheezes, reduced breath sounds, egophony, pectoriloquy, increased vocal fremitus, retractions, nasal flaring, cyanosis	Lobar or diffuse infiltrate, may have atelectasis
Endobronchial tuberculosis	Wheezes plus signs and symptoms of tuberculous pneumonia	Infiltrate, hyper-inflation, atelectasis
Chronic pulmonary tuberculosis ("reactivation")	Cough, crackles, rhonchi	Cavity, calcification, fibrosis
Miliary tuberculosis	None, cough, crackles, rhonchi, retractions, nasal flaring, cyanosis	Diffuse, bilateral 2-mm lesions
Tuberculous pleural effusion	Cough, unilateral reduced breath sounds, crackles, reduced vocal fremitus, friction rub	Pleural fluid; may have infiltrate, atelectasis, contralateral shift of mediastinum

forearm, forming a bleb. The size of indura-tion is measured 48–72 hours after injection, with interpretation of the skin test dependent on a history of the child having specific risk factors for acquisition of tuberculosis and the clinical status of the child (Table 30.2) (2, 27).

Although multiple-puncture tuberculin skin tests (i.e., tine, Mono-Vacc, Sclavotest, Aplitest, and Heaf) are popular for mass screening of populations because of their ease of administration, they are more likely to pro-duce both false-positive and false-negative results (Table 30.3) (2, 3, 14, 27). Except for the occurrence of vesiculation, any reaction with a multiple-puncture skin test must be

Table 30.2.
Interpretation of Mantoux Tuberculin Skin Test Reactions in Children

Risk Factors	Size of Induration	Interpretation
None known	≥15 mm	Positive
Moderate risk[a]	≥10 mm	Positive
High risk[b]	≥ 5 mm	Positive
BCG immunization[c]	≥15 mm	Positive

[a]Children born in high-prevalence areas (Africa, Asia, Latin America); using IV drugs; living in shelters for the homeless or institutions; or have malnutrition, diabetes mellitus, chronic renal failure, silicosis, Hodgkin disease, or leukemia, which predisposes to the development of tuberculosis.
[b]Children with radiographic evidence of tuberculosis, who are recent close contacts with someone with tuberculosis who is smear-positive for tubercle bacilli, or have cellular immune deficiency, such as HIV infection.
[c]If not in moderate or high-risk categories.

verified with a Mantoux intermediate-strength tuberculin skin test. The multiple-puncture tests are reserved for use in popula-tions at low risk for acquiring tuberculosis.

The bacillus Calmette-Guérin (BCG) vac-cine produces induration measuring ≤ 9 mm in diameter with a Mantoux tuberculin skin test (2, 3, 27). A reaction measuring ≥ 15 mm in a child immunized with BCG, regardless of the risk category for acquisition of *M. tb* (Table 30.2), indicates the occurrence of active tuberculosis and the necessity to investi-gate for disease.

A detailed history is required from the child with a positive tuberculin skin test reaction to identify the source of active tuberculosis with whom the child was in contact and to deter-mine if other family members, particularly children, have infection or disease (2, 3, 14). The source is usually an adult, rather than another child.

The child should also have a complete phys-ical examination, with evaluation of the extent of pulmonary involvement. In addition, detec-tion of extrapulmonary disease is important because its occurrence may alter the type and duration of antituberculous chemotherapy.

Laboratory studies include anteroposterior and lateral chest radiographs. If further evalu-ation of the extent of lung involvement is needed, such as with apical lesions or extensive

Table 30.3.
False-Positive and False-Negative Reactions with Multiple-Puncture Tuberculin Skin Tests

False-Positive	False-Negative
Incorrect administration	Incorrect administration
Incorrect interpretation	Incorrect Interpretation
Variable strength of tuberculin coating on prongs	Variable strength of tuberculin coating on prongs
Cross-reactivity with nontuberculous mycobacteria	Loss of potency of tuberculin
Sensitivity to testing material	Administration during incubation period
	Fading of tuberculin sensivity
	Anergy—massive tuberculous disease, corticosteroid use, malnutrition, certain infections (mumps, chicken pox, measles, pertussis), recent live virus immunization, sarcoidosis, cancer, immunosuppressive therapy, immunoincompetence

hilar adenopathy, then apical-lordotic and oblique films are helpful. Computerized tomography scans will aid in further delineation of extensive hilar adenopathy. A complete blood cell count, serum liver enzyme levels, erythrocyte sedimentation rate, and urinalysis are also performed. Culture material from gastric aspirates, sputum, pleural and cerebrospinal fluids, abscesses, blood, and bone marrow aspirates is obtained to identify the organism and evaluate drug sensitivity patterns. Gastric aspirates and urine specimens are collected on three successive mornings in concentrated samples (i.e., upon initially awakening) in order to enhance growth of *M. tb.* Blood culture media include the Löwenstein-Jensen and Middlebrook systems and the newer Bactec system, which allows growth, identification, and drug sensitivity studies of *M. tb* within 4 weeks (27). Although stains of specimens for acid-fast bacilli are helpful for rapid preliminary identification of mycobacteria, these stains may be falsely positive in gastric aspirates obtained in children living in areas with high prevalence rates of nontuberculous mycobacteria in drinking water, such as the southeastern United States (2, 3, 14). Tuberculosis is diagnosed definitively by culture and/or histologic examination of biopsy material obtained from bone marrow, liver, pleura, lymph nodes, and bone.

The newborn with tuberculosis usually has nonspecific signs and symptoms of disease (i.e., anorexia, poor suck reflex, poor weight gain, tachypnea, diarrhea, irritability, lethargy, hypotonia, and apnea) and is at increased risk for development of tuberculous meningitis. Therefore, the cerebrospinal fluid should be examined in the neonate in the following ways: cell count and type; glucose, protein, and chloride levels; acid-fast stain; *M. tb* culture; and turbidity upon standing, which is characteristic of elevated protein levels (2, 3).

Research tests used for identification of *M. tb* that may eventually be available clinically include DNA amplification of *M. tb* with the polymerase chain reaction, which can recognize the organism within 3–4 hours; fluorescence microscopy of acid-fast bacilli in gastric aspirates; serologic monoclonal antibody tests; enzyme-linked immunosorbent assays in serum and bronchial washings for antibodies to *M. tb*; and specific mycobacterial IgG antibodies in cerebrospinal fluid (2, 3, 27–31).

TREATMENT

Chemotherapy of pulmonary and most forms of extrapulmonary tuberculosis presently consists of either a 6-month or 9-month course of antituberculous drugs (2, 3, 14, 32–34). In these short-course chemotherapeutic regimens, multiple drugs, including at least two bactericidal agents, are used to kill tubercle bacilli in intracellular and extracellular lesions and prevent the development of drug resistance and complications of untreated disease. Either regimen is presently acceptable in children, provided the recommended numbers and dosages of drugs are followed.

The 6-month treatment schedule consists of isoniazid (10–20 mg/kg/day, maximum 300 mg/day, given in one dose, whether orally, intramuscularly, or intrathecally), rifampin (15–20 mg/kg/day, maximum 600 mg/day, in one dose, orally or intravenously), and pyrazinamide (15–30 mg/kg/day, maximum 2 g/day,

Table 30.5.
Toxicities, Drug Interactions, and Indications of Overdose of Antituberculous Chemotherapeutic Agents

Drug	Toxicity	Drug Interactions	Indications of Overdose
Isoniazid	Hepatotoxicity, peripheral neuritis, optic neuritis, encephalopathy, ataxia, arthralgia, bone marrow suppression, dermatitis, vasculitis, gastrointestinal irritation, gynecomastia, hypersensitivity, drug-induced fever	*Increases action of* alcohol, Antabuse, barbiturates, phenytoin, carbamazepine, vitamin D, acetaminophen; *decreases action of* pyridoxine, ketoconazole; delayed absorption with aluminum-containing antacids	Hyperglycemia, acetonuria, metabolic acidosis, slurred speech, visual hallucinations, convulsions, coma, urinary retention, photophobia, tachycardia, vomiting, hyperpyrexia, mydriasis. *Antidote:* pyridoxine in dose equivalent to amount of ingested isoniazid.
Rifampin	Hepatotoxicity; red-orange color of secretions; contact lens discoloration; dermatitis; bone marrow suppression; neurotoxicity; gastrointestinal irritation; cell-mediated immunosuppression; maternal and infant vitamin K-responsive postnatal hemorrhage if given late in pregnancy; hepatorenal syndrome, thrombocytopenia, autoimmune anemia with $\geq$1200 mg drug daily or administered less than twice weekly	*Decreases action of* beta blockers, verapimil, theophylline, ketoconazole, chloramphenicol, sulfonylureas, corticosteroids, cyclosporin, oral hypoglycemic agents, oral contraceptives, coumadin, quinidine, digoxin, methadone, narcotics, anticonvulsants; *increases action with* halothane, probenecid; reduced action with ketoconazole, para-aminosalicylic acid; *delayed absorption with* salicylic acid	Hepatitis, angioedema, headache, vomiting, lethargy, coma, facial edema, pruritis, red-orange color of skin and secretions
Pyrazinamide	Hepatotoxicity, gastrointestinal irritation, arthralgia, dermatitis, dysuria, hyper-uricemia, drug-induced fever	None known	—
Ethambutol	Retrobulbar and optic neuritis with loss of visual acuity, peripheral vision, red/green color vision; diplopia; central scotoma; neurotoxicity; pruritus; dermatitis; gastrointestinal irritation; hyper-uricemia; hyper-sensitivity	None known	—
Streptomycin	Auditory and vestibular ototoxicity, nephrotoxicity, peripheral neuritis, paresthesias, bone marrow suppression, dermatitis, hyper-sensitivity, anaphylaxis, drug-induced fever	*Increases action of* cephalosporins, aminoglycosides, polymyxin B, ethacrynic acid, neuromuscular blockers; *increases action with* probenecid	Neurotoxicity (stupor, hypotonia, coma, respiratory depression) in infants
Prednisone	Growth suppression, hypertension, neurotoxicity, hypokalemic alkalosis, electrolyte imbalance, peptic ulcer, pacreatitis, diabetes mellitus, osteoporosis, glaucoma, cataracts, myopathy, obesity, pituitary-adrenal axis inhibition	*Increases action of* neuromuscular blockers; *decreases action of* calcium salts; *decreases action with* barbiturates, phenytoin, rifampin	—

nization (3). The vaccine is also used in children with asymptomatic HIV infection who are at increased risk of developing tuberculosis (2, 24, 36).

BCG is injected intradermally in a dose of 0.10 ml for older children and 0.05 ml for neonates (2, 3). It forms a round, raised scar and, 6–8 weeks after immunization, results in a Mantoux tuberculin skin test reaction of 5–9 mm of induration (2, 3). If this reaction of the tuberculin skin test is not present, the immunization is repeated, and the tuberculin skin test is reapplied 6–8 weeks later. A magnetic, multiple-puncture disk technique of the vaccine is also available (2, 3).

Side effects of BCG immunization include local and disseminated infection, osteomyelitis, anaphylaxis, and death (3, 33, 36, 38, 39). Since BCG is a live, attenuated form of *M. bovis*, the vaccine is contraindicated in patients with immunosuppression, corticosteroid use, symptomatic HIV infection, burns, or skin infections, and in pregnant women (2, 3, 24, 36).

REFERENCES

1. Inselman LS, El-Maraghy NB, Evans HE. Apparent resurgence of tuberculosis in urban children. *Pediatrics* 1981; 68:647–649.
2. Inselman LS. Tuberculosis in children: An unsettling forecast. *Contemp Pediatr* 1990; 7:110–130.
3. Inselman LS, Kendig EL Jr. Tuberculosis. In Chernick V, ed. *Kendig's disorders of the respiratory tract in children*, 5th ed. Philadelphia, WB Saunders, 1990, pp 730–769.
4. Centers for Disease Control. Tuberculosis morbidity in the United States: final data, 1990. *Morbid Mortal Wkly Rpt* 1991; 40:23–27.
4a. Centers for Disease Control. Tuberculosis morbidity—United States, 1992. *Morbid Mortal Wkly Rpt* 1993; 42:363.
5. Centers for Disease Control. Division of Tuberculosis Elimination. 1989 tuberculosis statistics in the United States. Atlanta, August, 1991.
6. Centers for Disease Control. Division of Tuberculosis Elimination. Tuberculosis Cases and case rates, states and cities of 250,000 or more population, 1990 and 1989. Atlanta, August and September, 1991.
7. Centers for Disease Control. Tuberculosis in developing countries. *Morbid Mortal Wkly Rpt* 1990; 39:561–569.
8. Centers for Disease Control. A strategic plan for the elimination of tuberculosis in the United States. *Morbid Mortal Wkly Rpt* 1989; 38:269–272.
9. Centers for Disease Control. Prevention and control of tuberculosis in correctional institutions: Recommendations of the Advisory Committee for the Elimination of Tuberculosis. *Morbid Mortal Wkly Rpt* 1989; 38:313–325.
10. Centers for Disease Control. Tuberculosis control among homeless populations. *Morbid Mortal Wkly Rpt* 1987; 36:257–260.
11. Morris CDW. Pulmonary tuberculosis in the elderly: A different disease? *Thorax* 1990; 45:912–913.
12. Centers for Disease Control. Tuberculosis among foreign-born persons entering the United States. Recommendations of the Advisory Committee for Elimination of Tuberculosis. *Morbid Mortal Wkly Rpt* 1990; 39:1–21.
13. Center for Disease Control. Tuberculosis and human immunodeficiency virus infection: Recommendations of the Advisory Committee for the Elimination of Tuberculosis (ACET). *Morbid Mortal Wkly Rpt* 1989; 38:236–250.
14. Smith MHD, Starke JR, Marquis JR. Tuberculosis and other opportunistic mycobacterial infections. In Feigin RD, Cherry JD, eds. *Textbook of pediatric infectious diseases*, 3rd ed. Philadelphia, WB Saunders, 1992, pp. 1321–1362.
15. Lincoln EM, Sewell EM. *Tuberculosis in children*. New York, McGraw-Hill, 1963, pp. 12–15, 18–35.
16. Moulding T. Pathogenesis, pathophysiology, and immunology. Schlossberg D, ed. *Tuberculosis*, 2nd ed. New York, Springer-Verlag, 1988, pp. 13–22.
17. Dannenberg AM Jr. Pathogenesis of pulmonary tuberculosis. *Am Rev Respir Dis* 1982; 125:25–29.
18. Geppert EF, Leff A. The pathogenesis of pulmonary and miliary tuberculosis. *Arch Intern Med* 1979; 139:1381–1383.
19. Antony VB, Sahn SA, Harada RN, Repine JE. Lung repair and granuloma formation. Tubercle bacilli stimulated neutrophils release chemotactic factors for monocytes. *Chest* 1983; 83:85S–96S.
20. Dutt AK, Stead WW. Chemotherapy of tuberculosis for the 1980's. In Stead WW, Dutt AK, eds. *Tuberculosis*. Philadelphia, WB Saunders 1980, pp. 243–252.
21. Grosset J. Bacteriologic basis of short-course chemotherapy for tuberculosis. In Stead WW, Dutt AK, eds. *Tuberculosis*. Philadelphia, WB Saunders, 1980, pp. 231–241.
22. Murray JF. The white plague: Down and out, or up and coming? *Am Rev Respir Dis* 1989; 140:1788–1795.
23. Rieder HL, Snider DE Jr, Cauthen GM. Extrapulmonary tuberculosis in the United States. *Am Rev Respir Dis* 1990; 141:347–351.
24. Inselman LS. Pulmonary disorders in pediatric acquired immune deficiency syndrome. In Chernick V, ed. *Kendig's disorders of the respiratory tract in children*, 5th ed. Philadelphia, WB Saunders, 1990 pp. 991–1003.
25. Braun MM, Byers RH, Heyward WL, Ciesielski CA, Bloch AB, Berkelman RL, et al. Acquired immunodeficiency syndrome and extrapulmonary tuberculosis in the United States. *Arch Intern Med* 1990; 150:1913–1916.
26. Varteresian-Karanfil L, Josephson A, Fikrig S, Kauffman S, Steiner P. Pulmonary infection and cavity formation caused by *Mycobacterium tuberculosis* in a child with AIDS. *N Engl J Med* 1988; 319:1018–1019.
27. Bass JB Jr, Farer LS, Hopewell PC, Jacobs RF, Snider DE Jr. Diagnostic standards and classification of tuberculosis. *Am Rev Respir Dis* 1990; 142:725–735.
28. Brisson-Noel A, Aznar C, Chureau C, Nguyen S, Pierre C, et al. Diagnosis of tuberculosis by DNA

amplification in clinical practice evaluation. *Lancet* 1991; 338:364–366.

29. Lu C-Z, Qiao J, Shen T, Link H. Early diagnosis of tuberculous meningitis by detection of anti-BCG secreting cells in cerebrospinal fluid. *Lancet* 1990; 336:10–13.

30. Levy H, Wadee AA, Feldman C, Rabson AR. Enzyme-linked immunosorbent assay for the detection of antibodies against *Mycobacterium tuberculosis* in bronchial washings and serum. *Chest* 1988; 93:762–766.

31. Wilkins EGL, Ivanyi J. Potential value of serology for diagnosis of extrapulmonary tuberculosis. *Lancet* 1990; 336:641–644.

32. Starke JR. Multidrug therapy for tuberculosis in children. *Pediatr Infect Dis J* 1990; 9:785–793.

33. Bass JB Jr, Farer LS, Hopewell PC, Jacobs RF. Treatment of tuberculosis and tuberculosis infection in adult and children. *Am Rev Respir Dis* 1986; 134:355–363.

34. Snider DE Jr. TB in children: Time for short-course chemotherapy. *J Respir Dis* 1987; 8:70–76.

34a. Centers for Disease Control. Initial therapy for tuberculosis in the era of multidrug resistance. Recommendations of the Advisory Council for the Elimination of Tuberculosis. *Morbid Mortal Wkly Rpt* 1993;42:1–8.

35. Pellock JM, Howell J, Kendig EL Jr, Baker H. Pyridoxine deficiency in children treated with isoniazid. *Chest* 1985;87:658–661.

36. Centers for Disease Control. Use of BCG vaccines in the control of tuberculosis: A joint statement by the ACIP and the Advisory Committee for Elimination of Tuberculosis. *Morbid Mortal Wkly Rpt* 1988; 37:663–675.

37. Anonymous. Perinatal prophylaxis of tuberculosis [Editorial]. *Lancet* 1990; 336:1479–1480.

38. Rudin CH, Amacher A, Berglund A. Anaphylactoid reaction to BCG vaccination. *Lancet* 1991; 337:377.

39. Praveen KN, Smikle MF, Prabhakar P, Pande D, Johnson B, Ashley D. Outbreak of Bacillus Calmette-Guérin–associated lymphadenitis and abscesses in Jamaican children. *Pediatr Infect Dis J* 1990; 9:890–893.

31

Bronchopulmonary Dysplasia

VEDA L. ACKERMAN

Bronchopulmonary dysplasia (BPD) is the chronic respiratory insufficiency that follows an acute lung injury in the neonatal or infant lung. BPD is characterized by tachypnea, wheezing, and retractions with typical radiographic changes of hyper-inflation, increased linear densities, and cystic areas. As originally described by Northway in 1967 (1), BPD was thought to occur only in premature infants whose respiratory distress syndrome (RDS) was treated with mechanical ventilation and/or high levels of inspired oxygen. This chapter will focus on the comprehensive management of these infants once they have stabilized from their acute illness. A brief summary of predisposing factors, clinical manifestations, and pathophysiology will be followed by a practical approach to the respiratory, nutritional, cardiac, infectious, neurodevelopmental, psychosocial, and "well child" care of these children.

PATHOPHYSIOLOGY AND CLINICAL MANIFESTATIONS

The development of BPD starts with an acute insult to the neonatal lung—RDS/hyaline membrane disease, pneumonia, aspiration, pulmonary edema—that requires therapy with high concentrations of inspired oxygen and positive pressure ventilation over time (2). This results in cellular injury to the immature lung. The conducting airways develop metaplastic epithelial lesions which, in animal models, appear related to both hyperoxia and positive pressure (3). Direct cellular injury occurs from oxygen radicals that are not well handled by an immature antioxidant host defense system. Excessive pulmonary fluid is increasingly recognized as a major contributing factor. Van Marter et al., evaluating varia-

tions in clinical practice among neonatal units, found a more significant correlation between excessive hydration and the development of BPD than with variations in oxygen toxicity or barotrauma (4). Recurrent bacterial or viral infections may cause a persistent alveolitis, allowing continued damage to occur. Multiple markers of inflammation are shown to be elevated in this population including lipid mediators, proteolytic enzymes, oxygen radicals, and lymphokines (5–8). Genetic factors including race, gender, and family history of increased airway reactivity also play a significant role (9). The state of chronic undernutrition seen in these infants affects the ability of the lung to both resist damage and repair sloughed and damaged cells (10).

Because there are no formal diagnostic criteria for BPD, the incidence and prevalence are difficult to assess. Retrospective neonatal studies suggest a range from 12 to 70%, inversely related to birthweight (11). The impact of surfactant replacement on the incidence of BPD remains to be seen. Horbar et al. clearly document that a single dose of surfactant reduced the severity of RDS as evidenced by improved oxygenation and a decreased frequency of pneumothorax, but could show neither a decrease in mortality nor a decrease in serious morbidity such as BPD (12). Merritt et al., using human-derived surfactant, were able to document decreased mortality in the surfactant-treated group but no change in the number of survivors without BPD (13). Many clinicians suspect that there will be little decrease in the actual incidence of BPD in survivors, since surfactant therapy may allow infants to survive who previously would have died during their early neonatal course. Optimal use of surfactant remains under investigation, with the choice of preparation, dosing schedule, and patient selection criteria major areas of controversy (14).

The clinical manifestations of BPD reflect the multi-system involvement of this disease (15). Lung mechanics are significantly altered. Pulmonary compliance is diminished by a combination of (a) fibrosis, which occurs secondary to alveolar damage, (b) increased lung water, due to disruption of the alveolar-capillary membrane, and (c) overdistension, due to damage to alveolar supporting structures resulting in airway collapse and subsequent air-trapping. Airway resistance is increased by fibrosis, airway edema, and small airway constriction, the latter related to inflammation and bronchoconstriction. Decreased compliance and increased resistance increases the work of breathing, manifested as dyspnea and tachypnea, as well as wheezing, depending on the degree of airway narrowing. Pulmonary function testing of infants with BPD has demonstrated severe airway obstruction with some degree of reversibility with a bronchodilator (16). Lung volumes may range from low to increased depending on the degree of collapse and scar formation as compared to the degree of over-inflation.

Pulmonary gas exchange is impeded by several factors. Hypoxia occurs because of ventilation-perfusion mismatch in areas of alveolar collapse with poor ventilation but continued perfusion. Intrapulmonic shunts due to increased pulmonary vascular resistance also contribute to hypoxia. Hypercarbia is common and results from a combination of increased production, hypo-ventilation, and ventilation-perfusion mismatch. Increased CO_2 production results from an increased work of breathing from altered lung mechanics. Chest wall compliance is high, resulting in paradoxical chest wall movement during inspiration which then decreases the effective tidal volume. Damage to the airways results in long time constants with resultant air trapping and regional hypo-ventilation as the rapid respiratory rate of these infants allows insufficient time to empty (ventilate) these spaces. The large carbohydrate load needed for nutritional support may contribute to the increased work of breathing by increasing CO_2 production.

Large airway disease was not initially described as a common component of BPD,

but is now known to be a frequent occurrence as the disease progresses. Both tracheomalacia and bronchomalacia are well documented in this population and are postulated to be the cause of the acute, severe cyanotic episodes in the older BPD infant (17, 18).

Growth failure in BPD is almost universal, resulting from increased caloric needs caused by increases in the work of breathing and resting oxygen consumption (19). Growth failure is also complicated by gastroesophageal reflux with emesis, poor oral feeding skills, and recurrent respiratory infections.

Pulmonary hypertension can result from structural changes caused by fibrosis as well as those from chronic hypoxia. Infants with BPD develop excessive muscularization of the pulmonary arterioles early in the course of their disease with a resultant increase in the reactivity of the pulmonary vasculature to hypoxia (15). Data from cardiac catheterization of oxygen-dependent BPD infants document pulmonary hypertension, which responds at least in part to administration of the pulmonary vasodilator oxygen (20). Persistence of pulmonary hypertension can result in right ventricular hypertrophy. Right ventricular failure is uncommon but when present is often a terminal event.

Apnea can persist in the BPD infant long past the time of apnea of prematurity (22). The etiology is difficult to assess because of the multiple perinatal and ongoing insults these infants have sustained. Some investigators have documented abnormal arousal responses to hypoxia, suggesting abnormalities in the respiratory control centers (22). Pneumograms do not predict which infants will have prolonged apnea and bradycardia with hypoxia.

RESPIRATORY MANAGEMENT

Oxygen Therapy

The primary and most important aspect of therapy of infants with BPD is the management of hypoxia. It is essential to maintain adequate tissue oxygen levels in order to prevent significant morbidity and potential mortality. The goals of therapy are to promote growth and neurodevelopment and prevent or control pulmonary hypertension (Table 31.1). Hudak et al. document improved rate of weight gain in BPD infants discharged on

Table 31.1.
Oxygen Therapy in Bronchopulmonary Dysplasia

Goals	Provide adequate tissue oxygenation
	Prevent pulmonary hypertension
	Respond to changing oxygen needs
	Promote growth
	Promote neurodevelopment
Weaning criteria	
Awake O$_2$:	Adequate growth rate
	O$_2$ sat > 92% awake on room air for 15 minutes
	Echocardiogram without pulmonary HTN
Night O$_2$:	Stable off awake O$_2$ 4–6 weeks
	Continued growth and development
	O$_2$ sat > 92% asleep on room air
	EKG or echocardiogram unchanged
Follow-up:	Continued growth and development
	Follow-up echocardiogram in 4–6 months
	reassess O$_2$ needs during acute illness

home oxygen therapy to maintain O$_2$ saturation at least 95% (25). Data from cardiac catheterization suggests that by maintaining the Po$_2$ at at least 60 mm Hg or the O$_2$ saturation at at least 92%, pulmonary hypertension will be controlled (21). These parameters should be used once the premature infant's retinas are fully vascularized. It is also vital to respond to changing oxygen needs, especially during feeding, periods of increased activity, and sleep (26, 27). Episodes of desaturation during these times are sufficient in duration to contribute to pulmonary hypertension and cor pulmonale. Desaturation during sleep is more likely to occur if the infant's awake oxygen saturation is < 92%. Parents and other caretakers may sometimes be reluctant to use adequate oxygen therapy on the premise that oxygen is "toxic" to the lungs, but the data support the contention that the benefits far exceed any risk, once retinal vascularization occurs. Premature discontinuation of home oxygen therapy can have permanent negative effects on the infant. Groothuis et al. documented seven infants who had rapid deceleration in weight gain when their parents discontinued oxygen therapy, and even though weight gain increased when home oxygen

therapy was resumed, the infants never regained their original percentiles (28).

Administration of supplemental oxygen depends on the specific needs of the child. Infants with mild to moderate disease will tolerate the use of a nasal cannula provided there is adequate humidification. Children with tracheostomy tubes can use a tracheostomy collar. It is important to realize that in the very small infant that what appears to be a low liter flow (e.g., 1/8 L/minute) can actually be delivering an Fio$_2$ as great as 0.70–0.80 because of the small tidal volumes of these infants. Some more severely afflicted infants are best served with a free-standing system that can deliver higher flow rates and humidity. Lack of adequate humidification may result in increased mucus plugging and resultant bronchospasm, especially in patients with tracheostomies. Ongoing needs, especially during times of increased demands such as an acute illness, fever, increased activity, and stress, should be assessed by periodic oximetry.

Weaning of oxygen therapy is a staged event; the criteria are summarized in Table 31.1. Initially, oxygen is weaned during wakefulness once the child has achieved a period of medical stability and adequate growth. Oxygen saturation should be documented at 92% on room air for at least 15 minutes. A recently obtained EKG or echocardiogram should document stable or improving pulmonary hypertension or right ventricular hypertrophy. Nighttime oxygen (including naps) is continued until the child has remained stable off day oxygen for 4–6 weeks and has continued both adequate growth and adequate neurodevelopment. Most infants require supplemental oxygen at night for much longer than they require daytime therapy. Oxygen saturation should be documented to remain at least 92% during sleep on room air and should be evaluated for an extended period overnight, since failure to evaluate during deep sleep may underestimate hypoxia. In-home use of oxypneumocardiograms is an efficient and relatively inexpensive way to evaluate sleeping saturation. EKG or echocardiogram should also be unchanged from previous studies. Once supplemental night oxygen therapy is discontinued, the child should be monitored for continued growth and development and an EKG or echocardiogram should be checked in 4–6

candidates for long-term assisted ventilation if aggressive diuretic and bronchodilator therapy fail. The use of inhaled corticosteroids has not been evaluated, but their use may be considered in the older child with BPD who has persistent problems with bronchospasm.

The use of sodium cromolyn (Intal) as an anti-inflammatory agent may be beneficial in those BPD infants with significant airway reactivity but this has not been adequately evaluated. A single small study by Stenmark did demonstrate decreased oxygen requirement, wheezing, and ventilatory pressures in infants treated with nebulized cromolyn (54). However, since cromolyn therapy has minimal to no adverse effects, an empiric trial may be indicated (55).

Pulmonary Toilet

Excessive airway secretions resulting in mucus plugging and air-trapping are a difficult problem for the infant with BPD, because cough effectiveness is compromised because of airflow obstruction and tracheomalacia. Thus adequate pulmonary toilet is essential to ongoing management. Chest physiotherapy may improve secretion clearance and lessen atelectasis, but in some infants may actually potentiate bronchospasm.

Tracheostomy

Infants with BPD who should be considered candidates for tracheostomy include those who require assisted ventilation for more than 3 months as a neonate and those infants in whom chronic hypercarbia and increased work of breathing are problematic. A tracheostomy can reduce the work of breathing by as much as 50% and thus facilitate long-term management.

Home Mechanical Ventilation

For the infant with severe BPD, long-term assisted ventilation can be beneficial and safe (56). Home ventilation allows some degree of normalization of family structure while enhancing the developmental and social skills of the infant. Home ventilation also significantly reduces the cost of care without compromising care (57). Obviously the adverse effects include stresses on family dynamics (although generally less than the stress of a chronically hospitalized child), new environmental exposures for the BPD infant, and the potential for parental burn-out. Support with home nursing is critical to the success of home care (58) (see Chapter 58).

Cyanotic Spells in the BPD Infant

Evaluation and management of cyanotic episodes in the BPD infant have frustrated clinicians for quite some time, since spells are difficult to treat and generally do not respond well even to positive pressure ventilation. Mechanisms that may contribute to these spells include tracheomalacia, gastroesophageal reflux, pulmonary hypertension with pulmonary artery spasm, and seizures. Doppler echocardiography may be helpful, but can be normal if not obtained during an episode. Airway fluoroscopy can detect tracheomalacia, especially if the infant is deliberately agitated during the study. Flexible bronchoscopy is the definitive study for tracheomalacia and must be done with only light sedation so that the infant can be stimulated while the clinician is directly observing the trachea. Therapy depends on the etiology, but if tracheomalacia is discovered, the use of continuous positive airway pressure (CPAP) or positive end-expiratory pressure (PEEP) may be very helpful despite the potential to increase air-trapping. In addition, prevention of agitation may be needed through the use of sedation, stool softeners, and comfort measures. During severe episodes pharmacologic paralysis may necessary for short-term resolution. Improvement of tracheomalacia appears to be related to improved nutritional state.

NUTRITIONAL MANAGEMENT

Growth failure is common in BPD and is due to a number of factors: increased work of breathing with chronic marginal oxygenation, congestive heart failure, gastroesophageal reflux and emesis, acute and chronic infections, developmental delay and behavioral feeding problems (which both decrease intake), and polypharmacy, with many adverse effects pertaining to the gastrointestinal system. Growth failure thus results from an increased caloric requirement caused by high resting energy expenditure coupled with an inability to consume adequate calories because of gastroesophageal reflux, emesis, chronic illness, and poor feeding skills (59, 60).

Nutritional assessment of the infant with chronic respiratory disease is described in Chapter 61.

Strategies in nutritional support focus on optimizing the caloric intake to meet the individual needs of each infant. Most infants require 120–160 cal/kg/day, with infants on chronic ventilation requiring somewhat less. It is also important to optimize oxygen therapy and to control for gastroesophageal reflux and emesis. In mild to moderate growth failure, concentration of formula will allow increased caloric intake without necessitating an increase in fluid intake.

Nasogastric feeding tubes may be helpful for caloric supplementation in the BPD infant. However, the risk of aspiration is significant since prolonged passage of a nasogastric tube through the gastroesophageal junction can exacerbate reflux.

Infants who continue to require supplemental feeds should be considered for placement of a gastrostomy tube either percutaneously or surgically in conjunction with a Nissen fundoplication. Since gastroesophageal reflux and aspiration can exacerbate the lung injury in BPD, the presence of reflux should be evaluated by technetium-99m. If negative and clinical suspicion is high, a prolonged pH probe study should be done. Percutaneous gastrostomy tubes, if there is no underlying gastroesophageal reflux, require less anesthesia time and less time for postoperative recovery. A potential problem with gastrotomy tubes is that gastroesophageal reflux can develop after placement. Infants who have documented reflux or are at high risk of developing reflux—such as those who are significantly impaired neurologically—should receive a Nissen fundoplication (61).

Feeding dysfunction is common in the BPD infant and may be due to behavioral feeding aversion or dysfunctional swallowing. Behavioral aversion may be prevented by early intervention with positive oral stimulation and non-nutritive sucking during tube feedings. Prolonged endotracheal intubation can contribute to feeding dysfunction; this issue must be dealt with in the chronically ventilated infant. Once oral feedings can be initiated, evaluation for swallowing dysfunction is done and a behavior modification program is initiated to gradually decrease feeding resistance. Solids are introduced slowly by spoon to promote oral-motor skills and development but should not replace calorically dense formulas.

CARDIAC MANAGEMENT

Pulmonary Hypertension and Cor Pulmonale

The development of pulmonary hypertension and progression to cor pulmonale is one of the major causes of late mortality in the BPD infant. Pulmonary hypertension and mild cor pulmonale may be clinically silent until severe and irreversible. EKG is an adequate screen in mild disease, but Doppler echocardiography is more sensitive. It is important to remember that if pulmonary artery pressure is measured on supplemental oxygen, it may appear normal, but may be elevated if the oxygen is stopped. Therapy of pulmonary hypertension and cor pulmonale consists primarily of oxygen supplementation. In more severe disease, aggressive use of diuretics and fluid restriction may be needed. Digoxin may be useful clinically if right ventricular failure develops, but its use is not well studied. Calcium-channel blockers such as nifedipine have been proposed to decrease pulmonary vasoconstriction. Johnson studied nine BPD infants with pulmonary hypertension, demonstrating acute decreases in pulmonary artery pressure after administration of nifedipine (62). Use of nifedipine on a chronic basis remains under investigation. Anticipatory guidance is most important and consists of maintaining adequate oxygenation as documented by objective parameters such as oximetry. Infants with BPD who continue to require supplemental oxygen therapy should be assessed with echocardiography every 4–6 months in order to detect early changes consistent with pulmonary hypertension.

Systemic Hypertension

Systemic hypertension has been noted in some infants with BPD. The etiology is unclear; some investigators postulate a relationship to umbilical artery catheters, but this has never been proven (2). It is more likely that this hypertension results from lung damage and alterations in the angiotensin system. Obviously, with chronic pulmonary and cardiac disease, it is important to maintain a normal systemic blood pressure to decrease myocardial work. Once hypertension is diagnosed, concomitant renal disease should be excluded as a cause and then therapy should be initiated. Since most of these infants are already on diuretics, therapy with captopril may be helpful. Because of the risk of profound hypotension with the first dose, initiation of captopril requires careful monitoring. Systemic hypertension tends to develop later in the BPD course; thus regular assessment of blood pressure is required.

INFECTION

Infants and older children with BPD are prone to infections, which are the major cause of rehospitalization and the primary etiology of late morbidity and mortality (63). Rate of rehospitalization is directly related to time since initial discharge, with 80% of readmissions within 4 months of discharge and related to season (tripled increase if the patient is discharged in peak respiratory viral season). Most infections are respiratory and thus set off an acute exacerbation of the patient's respiratory disease with increased hypoxia, worsening of bronchospasm, and occasionally acute respiratory failure. The respiratory syncytial virus (RSV) and influenza predominate in those more seriously ill (64). Virally induced gastrointestinal infections can also be more severe in these infants since they are often fluid-restricted and on diuretics. Significant dehydration can occur secondary to increased fluid needs from fever, tachypnea, decreased intake, or diarrhea. Fever and infection also increase oxygen consumption, also potentiating cardiac compromise. In infants with severe dehydration, which can occur rapidly, cardiac arrhythmias such as ventricular fibrillation can occur.

Control of infection is possible by minimizing environmental exposures. Large crowds and individuals with upper respiratory infections should be avoided. In the very young or fragile infant with BPD, social isolation during RSV season may be beneficial. The primary key to decreasing viral transmission remains good hand-washing by all caretakers.

Some infants with BPD have recurrent fevers, the causes of which are usually undetermined. Diagnostic considerations include HIV infection, CMV, and endocarditis (65). The potential for bacterial sepsis must always be considered but is infrequent unless the child has an indwelling venous catheter.

Children with tracheostomies may undergo tracheal aspirate cultures, but the results are generally not helpful since all children with tracheostomies have chronic colonization with several nosocomially acquired organisms. There may be a limited use to tracheal aspirate cultures in the infant with overwhelming sepsis to aid in antibiotic choice, since those same nosocomial organisms should be treated if there is life-threatening infection. In addition, Gram stain may reveal increased polymorphonuclear neutrophils (PMNs), which suggests acute infection.

A few case reports of hypogammaglobulinemia have been reported in BPD infants that responds to intravenous replacement therapy (66). Prospective, randomized prophylactic treatment with intravenous immunoglobulin has been shown to be associated with a reduced number of infections, excluding sepsis (67). Verification with a larger trial is indicated before routine use. However, evaluation of immune function in the BPD infant with frequent infections should be undertaken, and replacement therapy should be considered if there is documented hypogammaglobulinemia.

NEURODEVELOPMENT

Seizures

It is not unusual for infants with BPD to have an underlying seizure focus. In evaluating neurodevelopmental outcome, Teberg et al. found a history of seizures in 27% of BPD infants (68). Seizures may be induced by electrolyte abnormalities or theophylline toxicity resulting from pharmacotherapy. Ventilatory support is often required for acute seizures. In infants with a known seizure disorder, theophylline products should be avoided if possible and diuretic therapy monitored closely, especially during concurrent illness, when theophylline pharmacokinetics and fluid balance may change dramatically.

Developmental Delay

The BPD population is at high risk for developmental delay and learning disorders. Primary predictors for poor developmental outcome are intracranial hemorrhage and periventricular leukomalacia with no correlation to duration of mechanical ventilation or oxygen therapy (69, 70). Early intervention with occupational therapy, physical therapy, and communication therapy is essential for the best possible outcome. Regular reassessment of developmental status and learning dysfunction is an ongoing process. Evaluation for auditory and visual impairment should be repeated at regular intervals.

PSYCHOSOCIAL ISSUES

Adaptation of the family to the BPD infant with a long-term chronic illness requires time and significant support (71). These infants have classically been described as having a negative temperament characterized by irritability, poor social interactions, and difficulty feeding. Many of these "traits" can be minimized by relief of hypoxia and hypercarbia and by early intervention with positive behavioral input (i.e., teaching the infant that not all touch is painful). Because the incidence of BPD is increased in lower socioeconomic groups and in those mothers who receive little or no prenatal care, parents are often young, single, and with few personal or financial resources. This obviously necessitates helping the parents to develop a social support system and achieve a source of funding, and makes extensive and early discharge planning essential. The use of a primary nurse and a social worker, both of whom are well versed in the long-term needs and problems of BPD, can be extremely helpful in promoting strong parent-child bonding and facilitating early and successful home management (72).

"WELL CHILD" CARE

Infants with BPD should receive regular immunizations according to schedule, including pertussis, unless there is a non-BPD contraindication. If the infant requires prolonged hospitalization prior to the initial discharge, these immunizations should begin in the hospital. IPV may be used in place of OPV while the infant is still hospitalized to prevent viral shedding. Once the child is 6 months of age (corrected for gestation), yearly influenza immunizations should be provided until the child is at least stable one winter off all medications, and should probably be continued for those children with moderate to severe dis-

ease, since they are likely to have persistent pulmonary function abnormalities.

After the initial hospital discharge, the BPD infant should be evaluated by the primary care physician within 2 weeks. Monthly visits during the first 4–6 months at home are important in order to monitor growth, respiratory status, and pharmacotherapy, as well to assess family adaptation to having the infant at home. Consultation with the tertiary care center will continue until the infant is stable on minimal to no medication. Blood pressure, weight, length, and ideally, oximetry (if the infant is on supplemental oxygen) should be documented each visit. Assessment of vision, hearing, and developmental status should continue on a regular basis. Hearing impairment appears to be increased in ventilator-dependent infants, and thus hearing should be assessed frequently in this subgroup (73).

PROGNOSIS AND OUTCOME

The pulmonary prognosis for long-term survivors of BPD is relatively good. Northway et al. evaluated 26 young adults with BPD born between 1964 and 1973. Seventy percent demonstrated airway obstruction, with 52% showing persistent airway hyper-reactivity. Only 6 of the 26 had persistent symptoms of respiratory difficulty (74). Studies of more recent survivors of BPD document persistent pulmonary function abnormalities and airway hyper-reactivity (75). However, continued improvement can occur, as shown by Blayney et al., who found that FEV_1 increased between ages 7 and 10 years, even when adjusted for somatic growth (76). Chest radiographs also continue to show abnormalities (linear shadows, peribronchial cuffing, hyper-expansion, interstitial thickening, and increased anteroposterior dimensions) years past the initial lung insults (74, 77). The impact of these findings on the older adolescents and young adults is unknown because the earliest survivors of BPD are just now in their early twenties. The potential to develop chronic obstructive pulmonary disease as adults warrants that these individuals be discouraged from smoking and exposure to other noxious environmental agents that might exacerbate these underlying abnormalities.

The "nonpulmonary" prognosis is somewhat more guarded, with most problems still related to a suboptimal pulmonary status.

Approximately 25% of BPD patients with severe disease die. Although early deaths are from unrelenting, untreatable respiratory failure, late deaths are associated with sepsis and infection or are "sudden" and appear to be related to pulmonary hypertension and cor pulmonale or frequent cyanotic "spells" (78). A significant proportion of infants with BPD who die are found to have substantial cor pulmonale (15). Unless there was a perinatal central nervous system (CNS) insult, neurodevelopmental outcome is surprisingly good. By 10–12 years of age, > 60% of patients are developmentally normal (79). Learning disabilities may surface during the school years and should be monitored. The majority of infants grow well once past 2 years of age, but approximately 35% remain below the 10th percentile for weight and 25% are below the 10th percentile for length (80). In addition, because of their protracted illness, these infants are at risk for the vulnerable child syndrome, and one must always watch for child abuse or neglect.

REFERENCES

1. Northway WH, Rosan RC, Porter DY. Pulmonary disease following respiratory therapy of hyaline membrane disease. *N Engl J Med* 1967; 276:357–368.
2. Katz R, McWilliams B. Bronchopulmonary dysplasia in the Pediatric Intensive Care Unit. *Crit Care Clin* 1988; 4:755–787.
3. Coalson JJ, Winter VT, Gerstmann DR, et al. Pathophysiologic, morphometric, and biochemical studies of the premature baboon with bronchopulmonary dysplasia. *Am Rev Respir Dis* 1992; 145:872–881.
4. Van Marter LJ, Pagano M, Allred EN, Leviton A, Kuban KCK. Rate of bronchopulmonary dysplasia as a function of neonatal intensive care practices. *J Pediatr* 1992; 120:938–946.
5. Stenmark KR, Eyzaguirre M, Westcott JY, et al. Potential role of eicosanoids and PAF in the pathophysiology of bronchopulmonary dysplasia. *Am Rev Respir Dis* 1987; 136:770–772.
6. Walti H, Tordet L, Gerbaut P, et al. Persistent elastase/proteinase inhibitor imbalance during prolonged ventilation of infants with bronchopulmonary dysplasia: Evidence for the role of nosocomial infections. *Pediatr Res* 1989; 26:351–355.
7. Gerdes JS, Harris MC, Polin RA. Effects of dexamethasone and indomethacin on elastase, α_1-proteinase inhibitor, and fibronectin in bronchoalveolar lavage fluid from neonates. *J Pediatr* 1988; 113:727–731.
8. Bruce MC, Schuyler M, Martin RJ et al. Risk factors for the degradation of lung elastic fibers in the ventilated neonate. *Am Rev Respir Dis* 1992; 146:204–212.
9. Motoyama EK, Fort MD, Llesh KW, et al. Early onset of airway reactivity in premature infants with

bronchopulmonary dysplasia. *Am Rev Respir Dis* 1987; 136:50–57.
10. Frank L and Sosenko IRS. Undernutrition as a major contributing factor in the pathogenesis of bronchopulmonary dysplasia. *Am Rev Respir Dis* 1988; 138:725–729.
11. Tooley WH. Epidemiology of bronchopulmonary dysplasia. *J Pediatr* 1979; 95:851–858.
12. Horbar JD, Soll RF, Sutherland JM, et al. A multicenter randomized, placebo-controlled trial of surfactant therapy for respiratory distress syndrome. *N Engl J Med* 1989; 320:959–965.
13. Merritt TA, Hallman M, Berry C, et al. Randomized, placebo-controlled trial of human surfactant given at birth versus rescue administration in very low birth weight infants with lung immaturity. *J Pediatr* 1991; 118:581–594.
14. Jobe A and Ikegami M. Surfactant for the treatment of respiratory distress syndrome. *Am Rev Respir Dis* 1987; 136:1256–1275.
15. Fiascone JM, Thodes TT, Grandgeorge SR, Knapp MA. Bronchopulmonary dysplasia: A review for the pediatrician. *Curr Probl Pediatr* 1989; 19:169–227.
16. Tepper RS, Morgan W, Cota K, Taussig L. Flow limitation in infants with bronchopulmonary dysplasia. *J Pediatr* 1986; 109:1040–1046.
17. McCubbin M, Frey EE, Wagener JS, Tribby R, Smith, WL. Large airway collapse in bronchopulmonary dysplasia. *J Pediatr* 1989; 114:304–307.
18. Miller RW, Woo P, Kellman RK, Slagle TS. Tracheobronchial abnormalities in infants with bronchopulmonary dysplasia. *J Pediatr* 1987; 111:779–792.
19. Kurzner SI, Garg M, Bautista BA, et al. Growth failure in infants with bronchopulmonary dysplasia: Nutrition and elevated resting metabolic expenditure. *Pediatrics* 1988; 81:379–384.
20. Abman SH, Wolfe RR, Accurso FJ, et al. Pulmonary vascular response to oxygen in infants with severe bronchopulmonary dysplasia. *Pediatrics* 1985; 75:80–84.
21. Goodman G, Perdin RM, Anas NG, et al. Pulmonary hypertension in infants with bronchopulmonary dysplasia. *J Pediatr* 1988; 112:67–72.
22. Sekar KC, Duke JC. Sleep apnea and hypoxemia in recently weaned premature infants with and without bronchopulmonary dysplasia. *Pediatr Pulmonol* 1991; 10:112–116.
23. Garg M, Kurzner SI, Bautista D, et al. Hypoxic arousal responses in infants with bronchopulmonary dysplasia. *Pediatrics* 1988; 82:59–63.
24. Werthammer J, Brown ER, Neff RK, et al. Sudden Infant Death Syndrome in infants with bronchopulmonary dysplasia. *Pediatrics* 1982; 69:301–304.
25. Hudak BB, Allen MC, Hudak ML et al. Home oxygen therapy for chronic lung disease in extremely low-birth-weight infants. *Am J Dis Child* 1989; 143:357–360.
26. Garg M, Kurzner SI, Bautista DB, et al. Clinically unsuspected hypoxia during sleep and feeding in infants with bronchopulmonary dysplasia. *Pediatrics* 1988; 81:635–642.
27. Zinman R, Blanchard P, Vachon F. Oxygen saturation during sleep in patients with bronchopulmonary dysplasia. *Biol Neonate* 1992; 61:69–75.

28. Groothuis JR, Rosenberg AA. Home oxygen promotes weight gain in infants with bronchopulmonary dysplasia. *Am J Dis Child* 1987; 141:992–995.
29. Wilkie RA, Bryan MH. Effect of bronchodilators on airway resistance in ventilator-dependent neonates with chronic lung disease. *J Pediatr* 1987; 111:278–282.
30. Rotschild A, Solimano A, Puterman M, et al. Increased compliance in response to salbutamol in premature infants with developing bronchopulmonary dysplasia. *J Pediatr* 1989; 115:984–991.
31. Denjean A, Guimaraes H, Migdal M, et al. Dose-related bronchodilator response to aerosolized salbutamol (albuterol) in ventilator-dependent premature infants. *J Pediatr* 1992; 120:974–979.
32. Blanchard PW, Brown TM, Coates AL. Pharmacotherapy in bronchopulmonary dysplasia. *Clin Perinatol* 1987; 14:881–910.
33. Nahata MC, Serafini D, Edwards R. Theophylline pharmacokinetics in patients with bronchopulmonary dysplasia. *J Clin Pharm Therap* 1989; 14:225–229.
34. Brundage KL, Moshsini KG, Froese AB, et al. Bronchodilator response to ipratropium bromide in infants with bronchopulmonary dysplasia. *Am Rev Respir Dis* 1990; 142:1137–1142.
35. Chemtob S, Kaplan B, Sherbotie JR, et al. Pharmacology of diuretics in the newborn. *Pediatr Clin North Am* 1989; 36:1231–1250.
36. Kao LC, Warburton D, Cheng MH, et al. Effect of oral diuretics on pulmonary mechanics in infants with chronic bronchopulmonary dysplasia: Results of a double-blind crossover sequential trial. *Pediatrics* 1984; 74:37–44.
37. Kao LC, Durand DJ, Phillips BL, et al. Oral theophylline and diuretics improve pulmonary mechanics in infants with bronchopulmonary dysplasia. *J Pediatr* 1987; 111:439–444.
38. O'Donovan BH, Bell EF. Effects of furosemide on body water compartments in infants with bronchopulmonary dysplasia. *Pediatr Res* 1989; 26:121–124.
39. Albersheim SG, Solimano AJ, Sharma AK, et al. Randomized, double-blind, controlled trial of long-term diuretic therapy for bronchopulmonary dysplasia. *J Pediatr* 1989; 115:615–620.
40. Giacoia GP and Pineda R. Diuretics, hypochloremia, and outcome in bronchopulmonary dysplasia patients. *Dev Pharmacol Ther* 1991; 4:212–220.
41. Ryan S, Congdon PJ, Horsman A, et al. Bone mineral content in bronchopulmonary dysplasia. *Arch Dis Child* 1987; 62:889–894.
42. Brem AS. Electrolyte disorders associated with respiratory distress syndrome and bronchopulmonary dysplasia. *Clin Perinatol* 1992; 19:223–232.
43. Rush MG, Engelhardt B, Parker RA, et al. Double-blind, placebo-controlled trial of alternate-day furosemide therapy in infants with chronic bronchopulmonary dysplasia. *J Pediatr* 1990; 117:112–118.
44. Segar JL, Robillard JE, Johnson KJ, et al. Addition of metolazone to overcome tolerance to furosemide in infants with bronchopulmonary dysplasia. *J Pediatr* 1992; 120:966–973.
45. Hufnagle KG, Khan SN, Penn D, et al. Renal calcifications: A complication of long–term furosemide therapy in preterm infants. *Pediatrics* 1982; 70:360–363.
46. Cummings JJ, D'Eugenio DB, Gross SJ. A controlled trial of dexamethasone in preterm infants at high risk for bronchopulmonary dysplasia. *N Engl J Med* 1989; 320:1505–1510.
47. Yoder MC, Chua R, Tepper R. Effect of dexamethasone on pulmoanry inflammation and pulmoanry function of ventilator-dependent infants with bronchopulmonary dysplasia. *Am Rev Respir Dis* 1991; 143:1044–1048.
48. Kazzi NJ, Brans YW, Poland RL. Dexamethasone effects on the hospital course of infants with bronchopulmonary dysplasia who are dependent on artificial ventilation. *Pediatrics* 1990; 86:722–727.
49. Arnold JD, Leslie GI, Williams G, et al. Adrenocortical responsiveness in neonates weaned from the ventilator with dexamethasone. *Aust Paediatr J* 1987; 23:227–229.
50. Blackburn ME, Brownlee KG, Buckler JMH, et al. Adrenal response in very low birthweight babies after dexamethasone treatment for bronchopulmonary dysplasia. *Arch Dis Child* 1989; 64:1721–1726.
51. Alkalay AL, Pomerance JJ, Puri AR, et al. Hypothalamic-pituitary-adrenal axis function in very low birth weight infants treated with dexamethasone. *Pediatrics* 1990; 86:204–210.
52. Rizvi ZB, Aniol HS, Myers TF, et al. Effects of dexamethasone on the hypotahalamic-pituitary-adrenal axis in preterm infants. *J Pediatr* 1992; 120:961–965.
53. Werner JC, Sicard RE, Hansen TWR, et al. Hypertrophic cardiomyopathy associated with dexamethasone therapy for bronchopulmonary dysplasia. *J Pediatr* 1992; 120:286–291.
54. Stenmark KR, Eyzaguirre M, Remigio L, et al. Recovery of platelet activating factor and leukotrienes from infants with severe bronchopulmonary dysplasia: Clinical improvement with cromolyn treatment [abstract]. *Am Rev Respir Dis* 1985; 131:236.
55. Davis JM, Sinkin RA, Aranda JV. Drug therapy for bronchopulmonary dysplasia. *Pediatr Pulmonol* 1990; 8:117–125.
56. Carpenter E, Watson J, Ackerman V, et al. Case management of home mechanical ventilation in children with severe bronchopulmonary dysplasia. *Am Rev Resp Dis* 1992; 145:A344.
57. Fields AI, Rosenblatt A, Pollack MM, et al. Home care cost-effectiveness for respiratory technology–dependent children. *Am J Dis Child* 1991; 145:729–733.
58. Eigen H, Zander J, Lemen RJ, et al. Home mechanical ventilation of pediatric patients. *Am Rev Respir Dis* 1990; 141:258–259.
59. Kurzner SI, Garg M, Bautista DB, et al. Growth failure in bronchopulmonary dysplasia: Elevated metabolic rates and pulmonary mechanics. *J Pediatr* 1988; 112:73–80.
60. Sindel BD, Maisels MJ, Ballantine TVN. Gastroesophageal reflux to the proximal esophagus in infants with bronchopulmonary dysplasia. *Am J Dis Child* 1989; 143:1103–1106.
61. Giuffre RM, Rubin S, Mitchell I. Antireflux surgery in infants with bronchopulmonary dysplasia. *Am J Dis Child* 1987; 141:648–651.
62. Johnson CE, Beekman RH, Kostyshak DA, et al. Pharmacokinetics and pharmacodynamics of nifedipine in children with bronchopulmonary dysplasia

and pulmonary hypertension. *Pediatr Res* 1991; 29:500–503.

63. Cunningham CK, McMilan JA, Gross SJ. Rehospitalization for respiratory illness in infants of less than 32 weeks gestation. *Pediatrics* 1991; 88:527–532.

64. Groothuis JR, Gutierrez KM, Lauer BA. Respiratory syncytial virus infection in children with bronchopulmonary dysplasia. *Pediatrics* 1988; 82:199–203.

65. Sawyer MH, Edwards DK, Spector SA. Cytomegalovirus infection and bronchopulmonary dysplasia in premature infants. *Am J Dis Child* 1987; 141:303–305.

66. Lederman HM, Metz SJ, Zuckerberg AL, et al. Antibody deficiency complicating severe bronchopulmonary dysplasia. *Pediatr Pulmonol* 1989; 7:52–54.

67. Malik S, Giacoia GP, West K. The use of intravenous immunoglobulin (IVIG) to prevent infections in bronchopulmonary dysplasia: Report of a pilot study. *J Perinatol* 1991; 11:239–244.

68. Teberg AJ, Pena I, Finello K, et al. Prediction of neurodevelopmental outcome in infants with and without bronchopulmonary dysplasia. *Am J Med Sci* 1991; 301:369–374.

69. Luchi JM, Bennett FC, Jackson JC. Predictors of neurodevelopmental outcome following bronchopulmonary dysplasia. *Am J Dis Child* 1991; 145:813–817.

70. Lifshitz MH, Seilheimer DK, Wilson GS. Neurodevelopmental status of low birth weight infants with bronchopulmonary dysplasia requiring prolonged oxygen supplementation. *J Perinatol* 1987; 7:127–132.

71. McElheny JE. Parental adaptation to a child with bronchopulmonary dysplasia. *J Pediatr Nurs* 1989; 4:346–352.

72. Embon CM. Discharge planning for infants with bronchopulmonary dysplasia. *J Perinat Neonat Nurs* 1991; 5:54–63.

73. Marsh RR and Handler SD. Hearing impairment in ventilator–dependent infants and children. *Int J Pediatr Otorhinolaryngol* 1990; 20:213–217.

74. Northway WH, Moss RB, Carlisle KB, et al. Late pulmonary sequelae of bronchopulmonary dysplasia. *N Engl J Med* 1990; 323:1793–1799.

75. Mallory GB, Chaney H, Mutich RL. Longitudinal changes in lung function during the first three years of premature infants with moderate to severe bronchopulmonary dysplasia. *Pediatr Pulmonol* 1991; 11:8–14.

76. Blayney M, Kerem E, Whyte H, et al. Bronchopulmonary dysplasia: Improvement in lung function between 7 and 10 years of age. *J Pediatr* 1991; 118:201–206.

77. Griscom NT, Wheeler WB, Sweezey NB, et al. Bronchopulmonary dysplasia: Radiographic appearance in middle childhood. *Radiology* 1989; 171:811–814.

78. Abman SH, Burchell MF, Schaffer MS, et al. Late sudden unexpected deaths in hospitalized infants with bronchopulmonary dysplasia. *Am J Dis Child* 1989; 143:815–819.

79. Vohr BR, Coll CG, Lobato D, et al. Neurodevelopmental and medical status of low-birthweight survivors of bronchopulmonary dysplasia at 10 to 12 years of age. *Develop Med Child Neurol* 1991; 33:690–697.

80. Robertson CMT, Etches PC, Goldson E, et al. Eight-year school performance, neurodevelopmental, and growth outcome of neonates with bronchopulmonary dysplasia: A comparative study. *Pediatrics* 1992; 89:365–372.

32

Interstitial Lung Disease

SUSAN M. BRUGMAN, HARRY WILSON, and LELAND L. FAN

Interstitial lung disease in childhood (ILD-C) is rare, and our current knowledge is fragmented. The term "interstitial lung disease" comprises a heterogeneous array of some 150 pulmonary disorders (Table 32.1). Carrington and Gaensler (1) proposed "diffuse infiltrative lung diseases" as a more generic term to describe disorders in which both alveolar walls and their adjacent spaces become inflamed and often fibrotic. Although this term may more accurately describe this diverse group of diseases, ILD has been an accepted designation in the literature, and we will continue to use it.

Much of our knowledge derives either from the adult literature or from limited series of pediatric patients with discreet histologic diagnoses. Both of these sources have significant limitations (2). The validity of extrapolating from adult data to the pediatric population is debatable. Likewise, knowledge of ILD-C gained from case reports or small series, although useful, provides details of only isolated parts of the whole spectrum of diseases.

It is our purpose to present a systematic clinical approach to the child with suspected ILD-C (Fig. 32.1), based on published observations in children and adults, and on our own experience (2a, 2b).

INCIDENCE

ILD is much less common in adults than chronic airflow obstruction, accounting for 15–20% of patients with a noninfectious etiology seen by pulmonary internists (3). Numbers of patients and types of diseases are considerably influenced by the regional prevalence of associated conditions (e.g., AIDS or organ transplantation) or by the special interest of any particular center. In children, the

incidence of ILD is unknown but perceived to be rare (4).

PATHOPHYSIOLOGY

The normal alveolar wall is composed of lining cells, a closely apposed network of capillaries, and a delicate fibroelastic matrix. A rich and varied array of cells normally populate the alveolar-capillary unit and can be divided into two subgroups:

1. *Intrinsic cells:* Epithelial lining cells of the type I or type II cells; endothelial cells; structural cells such as fibroblasts and smooth muscle cells; immune cells such as alveolar macrophages and lymphocytes.
2. *Extrinsic cells:* Monocytes, polymorphonuclear leukocytes, eosinophils, histiocytes, and plasma cells.

The alveolar-capillary unit responds in a stereotyped manner to a number of different insults. Thus, most injury is characterized by a chronic accumulation of inflammatory and immune effector cells within the alveolar wall and airspace ("alveolitis"), with resultant repair characterized by derangement of interstitial collagen ("fibrosis") and an alteration in pulmonary parenchymal cells (Fig. 32.2). The result of this process, if unbridled, is initially distortion, and then destruction, of the alveolar-capillary unit with its physiologic consequence of hypoxia (5–8).

The practice of categorizing ILD by histologic criteria has resulted in an "alphabet soup" nomenclature and subsequent confusion among clinicians caring for these patients. Labeling diseases by cellular content and pattern (e.g., desquamative interstitial pneumonitis [DIP], usual interstitial pneumonitis [UIP]) may not be consistent from one inter-

Table 32.1.
Potential Etiologies of Interstitial Lung Disease in Childhood

Infections

  Mycobacteria (especially miliary tuberculosis)
  Viruses
    Adenovirus
      influenza A_2
    Parainfluenza
    Cytomegalovirus
    Ebstein-Barr virus
    Respiratory suncytial virus
  Mycoplasma pneumoniae
  Legionella pneumonphila
  Pneumocystis carinii
  Fungi
  Chlamydia trachomatis
  Ureaplasma urealyticum
  Psittacosis
  Q fever

Environmental causes

  Organic dusts (hypersensitivity pneumonitis—e.g., "bird fancier's lung")
  Toxic gases
    NO_2
    SO_2
    Br
    Cl
  Fumes, vapors, aerosols
  Insecticides (e.g., paraquat)

Connective tissue disorders

  Systematic lupus erythematous
  Rheumatoid arthritis
  Progressive Systemic Sclerosis
  Sjögren syndrome
  Inflammatory bowel disease
  Ankylosing spondylitis

Sarcoidosis

Interstitial pneumonias

  Usual interstitial pneumonia (UIP)
  Desquamative interstitial pneumonia (DIP)
  Lymphocytic infiltrative disorder (with/without immunodeficiency)
    Lymphocytic interstitial pneumonia (LIP)
    Pulmonary lymphoid hyperplasia (PLH)
    Nodular lymphoid hyperplasia (NLH)
    Follicular bronchiolitis
  Idiopathic pulmonary fibrosis (IPF)
  Bronchiolitis obliterans (BO)
  Bronchiolitis obliterans with organizing pneumonia (BOOP)

Adverse effects of therapy

  Radiation fibrosis
  Drug toxicity
    Chemotherapy
      Busulfan
      Bleomycin
      Cyclophosphamide
      Methotrexate
      Nitrosourens (BCNU)
      Procarbazine
      Mitomycin

  Antibiotics
    Nitrofurantoin
    Sulfonamides
    Penicillin
  Others
    Propranolol
    Carbamazine
    Gold salts
    Diphenylhydantoin
    Hexamethonium
    Mecamylamine
    Methysergide
    Pentolinium
  Oxygen toxicity

Cardiopulmonary disease

  Multiple pulmonary emboli
  Chronic pulmonary edema
  Veno-occlusive disease
  Arteriolitis
  Congenital cardiovascular anomalies
    Anomalous pulmonary venous return
    Pulmonary vein stenosis

"Allergic" reactions

  Chronic eosinophilic pneumonia
  Churg-Strauss syndrome
  Hypersensitivity angiitis

Malignant neoplasms

  Leukemia/lymphoma
  Bronchoalveolar carcinoma
  Carcinomatosis, metastases

Aspiration syndromes

  Food, gastric acid
  Oil
  Talc

Unusual specific disorders

  Pulmonary hemosiderosis
  Alveolar proteinosis
  Histiocytosis X
  Pulmonary alveolar microlithiasis
  Wegener granulomatosis
  Lymphangiomyomatosis (LAM)
  Diffuse amyloidosis of lung
  Goodpasture syndrome
  Pulmonary telangiectasia
  Pulmonary lymphangiectasia/lymphangiomatous

ILD with associated disorders

  Cystic fibrosis
  Immunodefficiency diseases
  Whipple disease
  Weber-Christian disease
  Hermansky-Pudlak syndrome
  Neurofibromatosis
  Tuberous sclerosis

Unclassified/idiopathic

Evaluation of the Child with Interstitial Lung Disease (ILD)

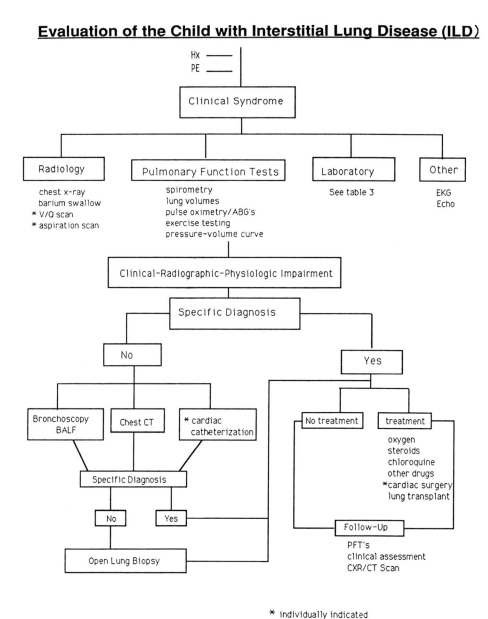

* individually indicated

Figure 32.1. Suggested scheme for evaluating a child suspected of having interstitial lung disease.

preter to the next, and it is unclear whether a specific histologic diagnosis is discreet or an expression of a continuum of disease. Furthermore, unlike the case in adults, there are scarce data in children as to therapeutic and prognostic implications of any particular histologic finding.

A standardized method of examining and reporting lung histology in ILD-C, as summarized in Table 32.2, provides a framework that will make the complicated terminology of pathologists understandable to clinicians. One must first determine which structures of the alveolar capillary unit are involved. Then specific infectious, environmental, or malignant agents should be sought when the etiology is not readily apparent. The findings are categorized by the pathologic process in evidence,

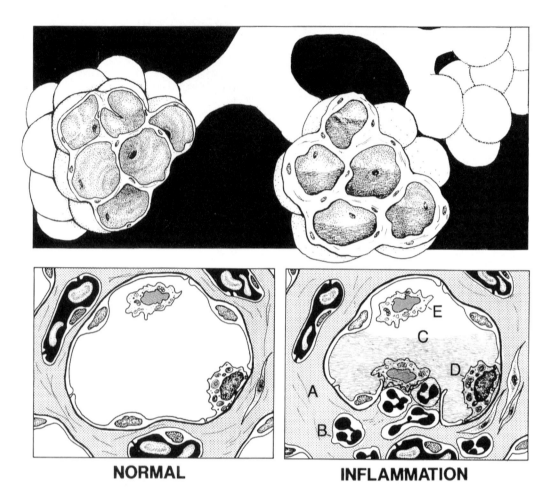

NORMAL   **INFLAMMATION**

Figure 32.2. Diagram of alveolar air spaces under normal *(left)* and acutely inflamed *(right)* conditions. The interstitium *(A)* is thickened with edema and acute inflammatory cells *(B)* that migrate from the capillaries. The alveolar epithelium is disrupted and fluid and cells have extravasated into the alveolar air space *(C)*. Type II cells *(D),* activated alveolar macrophages *(E),* neutrophils, and sometimes lymphocytes are present in increased numbers and release cytokines, growth factors, reactive oxygen species, and other mediators that perpetuate the inflammatory response. Collapse of the entire alveolus from fibrosis may ultimately occur.

by the cellular constituents and their patterns, by the cell products present, and by the distribution of lesions. More sophisticated cellular identification through immunohistochemical techniques will add further information on which therapeutic rationale can be based. Refining the approach to lung histology will result in a tighter and more orderly classification system for ILD-C and advance our understanding (Fig. 32.3) of this class of diseases.

CLINICAL SYNDROME

Children with ILD most often present in the first year of life with a characteristic pattern of signs and symptoms. Dry cough, tachypnea, dyspnea or "hard breathing," poor growth, and exercise intolerance are the most frequent complaints. Although cyanosis may not be recognized by the parents, low oxygen saturation is found at diagnosis in 80% of children. A history of repeated respiratory infections, wheezing and, rarely, hemoptysis, may also be elicited. Symptoms are insidious, resulting in a lag of many months between their onset and the seeking of medical care.

Some historical details may be particularly pertinent to the evaluation of ILD-C. Family members with similar respiratory complaints suggest entities such as DIP, UIP, sarcoidosis,

Table 32.2
A General Approach to Lung Histology in Childhood ILD

1. *Identify the structures involved*
   Alveolar space
   Interstitium (including lining cells and
      capillaries)
   Airways (small, medium or large)
   Vessels (arteries or veins)
   Lymphatics

2. *Categorize the pathologic process*
   Exudation/organization
   Granulomas
   Hemorrhage
   Atelectasis
   Hyperinflation
   Abnormal lymphoid tissue
   Fibrosis
   Airway obliteration
   Necrosis

3. *Search for specific etiologies*
   Infectious agents/inclusion bodies
   Lipid (aspiration)
   Hemosiderin (hemosiderosis)
   Dust
   Tumor

4. *Survey cells and their products*
   Intrinsic cells

      Pneumocytes (type I & type II)
      Fibroblasts
      Smooth muscle cells
      Alveolar macrophages
      Lymphocytes

   Extrinsic cells

      Neutrophils
      Eosinophils
      Histiocytes
      Monocytes
      Plasma cells

   Elaborated cell products

      Hyaline membranes
      Proteinaceous exudate
      Fibrin
      Edema
      Mucus

   Intracellular products

      Iron/hemosiderin
      Lipid
      Dust particles
      Birbeck granules (histiocytosis X)

   Specific patterning of cells
      UIP, DIP, LIP

5. *Ascertain the distribution of lesions*
   Diffuse or focal
   Random or targeted to specific normal
      structures
   Concentrated along lymphatics
   Pleural based
   Peripheral or central

or autoimmune etiologies. A careful environmental history should uncover exposure to birds or other organic sensitizing agents, asbestos, wood dust, or toxic gases, particularly chlorine, nitrous dioxide, or sulphur dioxide. Although most children are unlikely to contact such agents, thorough questioning of the parents' occupational or recreational activities may disclose an exposure source. In infants, questions regarding the use of baby powders, home or cultural remedies for common infantile conditions (e.g., mineral oil for constipation), and feeding practices are vital, since pulmonary aspiration is a frequent and readily treatable cause of ILD-C.

Previous infections, pulmonary or otherwise, are important clues to underlying immunodeficiency states or Wegener granulomatosis. A history of malignancy should direct attention to thoracic involvement in a primary or metastatic tumor or to the sequelae of treatment, such as radiation or drug-induced pulmonary toxicity. A history of blood transfusion or high-risk parental behavior should raise the possibility of AIDS.

Findings on physical examination are usually confined to the respiratory tract. Crackles are readily heard, and tachypnea is observed in over half the cases. Wheezing occurs occasionally. Chest retractions, clubbing, and evidence of poor growth are often present as well. Dyspnea may be indexed by observing how long an older child can count or speak before taking a breath. In the infant, similar information may be gained by assessing the crying pattern. Evidence of pulmonary hypertension is occasionally present.

Physical findings that point to specific etiologies are valuable if found. Dermal hemangiomas, tubers, or ash leaf lesions may signal the pulmonary involvement of hemangiomatosis, tuberous sclerosis, or neurofibromatosis, respectively. Likewise, pathognomonic skin and joint findings of autoimmune diseases such as systemic lupus erythematosus or Sjögren syndrome suggest pulmonary disease associated with these conditions. Sparse peripheral lymphadenopathy, splenomegaly, or lack of tonsillar tissue should raise concern for immune deficiency. The cardiovascular examination may disclose a prominent second heart sound, a murmur, or hepatomegaly, pointing to a previously undiagnosed intracardiac or intrapulmonary shunt.

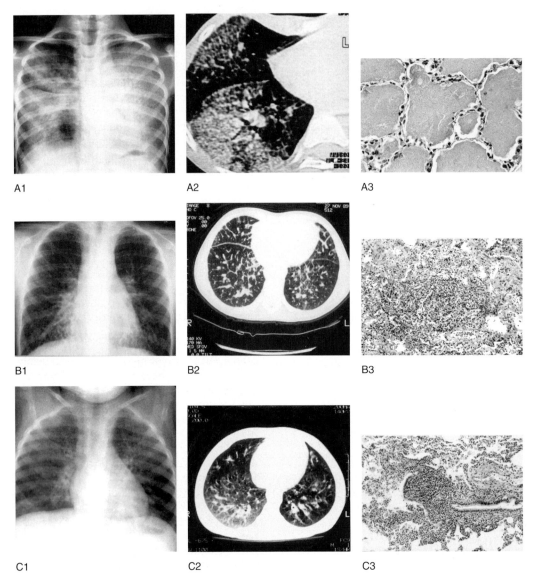

Figure 32.3. Illustrative cases of pediatric ILD. *A,* 8-year-old girl with alveolar proteinosis. *A1,* Chest radiograph shows diffuse, bilateral alveolar infiltrates with some sparing of the right upper and middle lobes. *A2,* Chest CT image of the right lung shows patchy areas of alveolar filling alternating with reticular densities and normal lung. *A3,* Histopathology confirms dense, air space filling with amorphous material and some areas of focal, interstitial hypercellularity. *B,* 8-year-old girl with pulmonary lymphangiomatosis. There are marked, bibasilar interstitial infiltrates evident on chest radiograph *(B1).* Intralobular septal thickening is apparent in all lung fields on this infrahilar slice of the chest CT *(B2).* Lung biopsy specimen shows nearly complete obliteration of alveolar spaces by fibrous tissue, cellular infiltrate of type II cells, macrophages and lymphocytes, and a marked proliferation of lymphatic channels *(B3).* *C,* 2-year-old male with hypogammaglobulinemia and pulmonary lymphoid hyperplasia. Lacy, interstitial infiltrates are seen on chest radiograph with greatest involvement of the right lower and middle lobes *(C1).* Chest CT reveals increased overall density of the right lower lobe with a prominence of the interstitial markings *(C2).* Histologic examination shows focal accumulations of B lymphocytes and dense fibrotic thickening in the peribronchiolar areas *(C3).* There is mild lymphocytic infiltration of the interstitium and the alveolar spaces are normal.

RADIOGRAPHIC EVALUATION—STAGE I

A pattern of linear or reticular shadows on plain chest radiograph is most typical of ILD and occurs in two-thirds of patients in our experience (Fig. 32.3). Other recognizable patterns may be seen alone or in combination. These include nodular (1–10 mm in size), reticulonodular, ground glass, homogeneous shadowing and honeycomb patterns (9). The type and distribution of these opacities in the upper, mid, and lower lung zones or in the perihilar or peripheral areas has been helpful in differentiating various ILD in adults. Plain chest radiographs can also yield valuable information about lung volumes, hilar adenopathy, pleural disease, and pulmonary hypertension. Despite this usefulness, the chest radiograph is a relatively insensitive measure of the presence or extent of disease. A well-controlled study of chest radiograph interpretation in ILD showed that a "confident" diagnosis could be made initially only 23% of the time (10). A normal chest radiograph should not discourage further evaluation when there is clinical suspicion of ILD-C (11).

The radiographic pattern of aspiration includes interstitial infiltrates; this potential etiology deserves consideration in most patients with suspected ILD-C. A barium esophagram is a cost-effective, diagnostic study in the evaluation of ILD-C, since aspiration that results from discoordinated swallowing, gastroesophageal reflux, or congenital anomalies such as tracheoesophageal fistula or laryngeal cleft is a common cause of interstitial lung disease (see Chapter 31).

Ventilation-perfusion (V/Q) scanning is useful in selected circumstances. In one study a pattern of matched defects reported in children with bronchiolitis obliterans was felt to be sufficiently diagnostic as to circumvent the need for lung biopsy confirmation (12).

RADIOLOGIC EVALUATION—STAGE II

Chest Computed Tomography

The ability to assess fine detail of the pulmonary parenchyma has been made possible by computed tomography (CT) of the chest. Radiographic images of lung "slices" can now be obtained on children since scan times of as little as 0.6 seconds result in diminished motion artifact. High-resolution CT (HRCT) of a single lung combining very thin sections (1–2 mm) with a high-frequency resolution algorithm significantly enhances the image, providing resolution of structures as small as 0.5 mm (13). Several patterns of CT abnormalities have been found to correspond with specific histologic diseases in adults: (a) *irregular linear pattern:* idiopathic pulmonary fibrosis, asbestosis, lymphatic tumor spread; (b) *cystic pattern:* lymphangiomatosis; (c) *nodular pattern:* silicosis, sarcoidosis, histiocytosis X, hypersensitivity pneumonitis; and (d) *ground glass pattern:* alveolar proteinosis, eosinophilic pneumonia, bronchiolitis obliterans with organizing pneumonia (13). The relevance of these CT patterns to ILD-C is not known, especially since the distribution of these diseases in children may be quite different than that found in adults. This technology should be used in ILD-C because chest CT is non-invasive and can be used to stage disease severity and follow response to therapy (14), CT is more sensitive than plain chest radiographs for detecting and defining radiographic abnormalities (10), and the precise localization of abnormalities can serve as a guide to optimal sites for open lung biopsy (15).

PULMONARY FUNCTION TESTING

Pulmonary function has been reasonably well characterized in ILD-C (16–23). As with adults, children most often present a physiologic picture of restrictive lung disease (Fig. 32.4A) (24). Vital capacity is the most significantly diminished, with inspiratory capacity and total lung capacity (TLC) also invariably reduced (18, 20–22). Functional residual capacity (FRC) and residual volume (RV) may be decreased or increased, and the ratios of FRC/TLC and RV/TLC are frequently larger than predicted, reflecting either the relatively greater contraction of the TLC or true hyperinflation (18, 22).

Evidence of airflow limitation has varied from study to study. The ratio of forced expiratory flow in the first second to the forced vital capacity (FEV_1/FVC) was abnormal in only 6% of Zapletal's group (18), 17% in our patients, and 43% of Diaz's study population (24). Airways resistance and conductance measurements, assumed to reflect flow in large airways, are usually normal to supernormal. However, flows at low lung volumes (FEF 25-75

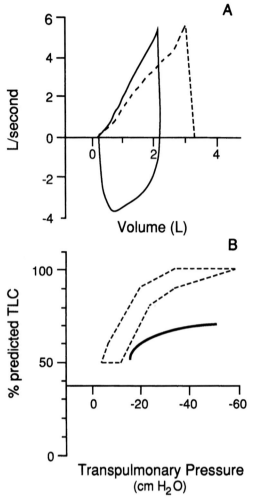

Figure 32.4. *A,* Flow–volume loop from a 12-year-old girl with pulmonary fibrosis. Total lung capacity is diminished whereas volume-corrected flows in early expiration are supranormal. *B,* Pressure–volume curve from same patient. Curve is shifted down and to the right, indicating loss of pulmonary compliance. *Dashed line* = predicted; *Unbroken line* = patient.

or V_{max} 25%, 50%, or 75%) are reduced in a substantial number of children (18). This finding corroborates the frequent histopathologic demonstration of small airways disease in many types of ILD in both children and adults (25). Thus, a mixed restrictive/obstructive pattern of pulmonary function is to be expected in ILD-C.

Alterations in the elastic properties of the lungs are particularly striking (Fig. 32.4B). The shape of the pressure-volume curve is typically flattened and displaced downward and to the right of normal, indicating stiffness or loss of compliance of the lung. Transpulmonary pressure at maximum inspiration is elevated to as much as 220% of the predicted value in nearly all children (18). In addition, measurements of specific static and dynamic compliance (SCL-dyn) are significantly reduced in most children, and there is evidence that the decrease in SCL-dyn correlates with the degree of pulmonary fibrosis (22). These measures of lung mechanics are useful in adults to identify physiologic abnormalities in patients with normal chest radiographs and in following responses to therapy and may have similar value in children.

Resting arterial oxygen tension is nearly always decreased in children with ILD, even when cyanosis is not detectable (16, 26, 27). Non-invasive assessment of hemoglobin saturation with pulse oximetry closely approximates arterial oxygen saturation, making it a valuable assessment tool in children. Arterial blood gas tensions should be measured, and the calculation of the alveolar-arterial oxygen difference (AaDo$_2$) should be calculated, since an increase in AaDo$_2$ of more than 10 mm Hg correlates with lung disease severity (28), presence of pulmonary hypertension (29), and diminished survival in adults with idiopathic pulmonary fibrosis (30). In adults the measurement of gas exchange during exercise, particularly when corrected for oxygen consumption, is the best index of overall physiologic dysfunction and correlates well with histopathologic abnormalities (31, 32). Diffusing capacity for carbon monoxide (DLCO) corrected for alveolar volume (DLCO/VA), is abnormal in 42–61% of patients with ILD-C (16, 18, 26, 27). However, it is technically problematic to perform in children and has not been useful in adults for predicting either histologic findings on lung biopsy or the cause of disease (33, 34).

Advances in the measurement of lung function in infants has broadened the physiologic assessment of ILD-C to include the youngest age group. In a single report of three cases, Kerem and colleagues found respiratory system compliance, measured by the multiple occlusion and end-inspiratory occlusion techniques, to improve following therapy for usual and desquamative interstitial pneumonitis (19).

LABORATORY TESTS

There are few laboratory tests of proven value in identifying specific etiologies in ILD-C. Exceptions might include the finding of microcytic anemia unresponsive to iron or a positive anti-neutrophil cytoplasmic antibody in pulmonary hemosiderosis and Wegener granulomatosis, respectively. A list of potentially useful laboratory investigations that may be applied on an individual basis appears in Table 32.3.

Quantification of white blood cells and immune function is useful is detecting malignancy, hypereosinophilic syndromes, immunodeficiency states, and occasionally UIP. Other helpful studies are angiotensin-converting enzyme, a marker for sarcoidosis, and circulating immune complexes, which are frequently elevated in both sarcoidosis and idiopathic pulmonary fibrosis (35, 36). Nonspecific measurements of systemic inflammation (e.g., erythrocyte sedimentation rate [ESR] and C-reactive protein) are often elevated. Unfortunately, none of these measurements are specific; nor do they necessarily reflect the severity or therapeutic responsiveness of the underlying lung disease.

Laboratory investigations for infectious etiologies are equally problematic. Serologic studies for viruses, mycoplasma, *Legionella* and fungi provide only circumstantial evidence of cause and effect. Such studies are typically not helpful in the most susceptible population, the immunocompromised hosts. Identification of specific organisms by histology, culture, or gene probing of lung biopsy or BAL fluid specimens remains the definitive diagnostic tool for infectious disorders.

GALLIUM SCANNING

Gallium-67, a radionuclide that is engulfed by activated macrophages and, to a lesser extent, neutrophils, can delineate areas of pulmonary inflammation by nuclear scintigraphic scanning. The gallium scan (GS) has been used in adults to quantify the interstitial and alveolar cellularity in idiopathic pulmonary fibrosis (37). There is a correlation of GS with inflammation detected by either open lung biopsy or BAL fluid analysis (32). However, there appears to be little relationship between GS and the patient's clinical course in either adults (32) or children (16). At present, GS cannot be recommended routinely in ILD-C.

BRONCHOALVEOLAR LAVAGE (BAL)

Although it has been frequently used in adults with a variety of ILDs (38–41), BAL fluid analysis in children is in a primitive state and is not often helpful, particularly in the nonimmunocompromised child with ILD (42–49). There are a number of reasons for this: (a) lack of "normal" values in children, (b) scarcity of large groups of pediatric patients with specific types of ILD, (c) inhomogeneity of lung involvement and consequent sampling errors, (d) uncertainty as to the comparison of BAL fluid results from adults with those from children, and (e) nonstandardized methodology for collecting, quantifying, and testing BAL fluid in children (16). BAL fluid analysis in children will only achieve clinical utility when a standardized method is widely applied. We propose one such scheme in Table 32.4.

In spite of these drawbacks, there is much to recommend BAL fluid analysis as a potentially useful tool. In the immunocompromised child, recovery of agents such as *Pneumocystis carinii*, cytomegalovirus, respiratory syncytial virus, *Legionella pneumophila*, and fungi can be diagnostic (42–48). A characteristic cellular profile in BAL fluid, derived from experience in immunocompetent adults, is supportive evi-

Table 32.3.
Useful Laboratory Studies in Childhood ILD

Complete blood count, differential, platelet count
Erythrocyte sedimentation rate
Alpha-1 antitrypsin level
Sweat test
Studies of immune function
  IgG, A, M, and E, including IgG subclasses
  Specific antibody levels (e.g., anti-tetanus
    antibody)
  Complement levels
  Immune complexes
  Delayed hypersensitivity skin testing
  T and B cell enumeration
  Lymphocyte stimulation (antigens/mitogens)
  HIV antibody or antigen
Autoimmune studies (ANA, RF, ANCA)
Anti-neutrophil cytoplasmic antibodies
Angiotensin converting enzyme
Studies for infectious etiology
  Nasal wash (RSV, pertussis, chlamydia)
  Sputum stains and cultures
  Serologies (EBV, CMV, RSV, adenovirus,
    Mycoplasma, Legionella)

DIP (20, 22, 59, 60, 62) and LIP (64, 65). The response rate in children is generally 60% for DIP (22, 62), although the familial and infantile forms of this disease are frequently fatal (59, 62). Precise dosing recommendations vary but 2 mg/kg of prednisone daily is reasonable on initiation, with gradual tapering of this dose based on clinical response and lung function measurements. An alternative treatment regimen is sequential, intravenous "pulse therapy" with high-dose solumedrol (30–50 mg/kg/dose to a maximum of 1 g) for 3–5 days at monthly intervals. This form of therapy, pioneered in transplant patients experiencing organ rejection, has the advantage of complete immune suppression with few long-term side effects (66). However, pulse therapy is, at present, untested in ILD-C. Overall, CSs may induce a remission of particular types of ILD-C, but continuous treatment is usually necessary to maintain improvement (21, 22).

In our own series, 40 of 68 patients with varying forms of ILD-C were treated with CSs. Approximately one-third of these patients were judged to have had a good response, whereas definite improvement could not be demonstrated in the remaining two-thirds. We could not identify clinical markers of CS responsiveness such as age at onset of ILD, duration of symptoms at initiation, or histologic type. Given the possibility of clinical improvement, it seems reasonable to institute a trial of CSs in any child with ILD, with careful monitoring of clinical response. The known suppressive effects of long-term CSs on bone mineralization, linear growth, and possibly lung maturation (67) certainly dictate caution in this approach.

Hydroxychloroquine

The grim specter of disabling side effects and the frequent resistance of any particular disease to CS has prompted consideration of other drugs. The use of hydroxychloroquine was first described by Tooley in an anecdotal report of a 3-year-old child with DIP (68). Since then, a small number of other pediatric patients with DIP and UIP have been treated successfully with hydroxychloroquine in combination with, or following, prednisone (19, 61, 69). The rationale for use of this drug stems from its anti-inflammatory effects and usefulness in rheumatoid arthritis, systemic

lupus erythematosus, and other diseases (70–72). Dosage recommendations in children are more problematic than with CSs, since serum levels reflect only a minuscule proportion of the drug concentrated in the lung (73). Furthermore, since retinopathy is a serious toxic effect of chloroquine, its use in very young children who cannot cooperate with vision testing is relatively contraindicated (74).

Other Drugs

Alternative pharmacologic interventions have been used in adults with ILD, mostly as rescue therapy when steroids have failed (58). Cyclophosphamide, azathioprine, penicillamine, vincristine, and chlorambucil have been used in individual cases with success (35). The use of these drugs in children is limited by concerns for long-term adverse effects, particularly secondary malignancies, sterility, and the induction of ILD. Less conventional forms of drug therapy are undertaken on a case-by-case basis, but definitive recommendations await further study.

Lung Transplantation

The ultimate therapeutic intervention for unremitting ILD-C is lung transplantation. This form of therapy has proven successful in end-stage, fibrotic lung disease, pulmonary hypertension, chronic obstructive lung disease, and cystic fibrosis (75, 76). Although the bulk of experience has been accumulated in adult patients, the age of eligible recipients has been lowered considerably, with children as young as 3 years undergoing successful transplantation (77). In patients with fibrotic, non-infected lung disease and recoverable right heart function, single-lung transplantation should be considered.

The hazards inherent in lung transplantation in ILD-C are legion and have been elaborated by Diaz (16). Patients who achieve some measure of clinical remission from steroids may experience rapid deterioration when therapy is withdrawn preoperatively as prophylaxis against bronchial anastomotic dehiscence. Secondly, the inertia of any particular ILD is unknown, and clinical stability over some years may suddenly give way to inexorable progression and death. The "window of opportunity" for lung transplantation in a given individual is thus difficult to ascertain and plan for. Thirdly, the expense, both financial and emotional, is enormous and out of reach of many otherwise eligible candidates. Lastly, there is no guarantee against recurrence of the original disease, and there is a 10–54% risk of obliterative bronchiolitis in the transplanted lung, which may itself be fatal (78). As with other therapies for this perplexing disease, lung transplantation holds both promise and problems.

LONGITUDINAL FOLLOW-UP

The overall outlook for children with ILD is less than encouraging. In Diaz's series of 17 patients, 19% died, 50% were classified as having a poor quality of life, and 31% were relatively well (16). Our 68 patients showed remarkably comparable outcomes, with a mortality rate of 16%, a static or deteriorating course in 50%, and improvement in 33%. Only two of our patients could actually be considered to have fully recovered, and late relapse of disease always remains a concern (79).

There are no well established parameters to monitor accurately the course of ILD-C. In adults, the following tests obtained serially have borne a reasonable relationship to exacerbations of disease and to therapeutic response: (a) pulmonary function tests, particularly measurements of resting and exercise gas exchange (80); (b) bronchoalveolar lavage fluid cellularity (81); (c) high-resolution CT scan (14); and (d) serum levels of circulating immune complexes (36). As previously mentioned, gallium scanning as a measure of lung inflammation has little utility in predicting clinical course. There are several new technologies, however, which are more promising. These include positron emission tomography (PET), which can measure extracellular lung density and glucose utilization, and ^{99m}Tc-diethylene-triminepenta-acetate (^{99m}Tc-DTPA) clearance (82, 83).

A practical approach to assessment of ILD that has great potential utility in pediatric patients is the clinical-radiographic-physiologic (CRP) scoring system devised by Watters and colleagues (31). A range of values is assigned to each of seven variables: dyspnea, chest radiography, spirometry, lung volumes, diffusion capacity, resting alveolar-arterial oxygen difference, and exercise oxygen satura-

tion. The CRP score, ranging from 0 to 100, correlated significantly with histopathologic findings on open lung biopsy and also with response to steroid therapy at 6 months. Such a scoring system, adapted for children, has great appeal for assessing severity of initial pathologic derangement and for longitudinal evaluation of functional status. Furthermore, such a tool could help standardize clinical assessment, thus promoting the multi-center cooperation necessary to study ILD-C.

COMPLICATIONS

The comprehensive care of the child with ILD requires vigilant monitoring for progress of the disease, its effect on other organs, and the adverse consequences of therapy. Primary among these concerns is pulmonary hypertension (84), which develops from progressive hypoxia, resulting initially from V/Q mismatch and then from obliteration of the pulmonary vascular bed. Periodic electrocardiograms and echocardiograms are indicated, although their sensitivity is debatable. Cardiac catheterization should be undertaken in any patient in whom there is a strong suspicion of pulmonary hypertension. Prompt recognition of hypoxia, particularly at night, should guide early and "enough" oxygen therapy to prevent or forestall this complication. An evaluation of hypoxia during sleep should be undertaken in any patient with borderline awake saturations or in a patient with adequate awake saturations who develops growth failure, polycythemia, or progressive pulmonary hypertension. In patients who develop right heart failure, diuretic therapy may be of some benefit, although the use of digoxin is controversial (85, 86).

The incidence of pulmonary infection is known to be increased in adults with ILD (87). Impaired macrophage function and altered local host defense of the airway may account for this. In the typical immunologically naive child, viruses may wreak havoc in the damaged lung. When significant pulmonary fibrosis is present, aspergillosis with mycetoma formation can occur. Likewise, suspicion should be raised of tuberculosis (typical and atypical) and endemic fungi whenever clinical or radiographic deterioration occurs. Of course, opportunistic infection is always a concern when profound immunosuppression occurs in concert with ILD-C.

plantation in adults. *Transplantation* 1984, 37:246–249.

67. Ferguson MA, Durmowicz AG, Dobyns EL, Hofmeister SE, Stenmark KR. Effect of dexamethasone on matrix protein production and cell proligeration in bovine and human lung cells. *Pediatr Res* 1991; 29:370A.

68. Barnett HL ed. *Pediatrics*, 15th ed. New York, Appleton-Century-Crofts, 1972, pp 1315–1316.

69. Leahy F, Pasterkamp H, Tal A. Desquamative interstitial pneumonia responsive to chloroquine. *Clin Pediatr* 1985; 24:230–232.

70. Salmeron G, Lipsky PE. Immunosuppressive potential of antimalarials. *Am J Med* 1983; 75:19–26.

71. Wollheim FA, Hanson A, Laurell C–B. Chloroquine treatment in rheumatoid arthritis. Correlation of clinical response to plasma protein changes and chloroquine levels. *Scand J Rheumatol* 1978; 7:171–176.

72. Leaksonen A–L, Koskiahde V, Juva K. Dosage of antimalarial drugs for children with juvenile rheumatoid arthritis and systemic lupus erythematosis. *Scand J Rheumatol* 1974; 3:103–108.

73. Webster LT. Drugs used in the chemotherapy of protozoal infections: Malaria. In Gilman AG, Goodman LS, Rall TW, Murad F, eds: *Goodman and Gilman: The pharmacological basis of therapeutics*, 7th ed. New York, Macmillan, 1985, pp 1029–1048.

74. Marks JS. Chloroquine retinopathy. Is there a safe daily dose? *Ann Rheum Dis* 1982; 41:512–558.

75. Morrison DL, Maurer JR, Grossman RF. Preoperative assessment for lung transplantation. *Clin Chest Med* 1990; 11:207–215.

76. Scott J, Hutter J, Stewart S, Higgenbottam T, Hodson M, Penketh A, Wallwork J. Heart-lung transplantation for cystic fibrosis. *Lancet* 1988; 2:192–194.

77. Palazzo RM. Pediatric lung and heart-lung transplantation. Seminar at the American Lung Association/American Thoracic Society International Conference, Anaheim, California, May 13, 1991.

78. Theodore J, Starnes VA, Lewiston NJ. Obliterative bronchiolitis. *Clin Chest Med* 1990; 11:309–321.

79. Lipworth B, Woolcock A, Addis B, Turner–Warwick M. Late relapse of desquamative interstitial pneumonia. *Am Rev Resp Dis* 1987; 136:1253–1255.

80. Gaensler EA, Carrington CB, Coutou RE, Fitzgerald MX. Radiographic, pathologic correlations in interstitial pneumonias. In Basset F, Georges R, eds. Alveolar interstitium of the lung. Pathological and physiologic aspects. *Prog Respir Res* 1974; 8:223–242.

81. Haslam PL, Turton CWG, Lukoszek A, et al. Bronchoalveolar lavage fluid cell counts in cryptogenic fibrosing alveolitis and their relation to therapy. *Thorax* 1980; 25:328–339.

82. Pantin CF, Valind SO, Sweatman M, et al. Measures of the inflammatory response in cryptogenic fibrosing alveolitis. *Am Rev Respir Dis* 1988; 138:1234–1241.

83. Rinderkuecht J, Shapiro L, Krauthammer M, et al. Accelerated clearance of small solutes from the lungs in interstitial lung disease. *Am Rev Respir Dis* 1980; 121:105–117.

84. Packe GE, Cayton RM, Edwards CW. Comparison of right ventricular size at necropsy in interstitial pulmonary fibrosis and in chronic bronchitis and emphysema [Abstract]. *Thorax* 1985; 40:712.

85. Green LH, Smith TW. The use of digitalis in patients with pulmonary disease. *Ann Intern Med* 1977; 87:459–465.

86. Mathur PN, Powles ACP, Pugsley SO, McEwan MP, Campbell EJM. Effects of digoxin on right ventricular function in severe chronic airflow obstruction. *Ann Intern Med* 1981; 95:283–288.

87. Snider GE. Interstitial pulmonary fibrosis. Clinical features, natural history and complications. *Semin Respir Med* 1984; 6:71–79.

88. Kerr JS. Nutrition and the lung. In Laraya-Cuasay LR, Hughes WT, eds. *Interstitial lung disease in children*, vol I. Boca Raton, FL, CRC Press, 1988, pp 129–138.

33

Cilia Dyskinesia Syndrome

PAUL C. STILLWELL

Mucociliary clearance is one of the primary lung defense systems. Its efficient function depends on a coordinated and integrated interaction between the cilia and mucus; abnormalities of either can impair host defenses to the point of producing chronic lung disease (1, 2). Abnormalities in mucus production and composition occur quite commonly (e.g., cystic fibrosis, asthma) whereas primary ciliary dysfunction is relatively uncommon. Although the triad of bronchiectasis, sinusitis, and situs inversus (Kartagener syndrome) has been recognized for some time, the unifying explanation has only recently been discovered during evaluation of infertile men with chronic respiratory syndromes (3). Studies of sperm and cilia revealed absent motility associated with ultrastructural defects, thereby establishing ciliary dysfunction as a cause of infertility and recurrent sinopulmonary disease. This chapter will focus on ciliary abnormalities leading to chronic respiratory diseases in children.

CILIARY PHYSIOLOGY AND BIOLOGY

The cilia are specific organelles found in several organ systems (Table 33.1). The nonmotile cilia are predominantly located in sensory organs. The cilia of the respiratory epithelium are motile and are present in the

middle ear, the sinuses, the nasopharynx, and the tracheobronchial tree. As expected, each of these areas becomes diseased with primary ciliary dysfunction syndromes. There are approximately 200 cilia projecting from the surface of each cell. A coordinated beat within and between cells propels mucus and other surface particles toward the oropharynx (metachronism). At body temperature the normal beat frequency is approximately 12–15 Hz (or 1000 beats per minute). During the "forward" or propelling stroke the cilia are fully extended; during the recovery stroke the cilia are close to the cell surface. The normal wave form resembles the arm stroke of a swimmer (1).

The energy source for ciliary motion is adenosine triphosphate (ATP). The complex ultrastructural protein arrangements within the cilia provide a flexible framework that allows organized movement. These ultrastructural proteins are remarkably constant between the cilia and flagella in many areas of nature. The central pair of tubules are surrounded by nine peripheral doublets, which produce the characteristic "9 + 2" configuration. The sheath around the central pair is connected to the outer doublets by radial spokes. There are small "arms" projecting off each outer doublet (inner and outer dynein arms) that contain ATP-ase, thus providing access to the energy for movement. The outer doublets are also connected by nexin links (Fig. 33.1). The cilia of a given cell (and usually those around it) are oriented in approximately the same direction. As the microtubules slide past one another during movement, it is postulated that these interprotein links detach and re-attach (1, 2).

Table 33.1.
Locations of Cilia in the Body

Motile	Immotile
Respiratory epithelia	Retina
Spermatozoa	Cochlea
Fallopian tubes	Olfactory bulb
Ependyma (embryo)	

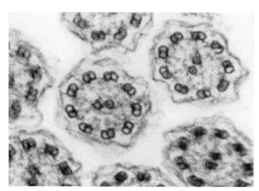

Figure 33.1.   Cross-sectional electron micrograph of normal respiratory cilia demonstrating the nine outer doublets, central pair, radial spokes, and dynein arms. Magnification × 225,000.

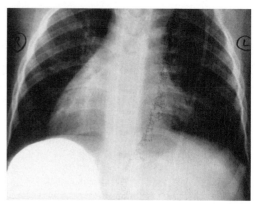

Figure 33.2.   Chest radiograph of an infant with primary ciliary dyskinesia and situs inversus. Barium clearly identifies the stomach on the right side. There are increased peribronchial markings in the left middle lobe region.

CILIARY DYSFUNCTION

The clinical presentation of the child with ciliary dysfunction is similar to that of any child with ineffective mucociliary transport or bronchiectasis (Table 33.2) (4). The severity of the pulmonary disease is related to the extent of the bronchiectasis. If the Kartagener triad is present (situs inversus, sinusitis, bronchiectasis), the diagnosis is often suspected early in life because of the dextrocardia (Fig. 33.2). It is estimated that only 50% of patients with primary ciliary dysfunction have dextrocardia, and the diagnosis may not be readily considered without such an obvious marker (2, 3). The heart is usually structurally and dynamically normal despite its mirror-image location (5).

Table 33.2.
Symptoms and Signs of Primary Ciliary Dyskinesia

Symptoms
Chronic/recurrent otitis media
Chronic sinusitis
Productive coughing
Recurrent pneumonia
  (male infertility)

Signs
Inspiratory crackles (may only be heard on deep
  inspiration)
Decreased intensity of breath sounds
Hyper-inflated chest
Prolonged expiratory phase
Expiratory wheeze
Digital clubbing
Nasal polyps
  (situs inversus totalis)

Just as the symptoms are related to the severity of the bronchiectasis, so are the radiographic and physiologic abnormalities. Early in the disease there may be recurrent areas of atelectasis on chest radiograph (CXR) with a relatively normal appearing film between acute illnesses. The CXR becomes more abnormal over time as the changes of bronchiectasis progress (see Chapter 25). Other radiographic procedures such as high-resolution computed tomography (CT) may better identify the bronchiectasis when the plain CXR shows mild or minimal abnormalities.

The pulmonary functions may be normal early in the disease process but will subsequently demonstrate an obstructive pattern; this usually responds poorly to inhaled bronchodilator although some patients seem to have a significant improvement in flows following bronchodilator treatment. The arterial blood gases generally become abnormal only after extensive lung damage has occurred. Mild hypoxia is the initial abnormality, with hypercarbia occurring only late in the progressive disease process (4).

DIAGNOSIS

In the child who does not have situs inversus or dextrocardia as a marker to suggest primary ciliary dyskinesia, more common diseases causing mucociliary defects (e.g., cystic fibrosis, immunodeficiency, aspiration) should be considered first. If a primary ciliary disorder is suspected, a comprehensive diagnostic evaluation should include wave form analysis, beat frequency, and quantified electron microscopy (EM) (Table 33.3) (6). The mucociliary transport rate should also be measured, which can be difficult in younger children since cooperation is required. The modified saccharine test in older children may document the absence of mucociliary transport (7, 8). A drop of saccharine solution is placed at the mucous junction of a nostril and the time elapsed to taste sweetness is measured; children with primary ciliary dysfunction never taste the sweetness because of absent transport. Radionucleotide insufflation and video bronchoscopy of teflon disks require specialized equipment and cooperation; these measurements of mucociliary transport are seldom done in children.

Cilia for EM and video microscopy are usually obtained from the nasopharynx. Brushing the mucosal surface with a cytology brush provides adequate cellular material about 80% of the time, and there are very few side effects from this procedure (9). Mucosal biopsy produces adequate cellular material slightly less often. Cells can also be obtained from the lower respiratory tract during bronchoscopy or from ejaculate in older subjects. A sample placed in nutrient media (i.e., HBSS or MEM) is used for phase-contrast microscopy of the living cells. EM samples are fixed in glutaraldehyde.

It is important to evaluate the wave form and beat frequency, not just the presence or absence of beating. Some ultrastructural defects have motile cilia, but the wave form and beat frequency are abnormal. Certain ultrastructural defects have been associated with specific wave form abnormalities (Table 33.4) (6). Failure to document the wave form and beat frequency abnormalities may lead to an incorrect diagnosis by assuming the beating

Table 33.3.
Comprehensive Ciliary Evaluation

Electron microscopy
Quantification of abnormalities

Ciliary beat frequency

Ciliary wave form

Mucociliary transport rate
Saccharin test
(Radionucleotide insufflation)
(Bronchoscopic video of teflon disks)

---

cilia are normal. Furthermore, for some patients with acquired ciliary dysfunction, the EM has no abnormalities, so EM study alone will fail to identify the abnormality in ciliary movement (10–12). Unfortunately, beat frequency and wave form analysis are not readily available in all institutions. Therefore it is common to initiate the evaluation by EM studies alone. If primary ciliary dyskinesia is suspected and the EM is nondiagnostic, the full comprehensive evaluation should be pursued.

It is also important to quantify the EM findings. Even in normal subjects it is uncommon to visualize the full complement of subunits within a single cilium (13). Therefore, unless the subject has a striking abnormality such as complete absence of all dynein arms or ciliary aplasia, the distinction between normal and abnormal may be subtle. In some congenital diseases, it is not uncommon to have protein abnormalities that are of variable severity and variable expression (i.e., alpha-1 antiprotease deficiency). Thus it is not surprising that an abnormal ciliary protein could be present in the cilia of some cells but not all cells. The occasional documentation of discordant ultrastructural abnormalities between the respiratory cilia and the spermatozoa of individual patients supports the concept that production of ciliary protein subunits may be under independent control, leading to partial or incomplete abnormalities that may be clinically significant. Correlating the EM findings with wave form analysis and beat frequency determination should allow a precise diagnosis in almost all cases. Repeated evaluation over time can also be helpful in establishing ciliary dysfunction as the cause of chronic lung disease.

Ciliary defects can be acquired or congenital (2, 12). The best characterized and most common congenital defect is the dynein arm defect (Fig. 33.3). Others include absent radial spokes, translocation of the peripheral tubules, ciliary dysplasia, and random orientation (3, 6, 12, 14, 15). Children with congenital defects are usually symptomatic from an early age (i.e., 1 month), whereas those with acquired defects usually begin having problems at a later age (12). The patients with acquired dysfunction generally have a slow beat frequency, abnormal mucociliary clearance, and normal or nonspecific ultrastructure

Table 33.4.
Structure and Dysfunction Associations with Primary Ciliary Dyskinesia

EM Abnormality	Wave Form	% Beating	Beat Frequency
Dynein arm	Vibrating	40–60	Decreaesd 50%
Radial spoke	Corkscrew	90–100	Decreased 20%
Translocation tubules	Grabbing	90–100	Normal to decreased 20%

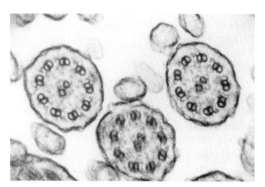

Figure 33.3. Cross-sectional electron micrograph of respiratory cilia with absent inner and outer dynein arms. Magnification × 225,000.

changes (i.e., compound cilia, extra microtubules). Many patients with acquired dysfunction will improve when re-evaluated at a later date. Congenital defects seen on EM are felt to be distinctly different than those found with chronic inflammation or infection (Table 33.5).

TREATMENT

The focus of treatment for ciliary dysfunction syndromes is on improving mucociliary transport. Beta agonists bronchodilators increase ciliary beat frequency in vitro and increase mucociliary transport in some disease such as cystic fibrosis. It is not clear that beta agonists

Table 33.5.
Ultrastructural Defects

Acquired
Compound cilia
Extranummary tubules
Deletion of tubules
Degenerating cells

Congenital
Absent dynein arms
Absent radial spokes
Translocation of tubules
Ciliary aplasia
Random orientation

correct the abnormal wave form seen with primary ciliary dyskinesia or that the overall mucociliary transport is improved. Beta agonists may improve transport by other mechanisms, however, such as bronchodilatation and promoting thinner secretions (2). Coupled with chest percussion and postural drainage, inhaled bronchodilators are a cornerstone of therapy for primary ciliary dyskinesia and related syndromes.

Generous use of antibiotics is another important therapy for ciliary dysfunction. Most patients have recurrent upper and lower respiratory tract infections with common pathogens such as *Haemophilus influenza*, *Streptococcus pneumonia*, and *Staphylococcus aureus* (4). Some patients have more virulent organisms such as *Pseudomonas aeruginosa*, increasing the confusion between ciliary dyskinesia and cystic fibrosis. Chronic prophylactic antibiotic therapy may be helpful in infants and toddlers, an age at which chronic ear disease is likely to be the predominant problem. For preschool and school age children, restricting antibiotic use to times of clinical exacerbations (increased cough, dyspnea, sputum production) may help decrease antibiotic resistance or colonization with more virulent organisms. With moderate to advanced bronchiectasis, treatment with chronic, rotating antibiotics may help decrease clinical symptoms.

Although the role of myringotomy tubes may still be somewhat controversial for "normal" children with recurrent purulent otitis media or chronic serous otitis, early otorhinolaryngology (ear-nose-throat, or ENT) consultation for children with primary ciliary dysfunction is recommended. Because chronic ear disease is almost universal in these children, efforts should be made to prevent hearing loss and delayed speech development. Because large controlled studies of ENT management in children with ciliary dysfunction are not available, management strategies need to be extrapolated from studies in other patients. Options to be considered are chronic prophylactic antibiotics (such as amoxicillin or sulfadiazine) and insertion of myringotomy tubes. After pneumatization of the sinuses, chronic sinus disease is also likely to be a problem. ENT evaluation of sinus disease should also be helpful.

The role of surgical participation in the management of bronchiectasis is less clear. Previous surgical dogma held that resection of isolated bronchiectasis might prevent "spread" to other areas by "spilling" infection into uninvolved areas. With generalized mucociliary dysfunction it seems that all areas of the lung are at risk, regardless of how diseased or well adjacent areas may be. Eventually no part of the lung will be spared. Therefore, surgical resection is seldom recommended for bronchiectasis due to generalized diseases such as primary ciliary dysfunction and cystic fibrosis. However, in a young child with well localized disease who is repeatedly ill and who does not respond to aggressive medical management, surgical resection may improve the quality of life (see also Chapter 25 on bronchiectasis).

Because of the risk for overwhelming pneumonia, children with primary ciliary dysfunction should receive the routine childhood immunizations (e.g., for pertussis, measles) as well as an annual influenza immunization. It is not clear that Haemophilus influenza B or pneumococcal vaccines will be protective in preventing lower airway infections in these patients. Patients who have a significant reactive airways disease component to their symptoms may benefit from standard asthma therapy in addition to the treatments for ciliary dysmotility. Newer treatments for bronchiectasis may also be helpful for these children (e.g., rhDNase).

PROGNOSIS

Although patients with primary ciliary dyskinesia can anticipate life-long problems with otitis, sinusitis, and bronchitis, their life span is generally not shortened (16). A few children seem to have an aggressive clinical disease that is more like cystic fibrosis (despite negative sweat tests); their life span may be shorter than expected. Thus for most patients, a vigorous

and effective cough (along with other treatments mentioned above) may compensate for a deficient mucociliary transport system.

REFERENCES

1. Sleigh MA, Blake JR, Liron N. The propulsion of mucus by cilia. *Am Rev Respir Dis* 1988; 137:726–741.
2. Rubin BK. Immotile cilia syndrome (primary ciliary dyskinesia) and inflammatory lung disease. *Clin Chest Med* 1988; 9:657–668.
3. Eliasson R, Mossberg B, Camner P, Afzelius BA. The immotile cilia syndrome: A congenital ciliary abnormality as an etiologic factor in chronic airway infection and male sterility. *N Engl J Med* 1977; 297:1–6.
4. Turner JAP, Corkey CWB, Lee JYC, Levison H, Sturgess J. Clinical expressions of immotile cilia. *Pediatrics* 1981; 67:805–810.
5. Engesaeth VG, Warner JO, Bush A. New associations of primary ciliary dyskinesia syndrome. *Pediatr Pulmonol* 1993; 16:9–12.
6. Rossman CM, Lee RMKW, Forrest JB, Newhouse MT. Nasal ciliary ultrastructure and function in patients with primary ciliary dyskinesia compared with that in normal subjects and in subjects with various respiratory diseases. *Am Rev Respir Dis* 1984; 129:161–167.
7. Corbo GM, Foresi A, Bonfitto P, Mugnano A, Agabiti N, Cole RJ. Measurement of nasal mucociliary clearance. *Arch Dis Child* 1989; 64:546–550.
8. Canciani M, Barlocco EG, Mastella G, de Santi MW, Gardi C, Lungarella G. The saccharin method for testing mucociliary function in patients suspected of having primary cilia dyskinesia. *Pediatr Pulmonol* 1988; 5:210–214.
9. Stillwell PC, Abell-Aleff P, Scheithauer BW. Electron microscopy of cilia obtained by nasal brushing. *Am Rev Respir Dis* 1990; 141:A626.
10. Carson JL, Collier AM, Shih-chin SH. Acquired ciliary defects in nasal epithelium of children with acute viral upper respiratory infection. *N Engl J Med* 1985; 312:463–468.
11. Corbeel L, Cornillie F, Lauweryns J, Boel M, van den Berghe G. Ultrastructural abnormalities of bronchial cilia in children with recurrent airway infections and bronchiectasis. *Arch Dis Child* 1981; 56:929–933.
12. Buchdahl RM, Reiser J, Ingram D, Rutman A, Cole PJ, Warner JO. Ciliary abnormalities in respiratory disease. *Arch Dis Child* 1988; 63:238–243.
13. Wilton LJ, Teichtahl H, Temple-Smith PC, de Krester DM. Structural heterogeneity of the axonemes of respiratory cilia and sperm flagella in normal man. *J Clin Invest* 1985; 75:825–831.
14. deBoeck K, Jorissen M Wouters K, van der Schueren, Eyssen M, Casteels-Van Daele M, Corbeel L. Aplasia of respiratory tract cilia. *Pediatr Pulmonol* 1992; 13:259–265.
15. Rutland J, Iongh RU. Random ciliary orientation: A cause of respiratory tract disease. *N Engl J Med* 1990; 323:1681–1684.
16. Miller RD, Divertie MB. Kartagener's syndrome. *Chest* 1972; 62:130–135.

34

Pulmonary Hemosiderosis

C. MICHAEL BOWMAN

Pulmonary hemosiderosis (PH) is a rare condition in pediatrics (0.24 cases per million children in one Swedish report) (1) that is actually a clinical syndrome rather than a specific disease. As suggested from the name, it is a condition of ongoing pulmonary bleeding in which iron from red blood cells collects as hemosiderin in the lung parenchyma. The iron remains sequestered in the lung, usually leading to iron deficiency anemia (2–4). The diagnosis of PH is descriptive rather than suggestive of a specific etiology. PH is, in fact, a "final common pathway" of chronic pulmonary bleeding. If a more specific diagnosis can be found to explain the pulmonary hemorrhage (e.g., Goodpasture syndrome [GS] or systemic lupus erythematosus [SLE]) that term is applied. If no other diagnosis is found, the classification of idiopathic pulmonary hemosiderosis (IPH) is given (5–7). Thus, IPH is probably a family of related conditions rather than a single entity. PH is important because patients require long-term, potentially toxic therapy in the hope of maintaining stability, yet there is often an unfavorable outcome in spite of therapy, with mortality as high as 50% in one series (8). PH affects primarily young children, usually age 6 months to 9 years (9), with males and females affected equally (in contrast to GS, which affects primarily young adult males.) PH is generally thought to be an immune disorder with no genetic component (5), although some reports suggest that genetic influences may participate in the expression of at least some cases of PH.

The clinical syndrome of PH is an important one to recognize. The classic PH syndrome is that of a young child with recurrent episodes of respiratory distress, patchy infiltrates on chest radiograph, and iron deficiency anemia. A child with more than two such episodes should be considered to have PH until proven otherwise. The key point is the temporal association of lung disease with anemia. However, pulmonary symptoms may be relatively mild with only episodic tachypnea, mild cough, or wheeze, and minimal fever (Fig. 34.1). New infiltrates may clear in a matter of days or weeks. The respiratory distress may be overshadowed by the anemia, which may become the focus of the diagnostic work-up. Because young children swallow their sputum, the gastrointestinal tract may even be the presumptive site of blood loss because of the presence of heme-positive stools. Only occasion-

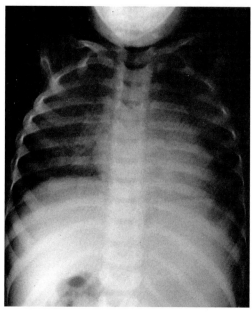

Figure 34.1. The chest radiograph at diagnosis of patient BA from 6/2/89.

417

ally do children with PH show hemoptysis or blood-stained sputum at diagnosis (9).

An absolute requirement for the diagnosis is the finding of hemosiderin-laden alveolar macrophages (Fig. 34.2). In young children who swallow their sputum, the finding of hemosiderin-laden macrophages in gastric aspirates may be sufficient for the diagnosis of PH (7). Lacking this finding, evaluation of the patient should include a bronchoalveolar lavage (BAL) or open lung biopsy. With the widespread availability of flexible fiberoptic bronchoscopy in pediatrics (10), BAL has become the diagnostic procedure of choice. Open lung biopsy (OLB) may be necessary to define the exact lung pathology, and immuno-fluorescent studies may allow differentiation of PH from other pulmonary hemorrhage syndromes (11, 12). A key differential diagnostic point for patients with possible PH is the presence or absence of glomerular involvement or of collagen vascular disease. Serum studies to assess the patient for possible GS, rheumatoid arthritis, SLE, mixed connective tissue disease, and Wegener granulomatosis (WG) should be undertaken during the initial evaluation, usually prior to the BAL. In addition to making an accurate diagnosis, such investigation is necessary because patients with extrapulmonary involvement may develop renal failure or other organ dysfunc-

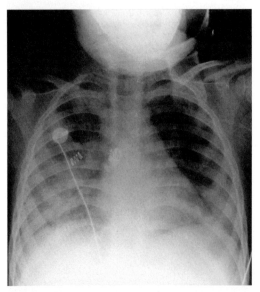

Figure 34.2. The chest radiograph from the same patient during an acute deterioration (caused by parainfluenza) dated 11/21/89.

tion while their pulmonary status (even if it was the initial problem) remains relatively stable. Patients with evidence of kidney disease may undergo a renal biopsy for diagnosis of GS rather than a BAL or OLB.

Once PH is diagnosed (meaning renal involvement and collagen vascular disease have been excluded for the present), it is necessary to look for a variety of contributing conditions that may present with PH. Multiple immune system abnormalities (usually humoral) have been associated with PH (7), but none is found uniformly in all cases of PH. The most widely held impression about the immunologic basis of PH is its frequent association with the presence of precipitins to milk protein (Heiner syndrome) or with other food sensitivities (13, 14). Milk precipitins and historical evidence of any food sensitivity should be identified in these patients. However, milk precipitins are neither specific nor sensitive for monitoring the course or defining the severity of PH. It is not clear why patients with precipitins and a presumed immune response to milk might manifest this as a pulmonary bleeding syndrome. One patient evaluated at our center is of interest. The patient had the classic syndrome of IPH. He had been given a bottle of milk in bed every night throughout most of his life, and was likely to have been depositing milk in his lungs routinely. He improved when this feeding practice was discontinued. Aspiration of milk, undenatured by gastric acid, may be an explanation for why an immune response to milk might develop in the lungs. Gastroesophageal reflux (GER) is known to be associated with chronic bronchitis and pulmonary disease, but few patients with GER are evaluated for the presence of milk precipitins.

Children with certain cardiac malformations such as mitral valve stenosis may develop PH. This is termed "secondary PH" rather than IPH. In this situation, it is presumed that the increased pulmonary flow and/or venous pressure leads to episodic oozing of blood from fragile capillaries into the pulmonary parenchyma. Cardiac conduction disturbances in association with PH have been reported as well (15), presumably related to capillary damage in the heart as well as lungs.

Once the diagnosis of PH is made, treatment falls into three general categories. General support should be given as clinically indicated, including oxygen, bronchodilators, iron replacement, and even transfusions when necessary. Since it may be difficult to distinguish the bleeding episode of PH from an acute pneumonia, antibiotics are frequently used. Next, there should be treatment of any associated condition such as treatment of GER, correction of inappropriate feeding practices, and minimizing left to right shunt. Removal of milk products from the diet may lead to a dramatic improvement of symptoms. Patients with PH should all be advised against taking aspirin (in all its forms) or other drugs that might promote bleeding. Third, treatment of PH usually includes the use of corticosteroids. There is no specific treatment protocol, although a dose of 2–4 mg/kg/day of methylprednisolone or prednisone lasting for 1–2 weeks is usually given (7). This is followed by gradual reduction to 1 mg/kg on alternate days, which is then maintained for several months. Patients who fail to improve or who show deterioration of their respiratory function while being treated with steroids are candidates for trials of other immune suppressing agents such as cyclophosphamide or azathioprine (16). Although anecdotal reports are encouraging, there have been no prospective randomized studies. Therefore, it is impossible to make specific recommendations at this time. Disease heterogeneity also makes it difficult to interpret the results of treatments of small groups of patients.

The clinical course of patients with PH is highly variable (Figs. 34.3, 34.4). Some patients improve after treatment begins, having no further pulmonary problems. Others have recurrent exacerbations throughout their lives (5, 17). New bleeds may appear spontaneously or may be associated with intercurrent viral illness. They may be mild or severe, with acute respiratory distress and respiratory failure related to exsanguinating hemorrhage sometimes occurring. In addition to recurrent bleeding, patients with PH may suffer long-term pulmonary scarring and pulmonary fibrosis (5), presumably due to the iron deposition in the lung. Some patients may also develop right heart failure (18) or cardiac arrhythmias (15). Complete pulmonary function tests should be performed at frequent intervals once the child can cooperate with the testing procedure (17). Carbon monoxide uptake has been shown to be a non-invasive

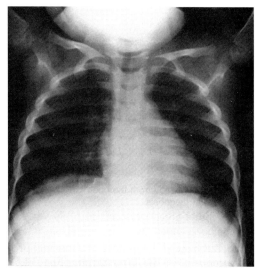

Figure 34.3. The CXR from the same patient dated 12/6/89, showing the rapid potential for clearing.

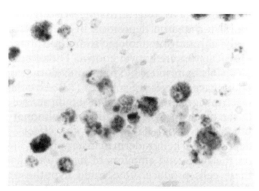

Figure 34.4. A slide of the BAL from patient BA at diagnosis.

indicator of acute bleeding in patients with Goodpasture syndrome (19), but has not been reported in young children with PH. In addition, since some patients with SLE, GS, or WG may initially present with only pulmonary involvement (12) mimicking PH, patients with presumed PH need careful long-term follow-up for the late appearance of progressive glomerulonephritis.

A detailed discussion of the pathology of PH and related syndromes is beyond the scope of this chapter (20, 21). However, typically there is evidence of diffuse pulmonary hemorrhage with mild disruption of pulmonary capillary basement membranes and degeneration of the epithelial surface. There is seldom evidence of a massive cellular pulmonary infil-

untary glottic closure prevents inspiration (15). The glottis subsequently opens and involuntary gasping respirations occur, which allows fluid to flood the lungs. Typically, near-drowning victims aspirate less than 4 ml/kg of fluid, but the volume can exceed 20 ml/kg (16). These events are modified when they occur in frigid water (17–20).

Aspiration of 1–2 ml/kg of fluid can produce significant impairment in gas exchange (21). Initially, P_{O_2} and pulmonary compliance decrease and P_{CO_2} increases. Often a component of metabolic acidosis compounds the respiratory acidosis. With appropriate resuscitation, P_{CO_2} may be returned to normal in less than 1 hour, but hypoxia persists, indicating ongoing V/Q mismatching and intrapulmonic shunting. Grossly the lungs appear edematous with focal hemorrhage, while microscopically there is severe injury to the alveoli and the pulmonary capillary endothelium. This injury increases permeability, causing the alveoli to fill with fluid and proteinaceous material (22).

Although clinical management is affected little, there is a distinct difference between the pathophysiology of fresh water and sea (salt) water drownings. In fresh water, pulmonary surfactant is denatured, leading to alveolar collapse and atelectasis, which causes intrapulmonary shunting (22). The hypotonicity of fresh water relative to plasma leads to a rapid uptake of this fluid into the intravascular space, increased blood volume, and subsequent hemodilution (23). In sea water drowning, pulmonary surfactant function appears to be lost secondary to dilution rather than denaturation, since it has been recovered in tracheal aspirates of drowning victims (22). The hypertonicity of salt water causes water and plasma protein components to be drawn across the disrupted pulmonary basement membranes into the alveolar space. This additional influx of proteinaceous fluid exacerbates the original problem of intrapulmonic shunting caused by the salt water aspiration (23). The movement of fluid from the intravascular space into the injured lung produces a hemoconcentration and loss of intravascular volume. However, in both fresh and salt water drownings, the effects of hemoconcentration or dilution and the changes in intravascular volume are transient and rarely have an impact clinically (21, 24).

The fluid shifts that occur in either fresh or sea water drowning can be substantial. Early literature on near drowning placed major emphasis on the effects this fluid had on sodium, chloride, potassium, and calcium concentrations in the plasma (25). However, animal studies have shown that, independent of the type of water aspirated, greater than 22 ml/kg of fluid must be aspirated before significant electrolyte abnormalities occur (21, 24). Less than 15% of near drowning victims aspirate enough fluid to produce persistent significant electrolyte abnormalities (16). Typically the minor changes seen resolve themselves within 1 hour of aspiration and are not life-threatening (21, 24).

The effect of the drowning episode on the central nervous system (CNS) depends on the severity and duration of the hypoxic episode. However, it appears that neuronal damage frequently continues to occur after restoration of oxygenation and perfusion. The ongoing neuronal loss is caused by a dramatic increase in cerebral vascular resistance and a decrease in cerebral flow that occurs following a transient period of vasodilatation after restoration of circulation. The mechanisms of this decreased flow are not clearly understood (26, 27). However, increases in intracranial pressure (ICP) do not appear to be causally related, since successful treatment of ICP does not correlate with favorable neurologic outcome. Rather, it would appear that increases in ICP are an indication of the severity of CNS injury produced by the drowning episode and that prolonged or marked elevations in ICP correlate with poor outcome (28–31).

Myocardial function may be impaired by hypoxia and metabolic acidosis. In addition, end diastolic pressure may be decreased because of volume loss secondary to pulmonary and systemic capillary leak (32). Ventricular dysrhythmias do not occur unless large quantities (22 ml/kg) of fresh water are aspirated (24). At the more typical volume of 6 ml/kg of aspirated fluid, only occasional premature ventricular beats are noted (33). Electrolyte abnormalities caused by fluid shifts after the aspiration of either fresh or salt water are very rarely severe enough to be dysrhythmogenic (21, 24).

Hypothermia during submersion in cold water is more common and of greater concern in children because of their relatively greater surface area. Skeletal muscle activity, such as attempts to swim, produces vasodilatation, which increases heat loss (34). Cerebral blood flow decreases by 6–7% per degree centigrade (35), which can produce unconsciousness in even mild to moderate hypothermia (30–34°C) (34). Significant hypothermia also decreases cerebral metabolism, which has a protective effect and allows for a better neurologic outcome than could otherwise be expected. Ventricular fibrillation may develop at temperatures less than 28°C and asystole at less than 22°C (34, 35). Adjustments must be made to the reported values for arterial blood gas to allow proper interpretation. For each degree the patient's temperature is below 37°C, measured pH should be increased by 0.015, and PO_2 and PCO_2 should be decreased by 7.2% and 4.4%, respectively (36). The oxygen dissociation curve is shifted to the left by hypothermia, thereby impairing oxygen delivery to the tissues. Insulin release and tissue sensitivity to its activity are also inhibited, resulting in hyperglycemia, which is exacerbated by the body's decreased glucose utilization (35).

Hydrocarbon Aspiration

Hydrocarbons are organic compounds found in nearly every household as components of gasoline, kerosene, furniture polish, charcoal lighter fluid, paint thinner, and turpentine; this ubiquity makes them a constant danger for accidental ingestion and aspiration. The risk is enhanced by the fact that these products are often brightly colored, possess fruity, pleasant aromas, and are often kept in unlabeled containers originally designed for other purposes, such as soft drink bottles. Hydrocarbons account for 5–7% of all reported poisonings, the majority of which occur in children less than 6 years of age. In 1990 alone there were over 30,000 exposures and at least 4 deaths (37, 38). Historically, kerosene was the most common offending substance, but it has now been replaced by charcoal lighter fluid (containing kerosene or naphtha) and furniture polish (39). The aliphatic group of hydrocarbons encompasses the large majority of the compounds involved in accidental exposures. The volume of hydrocarbon ingested is an important determinant in the severity of symptoms because the greater the volume, the greater the risk of aspiration. Although these

compounds look and smell appealing, their taste is quite unpleasant, and the typical ingestion amounts to only two or three swallows, or 10–15 ml. Except in a suicide attempt, a child rarely ingests more than 90 ml (40–42). Toxicity is directly related to viscosity, or resistance to flow; compounds with viscosities of less than 60 units, such as mineral seal oil (in furniture polish) and kerosene, present the greatest risk for pulmonary injury. Compounds with viscosities of greater than 100, such as lubricating oil and petroleum jelly, present little risk for lung injury (39). High volatility and low surface tension are other properties that increase the likelihood a hydrocarbon will damage the respiratory system (43).

The two areas most commonly affected by hydrocarbon ingestion are the CNS and the lungs. Originally, this constellation was attributed to a combination of aspiration and systemic effects following gastrointestinal absorption. However, multiple studies have shown that the aliphatic hydrocarbons have little or no gastrointestinal absorption, even when volumes of 20 ml/kg are ingested, and that the pulmonary and neurologic symptoms seen are the result of aspiration and hypoxia (44, 45).

The clinical picture of children who have ingested a hydrocarbon is varied. Frequently, there is a history of coughing, choking, and gasping at the time of the ingestion (not unexpected in light of the irritating effect that hydrocarbons have on mucosal surfaces). The absence of such events at the time of ingestion, however, does not preclude the possibility of symptomatic aspiration, because as little as 0.2 ml of a low-viscosity hydrocarbon can produce pulmonary symptoms (46). Spontaneous vomiting often occurs immediately following ingestion, which increases the aspiration risk. Pulmonary symptoms include tachypnea, wheezing, rales, cough, and retractions. Rarely, cyanosis is seen immediately after aspiration, which is thought to result from the displacement of alveolar oxygen by hydrocarbon vapors (47).

Pathologic changes in the lungs include hyperemia, alveolar cell damage, granulocyte infiltration, and edema consistent with inflammation. Focal areas of vascular thrombosis, hemorrhage, and necrosis are also seen in addition to areas of bronchospasm, emphysema, and atelectasis (47). Hydrocarbons are organic solvents; upon entering the alveolar space, they dissolve the surfactant lipid and impair the surface tension-reducing activity, leading to atelectasis (48). Examination of the brain is usually unremarkable.

Chest radiographs are abnormal in 65% of hospitalized patients and demonstrate findings typical of aspiration with mottled perihilar densities that progress to patchy bibasilar infiltrates and larger areas of consolidation (42, 47). Infiltrates may appear within 20 minutes but are usually present by 6 hours after ingestion. They reach a maximum by 72 hours and then resolve gradually (49). The degree of involvement on chest radiograph does not correlate with the severity of symptoms, which limits the clinical usefulness of the chest radiograph. Pneumatoceles and pseudotumors have been described but are rare and resolve spontaneously (50, 51).

The primary neurologic symptoms in hydrocarbon aspiration are somnolence and decreased mental status. Seizures or coma are rare. These effects are generally attributed to the hypoxia and acidosis caused by the pulmonary insult and not to direct neurologic toxicity (52, 53).

Although aromatic hydrocarbons sensitize the myocardium to catecholamines and increase the risk of dysrhythmias, the most common cardiac abnormality seen in aliphatic aspirations is mild myocardial fiber degeneration secondary to hypoxia and acidosis (54). Dysrhythmias are unusual but if they occur are most commonly ventricular in origin (55).

Nausea and vomiting are very commonly seen in association with hydrocarbon ingestion and are caused by the mucosal irritation these compounds produce. Abdominal pain, superficial ulcers, and diarrhea may also occur (56, 57). Renal lobule damage, intravascular hemolysis, hepatocellular damage, and hemoglobinuria have been reported (58, 59).

Fever is seen in 30% of hydrocarbon aspiration cases. The fever sometimes occurs within one hour of the aspiration, indicating that the hydrocarbon itself and not concomitant infection is responsible for a portion of the febrile reaction (39). In the absence of secondary bacterial infection, fever typically resolves spontaneously within 48 hours. Leukocytosis with a total white blood cell count of 15,000–20,000 is common (60). Onset of fever and leukocyto-

sis several days after the aspiration event suggests the occurrence of a secondary bacterial infection.

It is important to remember that hydrocarbons are rarely pure substances. One must be prepared to treat the symptoms that may be caused by additive substances, most commonly organophosphate pesticides and heavy metals.

Smoke Inhalation

More than 1 million people in the United States suffer burns each year; approximately 150,000 of these require hospitalization (61). With improvements in fluid and wound management, smoke inhalation has now become the leading cause of death in fire-related injuries. Approximately 60% of the 12,000 fire-related deaths that occur annually result from smoke inhalation, and more than 25% of patients with injuries severe enough to require hospitalization demonstrate evidence of smoke inhalation (55, 62). Children are less likely to suffer smoke inhalation than adults (63, 64). Smoke inhalation acts synergistically with surface burns to increase mortality above that expected for either alone by as much as 10 times (65).

The respiratory injuries produced by smoke inhalation are a combination of thermal burn, chemical irritation, and asphyxia. Thermal burns are rarely of significance below the upper airway because of the low heat capacity of dry air, but are more frequent in steam-inhalation injuries (66). The chemical irritants contained in smoke are a function of the materials that fuel the fire, the oxygen available, and the temperature at which it burns. Hydrochloric acid is the major irritant produced when polyvinyl chloride, a common component of household plastics, burns (67). Acrolein, along with the aldehydes, is of primary importance in fires involving wood or acrylics (68). Carbon particles themselves are not particularly irritating, but serve as vehicles to carry other toxins and irritants deep into the airways (69).

In the past, the process of diagnosing smoke inhalation focused on physical findings such as facial burns; singed nasal hair; carbonaceous particles in the nose, throat, or sputum; and decreased sensorium. A history of the victim having been in an enclosed space and findings on chest radiograph were also considered.

Taken together these findings imputed a 10–15% incidence of inhalation injury in fire victims (70, 71). The addition of fiberoptic laryngoscopy and bronchoscopy to visualize the airway mucosa and the use of Xenon ventilation-perfusion scanning to assess lower airway injury has increased the sensitivity of diagnosis of inhalation injury to the point that current incidence is thought to be approximately 25% (72, 73).

The thermal injury to the respiratory mucosa rarely extends beyond the level of the subglottic space because of the low heat capacity of dry air and the ability of the mucosa of the nasal passages and pharynx to cool and humidify the incoming air. The mucosa is typically diffusely reddened and edematous. Swelling and inflammation develop within the first 8 hours, peak within 48–72 hours, and have largely resolved by 4–5 days post insult (74). Symptoms include those of smoke inhalation in general with the addition of stridor or hoarseness.

The injury to the pulmonary parenchyma appears in three separate stages. Initially there is pulmonary insufficiency followed by pulmonary edema and finally by bronchopneumonia (75). Pulmonary insufficiency not secondary to upper airway edema is mediated through several routes. Anoxic injury leads to loss of epithelial cells in the bronchioles and alveoli. There is loss of ciliary function and severe mucosal edema, which impair secretion clearance (55). Products of incomplete combustion produce mucosal irritation and bronchospasm while rapid destruction of surfactant activity leads to widespread areas of atelectasis. Type II pneumocytes are often damaged, decreasing surfactant production and exacerbating atelectasis (76).

Carbon monoxide (CO) generated by the fire plays a major role in the acute respiratory insufficiency. Children are particularly vulnerable to CO poisoning because of their higher basal metabolic rate and their tendency for lower hemoglobin levels. CO has an affinity for hemoglobin 250 times that of oxygen, resulting in 50% saturation of hemoglobin with partial pressures of CO as low as 0.1 mm Hg (78). The blood carboxyhemoglobin (COHb) level is affected by the inspired CO concentration and duration of exposure, with prolonged exposure leading to further increases in blood COHb. The half-life of

COHb at room air and atmospheric pressure is approximately 5 hours, but this decreases to 90 minutes by administration of 100% oxygen and decreases further to approximately 23 minutes if hyperbaric oxygen of 3 atmospheres is delivered (79). Symptoms related to CO poisoning vary with COHb levels (Table 35.2) (80). Although COHb levels can be loosely associated with symptoms in this fashion, there is no direct correlation between COHb levels and symptom severity (79).

In addition to displacing oxygen from hemoglobin, CO shifts the oxyhemoglobin dissociation curve to the left, further reducing the amount of oxygen available to the tissues (78). CO also binds to myoglobin, impairing muscle cell utilization of oxygen, and to the cytochrome oxidases, although the significance of this latter effect is not known (81, 82). Symptoms of CO poisoning most commonly manifest themselves first in the areas most sensitive to oxygen deprivation, the CNS and the myocardium.

Noncardiogenic pulmonary edema is not evident in the first few hours after smoke inhalation but develops 6–72 hours later. There is an increase in tracheobronchial blood flow (83) and lymphatic flow through the injured lungs (84) while capillary permeability increases due to local smoke injury and mediators released by degranulating pulmonary macrophages (85). These mediators include histamine, prostaglandins, thromboxanes, oxygen radicals, and chemotactic factors that cause leukocytes to migrate to the damaged pulmonary tissue. Polymorphonuclear cells predominate and after activation release proteolytic enzymes and additional oxygen free radicals (86). This produces widespread cellular injury and loss of epithelial integrity with a flood of proteinaceous fluid into the airways. The pulmonary mucosa demonstrates marked edema and sloughing of cells (55, 87). The mixture of sloughed cells and edema fluid may

Table 35.2.
COHb Levels and Symptoms

COHb Level	Symptoms
< 10%	Impaired mentation
10–20%	Exertional dyspnea
20–40%	Nausea, weakness, dizziness
40–60%	Syncope, seizures
> 60%	Death

form casts that can produce areas of hyper-inflation or atelectasis. Although the processes that produce the injury have aspects requiring systemic responses, the injury itself is mediated locally, with the initial damage produced by the smoke almost certainly being the trigger (88). While bronchial blood flow is increased to the injured area, pulmonary blood flow decreases as pulmonary vascular resistance rises and there is preferential shunting of blood flow to the undamaged lung (89, 90).

Mortality increases dramatically when smoke inhalation is compounded by surface burns. The burns cause release of tissue mediators, consumptive coagulopathy, and microemboli, which exacerbate the pulmonary injury, as does the fluid resuscitation that burn treatment necessitates (55, 84). However, victims of combination surface and inhalation injury typically require more fluid than equivalent surface injury alone for resuscitation, and therefore attempts to limit resuscitation fluid may prove detrimental (91–93).

The bronchopneumonia stage of smoke inhalation injury typically occurs 4–10 days after exposure and is precipitated by the injury imparted on the lung by the inhalation, especially the mucosal disruption, and by mechanical ventilation. This injury, combined with the loss of protection afforded by the epidermis and the increased risk of infection that accompanies use of invasive devices (endotracheal tubes, central venous lines, arterial lines, and others), leaves the smoke inhalation victim at very high risk for development of pneumonia. Pneumonia appearing early in the clinical course typically is caused by gram-positive organisms, most commonly *Staphylococci*, whereas late-appearing pneumonia is usually gram-negative in origin, with *Pseudomonas* and *Klebsiella* predominating (94).

Neurologic sequelae of general hypoxic injury may appear as long as 4 weeks after the injury (95, 96). Cardiac dysfunction similarly arises largely due to hypoxic damage and presents with dysrhythmia and decreased contractility. Cardiac output may be further impaired by increases in peripheral and pulmonary vascular resistance because of local vasoconstriction in response to hypoxia, ischemia, and acidosis (55). Cardiac enzymes are rarely elevated (97).

The kidneys and other organ systems typically manifest dysfunction consistent with the degree of hypoxia unless the smoke contains a specific toxin to which that organ is sensitive (98).

TREATMENT

Although the causes of the initial insult to the respiratory tract are different and the pathophysiology varies, near-drowning, smoke inhalation, and hydrocarbon aspiration produce clinical conditions that appear very similar and call for management strategies that are common to all three—thus their inclusion as acute lung injuries. These areas of similarity in treatment will be discussed first, and then points of therapy specific to each of the entities will be reviewed.

Initial Evaluation and Prognostic Factors

Following acute lung injury, initial evaluation should include chest radiograph and arterial blood gas analysis to assess severity of hypoxia and acidosis. Serum electrolytes, blood urea nitrogen (BUN), creatinine, and complete blood count and platelet count may be helpful, especially if hypoxia and acidosis are severe. Measurement of COHb, bronchoscopy, and Xenon scanning, if available, should be included in the assessment of smoke inhalation victims. Since myocardial contractility and normal conduction may be disturbed, an echocardiogram and ECG should be included in the initial evaluation if concern about cardiac function exists (Table 35.3).

Following a near-drowning episode, pediatric patients should be observed for at least 6 hours. If the child was submerged less than 1 minute, was never apneic and never cyanotic, required no resuscitation at the scene, and

Table 35.3.
Acute Lung Injury Evaluation

- Chest radiograph
- Arterial blood gas analysis
- Serum electrolytes
- CBC
- BUN/creatinine
- Echocardiogram/EKG
- Evaluate for concomitant trauma

remains asymptomatic for 6 hours with normal chest radiograph (CXR), he or she can generally be released safely. However, if the episode is more serious by history, symptoms are present, or abnormalities exist on CXR or arterial blood gas analysis (ABG), then the child should be admitted for at least 24 hours of careful observation and therapy as needed (99). After a smoke inhalation, the child should be observed for at least 12 hours and admitted if symptoms or CXR abnormalities develop (79). In the case of hydrocarbon ingestion, the child should be observed for 6 hours. If the patient remains asymptomatic and CXR is clear, admission is not required. If symptoms are present 6 hours after ingestion, the patient should be admitted to the hospital (41). The management of asymptomatic patients with pathologic changes on CXR and symptomatic patients with clear CXR whose symptoms resolve within 6 hours is more difficult, but it would appear reasonable to release these children if careful home follow-up can be assured and to hospitalize them if follow-up is uncertain (100).

The ability to assess prognosis at presentation would be very helpful in counseling families and in making management decisions. However, no clear criteria to predict outcome have been identified in smoke inhalation or hydrocarbon aspiration, although the vast majority of hydrocarbon victims recover fully. Outcome in hydrocarbon aspiration is related to the amount ingested, but this is often not known. In near-drowning, five criteria have been noted to aid in determining prognosis (see Table 35.1). If two or fewer of these features are present, the child has a 90% likelihood for good recovery, but if three or more are present, the chance of good recovery is only 5% (101).

Common Aspects of Management

The cornerstones of management of acute lung injury are airway stabilization and rapid correction of hypoxia and acidosis. The majority of nonpulmonary organ dysfunction arises because of these problems, making prompt and aggressive treatment critical if the patient is to recover fully.

The airway should be assessed and cleared of any foreign material or debris. If the patient is unable to maintain a functional airway, either because of airway injury, edema, or

impaired neurologic status, endotracheal intubation should be performed. The ability of the patient to protect the airway, based on the presence of a gag reflex and strong cough, should also be considered. The decision for intubation is independent of whether there is a clear need for mechanical ventilation. Nasopharyngeal and oropharyngeal airways may be useful adjuncts but tend to be poorly tolerated and are of limited usefulness in children. Early intubation is particularly important in smoke inhalation because thermal injury to the upper airway may result in rapidly progressive edema and airway obstruction (74). Vigorous pulmonary toilet and frequent suctioning to facilitate clearance of secretions are also important.

Humidified supplemental oxygen should be initiated as soon as possible after the injury. Initially 100% oxygen is administered and then titrated to maintain $Po_2 > 90$ mm Hg based on arterial blood gas analysis. In smoke inhalation, carboxyhemoglobin levels should also be monitored and 100% Fio_2 should be continued until COHb falls below 10%. An alveolar-arterial oxygen gradient of greater than 300 or an Fio_2 requirement of 60% or more indicates severe ventilation-perfusion mismatch and is itself an indication for elective intubation even if the child is alert and the upper airway is stable. Typically, ABG analysis reveals hypocapnia as the child hyperventilates to compensate for the interstitial edema and hypoxia. In the presence of tachypnea, a normal or elevated Pco_2 indicates impending respiratory failure.

DISTENDING PRESSURE

Because of functional surfactant insufficiency, airways filled with cellular debris and pulmonary edema fluid, there is a predilection to atelectasis, reduced functional residual capacity (FRC), and low pulmonary compliance. The use of positive airway distending pressure, either as continuous positive airway pressure (CPAP) or positive end-expiratory pressure (PEEP), is very effective in decreasing intrapulmonary shunting and improving oxygenation (55, 102–104). Positive distending pressure is particularly indicated if an $Fio_2 \geq$ 60% is required or if the A-a gradient exceeds 300. CPAP may be delivered in a non-intubated patient via nasal prongs or face mask, although these methods tend to be less effective and poorly tolerated in children. Therefore, distending pressure is most commonly administered as PEEP in combination with mechanical ventilation in the intubated patient. PEEP aids in oxygenation by increasing FRC and recruiting additional alveoli for gas exchange. The amount of PEEP provided should be the minimum amount that maintains PaO_2 above 90 mm Hg and decreases required FiO_2 below 50%, thus reducing oxygen toxicity and atelectasis secondary to oxygen reabsorption. Patients with acute lung injury are prone to develop pulmonary air leaks (pneumothorax, pneumomediastinum, pneumopericardium) secondary to the lung injury and barotrauma. Extreme vigilance is required when PEEP of ≥ 10 cm H_2O is necessary. Emergency needle aspiration equipment should be readily available at the bedside. Pneumothorax should be the first diagnosis considered in any child on PEEP with an abrupt change in oxygenation or cardiovascular status. Tube thoracostomy is generally required for definitive treatment, since the air leak rarely seals spontaneously during positive-pressure ventilation. Initial use of PEEP at 4–6 cm H_2O and increasing or decreasing in increments of 2 is appropriate, with PEEP as high as 20 sometimes necessary. Cardiac output may be impaired at high levels of PEEP as central venous return is decreased, especially if circulating blood volume remains low because of inadequate fluid resuscitation. However, even with adequate intravascular volume, inotropic support may be necessary to maintain cardiac output. Dobutamine is generally preferred because it causes little pulmonary vasoconstriction, but dopamine may be indicated if blood pressure support is also desired.

MECHANICAL VENTILATION

The addition of mechanical ventilation to the regimen of supplemental oxygen and end-distending pressure is appropriate when the child's spontaneous ventilation is inadequate, as indicated by marked tachypnea, above-normal PCO_2 or, when the work of breathing causes acidosis, excessive caloric requirement or clinical distress. Typically, relatively large tidal volumes (12–15 ml/kg delivered volume) are most effective accompanied by a low rate to achieve a normal PCO_2. This pattern is preferable to higher rates and smaller tidal volumes because it provides improved expansion, helping to overcome the obstruction and atelectasis in acute lung injury. In severe episodes of lung injury, maintaining PO_2 and PCO_2 in the normal range may require ventilating pressures that increase risk of barotrauma and oxygen injury. Therefore it is prudent, assuming the patient does not become acidotic, to accept oxygen tensions less than normal and carbon dioxide tensions greater than normal in order to mitigate this additional risk. Allowing $PO_2 > 65$–70 and $PCO_2 < 50$–55 if the pH is > 7.28 should be considered in patients requiring $FiO_2 > 60\%$ and PEEP > 10.

Serial blood gas analysis and chest radiographs should be obtained in monitoring disease progression and response to therapy (Table 35.3). Treatment of acidosis should center on correction of the underlying cause (hypoxia, hypovolemia, hypoperfusion), with sodium bicarbonate used largely as a temporizing measure while the primary problem is being corrected. Chest physiotherapy may be beneficial for large areas of focal atelectasis and for secretion clearance. Many patients will demonstrate clinical symptoms of bronchospasm and require treatment with beta-2 agonists to improve air exchange and oxygenation.

MONITORING

All children should have continuous EKG monitoring because of the tendency for dysrhythmias, and most require an indwelling arterial catheter. Pulse oximetry provides valuable information as a continuous monitor of oxygenation. It is useful in demonstrating episodic desaturations, especially during stressful periods or painful procedures, and reduces the need for arterial blood gas analysis as support is being weaned. However, since it does not measure oxygen delivery, one may be misled by adequate saturation readings in a patient who is anemic, has significant COHb levels, or who has impaired cardiac output.

Pulmonary artery catheters (Swan-Ganz catheters) may be useful in monitoring pediatric patients during the early stages of acute lung injury (Table 35.4). Such catheters provide information on venous return, cardiac output, and pulmonary capillary wedge pressure, which can help guide decisions about ventilator, inotrope, and fluid management. However, in the face of abnormal pulmonary

Table 35.4.
Indications for Consideration of Pulmonary Artery Catheter Placement

- High mechanical ventilation requirements, especially PEEP $\geq$ 14
- Multisystem organ failure with unclear fluid status
- Shock or hemodynamic instability with $+/-$ response to fluid resuscitation

compliance, positive pressure ventilation, PEEP, and inotrope therapy, the measured values from the pulmonary artery catheter cannot be expected to be within the normal range, and therefore interpretation of a single set of values may be difficult. Observing data over a series of measurements may reveal trends that can be useful in management. Despite the large amount of information that pulmonary artery catheters provide, their use has not been proven to decrease mortality in pediatric acute lung injury (105).

FURTHER MANAGEMENT

With the resolution of the acute stages of the lung injury, ventilatory support can be withdrawn slowly. It is desirable to have PEEP $\leq$ 10, $Fio_2 \leq 40\%$, and the patient hemodynamically stable for 24–48 hours before reduction in ventilatory support is initiated. PEEP can be decreased by 2 cm H_2O every 12–24 hours to allow observation of the full effect of a change, which can take 6–8 hours to become evident. Decreases in ventilator rate and Fio_2 can be made in the interim as tolerated.

There has long been concern regarding the appropriateness of long-term endotracheal intubation in these patients, but it is now known that they can be extubated successfully even after 8 or more weeks of intubation. In light of increased risk of pulmonary infection, skin breakdown, and wound infection in patients receiving tracheostomies, especially in patients with surface burns, prolonged intubation is now the favored approach when extubation is still considered possible (106–108).

Patients with acute lung injury and global hypoxic injury often have depletion of intravascular volume secondary to widespread capillary leak. Fluid resuscitation should be adequate to maintain systemic blood pressure, good peripheral perfusion, and urine output. Although excessive fluid infusion can exacerbate the edema caused by the original injury,

evidence indicates that fluid restriction during the early stages of acute lung injury may be more deleterious (91–93).

Frequent neurologic examinations are vital for identifying changes in mental status that may result from the effects of hypoxia and acidosis on the CNS. Computed tomography (CT) scans and intracranial pressure monitoring are often used and can be helpful in determining prognosis, but treatment based on their results has not been shown to improve morbidity and mortality (28–31, 109, 110). EEG may identify subclinical seizure activity and may also provide prognostic information (111, 112).

Despite numerous studies investigating their possible benefits, prophylactic antibiotics have no proven utility in the treatment of acute lung injury. They may in fact select out resistant strains of bacteria that would make treatment more difficult (113–116). Antibiotics should be reserved for infections documented by positive blood cultures or by definite clinical evidence (fever, leukocytosis, new infiltrate on CXR). Tracheal aspirates in intubated patients typically reveal colonizing organisms, but not necessarily pathogenic ones. The choice of antibiotics should be guided by the clinical setting, with early infection after smoke inhalation more commonly caused by gram-positive organisms and late infection caused by gram-negative organisms, especially *Pseudomonas.* Near-drowning victims are at increased risk for infection with unusual organisms.

Corticosteroid therapy aimed at suppressing the inflammatory component of acute lung injury has been examined using both high and low doses, and prolonged and short courses. No study in humans has demonstrated a beneficial role for steroids, and the incidence of serious infection has been increased in some studies, especially those using longer courses of treatment (114–119). Therefore, at present, there is no role for steroids in the treatment of acute lung injury in children.

Sedation and pharmacologic paralysis are often necessary in the treatment of acute lung injury, especially if high levels of ventilatory support are necessary. Secobarbital and midazolam are commonly used for sedation, sometimes in combination with an analgesic such as morphine or butorphanol. Doses should be titrated for the minimum dose that produces

24. Modell J and Moya F. Effects of volume of aspirated fluid during chlorinated fresh water drowning. *Anesthesiology* 1966; 27:662–672.

25. Swann H, Brucer M, Moore C, Vezien B. Fresh water and sea water drowning: A study of the terminal cardiac and biochemical events. *Tex Rep Biol Med* 1947; 5:423–437.

26. Ames III A, Wright R, Kowada M, et al. Cerebral ischemia II. The no-reflow phenomenon. *Am J Pathol* 1968; 52:437–447.

27. White B, Gadzenski D, Hoehner P, et al. Effect of flunarizine on canine cerebral blood flow and vascular resistance post cardiac arrest. *Ann Emerg Med* 1982; 11:119–126.

28. Sarnaik A, Preston G, Lieh-Lai M, et al. Intracranial pressure and cerebral perfusion pressure in near drowning. *Crit Care Med* 1985; 13:224–227.

29. Allman F, Nelson W, Pacentive G, et al. Outcome following cardiopulmonary resuscitation in severe pediatric near-drowning. *Am J Dis Child* 1986; 140:571–575.

30. Nussbaum E, Galant S. Intracranial pressure monitoring as a guide to prognosis in the nearly drowned severely comatose child. *J Pediatr* 1983; 102:215–218.

31. Nussbaum E. Prognostic variables in nearly drowned comatose children. *Am J Dis Child* 1985; 139:1058–1059.

32. Sarnaik A, Vohra M. Near-drowning: Fresh, salt and cold water immersion. *Clin Sports Med* 1986; 5:33–46.

33. Karch A. Pathology of the heart in drowning. *Arch Pathol Lab Med* 1985; 109:176–178.

34. Conn A, Edmonds J, Barker G. Cerebral resuscitation in near drowning. *Pediatr Clin North Am* 1979; 26:691–701.

35. Reuler J. Hypothermia: Pathophysiology, clinical settings and management. *Ann Intern Med* 1978; 89:519–527.

36. Kelman G and Nunn J. Nomograms for correction of blood pO_2, pCO_2, pH and base excess for time and temperature. *J Appl Physiol* 1966; 21:1484–1490.

37. National Clearinghouse for Poison Control Centers Bulletin. April, 1980; 24:1–20.

38. Litovitz T, Bailey K, Schmitz B, et al. 1990 Annual Report of the American Association of Poison Control Centers National Data Collection System. *Am J Emerg Med* 1991; 9:461–509.

39. Kulberg A, Goldfrank L, Bresnitz E. Hydrocarbons. In Goldfrank L, Weisman R, Flomenbaum N, Howland M, Lewin N, Kulberg A, eds. *Goldfrank's toxicologic emergencies*, 3rd ed. Norwalk, CT, Appleton-Century-Croft, 1986; pp 672–685.

40. Press E, Adams W, Chittendon R, et al. Cooperative kerosene poisoning study: Evaluation of gastric lavage and other factors in the treatment of accidental ingestion of petroleum distillate products. *Pediatrics* 1968; 29:648–674.

41. Anas N, Namasonthi V, Ginsberg C. Criteria for hospitalizing children who have ingested products containing hydrocarbons. *JAMA* 1981; 246:840–843.

42. Foley J, Dreyer N, Soule A Jr, Woll E. Kerosene poisoning in young children. *Radiology* 1954; 62:817–829.

43. Bryson P. Hydrocarbons. In *Comprehensive review in toxicology*, 2nd ed. Rockville, MD, Aspen Publications, 1989, pp 553–560.

44. Wolfe B, Brodeur A, Sheilds J. The role of gastrointestinal absorption of kerosene in producing pneumonitis in dogs. *J Pediatr* 1970; 76:867–873.

45. Dice W, Ward G, Kelley J, et al. Pulmonary toxicity following gastrointestinal ingestion of kerosene. *Ann Emerg Med* 1982; 11:138–142.

46. Litovitz T. Hydrocarbon ingestion. *Ear Nose Throat J* 1983; 62:45–55.

47. Eade N, Taussig L, Marks M. Hydrocarbon pneumonitis. *Pediatrics* 1974; 54:351–357.

48. Giammona S. Effects of furniture polish on pulmonary surfactant. *Am J Dis Child* 1967; 113:658–663.

49. Karlson K. Hydrocarbon poisoning in children. *South Med J* 1982; 75:839–840.

50. Wolfe R, Adams F, Desilats D. Pneumatoceles complicating hydrocarbon pneumonitis. *J Pediatr* 1967; 71:711–714.

51. Scott P. Hydrocarbon aspiration: An unusual cause of multiple pulmonary pseudotumors. *South Med J* 1989; 82:1032–1033.

52. Wolfsdorf J. Kerosene intoxication: An experimental approach to the etiology of the CNS manifestations in primates. *J Pediatr* 1976; 88:1037–1040.

53. Mann M, Pirie D, Wolfsdorf J. Kerosene absorption in primates. *J Pediatr* 1977; 91:495–498.

54. James F, Kaplan S, Benzing G III. Cardiac complications following hydrocarbon ingestion. *Am J Dis Child* 1971; 121:431–433.

55. Trunkey DD. Inhalation injury. *Surg Clin North Am* 1978; 8:1133–1140.

56. Steiner M. Syndromes of kerosene poisoning in children. *Am J Dis Child* 1947; 74:32–44.

57. Deichmann W, Kitzmiller K, Witherup S, Johansmann R. Kerosene intoxication. *Ann Intern Med* 1944; 21:803–823.

58. Adler R, Robinson R, Binkin N. Intravascular hemolysis: An unusual complication of hydrocarbon ingestion. *J Pediatr* 1976; 89:679–680.

59. Stockman J. More on hydrocarbon-induced hemolysis. *J Pediatr* 1977; 90:848.

60. Beamon R, Siegel C, Landers G, et al. Hydrocarbon ingestion in children: A six-year retrospective study. *J Coll Emerg Phys* 1976; 5:771–775.

61. National Center for Health Statistics. Detailed diagnoses and surgical procedures for patients from short stay hospitals, United States, 1977. Hyattsville, MD, Department of HEW, Publication No. (PHS) 79–1274/G.

62. Herndon DN, Thompson PB, Linares HA, et al. Postgraduate course: Respiratory injury. I. Incidence, mortality, pathogenesis and treatment of pulmonary injury. *J Burn Care Rehabil* 1986; 7:184–191.

63. Herndon DN, Barrow RE, Linares HA, et al. Inhalation injury in burned patients: Effects and treatment. *Burns* 1988; 14:349–356.

64. Desai M, Rutan R, Herndon D. Managing smoke inhalation injury. *Postgrad Med* 1989; 86:69–76.

65. Herndon D, Thompson P, Traber D. Pulmonary injury in burned patients. *Crit Care Clin* 1985; 1:79–96.

66. Chu CS. New concepts of pulmonary burn injury. *J Trauma* 1981; 21:958–961.

67. Dyer RF, Esch VH. Polyvinyl chloride toxicity in fires. *JAMA* 1976; 235:393–397.

68. Terrill JB, Montgomery RR, Reinhardt CF. Toxic gases from fires. *Science* 1978; 200:1343–1347.

69. Stone JP, Hoglett RN, Johnson JE. The transport of hydrogen chloride by soot from burning polyvinyl chloride. *J Fire Flammability* 1973; 4:42–51.

70. Stone H and Martin J. Pulmonary injury associated with thermal burns. *Surg Gynecol Obstet* 1969; 129:1242–1246.

71. Venus A, Matsuda T, Copiozo J, et al. Prophylactic intubation and continuous positive airway pressure in the management of inhalation injury in burn victims. *Crit Care Med* 1981; 9:519–523.

72. Moylan JA, Adib K, Birnbaum M. Fiberoptic bronchoscopy following thermal injury. *Surg Gynecol Obstet* 1975; 140:541–543.

73. Moylan JA, Alexander G Jr. Diagnosis and treatment of inhalation injury. *World J Surg* 1978; 2:185–191.

74. Zikria BA, Sturner WQ, Astarjian NK, et al. Respiratory tract damage in burns: Pathophysiology and therapy. *Ann N Y Acad Sci* 1963; 150:618–626.

75. Stone HH, Rhame DW, Corbitt JD, et al. Respiratory burns: A correlation of clinical and laboratory results. *Ann Surg* 1967; 165:157–168.

76. Nieman GF, Clark WR Jr, Wax SD, et al. The effect of smoke inhalation on pulmonary surfactant. *Ann Surg* 1980; 191:171–181.

77. Zimmerman S and Truxal B. Carbon monoxide poisoning. *Pediatrics* 1981; 68:215–224.

78. Thom S. Smoke inhalation. *Emerg Med Clin North Am* 1989; 7:371–387.

79. Winter PM, Miller JN. Carbon monoxide poisoning. *JAMA* 1976; 236:1502–1504.

80. Coburn RF and Mayers LB. Myoglobin O_2 tension determined from measurements of carboxyhemoglobin in skeletal muscle. *Am J Physiol* 1971; 220:66–74.

81. Roth RA and Rubin RJ. Comparison of the effect of carbon monoxide and of hypoxic hypoxia II. Hexobarbital metabolism in the isolated, perfused rat liver. *J Pharmacol Exp Ther* 1976; 199:61–66.

82. Stothert J, Ashley K, Kramer G, et al. Intrapulmonary distribution of bronchial blood flow after moderate smoke inhalation. *J Appl Physiol* 1990; 69:1734–1739.

83. Demling RH. Burn edema Part I: Pathogenesis. *J Burn Care Rehabil* 1982; 3:138–148.

84. Staub NC, Schultz EL, Albertine KH. Leukocytes and pulmonary microvascular injury. *Ann N Y Acad Sci* 1982; 384:332–343.

85. Stein MD, Herndon DN, Stevens JM, et al. Production of chemotactic factors and lung cell changes following smoke inhalation. *J Burn Care Rehabil* 1986; 7:117–121.

86. Stone HH. Pulmonary burns in children. *J Pediatr Surg* 1979; 14:48–52.

87. Demling RA. Burns. *N Engl J Med* 1985; 313:1389–1397.

88. Prien T, Traber DL, Richardson JA, Traber LD. Early effects of inhalation injury on lung mechanics and pulmonary perfusion. *Intens Care Med* 1988; 14:25–29.

89. Prien T, Traber LD, Herndon DN, Stothert JC Jr, Lubbesmeyer HJ, Traber DL. Pulmonary edema with smoke inhalation undetected by indicator–dilution technique. *J Appl Physiol* 1987; 63:907–911.

90. Navar PD, Soffle JR, Worden GD. Effect of inhalation injury on fluid resuscitation requirements after thermal injury. *Am J Surg* 1985; 150:716–720.

91. Herndon DN, Burrow RE, Traber DL, Rutan TC, Rutan RL, Abston S. Extravascular lung water changes following smoke inhalation injury in massive burns. *Surgery* 1987; 102:341–349.

92. Herndon DN, Traber DL, Traber LD. The effect of resuscitation on inhalation injury. *Surgery* 1986; 100:248–250.

93. Stone H. Pulmonary burns in children. *J Pediatr Surg* 1979; 14:48–52.

94. Myers R, Snyder S, Emhoff T. Subacute sequelae of carbon monoxide poisoning. *Ann Emerg Med* 1985; 14:1163–1167.

95. Choi I. Delayed neurologic sequelae in carbon monoxide intoxication. *Arch Neurol* 1983; 40:433–435.

96. Anderson RF, Allensworth DC, de Groot WJ. Myocardial toxicity from CO poisoning. *Ann Intern Med* 1967; 67:1172–1182.

97. Linton A, Adams J, Lawson D. Muscle necrosis and acute renal failure in carbon monoxide poisoning. *Postgrad Med J* 1968; 44:338–341.

98. Orlowski J. Drowning, near-drowning and ice water submersions. *Pediatr Clin North Am* 1987; 34:75–92.

99. Klein B and Simon J. Hydrocarbon poisonings. *Pediatr Clin North Am* 1986; 33:411–419.

100. Orlowski J. Prognostic factors in pediatric cases of drowning and near-drowning. *Ann Emerg Med* 1979; 8:176–179.

101. Bergquist R, Vogelhut M, Modell J, et al. Comparison of ventilatory patterns in the treatment of freshwater near-drowning in dogs. *Anesthesiology* 1980; 52:142–148.

102. Modell J, Calderwood H, Ruiz B, et al. Effects of ventilatory patterns on arterial oxygenation after near-drowning in sea water. *Anesthesiology* 1974; 40:376–384.

103. Davies L, Poulton T, Modell J. Continuous positive airway pressure is beneficial in treatment of smoke inhalation. *Crit Care Med* 1983; 11:726–729.

104. Katz R, Pollack M, Spady D. Cardiopulmonary abnormalities in severe acute respiratory failure. *J Pediatr* 1984; 104:357–364.

105. Tranbaugh RF, Lewis FR, Christensen JM, Elings VB. Lung water changes after thermal injury: the effects of crystalloid resuscitation and sepsis. *Ann Surg* 1980; 192:479–488.

106. Walker HL, McLeod CG, McManus WL. Experimental inhalation injury in the goat. *J Trauma* 1981; 21:962–964.

107. Moylan JA Jr, West JT, Nash G, et al. Tracheostomy in thermally injured patients: A review of five years experience. *Am J Surg* 1972; 38:119–123.

108. Muira T, Mitomo M, Kawai R, et al. CT of the brain in acute carbon monoxide intoxication. *Am J Neuroradiol* 1982; 6:739–742.

109. Sawada Y, Ohashi N, Maemura K, et al. Computerized tomography as an indicator of long-term outcome after CO poisoning. *Lancet* 1980; 1:783–784.

110. Ginsburg R, Romano J. CO Encephalopathy: Need for appropriate treatment. *Am J Psychiatry* 1976; 133:317–320.

111. Kruus S, Bergström L, Suutarisên T, et al. The prognosis of near–drowned children. *Acta Paediatr Scand* 1979; 68:315–322.

112. Oakes D, Sherck J, Maloney J, et al. Prognosis and management of victims of near-drowning. *J Trauma* 1982; 22:544–549.

113. Wroblewski DA and Bower GC. The significance of facial burns in acute smoke inhalation. *Crit Care Med* 1979; 7:335–338.

114. Brown III J, Burke B, Dajani A. Experimental kerosene pneumonia: Evaluation of some therapeutic regimens. *J Pediatr* 1974; 84:396–401.

115. Steele R, Conklin R, Mark H. Corticosteroids and antibiotics for the treatment of fulminant hydrocarbon aspiration. *JAMA* 1972; 219:1434–1437.

116. Calderwood H, Modell J, Ruiz B. The ineffectiveness of steroid therapy for treatment of fresh–water near-drowning. *Anesthesiology* 1975; 43:642–649.

117. Moglan JA, Chan CK. Inhalation injury—An increasing problem. *Surgery* 1978; 188:34–37.

118. Wolfsdorf J, Kündig A. Dexamethasone in the management of kerosene pneumonia. *Pediatrics* 1974; 53:86–90.

119. Bergman I, Steeves M, Burckart G, Thompson A. Reversible neurologic abnormalities associated with prolonged intravenous midazolam and fentanyl administration. *J Pediatr* 1991; 119:644–649.

120. Lane JC, Tennison MB, Lawless ST, Greenwood RS, Zaritsky AL. Movement disorder after withdrawal of fentanyl infusion. *J Pediatr* 1991; 119:649–651.

121. Modell J. Treatment of near-drowning: Is there a role for HYPER therapy? [Editorial]. *Crit Care Med* 1986; 14:593–594.

122. Meyers P, Britten J, Cowley R. Hypothermia: Quantitative aspects of therapy. *J Am Coll Emerg Phys* 1979; 8:523–527.28. The Medical Letter: Treatment of hypothermia. *Med Lett* 1983:9–11.

123. Ng R, Darwish H, Stewart D. Emergency treatment of petroleum distillates and turpentine ingestion. *Can Med Assoc J* 1974; 111; 537–538.

124. Mathieu D, Nolf M, Durocher A, Saulnier F. Acute carbon monoxide poisoning risk of late sequelae and treatment by hyperbaric oxygen. *Clin Toxicol* 1985; 23:315–324.

125. Myers RA, Linberg SE, Cowley RA. Carbon monoxide poisoning: The injury and its treatment. *J Coll Emerg Phys* 1979; 8:479–484.

126. Bour H, Ledingham I, eds. *Carbon monoxide poisoning*. Amsterdam, NY, Elsevier, 1967, pp 123–182.

36

Adult Respiratory Distress Syndrome

JAMES A. ROYALL and STEVEN T. BALDWIN

Adult respiratory distress syndrome (ARDS) is a syndrome of acute hypoxemic respiratory failure following a severe physiologic insult. One or more of a large number of pulmonary and nonpulmonary pathologic processes may be the antecedent insult (Table 36.1). Respiratory failure with ARDS is characterized by the acute development of pulmonary edema and the rapid onset of severe hypoxia, which is poorly responsive to increased oxygen delivered at ambient pressure. The pathophysiologic hallmark of ARDS is increased permeability of the alveolar-capillary membrane. The term "adult" is of historical origin and is misleading since ARDS occurs in patients of all ages, including children and neonates (1, 2).

The first description of ARDS as a distinct entity with characteristic clinical, pathologic, and pathophysiologic features was from Ashbaugh et al. in 1967 (3). They described 12 adults with acute respiratory failure characterized by dyspnea, tachypnea, cyanosis refractory to oxygen therapy, decreased lung compliance, and diffuse infiltrates on chest radiograph following different initiating insults. Pulmonary pathologic specimens showed hyaline membranes similar to those seen in neonatal respiratory distress syndrome, and the term "adult respiratory distress syndrome" was adopted. Early reports of ARDS focused on patients with severe pulmonary injury, but it is clear that the same pathophysiologic events lead to a range of pulmonary dysfunction. Thus, ARDS is now considered the most severe clinical presentation of a process called "acute lung injury" (4). It is important to recognize that acute lung injury is one of a group of acute post-insult organ dysfunction syndromes including sepsis, multiple organ failure syndrome (MOFS), and post-traumatic hypermetabolism, having considerable similarities in the basic pathogenic mechanisms leading to tissue injury and clinical picture (5, 6). Pulmonary injury has a high profile among these organ dysfunction syndromes since the lungs are frequently the first and most severely affected organ.

CLINICAL COURSE

The clinical course of ARDS can be divided into four phases: (a) acute injury, (b) latent period, (c) acute respiratory failure, and (d) severe physiologic abnormalities. During the acute injury, clinical findings are related to the precipitating insult. Some patients may hyperventilate, developing hypocarbia and respiratory alkalosis despite an adequate Pao_2, but generally there are no signs of pulmonary dysfunction unless the lungs were involved in the initial insult. A latent period of 6–72 hours follows, during which the patient appears to be stable or recovering. In some patients hyperventilation will persist and fine reticular infiltrates, consistent with interstitial pulmonary fluid, may be noted on chest radiograph. The

Table 36.1.
Common Conditions Associated With ARDS

Direct pulmonary injury	Secondary pulmonary injury
Pulmonary infections	Shock of any cause
Noxious gas inhalation	Sepsis
Oxygen	Trauma
Smoke	Drug overdose/ingestion
Aspiration	Increased intracranial pressure
Gastric fluid	Post-cardiopulmonary bypass
Near drowing	Pancreatitis
Pulmonary contusion	Massive blood transfusion

diagnosis of ARDS is made during the phase of acute respiratory failure when there is the rapid onset of tachypnea, dyspnea, and hypoxia refractory to increased oxygen administration. Diffuse, hazy bilateral infiltrates are noted on chest radiograph due to interstitial and intra-alveolar fluid. Rales on auscultation are frequently but not universally noted (Fig. 36.1). Intrapulmonary shunting with hypoxia is the principle alteration in gas exchange, but hypercarbia is rare. Decreased pulmonary compliance, manifested clinically as tachypnea and labored respiration, becomes apparent as elevated airway pressures are required for adequate ventilation. During the phase of acute respiratory failure, some patients will recover, others will die of causes other than respiratory failure, and some will progress to the next phase. In the phase of severe physiologic abnormalities, there is development of a chronic, fibrotic lung disease. The transition from acute respiratory failure to this phase is not distinct but involves increasing difficulties with ventilation, such that CO_2 retention is an indication of progression. Patients in this phase may progress to intractable respiratory failure but also remain at risk for death due to factors not related directly to gas exchange. Those who recover from this phase usually

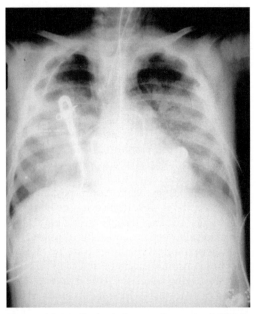

Figure 36.1. Typical chest radiograph of ARDS. (From Royall JA. *Essential guide to pediatric intensive care.* St. Louis, Quality Medical Publishing, 1990.)

require respiratory support for a prolonged period, often for months.

EPIDEMIOLOGY

More than 150,000 patients develop ARDS each year in the United States. The occurrence rate in pediatrics is 8–10 cases per 1000 pediatric intensive care unit admissions (1). The overall mortality rate with ARDS is approximately 60% in both the pediatric and adult populations. Outcome is even poorer in patients with gram-negative sepsis and with underlying malignancies. Since the introduction of positive-end expiratory pressure (PEEP) as therapy for ARDS, death is no longer caused primarily by the gas exchange abnormalities. Early deaths (in the first 3 days) are primarily related to the severity of the precipitating insult; death after this period is usually due to MOFS or secondary infection, or both. Intractable respiratory failure accounts for about 16% of deaths (7). Persistent respiratory dysfunction, secondary infection, and MOFS are interrelated such that the presence of one makes the occurrence of the others more likely. Initially in MOFS, ARDS is the only apparent organ failure followed by the sequential failure of other organ systems, but occasionally the entire MOFS picture including ARDS becomes apparent at once. Failure of any organ system occurs in association with ARDS. Gastrointestinal (GI) dysfunction has been emphasized from two perspectives. Colonization of the upper GI tract with gram-negative bacteria increases the risk of secondary bronchopneumonia (8). Altered mucosal barrier function allowing translocation of bacteria or there products into the circulation has been proposed as a pathogenic mechanism in ARDS (5). Hepatic dysfunction appears to be important as both a marker of MOFS and participant in injury (9).

For survivors of ARDS, the long-term prognosis for pulmonary function is good (10, 11). Abnormalities including reduced lung volumes, abnormal diffusing capacity, decreased PaO_2 with exercise, ventilation irregularities, and reversible airway obstruction have been identified. These tend to improve over 6–12 months, but abnormalities may remain. A rare patient has chronic impairment of pulmonary function with a significant negative effect on lifestyle, but generally a normal life can be anticipated. Our experience in children supports this general conclusion. The first year following ARDS there are problems with hypoxia and reversible airway obstruction requiring routine therapy. These problems improve over about 1 year such that no subsequent respiratory support or medication is required. Although there are persistent reductions in lung volumes, these patients have a normal lifestyle. Whether pulmonary sequelae will adversely influence pulmonary function in later life is a matter of concern.

PATHOPHYSIOLOGY

Under normal conditions, the hydrostatic pressure gradient across the pulmonary capillaries exceeds the opposing forces of the oncotic pressure gradient, which tend to move fluid from interstitium to vasculature, such that there is net fluid flux into the interstitium. This interstitial fluid is removed by the pulmonary lymphatics.

The primary derangement leading to pulmonary edema in ARDS is increased permeability of the alveolar-capillary membrane (permeability edema). Increased permeability of both the capillary endothelium and alveolar epithelium has been demonstrated. Fluid flux across a membrane is determined by the permeability and surface area of the membrane, net hydrostatic pressure across the membrane, and net oncotic pressure across the membrane. For the capillary endothelium, this relationship can be described by the Starling equation:

$$Q = L_pA \left[(P_{cap} - P_{int}) - \sigma (\pi_{cap} - \pi_{int})\right]$$

Where: Q = net transcapillary fluid flux; L_p = hydraulic conductance (ease of water passage); A = surface area available for fluid flux; P = hydrostatic pressure in the capillary (P_{cap}) and interstitium (P_{int}); σ = reflection coefficient (hinderance of macromolecule passage); π = colloid oncotic pressure in the capillary (π_{cap}) and the interstitium (π_{int}). The alteration in L_p and σ lead to increased movement of high protein fluid at lower P_{cap}. Because the interstitial fluid has a high protein content, the oncotic pressure gradient ($\pi_{cap} - \pi_{int}$) is reduced, exacerbating edema formation. This contrasts with hydrostatic pulmonary edema, seen with left ventricular failure, where despite an increased P_{cap} the function of the endothelial barrier remains largely intact. In this case edema fluid has a low protein content,

increases the colloid oncotic pressure gradient moving fluid into the vessel, and has a mitigating effect on pulmonary edema formation.

Decreased performance of both the right and left ventricles may occur because of the pathologic process of ARDS and the use of PEEP as therapy (12). Increased pulmonary vascular resistance occurs from alveolar hypoxia, mediator-induced vasoconstriction, and vascular occlusion from thrombosis and embolism. The magnitude and duration of elevated pulmonary vascular resistance correlates with the severity of ARDS (13). Right ventricular performance is adversely affected by increased afterload and possibly by myocardial ischemia. Vasodilators used to reduce pulmonary vascular resistance improve cardiac output but at the cost of worsened hypoxia from an increased intrapulmonary shunt caused by the inhibition of hypoxic pulmonary vasoconstriction. Thus, although elevated pulmonary vascular resistance is an important factor in cardiac suppression during ARDS, there is currently no therapy to alleviate this problem directly. Left ventricular function may be adversely affected by alteration of the diastolic pressure-volume relationship from a shift of the intraventricular septum into the left ventricle. PEEP may result in decreased venous return, and some data suggest a humorally mediated depression of contractility induced by PEEP. Cardiac suppression may not be manifested as shock or heart failure unless there is additional myocardial injury, or cardiac failure develops as part of MOFS. Commonly cardiac suppression results in an inability to increase cardiac function appropriately to meet metabolic demands.

In addition to increased metabolic demands for oxygen, defects in peripheral oxygen utilization have been identified in patients with ARDS (Fig. 36.2). Normally, oxygen delivery ($\dot{D}O_2$) is well above metabolic needs, and reduction in $\dot{D}O_2$ leads to a compensatory increase in O_2 extraction. Oxygen consumption ($\dot{V}O_2$) only becomes dependent on $\dot{D}O_2$ after $\dot{D}O_2$ is reduced markedly. In critically ill patients, $\dot{V}O_2$ is linearly related to $\dot{D}O_2$, implying inadequate DO_2 to meet metabolic needs, even when DO_2 is well above the normal range (14–16). An interdependence of VO_2 and DO_2 has been noted in ARDS, whereas no correlation of $\dot{V}O_2$ and $\dot{D}O_2$ was noted in non-ARDS patients (14). In retro-

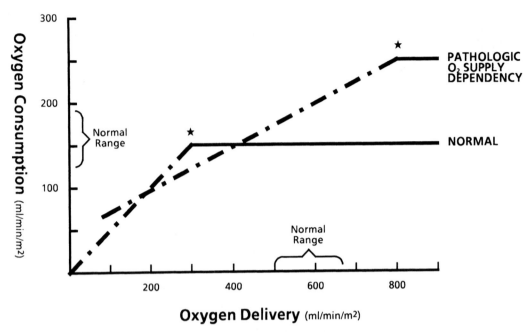

Figure 36.2. Altered oxygen utilization in critically ill patients. In patients with ARDS and other critical conditions, oxygen consumption (VO_2) becomes abnormally dependent on oxygen delivery (DO_2). (Modified from Royall JA. *Essential guide to pediatric intensive care.* St. Louis, Quality Medical Publishing, 1990.)

spective studies, survivors of sepsis and ARDS are those who tend to maintain $\dot{D}O_2 > 600$ ml O_2/min/m^2. Prospective studies in critically ill patients have shown an improved outcome when therapy was directed at maintenance of a high rather than normal $\dot{D}O_2$ (17, 18). Although questions remain about $\dot{V}O_2$ dependence on $\dot{D}O_2$ in ARDS, therapy directed at counteracting this abnormality appears to improve outcome.

PATHOLOGY

The pulmonary pathologic changes of ARDS can be divided into three stages; early exudative, cellular proliferative, and fibrotic proliferative (Fig. 36.3). The early exudative stage lasts up to 3 days and is characterized by inflammation and exudation of protein-rich fluid into the interstitium and alveoli. Alveoli contain a proteinaceous and often hemorrhagic fluid with acute inflammatory cells. Hyaline membranes are noted, especially in alveolar ducts. The vasculature may be occluded with microthrombi, fibrin, and sometimes aggregates of leukocytes. Alveolar epithelial cell degeneration and death is prominent, whereas capillary endothelial cells

appear relatively intact despite the marked alteration in endothelial barrier function. Proliferation of type II alveolar epithelial cells such that they cover the majority of the alveolar surface is characteristic of the cellular proliferative stage, which occurs between 3 and 10 days after the onset of ARDS. This appears to be a reparative process since these cells can transform into type I alveolar epithelial cells to regenerate a normal alveolar lining. Early fibrotic changes and progression of inflammation to a more chronic appearance are also noted. In the fibrotic proliferative stage, the alveolar fluid may organize to form intra-alveolar fibrosis, and alveolar duct fibrosis is seen with expanded terminal airways surrounded by a thick layer of fibrotic tissue; normal lung structure can be totally disrupted. The appearance of severe, extensive fibrosis correlates with the clinical development of intractable respiratory failure.

PATHOGENESIS

The pathogenic mechanisms responsible for initiation and perpetuation of ARDS can be divided into those that cause or amplify the initial lung injury, those that are the secondary

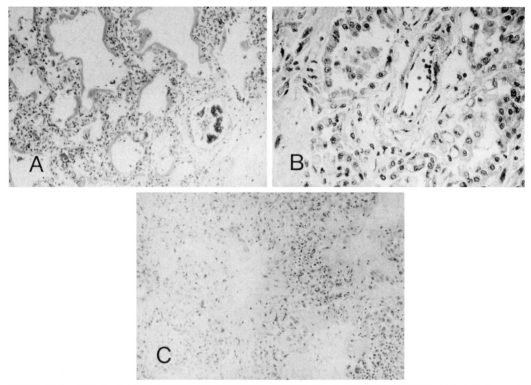

Figure 36.3. Diffuse alveolar damage, the pathologic appearance of ARDS. Photomicrograph *A* is the early exudative stage, *B* is the cellular proliferative stage, and *C* is the fibrotic proliferative stage. (Supplied by Joseph Rutledge, M.D., Dept. of Pathology, Children's Hospital and Medical Center, Seattle, Washington. From Royall JA, Levin DL. *Pediatric intensive care,* ed 2. Mount Kisco, NY, Futura Publishing, 1989.)

effects of lung injury, and those that are iatrogenic. In ARDS, as in the other post-injury organ dysfunction syndromes, there appears to be activation of endogenous systems including inflammatory cell activation, lipid mediator release, complement activation, and activation of the coagulation system. These endogenous responses would normally function to limit injury and protect the host, but in some cases they are not adequately localized or down-regulated, resulting in diffuse intravascular inflammation that frequently has the most pronounced affect on the lungs. Attempts to identify a specific marker for prediction of ARDS in a population at risk have not been successful, principally because there is widespread activation of endogenous systems after injury without universal progression to clinical ARDS. Also, individual systems may play a greater or lesser role in ARDS, depending on the precipitating insult and stage of ARDS. Despite advances in understanding the pathogenic mechanisms of

ARDS, there has to date been no direct application to improving therapy. Clinical trials of corticosteroids and prostaglandin E_1 have not improved outcome (19, 20). It is thought that a better understanding of the basic alterations in cellular metabolism will allow the early identification of developing intravascular inflammation and intervention before there is progression to organ system failure recognized clinically as ARDS and MOFS.

Initiation or Amplification of Acute Lung Injury

COMPLEMENT ACTIVATION AND POLYMORPHONUCLEAR LEUKOCYTES (PMNs)

In the 1980s studies suggested a correlation between activation of the complement system and the development of ARDS. Complement activation was proposed as inducing PMN aggregation and sequestration in the lung. Subsequent investigations found that complement activation occurs in a variety of inflammatory states but is not a specific inciter of ARDS (21). Complement activation has adverse effects, principally via inflammatory cells, although some data suggest a direct toxic effect of C5a on endothelial cells (22).

Substantial evidence suggests that PMNs and their products play a central role in ARDS, although ARDS can occur without substantial PMN participation (23). PMNs may be activated by exogenous substances (e.g., endotoxin) or by other endogenous systems. Participation of PMNs in the pathologic process involves recruitment to the area of injury, adherence to endothelial cells, migration between endothelial cells into the interstitium, and stimulated release of toxic substances to kill the offending agent (Fig. 36.4). Toxic substances released by the PMN include reactive O_2 species, lipid mediators, and proteolytic enzymes. Tissue injury seems to require a synergistic effect of reactive O_2 species and proteinases (24).

MONONUCLEAR PHAGOCYTES AND CYTOKINES

Although endothelial cells appear to be key targets of injury in ARDS, the macrophage

(and related cells of the mononuclear-phagocyte line including monocytes, Kupffer cells, and microglial cells) appear to be key cells mediating the endogenous response that amplifies a primary exogenous insult (25). Release of cytokines, particularly tumor necrosis factor-alpha (TNF), is central to this process (26). Alterations in both inflammatory cell and endothelial cell function occur after TNF exposure (Fig. 36.4). The hemostatic properties of the endothelium are altered, promoting intravascular coagulation. Release of lipid mediators from both inflammatory and endothelial cells is stimulated. Activation of PMNs results in chemotaxis, increased degranulation, and enhanced phagocytosis. Release of reactive O_2 species is not directly stimulated significantly with TNF, but PMNs are "primed" such that subsequent exposure to a PMN-activating stimulus results in markedly increased release. Both PMNs and endothelial cells are induced to produce adhesion molecules that regulate PMN adherence and migration across the endothelium (27). Increased permeability of the vascular endothelium occurs after TNF exposure, which may aid in PMN migration but also may

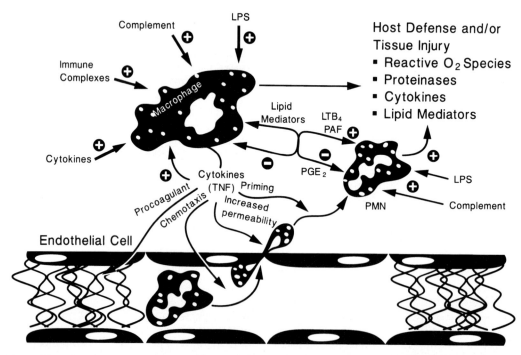

Figure 36.4. Acute intravascular inflammation. Interaction of the macrophage, polymorphonuclear leukocyte, and endothelium in inflammation and tissue injury.

increase edema formation. If this spectrum of events—(a) induced secretion of cytokines from macrophages, (b) recruitment of PMNs to the area of injury, (c) priming of PMNs such that a second stimulation by the offending agent leads to a maximum response, (d) alteration of endothelial function such that PMNs are maintained in the area and directed to migrate across the endothelium, and (e) stimulation of localized intravascular coagulation such that spread of potential harmful agents is limited—occurs in a limited microenvironment, it is protective. If these events occur throughout the circulation in multiple organs, the pathologic events of ARDS and MOFS are seen. Macrophages also release toxic substances similar to the PMN, and resident populations within the lung and pulmonary vasculature may participate directly in tissue injury.

OTHER MEDIATORS

Reactive O_2 Species. Potential sources of reactive O_2 species in acute lung injury include (a) the respiratory burst of inflammatory cells, (b) hyperoxia from increased FiO_2, (c) ischemia-reperfusion injury, and perhaps (d) endogenous endothelial production (22, 28, 29). Superoxide anion (O_2^-) and hydrogen peroxide (H_2O_2) are byproducts of normal cellular respiration, in addition to being produced in pathologic states. Reactions in the presence of transition metals (principally iron) may lead to formation of hydroxyl radical ($OH\bullet$), and reactions with membrane lipids may result in lipid hydroperoxide formation. The hydroxyl radical is a powerful oxidant, and the formation of lipid hydroperoxides occurs within the lipid bilayer sequestered from most cellular antioxidants. A recently described reaction between O_2^- and nitric oxide (endothelium-derived relaxing factor) produces peroxynitrite, which is a strong oxidant on the order of $OH\bullet$ (30). A group of enzymatic (superoxide dismutase, catalase, glutathione peroxidase) and non-enzymatic scavengers (vitamin E, ascorbate, urea, glutathione) protect against injury from reactive O_2 species. In pathologic states, toxicity is determined by the balance between the level of reactive O_2 species production and removal by antioxidant systems in a given cellular compartment.

Lipid Mediators. A number of products that function in the inflammatory response are formed from lipids released from cellular membranes by phospholipases (31). This process is controlled by phospholipase-activating protein synthesized in response to endotoxin, TNF, and other agents. Free arachidonic acid is metabolized through the cyclo-oxygenase pathway to prostaglandins and thromboxane, or via lipoxygenase pathway to LTB_4, LTC_4, LTD_4, and LTE_4. Laboratory investigations have suggested a role for cyclo-oxygenase products in increasing pulmonary vascular resistance, but clinical studies do not support an important role for thromboxane (32). Cyclo-oxygenase products may increase PMN adherence to the endothelium and induce platelet aggregation. The leukotrienes appear to have a more important role in ARDS (33). LTC_4, LTD_4, and LTE_4 (the sulfidopeptide leukotrienes) have their greatest effect in causing vasoconstriction, and LTB_4 is a potent agent in attracting and activating inflammatory cells.

The action of phospholipase on phosphatidylcholine results in lysophosphatidylcholine release and subsequent formation of platelet activating factor (PAF) (34). In addition to platelet activation, PAF has extensive proinflammatory effects including PMN chemotaxis and activation, vasoconstriction, and increased vascular permeability.

Coagulation System. Disseminated intravascular coagulation and thrombocytopenia are frequently associated with ARDS. Fibrin and fibrin-platelet microthrombi are common pathologic findings, and some data suggest that intravascular coagulation can occur isolated to the lungs. The products of increased coagulation may increase pulmonary vascular resistance by direct mechanical obstruction of the pulmonary circulation as well as by stimulation of vasoconstrictor lipid mediator release. Fibrin and fibrin degradation products cause cellular injury both directly and via activation of inflammatory cells.

Secondary Effects of Lung Injury

Factors that may result in surfactant deficiency in ARDS include injury to alveolar type II epithelial cells and inhibition of surfactant function by plasma proteins (35). Samples from patients with ARDS have normal or, in some cases, elevated levels of phospholipid.

However, the phospholipid composition is abnormal and has elevated minimum surface tension. The most obvious secondary abnormality of surfactant deficiency is alveolar collapse and impaired gas exchange. Increased alveolar edema formation, increased risk of secondary infection, and increased susceptibility to reactive O_2 species injury may also result from surfactant deficiency.

Alpha$_1$-proteinase inhibitor (alpha$_1$-PI; alpha$_1$-antitrypsin) is a major protection against proteolytic enzyme injury to the lung but is inactivated by oxidant and proteinase-mediated mechanisms. Bronchoalveolar lavage fluid from patients with ARDS generally has abnormally elevated proteolytic enzyme activity. However, if fluid is obtained just after onset of ARDS, no elastolytic activity is noted, but elastase is present by antigen testing and seems to be complexed with alpha$_1$-PI (36). Thus, alpha$_1$-PI may transiently serve a protective role against proteolytic injury early in the course of the syndrome, but this protection is lost as alpha$_1$-PI is inactivated. Additionally, alpha$_1$-PI may inhibit PMN migration until its inactivation allows enhanced PMN sequestration (37).

An extensive fibroproliferative response occurs secondary to the initial acute lung injury. Progression of fibrosis can be extensive and result in intractable respiratory failure. The mechanisms of this extensive fibrotic response are complex but, like the acute lung injury, the macrophage seems to be a key mediator cell in this process (38).

MANAGEMENT

To date, attempted specific therapies directed against the underlying mediators of ARDS have been disappointing. Clinical trials of corticosteroid and prostaglandin E$_1$ (PGE$_1$) infusion for patients with ARDS and sepsis have not improved outcome (19, 20). Indeed, some studies found an increased incidence of secondary infection with steroid use, possibly leading to increased mortality (39). Thus, therapy for ARDS remains primarily supportive but directed by an understanding of the pathophysiology and clinical issues discussed previously. Because ARDS is a multi-organ system insult, with the pulmonary injury being the most pronounced, management is directed not only at improving pulmonary gas exchange but also toward assuring adequate

tissue oxygenation, nutritional support, and intervention for potential secondary infection. Guidelines for management are given in Table 36.2. These should be viewed as a general framework within which care is individualized, especially considering the variety of precipitating insults associated with ARDS that will affect the overall therapeutic goals for the patient. Iatrogenic factors are part of the pathogenesis of ARDS, and consideration of the relative risks and benefits of a given therapeutic intervention is an ongoing issue throughout treatment.

Cardiorespiratory Support

TISSUE OXYGEN DELIVERY ($\dot{D}O_2$)

A primary treatment goal for ARDS is to maintain adequate levels of tissue oxygenation while minimizing the potentially detrimental aspects of therapy, particularly pulmonary oxygen toxicity. Although there are individual variations in sensitivity to O_2 toxicity, in general clinical practice an Fio$_2$ of less than 0.50–0.60 is considered to have minimal risk of O_2 toxicity. High airway pressures increase the risk of pulmonary air leak and cause alveolar injury (40). Adequate tissue oxygenation is accomplished by increasing $\dot{D}O_2$ and to a limited extent by minimizing $\dot{V}O_2$. One approach to assuring adequate $\dot{D}O_2$ is to increase $\dot{D}O_2$ until $\dot{V}O_2$ reaches a plateau. A distinct plateau can be difficult to define in individual patients; another approach is to achieve a $\dot{D}O_2$ level of > 600 ml O_2/min/m^2, a level noted to improve outcome (17, 18).

Tissue O_2 delivery is determined both by the oxygen content of arterial blood (Cao$_2$) and the cardiac index (CI):

$$\dot{D}O_2 \text{ (ml } O_2\text{/min/m}^2) = Cao_2 \text{ (ml } O_2\text{/dl blood)} \times CI \text{ (L/min/m}^2) \times 10 \text{ (dl/L)}$$

Arterial O_2 content is described by:

$$Cao_2 \text{ (ml } O_2\text{/dl blood)} = \text{[Hgb (g/dl)} \times 1.36 \text{ (ml } O_2\text{/g Hgb)} \times O_2 \text{ saturation of Hgb (\%)]} +$$

$$\text{[Pao}_2 \text{ (mm Hg)} \times 0.003 \text{ (ml } O_2\text{/dl blood/mm Hg)]}$$

The major portion of Cao$_2$ is due to O_2 bound to Hgb as described in the upper portion of this equation. The amount of O_2 bound to fully saturated Hgb is constant; thus Hgb and

Table 36.2.
General Guidelines for Management in ARDS

Therapy for the initiating insult
Maintain adequate DO_2 on a "nontoxic" Fio_2
   Hemoglobin of 12–15 g/dl (hematocrit ~ 40%)
   Arterial Sao_2 ≥ 90%
   Cardiac index ≥ 4.5 L/min/m²
   DO_2 > 600 ml/min/m²
   Fio_2 ≤ 0.50–0.60

Fluids initially at 70% maintenance; additional fluids as needed for cardiac or nutritional support
Nutritional support (see text)
Aggressive therapy for suspected secondary infection (see text)
Cardiorespiratory monitoring
   Arterial catheter
   Pulse oximetry
   Pulmonary arterial catheter helpful if:
     1. Therapeutic interventions are likely to suppress cardiac function (usually PEEP ≥ 15 cm H_2O)
     2. Initiating insult likely to cause myocardial dysfunction
     3. Clinical status indicates a low cardiac output state not easily corrected with fluid infusion
     4. Need to differentiate hydrostatic vs. permeability edema

Monitor for other organ system dysfunction:
   Renal, hepatic, gastrointestinal, coagulation

O_2 saturation (Sao_2) are available for therapeutic manipulation. The Hgb level should give adequate O_2 carrying capacity without increasing blood viscosity to the point where hyperviscosity adversely affects tissue perfusion. This is accomplished with a Hgb of 12–15 g/dl. For patients with severe respiratory failure requiring high levels of Fio_2 or PEEP, an Sao_2 of 90% is acceptable. With a large alveolar-arterial oxygen difference [$P(A-a)o_2$] gradient, potentially detrimental increases in respiratory support are required to increase the Sao_2 and Cao_2 further. The O_2-Hgb dissociation curve (Fig. 36.5) is often shifted in critically ill patients, and a direct measurement of Sao_2 (pulse oximeter or CO-oximeter) is preferred over a nomogram estimation of Sao_2 from the measured Pao_2. When the patient is improving such that Sao_2 measurements close to normal are attained on lower, nontoxic levels of Fio_2, then higher measurements of Sao_2 are acceptable since the respiratory support has minimal toxicity. With an Hgb of 12–15 g/dl and an Sao_2 of 90%, the DO_2 will be well within the adequate range of > 600 ml/min/m² if the CI is ≥ 4.5 L/min/m².

Ventilatory Support

Although isolated reports describe successful non-invasive respiratory support of patients with ARDS, most require endotracheal intubation for mechanical ventilation. Hypoxia is the most common indication for intubation. A general criterion would be an Sao_2 of less than 90% on an Fio_2 greater than 0.50 (an alveolar-arterial difference of 250 mm Hg or greater). Earlier intervention is reasonable and often available in the context of clearly progressive pulmonary dysfunction or the clinical appearance of distress. In the past, ventilation was usually accomplished by volume-limited ventilation with an initial tidal volume (V_T) of 12–15 ml/kg. Because of the predominantly restrictive nature of the pulmonary pathophysiology, effective ventilation can be accomplished with smaller tidal volumes and rapid respiratory rates (41, 42). The demonstration that large alveolar volumes and/or high alveolar pressures cause alveolar injury and that there is a portion of the lung with normal aeration in ARDS has led to the suggestion that smaller tidal volumes and lower pressures should be used. It is clear that the $Paco_2$ can be maintained above the normal level without adverse effect (permissive hypercarbia) with the limiting factor being the severity of the acidosis. Some suggest correction of acidosis with bicarbonate or other buffers. Therefore, rather than initiating ventilation with a traditional tidal volume of 10–15 ml/kg, 8–10 ml/kg can be used. It may be

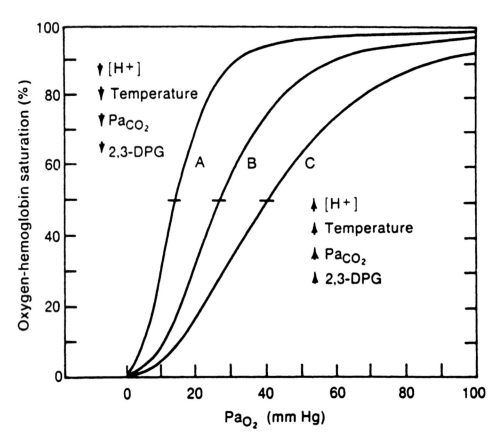

Figure 36.5. Oxygen-hemoglobin dissociation curve. (From Levin DL, Morris FC, Moore GC, eds. *A practical guide to pediatric intensive care,* ed 2. St. Louis, CV Mosby, 1984.)

desirable to keep the peak alveolar (plateau) pressure at less than 40 cm H_2O. A variety of ventilatory strategies have been proposed to accomplish this, including further reductions in tidal volume, pressure- or volume-controlled inverse ratio ventilation, constant oxygen insufflation, and airway pressure release ventilation (42a).

Alternative approaches to improving oxygenation have been successful but are not clearly superior to the traditional approach using PEEP. High-frequency ventilation (high-frequency positive pressure ventilation, high-frequency jet ventilation, high-frequency oscillatory ventilation) in general appears to offer no advantage in ARDS (43). High-frequency ventilation may reduce massive pulmonary air leak. Inverse ratio ventilation is a pressure-limited mode of ventilation in which reversed inspiratory/expiratory ratios of up to 4:1 are used. Increased alveolar

recruitment compared to traditional ventilation has been proposed but the mechanism may be no different from that of conventional PEEP. Inverse ratio ventilation has been evaluated in only a limited number of patients with ARDS and in an uncontrolled fashion (44–46). As with high-frequency ventilation, the routine use of inverse ratio ventilation for patients with ARDS cannot be recommended but may be used as a salvage attempt in individual patients who fail a traditional approach to respiratory support.

In some patients with severe respiratory failure, chest physical therapy (CPT) and other procedures can be associated with adverse events. Patients with ARDS are not likely to derive significant benefit from routine use of CPT (48). Therefore, CPT should not be used routinely or when associated with cardiorespiratory deterioration. Endotracheal suctioning is required to clear secretions from the endotracheal tube and trachea. Hyperventilation with 100% O_2 before and after suctioning and short duration of suctioning prevents hypoxia in most patients. Patients requiring high levels of PEEP are prone to rapid alveolar collapse and hypoxia if PEEP is removed for suctioning. The use of special adapters allows the continuation of PEEP and ventilatory support during suctioning. Pharmacologic neuromuscular blockade is occasionally needed to allow efficient respiratory support, especially in patients with severe respiratory failure. Paralysis may also decrease the patient's ventilatory work and decrease VO_2. Sedation should be ordered routinely for patients being paralyzed and given as needed for other intubated patients.

POSITIVE END-EXPIRATORY PRESSURE (PEEP)

The use of PEEP improves oxygenation in most patients with ARDS primarily by recruitment of collapsed or poorly ventilated alveoli, thereby reducing the intrapulmonary shunt (49). Pulmonary mechanics may also be improved by increasing functional residual capacity. The use of PEEP does not hasten the resolution of lung injury or decrease pulmonary edema, but an appropriate level of PEEP does allow the use of less toxic levels of FiO_2 (50). Adverse effects of PEEP include pulmonary barotrauma and airleak, air trapping with CO_2 retention, and decreased cardiac output. Patients requiring high levels of PEEP do have a high incidence of airleak, but factors such as peak airway pressure and the status of the lung itself may be more important than the level of PEEP (51). With the exception of massive airleak and inability to achieve adequate ventilation, PEEP should not be limited as prophylaxis against or therapy for pulmonary airleak. While PEEP is being adjusted in the range of continued alveolar recruitment, CO_2 retention should not be a factor in limiting PEEP. The major difficulty with PEEP in patients with ARDS is inhibition of cardiac function with a accompanying decrease in DO_2.

At initiation of mechanical ventilatory support, an FiO_2 of 1.0 is used. Short exposures to a high FiO_2 are not toxic. A "physiologic PEEP" of 2–4 cm H_2O should be used from initiation to termination of endotracheal intubation. The PEEP is then increased in increments of 2–3 cm H_2O, and the FiO_2 decreased to keep SaO_2 at approximately 90% until the FiO_2 is reduced below 0.50–0.60. In the early stages of ARDS, when the pathology is primarily one of acute inflammation and edema, improvement in oxygenation usually occurs within 15–30 minutes of an increase in PEEP. There is a critical opening pressure that must be exceeded before PEEP results in significant alveolar recruitment. Increasing PEEP in a low range may not result in improved oxygenation, but improvement may occur at higher levels of PEEP after this threshold pressure for recruitment is exceeded. In the later stages of ARDS, when fibrosis predominates, increases in PEEP are less likely to be effective and may take several hours to be noted. It is also possible to increase PEEP beyond the beneficial range, with alveolar overdistension resulting in decreased oxygenation, CO_2 retention, and cardiac suppression. Appropriate titration of PEEP requires sequential evaluation of respiratory and cardiac function associated with each alteration in the level of PEEP. Therefore, PEEP is increased incrementally until one of the following end-points is reached: (a) adequate DO_2 (90% SaO_2, Hgb 12–15 g/dl, CI ≥ 4.5 L/min/m^2) is achieved on an FiO_2 ≤ 0.50 to 0.60, (b) PEEP is beyond the beneficial range in that increases in PEEP result in decreased cardiac output (and therefore DO_2) that is not corrected by fluid infusion or inotropy (adjust therapy to give maximum DO_2; the adverse effects of high FiO_2 may carry less risk than the adverse effects of higher PEEP), or (c) PEEP is beyond the beneficial range in that increases in PEEP have an adverse effect on gas exchange that is not attributable to changes in cardiac function. There is no arbitrarily set upper limit for PEEP.

In patients with resolving ARDS, a common observation is the recurrence of hypoxia during weaning from PEEP. Generally this can be avoided if PEEP is decreased in increments of 2–3 cm H_2O and weaning from PEEP is attempted under the following conditions: (a) stable, nonseptic patient, (b) FiO_2 ≤ 0.40, (c) PaO_2 ≥ 80 mm Hg (SaO_2 about 95%), which has been stable or improving for 6–12 hours, and (d) pulmonary compliance is improving (lowered peak airway pressure on the same V_T).

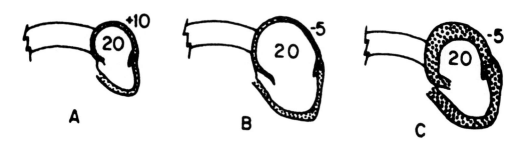

A   **B**   **C**

Figure 36.6. Interpretation of pulmonary wedge pressure (PWP). *A,* A high juxtacardiac pressure elevates the measured intravascular PWP with a normal transmural filling pressure. *B,* Juxtacardiac pressure is normal, as is ventricular compliance; the elevated PWP indicates elevated left ventricular end-diastolic volume. *C,* The ventricle has poor compliance and the elevated PWP is required to attain adequate left ventricular end-diastolic volume. (From O'Quin R, Marini JJ. Pulmonary artery occlusion pressure: Clinical physiology, measurement, and interpretation. *Am Rev Respir Dis* 1983; 123:319–326.)

Cardiovascular Support

Inhibition of cardiac function can occur by a variety of mechanisms as discussed previously. Suppression of cardiac function with inadequate DO_2 can occur without the overt signs of low cardiac output associated with shock or congestive heart failure (decreased urine output, prolonged capillary refill, cool extremities, hypotension). Patients with ARDS are relatively protected from cardiac suppression with PEEP because of less efficient transmission of airway pressure through edematous lung tissue. Pediatric patients without primary pathology involving the heart tolerate PEEP to about 15 cm H_2O without significant cardiac suppression (52). Often a pulmonary arterial catheter is helpful to measure directly cardiac output and to assess more accurately left ventricular preload (Table 36.2). Central venous pressure can also be used to evaluate left ventricular preload but may not be accurate in patients with cardiorespiratory disease (53). This is particularly a problem with ARDS considering the increased pulmonary vascular resistance and proportionally greater right ventricular dysfunction. Therefore, the pulmonary wedge pressure (PWP) is a preferred estimate of left ventricular preload in ARDS.

Hemodynamic monitoring measures intravascular pressure while left ventricular preload is left ventricular end-diastolic volume (LVEDV). With ARDS, left ventricular compliance may be decreased such that a higher than normal pressure is required to give a normal LVEDV (Fig. 36.6C). Additionally,

the effective filling pressure is the transmural pressure across the ventricle. With positive pressure ventilation, a portion of the elevated airway pressure is transmitted to the juxtacardiac space so that a higher than normal intravascular pressure may represent a normal transmural pressure (Fig. 36.6A). The effect of airway pressure on CVP and PWP measurement can be minimized by using end-expiratory values either from the lower values on a graphic display or from the diastolic values with a digital monitor (54). Because of the effect of airway pressure, measured PWP in an individual patient cannot be compared to published normal values to estimate intravascular volume status. Trends in PWP and CI related to changes in intravascular volume status are used to determine the position of left ventricular function on the ventricular function curve (Fig. 36.7). Usually intravascular volume is increased with a fluid infusion, but a similar evaluation can be performed by reducing intravascular volume. The pre-infu-

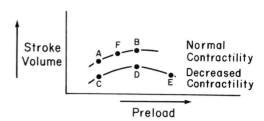

Figure 36.7. Ventricular function curve. See text for discussion. (From Perkin RM, Levin DL. Shock in the pediatric patient. Part II: Therapy. *J Pediatr* 1982; 101:319–322.)

sion PWP value is compared to the value about 15 minutes after completion of an infusion. If the post-infusion PWP is within 2–3 mm Hg of pre-infusion value and is accompanied by an increase in CI, then the ventricle is functioning on the ascending limb of the curve (Fig. 36.7C, D). If a further increase in CI is needed, another fluid infusion can be given with the new PWP as the pre-infusion value. If the post-infusion PWP exceeds the pre-infusion value by greater than 2–3 mm Hg and there is no increase in CI, the ventricle is functioning on the descending limb of the curve (Fig. 36.7D, E). Inotropic support is then needed to directly stimulate contractility and shift function to a higher curve (Fig. 36.7E, F). Dobutamine and dopamine are commonly used for inotropic support. There is no clear advantage between these agents, but dobutamine may be better except when greater blood pressure support or enhancement of renal blood flow are specifically desired (55).

Fluid Therapy

The volume and types of fluids to be used in ARDS, as well as in other pathologic states with loss of capillary endothelial integrity, continues to be an area of controversy. One controversy is whether crystalloid or colloid solutions should be used for acute intravascular volume expansion. The theoretical argument that colloids will leak into the interstitial space and draw additional fluid has not been demonstrated clinically. There is a report of increased pulmonary edema in adult patients using crystalloid resuscitation for shock potentially due to a decrease in plasma oncotic pressure (56). Since the outcome in ARDS is not directly related to the amount of extravascular lung water or magnitude of the gas exchange abnormality the effect of a given fluid on pulmonary edema may not be a major discriminating factor. Interstitial edema in the systemic circulation may have a more detrimental effect if tissue oxygenation is reduced because of limited O_2 diffusion. Some authors have suggested that crystalloid resuscitation may result in greater interstitial edema due to overhydration of the interstitial matrix with reduced ability to exclude protein (57). Additionally, two to four times greater volume of crystalloid compared to colloid is required for the same response in intravascular volume.

Because common goals of a fluid infusion are to increase rapidly intravascular volume and note the response to aid in further therapeutic decisions, colloid infusion would be preferred on this basis.

Another area of controversy is the overall goals for fluid administration. Because edema, both pulmonary and peripheral, will be increased with any elevation in intravascular volume, our goal for fluid administration is to maintain adequate DO_2 with the lowest effective intravascular volume. Initially, fluids are administered at 70% of maintenance, but additional volume is given as needed for cardiac or nutritional support. Experience from the 1970s indicated that reducing intravascular volume in an attempt to keep the lungs as dry as possible did not improve outcome (58). Two reports appear to bring this approach to fluid management into question. A prospective study found a correlation between positive fluid balance and poor outcome (59). Another retrospective study found improved survival in patients having a 25% reduction in PWP compared to those with less than 25% reduction (60). Pulmonary edema reduction with improved gas exchange would seem an unlikely explanation for any beneficial effect. Possible explanations for a beneficial effect include a view of the lungs as a perpetuator of ARDS either as a nidus of mediator generation or through secondary infection. Reduced edema might lessen this, either directly or because of a requirement for less vigorous respiratory support. Also, if peripheral edema is reduced, there may be some improvement in tissue oxygenation. These reasons are highly speculative; an equally plausible explanation is that the differences reflect severity of the injury with greater capillary permeability or cardiovascular dysfunction (61). These reports serve as an impetus for further investigation and may cause one to use inotropes more aggressively than volume infusion for cardiac support, but there are not sufficient data to support a change in the current approach to ARDS that emphasizes adequate DO_2 and deemphasizes reduction of pulmonary edema as a primary therapeutic goal.

Nutritional Support

Patients suffering a severe injury develop a hypermetabolic state that generally peaks at 3 days and lasts from 7 to 21 days (5). Persistence of post-injury hypermetabolism is associated with development of MOFS and poor outcome. During hypermetabolism energy expenditure is increased and supported by amino acid utilization, primarily from endogenous proteins, with inefficient use of glucose and fat. The goal of nutritional support during this time is to minimize depletion of endogenous proteins. Suggested guidelines include approximately 30 cal/kg/day in the adult with 4 to 5 g/kg/day glucose, 0.5–1 g/kg/day lipid, and protein at 1.5–2 g /kg/day, depending on the severity of injury. Older children should receive approximately 40 cal/kg/day, and infants 50 cal/kg/day. After resolution of hypermetabolism, nutrition can be supplied with standard substrate distribution. During this healing phase, a caloric intake of 25–50% above usual age requirements may be needed.

Administration of excessive nutrition does have risks. Lipogenesis occurs if glucose administration is given in excess of utilization with an associated and marked increase in CO_2 production. Limited ventilatory reserve may result in hypercapnia or inability to wean ventilatory support. Infusion of intravenous lipid can worsen hypoxia, perhaps because of altered prostaglandin production in the lung (62). Infusions at clinically applied rates are usually tolerated, but one should be aware than an occasional patient may experience significant hypoxia.

Secondary Infection

Secondary infection, particularly gram-negative bacterial bronchopneumonia, is a major cause of mortality in patients with ARDS. Bronchopneumonia develops secondary to oropharyngeal colonization with subsequent aspiration of small amounts of secretions. Although gram-negative bacteria, including *Pseudomonas*, are the most common organisms, gram-positive bacteria are a significant problem, and virtually any other infectious agent can cause bronchopneumonia. The definitive diagnosis of bronchopneumonia in patients with ARDS is difficult. The usual clinical findings that suggest pneumonia (infiltrates on chest radiograph, fever, abnormal white blood cell count, purulent secretions, and apparent response to antibiotic therapy) are not reliable and are associated with about 30% false-positive and false-negative diagnoses. New methods for diagnosis of bronchopneu-

monia, including quantitative bronchoalveolar lavage cultures, use of protected specimen brush for attaining lower airway samples, and evaluation of pulmonary secretions for elastin fibers and bacterial products, are being evaluated (63). One report suggests that once gram-negative pneumonia is established, antibiotic therapy has little effect on the eventual poor outcome. The investigators found that when secondary infection was diagnosed clinically and appropriate antibiotics were given for the infecting organism, the 29% survival rate was not different from the 23% survival rate when inadequate antibiotic therapy was given (64).

Another approach to preventing bronchopneumonia is to prevent the original oropharyngeal colonization. Use of systemic and topical antibiotics appears to reduce the incidence of bronchopneumonia but has not been shown to reduce mortality (65). Elevation of gastric pH by agents used for stress ulcer prophylaxis allows bacterial colonization of the stomach and increases oropharyngeal colonization. All pediatric patients may not require stress ulcer prophylaxis but, if prophylaxis is used, some data support the use of sucralfate, which does not alter gastric pH and may lessen the risk of secondary bronchopneumonia compared to use of antacids or H-2 blockers (66).

Dealing with secondary infection is one of the most difficult areas of management in ARDS. A reasonable approach is to maintain a high index of suspicion and initiate antibiotic therapy empirically, treating for both gram-negative (including *Pseudomonas*) and gram-positive bacteria (including *Staphylococcus*), once there is suspicion of secondary infection. An anti-staphylococcal penicillin in combination with an aminoglycoside and anti-pseudomonal penicillin, or in combination with a third-generation cephalosporin with anti-pseudomonal activity, can be used. This approach will put some patients at risk for secondary infection with resistant organisms, fungi, and other pathogens. Clearly, this area should continue to be an active area of research, because a better understanding of the mechanism, diagnosis, and therapy for secondary infection could yield substantial benefits in improved outcome.

New Approaches To Therapy

SUPPORTIVE CARE

An extracorporeal membrane oxygenation (ECMO) cooperative study of adults with severe acute respiratory failure in 1979 showed no improvement in survival (67). A variation of this technique, low-frequency positive-pressure ventilation with extracorporeal CO_2 removal, was used in an uncontrolled manner with a 49% survival rate in a group of patients with a predicted mortality of 90% based on the previous ECMO study (68). Retrospective analysis of mortality can be misleading. A randomized, controlled trial comparing this technique with conventional ventilation found no difference in outcome (69). Surfactant supplementation has been used to a limited extent in ARDS showing a transient improvement in oxygenation (35). The greater availability of surfactant has made supplementation for patients outside the neonatal period more feasible, and trials of surfactant replacement in adults with ARDS are currently in progress. Inhaled nitric oxide has been used in a small number of ARDS patients to reduce pulmonary vascular resistance (69a).

SPECIFIC THERAPY

A variety of specific therapies have been proposed for ARDS (34). Clinical efficacy has not been clearly demonstrated for a human monoclonal antibody against endotoxin (70). Other monoclonal antibodies against TNF, C5a, adhesion molecules, and other agents are of potential therapeutic benefit. Therapy aimed at limitation of reactive O_2 species–mediated injury includes supplementation of antioxidant enzymes. Several methods to prolong the circulating half-life and enhance intracellular enzyme levels, including entrapment of enzymes in liposomes and conjugation of enzymes with polyethylene glycol, have been described (71). Other agents that may modulate the inflammatory response, including pentoxifylline and ibuprofen, are of current interest. Hemofiltration has been proposed as a method to remove mediator substances from the circulation (72).

REFERENCES

1. Royall JA, Levin DL. Adult respiratory distress syndrome in pediatric patients: Part I. Clinical aspects, pathophysiology, pathology, and mechanisms of lung injury. Part II. Management. *J Pediatr* 1988; 112:169–180, 335–350.
2. Faix RG, Viscardi RM, DiPietro MA, Nicks JJ. Adult respiratory distress syndrome in full-term newborns. *Pediatrics* 1989; 83:971–976.
3. Ashbaugh DG, Bigelow DB, Petty TL, Levine BE. Acute respiratory distress in adults. *Lancet* 1967; 2:319–323.
4. Murray JF, Matthay MA, Luce JM, Flick MR. An expanded definition of the adult respiratory distress syndrome. *Am Rev Respir Dis* 1988; 138:720–723.
5. Barton R, Cerra FB. The hypermetabolism multiple organ failure syndrome. *Chest* 1989; 96:1153–1160.
6. Dorinsky PM, Gadek JE. Mechanisms of multiple nonpulmonary organ failure in ARDS. *Chest* 1989; 96:885–892.
7. Montgomery AB, Stager MA, Carrico J, Hudson LD. Causes of mortality in patients with the adult respiratory distress syndrome. *Am Rev Respir Dis* 1985; 132:485–489.
8. Johanson WG. Bacterial infection in ARDS: Pathogenic mechanisms and consequences. In Shoemaker WC, ed. *Critical care state of the art*, vol 5. Fullerton, CA, Society of Critical Care Medicine, 1984, pp H1–43.
9. Matuschak GM, Rinaldo JE. Organ interactions in the adult respiratory distress syndrome during sepsis: Role of the liver in host defense. *Chest* 1988; 94:400–406.
10. Alberts WM, Priest GR, Moser KM. The outlook for survivors of ARDS. *Chest* 1983; 84:272–274.
11. Fanconi S, Kraemer R, Weber J, Tschaeppler H, Pfenninger J. Long-term sequelae in children surviving adult respiratory distress syndrome. *J Pediatr* 1985; 106:218–222.
12. Sibbald WJ, Driedger AA, Myers ML, Short AIK, Wells GA. Biventricular function in the adult respiratory distress syndrome: Hemodynamic and radionuclide assessment, with special emphasis on right ventricular function. *Chest* 1983; 84:126–134.
13. Katz R, Pollack M, Spady D. Cardiopulmonary abnormalities in severe acute respiratory failure. *J Pediatr* 1984; 104:357–364.
14. Danek SJ, Lynch JP, Weg JG, Dantzker DR. The dependence of oxygen uptake on oxygen delivery in the adult respiratory distress syndrome. *Am Rev Respir Dis* 1980; 122:387–395.
15. Dorinsky PM, Costello JL, Gadek JE. Relationship of oxygen uptake and oxygen delivery in respiratory failure not due to the adult respiratory distress syndrome. *Chest* 1988; 93:1013–1019.
16. Vermeij CG, Feenstra BWA, Bruining HA. Oxygen delivery and oxygen uptake in postoperative and septic patients. *Chest* 1990; 98:415–419.
17. Shoemaker WC, Appel PL, Kram HB, Waxman K, Lee TS. Prospective trial of supranormal values of survivors as therapeutic goals in high-risk surgical patients. *Chest* 1988; 94:1176–1186, 1988.
18. Tuchschmidt J, Fried J, Astiz M, Rackow E. Supranormal oxygen delivery improves mortality in septic shock patients [Abstract]. *Crit Care Med* 1991; 19(Suppl):66.
19. Putterman C. Use of corticosteroids in the adult respiratory distress syndrome: A clinical review. *J Crit Care* 1990; 5:241–251.
20. Bone RC, Slotman G, Maunder RJ, et al. Randomized double-blind, multicenter study of prostaglandin E₁ in patients with the adult respiratory distress syndrome. *Chest* 1989; 96:114–119.
21. Duchateau J, Haas M, Schreyen L, et al. Complement activation in patients at risk of developing the adult

respiratory distress syndrome. *Am Rev Respir Dis* 1984; 130:1058–1064.

22. Friedl HP, Till GO, Ryan US, Ward PA. Mediator-induced activation of xanthine oxidase in endothelial cells. *FASEB J* 1989; 3:2512–2518.

23. Ognibene FP, Martin SE, Parker MM, et al: Adult respiratory distress syndrome in patients with severe neutropenia. *N Engl J Med* 1986; 315:547–551.

24. Weiss SJ. Tissue destruction by neutrophils. *N Engl J Med* 1989; 320:365–367.

25. Sibille Y, Reynolds HY. Macrophages and polymorphonuclear neutrophils in lung defense and injury. *Am Rev Respir Dis* 1990; 141:471–501.

26. Beutler B. Tumor necrosis, cachexia, shock, and inflammation: A common mediator. *Ann Rev Biochem* 1988; 57:505–518.

27. McEver RP. Role of the endothelium in the inflammatory response. Taylor RW, Shoemaker WC, eds. *Critical care state of the art*, vol 12. Fullerton, CA, Society of Critical Care Medicine, 1991, pp 121–139.

28. Saugstad OD. Oxygen radicals and pulmonary damage. *Pediatr Pulmonol* 1985; 1:167–175.

29. Brigham KL, Meyrick B, Berry LC, Repine JE. Antioxidants protect cultured bovine lung endothelial cells from injury by endotoxin. *J Appl Physiol* 1987; 63:840–850.

30. Beckman JS, Beckman TW, Chen J, Marshall PA, Freeman BA. Apparent hydroxyl radical production by peroxynitrite: Implications for endothelial injury from nitric oxide and superoxide. *Proc Natl Acad Sci U S A* 1990; 87:1620–1624.

31. Aderem AA, Rosen A, Barker KA. Modulation of prostaglandin and leukotriene biosynthesis. *Curr Opin Immunol* 1988; 1:56–62.

32. Leeman M, Boeynaems JM, Degaute JP, Vincent JL, Kahn RJ. Administration of dazoxiben, a selective thromboxane synthetase inhibitor, in the adult respiratory distress syndrome. *Chest* 1985; 87:726–730.

33. Bernard GR, Korley V, Chee P, Swindell B, Ford-Hutchinson AW, Tagari P. Persistent generation of peptido leukotrienes in patients with the adult respiratory distress syndrome. *Am Rev Respir Dis* 1991; 144:263–267.

34. Said SI, Foda HD. Pharmacologic modulation of lung injury. *Am Rev Respir Dis* 1989; 139:1553–1564.

35. Holm BA, Matalon S. Role of pulmonary surfactant in the development and treatment of adult respiratory distress syndrome. *Anesth Analg* 1989; 69:805–818.

36. Weiland JE, Davis WB, Holter JF, Mohammed JR, Dorinsky PM, Gadek JE. Lung neutrophils in the adult respiratory distress syndrome: clinical and pathophysiologic significance. *Am Rev Respir Dis* 1986; 133:218–225.

37. Stockley RA, Shaw J, Afford SC, Morrison HM, Burnerr D. Effect of alpha-1-proteinase inhibitor on neutrophil chemotaxis. *Am J Respir Cell Mol Biol* 1990; 2:163–170.

38. Snyder LS, Hertz MI, Harmon KR, Bitterman PB. Failure of lung repair following acute lung injury: Regulation of the fibroproliferative response (Parts 1 and 2). *Chest* 1990; 98:733–738, 989–993.

39. Weigelt JA, Norcross JF, Borman KR, Snyder WH. Early steroid therapy for respiratory failure. *Arch Surg* 1985; 120:536–540.

40. Kolobow T, Moretti MP, Fumagalli R, et al. Severe impairment in lung function induced by high peak

airway pressure during mechanical ventilation. *Am Rev Respir Dis* 1987; 135:312–315.

41. Lee PC, Helsmoortel CM, Cohn SM, Fink MP. Are low tidal volumes safe? *Chest* 1990; 97:425–490.

42. Leatherman JW, Lari RL, Iber C, Ney AL. Tidal volume reduction in ARDS: Effect on cardiac output and arterial oxygenation. *Chest* 1991; 99:1227–1231.

42a. Marini JJ. New approaches to the ventilatory management of the adult respiratory distress syndrome. *J Crit Care* 1992; 7:256–267.

43. Froese AB, Bryan AC. High frequency ventilation. *Am Rev Respir Dis* 1987; 135:1363–1374.

44. Tharratt RS, Allen RP, Albertson TE. Pressure controlled inverse ratio ventilation in severe adult respiratory failure. *Chest* 1988; 94:755–762.

45. Lain DC, DiBenedetto R, Morris SL, Nguyen AV, Saulters R, Causey D. Pressure control inverse ratio ventilation as a method to reduce peak inspiratory pressure and provide adequate ventilation and oxygenation. *Chest* 1989; 95:1081–1088.

46. Duncan SR, Rizk NW, Raffin TA. Inverse ratio ventilation: PEEP in disguise? *Chest* 1987; 92:390–391.

47. Rasanen J, Cane RD, Downs JB, et al. Airway pressure release ventilation during acute lung injury: A prospective multicenter trial. *Crit Care Med* 1991; 19:1234–1241.

48. Kirriloff LH, Owens GR, Rogers RM, Mazzocco MC. Does chest physical therapy work? *Chest* 1983; 83:621–627.

49. Shapiro BA, Cane RD, Harrison RA. Positive end-expiratory pressure therapy in adults with special reference to acute lung injury: Review of the literature and suggested clinical correlations. *Crit Care Med* 1984; 12:127–141.

50. Weisman IM, Rinaldo JE, Rogers RM. Positive end-expiratory pressure in adult respiratory failure. *N Engl J Med* 1982; 307:1381–1384.

51. Hakke R, Schlichtig R, Ulstad DR, Henschen RR. Barotrauma: Pathophysiology, risk factors, and prevention. *Chest* 1987; 91:608–613.

52. Pollack MM, Fields AI, Holbrook PR. Cardiopulmonary parameters during high PEEP in children. *Crit Care Med* 1980; 8:372–376.

53. Toussaint GPM, Burgess JH, Hampson LG. Central venous pressure and pulmonary wedge pressure in critical surgical illness. *Arch Surg* 1974; 109:265–269.

54. O'Quin R, Marini JJ. Pulmonary artery occlusion pressure: clinical physiology, measurement, and interpretation. *Am Rev Respir Dis* 1983; 128:319–326.

55. Shoemaker WC, Appel PL, Kram HB, Duarte D, Harrier HD, Ocampo HA. Comparison of hemodynamic and oxygen transport effects of dopamine and dobutamine in critically ill surgical patients. *Chest* 1989; 96:120–126.

56. Rackow EC, Falk JL, Fein IA, et al. Fluid resuscitation in shock: A comparison of cardiorespiratory effects of albumin, hetastarch and saline solutions in patients with hypovolemic shock. *Crit Care Med* 1983; 11:839–850.

57. Neumann M, Demling RH. Colloid vs crystalloid: A current perspective. *Intens Crit Care Dig* 1990; 9:3–6.

58. Bone RC. Treatment of adult respiratory distress syndrome with diuretics, dialysis, and positive end-expiratory pressure. *Crit Care Med* 1978; 6:136–139.

59. Simmons RS, Berdine GC, Seidenfeld JJ, et al. Fluid balance and the adult respiratory distress syndrome. *Am Rev Respir Dis* 1987; 135:924–929.

60. Humphrey H, Hall J, Sznajder I, Silverstein M, Wood L. Improved survival in ARDS patients asscoiated with a reduction in pulmonary capillary wedge pressure. *Chest* 1990; 97:1176–1180.

61. Russell JA, Ronco JJ, Lockhat D, Belzberg A, Kiess M, Dodek PM. Oxygen delivery and consumption and ventricular preload are greater in survivors than in nonsurvivors of the adult respiratory distress syndrome. *Am Rev Respir Dis* 1990; 141:659–665.

62. Mathru M, Cries DJ, Zecca A, Fareed J, Rooney MW, Rao TLK. Effect of fast vs slow intralipid infusion on gas exchange, pulmonary hemodynamics, and prostaglandin metabolism. *Chest* 1991; 99:426–429.

63. Faling LJ. New advances in diagnosing nosocomial pneumonia in intubated patients. Part I. *Am Rev Respir Dis* 1988; 137:253–255.

64. Seidenfeld JJ, Pohl DF, Bell RC, Harris GD, Johanson WG. Incidence, site, and outcome of infections in patients with the adult respiratory distress syndrome. *Am Rev Respir Dis* 1986; 134:12–16.

65. Hartenauer U, Thulig B, Diemer W, et al. Effect of selective flora suppression on colonization, infection, and mortality in critically ill patients: A one-year, prospective consecutive study. *Crit Care Med* 1991; 19:463–473.

66. Driks MR, Craven DE, Celli BR, et al. Nosocomial pneumonia in intubated patients given sucralfate as compare with antacids or histamine type 2 blockers. *N Engl J Med* 1987; 317:1376–1382.

67. Zapol WM, Snider MT, Hill JD, et al. Extracorporeal membrane oxygenation in severe acute respiratory failure: A randomized prospective study. *JAMA* 1979; 242:2193–2196.

68. Gattinoni L, Pesenti A, Mascheroni D, et al. Low-frequency positive–pressure ventilation with extracorporeal CO_2 removal in severe acute respiratory failure. *JAMA* 1986; 256:881–886.

69. Suchyta MR, Clemmer TP, Orme JF, Morris AH, Elliott CG. Increased survival of ARDS patients with severe hypoxemia (ECMO criteria). *Chest* 1991; 99:951–955.

69a. Rossaint R, Falke KJ, Lopez F, Slamak, Pison V, Zapol WM. Inhaled nitric oxide for the adult respiratory distress syndrome. *N Engl J Med* 1993; 328:399–405.

70. Ziegler ZJ, Fisher CJ, Sprung CL, et al. Treatment of gram–negative bacteremia and septic shock with HA-1A human monoclonal antibody against endotoxin. *N Engl J Med* 1991; 324:429–436.

71. Heffner JE, Repine JE. Pulmonary strategies of antioxidant defense. *Am Rev Respir Dis* 1989; 140:531–554.

72. Gotloib L, Barzilay E. The impact of using the artificial kidney as an artificial endocrine lung upon severe septic ARDS. *Intens Crit Care Dig* 1986; 5:3–5.

37

Pleural Effusions and Empyema

PAMELA L. ZEITLIN

ANATOMY AND PHYSIOLOGY OF THE PLEURAL SPACE

The accumulation of excess fluid in the pleural space can occur in both noninfectious and infectious disorders. Despite the large body of literature available on etiology and therapy of pleural effusions in the adult patient, the diagnosis and management of pleural effusions in the infant and child remain controversial.

DEVELOPMENT AND CELL BIOLOGY OF THE PLEURA

The pleural space is lined by membranes that form from the mesenchyme to separate the lungs from the chest wall, mediastinum, and diaphragm (1). The visceral pleural membrane covers the lungs, and the parietal pleural membrane lines the chest wall, mediastinum, and diaphragm. Both membranes are composed of a mesothelial cell layer with microvilli that lie enmeshed in a glycoprotein matrix that acts as a lubricant for the two surfaces (1, 2).

Lying beneath the mesothelial layer of the parietal pleura is a connective tissue layer supplied by pain fibers and systemic arteries. The submesothelial connective tissue of the visceral pleura is not innervated by pain fibers and is supplied by bronchial or pulmonary arteries. The visceral pleura is richly supplied with lymphatics that do not communicate with the pleural space but drain the lung parenchyma. The lymphatics of the parietal pleura recover pleural space protein through stomal pores (3).

PLEURAL FLUID PRODUCTION AND FUNCTION

The pleural space is normally filled with between 1 and 15 ml of an ultrafiltrate of plasma (4) that has a reduced protein level (5). The function of the pleura has been thought to couple the lungs to the chest wall, but pleurectomy alone has been shown to have no effect on pulmonary function (5).

Pleural fluid is produced by forces described by Starling in 1896. In this assumption bulk fluid movement is a consequence of a balance between filtration and reabsorption and can be described by Starling's law of transcapillary exchange (6):

$$F = k[(P_{cap}-P_{pl})-\sigma(p_{cap}-p_{pl})]$$

where F = rate of fluid movement, P and p = the hydrostatic and oncotic pressures, respectively, k = the filtration coefficient, s = the osmotic reflection coefficient for protein, cap = capillary, and pl = pleural space.

Classic measurements estimate that fluid is formed at about 100 ml/hour on the parietal side. The visceral pleura has the capacity to reabsorb a maximum of 300 ml/hour and lymphatics a maximum in the range of 250–500 ml/24 hours. A pleural effusion forms whenever the formation of fluid exceeds the removal. According to most sources, pleural fluid normally turns over at a rate of 1–2 L/day, but a very slow rate of 7 ml/day has been proposed (7).

Experimental work in sheep (8) supports the idea of systemic microcirculation as the source of pleural liquid. During fetal lung development, systemic arterial blood pressure increases and pulmonary artery pressure decreases. The microvascular protein barrier remains constant during development. Pleural/plasma protein concentration decreases as would be predicted for a model in which the microvascular protein barrier remained unchanged. Interestingly, the volume of pleu-

Table 37.2.
Procedure for Thoracentesis

Confirm presence of pleural fluid with decubitus radiograph

Position:	Seated, leaning forward over a pillow
Monitoring:	Pulse oximetry, person assigned to monitor vital signs and patient's status and to coach the child during the procedure.
Preparation:	Sterile field—universal precautions
Sedation:	Chloral hydrate Midazolam
Analgesia:	Local infiltration with xylocaine

Technique:	Use a large bore angiocath with a three-way stopcock attached. A 5- to 10-ml needle is attached to the stopcock.
	    Arrange so that stopcock is held in the palm and the thumb is placed 2–3 cm from the tip of the needle. This allows the thumb to act as stop when the needle enters the pleural space.
	    Identify the appropriate interspace. Usually, the 7th interspace is used and lies at the tip of the scapula in the posterior axillary line when the arm is elevated. The needle is aimed toward the center of the rib below the interspace. Make certain that the angle of insertion is perpendicular to the chest wall. Deviation from this angle can result in the needle passing along the outside of the pleural space. Upon entering the skin move the needle and skin up so the needle passes over the top of the rib and into the pleural space. Aspirate a small amount of fluid. Advance slightly to get the tip of the catheter into pleural space and then advance the catheter over the needle while holding the needle still. This places the catheter but not the needle deep into the pleural space. As the needle is withdrawn from the catheter place the left thumb over the catheter to prevent air leak. Reattach the stopcock and syringe to the catheter.
	    Aspirate several syringes of fluid for diagnostic tests and culture. The child may need to lean back to allow sufficient sample to be obtained. Once the sample is obtained, pull the catheter out and break up the tract. This technique creates "Z" tract and minimizes leakage.
	    Cover with sterile dressing of appropriate size.
	    Chest radiograph should be obtained following the procedure.

Specimen:	
Chemistry:	Protein, LDH, lipids, glucose
Cytology:	Cell count Cell block if malignancy is a consideration Gram stain
Culture:	*Bacteria:* Aerobes and anaerobes *Mycobacteria*

ered when tuberculosis and malignancy are under consideration or the pleural fluid contains a preponderance of monocytes.

MANAGEMENT OF TRANSUDATES

Nonspecific Effusions

Transudates accompany many common non-pulmonary clinical disorders (Table 37.1). Recognition of the systemic disease is essential since treatment of the effusion is based on treatment of the systemic disorder. The mechanisms underlying effusions varies with the condition. In patients with cirrhosis and ascites, a pleural effusion arises from penetration of the ascites fluid through defects in the diaphragm. There is also a high incidence of pleural effusion in the nephrotic syndrome (21%) (16). The predominant mechanism is believed to be pulmonary emboli.

Fetal and Neonatal Transudates

Pleural transudates can develop both pre- and post-natally. In the fetus, primary effusions are usually chylous, whereas secondary effusions are seen with the generalized fluid retention of non-immune hydrops. In utero, large pleural effusions prevent lung growth, and the degree of subsequent pulmonary hypoplasia is probably related to the time of onset (early onset is more critical), size, and duration of the pleural effusion. Longaker et al. (17) reviewed 32 cases to determine criteria for successful intervention. The presence of a unilateral effusion without a mediastinal shift, spontaneous resolution, and the absence of non-immune hydrops were associated with superior survival. Placement of thoraco-amniotic shunts provided better long-term drainage than serial aspirations and was associated with better survival (17, 18).

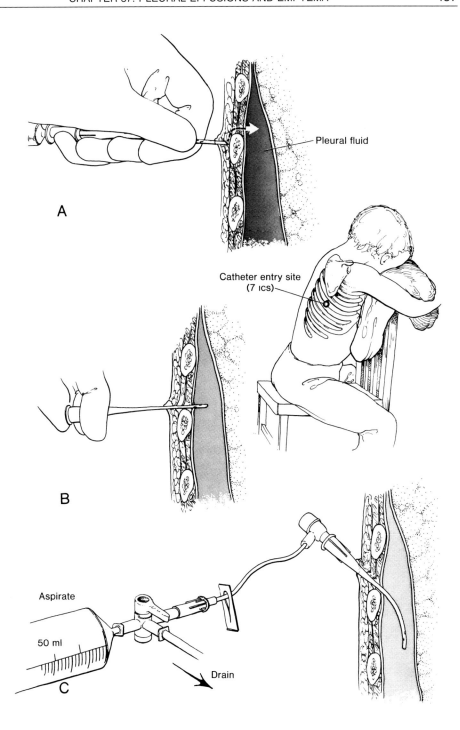

Figure 37.2. Approach to thoracentesis in a child. See Table 37.2 for detailed description.

Table 37.3.
Pleural Fluid Analysis

Test	Transudate	Exudate
pH	> 7.2	< 7.2
Protein P/S	< 0.5	> 0.5
LDH P/S	< 0.6	> 0.6
LDH IU	< 200	> 200
Amylase P/S	< 1	> 1
Glucose mg/dl	> 40	< 40
RBC	< 5000	> 5000
WBC	< 1000 monos	> 10,000 polys

P/S: pleural/serum.

Table 37.4.
Surgical Management of Pleural Effusions

Procedure	Objective
Thoracentesis	Diagnosis
Chest tube drainage, continuous	Reduce reaccumulation, drain empyema
Open thoracotomy with rib resection	Control of empyema
Decortication	Symptomatic chronic empyema, relief of thick fibrous peel
Pleurectomy	Control of chylothorax, malignant effusion

Extralobar pulmonary sequestration is associated with pleural effusion and fetal hydrops. It has been hypothesized (19) that obstruction of efferent lymphatic channels and veins leads to fluid accumulation, which then worsens lung compression and fetal hydrops through systemic venous obstruction.

Chylothorax in childhood is an uncommon, but potentially life-threatening condition, most often seen in association with surgical repair of congenital heart disease (20) and with trauma (21). It has been described after an event as trivial as coughing (22). Nontraumatic causes include neoplasia, subclavian vein thrombosis, mediastinal lymphangiectasia, generalized lymphangiomatosis (23), and parasitic infection.

As chyle accumulates in the pleural space, it compresses the lungs and compromises ventilation (Fig. 37.3). There is continuing debate over the relative efficacy of surgical and conservative medical management. Fluid should be removed for diagnosis, and a chest tube should be placed if it reaccumulates. If the patient is not on enteral feeding, the usually milky fluid will appear serous. In this case, the protein content will be similar to plasma and there will be an abundance of lymphocytes.

Conservative medical management consists of thoracentesis, chest tube drainage, and dietary modification usually consisting of a low-fat, high-protein diet supplemented with medium-chain triglycerides. The goal is to reduce thoracic duct lymph flow and allow the injury to heal. In one series of 15 children with chylothorax from a variety of causes, conservative management was successful in 10 (22). The median duration of leak was 12 days (varying from 4 to 64). Complications of this form of management as a consequence of persistent chyle drainage include nutritional depletion and weight loss, hypoproteinemia and hyponatremia, and immune deficiency secondary to lymphopenia.

Presence of an underlying lymphatic disorder, failure of conservative management after 3 weeks, or reaccumulation of chyle upon return to a normal diet are indications for surgical repair. When the site of the leak can be visualized, the thoracic duct is ligated. When the point of leakage is unclear, pleurodesis has been successful (22).

Iatrogenic Pleural Effusions

Pleural effusions are relatively common complications of a variety of routine therapeutic measures. Central venous catheters for intravenous access are associated with a risk of hydrothorax in adults and children. Perforation of the vessel is a well recognized complication at time of placement, but late perforations have been described (23). Hyper-osmolar fluid during the administration of total parenteral nutrition may contribute to vessel perforation (23). Therapy consists of pleural fluid drainage and removal of the central venous catheter. Ventriculopleural shunts placed for the treatment of hydrocephalus have also been associated with pleural effusions (Fig. 37.4) in the pediatric population.

An effusion that develops following surgical treatment of gastroesophageal reflux suggests the possibility of esophageal perforation, a complication of the Nissen fundoplication procedure (24). It has been suggested that it occurs more frequently in children < 2 years of age and in those with neurologic impairment. Although not all series bear this out (24), a high degree of suspicion in these groups should lead to immediate thoracentesis and radiographic studies. Fluid arising from esophageal perforation initially is a transudate,

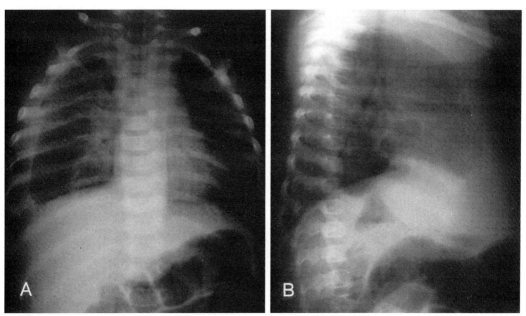

Figure 37.3. This right-sided pleural effusion was an incidental discovery on an abdomenal radiograph performed on a 2-month-old white male with a complaint of colic. There was no evidence of respiratory distress, and the patient was acyanotic when this chest radiograph was obtained. Fluid obtained by thoracentesis contained numerous mature lymphocytes. A diagnosis of congenital chylous effusion was made. The patient was managed by diet and the effusion had completely resolved by age 5 months.

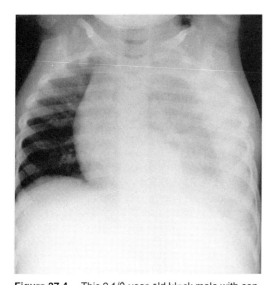

Figure 37.4. This 2 1/2-year-old black male with congenital hydrocephalus had a ventriculopleural shunt placed. One day later, a massive pleural effusion developed. This chest radiograph demonstrates a large left-sided effusion with mediastinal shift. The fluid obtained by thoracentesis was consistent with a transudate. Repeated drainage procedures were necessary.

but if it becomes infected, attains features of an exudate.

Continuous ambulatory peritoneal dialysis (CAPD) is complicated by the development of hydrothorax in 2% of pediatric cases (25, 26). In these patients, pleural effusion involves a combination of diaphragmatic defect (either eventration, gross defect, or microscopic perforations), lymphatic obstruction, and increased intraperitoneal pressures and volumes (27). Diagnosis is made by nuclear medicine scans or radiographic studies. In adults, repeated thoracentesis has been used successfully, but children may not tolerate repeated thoracentesis. If a trial of reduced dialysate volume is not immediately effective and a diaphragmatic defect has been identified, thoracotomy and diaphragm repair has been successful in controlling pleural effusion so that CAPD can be continued (27).

EXUDATES

Hemothorax

The most common cause of hemothorax in children is trauma, but hemothorax is also seen as a complication of subpleural pulmonary arteriovenous malformations (PAVMs) and malignancy. Treatment of choice for the PAVM is surgical resection or ligation. Embolotherapy has been used successfully (28–30).

Empyema

There are three phases in the natural history of an empyema. The *exudative phase* involves rapid accumulation of fluid with relatively low cell count and viscosity. The *fibrinopurulent phase* marks the appearance of pus and fibrin, during which loculation of fluid and compression of lung occur. The *organizing phase* is characterized by fibroblast activity on both pleural surfaces that induces a fibrous inelastic membrane (pleural peel) that encases the lung. If untreated, an empyema in this stage could spontaneously drain into the lung through a bronchopleural fistula or out through the chest wall (empyema necessatans).

MICROBIOLOGY OF EMPYEMA IN CHILDREN

The presence of a pleural exudate implies an active inflammatory process in the pleural space. When this becomes acutely infected with pathogenic bacteria, it can progress rapidly to an empyema. Empyema is recognizable by highly viscous material, white blood cell count greater than 100,000, and bacteria present on Gram stain. It must be drained as well as treated with antibiotics.

The three major organisms responsible for empyema in children and adolescents are *Staphylococcus aureus*, *Streptococcus pneumoniae*, and *Haemophilus influenzae*. These organisms account for 28%, 20%, and 13% of pleural fluid cultures in children and adolescents (32–48). Anaerobic bacteria have been demonstrated only rarely, and usually as a consequence of trauma, aspiration pneumonia, or extension of lung or subdiaphragmatic abscesses. Of anaerobic organisms detected, *Bacteroides* species were most frequently isolated, and the infections were often mixed. This is in marked contrast to parapneumonic effusions in adults where anaerobic organisms are those most frequently isolated from pleural fluid (49).

Pneumonia secondary to *Staphylococcus aureus* in children is very likely to have a culture-positive pleural effusion (80%) (49). *Streptococcus pyogenes*, although uncommon, is also likely to develop a culture positive effusion (33%) (Fig. 37.5). *Haemophilus influenzae* pneumonia in children is associated with a culture positive pleural fluid in 75% (49). Ten percent of children with *H. influenzae* pneumonia also develop empyema (50).

In every patient with pneumonia and an associated effusion, it is mandatory to evaluate the pleural fluid, since any delay in the institution of appropriate therapy for infected effusions substantially increases morbidity.

Most parapneumonic effusions will resolve with antibiotic administration alone (Fig. 37.6). Early identification of those children who require chest tube drainage is desirable. The factors that contribute to a complicated parapneumonic effusion requiring drainage include immunologic incompetence, the presence of staphylococcal or anaerobic infection, the presence of bacteria in the pleural space, the amount of fluid, and the presence of loculations.

There is no question that frank pus on diagnostic thoracentesis should be drained by thoracostomy tube. When the pleural fluid Gram stain is positive, the glucose is less than 40, or the pH is less than 7.00, a chest tube is almost certain to be required to facilitate clinical improvement. In the gray zone (pH 7.00–7.20, LDH over 1000) it is possible to succeed with serial thoracenteses and avoid a chest tube. If the child has a negative pleural fluid culture, a glucose over 40, and a pH over 7.2, a chest tube is rarely necessary.

The complications of chest tube drainage in children are formation of a bronchopleural fistula, exit site wound infections, and repeated replacement of tubes for failure to drain the effusion. In addition, a chest tube limits mobility and may interfere with effective coughing.

The usual course of empyema treated with chest tube drainage and antibiotics is resolution of the infection and reabsorption of the inflammatory material. Failure of conventional treatment is associated with major accompanying medical problems, cancer, esophageal perforation, and infradiaphragmatic abscess (47, 48). In children with refractory, symptomatic postpneumonic empyema, the role of lung decortication has been widely debated. Decortication consists of a thoracotomy, evacuation of intrapleural gelatinous debris and fibrin, and removal of the fibrinous

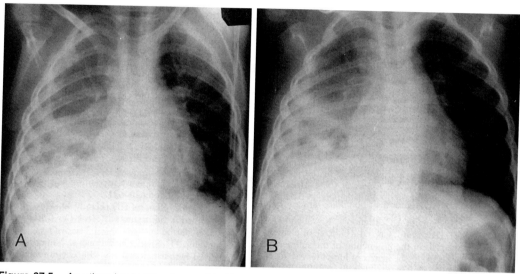

Figure 37.5. An otherwise healthy 3-year-old white female developed fever, pneumonia, and pleural effusion. The fluid obtained by thoracentesis was purulent, and both the fluid and blood cultures grew *Streptococcus pyogenes*. She responded to intravenous penicillin and continuous chest tube drainage. *A,* Left side down. *B,* Right side down. Note that the fluid was loculated in the right chest and did not significantly redistribute with changes in position of the patient.

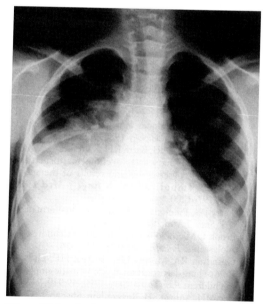

Figure 37.6. An 8-year-old black female with hemoglobin SC disease developed *Mycoplasma* pneumonia. Despite treatment with erythromycin and cefuroxime, she eventually required an exchange transfusion. Twelve days later, she had a persistent left pleural effusion and resolving bilateral pneumonia on chest radiograph. The patient improved on intravenous antibiotic therapy without continuous chest tube drainage. No organism was ever isolated.

peel from both pleural surfaces. This peel has been associated with prolonged tachypnea, asymmetric chest wall expansion, scoliosis, lung compression or atelectasis, slow resolution of parenchymal infiltrates, increased hospital stays, and prolonged febrile periods (38, 48). In more recent pediatric surgical reports, decortication has been shown to reduce hospital stays (35, 36). Mortality in pediatric patients managed by decortication has varied between 0 and 10% (37, 48). Nonetheless, since in most instances simple drainage and patience result in a complete recovery, decortication should be reserved for those pediatric cases complicated by associated major medical problems and refractory to conventional therapies.

LONG-TERM FOLLOW-UP

Studies of pulmonary function in children who have recovered from empyema have demonstrated essentially normal respiratory function. McLaughlin et al. (43) found some evidence of mild restrictive disease (reduced total lung capacity by plethysmography in five of eight children) and no obstructive lung disease. None had undergone thoracotomy or decortication. Redding et al. (44) performed spirometry and exercise testing in 15 children

be carried out with sensitivity to the feelings of the bereaved family and caregivers, and with appreciation that the incidence of infanticide among infants dying suddenly and unexpectedly is probably very low. The death scene investigators must be well informed about SIDS, child abuse, and grief reactions of parents, and must be aware of any bias they may have for or against any socioeconomic or ethnic groups or practices. Such personal bias must not influence the sensitivity, thoroughness, or conclusions of the death scene investigation.

INCIDENCE

The incidence of SIDS in the general population in the United States is between 1.5 and 2.0 per 1000 live births. As with total infant mortality, the risk of SIDS is significantly higher in African-American infants (3.7 per 1000 live births) than in Caucasian infants (1.1 per 1000 live births) (7). The incidence among Hispanic infants in the Chicago area was similar to the SIDS incidence in the non-Hispanic Caucasian infants in that population. Most studies have reported an increased incidence among American Indians (8).

The SIDS incidence reported for different populations worldwide demonstrates a variability of approximately 10 times. The highest rates are in the populations from the Antipodes in New Zealand, where the reported incidence is 4.9 per 1000 live births (3) and 4.4 per 1000 live births in the Australian state of Tasmania (14). The rate in Japan (1.2 per 1000 live births [1]) is lower than the rate in the United States, whereas the SIDS incidence in Great Britain is usually reported to be slightly higher (2.5 per 1000 live births [16]).

Table 38.1.
Risk Factors for SIDS

Maternal

Cigarette smoking
Young maternal age
Less prenatal care
Social deprivation

Infant

Low birth weight
Prematurity
Male
Sleeping prone
Multiple births

The age at death for SIDS cases shows a characteristic peak incidence during the 3rd month of life (17). Approximately 5% of SIDS cases occur in the first month, approximately 60% by the end of the third month, 85% by 6 months of age, and 99% by 1 year of age. The true incidence of SIDS in the first month of life has not been clearly established, since most studies omit death in the first week of life. Of the 1–10% of neonatal deaths that remain unexplained after careful autopsy examination (18), some may be SIDS cases.

An early winter peak in SIDS incidence is reported in almost all studies of the epidemiology of SIDS. More SIDS cases occur during the colder months of the year in both the northern and southern hemispheres. No correlation has been found between latitude and SIDS incidence (19, 20). The explanation of the seasonal variation is unknown, but it could be related to the increased rate of respiratory infections or the lower environmental temperature in the winter, or to the increased incidence of pre-term deliveries in the fall (21). This seasonal pattern of SIDS incidence persists even after controlling for the infant's race, sex, and age at death (22).

Although the incidence of SIDS can vary significantly from year to year, particularly in smaller populations, the overall incidence of SIDS has not changed significantly in the past 20 years (23, 24). Reports from Scandinavia suggest a slight increase in SIDS incidence recently (25), but this must be examined over a period of at least 5 years before definite conclusions can be drawn.

ETIOLOGY

Neither the etiology of SIDS nor the mechanisms by which SIDS infants die is known (26). The leading hypothesis involves primary failure of respiration due either to upper airway obstruction with or without impaired arousal, acute hypoventilation due to rebreathing of expired air (27), or prolonged central apnea. There is little support for primary cardiac arrythmia, although neurally mediated bradycardia as the primary event is a possibility (28). Although unlikely to explain most SIDS cases, it is thought that the rare infants whose death is attributed to SIDS may have died from botulism (29) or infanticide (30). The contribution of a metabolic disorder such as medium-chain acyl-coenzyme A dehydrogenase deficiency (MCAD deficiency) is unclear, but recent studies have suggested that it may contribute to 3% of SIDS cases (31, 32). There is recent interest in the as yet unsubstantiated hypothesis that hyperthermia may contribute to the death of SIDS infants (33).

Rather than considering that only a subgroup of the infant population as particularly vulnerable, a different approach to considering the etiology of SIDS is to view the 2- to 4-month age range as a time when all infants are more vulnerable to death. In other words, SIDS may occur because of a vulnerable stage in the development of all infants when they are particularly susceptible to small insults that would not be life-threatening at other ages. This vulnerable period would most likely be explained by desynchronous functional development of various components of the central nervous system (CNS), resulting in windows of particular vulnerability to cardiorespiratory depression, particularly during sleep.

Postmortem Studies of SIDS Victims

ROUTINE AUTOPSY

An autopsy must be performed to establish a diagnosis of SIDS. Ten to twenty percent of sudden unexpected deaths are explained by a careful routine autopsy. The autopsy is performed to rule out identifiable causes of sudden unexpected death such as intracranial hemorrhage, sepsis, meningitis, dehydration, myocarditis, severe pneumonia, and trauma. Among those cases in which no obvious cause of death is apparent from the clinical history, death scene investigation, or autopsy, there is a spectrum of histologic abnormality ranging from none, to minor localized inflammation in the upper or lower respiratory tract, to a positive viral culture for rhinovirus or CMV, to significant but localized evidence of inflammation and/or infection that is not felt to be a sufficient cause of death. For purposes of family counseling, it is best to err on the side of overusing the SIDS diagnosis in these unclear cases, to avoid falsely implying to the family that if they had been more observant they might have been able to avoid the infant's death. From the perspective of public health, it is less critical whether a death is completely unexplained than whether it is sudden and unexpected, since the goal is to identify an appropriate system or intervention that will decrease the risk of all sudden unexpected deaths. From the perspective of SIDS research, however, it is very important to establish standardized criteria by which the SIDS diagnosis is to be established in cases with minor or moderate histologic abnormality but no obvious cause of death, so that the similarities or dissimilarities between different study populations can be appreciated.

There are no findings diagnostic of SIDS on routine autopsy (34). Nonspecific findings such as mild pulmonary edema, vascular congestion, or pulmonary inflammation are commonly found. Intrathoracic petechiae are present by visual inspection on the visceral surfaces of the heart, lungs, and thymus in approximately 80% of SIDS victims (35). Microscopic examination reveals intrathoracic petechiae in an even higher percentage of SIDS victims. Although intrathoracic petechiae are not unique to SIDS, their localization to the thoracic cavity has led to the unproven hypothesis that they result from inspiratory efforts against an occluded upper airway. Krous and Jordan analyzed the thoraco-abdominal distribution of petechiae in patients dying of a variety of different causes and found that, with few exceptions, petechiae were limited to the thoracic cavity only in SIDS and cases of lethal upper airway obstruction (36). Failure of the left ventricle could also theoretically explain the thoracic distribution of petechiae in SIDS victims.

SPECIALIZED POSTMORTEM STUDIES

Studies of autopsy material from SIDS victims have demonstrated some group postmortem differences between SIDS victims and control infants who have died of other causes. The most appropriate control infants are healthy infants who have an abrupt accidental death. Since such tragedies are rare, many investigators have used less appropriate controls. Of the many reported histologic or biochemical differences between SIDS and controls, only a small number have been well established and consistently confirmed. These "tissue markers" of SIDS have no role in the diagnosis of SIDS since they do not occur in all cases of SIDS, nor are they specific to SIDS. They are, however, statistically more common in SIDS cases than in control infants.

None of the tissue differences between SIDS and control infants have been unequivocally confirmed. However, those which are most consistently reported include increased extramedullary hematopoiesis, prolonged retention of periadrenal brown fat, qualitative abnormalities of pulmonary surfactant, brain stem gliosis, and a greater density of dendritic spines in the CNS of SIDS infants than in controls (37). Each of these findings is consistent with the hypothesis that a SIDS death is preceded by recurrent or chronic hypoxia, but this hypothesis remains unproven. SIDS victims also have a higher incidence of minor dysmorphic lesions and minor congenital anomalies (38).

Although the CNS findings are intriguing, since some of them involve structures active in the control of respiration, it is not known whether these CNS changes are the cause of respiratory control abnormalities, the results of recurrent hypoxia or ischemia, or merely a chance association due to the presence of some other confounding variables (39). Surfactant abnormalities (e.g., lower concentration of phosphatidylcholine), although not consistent, have been confirmed in several studies (40). However, in a study of the pressure volume characteristics of lungs from SIDS infants, there was no evidence of any functional correlate of this biochemical abnormality; thus the significance of the surfactant difference remains unclear (41).

No single organism has been consistently found to be more frequent in SIDS victims than in an appropriate control population (42), so the role of infection in SIDS is yet to be elucidated.

Studies of growth in SIDS victims have rather consistently demonstrated that the SIDS victims have lower birth weights than controls (43, 44). This difference, which averages about 300 g, persists after controlling for race, maternal smoking, and, in some studies, gestational age. There is conflicting data as to whether postnatal growth of SIDS victims is normal, although it appears most likely that when controlled for confounding variables, the postnatal growth rate of SIDS infants is slightly slower than that of controls (44).

Although none of the tissue differences have been incontrovertibly established, it is likely that as a group, SIDS infants do have some tissue differences from appropriate controls.

It is unclear whether these differences are primarily related to the cause or mechanism of SIDS.

EPIDEMIOLOGY

Epidemiologic studies have identified a variety of environmental, clinical, and demographic characteristics of mothers, infants, and the events themselves that are associated with an increased incidence of SIDS (45). Although some studies were well designed, implemented, and analyzed, there is a larger number of studies that are sufficiently defective as to invalidate the results. The minimal criteria for an acceptable, epidemiologic SIDS study are as follows:

1. It is population based.
2. The SIDS definition must be clearly stated and acceptable.
3. All SIDS cases must be confirmed by autopsy.
4. There must be appropriately selected control infants.
5. The study group should consist of SIDS infants, not simply all sudden unexpected infant deaths.

The SIDS risk factors summarized below and in Table 38.2 are those that have been most consistently identified and are most likely to be independent risk factors. An increase in SIDS incidence is consistently associated with younger maternal age (46, 47) and, independently, with increasing parity (48). Both of these risk factors retain their statistical significance after controlling for socioeconomic status and race. Maternal smoking is another one of the most consistent and strong risk factors for SIDS, conferring a relative risk of 2.5 to 3.0 in comparison to nonsmoking mothers (12). Although slightly weaker, the association remains significant after adjustment for birth weight and social factors. The effect of

Table 38.2.
Clinical Populations at High Risk for SIDS

Percentage of SIDS Population		SIDS per 1000 Infants
5%	Apparent life-threatening event (ALTE)	20–70
25%	Low birth weight	5–10
<1%	SIDS siblings	7–8

maternal smoking is stronger for SIDS infants who die in the first 3 months of life than for older SIDS infants, in contrast to most of the other risk factors, which confer higher risks in older SIDS. Smoking by the mother's partner confers a lesser but statistically significant increased risk, suggesting that postnatal exposure to cigarette smoke (passive smoking) contributes in some way to the occurrence of SIDS. Maternal anemia is a risk factor for SIDS in smoking mothers but not in nonsmoking mothers. (49) Other maternal factors that have been consistently associated with SIDS include social deprivation (50) and less parental care (50).

Approximately 60% of SIDS infants are male. Other risk factors, related to the infant, include low birth weight (48), prematurity (16), and being one of a multiple birth (51). Both prematurity and multiple birth remain significantly associated with SIDS after adjustment for birthweight and race. Adjustment for smoking does not eliminate the significant association of SIDS with low birth weight or prematurity. Low birth weight also remains significant after adjustment for race and gestational age. Although breast feeding probably conveys a slight protection against SIDS (52), maternal use of illicit drugs during pregnancy probably increases SIDS risk (53). It has not been clearly established that these associations are primary and not due to some confounding variable.

A number of prenatal, neonatal, maternal, and postnatal risk factors have been found to be significantly associated with increased SIDS risk. One of the most controversial factors deals with sleeping position. In the West, infants are placed in the prone position because of a fear of vomiting and aspiration during sleep. However, in Hong Kong, fear of suffocation has prompted use of the supine position for sleeping infants. Interestingly, a study from Hong Kong reported an incidence of SIDS which was one of the lowest in the world (9). SIDS victims were more likely to sleep in the prone position than control infants. Similarly, two large controlled studies from Australia and New Zealand have demonstrated an association between the prone position and an increased risk of SIDS (odds ratio = 3.14 and 3.53). After adjusting for confounding variables, the adjusted odds ratio for SIDS risk and prone sleeping position was

increased (54, 55). The mechanisms underlying this association are unknown but may involve nasopharyngeal airway obstruction or altered heat loss capabilities of the infant. Clearly, more research is needed (56). Nonetheless, a recent statement by the American Academy of Pediatrics supported placing healthy infants in the supine or side-lying position, except for premature infants with respiratory disease, infants with gastroesophageal reflux, and infants with upper airway obstruction or anomalies.

In the most developed countries, approximately 65% of all SIDS deaths occur during the winter months (14). Despite anecdotal reports to the contrary, SIDS is not associated with DPT immunization (58, 59). Similarly, the presence of minor clinical symptoms has no role in identifying infants at high risk for SIDS, because of the high prevalence of minor clinical symptoms and the low occurrence of SIDS (60).

The incidence of SIDS among subsequent siblings of SIDS victims is consistently reported to be three to five times greater than the SIDS risk in the general population (61, 62). It is not known whether this increased risk is due to a greater frequency of adverse social and environmental influences, due to a very small subgroup of SIDS cases with a strong genetic influence, or due to a small genetic influence on the overall population of SIDS siblings. Although still unresolved, it seems most likely that there is not a general genetic predisposition to SIDS.

Definition of true SIDS risk factors have important implications for the identification of the etiology of SIDS, and for identification of appropriate interventions that might decrease the incidence of SIDS. There is much similarity between the risk factors for SIDS and the risk factors for other pediatric morbidity and mortality (63). In Seattle (23) and in Copenhagen (24), there are good data to indicate that over a period of approximately 20 years, the SIDS incidence was constant despite decreases in some important risk factors (e.g., births to teenage mothers, multiple births, and low-birth-weight infants). Therefore, diminishing the frequency of adverse risk factors will not necessarily diminish the incidence of SIDS.

Physiologic Studies

A limited number of recordings of cardiorespiratory function have been obtained on infants who subsequently succumbed to SIDS. Most of the papers published on this subject use data from some of the 16 full-term SIDS victims and the control infants selected from Southall's study of 6914 normal full-term infants who had 24-hour cardiorespiratory recordings made in the first 6 weeks of life (64). In comparison to controls, the SIDS victims recordings demonstrated fewer short apneas in the second month of life, increased heart rate in the first 2 months of life, and decreased heart rate variability (65, 66).

Prospective Identification of Infants at High Risk for SIDS

Three approaches to prospective, clinically feasible identification of infants at high risk for SIDS have been used. The first of these was the rather widespread analysis of 2- to 24-hour hardcopy cardiorespiratory recordings (pneumograms) to identify infants with increased breathing pattern irregularities or bradycardia (68). The fallacy of this approach is that there has never been any definitive demonstration that increased amounts of periodic breathing or increased numbers of respiratory pauses are associated with an increased risk of subsequent SIDS. In fact, the physiologic studies reviewed above indicate that premortem respiratory studies on SIDS victims would not demonstrate increased respiratory irregularity. Thus, there is no basis for the use of pneumograms to identify infants at high risk for SIDS.

A second approach has been to develop, based on the epidemiologic studies reviewed above, scoring systems that could be used in early life to identify those infants who are at significantly increased risk of SIDS. The two systems that have been most widely used, the Sheffield Birth Score (69) and the Oxford score (66, 70), identify populations with a twofold to fourfold increased risk of SIDS compared to the general population. Approximately 20% of all births are identified as high risk. In the absence of any intervention with proven efficacy for SIDS prevention, these high rates of false positivity and false negativity argue against clinical usefulness for these scoring systems at this time.

The third approach to clinically useful, prospective identification of infants at high risk for SIDS has been to evaluate the SIDS risk in infants with specific clinical diagnoses (Table 38.2). It is of particular clinical usefulness if subgroups of infants within these diagnostic groups can be identified with very high or low risk of SIDS. For example, infants who experience apparent life-threatening events that occur during sleep and are reported to require resuscitation have an 8–10% risk of dying subsequently despite the prescription of home monitors (71). Infants who have more than one of these severe spells may have a risk as high as 28% (72). Although premature infants as a group have an increased risk of SIDS (16), the greatest risk is in infants with birth weights under 1 kg. Neither apnea of prematurity (53) nor bronchopulmonary dysplasia are risk factors for SIDS, although bronchopulmonary dysplasia is a risk factor for postneonatal mortality (73). Although some of these subgroups have quite high risks of SIDS, they do not account for the majority of SIDS cases (74) (Fig. 38.1). Only about 5% of SIDS victims have been noted to experience apparent life-threatening events; less than 1% of SIDS are subsequent siblings of SIDS victims; and about 18% of SIDS cases have been born prematurely.

SIDS PREVENTION

There is no intervention that has been proven to decrease the incidence of SIDS. Home cardiorespiratory monitors, usually employing the thoracic impedance technology, have been used most widely. The explanation for the absence of any decrease in SIDS incidence with the use of home monitoring may be that adequate numbers of the appropriate infants have not been monitored, or that some significant percentage of SIDS victims will succumb despite resuscitative efforts, or that home monitor use is not effective in decreasing infant deaths (75). In at least half of the reported cases wherein infants died despite the prescription of home monitors, the monitor was not being used properly or the resuscitative efforts were not properly initiated (76), although some infants have died despite prompt initiation of apparently correct cardiopulmonary resuscitation, even in hospitals. Other interventions such as increased home visits by community health nurses (77) and

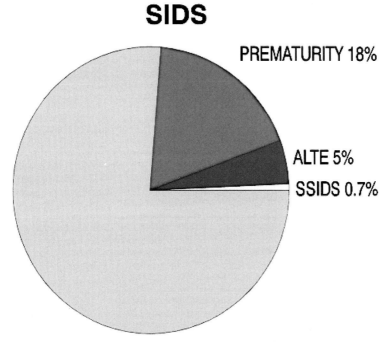

Figure 38.1. Representation of the contribution of certain at-risk populations to the overall incidence of SIDS.

the practice of carefully weighing the infant each day have not been validated (78).

MANAGEMENT OF THE FAMILY AFFECTED BY SIDS

The loss of an infant to SIDS is a devastating experience for family, caretakers, and health providers (79). The physician's role is to remain informed about SIDS, to ensure that a thorough autopsy is performed on all sudden unexpected infant deaths, to see that the family is provided with accurate, appropriate information about SIDS, and to see that opportunities for ongoing support and counseling are offered. Appropriate discussions and support should be provided to all family members, including the father (80). The common bereavement reaction of shock, denial, anger, and sadness should be discussed with the family. Current information about SIDS and local counseling and support groups can be obtained through the National SIDS Alliance (1-800-221-SIDS).

REFERENCES

1. Bergman, et al. *Proceedings of the Second International Conference on Causes of Sudden Death in Infants.* Seattle, University of Washington Press, 1970, p 18.
2. Taylor EM, Emery JL. Categories of preventable unexpected infant deaths. *Arch Dis Child* 1990; 65:535–539.
3. Jones AM, Weston JR. The examination of the sudden infant death syndrome infant: Investigative and autopsy protocols. *J Forens Sci* 1976; 21:833–841.
4. Wigglesworth JS, et al. Pathological investigations in cases of sudden infant death. J Clin Pathol 1987; 40:1481–1483.
5. Zylke JW. Sudden infant death syndrome: resurgent research offers hope. *JAMA* 1989; 262:1565–1566.
6. Smialek JE, Lambros Z. Investigation of Sudden Infant Deaths. *Pediatrician* 1988; 15:191–197.
7. Black L, David RJ, Brouillette RT, Hunt CE. Effects of birth weight and ethnicity on incidence of sudden infant death syndrome. *J Pediatr* 1986; 108:209–214.
8. Bulterys M. High incidence of sudden infant death syndrome among northern Indians and Alaska natives compared with southwestern Indians: Possible role of smoking. *J Commun Health* 1990; 15.
9. Davies DP: Cot death in Hong Kong: A rare problem? *Lancet* 1985; 2:1346–1349.
10. Winter ST, Emetarom NB. Sudden Infant Death: A pilot inquiry into its frequency in Israel. *Isr J Med Sci* 1973; 9:447.
11. Bloch A: SIDS in the Ashelon district: A 10–year survey. *Isr J Med Sci* 1973; 9:452.
12. Haglund B, Cnattingius S. Cigarette smoking as a risk factor for sudden infant death syndrome: A population-based study. *Am J Public Health* 1990; 80:29–32.
13. Hassal LB. SIDS, a serious New Zealand health problem. *N Z Med J* 1986; 99:233–234.

14. McGlashan ND. Sudden infant death in Tasmania, 1980–86: A seven year prospective study. *Soc Sci Med* 1989; 19:1015–1026.

15. Naito J. Study on infants' sudden death: Infants' sudden death in Hokkaido and Kyushu [Japanese]. Report of the studies of the Nippon Auku Research Institute, No. 12, pp. 83–93, 1976.

16. Golding J, Limerick S, Macfarlane A. *Sudden infant death: Patterns, puzzles and problems.* Seattle, University of Washington Press, 1985.

17. Goldberg J, Hornung R, Yamashita T, Wehrmacher W. Age at death and risk factors in sudden infant death syndrome. *Aust Paediatr J* 1986; Suppl:21–28.

18. Valdes-Dapena MA, Arey JB. The causes of neonatal mortality: An analysis of 501 autopsies on newborn infants. *J Pediatr* 1970; 77:366–375.

19. Spiers PS, Schlesselman JJ, Wright SG. Sudden infant death syndrome in the United States: A study of geographic and other variables. *Am J Epidemiol* 1974;100:380.

20. Peterson DR, Thompson DJ, Chinn NM. A method of assessing the geographic distribution and temporal trends of the sudden infant death syndrome from vital statistics data. *Am J Epidemiol* 1974; 100:373.

21. Cooperstock M, Wolfe RA. Seasonality of preterm birth in the Collaborative Perinatal Project: Demographic factors. *Am J Epidemiol* 1986; 124:234.

22. Anonymous. Seasonality in Sudden Infant Death Syndrome [Editorial]. *JAMA* 1990; 265:708.

23. Peterson DR. Clinical implications of Sudden Infant Death Syndrome: Epidemiology. *Pediatrician* 1988; 15:198–203.

24. Jorgensen T, Biering-Sorensen Hilden J. Sudden infant death in Copenhagen 1956–1971. III. Perinatal and perimortal factors. *Acta Paediatr Scand* 1979; 68:11.

25. Irgens LM, et al. Secular trends of SIDS & other causes of post perinatal mortality in Norweigian birth cohorts 1967–84. *Acta Paediatr Scand* 1989; 78:228–32.

26. Willinger M. Research reviews: SIDS—A challenge. *J NIH Res* 1989; 1:73–80.

27. Kemp JS, Thach BT. Sudden death in infants sleeping on polystyrene-filled cushions. *N Engl J Med* 1991; 324:1858–1864.

28. Kelly DH, Pathak A, Meny R. Sudden severe bradycardia in infancy. *Pediatr Pulmonol* 1991; 10:199–204.

29. Sonnabend OA, Sonnabend WF, Krech U, Molz G, Sigrist T. Continuous microbiological and pathological study of 70 sudden and unexpected infant deaths: Toxigenic intestinal Clostridium botulinum infection in 9 cases of SIDS. *Lancet* 1985; 1:237.

30. Meadow R. Suffocation, recurrent apnea, and sudden infant death. *J Pediatr* 1990; 117:351–357.

31. Rinaldo P, O'Shea JJ, Coates PM, Hale DE, Stanley CA, Tanaka K. Medium-chain ACYL-CoA dehydrogenase deficiency—Diagnosis by stable-isotope dilution measurement of urinary n-Hexanoylglycine and 3-Phenylpropionylclycine. *N Engl J Med* 1988; 319:1308–1313.

32. Bennett MJ, Allison F, Pollit CJ, Varend S. Fatty acid oxidation defects as causes of unexpected death in infancy. In Tanaka R, Coates PM, eds. *Fatty acid oxidation: Clinical, biochemical and molecular aspects.* New York, Alan R. Liss, 1990, pp 349–364.

33. Fleming PJ, Gilbert R, Azaz Y, et al. Interaction between bedding and sleeping position in the sudden infant death syndrome: A population-based case-control study. *Br Med J* 1990; 301:85–89.

34. Krous HF. Pathological considerations of sudden infant death syndrome. *Pediatrician* 1988; 15:231–239.

35. Krous HF, Catron AC, Farber JP. The microscopic distribution of intrathoracic petechiae in SIDS. *Arch Pathol Lab Med* 1984; 108:77.

36. Krous HF, Jordan J. A necropsy study of distribution of petechiae in non-sudden infant death syndrome. *Arch Pathol Lab Med* 1984; 108:75–76.

37. Molz G, Hartman H. Dysmorphism, dysplasia and anomaly in sudden infant death [Letter]. *N Engl J Med* 1984; 26:259.

38. Krous HF. The pathology of sudden infant death syndrome: An overview. In Culbertson JL, Krows HF, Bendell RD, eds. Sudden infant death syndrome. Baltimore, Johns Hopkins University Press, 1989, pp 18–47.

39. Kinney HC, Filiano JJ. Brainstem research in sudden infant death syndrome. *Pediatrician* 1988; 15:240–250.

40. James D, Berry PJ, Fleming P, Hathaway M. Surfactant abnormality and the sudden infant death syndrome—A primary or secondary phenomenon? *Arch Dis Child* 1990; 65:774–778.

41. Fagan DG, Milner AD. Pressure volume characteristics of the lungs in sudden infant death syndrome. *Arch Dis Child* 1985; 60:471–485.

42. Anonymous. Respiratory infection and sudden infant death [Editorial]. *Lancet* 1989; 2:1191–1192.

43. Buck GM, Cookfair DL, Michalek AM, et al. Intrauterine growth retardation and risk of sudden infant death syndrome (SIDS). *Am J Epidemiol* 1989; 129:874–884.

44. Williams SM, Taylor BJ, Ford RPK, Nelson AS. Growth velocity before sudden infant death. *Arch Dis Child* 1990; 65:1315–1318.

45. Kraus FJ, Bulterys M. The epidemiology of sudden infant death syndrome. In Kiely M, ed. *MDIU Reproductive and perinatal epidemiology.* Ann Arbor, Boston, CRC Press, 1990, pp 220–243.

46. Peterson DR, van Belle G, Chinn NM. Sudden infant death syndrome and maternal age: Etiologic implications. *JAMA* 1982; 247:2250.

47. Arsenault PS. Maternal and antenatal factors in the risk of sudden infant death syndrome. *Am J Epidemiol* 1980; 111:279–284.

48. Kraus JF, Franti CE, Borhani NO. Discriminatory risk factors in post-neonatal sudden unexplained death. *Am J Epidemiol* 1972; 96:328.

49. Bulterys MG, Greenland S, Kraus JF. Chronic fetal hypoxia and sudden infant death syndrome: Interaction between maternal smoking and low hematocrit during pregnancy. *Pediatrics* 1990; 86:535–540.

50. Standfast SJ, Jereb S, Janerich DT. The epidemiology of sudden infant death in Upstate New York. II: Birth characteristics. *Am J Public Health* 1980; 70:1061–1067.

51. Kraus JF, Borhani NO. Post-neonatal sudden unexplained death in California: A cohort study. *Am J Epidemiol* 1972; 95:497.

52. Damus K, Pakter J, Krongrad E, Standfast SJ, Hoffman HF: Postnatal medical and epidemiological risk

factors for the sudden infant death syndrome. In Harper RM, Hoffman HJ, eds. *MDIU Sudden infant death syndrome: Risk factors and basic mechanisms.* New York, PMA Publishing, 1988, pp 187–201.

53. Hillman L, Hoffman HF. Maternal and newborn medical risk factors for the sudden infant death syndrome. In Harper RM, Hoffman HJ, eds. *MDIU Sudden infant death syndrome: Risk factors and basic mechanisms.* New York, PMA Publishing, 1988, pp 177–186.

54. Dwyer T, Ponsonby AB, Newman NM, Gibbons LE. Prospective cohort study of prone sleeping position and sudden infant death sysndrome. *Lancet* 1991; 337:1244–1247.

55. Mitchell EA, Scragg R, Stewart AW, et al. Cot death supplement: Results from the first year of the New Zealand cot death study. *N Z Med J* 1991; 104:71–76.

56. Guntheroth WG, Spiers PS. Sleeping prone and the risk of sudden infant death syndrome. *JAMA* 1992; 267:2359–2362.

57. AAP Task Force on Infant Positioning and SIDS. Positioning and SIDS. *Pediatrics* 1992; 89:1120–1126.

58. Hoffman HF, Hunter JC, Damus K, et al. Diphtheria-Tetanus-Pertussis immunization and sudden infant death: results of the National Institute of Child Health and Human Development Cooperative Epidemiological Study of sudden infant death syndrome risk factors. *Pediatrics* 1987; 79:598–611.

59. Griffin MR, Ray WA, Livengood JR, Schaffner W. Risk of sudden infant death syndrome after immunization with the Diphtheria Tetanus Pertussis vaccine. *N Engl J Med* 1988; 319:618–623.

60. Gilbert RE, Fleming FJ, Azaz Y, Rudd PT. Signs of illness preceding sudden unexpected death in infants. *Br Med J* 1990; 300:1237–1239.

61. Peterson DR, et al. Infant mortality among subsequent siblings of infants who died of sudden infant death syndrome. *J Pediatr* 1986; 108:911–914.

62. Guntheroth WG, Lohmann R, Spiers PS. Risk of sudden infant death syndrome in subsequent siblings. J Pediatr 1990; 116:520–524.

63. Golding J, Peters TJ. What else do SIDS risk prediction scores predict? Early Hum Develop 1985; 12:247–260.

64. Southall DP, et al. Identification of infants destined to die unexpectedly during infancy: Evaluation of predictive importance of prolonged apnea and disorders of cardiac rhythm or conduction. Br Med J 1983; 286:1092–1096.

65. Kahn A, Blum D, Rebuffat E, et al. Polysomnographic studies of infants who subsequently died of sudden infant death syndrome. *Pediatrics* 1988; 82:721–727.

66. Schectman VL, Harper RM, Kluge KA, Wilson AJ, Hoffman HF, Southall DP. Cardiac and respiratory patterns in normal infants and victims of the sudden infant death syndrome. In *MDIU Sleep.* New York, Raven Press, 1988; 11:413, 424.

67. Schechtman VL, Harper RM, Wilson AJ, Southhall DP. Sleep apnea in infants who succumb to the sudden infant death syndrome. *Pediatrics* 1991; 87:841–846.

68. Rahilly RM. Pneumographic studies: predictors of future apneas but not sudden infant death in asymptomatic infants. *Aust Paediatr J* 1989; 25:211–214.

69. Carpenter RG, Emery JL. Identification and follow-up of infants at risk of sudden death in infancy. *Nature* 1974; 250:729.

70. Peters TJ, Golding J. Prediction of SIDS: An independent evaluation of four scoring methods. *Stat Med* 1986; 5:113.

71. Kelly DH, Shannon DC. Sudden infant death syndrome and near sudden infant death syndrome: A review of the literature, 1964–1982. *Pediatr Clin North Am* 1982; 29:1241–1261.

72. Oren J, et al. Identification of high risk group for sudden infant death syndrome among infants who were resuscitated for sleep apnea. *Pediatrics* 1986; 77:495–499.

73. Abman SH, Burchell MF, Schaffer MS, Rosenberg AA. Late sudden unexpected deaths in hospitalized infants with bronchopulmonary dysplasia. *Am J Dis Child* 1989; 143:815–819.

74. Brooks JG. Infantile apnea and home monitoring. *Pediatrician* 1988; 15:212–216.

75. Davies PA, Milner AD, Silverman M, Simpson H. Monitoring and sudden infant death syndrome: An update. *Arch Dis Child* 1990; 65:238–240.

76. Ward SL, Keens TG, Chan LS, et al. Sudden infant death syndrome in infants evaluated by apnea programs in California. *Pediatrics* 1986; 77:451–458.

77. Madeley RJ, Hull D, Holland T. Prevention of postneonatal mortality. *Arch Dis Child* 1986; 61:459–463.

78. Emery JL, Waite AJ, Carpenter RG, Limerick SR, Blake D. Apnea monitors compared with weighing scales for siblings after cot death. *Arch Dis Child* 1985; 60:1055–1060.

79. Mandell F, McClain M. Supporting the SIDS family. *Pediatrician* 1988; 15:179–182.

80. Mandell F, Dirks-Smith T, Fallon-Smith M. The surviving child in the SIDS family. *Pediatrician* 1988; 15:217–221.

39

Obstructive Sleep Apnea Syndrome

CAROLE L. MARCUS and JOHN L. CARROLL

When the first detailed description of the obstructive sleep apnea syndrome (OSAS) was published in 1976, it was considered to be rare (1). However, since that time it has become apparent that OSAS is a common condition in children, and an important cause of morbidity. The classic condition was described by William Osler in 1892: "Chronic enlargement of the tonsillar tissues is an affectation of great importance, and may influence in an extraordinary way the mental and bodily development of children. . . At night the child's sleep is greatly disturbed; the respirations are loud and snorting, and there are sometimes prolonged pauses, followed by deep, noisy inspirations. The child may wake up in a paroxysm of shortness of breath" (2).

OSAS in children differs significantly from that in adults (Table 39.1). These differences must be kept in mind when applying to children data derived from studies in adults.

TERMINOLOGY

Apnea may be central or obstructive. *Obstructive apnea* is the cessation of airflow at the nose and mouth despite respiratory efforts. This is distinct from *central apnea*, wherein cessation of airflow is not accompanied by respiratory effort. Many children with this disorder actually exhibit partial airway obstruction, associated with hypoxia and hypoventilation, rather than complete airway obstruction; this has been termed *obstructive hypoventilation*. In the pediatric literature, the term "obstructive hypoventilation" is used in preference to *hypopnea*, which means a reduction in airflow. The spectrum of abnormalities, from obstructive hypoventilation to obstructive apnea, is referred to as the *obstructive sleep apnea syndrome (OSAS)*. The term *primary snoring* is used to describe children with habitual snoring not associated with obstructive apnea, hypoxia, or hypoventilation. The phrase *sleep-disordered breathing* is often used to describe any ventilatory abnormalities occurring during sleep, including but not limited to OSAS.

EPIDEMIOLOGY

Age has an important effect on breathing during sleep. OSAS is more common in adults than in children, and the prevalence of OSAS in adults increases with age. Habitual snoring is common in childhood, and occurs in 7–9% of preschool and school-aged children (3, 4). A preliminary report suggests that OSAS is present in approximately 2% of 4- to 5-year-old children (4). OSAS occurs in children of all ages, including neonates. The peak incidence, mirroring the peak age of adenotonsillar hypertrophy, occurs between 3 and 6 years of age. In prepubertal children, it occurs equally among boys and girls (5). However, OSAS in adults occurs predominantly in males and postmenopausal females (6, 7). The administration of exogenous testosterone is known to result in OSAS (8, 9), suggesting that androgens play a role in the pathophysiology of OSAS, and that female sex hormones may play a protective role. The mechanism of androgen action in this respect is unknown. There is a familial tendency to OSAS (10–13). A preliminary report in a Japanese cohort described an association between OSAS and a specific HLA type (HLA-A2) (14). The prevalence of OSAS in different ethnic groups is not known.

NORMAL UPPER AIRWAY ANATOMY AND PHYSIOLOGY DURING SLEEP

In order to understand OSAS, it is necessary to have an understanding of sleep architecture,

475

and the normal ventilatory changes associated with sleep.

The normal upper airway is a complex area consisting of more than 30 pairs of muscles (38). Nasal resistance accounts for nearly half of the total airway resistance. The pharynx is collapsible, in order to facilitate phonation and swallowing. However, other than the transient closure associated with the above functions, the pharynx normally remains patent.

Sleep Architecture

At sometime between 2 and 6 months of age, sleep can be divided into *non-rapid eye movement (NREM)* and *rapid eye movement (REM)* sleep. Younger infants have less well-defined electroencephalogram (EEG) patterns. The proportion of each stage of sleep varies with age. NREM sleep is subdivided into stage 1 (drowsiness), stage 2, and slow wave sleep (stages 3 and 4). REM sleep, during which dreaming occurs, is associated with rapid eye movements, skeletal muscle hypotonia (except for occasional muscle twitches), and irregular ventilation. In the neonate, sleep is divided into active, quiet, and indeterminate sleep, with active sleep being similar to REM sleep and quiet sleep being similar to NREM sleep (15). Active sleep occurs for approximately 50% of total sleep time in the term neonate (16), whereas REM sleep occurs for 15–25% of total sleep time in the older child and adolescent (17–19). Slow wave sleep accounts for approximately 20–28% of total sleep time in the older child and adolescent (17–19). During the course of the night, sleep progresses through the different stages in four to six cycles (20, 21).

Ventilation During Sleep

During sleep, neural control of ventilation is altered. The behavioral influence on ventilation is absent during NREM sleep, and ventilation is governed by metabolic factors. Breathing is regular, and tidal volume and respiratory rate are decreased. In adolescents and adults, the minute ventilation during sleep decreases by 8–15% compared to wakefulness (22, 23). Functional residual capacity (FRC) decreases (24), and upper airway resistance increases (25, 26). During REM sleep, breathing is erratic, with variable respiratory rate

and tidal volume, and frequent central apneas. Abolition of tonic activity of the intercostal muscles during REM results in a further decrease in FRC (24, 27). Hypotonia of the upper airway muscles occurs in the presence of unchanged diaphragmatic contraction, predisposing the subject to obstructive apnea.

Compared to the awake state, hypoxic and hypercapnic ventilatory drives decrease during NREM sleep, and decrease even further during REM sleep (28–31). Hypercapnia and airway occlusion are potent stimuli to arousal in humans of all ages (30–34). In contrast, hypoxia is a poor stimulus to arousal (29–31, 35).

During sleep in normal adults, there is an increase in P_{CO_2} of 3–7 mm Hg, a decrease in P_{O_2} of 3–9 mm Hg, and a decrease in Sa_{O_2} of 2%, as compared to wakefulness (22). Similar changes occur in normal children and adolescents, with a mean increase in $P_{ET}CO_2$ of 7 mm Hg (36), and a decrease in Sa_{O_2} of 1–4% (22, 36, 37). These normal phenomena are magnified in patients with pulmonary disease or upper airway dysfunction.

PATHOGENESIS OF OSAS

The pathogenesis of OSAS in adults is not fully understood, and even less is known about OSAS in children. OSAS occurs when the relationship between the factors maintaining airway patency (the central ventilatory response to hypoxia, hypercapnia, and airway occlusion; the effect the central drive has on augmenting upper airway neuromuscular tone; and the effects of sleep state and arousal) and the components of the upper airway load (such as anatomic size) that promote airway collapse is perturbed. Basically, there are two theories that have been developed to explain the pathophysiology of airway collapse.

The "balance of forces" theory proposed by Remmers et al. (39) hypothesizes that the size of the pharyngeal lumen depends on the balance between the negative intrapharyngeal pressure generated during inspiration, and the outward dilating action of the upper airway muscles. The transmural pressure at which upper airway collapse occurs has been termed the "closing pressure." During wakefulness, activation of the upper airway muscles maintains transmural pressure above the closing pressure, and the upper airway remains patent. As sleep commences, neuromuscular tone decreases, resulting in a decreased pharyngeal luminal cross-sectional area. This results in flow-limitation/obstruction. An alternative theory is that the upper airway acts as a Starling resistor (40–42))—that is, that pressure changes upstream rather than downstream to the collapsible pharyngeal locus govern flow through the upper airway.

A number of factors effecting both intraluminal pressures and upper airway muscle function have been identified that contribute to the development of airway collapse during sleep. Sleep is key to the problem. OSAS develops when factors that result in increased airways resistance are coupled with an abnormality in central nervous system (CNS) control of upper airway muscle function. The necessity of this combination of factors most likely explains why some children with structural abnormalities develop OSAS whereas others with similar degrees of airway narrowing have normal respiration during sleep. Factors that appear to be important follow.

Structural Narrowing

In children, adenotonsillar hypertrophy is the most common condition leading to OSAS. The severity of OSAS is not always proportional to the size of the tonsils and adenoids (43), and although many children have adenotonsillar hypertrophy, few develop OSAS. Thus, a child with moderately enlarged tonsils and adenoids may have severe OSAS, whereas another child with the same degree of adenotonsillar hypertrophy may be asymptomatic. Adenotonsillar hypertrophy may also complicate the status of children with underlying bony abnormalities. Although in most children OSAS resolves following adenotonsillectomy, in a minority it persists postoperatively. A few children with OSAS who were successfully treated by adenotonsillectomy later developed a recurrence of their symptoms during adolescence in one study (44).

Adults with OSAS have a narrow pharyngeal airway (45–50). Similar data are not available in children other than in those with craniofacial anomalies who have obvious structural airway narrowing (micrognathia and midface hypoplasia) (Table 39.2). In children with grossly normal craniofacial anatomy, the most common cause of upper airway narrowing is adenotonsillar hypertrophy. However, it is possible that children with

Table 39.2.
Medical Conditions Associated with OSAS

Achondroplasia (232–236)
Apert's syndrome (81,180,236)
Beckwith-Wiedemann syndrome (237)
Cerebral palsy (179,238)
Choanal stenosis (239)
Crouzon syndrome (81,180,211)
Cystic hygroma (240)
Down syndrome (181–187,241)
Hallermann-Streiff syndrome (242)
Hypothyroidism (79,243)
Klippel-Feil syndrome (244)
Mucopolysaccharidosis (245–251)
Obesity (50,79,107,258)
Osteopetrosis (252)
Papillomatosis (oropharyngeal) (253)
Pierre Robin sequence (16,67,213,239)
Pfeiffer syndrome (81)
Prader Willi syndrome (254,255)
Sickle cell disease (188–190,256)
Treacher-Collins syndrome (175,180,257)

This table lists some of the medical conditions that have been reported in association with obstructive sleep apnea syndrome in children. There may be other conditions that are not listed that may be associated with obstructive sleep apnea syndrome.

adenotonsillar hypertrophy and OSAS may also have a subtle underlying small or abnormally shaped upper airway (51), since some children may have persistent signs of OSAS following adenotonsillectomy.

Although not as common a cause of OSAS in children as it is in adults, obesity is a factor in the pathogenesis of OSAS in children (52). Upper airway narrowing results from deposition of adipose tissue within the muscles and soft tissue surrounding the airway (53, 54), as well as external compression from the neck and jowls. Restrictive lung disease can contribute to hypoxia, and the small lung volumes reflexively result in a narrowed upper airway. In these patients, the supine position alone may result in hypoxia. Additionally, the central ventilatory drive may be blunted in obese patients. Similar data in obese children and adolescents are lacking, but one can assume that marked obesity is quite likely to have a similar effect in children.

Control of Upper Airway Patency

Although a specific defect in control of airway function during sleep has not been determined in either adults or children with OSAS, it seems quite likely that some abnormality exists in control of breathing during sleep in patients with OSAS. In support of this are observations that OSAS may be caused or aggravated by drugs that affect the reticular activating system, reduce the central ventilatory drive, or directly depress upper airway muscle tone, such as sedatives, general anesthesia, and alcohol (55–58). Although chloral hydrate has been used to induce sleep for polysomnography without worsening of OSAS (59), it does depress genioglossus tone, and has been reported to precipitate obstructive sleep apnea in isolated cases (60).

Adults with OSAS have decreased ventilatory responses to hypercapnia and hypoxia (11, 61–64), which is probably a secondary phenomenon resulting from chronic hypercapnia and hypoxia. In addition, since most adults with OSAS are obese, the decreased ventilatory responses may be due to the obesity-hypoventilation syndrome. In children with OSAS, however, ventilatory responses are usually preserved (65).

PATHOPHYSIOLOGY

Patients with OSAS are able to maintain a patent upper airway during wakefulness because of augmentation of airway muscle tone by input from higher cortical centers. During sleep, upper airway collapse occurs on inspiration despite continued and at times increased respiratory effort. In contrast to adults, in whom numerous and prolonged obstructive apnea dominants breathing during sleep, children are more likely to have protracted periods of partial airway obstruction and hypoventilation. Apnea events are less frequent and generally of shorter duration than in adults. Hypoxia and hypercapnia result from this cycle of partial and complete obstruction. Obstructive apnea results in increased activity of upper airway dilating muscles resulting in termination of apnea, usually by gasping. In adults with OSAS, this increase in airway tone terminating an apnea episode is associated with arousal. Arousals are usually manifested as transient changes in sleep state (detected by EEG) rather than by frank awakenings. In adults, these arousals may occur hundreds of times a night, resulting in sleep fragmentation. In children, with OSAS, however, arousals are far less common

(66), and partial obstruction may continue for hours without interruption (67–70). The mechanism by which children re-establish airway patency is unknown but may involve a brainstem pathway not detected by classic polysomnographic EEG detection or behavioral changes. In adults with OSAS, sleep disruptions occur secondary to these arousals, resulting in decreased slow wave and REM sleep as well as excessive daytime somnolence (71, 72). In contrast, children have normal sleep architecture and daytime hypersomnolence is uncommon (10, 73).

Some patients with OSAS have associated central and mixed apnea (apneas with both a central and obstructive component) (65, 73, 74). The mechanism underlying this is unknown but appears to be related to partial airway obstruction, since it resolves following relief of obstructive hypoventilation (73).

CLINICAL MANIFESTATIONS

History

Most children present with a history of difficulty in breathing during sleep. The onset of breathing difficulty is usually insidious. Parents often do not have regular or extended opportunities to observe their child asleep, and the significance of the snoring is often not appreciated. Although normal children may snore intermittently (3), children with OSAS snore loudly (snoring can often be heard from outside the bedroom) and habitually. Some children do not have classic snoring, but rather have grunting, snorting, or gasping; some form of noisy breathing is always present. Parents frequently note the presence of retractions, and can often describe episodes of increased respiratory effort associated with lack of airflow. These episodes are followed by gasping, "choking noises," movement, or arousal. It is useful to request parents to mimic their child's breathing pattern. Restlessness and diaphoresis occur commonly in association with OSAS. Although cyanosis or pallor may occur, most children sleep in darkened rooms, and therefore color changes are not appreciated. Children with OSAS frequently sleep in positions to promote airway patency, such as prone, seated, or with hyper-extension of the neck. Occasionally, bizarre postures are adopted. Parents of a child with OSAS may be so concerned about their child's breathing that they sit at their child's bedside all night, or stimulate their child to terminate the apneas.

Despite dramatic breathing difficulties during sleep, breathing during wakefulness is usually normal, although it may be noisy. Daytime symptoms related to adenotonsillar hypertrophy may be present. These include mouth breathing, frequent episodes of upper respiratory tract infections, and otitis media. Children with very large tonsils may have dysphagia or articulation difficulties. There is often a family history of snoring or OSAS.

Physical Examination

In the majority of children with OSAS, physical examination during wakefulness is entirely normal. This commonly leads to a delay in diagnosis, since the physician rarely has the opportunity to see the child asleep. Children with massive adenotonsillar hypertrophy, or with other causes for OSAS, may *very rarely* demonstrate obstructed breathing during wakefulness.

Physical examination should include an assessment of the child's growth, and obesity or failure to thrive should be noted. Allergic stigmata, such as "allergic shiners" or a horizontal nasal crease, may be present. The presence of mouth breathing, an adenoidal facies, midfacial hypoplasia, retro/micrognathia, or other craniofacial abnormalities is a key to diagnosis. The patency of the nasal passages should be assessed, and septal deviation, edematous turbinates, or nasal polyps noted. Tongue size, palatal integrity, oropharyngeal cross-sectional area, redundant palatal mucosa, size of the tonsils, and size of the uvula are important to observe. Pectus excavatum may be present (76). The lungs are usually clear to auscultation. Cardiac examination may reveal signs of pulmonary hypertension, such as an increased pulmonic component of the second heart sound, and a right ventricular heave. Congestive heart failure is occasionally present. Neurologic examination should be performed to evaluate muscle tone and developmental status.

When possible, the patient should be observed while asleep. During sleep, the child will be heard to snore. Breathing is labored, and tachypnea, nasal flaring, retractions (particularly suprasternal), and paradoxical inward motion of the chest during inspiration are present. During periods of complete obstruc-

tion, the patient will be noted to make respiratory efforts, but no snoring is heard, no airflow is detected, and breath sounds cannot be auscultated. Apneic episodes may be terminated by body movements or awakening.

COMPLICATIONS

The complications of OSAS result from chronic nocturnal hypoxia, acidosis, and sleep fragmentation.

Cardiovascular Complications

Pulmonary hypertension, resulting from recurrent nocturnal hypoxia, hypercarbia, and respiratory acidosis (77) is a major cause of morbidity in patients with OSAS, and if untreated will progress to cor pulmonale. Left ventricular dysfunction has also been reported (78–80), and may be secondary to right-sided failure, or to systemic hypertension (see below). The prevalence of pulmonary hypertension in children with OSAS is not known. Brouillette et al. reported cor pulmonale in 55% of 22 patients with OSAS (69), and Guilleminault et al. reported cardiac or cardiorespiratory failure in 20% of 50 patients (81). These statistics probably do not reflect current medical care, since the increased level of awareness of OSAS among pediatricians has resulted in earlier diagnosis. Tal et al. (78) used radionuclide ventriculography to demonstrate a lower than normal right ventricular ejection fraction in 10 of 27 children with a history consistent with OSAS. Children with significant OSAS should undergo cardiac evaluation prior to anesthesia. Sudden death has been reported (82, 83), as has peri-anesthetic (84, 85) or perioperative cardiac arrest or death (86, 87). Cor pulmonale may respond temporarily to treatment with supplemental oxygen, diuretics, and digitalis. However, relief of the airway obstruction is the only definitive treatment, and will effectively reverse the cor pulmonale (67, 84, 88–90).

Systemic hypertension is a frequent complication of OSAS in adults (91). Transient cyclical increases in blood pressure may occur during sleep, possibly related to the fluctuations in intrathoracic pressure, vagal activity, or catecholamine release (92). This is in contrast to the decrease in arterial blood pressure seen during sleep in normal individuals. There may also be an association between OSAS and sustained waking hypertension in adults (91), although the presence of obesity makes this difficult to evaluate (93). Case reports have described awake systemic hypertension in children with OSAS (80, 94), and Guilleminault and colleagues reported systemic hypertension in 8% of 50 children with OSAS (81).

Arrhythmia is a likely result of the combination of hypoxemia and underlying coronary artery disease, and is a common complication of OSAS in adults. Arrhythmias are far less common in children, although cyclical sinus bradycardia and tachycardia may occur in conjunction with obstructive apneas. Isolated bradycardia during obstructive apneas is often seen in infants (202, 205, 206). Children with significant hypoxia during sleep may have frequent premature ventricular contractions.

Neurobehavioral Complications

Neurobehavioral complications result from chronic nocturnal hypoxia and sleep fragmentation (95–97). Excessive daytime somnolence is reported to occur in 31–84% of children with OSAS (10, 81, 98). Developmental delay, poor school performance, hyperactivity, aggressive behavior, and social withdrawal may accompany OSAS (10, 69, 81, 99), but a causal relationship has not been established and the association has not been studied systematically. Brouillette (69) reported severe asphyxial brain damage in two children with OSAS, and neurologic dysfunction in another five. Although children have been reported to have seizures and coma associated with severe OSAS (69, 86, 100), these occurrences are infrequent. More subtle manifestations of cognitive impairment, however, probably occur frequently. Anecdotal reports suggest that relief of severe OSAS can result in a marked improvement in some patient's level of cognitive functioning.

Poor Growth

Failure to thrive is a frequent complication of OSAS in children, occurring in 27–56% of patients (69, 81). As with cardiovascular complications, this statistic most likely does not reflect current medical practice. Causes for poor growth in children with OSAS include anorexia or dysphagia secondary to adenotonsillar hypertrophy, increased work of breathing, hypoxia, or abnormal nocturnal growth

hormone secretion (101). Catch-up growth occurs following adenotonsillectomy (69, 102, 103).

Enuresis

Enuresis can be a complication of OSAS (69, 81, 98), although there is question as to whether this is a cause and effect relationship, since enuresis has not been a consistent finding. Possible etiologies include disrupted and restless sleep affecting arousal, or abnormalities in hormonal fluid regulation (104). Enuresis, particularly secondary enuresis, may improve following the relief of upper airway obstruction (105).

Other Respiratory Tract Disease

Atopic children frequently have adenoidal hypertrophy, and associated sinusitis, asthma, or bronchitis. Therefore, lower respiratory tract disease may coexist with OSAS. Patients with OSAS are more likely to aspirate upper respiratory tract secretions (106), which may result in bronchitis. In our experience, this may improve following adenotonsillectomy. Some children with kissing tonsils have dysphagia or frequent choking episodes (98), and are at risk for aspiration pneumonia.

Respiratory Failure and Death

Case reports have described respiratory failure or arrest in patients with severe OSAS (90, 107, 182) or as a perioperative complication (86). Sudden death has been reported (82–85, 108).

LABORATORY TESTING
Establishing the Diagnosis

POLYSOMNOGRAPHY

The definitive method of establishing the diagnosis of OSAS is overnight polysomnography. The international classification of sleep disorders diagnostic and coding manual currently states that "In the young child, the signs and symptoms of obstructive sleep apnea are more subtle than in the adult; therefore, the diagnosis is more difficult and should be confirmed by polysomnography" (109). Polysomnography will also exclude other causes of disordered breathing during sleep. It provides objective measures of severity, and provides a baseline for those children whose condition does not resolve postoperatively.

Techniques

The use of appropriate equipment and personnel will assure the successful performance of polysomnography in infants and children of all ages. It should be performed in a quiet, dark area that is nonthreatening and conducive to sleep—ideally in a pediatric laboratory dedicated to this purpose. Provision should be made for a parent to stay with the child. The technician should be skilled at working with children and understand that children frequently displace monitoring leads. It is preferable to study children during natural sleep, rather than sleep induced by sleep deprivation or sedation, since sleep-disordered breathing may increase (110) following sleep deprivation. Some laboratories use chloral hydrate to induce sleep. Although chloral hydrate does not affect ventilatory drive (111), and in one study did not affect polysomnogram results (59), animal data suggest that it may depress upper airway muscle tone (60).

During polysomnography, a wide variety of physiologic variables can be assessed (20, 112, 113). At a minimum, sleep state, airflow, chest and abdominal wall motion, arterial oxygen saturation (SaO_2), CO_2 tension, and electrocardiogram should be monitored. Sleep state is monitored with at least one EEG lead (C3/A2), two electro-oculogram leads (right and left), and a submental electromyogram. Airflow should be monitored at both the nose and mouth, which can be accomplished qualitatively via a thermistor or capnography, or quantitatively via a mask and pneumotachometer. Monitoring of respiratory pattern should include measurement of both chest and abdominal wall motion in order to detect paradoxical inward motion of the chest during inspiration. This can be accomplished with the use of respiratory inductance plethysmography (Respitrace), mercury-filled strain gauges, or impedance plethysmography. Although impedance plethysmography is used frequently to monitor breathing in children, thoracic impedance monitors have been reported to detect cardiac artifact as chest wall motion, resulting in false classification of central apneas as obstructive apneas (114). Oxygenation is best assessed by pulse oximetry. It is essential to record an oximeter pulse waveform in order to distinguish motion artifact. Monitoring of PCO_2 is necessary to detect obstructive hypoventilation. End-tidal capnometry is an accurate and rapidly-responsive technique for assessing PCO_2. In patients with ventilation-perfusion mismatching, the difference between arterial and end-tidal PCO_2 is increased, limiting capnography's usefulness in a small number of patients. Transcutaneous CO_2 monitoring is a less satisfactory technique, since it responds slowly to changes in PCO_2 and requires frequent calibration and changing of the sensor site, which may disrupt sleep. It has a wide interindividual variation. Transcutaneous PCO_2 monitoring may occasionally be useful in patients who do not tolerate the nasal cannula used in monitoring. Video recording of the patient is an invaluable adjunct to physiologic monitoring. Other parameters that may be useful to monitor in selected patients include esophageal pH (to assess for gastroesophageal reflux) and intrapleural pressure (using an esophageal balloon).

Interpretation

The standards used in the interpretation of polysomnography in adults cannot be extrapolated to infants and children.

Sleep Architecture

When interpreting polysomnograms, it is necessary to ensure that an adequate and representative night's sleep was recorded. If a patient sleeps poorly in the laboratory environment, sleep-disordered breathing may be underestimated. Occasionally, a child with a history highly suggestive of OSAS has a normal polysomnogram, but a repeat polysomnogram is abnormal. This may be due to a "first night effect," with the patient sleeping poorly in the unusual surroundings of the sleep laboratory; or to night-to-night variability in OSAS. In particular, sufficient total sleep time, sleep efficiency (total sleep time divided by total recording time), and REM time must be obtained. A polysomnogram can be considered adequate if total sleep time is $\geq$ 5 hours, sleep efficiency is $\geq$ 85%, and REM time is $\geq$ 15%.

Respiratory Parameters

Standards for normal pediatric respiratory parameters during sleep have not been established. Suggested normal values, based on the literature, are listed in Table 39.2. Statistically abnormal results are not necessarily clinically significant, and must be assessed in conjunction with each patient's clinical picture.

Since obstructive apneas of any length are rare in normal infants and children (16, 67, 68, 202, 208, 209, 216, 258), all obstructive events regardless of duration should be counted. An apnea index (number of obstructive apneas per hour sleep) > 1 is abnormal (36). Episodes of apparent obstructive apnea detected during routine polysomnography in infants without an esophageal balloon may not always represent airway obstruction, since episodes of movement with a closed glottis may simulate OSAS (116). An esophageal balloon is occasionally useful when OSAS and central apnea cannot be distinguished, by detecting respiratory effort that was not apparent by measurement of chest and abdominal wall motion. In addition, a subset of children have symptoms suggestive of OSAS and increased intrapleural pressure swings during sleep, but no abnormalities detectable by routine polysomnography (117).

As children with OSAS frequently demonstrate prolonged obstructive hypoventilation rather than discrete obstructive apneas, assessment of end-tidal CO_2 is essential. Hypoventilation cannot be detected accurately when qualitative measures such as thermistors are used to detect airflow (112). Conventionally, an end-tidal CO_2 > 45 mm Hg has been considered abnormal during sleep (115). However, the end-tidal CO_2 in normal sleeping children older than infancy frequently exceeds 45 mm Hg, and may exceed 50 mm Hg (36). P_{CO_2} in sleeping infants is usually < 40 mm Hg (7), although a recent study suggests that transcutaneous P_{CO_2} may exceed 45 mm Hg in normal infants (118). Both the total sleep time during which end-tidal CO_2 is elevated, and the peak end-tidal CO_2, should be determined (Table 39.3). Sa_{O_2} during wakefulness, baseline Sa_{O_2} during REM and nonREM sleep, and the frequency, degree, and duration of desaturation should be assessed. Conventionally, an Sa_{O_2} < 90% during sleep has been considered abnormal (115). However, several studies (23, 36, 37) suggest that the lower limit of Sa_{O_2} during sleep in normal children and adolescents is 92%. Age-appropriate normative data should be used in the evaluation of infants. At the present time there are no data on what constitutes mild, moderate, and severe disease. The clinical significance of brief severe episodes of desaturation, or for that matter prolonged periods of less severe desaturation (values in the high eighties), is not known. Oxygenation is lowest during the first week of life (119), and increases over the next 1–3 months (118). After several months of age, baseline Sa_{O_2} is ≥ 97% (120). Preterm infants (29–34 weeks' gestation) without cardiorespiratory disease have a mean sleeping Sa_{O_2} of 92 ± 3% (range 86–96%) (121). Oxygenation improves with increasing postconceptional age, rather than postnatal age (121), and baseline sleeping Sa_{O_2} of pre-term infants measured at term is usually the same as that of normal full-term infants (115, 121). Brief desaturation frequently occurs in association with central apnea or periodic breathing in normal infants (119, 120). Stebbens et al. (120) reported that hourly transient desaturations to < 80% occurred in conjunction with short central apneas in 81% of the 1- to 2-month-old infants studied.

SCREENING TESTS

Overnight polysomnography is not routinely available, is time-consuming, disruptive to a family's lifestyle, and expensive. Sleep laboratories can perform only one overnight study per 24-hour period per bed. Thus, although it is recognized that overnight polysomnography is the ideal diagnostic method, it is not always feasible or desirable, and a number of screening approaches have been suggested in order to reduce the number of children who need polysomnography.

History

A study conducted by Brouillette et al. (98) suggested that an abnormal sleep study could be predicted by a questionnaire score. However, those children receiving an intermediate score would still need polysomnography to establish a diagnosis. Furthermore, preliminary data from another center suggests that this method may not be applicable to all populations (122, 123). Therefore, the use of a

Table 39.3.
Suggested Normal Polysomnography Values

Measurement	Children	Comments
TST (hours)	≥ 5	"Acceptable" values during laboratory
Sleep efficiency (%)	≥ 85	conditions
REM sleep (% TST)	15–30	REM sleep increased during infancy
Slow wave sleep (% TST)	10–40	
Apnea index (N/hour)	≤ 1	
Peak $P_{ET}CO_2$ (mm Hg)	≤ 53	Normal peak CO_2 may be lower during infancy
$\Delta P_{ET}CO_2$ (mm Hg)	≤ 13	
Duration of hypoventilation ($P_{ET}CO_2$ > 45 mm Hg) % TST)	≤ 60	
S_aO_2 nadir (%)	≥ 92	Transient desaturations associated with central apnea occur during infancy
Desaturation > 4% (N/hour TST)	≤ 1.4	
ΔSaO_2 (%)	≤ 8	

Sleep efficiency: TST as percentage of total recording time. Apnea index defined as the number of obstructive apneas of any length per hour of sleep in infants and children, and number of obstructive apneas > 10 seconds duration per hour of sleep in adults. ΔS_aO_2 and $\Delta P_{ET}CO_2$ defined as the differences between the peak and nadir values during sleep. TST, total sleep time; $P_{ET}CO_2$, end-tidal carbon dioxide tension; S_aO_2, arterial oxygen saturation.

screening questionnaire without polysomnography cannot be recommended.

Laboratory Tests

Markers of chronic hypoxia, such as polycythemia or increased excretion of adenosine triphosphate (ATP) metabolites (124), are sometimes used as nonspecific indicators of OSAS. In our experience, polycythemia is seen rarely, especially in populations with a high incidence of iron-deficiency anemia. Patients with chronic hypercapnia during sleep may have a persistently elevated serum bicarbonate due to a compensatory metabolic alkalosis. The sensitivity and specificity of these measures in children have not been established.

Adults with OSAS may have characteristic flow-volume loops on pulmonary function testing, with signs of extrathoracic obstruction as well as saw-tooth flow oscillations. The sensitivity and specificity of this test has not yet been fully investigated (125–127). Most children with OSAS are too young to cooperate with pulmonary function testing.

Observation During Sleep

OSAS may be diagnosed by direct observation of the sleeping child in the doctor's office. Similarly, OSAS can be diagnosed by reviewing audiotapes or videotapes that can be made in the home. These techniques are inexpensive, simple, and effective, although they will not allow a full assessment of the severity of the illness, and have a high false-negative rate. It is important to note that an isolated, brief observation may not reflect a child's usual status. Audiotapes do not allow the differentiation of primary snoring from persistent obstructive hypoventilation. OSAS confined to REM sleep will not be appreciated unless the child is observed for prolonged periods.

Laboratory Tests During Sleep

Nocturnal cardiorespiratory monitoring without assessment of sleep state is a commonly used method from which substantial information can be obtained. However, the inability to assess sleep architecture precludes assurance that sufficient REM time occurred during the study and prevents assessment of the effects of OSAS on arousal and sleep fragmentation. Continuous recording of pulse oximetry alone, during sleep, has been advocated as a screening test and may show a characteristic cyclical desaturation suggestive of OSAS but will not detect patients with OSAS that is not associated with hypoxia. Arterial blood gas analysis during sleep, obtained either by direct arterial puncture (by an experienced and dexterous person) or from an indwelling arterial catheter, may aid in the diagnosis of OSAS. However, it is invasive and does not permit continuous physiologic monitoring.

Daytime nap polysomnography is an alternative to overnight polysomnography, but it has a high false-negative rate and frequently underestimates sleep-disordered breathing (59). Nap polysomnography is of shorter duration, may not include REM sleep, and may be altered by circadian variations in sleep patterns. In addition, sedation or sleep-deprivation is frequently necessary to induce sleep for nap studies.

Commercial computerized polysomnography systems are now available, some of which are marketed for use in the home. These currently cannot be recommended because home monitoring is rarely done in the presence of a trained technician and is complicated by artifacts. At this time, there are no reliable computerized scoring systems suitable for use in children.

Tests to Determine the Etiology of OSAS

OSAS is secondary to adenotonsillar hypertrophy in most children. Direct visualization of the oropharynx and the use of the flexible fiberoptic nasopharyngoscope is recommended in order to evaluate airway patency and anatomy. If these techniques are not available, adenoidal size can be demonstrated by lateral neck radiograph. In patients with craniofacial abnormalities or other underlying disease, fluoroscopy may be necessary to delineate the site of obstruction (128a). In patients with complex craniofacial anomalies, airway computed tomography (CT) or magnetic resonance imaging (MRI)—or cephalometry (129), when available—can aid the planning of the surgical approach.

Tests to Assess Complications of OSAS

EXCESSIVE DAYTIME SOMNOLENCE

The multiple sleep latency test (MSLT) is used to quantitate excessive daytime somnolence and to diagnose narcolepsy. This test is performed the day after a nocturnal polysomnograph is taken so that the adequacy of the preceding night's sleep can be determined. A standardized protocol involves asking the patient to take a series of naps spaced 2 hours apart. The time to onset of stage 1 sleep and the presence of REM onset naps is recorded (130). Although widely used in adults, the applicability of the MSLT to children has not yet been established. Normative data for children are available (18, 19, 131), but are based on small sample sizes and specific circumstances, and may not be applicable to the general population.

CARDIOVASCULAR COMPLICATIONS

Pertinent laboratory examinations include electrocardiogram, chest radiograph, and echocardiogram. Noninvasive assessment of pulmonary hypertension should be adequate in uncomplicated cases (89, 132). Doppler echocardiography is the most sensitive method for detecting early pulmonary hypertension, and is recommended for any patient with significant nocturnal hypoxia or OSAS, especially if the patient is to be subjected to general anesthesia.

NEUROBEHAVIORAL COMPLICATIONS

Specific abnormalities of cognitive function or hyperactivity characteristic of OSAS have not been determined in children. Although it has been suggested that neurobehavioral abnormalities may be secondary to OSAS (117), routine referral of patients with suspected OSAS for testing of cognitive function or assessment of hyperactivity cannot be recommended at this time. As experience with the full spectrum of the complications of OSAS in children increases it is quite likely that confirmation of neurobehavioral abnormalities on formal testing will become an indication for surgery in an otherwise asymptomatic child. Moreover, a complete sleep history should be included in the evaluation of children with neurobehavioral problems in order to determine if abnormal respiration during sleep may be a contributing factor.

TREATMENT

When to Treat?

An approach to management of the child with suspected OSAS is presented in Figure 39.3.

Children with severe OSAS (apnea index > 5 and or desaturation -SaO_2 < 85%, coupled with one or more of the complications discussed) should always be treated, and the effect

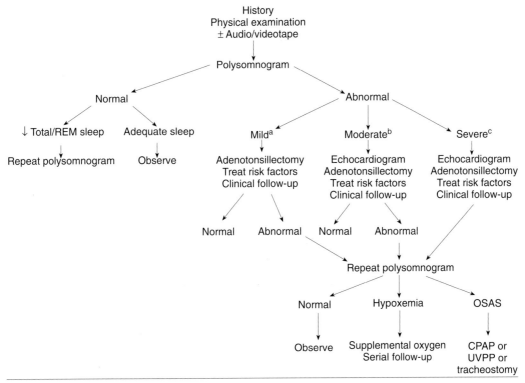

Figure 39.3.   Suggested management chart for a child with suspected OSAS.

[a]Mild OSAS: Normal growth; normal development; normal cardiac function. Polysomnogram shows apnea index 1-3; end-tidal CO_2 <55 mm Hg; $S_aO_2 \geq$ 92% except for transient dips to high 80's.

[b]Moderate OSAS: Poor growth (crossing percentiles); subtle neurological changes (behavioral abnormalities, poor school performance, excessive daytime sleepiness); mild ECG/echocardiographic abnormalities. Polysomnogram shows apnea index of 4-9; end-tidal CO_2 55-60 mm Hg; S_aO_2 dips 80%.

[c]Severe OSAS: Failure to thrive; developmental delay; cor pulmonale. Polysomnogram shows apnea index $\geq$ 10; end-tidal $CO_2 > 60$ mm Hg; S_aO_2 dips < 80%.

of treatment should be evaluated by repeat polysomnography. Treatment decisions for the child with mild OSAS are not as straightforward, as little is known about the natural course of untreated, mild OSAS in children. If a child is mildly symptomatic, and has a normal polysomnogram, then reassurance and follow-up are sufficient. If symptoms persist, the polysomnogram should be repeated. It is difficult to know when to treat a child with a mildly abnormal polysomnogram (i.e., one with few obstructions and minimal desaturation or hypoventilation). Treatment decisions should be based on the constellation of symptoms, physical examination, and polysomnography. If the child is not treated, repeat polysomnography is mandatory. Because most

children initially present because they are symptomatic, and there is concern that symptoms may progress, treatment of the children with mild disease is recommended. Children with primary snoring (isolated snoring without either symptoms or an abnormal polysomnogram) should not be subjected to surgery.

Emergency Stabilization and Treatment

Occasionally, children present with complications of severe OSAS requiring emergency admission. Monitoring in the hospital depends on pulse oximetry to detect the consequences of obstructed breathing. The administration of supplemental oxygen without simultaneous monitoring of P_{CO_2} may prolong obstructive apneas or precipitate respiratory failure (79, 133–136). Placement of a nasopharyngeal tube may provide temporary relief pending definitive treatment (128, 137). Vigilant nursing is necessary, as the tubes frequently clog with mucus. If a nasopharyngeal tube is unsuccessful in relieving the obstruction, elective placement of an endotracheal tube is necessary. Alternatively, nasal continuous positive airway pressure (CPAP) may be administered. Steroids shrink adenoidal tissue, and may relieve OSAS within 24 hours. This effect usually lasts only a few weeks, but may be useful in patients who cannot undergo surgery immediately.

Adenotonsillectomy

The definitive treatment of childhood OSAS is adenotonsillectomy (102, 103, 138). OSAS results from the relative size and structure of the upper airway components, rather than the absolute size of the tonsils and adenoids. Therefore, both tonsils and adenoids should be removed, even if one or the other appears to be the primary abnormality. Some surgeons prefer to perform adenoidectomy alone; but our experience and that of others suggests that this approach is unlikely to cure the patient (139–142). Even infants will improve dramatically postoperatively (142, 143). By the same logic, adenotonsillectomy should be the initial treatment of OSAS in children with other predisposing factors (e.g., obesity, Down syndrome), although further treatment may be necessary. In children with a submucous cleft palate, adenoidectomy may result in velopharyngeal incompetence; in this group, tonsillectomy alone is a consideration.

Adenotonsillectomy, though frequently considered to be minor surgery, may be associated with significant complications. In one study, adenotonsillectomy in the general population carried a complication rate of 7.9% (144). Complications are more common in patients with OSAS (145, 146) and in those < 3 years of age (145–147). The mortality rate for adenotonsillectomy is 1:16,000 (148, 149). Other complications include hemorrhage (2.7% of patients) (150), anesthetic complications, respiratory complications, dehydration, and pain (146, 151). *Patients with cor pulmonale may be at risk for arrhythmias and congestive heart failure.* Preoperative sedation may precipitate upper airway obstruction (152). Postoperative complications in children

with OSAS include upper airway edema, post airway obstruction, pulmonary edema (153, 154), and respiratory failure (147). Children with chronic sleeping hypercapnia may be relatively hyperventilated during anesthesia, and thus fail to breathe spontaneously postoperatively (147). The current economic climate promoting outpatient surgery makes it imperative that each child be evaluated carefully to determine their need for postoperative monitoring.

Although OSAS may not resolve fully until 6–8 weeks postoperatively, immediate improvement occurs in some patients (155). In patients with severe OSAS, hypoxia during sleep may persist for several weeks postoperatively, and supplemental oxygen may be necessary.

Continuous Positive Airway Pressure

Nasal CPAP is the mainstay of treatment of OSAS in adults. It has been used successfully in children (156, 157), including infants (158), obese children (156), and children with Down syndrome (157), achondroplasia (156), and craniofacial anomalies (156, 157, 159). In the pediatric age group, CPAP is particularly useful in obese patients and patients with persistent OSAS following adenotonsillectomy. Effective CPAP use is difficult in young, uncooperative, or developmentally delayed children. The key to successful CPAP treatment is good compliance, and the key to good compliance is adequate patient preparation and education, and aggressive follow-up. Many CPAP devices have an hour meter for assessing compliance.

CPAP is delivered by a positive pressure generator connected to a snug-fitting nasal mask. Home CPAP units are small, mobile, and simple to operate. Pediatric-sized masks are now commercially available, and infant masks are being developed. CPAP use is instituted in the sleep laboratory in a separate CPAP titration study following the initial diagnostic polysomnogram. Children and their families should be instructed in the use of the CPAP equipment during a separate daytime visit preceding the CPAP study. The child is given the opportunity to handle the equipment while awake and calm. During the CPAP titration study, mask pressure is gradually increased until an optimal CPAP level is attained (i.e., a pressure that is tolerable to the patient, and at which snoring, retractions, and desaturation are decreased or abolished). Airflow can be quantitated during the study by attaching a pneumotachometer to the nasal mask. In our experience, optimal CPAP levels usually range from 8 to 16 cm H_2O. Patients with mouth-breathing will frequently change to nasal breathing as the CPAP level is increased. Occasionally, supplemental oxygen is also required and can be delivered via the CPAP circuit. The use of a CPAP system with a gradual increase in inspiratory pressure, or with a lower expiratory pressure (BIPAP) (160), can increase patient comfort. CPAP side effects are usually minor, and related to air leak around a poorly fitted mask. This can result in dry eyes, conjunctivitis, skin rashes, and pressure sores. Nasal dryness or congestion is frequent, but usually resolves spontaneously within 2 weeks of therapy. Decongestants, saline nose drops, or the use of a CPAP system with a humidifier can be helpful. Serious complications are unusual and include rupture of the tympanic membrane in patients with otitis media and central apnea with high levels of CPAP. Aspiration is theoretically a complication; for this reason, nasal masks should be used rather than full face masks. Pneumothorax and a reduction in cardiac output are possible, but are rarely seen in the pressure ranges used (161), unless the patient has severe underlying cardiorespiratory disease.

Weight loss

In obese patients, weight loss usually results in resolution of OSAS. In the morbidly obese patient, a relatively small weight loss can result in a significant improvement (162). Unfortunately, weight reduction may be extraordinarily difficult in such children. Nasal CPAP should be used until sufficient weight loss has been achieved. In the patient with severe OSAS and potentially life-threatening complications, hospital admission for weight loss is justified.

Drugs

Nasal obstruction is a common contributing factor in children with OSAS, and can be treated with nasal decongestants or topical steroids. Progesterone has been used as a respiratory stimulant in pediatric patients with the obesity-hypoventilation syndrome (163), and has been used with mixed success in adults with OSAS (164–166). The effects of long-term hormonal therapy in developing children are not known. Protriptyline has been used to ameliorate OSAS in adults, and acts primarily by reducing REM sleep rather than by reducing airway obstruction (167). Its use in children has not been evaluated. Sedative drugs and alcohol-containing medications should be avoided, as these may aggravate OSAS.

Intra-Oral Appliances

Various types of intra-oral appliances (e.g., tongue-retaining devices) have been used to treat OSAS (168, 169). However, children do not usually tolerate these devices.

Surgery other than Adenotonsillectomy

Appropriate surgical techniques should be tailored to the site of the obstruction in selected patients. These include nasal septoplasty in patients with deviated nasal septums, lip-tongue adhesion procedures in patients with Pierre Robin sequence (170), epiglottoplasty in patients with severe laryngomalacia (171), and uvulopharyngopalatoplasty with tongue wedge resection in patients with Down syndrome (172, 173). Maxillofacial surgery has been used successfully in some adults with OSAS (174); it has been reported to be successful in the treatment of a few children with OSAS secondary to maxillofacial abnormalities (175).

Uvulopharyngopalatoplasty (UVPP) is widely used to treat adults with OSAS. UVPP involves resection of the uvula, tonsils, and redundant palatal and pharyngeal mucosa. It is major surgery, and postoperative intubation or temporary tracheotomy may be necessary. The cure rate using UVPP in unselected adults is approximately 50% (176), and depends on such factors as the site of airway collapse (177) and the degree of surgical expertise. UVPP has not been fully evaluated in children. It has been reported to be successful in the treatment of an otherwise normal 3-year old with OSAS (178), as well as in children with Down syndrome (172) and cerebral palsy (179). Currently, UVPP for children with OSAS should only be considered in those children who are unresponsive to either adenotonsillectomy or nasal CPAP, especially those children with redundant palatal soft tissue (179).

Tracheotomy

The use of CPAP and innovative types of airway surgery have resulted in a decrease in the number of children requiring tracheotomy for OSAS. Nevertheless, some children still require tracheotomy. These include children with uncorrectable craniofacial anomalies (83, 180), obese children with severe OSAS who are unable to lose weight or to cooperate with CPAP therapy, and infants with severe OSAS who either do not respond to adenotonsillectomy or are thought not to be candidates for this procedure. A tracheotomy should be considered a temporizing measure in children with severe, life-threatening OSAS, and for children living in areas where the surgical expertise for more complex procedures is unavailable.

PROGNOSIS AND NATURAL COURSE

The natural course and long-term prognosis of OSAS in children is not known. Specifically, it is not known whether childhood OSAS is a precursor of adult OSAS, or if it is an independent entity. Guilleminault reported recurrence of OSAS in three male adolescents who had been successfully treated by adenotonsillectomy during childhood (44). It has been conjectured that children "cured" of their OSAS by adenotonsillectomy are at risk for recurrence of OSAS during late adolescence or adulthood because of the influence of testosterone on the upper airway (in males) and the acquisition of additional risk factors such as obesity or alcohol ingestion.

SPECIFIC DISEASE CONDITIONS COMPLICATED BY OSAS

OSAS is associated with many pediatric conditions. Some of the more common conditions are discussed below.

Obesity

The majority of adults with OSAS are obese. Children with OSAS are less likely to be obese than adults with OSAS; indeed failure to thrive may be noted (69, 81). However, a group of children with obesity and OSAS exists (52, 81). Obese infants *without other symptoms of*

OSAS have been shown to have an increased frequency of obstructive apneas (258). OSAS occurs in children with primary obesity, as well in as those with obesity secondary to other conditions such as Prader-Willi syndrome. Treatment involves resection of adenotonsillar tissue if enlarged, CPAP if the patient is of sufficient age, and weight loss. How much weight must be lost to produce resolution of OSAS in a child is not known, but in adults a relatively small amount of weight loss may result in significant improvement (162).

Down Syndrome

Children with Down syndrome have many predisposing factors for OSAS. These include midfacial and mandibular hypoplasia (181), glossoptosis, a small upper airway with superficially positioned tonsils and relative tonsillar and adenoidal encroachment (172, 182), increased secretions, an increased incidence of lower respiratory tract anomalies (172), obesity, hypothyroidism, and generalized hypotonia. OSAS occurs in patients with Down syndrome of all ages, with an estimated prevalence of 31–72% (183, 184). Although adenotonsillectomy usually results in an improvement, it is usually not curative (184, 185). OSAS is probably a major contributor to the development or exacerbation of the pulmonary hypertension seen frequently in children with Down syndrome (186, 187). Because children with Down syndrome are "expected" to have pulmonary hypertension, growth failure, and developmental delay, the role of OSAS in these problems is frequently underestimated. A history of sleep and breathing patterns should always be obtained in a child with Down syndrome.

Other conditions

Some of the conditions associated an increased incidence of OSAS are listed in Table 39.2. OSAS is common in children with craniofacial anomalies, particularly if midfacial hypoplasia, micrognathia, developmental delay, hypotonia, or obesity is present. OSAS is especially problematic in children with sickle cell anemia, since these patients already have a decreased oxygen-carrying capacity secondary to their anemia. In addition, the hypoxia and acidosis associated with OSAS may exacerbate vaso-occlusive crises (188–190). Iatrogenic obstructive sleep apnea syndrome occurs in the majority of patients following pharyngeal flap surgery for correction of hypernasal speech (191–193). Obstructive apnea may occur in conjunction with stridor in infants with laryngeal anomalies or vocal cord paralysis (194–199).

OSAS IN INFANCY

Obstructive sleep apnea in neonates and infants may be misinterpreted as central apnea, or may coexist with central apnea (200). Some cases of so-called SIDS are actually due to OSAS (201–204). Routine cardiorespiratory monitoring of premature infants or infants with a history of apparent life-threatening events (ALTEs) will not detect obstructive apnea. Isolated bradycardia in an infant warrants an evaluation for obstructive apnea (202, 205, 206).

Infants are prone to OSAS for a variety of reasons related to developmental immaturity of the airway. Infants are predominantly nasal breathers (207–210), and are prone to develop OSAS whenever mild nasal obstruction is present. Nasal congestion alone may lead to severe respiratory distress in otherwise healthy infants (211). Central nervous system immaturity, and poor coordination between the muscles of the upper airway and diaphragm, contribute to sleep-disordered breathing (212). Airway stability improves with increasing maturity (213). Body position (supine versus prone) does not appear to be an important factor (206, 214), but neck flexion significantly increases airway collapsibility in infants (214, 215), possibly by inducing posterior displacement of the tongue. Because infants have a very compliant chest wall, negative inspiratory intrapleural pressure results in chest wall deformation; this is exaggerated during REM sleep (26). However, some degree of chest wall distortion and paradoxical inward motion of the chest during inspiration is normal during active sleep. Infants have a reduced FRC, and thus even brief apneas may be associated with desaturation. Infants also have an increased proportion of active/REM sleep, which is the sleep state during which breathing is most likely to be disturbed. Gastroesophageal reflux is another factor that may be associated with obstructive apneas during infancy (216, 217).

Prematurity

The association between prematurity and central apnea is well known. It is evident, however, that premature infants are also predisposed to airway obstruction (205, 218), especially in association with neck flexion (215) and feeding. In addition, premature infants usually have lower arterial oxygen levels than full-term infants, partly because of increased chest wall compliance with a resultant decrease in FRC. Episodes of desaturation during sleep are frequent, and may occur independently of apnea (219, 220).

SLEEP-DISORDERED BREATHING IN CHILDREN WITH CHRONIC LUNG DISEASE

The normal changes in ventilation associated with sleep were described in an earlier section. These changes are magnified in children with chronic lung disease. Sleeping hypoventilation is increased because of increased physiologic dead space. Patients with a low FRC have little functional reserve, and are more likely to desaturate as a result of REM-related intercostal muscle hypotonia (221). Mucociliary clearance is decreased during sleep, resulting in increased pulmonary secretions (222).

Patients with adequate oxygenation during wakefulness may desaturate during sleep (223, 224). Desaturation during sleep has been reported in patients with cystic fibrosis (221, 223), bronchopulmonary dysplasia (225, 226), asthma (224), and neuromuscular disease (226, 227). Hypercarbia may also worsen (224). Sleeping desaturation is especially important in infants, who spend a large proportion of their time asleep. Our experience with infants recovering from BPD has suggested that maintenance of hemoglobin saturation above 92% facilitates growth and development as well as the resolution of cor pulmonale (227a). Correction of hypoxia during sleep may improve growth in infants with bronchopulmonary dysplasia (228). Infants with bronchopulmonary dysplasia may also have OSAS secondary to morphologic changes induced by prolonged intubation (a high-arched or grooved palate), midfacial hypoplasia (229), or sinusitis. Failure of a patient with bronchopulmonary dysplasia to improve with age, increasing pectus excavatum, or severe chronic nasal congestion should raise the suspicion of OSAS. Concomitant OSAS also occurs relatively frequently in patients with neuromuscular disease (227, 230).

Patients with pulmonary disease and snoring, morning headaches, or unexpected polycythemia, growth failure, or cor pulmonale should be assessed for hypoxia during sleep. The sleep laboratory provides the ideal environment for assessing and monitoring gas exchange in those patients requiring oxygen supplementation or home ventilatory support (231).

REFERENCES

1. Guilleminault C, Eldrige F, Simmons FB, Dement WC. Sleep apnea in eight children. *Pediatrics* 1976; 58:23–30.
2. Osler W. Chronic tonsillitis. In *The principles and practice of medicine*. New York, Appleton and Co., 1892, pp 335–339.
3. Corbo GM, Fuciarelli F, Foresi A, De-Benedetto F. Snoring in children: Association with respiratory symptoms and passive smoking. *Br Med J* 1989; 299:1491–1494.
4. Ali NJ, Pitson D, Stradling JR. The prevalence of snoring, sleep disturbance and sleep related breathing disorders and their relation to daytime sleepiness in 4–5 year old children. *Am Rev Resp Dis* 1991; 143:381A.
5. Gozal D, Marcus CL, Keens TG, Ward SLD. Characteristics and polysomnographic abnormalities of children with the obstructive sleep apnea syndrome [Abstract]. *Pediatr Pulmonol* 1991; 11:372.
6. Block AJ, Wynne JW, Boysen PG. Sleep-disordered breathing and nocturnal oxygen desaturation in postmenopausal women. *Am J Med* 1980; 69:75–79.
7. Block AJ, Boysen PG, Wynne JW, Hunt LA. Sleep apnea, hypopnea and oxygen desaturation in normal subjects. *N Engl J Med* 1979; 300:513–517.
8. Johnson MW, Anch AM, Remmers JE. Induction of the obstructive sleep apnea syndrome in a woman by exogenous androgen administration. *Am Rev Resp Dis* 1984; 129:1023–1025.
9. Schneider BK, Pickett CK, Zwillich CW, et al. Influence of testosterone on breathing during sleep. *J Appl Physiol* 1986; 61:618–623.
10. Frank Y, Kravath RE, Pollak CP, Weitzman ED. Obstructive sleep apnea and its therapy: clinical and polysomnographic manifestations. *Pediatrics* 1983; 71:737–742.
11. Bayadi S, Millman RP, Tishler PV, et al. A family study of sleep apnea. Anatomic and physiologic interactions. *Chest* 1990; 98:554–559.
12. Strohl KP, Saunders NA, Feldman NT, Hallett M. Obstructive sleep apnea in family members. *N Engl J Med* 1978; 299:969–973.
13. Redline S, Tosteson T, Tishler PV, Carskadon MA, Milliman RP. Studies in the genetics of obstructive sleep apnea. *Am Rev Resp Dis* 1992; 145:440–444.
14. Yoshizawa T, Kurashina K, Sasaki I, et al. Analysis of HLA antigens in patients with obstructive sleep apnea syndrome. *Am Rev Resp Dis* 1991; 143:A381.

15. Anders T, Emde R, Parmalee A, eds. *A manual of standardized terminology: Techniques and criteria for scoring of states of sleep and wakefulness in newborn infants*. Los Angeles, UCLA Brain Information Service/Brain Research Institute, 1971.
16. Gaultier C. Respiratory adaption during sleep from the neonatal period to adolescence. In Guilleminault C, ed. *Sleep and its disorders in children*. New York, Raven Press, 1987, pp 67–97.
17. Coble PA, Kupfer DJ, Reynolds CF, Houck P. EEG sleep of healthy children 6 to 12 years of age. In Guilleminault C, ed. *Sleep and its disorders in children*. New York, Raven Press, 1987, pp 29–41.
18. Carskadon MA, Harvey K, Duke P, Anders TF, Litt IF, Dement WC. Pubertal changes in daytime sleepiness. *Sleep* 1980; 2:453–460.
19. Carskadon MA, Keenan S, Dement WC. Nighttime sleep and daytime sleep tendency in preadolescents. In Guilleminault C, ed. *Sleep and its disorders in children*. New York, Raven Press, 1987, pp 43–52.
20. Carskadon MA, Rechtschaffen A. Monitoring and staging human sleep. In Kryger MH, Roth T, Dement WC, eds. *Principles and practice of sleep medicine*. Philadelphia, WB Saunders, 1989, pp 665–683.
21. Rechtschaffen A, Kales A (eds). *A manual of standardized terminology: Techniques and scoring systems for sleep stages of human subjects*. Los Angeles, UCLA Brain Information Service/Brain Research Institute, 1968.
22. Krieger J. Breathing during sleep in normal subjects. In Kryger MH, Roth T, Dement WC, eds. *Principles and practice of sleep medicine*. Philadelphia, WB Saunders, 1989, pp 257–268.
23. Tabachnik E, Muller NL, Bryan AC and Levison H. Changes in ventilation and chest wall mechanics during sleep in normal adolescents. *J Appl Physiol* 1981; 51:557–564.
24. Hudgel DW, Devadatta P. Decrease in functional residual capacity during sleep in normal humans. *J Appl Physiol* 1984; 57:1319–1322.
25. Hudgel DW, Martin RJ, Johnson B, Hill P. Mechanics of the respiratory system and breathing pattern during sleep in normal humans. *J Appl Physiol* 1984; 56:133–137.
26. Lopes JM, Tabachnik E, Muller NL, Levison H, Bryan AC. Total airway resistance and respiratory muscle activity during sleep. *J Appl Physiol* 1983; 54:773–777.
27. Henderson–Smart DJ, Read DJC. Reduced lung volume during behavioral active sleep in the newborn. *J Appl Physiol* 1979; 46:1081–1085.
28. Berthon-Jones M, Sullivan CE. Ventilatory and arousal responses to hypoxia in sleeping humans. *Am Rev Respir Dis* 1982; 125:632–639.
29. Gothe B, Goldman MD, Cherniack NS, Mantey P. Effect of progressive hypoxia on breathing during sleep. *Am Rev Respir Dis* 1982; 126:97–102.
30. Douglas NJ, White DP, Weil JV, Pickett CK, Zwillich CW. Hypercapnic ventilatory response in sleeping adults. *Am Rev Respir Dis* 1982; 126:758–762.
31. Hedemark LL, Kronenberg RS. Ventilatory and heart rate responses to hypoxia and hypercapnia during sleep in adults. *J Appl Physiol* 1982; 53:307–311.
32. van der Hal AL, Rodriguez AM, Sargent CW, Platzker ACG, Keens TG. Hypoxic and hypercapneic arousal responses and prediction of subsequent

apnea in apnea of infancy. *Pediatrics* 1985; 75:848–854.

33. Marcus CL, Bautista DB, Ammahyia A, Ward SLD, Keens TG. Hypercapneic arousal responses in children with congenital central hypoventilation syndrome. *Pediatrics* 1991; 88:993–998.

34. Issa FG, Sullivan CE. Arousal and breathing responses to airway occlusion in healthy sleeping adults. *J Appl Physiol* 1983; 55:1113–1119.

35. Ward SLD, Bautista DB, Keens TG. Hypoxic arousal responses in normal infants. *Pediatrics* 1992; 89:860–864.

36. Marcus CL, Omlin KJ, Basinski DJ, Bailey SL, Rachal AB, von Pechmann WS, Keens TG, Ward SLD. Normal polysomnographic values for children and adolescents. *Am Rev Respir Dis* 1992; 146:1235–1239.

37. Chipps BE, Mak H, Schuberth KC, Talamo JH, Menkes HA, Scherr MS. Nocturnal oxygen saturation in normal and asthmatic children. *Pediatrics* 1980, 65:1157–1160.

38. van Lunteren E, Strohl KP. Striated respiratory muscles of the upper airways. In Mathew OP, Sant'Ambrogio G, eds. *Respiratory function of the upper airway.* New York, Marcel Dekker, 1988, pp 87–123.

39. Remmers JE, DeGroot WJ, Sauerland EK, Anch AM. Pathogenesis of upper airway occlusion during sleep. *J Appl Physiol* 1978; 44:931–938.

40. Smith PL, Wise RA, Gold AR, Schwartz AR, Permutt S. Upper airway pressure-flow relationships in obstructive sleep apnea. *J Appl Physiol* 1988; 64:789–795.

41. Schwartz AR, Smith PL, Wise RA, Gold AR, Permutt S. Induction of upper airway occlusion in sleeping individuals with subatmospheric nasal pressure. *J Appl Physiol* 1988; 64:535–542.

42. Schwartz AR, Smith PL, Wise RA, Bankman I, Permutt S. Effect of positive nasal pressure on upper airway pressure-flow relationships. *J Appl Physiol* 1989; 66:1626–1634.

43. Laurikainen E, Erkinjuntti M, Alihanka J, Rikalainen H, Suonpaa J. Radiological parameters of the bony nasopharynx and the adenotonsillar size compared with sleep apnea episodes in children. *Int J Pediatr Otorhinolaryngol* 1987; 12:303–310.

44. Guilleminault, C. Treatments in obstructive sleep apnea. In Guilleminault C, Partinen M, eds. *Obstructive sleep apnea syndrome.* New York, Raven Press, 1990, pp 99–118.

45. Rodenstein DO, Dooms G, Thomas Y, Liistro G, Stanescu DC, Culee C, Aubert–Tulkens G. Pharyngeal shape and dimensions in healthy subjects, snorers, and patients with obstructive sleep apnoea. *Thorax* 1990; 45:722–727.

46. Bradley TD, Brown IG, Grossman RF, et al. Pharyngeal size in snorers, nonsnorers, and patients with obstructive sleep apnea. *N Engl J Med* 1986; 315:1327–1331.

47. Rivlin J, Hoffstein V, Kalbfleisch J, McNicholas W, Zamel N, Bryan AC. Upper airway morphology in patients with idiopathic obstructive sleep apnea. *Am Rev Resp Dis* 1984; 129:355–360.

48. Galvin JR, Rooholamini SA, Stanford W. Obstructive sleep apnea: diagnosis with ultrafast CT. *Radiology* 1989; 171:775–778.

49. Suratt PM, Dee P, Atkinson RL, Armstrong P, Wilhoit SC. Fluoroscopic and computed tomographic features of the pharyngeal airway in obstructive sleep apnea. *Am Rev Respir Dis* 1983; 127:487–492.

50. Haponik EF, Smith PL, Bohlman ME, Allen RP, Goldman SM, Bleecker ER. Computerized tomography in obstructive sleep apnea. *Am Rev Respir Dis* 1983; 127:221–226.

51. Brodsky L, Adler E, Stanievich JF. Naso- and oropharyngeal dimensions in children with obstructive sleep apnea. *Int J Pediatr Otorhinolaryngol* 1989; 17:1–11.

52. Mallory GB, Fiser DH, Jackson R. Sleep-associated breathing disorders in morbidly obese children and adolescents. *J Pediatr* 1989; 115:892–897.

53. Horner RL, Mohiaddin RH, Lowell DG et al. Sites and sizes of fat deposits around the pharynx in obese patients with obstructive sleep apnoea and weight matched controls. *Eur Respir J* 1989; 2:613–622.

54. Stauffer JL, Buick MK, Bixler EO, et al. Morphology of the uvula in obstructive sleep apnea. *Am Rev Respir Dis* 1989; 140:724–728.

55. Kahn A, Hasaerts D, Blum D. Phenothiazine-induced sleep apneas in normal infants. *Pediatrics* 1985; 75:844–847.

56. Krol RC, Knuth SL, Bartlett D. Selective reduction of genioglossal muscle activity by alcohol in normal human subjects. *Am Rev Respir Dis* 1984; 129:247–250.

57. Sahn SA, Lakshminarayan, Pierson DJ, et al. Effect of ethanol on the ventilatory responses to oxygen and carbon dioxide in men. *Clin Sci Mol Med* 1975; 49:33–38.

58. Berry RB, Bonnet MH, Light RW. Effect of ethanol on the arousal response to airway occlusion during sleep in normal subjects. *Am Rev Respir Dis* 1992; 145:445–452.

59. Marcus CL, Keens TG, Ward SLD. Comparison of nap and overnight polysomnography in children. *Pediatr Pulmonol* 1992; 13:16–21.

60. Hershenson M, Brouillette RT, Olsen E, Hunt CE. The effect of chloral hydrate on genioglossus and diaphragmatic activity. *Pediatr Res* 1984; 18:516–519.

61. Rochester DF, Enson Y. Current concepts in the pathogenesis of the obesity-hypoventilation syndrome. *Am J Med* 1974; 57:402–420.

62. Zwillich CW, Sutton FD, Pierson DJ, Creagh EM, Weil JV. Decreased hypoxic ventilatory drive in the obesity-hypoventilation syndrome. *Am J Med* 1975; 59:343–348.

63. Garay SM, Rapoport D, Sorkin B, Epstein H, Feinberg I, Goldring RM. Regulation of ventilation in the obstructive sleep apnea syndrome. *Am Rev Respir Dis* 1981; 124:451–457.

64. Sullivan CE, Issa FG. Pathophysiological mechanisms in obstructive sleep apnea. *Sleep* 1980; 3:235–246.

65. Marcus CL, Gozal D, Basinski DJ, Omlin KJ, Keens TG, Ward SLD. Ventilatory and cardiac responses to hypercapnea and hypoxia during wakefulness in children with the obstructive sleep apnea syndrome [Abstract]. *Am Rev Respir Dis* 1992; 145:A176.

66. McGrath–Morrow SA, McColley SA, Carroll JL, Pyzik P, Cybulski M, Loughlin GM. Termination

of obstructive apnea in children is not associated with arousal. *Am Rev Respir Dis* 1990; 141:A195.

67. Guilleminault C. Obstructive sleep apnea and its treatment in children: Areas of agreement and controversy. *Pediatr Pulmonol* 1987; 3:429–436.

68. Rosen CL, D'Andrea L, Haddad GG. Adult criteria for obstructive sleep apnea do not identify children with serious obstruction. *Am Rev Respir Dis* 1992; 146:1231–1234.

69. Brouillette RT, Fernbach SK, Hunt CE. Obstructive sleep apnea in infants and children. *J Pediatr* 1982; 100:31–40.

70. Jeffries B, Brouillette RT, Hunt CE. Electromyographic study of some accessory muscles of respiration in children with obstructive sleep apnea. *Am Rev Respir Dis* 1984; 129:696–702.

71. Weitzman ED, Kahn E, Pollak CP. Quantitative analysis of sleep and sleep apnea before and after tracheostomy in patients with the hypersomnia–sleep apnea syndrome. *Sleep* 1980; 3:407–423.

72. Bradley TD, Phillipson EA. Pathogenesis and pathophysiology of the obstructive sleep apnea syndrome. *Med Clin North Am* 1985; 69:1169–1185.

73. McGrath SA, Carroll JL, McColley SA, et al. Normal sleep structure found in children with obstructive sleep apnea. Am Rev Respir Dis 1992; 145:A176.

74. Guilleminault C, Quera–Salva MA, Nino–Murcia G, Partinen M. Central sleep apnea and partial obstruction of the upper airway. *Ann Neurol* 1987; 21:465–469.

75. Sullivan CE, Issa FG. Obstructive sleep apnea. *Clin Chest Med* 1985; 6:633–650.

76. Fan L, Murphy S. Pectus excavatum from chronic upper airway obstruction. *Am J Dis Child* 1981; 135:550–552.

77. Perkin RM, Anas NG. Pulmonary hypertension in pediatric patients. *J Pediatr* 1984; 105:511–522.

78. Tal A, Leiberman A, Margulis G, Sofer S. Ventricular dysfunction in children with obstructive sleep apnea: radionuclide assessment. *Pediatr Pulmonol* 1988; 4:139–143.

79. Levin DL, Muster AJ, Pachman LM, Wessel HU, Paul MH, Koshaba J. Cor pulmonale secondary to upper airway obstruction: cardiac catheterization, immunologic, and psychometric evaluation in nine patients. *Chest* 1975; 68:166–171.

80. Ross RD, Daniels SR, Loggie JM, Meyer RA, Ballard ET. Sleep apnea-associated hypertension and reversible left ventricular hypertrophy. *J Pediatr* 1987; 111:253–255.

81. Guilleminault C, Korobkin R, Winkle R. A review of 50 children with obstructive sleep apnea syndrome. *Lung* 1981; 159:275–287.

82. Kravath RE, Pollak CP, Borowiecki B, Weitzman ED. Obstructive sleep apnea and death associated with surgical correction of velopharyngeal incompetence. *J Pediatr* 1980; 96:645–648.

83. Lauritzen C, Lilja J, Jarlstedt J. Airway obstruction and sleep apnea in children with craniofacial anomalies. *Plast Reconstruct Surg* 1986; 77:1–5.

84. Wilkinson AR, McCormick MS, Freeland AP, Pickering D. Electrocardiographic signs of pulmonary hypertension in children who snore. *Br Med J* 1981; 282:1579–1581.

85. Massumi RA, Sarin RK, Pooya M, Reicheldefern TR, Fraga JR, Rios JC, Ayesterian E. Tonsillar

hypertrophy, airway obstruction, alveolar hypoventilation, and cor pulmonale in twin brothers. *Dis Chest* 1969; 55:110–114.

86. Ainger LE. Large tonsils and adenoids in small children with cor pulmonale. *Br Heart J* 1968; 30:356–362.

87. Talbot AR, Robertson LW. Cardiac failure with tonsil and adenoid hypertrophy. *Arch Otolaryngol* 1973; 98:277–281.

88. Hunt CE, Brouillette RT. Abnormalities of breathing control and airway maintenance in infants and children as a cause of cor pulmonale. *Pediatr Cardiol* 1982; 3:249–256.

89. Nussbaum E, Hirschfeld SS, Wood RE, Boat TF, Doershuk CF. Echocardiographic changes in children with pulmonary hypertension secondary to upper airway obstruction. *J Pediatr* 1978; 93:931–936.

90. Brown OE, Manning SC, Ridenour B. Cor pulmonale secondary to tonsillar and adenoidal hypertrophy: management considerations. *Int J Pediatr Otorhinolaryngol* 1988; 16:131–139.

91. Levinson PD, Millman RP. Causes and consequences of blood pressure alterations in obstructive sleep apnea. *Arch Intern Med* 1991; 151:455–462.

92. Shepard JW. Cardiopulmonary consequences of obstructive sleep apnea. *Mayo Clin Proc* 1990; 65:1250–1259.

93. Millman RP, Redline S, Carlisle CC, Assaf/AR, Levinson PD. Daytime hypertension in obstructive sleep apnea. *Chest* 1991; 99:861–866.

94. Serratto M, Harris VJ, Carr I. Upper airways obstruction: Presentation with systemic hypertension. *Arch Dis Child* 1981; 56:153–155.

95. Greenberg GD, Watson RK, Deptula D. Neuropsychological dysfunction in sleep apnea. *Sleep* 1987; 10:254–262.

96. Bedard MA, Montplaisir J, Richer F, Malo J. Nocturnal hypoxemia as a determinant of vigilance impairment in sleep apnea syndrome. *Chest* 1991; 100:367–370.

97. Colt HG, Haas H, Rich GB. Hypoxemia vs sleep fragmentation as cause of excessive daytime sleepiness in obstructive sleep apnea. *Chest* 1991; 100:1542–1548.

98. Brouillette R, Hanson D, David R et al. A diagnostic approach to suspected obstructive sleep apnea in children. *J Pediatr* 1984; 105:10–14.

99. Weissbluth M, Davis AT, Poncher J, Reiff J. Signs of airway obstruction during sleep and behavioral, developmental, and academic problems. *J Dev Behav Pediatr* 1983; 4:119–121.

100. Cayler GG, Johnson EE, Lewis BE, Kortzeborn JD, Jordan J, Fricker GA. Heart failure due to enlarged tonsils and adenoids. *Am J Dis Child* 1969; 118:708–717.

101. Goldstein SJ, Wu RHK, Thorpy MJ, Shprintzen J, Marion RE, Saenger P. Reversibility of deficient sleep entrained growth hormone secretion in a boy with achondroplasia and obstructive sleep apnea. *Acta Endocrinol* 1987; 116:95–101.

102. Stradling JR, Thomas G, Warley ARH, Williams P, Freeland A. Effect of adenotonsillectomy on nocturnal hypoxaemia, sleep disturbance, and symptoms in snoring children. *Lancet* 1990; 335:249–253.

103. Williams EF, Woo P, Miller R, Kellman RM. The effects of adenotonsillectomy on growth in young children. *Otolaryngol Head Neck Surg* 1991; 104:509–516.

104. Krieger J. Mechanisms of daytime pulmonary hypertension and altered renal function in obstructive sleep apnea. In Guilleminault C, Partinen M, eds. *Obstructive sleep apnea syndrome.* New York, Raven Press, 1990, pp 71–79.

105. Weider DJ, Sateia MJ, West RP. Nocturnal enuresis in children with upper airway obstruction. *Otolaryngol Head Neck Surg* 1991; 105:427–432.

106. Konno A, Hoshino T, Togawa K. Influence of upper airway obstruction by enlarged tonsils and adenoids upon recurrent infection of the lower airway in childhood. *Laryngoscope* 1980; 90:1709–1716.

107. Luke MJ, Mehrizi A, Folger GM, Rowe RD. Chronic nasopharyngeal obstruction as a cause of cardiomegaly, cor pulmonale, and pulmonary edema. *Pediatrics* 1966; 37:762–768.

108. Lind MG, Lundell BPW. Tonsillar hyperplasia in children. A cause of obstructive sleep apneas, CO_2 retention, and retarded growth. *Arch Otolaryngol* 1982; 108:650–654.

109. Diagnostic Classification Steering Committee, Thorpy MJ, Chairman. *International classification of sleep disorders: Diagnostic and coding manual.* Rochester, MN, American Sleep Disorders Association, 1990.

110. Canet E, Gaultier C, D'Allest AM, Dehan M. Effects of sleep deprivation on respiratory events during sleep in healthy infants. *J Appl Physiol* 1989; 66:1158–1163.

111. Hunt CE, Hazinski TA, Gora P. Experimental effects of chloral hydrate on ventilatory response to hypoxia and hypercarbia. *Pediatr Res* 1982; 16:79–81.

112. American Thoracic Society. Indications and standards for cardiopulmonary sleep studies. *Am Rev Respir Dis* 1989; 139:559–568.

113. Kryger MH. Monitoring respiratory and cardiac function. In Kryger MH, Roth T, Dement WC, eds. *Principles and practice of sleep medicine.* Philadelphia, WB Saunders, 1989, pp 702–708.

114. Brouillette RT, Morrow S, Weese-Mayer DE, Hunt CE. Comparison of respiratory inductive plethysmography and thoracic impedance for apnea monitoring. *J Pediatr* 1987; 111:377–383.

115. Brouillette RT, Weese-Mayer DE, Hunt CE. Disorders of breathing during sleep in the pediatric population. *Semin Respir Med* 1988; 9:594–606.

116. van Someren V, Stothers JK. A critical dissection of obstructive apnea in the human infant. *Pediatrics* 1983; 71:721–725.

117. Guilleminault C, Winkle R, Korobkin R, Simmons B. Children and nocturnal snoring: Evaluation of the effects of sleep related respiratory resistive load and daytime functioning. *Eur J Pediatr* 1982; 139:165–171.

118. Hoppenbrouwers T, Hodgman JE, Arakawa A, Durand M, Cabal LA. Transcutaneous oxygen and carbon dioxide during the first half year of life in premature and normal term infants. *Pediatr Res* 1992; 31:73–79.

119. Mok JYQ, McLaughlin FJ, Pintar M, Hak H, Amaro-Galvez R, Levison H. Transcutaneous monitoring of oxygenation: What is normal? *J Pediatr* 1986; 108:365–371.

120. Stebbens VA, Poets CF, Alexander JR, Arrowsmith WA, Southall DP. Oxygen saturation and breathing patterns in infancy. 1: Full term infants in the second month of life. *Arch Dis Child* 1991; 66:569–573.

121. Mok JYQ, Hak H, McLaughlin FJ, Pintar M, Canny GJ, Levison H. Effect of age and state of wakefulness on transcutaneous oxygen values in preterm infants: A longitudinal study. *J Pediatr* 1988; 113:706–709.

122. Carroll JL, McColley SA, Marcus CL, Pyzik P, Curtis S, Loughlin GM. Can childhood obstructive sleep apnea syndrome (OSA) be diagnosed by a clinical symptom score? *Am Rev Respir Dis* 1992; 145:A179.

123. Carroll JL, McColley SA, Marcus CL, Curtis S, Pyzik P, Loughlin GM. Reported symptoms of childhood obstructive sleep apnea syndrome (OSA) vs primary snoring. *Am Rev Respir Dis* 1992; 145:A177.

124. Hasday JD, Grum CM. Nocturnal increase of urinary uric acid:creatinine ratio. A biochemical correlate of sleep-associated hypoxemia. *Am Rev Respir Dis* 1987; 135:534–538.

125. Tammelin BR, Wilson AF, Borowiecki BDB, Sassin JF. Flow-volume curves reflect pharyngeal airway abnormalities in sleep apnea syndrome. *Am Rev Respir Dis* 1983; 128:712–715.

126. Katz I, Zamel N, Slutsky AS, Rebuck AS, Hoffstein V. An evaluation of flow-volume curves as a screening test for obstructive sleep apnea. *Chest* 1990; 98:337–340.

127. Sanders MH, Stiller RA. Still going around on the flow-volume loop. *Chest* 1992; 101:301–303.

128. Guilleminault C, Partinen M, Penzel T, et al. Technical issues related to obstructive sleep apnea syndrome. In Guilleminault C, Partinen M, eds. *Obstructive sleep apnea syndrome.* New York, Raven Press, 1990, pp 183–207.

128a Felman AH, Loughlin GM, Leftridge CA, et.al. Upper airway obstruction during sleep in children. *Am J Roentgenol* 1979, 133:213–216.

129. Partinen M, Guilleminault C, Quera-Salva MA, Jamieson A. Obstructive sleep apnea and cephalometric roentgenograms. *Chest* 1988; 93:1199–1205.

130. Carskadon MA, Chairman: Association of Sleep Disorders Centers Task Force on Daytime Sleepiness. *Sleep* 1986; 9:519–524.

131. Carskadon MA, Dement WC. Sleepiness in the normal adolescent. In Guilleminault, ed. *Sleep and its disorders in children.* New York, Raven Press, 1987, pp 53–66.

132. Sofer S, Weinhouse E, Tal A, Wanderman KL, Margulis G, Leiberman A, Gueron M. Cor pulmonale due to adenoidal or tonsillar hypertrophy or both in children. Noninvasive diagnosis and follow-up. *Chest* 1988; 93:119–122.

133. Hudgel DW, Hendricks C, Dadley A. Alteration in obstructive apnea pattern induced by changes in oxygen- and carbon-dioxide–inspired concentrations. *Am Rev Respir Dis* 1988; 138:16–19.

134. Kravath RE, Pollak CP, Borowiecki B. Hypoventilation during sleep in children who have lymphoid airway obstruction treated by nasopharyngeal tube and T and A. *Pediatrics* 1977; 59:865–871.

135. Macartney FJ, Panday J, Scott O. Cor pulmonale as a result of chronic nasopharyngeal obstruction due to hypertrophied tonsils and adenoids. *Arch Dis Child* 1969; 44:585–592.

136. Fletcher EC, Munafo DA. Role of nocturnal oxygen therapy in obstructive sleep apnea. *Chest* 1990; 98:1497–1504.

137. Edison BD, Kerth JD. Tonsilloadenoid hypertrophy resulting in cor pulmonale. *Arch Otolaryngol* 1973; 98:205–207.

138. Croft CB, Brockbank MJ, Wright A, Swanston AR. Obstructive sleep apnoea in children undergoing routine tonsillectomy and adenoidectomy. *Clin Otolaryngol* 1990; 15:307–314.

139. Weninger M, Saletu B, Popow C, Gotz M, Haschke F. Obstructive sleep apnea: A polysomnographic study of sleep apnea before and after tonsillectomy and adenoidectomy. *Helv Paediatr Acta* 1988; 43:203–210.

140. Maw AR, Jeans WD, Cable HR. Adenoidectomy. A prospective study to show clinical and radiological changes two years after operation. *J Laryngol Otol* 1983; 97:511–518.

141. Goodman RS, Goodman M, Gootman N, Cohen H. Cardiac and pulmonary failure secondary to adenotonsillar hypertrophy. *Laryngoscope* 1976; 86:1367–1374.

142. Leiberman A, Tal A, Brama I, Sofer S. Obstructive sleep apnea in young infants. *Int J Pediatr Otorhinolaryngol* 1988; 16:39–44.

143. Derkay CS, Bray G, Milmoe GJ, Grundfast KM. Adenotonsillectomy in children with sickle cell disease. *South Med J* 1991; 84:205–208.

144. Reiner SA, Sawyer WP, Clark KF, Wood MW. Safety of outpatient tonsillectomy and adenoidectomy. *Otolaryngol Head Neck Surg* 1990; 102:161–168.

145. McColley SA, April MM, Carroll JL, Naclerio RM, Loughlin GM. Respiratory compromise after adenotonsillectomy in children with obstructive sleep apnea. *Arch Otolaryngol Head Neck Surg* 1992; 118:940–943.

146. Carithers JS, Gebhart DE, Williams JA. Postoperative risks of pediatric tonsilloadenoidectomy. *Laryngoscope* 1987; 97:422–429.

147. Wiatrak BJ, Myer CM, Andrews TM. Complications of adenotonsillectomy in children under 3 years of age. *Am J Otolaryngol* 1991; 12:170–172.

148. Pratt LW, Gallagher RA. Tonsillectomy and adenoidectomy: Incidence and mortality. *Otolaryngol Head Neck Surg* 1979; 87:159–166.

149. National Center for Health Statistics, Dennison CS: 1984 Summary: National Hospital Discharge Survey. Advance Data from Vital and Health Statistics. No. 112. DHHS Pub. No. (PHS) 85–1250. Public Health Service, Hyattsville, MD, Sept. 27, 1985.

150. Tami TA, Parker GS, Taylor RE. Post-tonsillectomy bleeding: an evaluation of risk factors. *Laryngoscope* 1987; 97:1307–1311.

151. Rasmussen N. Complications of tonsillectomy and adenoidectomy. *Otolaryngol Clin North Am* 1987; 20:383–390.

152. Yates DW. Adenotonsillar hypertrophy and cor pulmonale. *Br J Anaesth* 1988; 61:355–359.

153. Galvis AG. Pulmonary edema complicating relief of upper airway obstruction. *Am J Emerg Med* 1987; 5:294–297.

154. Feinberg AN, Shabino CL. Acute pulmonary edema complicating tonsillectomy and adenoidectomy. *Pediatrics* 1985; 75:112–114.

155. Helfaer MA, McColley SA, Pyzik PL, et al. Polysomnography after adenotonsillectomy in pediatric obstructive sleep apnea. *Am Rev Respir Dis* 1992; 145:180A.

156. Guilleminault C, Nino-Murcia G, Heldt G, Baldwin R, Hutchinson D. Alternative treatment to tracheostomy in obstructive sleep apnea syndrome: Nasal continuous positive airway pressure in young children. *Pediatrics* 1986; 78:797–802.

157. Crowe-McCann C, Nino-Murcia G, Guilleminault C. Nasal CPAP: the Stanford experience. In Guilleminault C, Partinen M, eds. *Obstructive sleep apnea syndrome*. New York, Raven Press, 1990, pp 119–127.

158. Miller MJ, Carlo WA, Martin RJ. Continuous positive airway pressure selectively reduces obstructive apnea in preterm infants. *J Pediatr* 1985; 106:91–94.

159. Ryan CF, Lowe AA, Fleetham JA. Nasal continuous positive airway pressure (CPAP) therapy for obstructive sleep apnea in Hallermann-Streiff syndrome. *Clin Pediatr* 1990; 29:122–124.

160. Sanders MH, Kern N. Obstructive sleep apnea treated by independently adjusted inspiratory and expiratory airway pressures via nasal mask. *Chest* 1990; 98:317–324.

161. Leech JA, Ascah CJ. Hemodynamic effects of nasal CPAP examined by Doppler echocardiography. *Chest* 1991; 99:323–326.

162. Smith PL, Gold AR, Meyers DA, Haponik EF, Bleecker ER. Weight loss in mildly to moderately obese patients with obstructive sleep apnea. *Ann Intern Med* 1985; 103:850–854.

163. Orenstein DM, Boat TF, Stern RC, Doershuk CF, Light MS. Progesterone treatment of the obesity hypoventilation syndrome in a child. *J Pediatr* 1977; 90:477–479.

164. Sutton FD, Zwillich CW, Creagh CE, Pierson DJ, Weil JV. Progesterone for outpatient treatment of Pickwickian syndrome. *Ann Intern Med* 1975; 83:476–479.

165. Cook WR, Benich JJ, Wooten SA. Indices of severity of obstructive sleep apnea syndrome do not change during medroxyprogesterone acetate therapy. *Chest* 1989; 96:262–266.

166. Orr WC, Imes NK, Martin RJ. Progesterone therapy in obese patients with sleep apnea. *Arch Intern Med* 1979; 139:109–111.

167. Brownell LG, West P, Sweatman P, Acres JC, Kryger MH. Protriptyline in obstructive sleep apnea. *N Engl J Med* 1982; 307:1037–1042.

168. Cartwright RD, Samelson CF. The effects of a nonsurgical treatment for obstructive sleep apnea. *JAMA* 1982; 248:705–709.

169. Schmidt–Nowara WW, Meade TE, Hays MB. Treatment of snoring and obstructive sleep apnea with a dental orthosis. *Chest* 1991; 99:1378–1385.

170. Bull MJ, Givan DC, Sadove AM, Bixler D, Hearn D. Improved outcome in Pierre Robin sequence: Effect of multidisciplinary evaluation and management. *Pediatrics* 1990; 86:294–301.

171. Marcus CL, Crockett DM, Ward SLD. Evaluation of epiglottoplasty as treatment for severe laryngomalacia. *J Pediatr* 1990; 117:706–710.

172. Strome M. Obstructive sleep apnea in Down syndrome children: A surgical approach. *Laryngoscope* 1986; 96:1340–1342.

173. Donaldson JD, Redmond WM. Surgical management of obstructive sleep apnea in children with Down syndrome. *J Otolaryngol* 1988; 17:398–403.

174. Powell NB, Riley RW, Guilleminault C. Maxillofacial surgery for obstructive sleep apnea. In Guilleminault C, Partinen M, eds. *Obstructive sleep apnea syndrome.* New York, Raven Press, 1990, pp 153–183.

175. Johnston C, Taussig LM, Koopmann C, Smith P, Bjelland J. Obstructive sleep apnea in Treacher-Collins syndrome. *Cleft Palate J* 1981; 18:39–44.

176. Fujita S, Conway WA, Zorick FJ, et al. Evaluation of the effectiveness of uvulopalatopharyngoplasty. *Laryngoscope* 1985; 95:70–74.

177. Hudgel DW, Harasick T, Katz RL, Witt WJ, Abelson TI. Uvulopalatopharyngoplasty in obstructive apnea. Value of preoperative localization of site of upper airway narrowing during sleep. *Am Rev Respir Dis* 1991; 143:942–946.

178. Abdu MH, Feghali JG. Uvulopalatopharyngoplasty in a child with obstructive sleep apnea. A case report. *J Laryngol Otol* 1988; 102:546–548.

179. Seid AB, Martin PJ, Pransky SM, Kearns DB. Surgical therapy of obstructive sleep apnea in children with severe mental insufficiency. *Laryngoscope* 1990; 100:507–510.

180. Schafer ME. Upper airway obstruction and sleep disorders in children with craniofacial anomalies. *Clin Plast Surg* 1982; 9:555–567.

181. Fink GB, Madaus WK and Walker GF. A quantitative study of the face in Down's syndrome. *Am J Orthodont* 1975; 67:540–553.

182. Southall DP, Stebbens VA, Mirza R, Lang MH, Croft CB, Shinebourne EA. Upper airway obstruction with hypoxaemia and sleep disruption in Down syndrome. *Dev Med Child Neurol* 1987; 29:734–742.

183. Stebbens VA, Dennis J, Samuels MP, Croft CB, Southall DP. Sleep related upper airway obstruction in a cohort with Down's syndrome. *Arch Dis Child* 1991; 66:1333–1338.

184. Marcus CL, Keens TG, Bautista DB, von Pechmann WS, Ward SLD. Obstructive sleep apnea in children with Down syndrome. *Pediatrics* 1991; 88:132–139.

185. Levine OR, Simpser M. Alveolar hypoventilation and cor pulmonale associated with chronic airway obstruction in infants with Down syndrome. *Clin Pediatr* 1982; 21:25–29.

186. Loughlin GM, Wynne JW, Victorica BE. Sleep apnea as a possible cause of pulmonary hypertension in Down syndrome. *J Pediatr* 1981; 98:435–437.

187. Kasian GF, Duncan WJ, Tyrrell MJ, Oman-Ganes LA. Elective oro-tracheal intubation to diagnose sleep apnea syndrome in children with Down's syndrome and ventricular septal defect. *Can J Cardiol* 1987; 3:2–5.

188. Sidman JD, Fry TL. Exacerbation of sickle cell disease by obstructive sleep apnea. *Arch Otolaryngol Head Neck Surg* 1988; 114:916–917.

189. Ijaduola CA, Akinyanju OO. Chronic tonsillitis, tonsillectomy and sickle cell crises. *J Laryngol Otol* 1987; 101:467–470.

190. Robertson PL, Aldrich MS, Hanash SM, Goldstein GW. Stroke associated with obstructive sleep apnea in a child with sickle cell anemia. *Ann Neurol* 1988; 23:614–616.

191. Orr WC, Levine NS, Buchanan RT. Effect of cleft palate repair and pharyngeal flap surgery on upper airway obstruction during sleep. *Plast Reconstr Surg* 1987; 80:226–230.

192. Robson MC, Stankiewicz JA, Mendelsohn JS. Cor Pulmonale secondary to cleft palate repair. *Plast Reconstr Surg* 1977; 59:254.

193. Ruddy J, Stokes M, Pearman K. Pharyngoplasty surgery and obstructive sleep apnea. *J Laryngol Otol* 1991; 105:195–197.

194. Kahn A, Baran D, Spehl M, Dab I, Blum D. Congenital stridor in infancy. *Clin Pediatr* 1977; 16:19–26.

195. Holinger LD. Etiology of stridor in the neonate, infant and child. *Ann Otol* 1980; 89:397–400.

196. Holinger PC, Holinger LD, Reichert TJ, Holinger PH. Respiratory obstruction and apnea in infants with bilateral abductor vocal cord paralysis, meningomyelocele, hydrocephalus, and Arnold-Chiari malformation. *J Pediatr* 1978; 92:368–373.

197. Cox MA, Schiebler GL, Taylor WJ, Wheat MW, Krovetz LJ. Reversible pulmonary hypertension in a child with respiratory obstruction and cor pulmonale. *J Pediatr* 1965; 67:192–197.

198. Cohen SR, Geller KA, Birns JW, Thompson JW. Laryngeal paralysis in children. A long-term retrospective study. *Ann Otol Rhinol Laryngol* 1982; 91:417–424.

199. Belmont JR, Grundfast K. Congenital laryngeal stridor (laryngomalacia): Etiologic factors and associated disorders. *Ann Otol Rhinol Laryngol* 1984; 93:430–437.

200. Rosen CL, Frost JD, Harrison GM. Infant apnea: Polygraphic studies and follow-up monitoring. *Pediatrics* 1983; 71:731–736.

201. Guilleminault C, Souquet M, Ariagno RL, Korobkin R, Simmons FB. Five cases of near-miss sudden infant death syndrome and development of obstructive sleep apnea syndrome. *Pediatrics* 1984; 73:71–78.

202. Kahn A, Blum D, Rebuffat E, et al. Polysomnographic studies of infants who subsequently died of sudden infant death syndrome. *Pediatrics* 1988; 82:721–727.

203. Guilleminault C, Ariagno RL, Forno LS, Nagel L, Baldwin R, Owen M. Obstructive sleep apnea and near miss for SIDS: 1. Report of an infant with sudden death. *Pediatrics* 1979; 63:837–843.

204. Guilleminault C, Ariagno R, Korobkin R, Nagel L, Baldwin R, Coons S, Owen M. Mixed and obstructive sleep apnea and near miss for sudden

infant death syndrome. 2. Comparison of near miss and normal control infants by age. *Pediatrics* 1979; 64:882–891.

205. Dransfield DA, Spitzer AR, Fox WW. Episodic airway obstruction in premature infants. *Am J Dis Child* 1983; 137:441–443.

206. Orr WC, Stahl ML, Duke J, et al. Effect of sleep state and position on the incidence of obstructive and central apnea in infants. *Pediatrics* 1985; 75:832–835.

207. Miller MJ, Martin RJ, Carlo WA, Fouke JM, Strohl KP, Fanaroff AA. Oral breathing in newborn infants. *J Pediatr* 1985; 107:465–469.

208. Purcell M. Response in the newborn to raised upper airway resistance. *Arch Dis Child* 1976; 51:602–607.

209. Martin RJ, Miller MJ, Siner B, DiFiore JM, Carlo WA. Effects of unilateral nasal occlusion on ventilation and pulmonary resistance in infants. *J Appl Physiol* 1989; 66:2522–2526.

210. Harding R. Nasal obstruction in infancy. *Aust Paediatr J* 1986; Suppl:59–61.

211. Roloff DW, Aldrich MS. Sleep disorders and airway obstruction in newborns and infants. *Otolaryngol Clin North Am* 1990; 23:639–649.

212. Southall DP, Croft CB, Stebbens VA, et al. Detection of sleep associated dysfunctional pharyngeal obstruction in infants. *Eur J Pediatr* 1989; 148:353–359.

213. Roberts JL, Reed WR, Mathew OP, Menon AA, Thach BT. Assessment of pharyngeal airway stability in normal and micrognathic infants. *J Appl Physiol* 1985; 58:290–299.

214. Wilson SL, Thach BT, Brouillette RT, Abu-Osba YK. Upper airway patency in the human infant: Influence of airway pressure and posture. *J Appl Physiol* 1980; 48:500–504.

215. Thach BT, Stark AR. Spontaneous neck flexion and airway obstruction during apneic spells in preterm infants. *J Pediatr* 1979; 94:275–281.

216. Pickens DL, Schefft G, Thach BT. Prolonged apnea associated with upper airway protective reflexes in apnea of prematurity. *Am Rev Respir Dis* 1988; 137:113–118.

217. Herbst JJ, Minton SD, Book LS. Gastroesophageal reflux causing respiratory distress and apnea in newborn infants. *J Pediatr* 1979; 95:763–768.

218. Milner AD, Boon AW, Saunders RA, Hopkins IE. Upper airways obstruction and apnea in preterm babies. *Arch Dis Child* 1980; 55:22–25.

219. Poets CF, Stebbens VA, Alexander JR, Arrowsmith WA, Salfield SAW, Southall DP. Oxygen saturation and breathing patterns in infancy. 2: Preterm infants at discharge from special care. *Arch Dis Child* 1991; 66:574–578.

220. Poets CF, Stebbens VA, Alexander JR, Arrowsmith WA, Salfield SAW, Southall DP. Arterial oxygen saturation in preterm infants at discharge from the hospital and six weeks later. *J Pediatr* 1992; 120:447–454.

221. Muller NL, Francis PW, Gurwitz D, Levison H, Bryan AC. Mechanism of hemoglobin desaturation during rapid-eye-movement sleep in normal subjects and in patients with cystic fibrosis. *Am Rev Respir Dis* 1980; 121:463–469.

222. Bateman JRM, Pavia D, Clarke SW. The retention of lung secretions during the night in normal subjects. *Clin Sci Mol Med* 1978; 55:523–527.

223. Coffey MJ, Fitzgerald MX, McNicholas WT. Comparison of oxygen desaturation during sleep and exercise in patients with cystic fibrosis. *Chest* 1991; 100:659–662.

224. Gaultier C, Praud JP, Clement A. Respiration during sleep in children with COPD. *Chest* 1985; 87:168–173.

225. Garg M, Kurzner SI, Bautista DB, Keens TG. Clinically unsuspected hypoxia during sleep and feeding in infants with bronchopulmonary dysplasia. *Pediatrics* 1988; 81:635–642.

226. Bye PTP, Ellis ER, Issa FG, Donnelly PM, Sullivan CE. Respiratory failure and sleep in neuromuscular disease. *Thorax* 1990; 45:241–247.

227. Smith PEM, Calverley PMA, Edwards RHT. Hypoxemia during sleep in Duchenne muscular dystrophy. *Am Rev Respir Dis* 1988; 137:884–888.

227a. Hudak B, Allen MC, Hudak ML, Loughlin GM. Home O$_2$ therapy for chronic lung disease in extremely low birth weight infants. *Am J Dis Child* 1989; 143:357–360.

228. Mileur LM, Pfeffer KD, Witte MK, Chapman D, Nielson D. Eliminating sleep associated hypoxemia improves growth in infants with BPD. *Clin Res* 1991; 39:111A.

229. Rotschild A, Dison PJ, Chitayat D, Solimano A. Midfacial hypoplasia associated with long-term intubation for bronchopulmonary dysplasia. *Am J Dis Child* 1990; 144:1302–1306.

230. Kahn Y, Heckmatt JZ. Breathing during sleep in Duchenne muscular dystrophy and normal subjects. *Am Rev Respir Dis* 1992; 145:A863.

231. Keens TG, Jansen MT, DeWitt PK, Ward SLD. Home care for children with chronic respiratory failure. *Semin Respir Med* 1990; 11:269–281.

232. Nelson WF, Hecht JT, Horton WA, Butler IJ, Goldie WD, Miner M. Neurological basis of respiratory complications in achondroplasia. *Ann Neurol* 1988; 24:89–93.

233. Reid CS, Pyeritz RE, Kopits SE, et al. Cervicomedullary compression in young patients with achondroplasia: Value of comprehensive neurologic and respiratory evaluation. *J Pediatr* 1987; 110:522–530.

234. Mador MJ, Tobin MJ. Apneustic breathing. A characteristic feature of brainstem compression in achondroplasia? *Chest* 1990; 97:877–883.

235. Stokes DC, Phillips JA, Leonard CO, et al. Respiratory complications of achondroplasia. *J Pediatr* 1983; 102:534–541.

236. Mixter RC, David DJ, Perloff WH, Green CG, Pauli RM, Popic PM. Obstructive sleep apnea in Apert's and Pfeiffer's syndromes: More than a craniofacial abnormality. *Plast Reconstr Surg* 1990; 86:457–463.

237. Smith DF, Mihm FG, Flynn M. Chronic alveolar hypoventilation secondary to macroglossia in the Beckwith-Wiedemann syndrome. *Pediatrics* 1982; 70:695–697.

238. Grundfast K, Berkowitz R, Fox L. Outcome and complications following surgery for obstructive adenotonsillar hypertrophy in children with neuro-

muscular disorders. *Ear Nose Throat J* 1990; 69:756–760.

239. Cozzi F, Pierro A. Glossoptosis-apnea syndrome in infancy. *Pediatrics* 1985; 75:836–843.

240. Kahn A, Blum D, Hoffman A, et al. Obstructive sleep apnea induced by a parapharyngeal cystic hygroma in an infant. *Sleep* 1985; 8:363–366.

241. Clark RW, Schmidt HS and Schuller DE. Sleep-induced ventilatory dysfunction in Down's syndrome. *Arch Intern Med* 1980; 140:45–50.

242. Friede H, Lopata M, Fisher E, Rosenthal IM. Cardiorespiratory disease associated with Hallermann-Streiff syndrome: Analysis of craniofacial morphology by cephalometric roentgenograms. *J Craniofac Genet Dev Biol* 1985; 1(Suppl):189–198.

243. Rajagopal KR, Abbrecht PH, Derderian SS, et al. Obstructive sleep apnea in hypothyroidism. *Ann Intern Med* 1984; 101:491–494.

244. Puckett CL, Pickens J, Reinisch JF. Sleep apnea in mandibular hypoplasia. *Plast Reconstr Surg* 1982; 70:213–216.

245. Semenza GL, Pyeritz RE. Respiratory complications of mucopolysaccharide storage disorders. *Medicine* 1988; 67:209–219.

246. Myer CM. Airway obstruction in Hurler's syndrome—Radiographic features. *Int J Pediatr Otorhinolaryngol* 1991; 22:91–96.

247. Perks WH, Cooper RA, Bradbury S, et al. Sleep apnoea in Scheie's syndrome. *Thorax* 1980; 35:85–91.

248. Shapiro J, Strome M, Crocker AC. Airway obstruction and sleep apnea in Hurler and Hunter syndromes. *Ann Otol Rhinol Laryngol* 1985; 94:458–461.

249. Ruckenstein MJ, MacDonald RE, Clarke JTR, Forte V. The management of otolaryngological problems in the mucopolysaccharidoses: A retrospective review. *J Otolaryngol* 1991; 20:177–183.

250. Ginzburg AS, Onal E, Aronson RM, Schild JA, Mafee MF, Lopata M. Successful use of nasal-CPAP for obstructive sleep apnea in Hunter syndrome with diffuse airway involvement. *Chest* 1990; 97:1496–1498.

251. Malone BN, Whitley CB, Duvall AJ, et al. Resolution of obstructive sleep apnea in Hurler syndrome after bone marrow transplantation. *Int J Pediatr Otorhinolaryngol* 1988; 15:23–31.

252. Carter M, Stokes D, Wang W. Severe obstructive sleep apnea in a child with osteopetrosis. *Clin Pediatr* 1988; 27:108–110.

253. Brodsky L, Siddiqui SY, Stanievich JF. Massive oropharyngeal papillomatosis causing obstructive sleep apnea in a child. *Arch Otolaryngol Head Neck Surg* 1987; 113:882–884.

254. Vela–Bueno A, Kales A, Soldatos CR, et al. Sleep in the Prader-Willi syndrome. *Arch Neurol* 1984; 41:294–296.

255. Cassidy SB, McKillop JA, Morgan WJ. Sleep disorders in Prader-Willi syndrome. *Dysmorphol Clin Genet* 1990; 4:13–17.

256. Maddern BR, Reed HT, Ohene-Frempong K, Beckerman RC. Obstructive sleep apnea syndrome in sickle cell disease. *Ann Otol Rhinol Laryngol* 1989; 98:174–178.

257. Colmenero C, Esteban R, Albarino AR, Colmenero B. Sleep apnoea syndrome associated with maxillofacial abnormalities. *J Laryngol Otol* 1991; 105:94–100.

258. Kahn A, Mozin MJ, Rebuffat E, Sottiaux M, Burniat W, Shepherd S, Muller MF. Sleep pattern alterations and brief airway obstructions in overweight infants. *Sleep* 1989; 12:430–438.

40

Congenital Malformations of the Lung and Airways

BONNIE B. HUDAK

Congenital abnormalities of the lungs and airways should be included in the differential diagnosis of most signs and symptoms referable to the respiratory tract throughout infancy and childhood (Table 40.1). Although some malformations are apparent early in life, others may not be distinguished from routine pediatric illnesses until adolescence or adulthood. Not only can congenital malformations be difficult to diagnose, they may continue to be a source of respiratory problems that persist after diagnosis and treatment.

Several excellent references exist that catalogue the congenital malformations of the

Table 40.1.
Signs and Symptoms of Congenital Malformations Presenting in Infancy

Malformation	Additional Findings
Respiratory distress at birth	
Laryngeal webs	Hoarse, weak, or absent cry
Laryngeal cysts	Stridor, hoarseness, aphonia
Laryngeal atresia	Voiceless cry, absent breath sounds
Bilateral vocal cord paralysis	Abnormal cry, stridor, aspiration
Subglottic stenosis	Stridor
Tracheal agenesis	Voiceless cry, absent breath sounds
Tracheal stenosis	Stridor
Pulmonary hypoplasia	Small thorax, orthopedic deformities
Cystic adenomatoid malformation	Anasarca, asymmetric breath sounds
Congenital lobar emphysema	Asymmetric breath sounds
Congenital diaphragmatic hernia	Scaphoid abdomen, asymmetric breath sounds, other anomalies
Pulmonary lymphangiectasia	Hydrops, congenital heart disease
Diaphragmatic paralysis	Paradoxical respirations
Vascular ring	Apnea, cyanosis
Bronchogenic cyst	Asymmetric breath sounds
Feeding problems and aspiration	
Vocal cord paralysis	Weak or hoarse cry, stridor
Laryngotracheoesophageal cleft	Other anomalies, apnea, stridor
Tracheoesophageal fistula	Copious oral secretions
Vascular ring	Apnea, cyanosis
Stridor	
Laryngomalacia	Exertional distress, normal cry
Laryngeal cysts, webs	Abnormal cry
Subglottic stenosis	Exertional distress, croup
Subglottic hemangiomas	Exertional distress, croup, hoarse cry
Tracheal stenosis or compression	Exertional distress, wheezing
Tracheomalacia	Wheezing, exertional distress
Vocal cord dysfunction	Abnormal voice or cry, aspiration

501

respiratory tract (1–6). This chapter is intended for use by the clinician in establishing a differential diagnosis, targeting the laboratory and radiologic evaluation, and directing the immediate and long-term management. The information contained in the following sections is summarized for quick reference in the Tables.

LARYNGEAL ANOMALIES

Congenital anomalies of the larynx are relatively common, occurring in 1 of every 2000 live births; they include laryngomalacia, laryngeal and laryngotracheoesophageal clefts, laryngeal atresia, laryngeal cysts, and laryngeal webs and subglottic stenosis. Although not a true anatomic abnormality, congenital vocal cord paralysis will also be considered in this section since it may present similarly to these other conditions. The malformations usually cause symptoms in the first days or weeks of life with respiratory distress or stridor and may result in life-threatening upper airway obstruction (Table 40.1).

Laryngomalacia

Laryngomalacia is the most common congenital abnormality of the larynx. It is not a true malformation but rather represents a delay in maturation of the supporting structures of the larynx. The most common and most notable symptom is inspiratory stridor, which is usually unaccompanied by significant airway obstruction and often resolves in the first 2 years of life. However, it is the usual reason for referral and is a great cause of concern for parents.

Most patients with laryngomalacia present before 6 weeks of age, with symptoms apparent in virtually all cases by 4 months (7–10). Inspiratory stridor, worse with the increased ventilation associated with crying and feeding and in the supine position, is characteristic. Some patients have stridor at rest, and 10% may have a minor expiratory component as well. The tone of the cry and voice is normal.

Diagnosis is suspected based on the clinical history and physical examination. High-voltage neck radiographs or airway fluoroscopy to rule out major airway abnormalities may be sufficient in patients with mild symptoms compatible with the diagnosis of laryngomalacia. Laryngomalacia is associated with laryn-

geal anomalies in as many as 15% of cases, some of which may cause progressive respiratory obstruction or require intervention (10). Therefore, evaluation is warranted in all patients with high-pitched stridor, marked retractions at rest, atypical presentations (e.g., worsening of symptoms at night), or persistence of stridor beyond the first year of life.

The classic findings include a long, flaccid, tubular-appearing ("omega-shaped") epiglottis that folds into the glottis on inspiration; poorly supported, prominent-appearing arytenoids that prolapse forward during inspiration; and short aryepiglottic folds (7). Evaluation of the subglottic space and lower respiratory tract with bronchoscopy is required for patients with severe or atypical symptoms to rule out an additional lesion (10).

Laryngomalacia is usually a benign, self-limited condition with an excellent prognosis. Although early series of infants with laryngomalacia suggested an increased incidence of cerebral palsy and mental retardation, more recent studies have not confirmed this finding (9). Usually, laryngomalacia occurs as an isolated finding but may be seen in association with tracheomalacia. Occasionally, there may be accompanying feeding difficulties, aspiration, or failure to thrive. Although awake symptoms dominant the clinical picture, polysomnography performed in infants with isolated laryngomalacia have demonstrated mild, brief obstructive events and decreased periodic breathing when compared to age-matched controls (11). Transcutaneous oxygen ($TCPO_2$) and carbon dioxide ($TCPCO_2$) monitoring during sleep has shown more episodes of increase in $TCPCO_2$ and decrease in $TCPO_2$ than in controls. However, these episodes accounted for a median of only 2.6% of sleep time (12). Typically, laryngomalacia can be thought of as a benign condition without clinical consequence except for parental anxiety. Severe laryngomalacia may result in cor pulmonale and sudden death (13). Treatment almost always consists of simple observation. Occasionally, surgical intervention with either epiglottoplasty or tracheotomy may be required for infants with severe airway obstruction as evidenced by high-pitched stridor, marked retractions, significant nocturnal symptoms confirmed by polysomnography, and interference with normal growth and development (14, 15) (see Chapter 27).

Several studies have addressed the natural history and pulmonary function outcome of children with laryngomalacia in childhood. Although symptoms do resolve in many children before the age of 2 years (40–53%), many have persistent stridor for longer periods (8, 9). Pulmonary function testing performed in asymptomatic children with a history of isolated laryngomalacia has demonstrated abnormalities of inspiratory flow. Flow-volume loops yield the pattern characteristic of a variable extrathoracic airway obstruction with a decreased mid vital capacity (mid-VC) ratio and maximal inspiratory flow at 50% of vital capacity ($V_{max}50_I$) (8, 16).

Laryngeal and Laryngotracheoesophageal Clefts

Congenital laryngeal and laryngotracheoesophageal (LTE) clefts are uncommon anomalies that are often considered late in the differential diagnosis, are hard to demonstrate, and are difficult to repair. Of all laryngeal anomalies, 0.3–1.0% are LTE clefts (17). Postmortem studies have demonstrated a rate as high as 0.2% of pediatric autopsies. However, this probably reflects the common association with other congenital anomalies including tracheoesophageal fistula (TEF) (12–20%) and other gastrointestinal, genitourinary, and cardiovascular malformations (17, 18). In one series of patients with laryngeal and LTE clefts, 67% of the fatalities were in patients with other anomalies. The mortality rate for laryngeal and LTE clefts is high, approximately 50% overall, with severe LTE clefts carrying a greater than 90% mortality rate (18).

Although there are several classification schemes for the different types of laryngeal and LTE clefts, simplistically, there are laryngeal clefts without tracheal involvement, and laryngotracheoesophageal clefts. The latter may range in severity from those involving only the larynx and proximal trachea to those that extend along the entire length of the trachea and into the mainstem bronchi. They occur as a result of failure of closure of the dorsal cricoid plates and development of the tracheoesophageal septum in the first trimester of gestation (19).

Isolated laryngeal clefts involve absence of intra-arytenoid muscles above the glottis.

They present with apnea, aspiration, and/or stridor. In many cases, a barium swallow study has already demonstrated aspiration of barium into the tracheobronchial tree prior to consideration of the diagnosis. More complex lesions, involving direct communication between the trachea and the esophagus, usually present at or shortly after birth. Symptoms include copious secretions, respiratory distress, and aspiration. The differential diagnosis is that of tracheoesophageal fistula, direct aspiration from abnormal swallowing function, and LTE cleft. Usually, the work-up is initiated with a barium esophagram, which often demonstrates spillage of contrast into the trachea, although, with small lesions, the type of communication may not be apparent. If the esophagram is done via a catheter, it must be gradually withdrawn as contrast is injected to ensure adequate study of the upper trachea. Flexible fiberoptic laryngoscopy and bronchoscopy may not demonstrate the presence of a cleft since esophageal mucosa may balloon through the cleft and disguise it. Suspension microlaryngoscopy and rigid bronchoscopy with probing of the posterior wall of the larynx and trachea is often required in order to make the diagnosis (17, 18, 20, 21).

Although LTE clefts were first described in the 1700s, correction of this type of defect was not attempted until 1955. A number of surgical approaches have been advocated, and none is universally accepted at this time. The most difficult aspect of all procedures remains maintenance of an adequate airway while separation of the trachea and esophagus is achieved. Virtually all such procedures require tracheostomy, often with custom-made tubes, and gastrostomy. Surgical repair can usually be accomplished by an anterior laryngofissure or an endoscopic approach. Even if separation of the respiratory and digestive tracts is accomplished, chronic respiratory problems persist related to tracheomalacia, ventilation prior to surgery, lung injury secondary to repeated episodes of aspiration, esophageal dysmotility, and/or recurrent laryngeal nerve injury. Gastroesophageal reflux is a common problem, frequently requiring an anti-reflux procedure (17, 18, 20, 21).

The association of both laryngeal and LTE clefts with esophageal atresia and tracheoesophageal fistula is an important but not surprising one. These anomalies all result from incomplete formation of the tracheoesophageal septum. With a reported simultaneous occurrence of 12–37% in patients with laryngeal or LTE clefts, an evaluation for a TEF is warranted at the time of diagnosis. In addition, 6% of patients with esophageal atresia and tracheoesophageal fistula were noted to have an associated laryngeal or LTE cleft in one study (17).

Laryngeal Atresia and Laryngeal Webs

The most immediately life-threatening laryngeal malformation is laryngeal atresia. The lumen of the normally developing larynx is occluded by proliferating epithelium until 6 weeks' gestation. Laryngeal atresia results when normal recanalization fails to occur at 10 weeks. The atresia may be supraglottic, infraglottic, or both. Lung development usually proceeds without significant abnormality, although hyperplasia of the lungs has been reported (22). Affected infants thrive in utero but develop respiratory distress at birth. At delivery, these infants attempt to breathe with vigorous chest wall movement and a "tracheal tug" but have a voiceless cry and absence of breath sounds on auscultation. The diagnosis is confirmed on laryngoscopy when there is a fibrous membrane or mass present in the larynx preventing the placement of an endotracheal tube. Treatment is perforation of the membrane or immediate tracheostomy accomplished by percutaneous placement of a large-bore intravenous catheter into the trachea. Most infants with this abnormality die shortly after birth because of failure to establish an airway. Long-term prognosis depends on the presence of other anomalies, consequences related to delay in initiating ventilation, and precise anatomy of the individual lesion. In some cases, reconstructive surgery may allow for the development of speech (23).

When partial recanalization or the larynx occurs, the result is a laryngeal web. Most webs (75%) are glottic in location, though they may also occur in the supraglottic or subglottic regions. They are usually anterior with a concave posterior glottic opening. Infants with complete laryngeal webs have symptoms at birth similar to those of laryngeal atresia. Those with partial webs have stridor and a hoarse or weak cry. The diagnosis of a laryngeal web can be made by laryngoscopy. Complete webs require immediate perforation or placement of an emergency tracheostomy (24). Treatment of thick partial webs involves lysis or excision and may require tracheostomy. Thin partial webs can usually be divided with a scalpel or laser. If time and clinical status permit, partial subglottic webs may be dilated.

Laryngeal Cysts

Cysts of the larynx are usually supraglottic in location and cause respiratory distress with hoarseness, muffled voice, aphonia, and stridor. There may be positional variation in the occurrence and severity of symptoms. Lateral neck radiographs show a large, smooth supraglottic swelling. Direct laryngoscopy reveals a bluish, fluid-filled cyst, usually in the area of the epiglottic fold. Complete airway occlusion requiring emergency tracheostomy is a potential complication of laryngoscopy in these infants. Although aspiration or incision of the cyst offers immediate relief, resection is required to prevent recurrence. This can usually be accomplished endoscopically. Postoperatively, patients are supported with an endotracheal tube until edema resolves (24, 25).

Vocal Cord Dysfunction

Congenital paralysis of the vocal cords is more common than generally appreciated, accounting for 10–15% of cases of neonatal stridor (26). Unilateral paralysis may occur in association with congenital heart disease, in particular anomalies of the great vessels. More frequently, unilateral vocal cord paralysis is acquired as the result of injury during cardiothoracic surgery, secondary to mediastinal lesions (e.g., lymphoma) or secondary to birth trauma. In the latter case, accompanying involvement of other cranial or cervical nerves suggests the etiology. Many cases of unilateral vocal cord paralysis are "idiopathic" (27). Paralysis of one vocal cord results in a weak cry, perhaps accompanied by stridor during exertion. Swallowing and breathing are generally normal since the other is unaffected. The left vocal cord is affected more frequently than the right because of the lengthy course of the left recurrent laryngeal nerve into the thorax.

The presence of bilateral vocal cord paralysis should immediately raise the suspicion of neurologic lesions, including hydrocephalus, 4th ventricle lesions, bulbar injury, and

Arnold-Chiari malformations. The symptoms of bilateral vocal cord dysfunction depend on the position of the vocal cords. Usually they are in a paramedian position, obstructing respiration and allowing aspiration. Bilateral abduction of the vocal cords results in a weak, breathy voice and aspiration. Diagnosis of vocal cord dysfunction requires laryngoscopy with the patient awake. An excellent view of the larynx can be achieved by having the infant sit on a parent's lap while the fiberscope is passed through a well-anesthetized nostril. Improper positioning of the laryngoscope or deep sedation may inhibit vocal cord movement (24).

Congenital Subglottic Stenosis

The congenital form of subglottic stenosis occurs as a consequence of an abnormality of the cricoid cartilage or the subglottic tissue, resulting in a decreased anterior-posterior dimension. The most common location of a congenital subglottic stenosis is approximately 2–3 mm below the glottis. Presentation may range from stridor apparent at birth to "croup," with recurrent or persistent episodes of stridor associated with respiratory infections. The diagnosis can often be suspected on high-voltage radiographs of the neck and confirmed by laryngoscopy. Bronchoscopy is also required to assure that there is no accompanying anomaly of the lower airway. Mild cases require only supportive therapy for intermittent episodes of croup. More severely affected infants may require tracheostomy and dilation, cricoid reconstruction, or cricoid split (see Chapter 27). Since most cases of subglottic narrowing improve with laryngeal growth, children requiring tracheostomy can usually be decannulated by 2–3 years of age (28, 29).

Subglottic Hemangioma

Subglottic hemangioma should be considered in the differential diagnosis of chronic or recurrent stridor, especially if the child also has a cutaneous hemangioma. However, a hemangioma may be absent in more than half the cases. In addition to stridor, affected infants have a hoarse cry and dyspnea, worsened by crying and respiratory tract infections. Usually symptoms are absent at birth and become apparent over the first 6–18 months of life, causing confusion with croup or subglottic stenosis. There is a female predominance of 2:1.

Radiographic findings include an irregular subglottic mass. On endoscopy, the hemangioma is visible as a soft, blue, compressible lesion in the posterior subglottic space. Small lesions can be managed without intervention since the natural history is one of gradual progression over the first 6–18 months of life, followed by regression. Treatment with surgical laser and steroids can be used to avoid tracheostomy in most other instances. Occasionally, tracheostomy or open resection are required (24, 30).

TRACHEAL MALFORMATIONS

The lesions discussed in this section are a combination of primary anomalies of the trachea and malformations of other thoracic structures that either concurrently or secondarily involve the trachea. Among the primary tracheal abnormalities are tracheal agenesis, tracheal stenosis, and tracheomalacia. Tracheoesophageal fistulas and vascular rings are examples of multi-organ system abnormalities involving the trachea. Although some malformations of the trachea are apparent early in life, others may result in chronic pulmonary disease before the diagnosis of a congenital anomaly involving the trachea is entertained (Tables 40.1–40.3).

Tracheomalacia

Tracheomalacia occurs as the consequence of inadequate cartilaginous support of the trachea, allowing collapse of the intrathoracic trachea with expiration. It may occur as a primary disorder in which the cartilage rings of the trachea are absent, hypoplastic, or insufficiently rigid, or in conjunction with other congenital anomalies that involve the trachea, such as a tracheoesophageal fistula or vascular ring. Similarly, lack of sufficient cartilaginous support may occur in the bronchi, resulting in bronchomalacia, a process implicated as a cause of congenital lobar emphysema (31–33). Tracheobronchomalacia can also develop as a consequence of recurrent airway trauma from prolonged intubation or aspiration.

Patients with primary tracheomalacia present in infancy with barking cough and expiratory wheezing that is worse with high flow

decreasing large airway tone, assistance in clearing secretions, accomplished by providing humidification and chest physiotherapy, may be helpful. Symptoms may worsen following inhalation of beta agonists because of additional decreases in airway tone. Patients with severe tracheomalacia may require tracheostomy with or without positive pressure support with CPAP (34, 35). Aortopexy has been performed in patients with severe tracheomalacia in an attempt to avoid tracheostomy. Over half of the patients had short-term resolution of their symptoms after aortopexy and successful treatment of any gastroesophageal reflux (36). Aortopexy is reserved for infants who have failed a trial of CPAP with a pressure of 10 cm H_2O. The need for tracheostomy should be based on the severity of the resting respiratory dysfunction. The response to stress, including agitation, infection, the effects on growth and development, and oxygen saturation measurements at rest and during periods of agitation should be considered in the decision making process.

Tracheal Stenosis

Isolated tracheal stenosis is an uncommon congenital malformation. Three types have been described: localized stenosis, diffuse long-segment hypoplasia, and funnel-shaped narrowing. Stenosis may result from the presence of complete tracheal rings ("napkin ring"), external compression, or incomplete recanalization of the developing trachea. Most patients present with stridor and varying degrees of respiratory distress shortly after birth. Milder cases may have recurrent bronchitis or croup (37). Congenital tracheal stenosis should also be considered in newborns with respiratory distress who have failed extubation (38). In fact, the stenosis may prevent passage of the endotracheal tube to an appropriate position. The finding of a persistent high position of the tip of the endotracheal tube (Fig. 40.2A) should alert clinicians to the presence of a stenotic tracheal segment. Other congenital anomalies of the tracheobronchial tree (bronchial stenosis, tracheomalacia, tracheal web, tracheoesophageal fistula), vascular rings, and congenital heart disease may be associated.

The differential diagnosis of tracheal stenosis is that of congenital stridor (Table 40.1). Initial evaluation includes high-kilovoltage neck radiographs and a barium esophagram. In many cases, the diagnosis can be made by computerized tomography (CT), foregoing the need for bronchoscopy or bronchography. A three-dimensional reconstruction of the trachea can be quite helpful in determining the extent and severity of the tracheal stenosis (Fig. 40.2B). Bronchoscopy will confirm the diagnosis. It is rarely necessary to pass the bronchoscope beyond the point of the stenotic segment since instrumentation of the narrowed area may result in post procedure edema and worsening obstruction.

Management of the infant with a tracheal stenosis is difficult at best. Endotracheal intubation or tracheostomy will not always establish a stable airway in distal lesions. Surgical options include tracheal resection with end-to-end anastomosis, which may be effective in correcting short-segment stenosis but may require repeated tracheal dilations. Long-segment stenosis may be repaired by splitting the stenotic tracheal rings and reconstructing with a rib graft or pericardial patch (37, 39, 40). For those infants surviving the postoperative period, residual bronchial stenosis and long-term growth of the anastomosis remains a concern.

Tracheal Agenesis

Tracheal agenesis is a rare and universally fatal congenital anomaly of the airway arising from either failure of normal development of the tracheoesophageal septum during the 4th week of gestation or of recanalization of the airway at approximately 10 weeks. As many as 65% of the infants (31/48) will also have two or more anomalies associated with the VATER syndrome (43, 44).

Affected children present with severe respiratory distress at birth, although some aeration of the lungs may be possible through a bronchoesophageal communication. Laryngoscopy most often reveals a grossly distorted larynx and/or subglottic space. Although surgical repair has been attempted by creating an airway from the esophagus, none survive more than 6 weeks (41, 42). Currently, attempts at operative repair can not be recommended. These infants are most often managed with appropriate counseling of the parents and withdrawal of support.

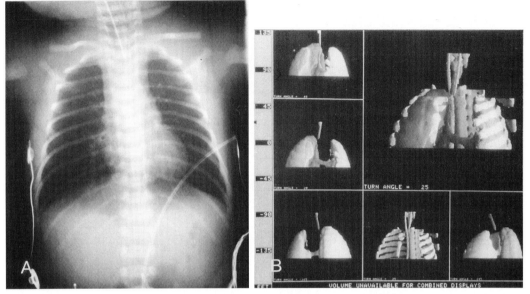

Figure 40.2. *A,* AP radiograph of an infant with severe tracheal stenosis. Note the very high position of the endotracheal tube. Chart notes confirmed difficulty advancing the tube beyond this point. *B,* A three-dimensional CT reconstruction of the tracheobronchial tree of this infant. The area in which the signal disappears denotes the area of the severe stenosis. The resolution capability of this technique is such that airway dimensions less than 2 mm in diameter cannot be detected, thus defining crudely the dimensions of the stenosis.

Vascular Ring

Anomalies of the aortic arch, often referred to as vascular rings and slings, account for 1–3% of congenital cardiovascular anomalies. They can cause a wide range of symptoms related to compression of the trachea and esophagus. Although the more severe cases present in infancy, diagnosis is often made in childhood after long-standing respiratory problems.

The aortic arch and its branches form in the first 8 weeks of fetal life from the dorsal aorta and the six paired aortic arches. In normal development, the left dorsal aorta is the primary structure giving rise to the transverse and descending aortic arch, and the right dorsal aorta largely disappears (45, 46). If the right dorsal aorta persists, a double aortic arch is formed, in which case the left arch is usually smaller than the right (80% of cases) and anterior to the trachea (47). The right arch passes posteriorly. Together these structures encircle and compress both the trachea and the esophagus (Fig. 40.3A). The double aortic arch is the most common type (30–65% of cases) of vascular ring (47–52).

When the right dorsal aorta persists in place of the left, the trachea and esophagus are then encircled by the right arch posteriorly, the pulmonary artery anteriorly and to the right, and the ductus (or ligamentum) arteriosus to the left. Right aortic arches represent 8–30% of vascular rings (47–51). Anomalous courses of other structures, including the right subclavian artery (6–20%) (49, 50), can also entrap the esophagus and trachea between vascular structures. An aberrant innominate artery (6–35%), overlying the anterior wall of the trachea, may cause tracheal narrowing without esophageal obstruction (47, 49–51). In addition, an aberrant course of the left pulmonary artery around the right side of the trachea and then between the trachea and esophagus results in a vascular sling (4–12%) (47, 49–53) with compression of the both trachea and esophagus.

The presentation of a vascular ring varies with the type of anomaly, the severity of compression of the trachea and/or the esophagus, and the age of the patient. Patients with a double aortic arch or pulmonary artery sling usually present in the first 6 months of life, whereas those children with a right aortic arch are seen later in infancy or in childhood. An anomalous innominate artery may not be recognized until adulthood (49). Symptoms lead-

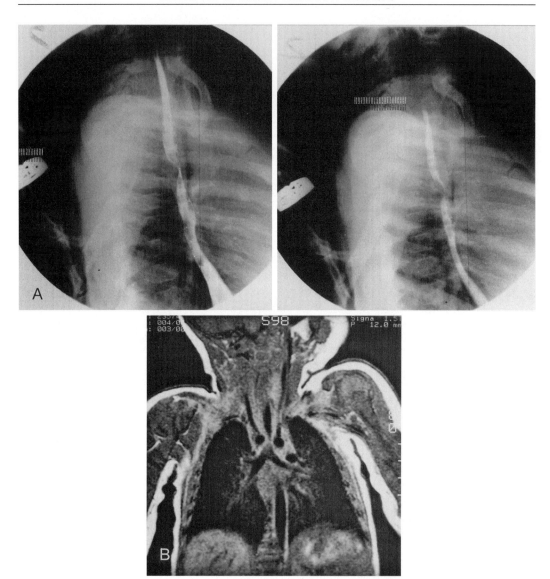

Figure 40.3. *A,* A barium esophagram from an infant with cystic fibrosis who presented with chronic wheezing. Note the posterior indentation of the esophagus consistent with a diagnosis of a vascular ring, in this instance a double aortic arch. *B,* An MRI scan from above the patient: the double aortic arch and its impact on the trachea is demonstrated.

ing to diagnosis in infancy may include respiratory distress (90–100%), stridor (92–100%), swallowing dysfunction (50–72%), cyanosis (26–69%) or apnea (17–21%). Apnea may result from reflexes stimulated by tracheal compression or esophageal dysfunction.

In children and adults, the most common complaints include recurrent wheezing, frequent respiratory tract infections, and dysphagia (54). Pulmonary function testing usually shows a decreased FEV_1 and $FEF_{25-75\%VC}$, simi-

lar to the findings in asthma, but with little response to bronchodilators. Flow-volume curves may show the flattening of both the inspiratory and expiratory limbs (55).

If a vascular ring is suspected, a barium esophagram is the recommended initial diagnostic study (49, 51, 54). With the exception of an anomalous innominate artery, the more common lesions appear as a fixed indentation in the barium column (Fig. 40.3A). Magnetic resonance imaging (MRI) (56) or a chest CT with contrast can then be performed to define the anatomy prior to operative repair (Fig. 40.3B). Arteriography is usually not needed prior to surgery unless questions regarding vascular anatomy remain unanswered (57). Fiberoptic bronchoscopy may be useful in identifying an anomalous innominate artery (49) or in evaluating a patient with persistent respiratory distress postoperatively.

Management of a symptomatic patient with a vascular ring requires surgical treatment. In general, perioperative morbidity and mortality are low and associated with severe tracheal compression or other congenital anomalies (50, 51).

Following surgery, there is usually some immediate improvement in symptoms, but full resolution proceed gradually over months to years. However, some patients may have residual tracheomalacia or tracheal stenosis. Rehospitalization for respiratory illnesses is common in the first 3 years following corrective surgery (47). Up to 30% of patients have persistent wheezing, abnormal cough, recurrent infections, or stridor (47, 49–51). The incidence of postoperative abnormalities ranges from 8% of patients examined with clinical follow-up alone to 53% evaluated with flow-volume curves (51, 47).

Tracheoesophageal Fistula

Tracheoesophageal fistula (TEF) occurs in approximately 1 per 25,000 live births. A TEF arises from failure of the normal division of the proximal foregut into separate respiratory and digestive tracts at 4 weeks' gestation. As many as 70% of children with TEF will have some type of skeletal abnormality (58, 59), 25% will have an additional gastrointestinal malformation (imperforate anus, duodenal atresia), and 25% will have a cardiovascular abnormality (PDA, VSD, ASD). The incidence of fatal cardiac or chromosomal anomalies may be as high as 11% in infants with TEF (58). Fifty percent of infants with TEF are small for gestational age or premature (58).

Esophageal atresia is present in nearly all TEFs. Eighty-five percent of TEFs involve atresia of the proximal esophagus and a fistula connecting the distal esophagus to the lower trachea at the level of the carina. These are usually diagnosed before or shortly after birth. Esophageal atresia leads to polyhydramnios during pregnancy and copious oral secretions following delivery. Chest radiograph may show a nasogastric tube coiling in the esophageal pouch. Usually the lungs appear normal, although there may be increased markings if aspiration of oral secretions has occurred. These infants require surgery in the newborn period. In most cases, an anastomosis of the proximal and distal portions of the esophagus can be performed with excision of the tracheoesophageal fistula. Rarely, repair of the atretic segment of esophagus may require colonic interposition.

Those cases in which there is an intact esophagus can pose a diagnostic dilemma. Usually, they involve one fistula arising from the esophagus near the thoracic inlet that courses anteriorly and superiorly to connect with the trachea, thus the term "H-type" fistula. Rarely, two or more fistulas are present. This type of malformation may be diagnosed at varying times during infancy and childhood. Infants present with choking and coughing with feeds, often with accompanying cyanosis. Abdominal distention may occur as air passes from the trachea to the digestive tract. In undiagnosed older infants and children, the common presentation is one of recurrent, severe pneumonia (60). However, the diagnosis should be suspected in a child with chronic cough or congestion, especially if these symptoms are associated with oral feeding. It should also be considered in the differential diagnosis of an infant or young child with recurrent pulmonary infiltrates or difficult-to-control asthma symptoms.

The diagnosis of an H-type TEF can be extremely difficult to make. Unlike the more common form of TEF, in which the fistula is usually located near the carina, H-type fistulas can occur at any level. In one series of 23 cases of H-type TEF, two (9%) involved fistulas communicating with the right mainstem bronchus, six (26%) within 2 cm of the carina, six (26%) between the thoracic inlet and the lower trachea, and nine (39%) in the cervical trachea (60). The chest radiograph demonstrates a pattern consistent with recurrent aspiration (Fig. 40.4A). The initial evaluation is best done with an esophagram (Fig. 40.4B). Continuous imaging and video taping during swallowing are essential since movement of the contrast material into a fistula may be brief and intermittent (61). Images obtained with the patient in a prone position and with the

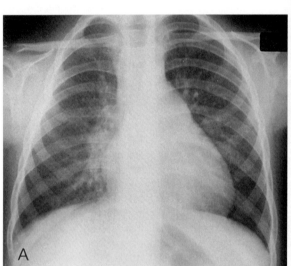
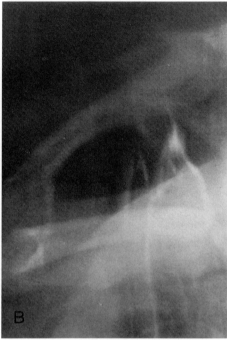

Figure 40.4. *A,* This 5-year-old girl had a tracheoesophageal fistula repaired in the newborn period. Over the next 5 years she developed chronic lung disease secondary to multiple pneumonias believed to be related to aspiration. *B,* On her fifth barium swallow, an oblique view demonstrated an H-type tracheoesophageal fistula near the level of the thoracic inlet. Despite repair, she remained oxygen-dependent at 8 years of age.

esophagus filled with contrast under pressure further increase the likelihood of obtaining a positive study. Bronchoscopy is occasionally useful in locating a suspected fistula not demonstrated radiographically. Esophageal endoscopy alone is rarely helpful in establishing the diagnosis. However, a combined procedure in which methylene blue is injected into the esophagus while a bronchoscopist watches for the presence of dye in the trachea may be diagnostic. In some patients, multiple examinations, including radiographic studies and combined bronchoscopy and esophagoscopy, are necessary before the diagnosis of an H-type TEF can be made (60).

Despite surgical correction of the TEF, recurrent respiratory symptoms are common. Three-quarters of children experience recurrent bronchitis in the first 3 years of life following repair of their TEF. Half have bronchitic symptoms that persist beyond 8 years of age. This bronchitis is accompanied by wheezing in approximately two-thirds of these children. Esophageal dysmotility may allow for reflux of swallowed material and aspira-

tion. Abnormalities of tracheal clearance mechanisms may also contribute (62).

A syndrome of severe apnea, hypoxia, and respiratory arrest has been reported in patients following TEF repair. It has been variably attributed to reflex apnea induced by tracheal obstruction from food boluses, compression of the trachea occurring between a food-filled esophagus posteriorly and normal vascular structure anteriorly, and tracheomalacia. Symptoms have been relieved and episodes eliminated by aortosternopexy (63, 64).

Tracheomalacia is another long-term problem following TEF repair. As with tracheomalacia of other causes, the clinical presentation includes a barking cough, expiratory wheezing, and/or episodes of respiratory distress. It can be documented by airway fluoroscopy, bronchoscopy, and/or flow-volume loop analysis. Autopsy studies have demonstrated deficiency of tracheal cartilage in up to 75% of pediatric cases of TEF. These abnormalities were not restricted to the area of the TEF. In 75% of patients with tracheal abnormalities, the degree of tracheal involvement ranged from half to the entire length of the trachea. Histologically, squamous metaplasia of the trachea were also noted with a loss of ciliated cells, suggesting an abnormality of mucociliary clearance (65).

Long-term pulmonary function outcome is neither well-documented nor conclusive. Patients in whom a TEF has been repaired may demonstrate restrictive or obstructive lung disease. Some have an increased responsiveness to methacholine challenge. Others demonstrate residual lung function abnormalities suggestive of an upper airway obstruction (66).

CONGENITAL MALFORMATIONS OF THE LUNG

Although some congenital malformations of the lung are diagnosed in the newborn period, others frequently are not recognized until later in life. They are associated with a complex of chronic and recurrent respiratory symptoms similar to those commonly seen in a variety of acquired respiratory diseases of children (Tables 40.1, 40.2). Establishing the correct diagnosis requires a high degree of suspicion, especially in the older child since congenital malformations are frequently overlooked outside of infancy.

Pulmonary Hypoplasia

Pulmonary hypoplasia may occur as the result of fetal anomalies (including renal, genitourinary, musculoskeletal, neuromuscular, and pulmonary) or prolonged oligohydramnios (Table 40.4). Lung hypoplasia may develop when there are alterations in the normal pressure relationships between the fetal lung, trachea, and amniotic fluid, as occurs with oligohydramnios (67, 68). Fetal breathing movements are also necessary for normal lung development as demonstrated by the occurrence of lung hypoplasia in the presence of neuromuscular or skeletal disease that prohibits or limits respiration in utero (69). Unilateral hypoplasia results when there is abnormal development of the pulmonary artery or bronchus to a lung, or in the presence of a space-occupying lesion of the chest such as occurs in congenital diaphragmatic hernia or cystic adenomatoid malformation. A severe injury at an early developmental stage may result in agenesis of the affected side (Fig. 40.5). In some cases, a cause is not identified.

Hypoplastic lungs are not only smaller but have a reduced alveolar number and low lung DNA content, which suggests reduced cell number. Onset earlier in gestation results in more severe hypoplasia with a decrease in bronchiolar branching, pulmonary vascularity, and histologic maturity. There is also an extension of the vascular smooth muscle toward the periphery, resulting in pulmonary hypertension.

At birth, infants with bilateral severe pulmonary hypoplasia have respiratory distress with hypoxia and hypercarbia. The thorax may appear small, and other anomalies may be present. In patients with no known predisposing factors, no other apparent anomalies and bilateral involvement, pulmonary hypoplasia may be difficult to distinguish from other neonatal respiratory disorders. The course is often characterized by persistent pulmonary hypertension of the newborn and persistent respiratory failure despite assisted ventilation. Barotrauma and pneumothoraces develop as a consequence of positive pressure ventilation.

The clinical course is extremely variable, depending on the extent of hypoplasia. Some infants with minimal involvement require brief periods of supplemental oxygen or assisted ventilation, whereas others die from unremitting respiratory insufficiency or associated congenital anomalies. Despite advances in neonatal care, the syndrome termed the oligohydramnios tetrad (pulmonary hypoplasia [Fig. 40.6], positional deformities of the extremities, Potter facies, and intrauterine growth retardation) is almost universally fatal. Some patients may develop chronic lung disease similar to severe bronchopulmonary dysplasia (70). Some children with unilateral hypoplasia or agenesis do reasonably well, compensating with increased volume and/or growth of the unaffected lung, resulting in nearly normal lung function (71, 72).

Survival and pulmonary prognosis depend on the severity of hypoplasia and associated anomalies. The recognition of the factors influencing the development and degree of lung hypoplasia has lead to therapeutic approaches aimed at preventing or ameliorating lung hypoplasia. Thus far restoration of amniotic fluid volume has been attempted but has not proved successful in preventing pulmonary hypoplasia secondary to oligohydramnios (68). Correction of surgical lesions

Table 40.4.
Causes of Pulmonary Hypoplasia

Bilateral	Unilateral
Idiopathic	Idiopathic
Oligohydramnios	Scimitar syndrome
Prolonged rupture of membranes	
Fetal renal disease:	Pulmonary artery agenesis
Posterior urethral valves	Congenital diaphragmatic hernia
Bilateral ureteropelvic junction	Unilateral phrenic nerve agenesis
obstruction	Accessory diaphragm
Bilateral renal dysplasia	Intrathoracic masses:
Bilateral cystic kidneys	Extralobar sequestration
Neuromuscular disease:	Cystic adenomatoid malformation
Congenital myotonic dystrophy	Congenital tumors of the thorax
Werdnig-Hoffman	
Arthrogryposis multiplex congenita	
Bilateral phrenic nerve agenesis	
Thoracic deformities:	
Thanatophoric dwarfism	
Asphyxiating thoracic dystrophy	
Osteogenesis imperfecta	
Ellis van Crevald	
Fetal hydrops	
Massive ascites	
Giant omphalocele	
Trisomy 13, 18, or 21	

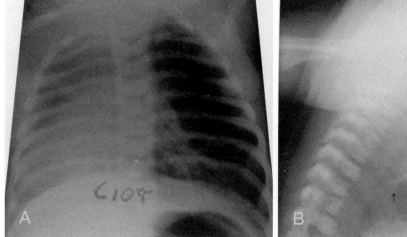
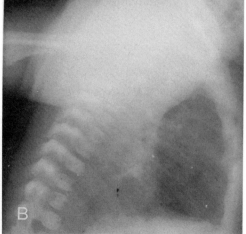

Figure 40.5. AP *(A)* and lateral *(B)* chest radiographs from an infant with complete agenesis of the right lung.

in utero, such as repair of a congenital diaphragmatic hernia or relief of urinary obstruction, may eventually ameliorate lung hypoplasia, but have not yet been perfected.

Bronchial Stenosis and Atresia

Bronchial stenosis occurs in association with other malformations, particularly those leading to extrinsic compression of the airway.

Isolated congenital bronchial stenosis is a rare anomaly. Recurrent bouts of respiratory infection and atelectasis confined to a single lobe is seen in the few reported cases. Pathologic findings include bronchomalacia and conical narrowing of the bronchus (73). Treatment consists of excision of the affected lobe.

Atresia of a segmental bronchus with hyperinflation of the distal lung parenchyma is another rare congenital anomaly of bronchial

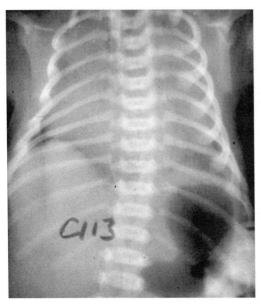

Figure 40.6. AP chest radiograph from an infant with bilateral pulmonary hypoplasia secondary to oligohydramnios.

development. It is believed to occur after the 15th week of gestation as the result of a vascular accident (74). Lung parenchyma distal to the atresia may receive ventilation from adjacent segments via collateral pathways. Obstruction of these pathways on expiration leads to hyper-inflation (75). The pathology consists of hyper-inflated lung with a central mucocele arising at the termination of the bronchus.

Patients with bronchial atresia are often asymptomatic. Others have shortness of breath, recurrent pneumonia, or chronic cough. Physical findings may be absent or include diminished breath sounds in the involved lobe. Chest radiographs reveal hyper-inflation of the involved lobe and, in two-thirds of cases, an extrahilar mass (76). Most frequently (73%) the left upper lobe is involved. Although bronchoscopy and bronchography have traditionally been considered the standard diagnostic procedures, CT scan with rapid imaging (0.1 seconds/image) may establish the diagnosis. Most reported patients in whom the diagnosis has been confirmed have undergone excision of the involved segment.

Bronchogenic Cyst

Bronchogenic cysts arise from abnormal lung budding early in the first trimester of gestation. Mediastinal bronchogenic cysts occur when the aberrant lung bud forms early, during branching of the proximal tracheobronchial tree. They are usually located along the trachea and the mainstem bronchi, commonly in the subcarinal region. They are often firmly attached to the airways but rarely communicate with them. Symptoms are related to compression of the trachea or a lobar bronchus. Infection of the cyst itself is uncommon.

Intraparenchymal or pulmonary bronchogenic cysts arise when there is an anomalous lung budding later in bronchial branching. These lesions can occur in any lobe but are more common in the lower lobes. Communications with the tracheobronchial tree, if present, are small and will allow bacterial contamination if there is impaired mucociliary clearance. Consequently, pulmonary bronchogenic cysts may cause recurrent and persistent symptoms of respiratory infection (77–79). If a bronchogenic cysts loses attachment to other lung structures it may migrate to extrathoracic locations including the chin, neck, thoracic wall, and abdomen. Occasionally these extrathoracic cysts maintain an extension into the mediastinum (80).

Bronchogenic cysts are lined by ciliated mucus-secreting cells. The epithelium varies from pseudostratified columnar to cuboidal epithelium, depending on the origin of the abnormal lung bud. Similarly, the wall contains smooth muscle, fragments of cartilage, and fibrous tissue corresponding to that found in the normal tracheobronchial tree at the level of abnormal branching. Bronchogenic cysts are usually singular and unilocular. Although they may range in size from several millimeters to many centimeters, most are between 2 and 10 cm in diameter. They are filled with mucus of a homogeneous consistency. Infected cysts may contain air or pus in addition.

Infants presenting with respiratory distress secondary to airway compression and hyperinflation of the distal lung are usually diagnosed promptly and treated with removal of the cyst. Older infants and children may develop recurrent cough, pneumonia, wheezing, or hemoptysis. It may be months or years before patients with these symptoms are correctly diagnosed (79). The diagnosis is occasionally made in adults with recurrent infections, dyspnea, or a mass on chest radiograph.

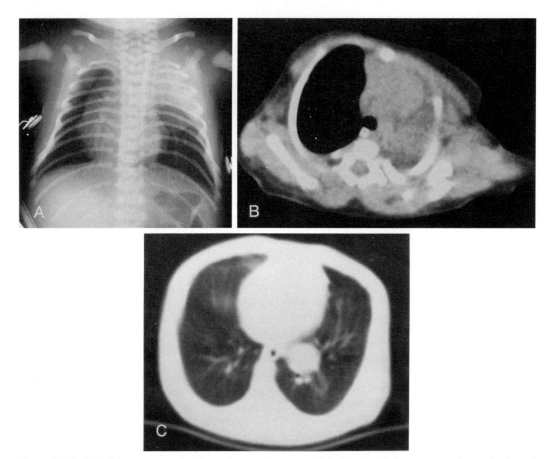

Figure 40.7. This infant presented with respiratory distress at birth. Chest radiograph showed opacification of the left upper lobe *(A)*. CT scan confirmed this and additionally demonstrated a mass obliterating the left upper lobe bronchus *(B, C)*. A diagnosis of bronchogenic cyst with bronchial atresia was made from pathology specimens obtained at operation.

Most patients presenting with a symptomatic bronchogenic cyst have diagnostic chest radiograph findings at the time of initial evaluation (Fig. 40.7A). Cysts that do not communicate with the tracheobronchial tree and are not infected have an oval, smooth-bordered appearance and a homogeneous fluid density. Infected cysts may contain air and have air-fluid levels. In some cases the findings may be indistinguishable from those of pneumonia. CT scan is the next imaging study in the evaluation. When performed with vascular contrast, it can establish the diagnosis and demonstrate the relationship of the cysts to the surrounding structures (Fig. 40.7B, C). MRI provides better resolution and sagittal images but is not required for most patients (77, 78). Barium esophagram contributes little information. Bronchoscopy may reveal a non-pulsatile fixed compression in the region of the carina, but is not diagnostic.

Treatment of a symptomatic bronchogenic cyst, regardless of location, is excision. Mediastinal lesions can be surgically excised via thoracotomy or sternotomy without resection of lung tissue. Endoscopic resection of tracheal bronchogenic cysts (81) and thoracoscopic removal of small extralobar cysts (79) may be performed in selected patients. For intrapulmonary cysts, the merits of segmental versus lobar resection are debated. Similarly, there is controversy regarding the need for resection of the asymptomatic bronchogenic cyst. Advocates for resection cite the possibility for infection and subsequent malignancy as indications for surgery (82). However, the true incidence of either complication is unknown.

Congenital Lobar Emphysema

Congenital lobar emphysema (CLE) accounts for about 15% of congenital bronchopulmonary malformations. It most frequently occurs on the left side and involves a single upper lobe (50% occur in the left upper lobe). Middle lobe and multilobe lesions do occur; lower lobe lesions are rare. Several pathogenetic mechanisms have been proposed. These include an underlying abnormality of a lobar bronchus leading to partial obstruction, overdistension and secondary alveolar abnormalities, or an abnormality of elastic properties in the involved lobe, leading to overdistension of alveoli and development of emphysema. The polyalveolar lobe is considered a form of CLE. These lobes have alveolar numbers that are three to five times normal. The number of terminal bronchioles remains normal with an increased number of alveoli distributed throughout the acini of the involved region. Portions of a polyalveolar lobe become emphysematous, probably secondary to air trapping. Clinically, these patients are indistinguishable in presentation and pulmonary function outcome from those with other forms of CLE (72, 88, 89).

The affected lobes are grossly overdistended and slow to deflate once excised. Diffuse alveolar emphysema and rupture with subpleural bleb formation is common. Hypoplasia or absence of bronchial cartilage plates has been noted in up to 79% of cases (83, 84).

Infants with CLE usually present in the first 4 months of life, often in the newborn period, with respiratory distress or poor feeding. Occasionally, the presentation is more insidious, consisting of tachypnea, dyspnea, wheezing, cough, poor feeding, intermittent cyanosis, or exercise intolerance. In some patients CLE is identified incidentally during routine health care. Physical examination may reveal retractions, hyper-inflation evidenced by increased resonance on percussion, decreased breath sounds, wheezing, or shift of the cardiac impulse.

Initial evaluation with a chest radiograph demonstrates a hyper-lucent, hyper-inflated lung field with shift of the mediastinum and cardiac silhouette (Fig. 40.8A). The differential diagnosis includes tension pneumothorax, foreign body with bronchial obstruction, and other rare forms of congenital lung cysts. In the typical setting of an infant under 4 months of age with characteristic clinical features and chest radiograph, no further work-up is needed. In the older child with an atypical presentation, a CT scan may be useful in delineating the lesion (85) (Fig. 40.8B, C). A V/Q scan can assess the function of the involved lobe(s) (86), but is generally not required. CLE can be associated with other anomalies including congenital heart disease (14–36% of cases) (83, 84).

Newborns presenting with severe respiratory distress require immediate surgical excision. Arguments for resection of CLE in all infants and young children have been made based on the assumption that early resection will relieve compression of the contralateral lung, allow opportunity for compensatory lung growth, remove a nidus for infection, and avoid episodes of increased hyper-inflation or rupture of the abnormal lung. However, recent reports demonstrate that children with mild or absent symptoms can be managed medically without significant progression of their respiratory symptoms. Intermittent worsening of hyper-inflation may occur in association with intercurrent illnesses or reactive airway disease but resolves naturally or with symptomatic treatment, allowing return to baseline pulmonary status (71, 87).

The results of pulmonary function in patients who have undergone resection of a CLE is controversial. One study suggests that there is compensatory hyper-inflation and normal growth of the remaining lobes rather than a compensatory increase in lung growth. In contrast, other data suggests that resection of a CLE in infancy allows for compensatory lung growth (72). However, in asymptomatic patients managed without surgery, CLE does not appear to inhibit growth of the remaining lung (71). There remains controversy as to the need for routine resection of CLE in asymptomatic or mildly affected patients. If surgery is required, all involved lobes should be resected during the initial procedure. Failure to remove apparently mildly affected areas can result in postoperative hyper-expansion of those areas, necessitating a second procedure (83).

Cystic Adenomatoid Malformation

Cystic malformations of the lung, including cystic adenomatoid malformation (CAM),

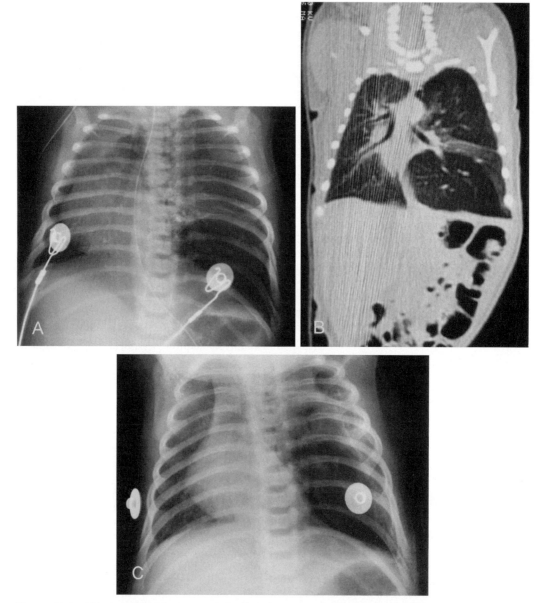

Figure 40.8. This 1-day-old infant presented with tachypnea and difficulty feeding. Chest radiograph showed marked hyper-inflation on the left with a shift of the mediastinum *(A)*. CT scan suggested diffuse hyper-inflation of both the left upper and lower lobes with sparing of the lingula *(B)*. At the time of operation, the left upper lobe was resected and confirmed the diagnosis of congenital lobar emphysema. However, the left lower lobe appeared normal and was not resected. Subsequently, it became markedly hyper-inflated, resulting in a continued mediastinal shift *(C)*.

congenital lobar emphysema (CLE), bronchogenic cysts, and pulmonary lymphangiectasia, account for 25% of lung malformations. Of these, about 20% are CAMs (90) that result from an abnormality of alveolar development with an overgrowth of terminal bronchiolar structures. They are composed of cystic structures of varying size enclosed within a wall lined by mucogenic cells. The individual cysts are lined by ciliated columnar epithelium but are without systematic architecture. No cartilage is contained within a CAM. Although an entire lung may be affected, most commonly a single lobe is involved. Lower lobes are more frequently involved than upper lobes. CAM may occur with other anomalies including pulmonary sequestration, bronchial atresia, cleft hand abnormalities, and congenital diaphragmatic hernia (90, 91).

Three histologically distinct types of CAM are described. Type I accounts for 70% of all CAMs and consists of one or a few large cysts, occurring primarily on the right side. These are rarely associated with other anomalies and carry a good prognosis with prompt intervention. Type II CAM is made up of multiple individual cysts ranging in size from 0.5 to 1.2 cm and has the worst prognosis of the three forms. It is associated with preterm delivery (75% of cases), is more likely to be accompanied by other anomalies (60%), and has a 60% mortality rate. Type III CAMs, representing about 10% of all CAMs, are composed of multiple small (0.5 cm) cysts. They occur exclusively in boys and are not associated with other anomalies. A 50% survival rate has been reported (92).

Eighty percent of CAMs are diagnosed prenatally or in the neonatal period (Fig. 40.9A). One presentation is that of fetal anasarca, prematurity, and polyhydramnios with fetal or neonatal death. Other infants present with respiratory distress or feeding difficulty. Chest radiograph demonstrates a cystic appearance of one or more lobes (Fig. 40.9B). The differential diagnosis includes CAM, congenital diaphragmatic hernia, CLE, pulmonary lymphangiectasia, and bronchogenic cysts. A CAM and a right-sided diaphragmatic hernia may be difficult to distinguish on the basis of a chest radiograph alone. Accurate preoperative diagnosis is important since the operative approach for resection of a CAM is through a thoracotomy rather than the laparotomy approach required for repair of a congenital diaphragmatic hernia. Computerized tomography (Fig. 40.9C), ultrasonography of the chest, or gastrointestinal (GI) contrast study can be used to differentiate between these two conditions. Usually, congenital lobar emphysema can be distinguished on chest radiograph because the affected side of the chest appears hyper-inflated and hyperlucent without distinct cysts. Extensive work-up to differentiate between these two lesions is not usually necessary since both require resection in symptom-

atic patients. Extracorporeal membrane oxygenation (ECMO) has been used as an adjunctive therapy for neonatal patients in whom the postoperative course is complicated by persistent pulmonary hypertension of the newborn (93). Recently, antenatal resection of a CAM in a 23-week fetus with mild polyhydramnios and ascites was successfully carried out. The child had an uncomplicated course after delivery at 30 weeks (94). However, the indications for and advantages of fetal intervention are unclear since CAMs diagnosed in utero may decrease in size relative to thoracic size prior to delivery (95).

Prognosis for infants undergoing surgical excision of a CAM in the neonatal period is excellent. Although long-term pulmonary function data are limited, the remaining lung expands to fill the thoracic cavity, leaving patients without significant respiratory symptoms. The degree to which this represents alveolar distension versus compensatory lung growth is unknown.

In 10% of cases, the diagnosis is made after 1 year of age. Older children present with recurrent respiratory infections or, more rarely, with other problems such as pneumothorax. In these patients, differential diagnosis includes CLE, diaphragmatic hernia, and pneumatoceles secondary to pneumonia. Clinical history and chest radiographs usually suggest the diagnosis. Computerized tomography is the next diagnostic study in the evaluation. Bronchoscopy or bronchography are of little value. As in neonatal cases, the definitive treatment is surgical excision of the involved lobe(s). This is recommended in asymptomatic patients because of the potential for infection and malignant degeneration (96).

Pulmonary Sequestration

A pulmonary sequestration is a mass of nonfunctioning, primitive pulmonary tissue separated from both the tracheobronchial tree and the pulmonary circulation. The sequestration is usually cystic and has disorganized fetal respiratory elements including bronchi, cartilage, alveoli, and respiratory epithelium. It receives its blood supply directly from the systemic circulation with multiple feeding vessels in 15–20% of cases (97, 98).

Intralobar sequestrations are contained within normal lung tissue and are encased by the same pleura. The boundaries of an intralo-

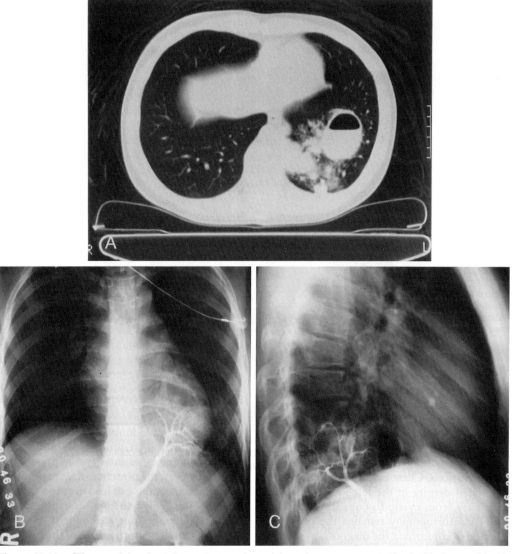

Figure 40.11. CT scan of the chest demonstrates a lower lobe pulmonary sequestration in this 8-year-old with recurrent pneumonia *(A)*. An aortogram delineated the systemic, subdiaphragmatic blood supply *(B, C)*.

telangiectasia (HHT) in 36% of patients with single and 57% with multiple lesions. Conversely, 15% of patients with HHT have PAVM (103). This is significant, since patients with both diseases have more symptoms, are more likely to have multiple lesions, have a faster rate of progression, and have more complications. However, HHT may not be apparent in childhood and may be unrecognized at the time of presentation with a PAVM.

The triad of cyanosis, digital clubbing, and polycythemia is characteristic of PAVM in children and adults. Despite symptoms dating

to childhood, only 10% of patients with PAVM are diagnosed before adolescence or adulthood. Symptoms can include dyspnea, cough, or chest pain. Vascular necrosis may predispose to pulmonary hemorrhage and hemoptysis. Neurologic symptoms may be present as the result of polycythemia, intracranial telangiectasia, or a brain abscess in patients with HHT. In addition to cyanosis and clubbing, physical examination may reveal telangiectasia, a bruit, a thrill, or systolic murmur. Pulmonary or gastrointestinal bleeding may lead to anemia (104–107). In neonates,

PAVM is one cause of cyanosis and congestive heart failure.

Initial laboratory evaluation requires documentation of reduced arterial oxygenation, a finding present in over 80% of cases. The lack of an increase in Pao$_2$ while breathing 100% oxygen will help identify the presence of a right-to-left shunt. Polycythemia offers further confirmatory evidence, but is also present in cases with intracardiac shunting secondary to congenital heart disease. Chest radiographs demonstrate cardiac enlargement, tortuosity of pulmonary vessels, or peripheral non-calcified lesions connected to the hilum by a blood vessel. An electrocardiogram and an echocardiogram should be obtained to differentiate PAVM from congenital heart disease.

Once suspected, screening for a PAVM is best done by CT scan, which can confirm the presence of a blood-density structure in the thorax. However, it may not distinguish highly vascular lesions from lesions of vascular origin (104). Radionuclide angiocardiography and contrast echocardiography may confirm the presence of a right-to-left shunt but are nonspecific (104, 107). Pulmonary angiography remains the definitive diagnostic technique and is essential to determine the number, extent, and location of lesions, as well as the suitability for therapy (104, 106, 107).

Once a diagnosis of PAVM is confirmed and the location and extent of the lesion(s) are determined, a decision must be made regarding intervention. In patients with minimal symptoms, treatment may not be required, and a course of regular reassessment may be chosen. However, because of the high rate of complications in untreated symptomatic patients (26% over 6-year follow-up), intervention must be strongly considered (108). The therapeutic modalities available include ligation of feeding vessels, excision of the lesion and surrounding segment, lobe, or lung, and embolization.

Ligature of a feeding vessel can be successful in the case of a single, discrete lesion with a well-defined arterial supply. More often, however, the lesions are multiple or the arterial supply is extensive, rendering this approach unsuitable. For single lesions, excision of the involved segment or lobe can be curative. Occasionally, pneumonectomy or ligature of the pulmonary artery has been performed when there is extensive unilateral disease. Bilateral disease has required staged procedures for resection of involved areas. The use of balloon embolization for treatment of PAVM in adults was first reported in 1980 (109). It has since become the preferred therapy in centers with the necessary facilities and expertise. In the case of diffuse, bilateral lesions, involvement may be so extensive as to preclude any therapy, although lung transplantation may be an option.

Prognosis depends on the type of PAVM(s) and the success of intervention. There is little follow-up information available regarding the outcome of untreated patients with small, asymptomatic lesions. The natural history in untreated symptomatic patients is one of frequent complications including pulmonary hemorrhage, hemoptysis, cerebral embolism, cerebral abscess, bacterial endarteritis, and progressive hypoxia leading to death.

An acquired form of PAVM has been well described in both adult and pediatric patients with acute and chronic liver disease. Cyanosis and digital clubbing may appear after resolution of hepatic symptoms. Lesions are usually diffuse and not amenable to treatment. Hypoxia may be progressive and ultimately fatal (110, 111). However, the arteriovenous malformation may regress following successful liver transplantation (112).

Pulmonary Lymphangiectasia

Congenital pulmonary lymphangiectasia (CPL) is an uncommon and often fatal lung anomaly. In the normal lung, there are two separate systems of lymphatic drainage. One is present in the subpleural area, running along the pleura, to the interlobular septa, and along the venous system to the hila. The other drains the central region of the lung, along the bronchi to the hilum. The lymphatic channels are very prominent early in gestation but normally regress between the 16th and 20th weeks of gestation (113). CPL is felt to arise when there is failure of regression of these channels.

Three forms of CPL have been described: one associated with generalized lymphangiectasia, another occurring with congenital heart disease, and the third arising as a primary abnormality of lung development (114). Those patients presenting in the newborn period may have other congenital anomalies as well, including cardiac malformations, abnormalities of gut rotation, and asplenia. All forms involve abnormalities of the lymphatic drainage of the lung with dilation of lymphatic channels and/or proliferation of pulmonary lymphatics (115–117). CPL occurring in association with obstruction of pulmonary venous return to the left atrium accounts for approximately one-third of cases (114, 115, 117). This obstruction is thought to interfere with normal regression of fetal lymphatics, thereby leading to CPL. Infants with this form usually present shortly after birth with tachypnea, retractions, and cyanosis. Chest radiographs may show cardiomegaly, hyper-inflation, cystic changes, increased interstitial markings, and/or segmental atelectasis. Diagnosis is suspected on the basis of clinical presentation, chest radiograph findings, and identification of obstruction of the pulmonary veins. Confirmation requires open lung biopsy. The prognosis is extremely poor with death in the first weeks or months of life.

Primary pulmonary lymphangiectasia occurs with a wide spectrum of severity. When presenting in the neonatal period, the findings are similar to those in CPL with obstructed venous return. Involvement is often diffuse, bilateral, and severe. Infants may be stillborn or hydropic. Death occurs in the first days of life. However, isolated primary CPL has been reported in otherwise healthy adolescents presenting with abnormalities on routine radiographs. When resected, these lesions were localized to one or two lobes and were histologically consistent with CPL. No obstruction of venous return was noted. There was no recurrence at follow-up 3–8 years later (118).

Pulmonary lymphangiectasia also occurs as part of a syndrome of generalized lymphangiectasia with intestinal and bony involvement and hemihypertrophy. In this diffuse form, the lung disease is usually less severe than in the other two forms. The prognosis is somewhat better but depends on the severity of involvement of other organ systems (114).

Scimitar Syndrome

The scimitar syndrome is a constellation of respiratory tract anomalies involving primarily the right lung and its vascular supply. The common features include a small right lung and hemithorax, a hypoplastic right pulmonary artery, anomalous return of the pulmonary vein to the inferior vena caval–right atrial junction, anomalous arterial supply to the right lung from the descending aorta, and varying degrees of bronchial sequestration on the right. Congenital heart disease and dextrocardia are also common (119–121). In some cases there may be fusion of the right and left lungs posterior to the cardiac apex ("horseshoe lung") (122–124). This syndrome usually comes to attention because of recurrent pulmonary infections or concern about a relative decrease in size of the right hemithorax. Symptoms range from none to severe respiratory distress (119–121).

A variety of radiographic imaging techniques suggest and confirm the diagnosis of scimitar syndrome. A chest radiograph will show a small right hemi-thorax, the scimitar sign (anomalous venous return to the inferior vena cava) and, perhaps, dextrocardia (Fig. 40.10). A ventilation-perfusion scan will demonstrate filling defects in the areas of systemic arterial supply. Vascular anatomy can also be documented by pulmonary artery and aortic angiography. The presence of a horseshoe lung can be detected by CT scan, which documents an isthmus of lung parenchyma between the pericardium and the spine. Often there are insufficient symptoms to warrant attempt at surgical correction. In patients with severe symptoms, resection of the sequestered lobe and/or correction of venous return may be indicated (120, 122).

Horseshoe Lung

Although most cases of horseshoe lung occur in association with the scimitar syndrome (79%), it may occur as an isolated anomaly consisting of a hypoplastic right lung with fusion of the right and left lungs posteriorly (122). The diagnosis of horseshoe lung should be considered in patients with recurrent respiratory infections, a hypoplastic right lung, and dextrocardia. Because of the association of horseshoe lung and scimitar syndrome, documentation of the arterial supply and venous drainage of the right lung should be obtained. Management has been targeted at preventing respiratory tract infections and aggressive treatment with antibiotics. However, when this has been unsuccessful, resection of the hypoplastic right lung has been performed (122).

CONGENITAL MALFORMATIONS OF THE DIAPHRAGM

Congenital Diaphragmatic Paralysis and Eventration

Congenital anomalies of the diaphragm produce more marked symptoms in the infant than in the older child or adult. In the infant, respiration requires more participation of the diaphragm because of the increased compliance of the chest wall and the relative weakness of other respiratory muscles. In addition, the mediastinum of the infant is mobile, allowing bilateral pulmonary compromise with unilateral diaphragmatic lesions. Supine positioning further compromises respiratory effort. Infants with diaphragmatic paralysis or eventration frequently present with respiratory distress or respiratory failure shortly after birth (125, 126).

Unilateral diaphragmatic paralysis is a well-recognized birth injury. It can occur after difficult vaginal deliveries, particularly those from a breech presentation and those requiring forceps, but rarely as a complication of caesarean delivery. The paralysis may be due to stretching of the phrenic nerve or edema along the course of the nerve. In these cases, the paralysis is usually transient with improvement occurring over the first 2 months of life (127, 128). However, there are reports of resolution occurring as late as 8 months of age (129, 130). Unfortunately, most series have not reported serial assessments of diaphragmatic function, instead reporting recovery on follow-up at 6–12 months (127, 130). Avulsion or agenesis of the phrenic nerve results in complete paralysis of the ipsilateral hemidiaphragm without recovery. Bilateral phrenic nerve agenesis is associated with pulmonary hypoplasia (131).

Acquired diaphragmatic paralysis may be seen in infants and children following cardiothoracic surgery, or as a consequence of transection, crush injury, or freeze injury. The prognosis depends on the specific etiology, and recovery usually occurs within 6 months, if at all (128, 132). Infants with spinal muscle atrophy and acid maltase deficiency may also develop diaphragmatic paralysis. In fact, respiratory failure secondary to diaphragmatic palsy may be the earliest manifestation of a genetic neuromuscular disease (133, 134).

Eventration of the diaphragm results when the muscular component of the diaphragm fails to develop. The affected hemidiaphragm consists only of a membrane of fascia, parietal pleura, and peritoneum. This is also referred to as a congenital diaphragmatic hernia with a sac (130).

In order to assess prognosis and plan therapy, it is necessary to differentiate among eventration of the diaphragm, diaphragmatic paralysis due to phrenic nerve trauma, and that secondary to complete avulsion of the phrenic nerve. An infant with unilateral diaphragmatic paralysis may by asymptomatic or have marked respiratory distress requiring ventilatory assistance. In most cases, there is an accompanying ipsilateral Erb palsy, signifying birth injury and likely recovery of diaphragmatic function. Nonspecific signs and symptoms include tachypnea, retractions, and cyanosis. There is paradoxical motion of the affected hemidiaphragm, ascending on inspiration and descending on expiration, apparent as asymmetric movements of the chest and abdominal walls. However, in patients under treatment with positive pressure mechanical ventilation, paradoxical motion will not be present.

Radiographic findings of right hemidiaphragm elevation two intercostal spaces above the left, or the left hemidiaphragm elevated one intercostal space above the right, suggests abnormal diaphragm function (Fig. 40.12). Unilateral elevation of the diaphragm on chest radiograph, in the absence of other evidence of birth trauma, points to either agenesis of a phrenic nerve or eventration of the diaphragm. Partial involvement of a diaphragm signifies eventration. Ultrasonography or fluoroscopy can confirm the presence of paradoxical movement of the diaphragm on the involved side (129, 135). Stimulation of the ipsilateral phrenic nerve with resultant contraction of the hemidiaphragm suggests that recovery is likely to occur. The response can be assessed by electromyography, ultrasonography, or fluoroscopy of the diaphragm (136, 137). There is no contraction of the diaphragm in response to phrenic nerve stimulation when there is avulsion or agenesis of the phrenic nerve or in cases of diaphragmatic eventration. Crying vital capacity has also been suggested as a means of assessing diaphragm function (138), but the findings are

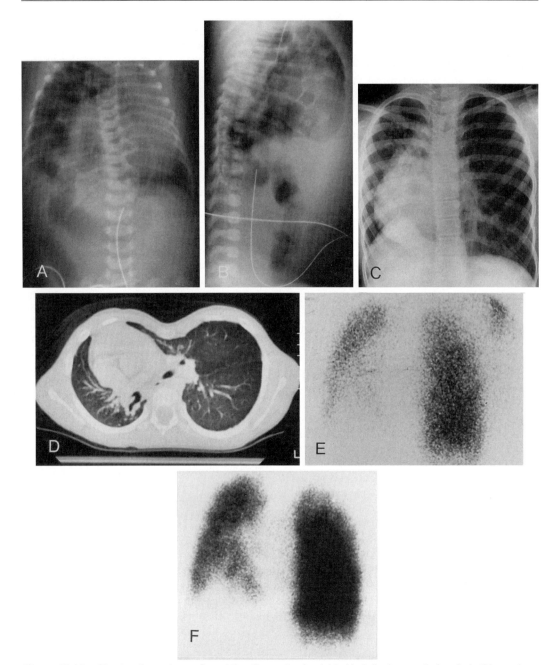

Figure 40.12. Chest radiographs confirmed the diagnosis of a right-sided diaphragmatic hernia in this newborn with respiratory distress *(A, B)*, which was surgically repaired in the first day of life. On follow-up at 8 years of age, chest radiograph and CT scan demonstrated hypoplasia of the right lung with compensatory hyperinflation on the left *(C, D)*. V/Q scan showed a matched decrease in ventilation *(E)* perfusion *(F)* on the right.

not specific and these studies are limited to facilities to measure infant lung function.

In those infants who have sufficient lung function to maintain adequate ventilation on their own, cautious observation for up to 12 months is warranted since recovery may occur at a later time (129, 130). Close follow-up is necessary since diaphragmatic paralysis is associated with atelectasis, pneumonia, and poor tolerance of upper respiratory illnesses. If there is no clinical or radiographic improvement after this period, plication is required in these infants to prevent respiratory complications and allow normal lung growth. In infants who are unable to support themselves, positive pressure respiration and plication of the diaphragm are the most commonly employed therapies. Failure to recover sufficient diaphragmatic function to allow weaning from mechanical ventilation by 2 weeks of age is a commonly used criterion for plication of the diaphragm (132, 137). Plication improves ventilation by allowing expansion of the ipsilateral lung and return of the mediastinum to a midline position. It also offers the theoretic advantage of preventing the development of lung hypoplasia on the affected side because of compression. When there is nerve stimulation evidence of residual diaphragmatic contractility, recovery may be complete, and thus a longer period of mechanical ventilation is indicated before proceeding with surgical correction.

Congenital Diaphragmatic Hernia

Diaphragmatic hernias arise when the pleuroperitoneal membrane, which normally separates the peritoneal and thoracic cavities at 7 weeks' gestation, fails to form completely prior to the return of the abdominal viscera to the peritoneal cavity at 10 weeks (139). Bochdalek hernias involve the posterolateral portion of the diaphragm, the last portion to close, and account for about 90% of all congenital diaphragmatic hernias. They occur five times more frequently on the left than the right and are slightly more common in males. The less common Morgagni hernia occurs in the retrosternal space. Diaphragmatic hernias are associated with significant abnormalities of lung growth, including a decrease in radial alveolar count and in lung maturity. Although both lungs appear morphologically immature

for gestational age, this finding is more striking in the ipsilateral lung (140).

Most newborns with congenital diaphragmatic hernias are diagnosed prenatally or shortly after delivery. The immediate management consists of establishing ventilation through an endotracheal tube and placement of a gastric catheter to suction, thus preventing gaseous distension of the displaced abdominal organs. The timing of surgical repair depends on the stability of the patient. Approximately 40% of infants with CDH will have another congenital anomaly, with 16–18% having a chromosomal anomaly or a recognized pattern of malformation. Cardiac malformations are present in 18% of infants with CDH (141). Since the presence of some of these conditions (e.g., trisomy 18) may preclude surgery, it is important to evaluate for other malformations prior to initiating surgical correction.

For decades, the mortality associated with CDH has remained high (approximately 40%) despite advances in neonatal transport, neonatology, and pediatric surgery (142, 143). However, there are several therapies on the horizon that appear likely to improve survival. Some data suggest that the group of infants in whom the CDH is recognized prior to 25 weeks' gestation has an relative increase in neonatal mortality (144). This is attributed to impingement upon lung growth and the development of severe pulmonary hypoplasia. Therefore, correction of the diaphragmatic defect in utero has been proposed. The success of this approach has been limited thus far (145, 146). However, the experience suggests that fetal repair of a CDH may allow more normal lung growth during gestation (145).

Animal and human evidence indicate that infants with CDH have a physiologic as well as structural immaturity of the lungs. Surfactant replacement therapy may have a role in the preoperative stabilization of these patients, but has not yet been evaluated in a controlled study (147).

Extracorporeal membrane oxygenation (ECMO) appears to have had an impact on the outcome of infants with CDH. Although there have been no controlled trials of ECMO compared to conventional therapy, it results in an improved outcome when compared with historical data obtained using conventional ventilation. It seems to be beneficial in both the preoperative stabilization and postoperative support of the most critically ill infants. Of 1543 patients with CDH in the ECMO registry, 980 (58%) survived following treatment with ECMO after "failing" conventional ventilation (148). No good predictors for failure of management with ECMO have been reported, leading proponents of this therapy to advocate its use in all infants with CDH (without other lethal anomalies or syndromes) failing conventional therapy. However, since in most studies ECMO was compared to historical controls, enthusiasm for this form of therapy should be tempered until it can be compared to infants managed with modern conventional therapy (149, 150).

Abnormalities of lung function persist following repair of a CDH. These infants frequently require rehospitalization with respiratory tract infections. They have increased respiratory symptoms including cough and exercise intolerance. Available studies suggest that patients with left-sided CDH have persistent abnormalities of ventilation and perfusion and expiratory flow. On V/Q scan, perfusion remains decreased to the left lung in the case of left-sided diaphragmatic hernias, whereas it is normal in right-sided lesions. The V/Q ratio is elevated secondary to a disproportionate decrease in perfusion. The relatively large ventilation (in relation to perfusion) may actually represent lung distension rather than lung growth. Pulmonary function testing in CDH survivors demonstrates decreased expiratory flow rates without a decrease in FVC when compared to age-matched controls (151, 152).

As many as 5% of diaphragmatic hernias may not be diagnosed until infancy or childhood. In these cases, the symptoms are varied and do not immediately suggest the diagnosis. Such patients may be asymptomatic or have complaints including recurrent respiratory illnesses, acute respiratory distress, failure to thrive, or GI problems (vomiting, diarrhea, intermittent abdominal pain, bowel obstruction). Clinical findings may include tachypnea, diminished breath sounds, shifted heart sounds, bowel sounds in the chest, cyanosis, or a scaphoid abdomen. The initial chest radiograph may be falsely interpreted as showing pneumothorax, infection with pneumatoceles, or congenital lung cysts. The presence of the stomach in the thorax, documented by nasogastric tube placement, is diagnostic. The

diagnosis can be confirmed quite simply with a barium swallow study. Although a CT scan or ultrasonography can also confirm the diagnosis, they are generally not needed. Patients who present late tolerate surgery well and seem to have few significant sequelae (153).

REFERENCES

1. Landing BH. Congenital malformations and genetic disorders of the respiratory tract (larynx, trachea, bronchi, and lungs). State of the art. *Am Rev Respir Dis* 1979; 120:151–185.
2. Boyd GL. Solid intrathoracic masses in children. *Pediatrics* 1955; 19:142–155.
3. Silverman FN, Kuhn JP. *Essentials of Caffey's pediatric x-ray diagnosis.* Chicago, Year Book, 1990.
4. Welch KJ, Randolph JG, Ravitch MM, O'Neill JA, Rowe MI. *Pediatric surgery,* ed 4. Chicago, Year Book, 1986.
5. Thurlbeck WM. *Pathology of the lung.* New York, Thieme, 1987.
6. Bluestone CD, Stool SE, Scheetz MD, eds. *Pediatric otolaryngology.* Philadelphia, WB Saunders, 1990.
7. Nussbaum E, Maggi, JC. Laryngomalacia in children. *Chest* 1990; 98:942–944.
8. Smith GJ, Cooper DM. Laryngomalacia and inspiratory obstruction in later childhood. *Arch Dis Child* 1981; 56:345–349.
9. McSwiney PF, Cavanagh NPC, Languth P. Outcome in congenital stridor (laryngomalacia). *Arch Dis Child* 1977; 52:215–218.
10. Wood RE. Spelunking in the pediatric airways: Explorations with the flexible fiberoptic bronchoscope. *Pediatr Clin North Am* 1984; 31:785–799.
11. Abreu FA, Silva E, Williams A, Simpson H. Sleep apnoea in infants with congenital stridor. *Arch Dis Child* 1986; 61:1125–1137.
12. McCray PB, Crockett DM, Wagener JS, Thies DJ. Hypoxia and hypercapnia in infants with mild laryngomalacia. *Am J Dis Child* 1988; 142:896–899.
13. Cox MA, Schiebler GL, Taylor WJ, Wheat MW, Krovetz LJ. Reversible pulmonary hypertension in a child with respiratory obstruction and cor pulmonale. *J Pediatr* 1965; 67:192–197.
14. Holinger LD, Konior RJ. Surgical management of severe laryngomalacia. *Laryngoscope* 1989; 99:136–142.
15. Marcus CL, Crockett DM, Davidson–Ward S. Evaluation of epiglottoplasty as treatment for severe laryngomalacia. *J Pediatr* 1990;117:706–710.
16. Macfarlane PI, Olinsky A, Phelan PD. Proximal airway function 8 to 16 years after laryngomalacia: Follow-up using flow-volume loop studies. *J Pediatr* 1985; 107:216–218.
17. Dubois JJ, Pokorny WJ, Harberg FJ, Smith RJH. Current management of laryngeal and laryngotracheoesophageal clefts. *J Pediatr Surg* 1990; 25:855–860.
18. Eriksen C, Zwillenberg D, Robinson N. Diagnosis and management of cleft larynx. Literature review and case report. *Ann Otol Rhinol Laryngol* 1990; 99:703–708.

19. Zaw-Tun HIA. Development of congenital laryngeal atreasias and clefts. *Ann Otol Rhinol Laryngol* 1988; 97:353–358.

20. Myer CM, Cotton RT, Holmes DK, Jackson, RK. Laryngeal and laryngotracheo-esophageal clefts: role of early surgical repair. *Ann Otol Rhinol Laryngol* 1990; 99:98–104.

21. Ogawa T, Yamataka A, Miyano T, Kohno S, Uemura S, Ichikawa G. Treatment of laryngotracheoesophageal cleft. *J Pediatr Surg* 1989; 24:341–342.

22. Silver MM, Thurston WA, Patrick JE. Perinatal pulmonary hyperplasia due to laryngeal atresia. *Hum Pathol* 1988; 19:110–113.

23. Fang SH, Ocejo R, Sin M, Finer NN, Wood BP. Congenital laryngeal atresia. *Am J Dis Child* 1989; 143:625–627.

24. Cotton TR, Richardson MA. Congenital laryngeal anomalies. *Otolaryngol Clin North Am* 1981; 14:203–218.

25. Booth JB, Birck HG. Operative treatment and postoperative management of saccular cyst and laryngocele. *Arch Otolaryngol* 1981; 107:500–502.

26. Holinger LD. Etiology of stridor in the neonate, infant and child. *Ann Otol Rhinol Laryngol* 1980; 89:397.

27. Ferguson CG. Congenital anomalies of the infant larynx. *Otolaryngol Clin North Am* 1970; 3:185.

28. Holinger PH, Kutnick SL, Schild JA, Holinger LD. Subglottic stenosis in infants and children. *Ann Otol* 1976; 85:591–599.

29. Cotton RT, Myer CM, Bratcher GO, Fitton CM. Anterior cricoid split, 1977–1987. *Arch Otolaryngol Head Neck Surg* 1988; 114:1300–1302.

30. Healy G, McGill T, Friedman EM. Carbon dioxide laser in subglottic hemangioma. An update. *Ann Otol Rhinol Laryngol* 1984; 93:370–373.

31. Cox WL, Shaw RR. Congenital chondromalacia of the trachea. *J Thorac Cardiovasc Surg* 1965; 49:1033–39.

32. Lynch JI. Bronchomalacia in children. Considerations governing medical vs surgical treatment. *Clin Pediatr* 1970; 9:279–282.

33. Benjamin B. Tracheomalacia in infants and children. *Ann Otol Rhinol Laryngol* 1984; 93:438–442.

34. Cogbill TH, Moore FA, Accurso FJ, Lilly JR. Primary tracheomalacia. *Ann Thorac Surg* 1983; 35:538–541.

35. Wiseman NE, Duncan PG, Cameron CB. Management of tracheobronchomalacia with continuous positive airway pressure. *J Pediatr Surg* 1985; 20:489–493.

36. Malone PS, Kiely EM. Role of aortopexy in the management of primary tracheomalacia and tracheobronchomalacia. *Arch Dis Child* 1990; 65:438–440.

37. Benjamin B, Pitkin J, Cohen D. Congenital tracheal stenosis. *Ann Otol* 1981; 90:364–371.

38. Hauft SM, Perlman JM, Siegel MJ, Muntz HR. Tracheal stenosis in the sick premature infant. Clinical and radiological features. *Am J Dis Child* 1988; 142:206–209.

39. Harrison MR, Heldt GP, Brasch RC, deLorimier AA, Gregory GA. Resection of distal tracheal stenosis in a baby with agenesis of the lung. *J Pediatr Surg* 1980; 15:938–943.

40. Healy GB, Schuster SR, Jonas RA, McGill TJI. Correction of segmental tracheal stenosis in children. *Ann Otol Rhinol Laryngol* 1988; 97:444–447.

41. Buchino JJ, Meagher DP, Cox JA. Tracheal agenesis: A clinical approach. *J Pediatr Surg* 1982; 17:132–137.

42. Altman RP, Randolph JG, Shearin RB. Tracheal agenesis: Recognition and management. *J Pediatr Surg* 1972; 7:112–117.

43. Holinger LD, Volk MS, Tucker GF. Congenital laryngeal anomalies associated with tracheal agenesis. *Ann Otol Rhinol Laryngol* 1987; 96:505–508.

44. Diaz EM, Adams JM, Hawkins HK, Smith RJH. Tracheal agenesis. A case report and literature review. *Arch Otolaryngol Head Neck Surg* 1989; 115:741–745.

45. Moore KL. *The developing human*, 4th ed. Philadelphia, WB Saunders, 1988, pp 314–325.

46. Harley HRS. The development and anomalies of the aortic arch and its branches. *Br J Surg* 1959; 46:561–573.

47. Marmon LM, Bye MR, Haas JM, Balsara RK, Dunn JM. Vascular rings and slings: Long-term follow-up of pulmonary function. *J Pediatr Surg* 1984; 19:683–692.

48. Vallette RC, Arensman RM, Falterman KW, Ochsner JL. Tracheoesophageal compression syndromes related to vascular ring. *South Med J* 1989; 82:338–340.

49. Bertolini A, Pelizza A, Panizzon G, et al. Vascular rings and slings. Diagnosis and surgical treatment of 49 patients. *J Cardiovasc Surg* 1987; 28:302–312.

50. Roesler M, de Leval M, Chrispin A, Stark J. Surgical management of vascular ring. *Ann Surg* 1983; 197:139–146.

51. Backer CL, Ilbawi MN, Idriss FS, DeLeon SY. Vascular anomalies causing tracheoesophageal compression. *J Thorac Cardiovasc Surg* 1989; 97:725–731.

52. Blumenthal S, Ravitch MM. Seminar on aortic vascular rings and other anomalies of the aortic arch. *Pediatrics* 1957; 22:896–906.

53. Sade RM, Rosenthal A, Fellows K, Castaneda AR. Pulmonary artery sling. *J Thorac Cardiovasc Surg* 1975; 69:333–346.

54. Keith HK. Vascular rings and tracheobronchial compression in infants. *Pediatr Ann* 1977; 6:541–549.

55. Loren ML, Cooley RL, Rohr C, Buck RO. Vascular ring presenting as asthma: The value of a flow-volume curve. *J Pediatr* 1979; 94:610–611.

56. Julsrud PR, Ehman RL. Magnetic resonance imaging of vascular rings. *Mayo Clin Proc* 1986; 61:181–185.

57. Otero-Cagide M, Moodie DS, Sterba R, Gill CC. Digital subtraction in the diagnosis of vascular rings. *Am Heart J* 1986; 112:1304–1308.

58. Ein SH, Shandling B, Wesson D, Filler RM. Esophageal atresia with distal tracheoesophageal fistula: Associated anomalies and prognosis in the 1980s. *J Pediatr Surg* 1989; 24:1055–1059.

59. Weigel W, Kaufmann HJ. The frequency and types of other congenital anomalies in association with tracheoesophageal malformations. Radiologic studies of 83 such infants. *Clin Pediatr* 1976; 15:819–834.

60. Bedard P, Girvan DP, Shandling B. Congenital H-type tracheoesophageal fistula. *J Pediatr Surg* 1974; 9:663–668.

61. Frates MC, terMeulen DC, Yee WFH. Congenital tracheoesophageal fistula (H-type) in a six-year-old. *Clin Pediatr* 1990; 29:117–119.

62. Dudley NE, Phelan PD. Respiratory complications in long-term survivors of oesophageal atresia. *Arch Dis Child* 1976; 51:279–282.

63. Filler RM, Rossello PJ, Lebowitz RL. Life-threatening anoxic spells caused by tracheal compression after repair of esophageal atresia: Correction by surgery. *J Pediatr Surg* 1976; 11:739–748.

64. Kimura K, Soper RT, Kao SCS, Sato Y, Smith WL, Franken EA. Aortosternopexy for tracheomalacia following repair of esophageal atresia: Evaluation by Cine-CT and technical refinement. *J Pediatr Surg* 1990; 25:769–772.

65. Wailoo MP, Emery JL. The trachea in children with tracheo-oesophageal fistula. *Histopathology* 1979; 3:329–338.

66. Milligan DWA, Levision H. Lung function in children following repair of tracheoesophageal fistula. *J Pediatr* 1979; 95:24–27.

67. Moessinger AC, Harding R, Adamson TM, Singh M, Kiu GT. Role of lung fluid volume in growth and maturation of the fetal sheep lung. *J Clin Invest* 1990; 86:1270–77.

68. Nicolini U, Fisk NM, Rodeck CH, Tabert D, Wigglesworth JS. Low amniotic pressure in oligohydramnios—Is this the cause of pulmonary hypoplasia? *Am J Obstet Gynecol* 1989; 161:1098–1101.

69. Wigglesworth JS, Desai R. Is fetal respiratory function a major determinant of perinatal survival? *Lancet* 1982; 1:264–267.

70. Bell JB, Gerdes JS, Bhutani VK, Wilmott RW. A chronic lung disorder following abdominal pregnancy. *Am J Dis Child* 1987; 141:1111–1113.

71. Eigen H, Lemen RJ, Waring WW. Congenital lobar emphysema: Long-term evaluation of surgically and conservatively treated children. *Am Rev Respir Dis* 1976; 113:823–831.

72. McBride JT, Wohl ME, Strieder DJ, et al. Lung growth and airway function after lobectomy in infancy for congenital lobar emphysema. *J Clin Invest* 1980; 66:962–970.

73. Chang N. Hertzler JH, Gregg RH, Lofti MW, Brough AJ. Congenital stenosis of the right mainstem bronchus. A case report. *Pediatrics* 1968; 41:739–742.

74. Lacquet LK, Fornhoff M, Dierickx R, Buyssens N. Bronchial atresia with corresponding segmental pulmonary emphysema. *Thorax* 1971; 26:68–73.

75. Robotham JL, Menkes HA, Chipps BE, et al. A physiologic assessment of segmental bronchial atresia. *Am Rev Respir Dis* 1980; 121:533–540.

76. Meng RL, Jensik RJ, Faber LP, Matthew GR, Kittle CF. Bronchial atresia. *Ann Thoracic Surg* 1978; 25:184–192.

77. DiLorenzo M, Collin PP, Vaillancourt R, Duranceau A. Bronchogenic cysts. *J Pediatr Surg* 1989; 24:988–991.

78. Defossez SM, Deluca SA. Bronchogenic cysts. *Am Fam Physic* 1989; 39:129–132.

79. Ramenofsky ML, Leape LL, McCauley RGK. Bronchogenic cyst. *J Pediatr Surg* 1979; 14:219–224.

80. Bagwell CE, Schiffman RJ. Subcutaneous bronchogenic cysts. *J Pediatr Surg* 1988; 23:993–995.

81. Wenig BL, Abramson AL. Tracheal bronchogenic cyst: A new clinical entity? *Ann Otol Rhinol Laryngol* 1987; 96:58–60.

82. Krous HF, Sexauer CL. Embryonal rhabdomyosarcoma arising within a congenital bronchogenic cyst in a child. *J Pediatr Surg* 1981; 16:506–508.

83. Lincoln JCR, Stark J, Subramanian S, et al. Congenital lobar emphysema. *Ann Surg* 1971; 173:55–62.

84. Murray GF. Congenital lobar emphysema. Collective review. *Surg Gynecol Obstet* 1967; 124:611–625.

85. Man DWK, Hamdy MH, Hendry GMA, Bisset WH, Forfar JO. Congenital lobar emphysema: Problems in diagnosis and management. *Arch Dis Child* 1983; 58:709–712.

86. Markowitz RI, Mercurio MR, Vahjen GA, Gross I, Touloukian RJ. Congenital lobar emphysema. The role of CT and V/Q scan. *Clin Pediatr* 1989; 28:19–23.

87. Morgan WJ, Lemen RJ, Rojas R. Acute worsening of congenital lobar emphysema with subsequent spontaneous improvement. *Pediatrics* 1983; 71:844–848.

88. Tapper D, Schuster S, McBride J, et al. Polyalveolar lobe: Anatomic and physiologic parameters and their relationship to congenital lobar emphysema. *J Pediatr Surg* 1980; 15:931–937.

89. Cooney TP, Dimmick JE, Thurlbeck WM. Increased acinar complexity with polyhydramnios. *Pediatr Pathol* 1986; 5:183–197.

90. Bailey PV, Tracy T, Connors RH, deMello D, Lewis JE, Weber TR. Congenital bronchopulmonary malformations. *J Thorac Cardiovasc Surg* 1990; 99:597–603.

91. Heij HA, Ekkelkamp S, Vos A. Diagnosis of congenital cystic ademomatoid malformation of the lung in newborn infants and children. *Thorax* 1990; 45:122–125.

92. Turcios NL, Cunningham F, Zarzuela AT. When a neonate has cystic lung disease. *J Respir Dis* 1987: 8:85–96.

93. Rescorla FJ, West KW, Vane DW, Engle W, Grosfeld JL. Pulmonary hypertension in neonatal cystic lung disease: Survival following lobectomy and ECMO in two cases. *J Pediatr Surg* 1990; 25:1054–1056.

94. Harrison MR, Adzick NS, Jennings RW, et al. Antenatal intervention for congenital cystic adenomatoid malformation. *Lancet* 1990; 336:965–967.

95. Saltzman DH, Adzick NS, Benacerraf, BR. Fetal cystic adenomatoid malformation of the lung: Apparent improvement in utero. *Obstet Gynecol* 1988; 71:1000–1002.

96. Ueda K, Gruppo R, Unger F, Martin L, Bove K. Rhabdomyosarcoma of lung arising in congenital cystic adenomatoid malformation. *Cancer* 1977; 40:383–388.

97. Collin PP, Desjardins JG, Khan AH. Pulmonary sequestration. *J Pediatr Surg* 1987; 22:750–753.

98. Ikezoe J, Murayama S, Godwin JD, Done SL, Verschakelen JA. Bronchopulmonary sequestration: CT assessment. *Radiology* 1990; 176:375–379.

99. Levine MM, Nudel DB, Gootman N, Wolpowitz A, Wisoff BG. Pulmonary sequestration causing congestive heart failure in infancy: A report of two

cases and review of the literature. *Ann Thorac Surg* 1982; 34:581–585.

100. Gustafson RA, Murray GF, Warden HE, Hill RC, Rozar GE. Intralobar sequestration. A missed diagnosis. *Ann Thorac Surg* 1989; 47:841–847.

101. DeParedes CG, Pierce WS, Johnson DG, Waldhausen JA. Pulmonary sequestration in infants and children: A 20-year experience and review of the literature. *J Pediatr Surg* 1970; 5:136–147.

102. Rodgers BM, Harman PK, Johnson AM. Bronchopulmonary foregut malformations. The spectrum of anomalies. *Ann Surg* 1986; 203:517–524.

103. Weinberg AG, Currarino G, Moore GC, Votteler TP. Mesenchymal neoplasia and congenital pulmonary cysts. *Pediatr Radiol* 1980; 9:179–182.

104. Burke CM, Safai C, Nelson DP, Raffin TA. Pulmonary arteriovenous malformations: A critical update. *Am Rev Respir Dis* 1986; 134:334–339.

105. Utzon F, Brandrup F. Pulmonary arteriovenous fistulas in children. Review article. *Acta Paediatr Scand* 1973; 62:422–432.

106. Dines DE, Seward JB, Bernatz PE. Pulmonary arteriovenous fistulas. *Mayo Clin Proc* 1983; 58:176–181.

107. Stringer CJ, Stanley AL, Bates RC, Summers JE. Pulmonary arteriovenous fistula. *Am J Surg* 1955; 89:1954–1080.

108. Higgins CB, Wexler L. Clinical and angiographic features of pulmonary ateriovenous fistulas in children. *Radiology* 1976; 119:171–175.

109. Terry PB, Barth KH, Kaufman SL, White RI: Balloon embolization for treatment of pulmonary arteriovenous fistulas. *N Engl J Med* 1980; 302:1189–1190.

110. Kravath RE, Scarpelli EM, Bernstein J. Hepatogenic cyanosis: Arteriovenous shunts in chronic active hepatitis. *J Pediatr* 1971; 78:238–245.

111. Silverman A, Cooper MD, Moller JH, Good RA. Syndrome of cyanosis, digital clubbing, and hepatic disease in siblings. *J Pediatr* 1968; 72:70–80.

112. McCloskey JJ, Schlein C, Schwarz K, Klein A, Colombani P. Severe hypoxia and intrapulmonary shunting resulting from cirrhosis reversed by liver transplantation in a pediatric patient. *J Pediatr* 1991; 118:902–904.

113. Murray JF. *The normal lung.* Philadelphia, WB Saunders, 1986, pp 61, 69.

114. Noonan JA, Walters LR, Reeves JT. Congenital pulmonary lymphangiectasis. *Am J Dis Child* 1970; 120:314–319.

115. Felman AH, Rhatigan RM, Pierson KK. Pulmonary lymphangiectasia. *AJR* 1972; 116:548–558.

116. Esterly JR, Oppenheimer EH. Lymphangiectasis and other pulmonary lesions in the asplenia syndrome. *Arch Pathol* 1970; 90:553–560.

117. France NE, Brown RJK. Congenital pulmonary lymphangiectasis. Report of 11 examples with special reference to cardiovascular findings. *Arch Dis Child* 1971; 46:528–532.

118. Wagenaar SJ SC, Swierenga J, Wagenvoort CA. Late presentation of primary pulmonary lymphangiectasis. *Thorax* 1978; 33:791–795.

119. Neill CA, Ferenca C, Sabiston DC, Shelton J. The familial occurrence of hypoplastic right lung with systemic arterial supply and venous drainage: "Scimitar syndrome." *Johns Hopkins Med J* 1960; 107:1–15.

120. Farnsworth AE, Ankeney JL. The spectrum of scimitar syndrome. *J Thorac Cardiovasc Surg* 1974; 68:37–42.

121. Mardini MK, Sakati NA, Lewall DB, Christie R, Nyhan WL. Scimitar syndrome. *Clin Pediatr* 1982; 21:350–354.

122. Frank JL, Poole CA, Rosas G. Horseshoe lung: Clinical, pathologic, and radiologic features and a new plain film finding. *AJR* 1986; 146:217–226.

123. Cipriano P, Sweeney LJ, Hutchins GM, Rosenquist GC. Horseshoe lung in an infant with recurrent pulmonary infections. *Am J Dis Child* 1975; 129:1343–45.

124. Freedom RM, Burrows PE, Moes CAF. "Horseshoe" lung: Report of five new cases. *AJR* 1986; 146:211–215.

125. Gibson GJ. Diaphragmatic paresis: Pathophysiology, clinical features, and investigation. *Thorax* 1989; 44:960–970.

126. Robotham JL. A physiological approach to hemidiaphragm paralysis. *Crit Care Med* 1979; 7:563–566.

127. Greene W, L'Heureux P, Hunt CE. Paralysis of the diaphragm. *Am J Dis Child* 1975; 129:1402–1405.

128. Haller JA, Pickard LR, Tepas JJ, et al. Management of diaphragmatic paralysis in infants with special emphasis on selection of patients for operative plication. *J Pediatr Surg* 1979; 14:779–785.

129. Ambler R, Gruenewald S, John E. Ultrasound monitoring of diaphragm activity in bilateral diaphragmatic paralysis. *Arch Dis Child* 1985; 60:170–172.

130. Wayne ER, Campbell JB, Burrington JD, Davis WS. Eventration of the diaphragm. *J Pediatr Surg* 1974; 9:643–651.

131. Goldstein JD, Reid LM. Pulmonary hypoplasia resulting from phrenic nerve agenesis and diaphragmatic amyoplasia. *J Pediatr* 1980; 97:282–287.

132. Mickell JJ, Oh KS, Siewers RD, Galvis AG, Fricker FJ, Matthews RA. Clinical implications of postoperative unilateral phrenic nerve paralysis. *J Thorac Cardiovasc Surg* 1978; 76:297–304.

133. Sivan Y, Galvis A. Early diaphragmatic paralysis in infants with genetic disorders. *Clin Pediatr* 1990; 29:169–171.

134. McWilliam RC, Gardner-Medwin D, Doyle D, Stephenson JBP. Diaphragmatic paralysis due to spinal muscular atrophy. *Arch Dis Child* 1985; 60:145–149.

135. Oh KS, Newman B, Bender TM, Bowen A. Radiologic evaluation of the diaphragm. *Radiol Clin North Am* 1988; 26:355–364.

136. Markand ON, Kincaid JC, Pourmand RA, et al. Electrophysiologic evaluation of diaphragm by transcutaneous phrenic nerve stimulation. *Neurology* 1984; 34:604–614.

137. McCauley RGK, Labib KB. Diaphragmatic paralysis evaluated by phrenic nerve stimulation during fluoroscopy or real–time ultrasound. *Radiology* 1984; 153:33–36.

138. Andreou A, Keh E, Vidyasagar D. Critical care problems of the newborn: neonatal diaphragmatic paralysis and crying vital capacity. *Crit Care Med* 1976; 4:308–310.

139. Moore KL. *The developing human*, 4th ed. Philadelphia, WB Saunders, 1988, pp 314–325.

140. George DK, Cooney TP, Chiu BK, Thurlbeck WM. Hypoplasia and immaturity of the terminal

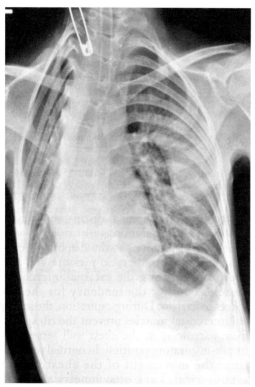

Figure 41.1. Chest radiograph showing distorted thorax in a patient with scoliosis due to severe muscle weakness. Identification of anatomical landmarks is often difficult in such cases.

muscular dystrophy affect both hemithoraces equally and do not cause alterations in the shape of the thorax despite marked dysfunction. Although marked obesity causes restrictive lung disease it does not alter the shape of the bony thorax.

Significant differences in the volumes of the lungs may cause asymmetry of the bony thorax. Relative hyper-inflation of one lung causes the affected hemi-thorax to bulge. Conversely, agenesis or hypoplasia of a lung may cause crowding of the ribs on the affected side, resulting in a flattened hemithorax. A similar situation may take place following pneumonectomy, especially if performed early in life or if scoliosis develops.

SHAPE RELATED TO FUNCTION

Inspection of the thorax provides valuable information about the function of the chest wall and underlying lungs. The thoracic index (ratio of widest anteroposterior plane, or AP

diameter, to the widest dimension of the transverse plane) can be estimated by visual inspection (Fig. 41.2). In normal infants, the chest wall appears to have an increase AP diameter and has a thoracic index of approximately 0.85. With growth, the shape of the chest changes. The growth of the thorax in the AP plane is relatively less than that in the transverse plane, and the chest flattens out. Thus, the thoracic index falls to about 0.72 at age 1–2 years and remains at that level throughout childhood (4).

Some children appear to have a large thorax proportionate to their body habitus; estimating thoracic index is useful when trying to determine if the shape of the chest is normal. Children who have a "barrel chest" have an increased thoracic index as a result of increased total lung capacity. Although this finding is often obvious, a mildly increased AP diameter can be subtle and is easily overlooked. This finding should alert clinicians that acute or chronic airway obstruction (e.g., asthma, cystic fibrosis) may be present and that further investigation is warranted. Severe hyper-inflation may cause a pectus carinatum, although most cases of pectus carinatum are congenital or associated with other underlying conditions such as scoliosis, Poland syndrome, neuromuscular disease, and rickets (5, 6). Children with marked hyper-inflation may have abnormalities in the mechanics of chest movement during respiration, which in association with low pulmonary compliance can cause intercostal retractions. When severe, costal or subcostal depressions or grooves give the chest an hourglass appearance (Fig. 41.3). Advanced cases of chronic hyper-inflation may also lead to mild kyphosis of the spine.

A low thoracic index is less common. If present at birth, abnormal rib structure or hypoplastic lungs should be suspected. This may not be evident until further somatic growth occurs. Although serial measurements of the chest circumference may aid in detecting inadequate thoracic growth, chest circumference is not a good indicator of thoracic shape. In children with conditions that cause pulmonary fibrosis associated with contraction scarring of the lung, one may see a reduction of the AP diameter. Although loss of one lobe does not appear to cause a change in chest shape because compensatory hyper-inflation of the remaining lobe(s) maintains lung vol-

Infant   ## Child

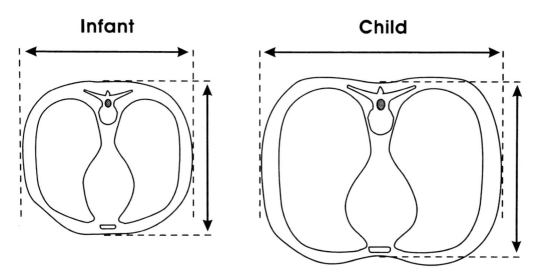

Figure 41.2. Thoracic index is estimated by dividing the largest anteroposterior plane by the widest transverse plane.

Table 41.1.
General Association of Abnormal Thoracic Shape and Abnormal Lung Function

	Function	
	Obstructive Lung Disease	Restrictive Lung Disease
Asymmetrical	- Regional hyper-inflation - Subcostal groove	- Pneumonectomy - Unilateral hypoplastic or absent rib(s) or lung(s) - Localized neuromuscular weakness - Pectus exvavatum (congenital)
Symmetrical	- Barrel chest - Pectus carinatum (acquired) - Pectus excavatum (acquired) - Sternal cleft	- Generalized muscle weakness - Obesity - Asphyxiating thoracic dystrophy - Pectus excavatum (congenital)

ume, loss of large portions of lung may reduce AP diameter.

A small thorax secondary to very short ribs is the hallmark of asphyxiating thoracic dystrophy (Jeune syndrome) (7) (Fig. 41.4A). In severe cases this condition is fatal because of progressive respiratory failure. In children who survive, the thorax grows but remains relatively small throughout life. The small thorax will not allow the lungs to expand fully, and restrictive lung disease ensues. Some of these infants may also have hypoplastic lungs. Thoracic cage expansion may be attempted surgically by a variety of approaches such as inserting a support strut between ribs on each side (Fig 41.4B). The approach to this problem is analogous to that used in craniosynos-

tosis. Freeing the ribs from the sternum is thought to improve chest wall compliance and allow the growing lungs to continue to expand the thoracic cavity. Although such procedures may hold promise for these patients, it is unclear that normal lung growth will occur. Each case must be considered individually with the severity of the deformity and associated anomalies factored into the decision to proceed with surgical intervention.

STERNAL DEFECTS

Sternal defects range from relatively minor defects such as a displaced or bifid xiphoid to large defects or even absence of the sternum. Included in this group are two important con-

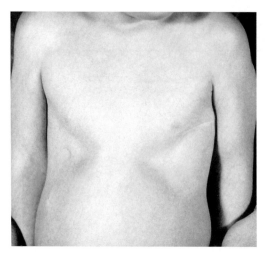

Figure 41.3. Costal grooves that have resulted from chronic retractions of costal/subcostal area during inspiration in a boy with severe hyper-inflation.

experience difficulty breathing, and noisy respiration is common. Surgical repair is usually indicated in the neonatal period (8–11).

One of the most common thoracic cage disorders is congenital pectus excavatum. A typical pectus excavatum is characterized by a depression of the mid-sternum between the manubrium and the xiphoid (Fig. 41.5) and may be noted in more than one family member. The depression is usually deepest at the junction between the gladiolus and the xiphoid. The sternum may lie at an angle, resulting in flattening of the ribs on one side. This may contribute to the development of a thoracic scoliosis as the chest wall grows asymmetrically. Although the etiology of this deformity is not well understood, it has been suggested that defects in osteogenesis and chondrogenesis cause the mid-portion of the sternum to become misaligned. The increased frequency of the pectus deformity in Marfan syndrome

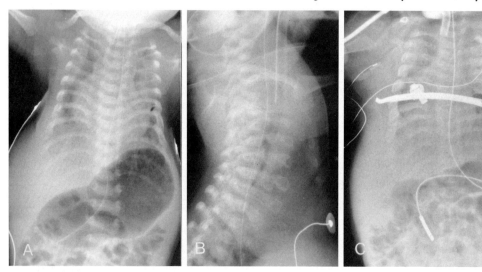

Figure 41.4. Chest radiographs (A, and B, lateral) in an infant with asphyxiating thoracic dystrophy (Jeune syndrome). Patient is intubated for respiratory failure. Note short ribs and narrow thorax. C, Same patient following placement of a strut to expand ribs.

ditions, namely, cleft sternum and pectus excavatum.

Sternal clefts likely result from incomplete embryonic union of sternal cartilage bars. Although total clefts may occur, partial clefts are more common, occurring at either the superior or the inferior end of the sternum. Ectopia cordis may be present. A large sternal defect results in poor support for the trachea and accentuates the dynamic narrowing of the trachea and possibly the bronchi. Patients may

(12) lends support to the presence of a connective tissue disorder as the cause of pectus deformity. Although most cases of pectus excavatum are congenital, pectus excavatum may also be acquired. This can occur in infants and young children whose thoracic compliance is high. In the presence of airway obstruction, generation of high negative intrathoracic pressures on inspiration causes the sternum to be pulled inward (13–15). The recurrent nature of the sternal deformation results in

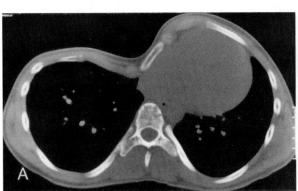
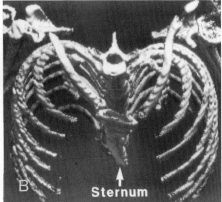

Figure 41.5. *A*, Chest CT of pectus excavatum. Note flattened hemithorax and alignment of sternum. *B*, Computerized reconstruction of thorax in same patient. Note relationship of sternum to ribs. (Courtesy Ehsan Afshani, M.D.)

the eventual remodelling of the chest wall. Appropriate treatment for the airway obstruction generally resolves this, but chronic airway obstruction may be associated with a residual pectus excavatum.

The diagnosis of pectus excavatum is typically made by visual inspection. Some children with a small pectus excavatum are diagnosed only after careful inspection or palpation of the sternum, whereas other children with severe depression of the sternum are identified easily, usually by concerned parents. There is usually no need for a routine radiograph or computed tomography (CT) of the chest in order to make the diagnosis. Some have advocated chest CT in order to quantitate the severity of the defect (16), but the value of chest CT to predict the effect of pectus excavatum on cardiopulmonary function and prognosis is untested.

Despite the appearance of the chest wall, pectus excavatum alone generally does not cause significant cardiac or respiratory dysfunction. Echocardiographic evidence of prolapse of the mitral valve is seen in 18–65% of children with pectus excavatum, but this finding is nonspecific (17, 18). Although surgical repair of pectus excavatum may resolve a prolapsing mitral valve, the clinical significance of this is not known (19). Moderately severe pectus excavatum shifts the heart leftward, but it is not known what degree of shift, if any, will result in altered cardiac function. Although the cardiac silhouette appears displaced and flattened on the AP chest radiograph, the electrocardiogram is normal or

shows minor abnormalities (19, 20). Resting cardiac function is typically within normal limits. Alterations in cardiac function have been reported in adults with pectus excavatum, primarily following strenuous exercise (21, 22). These findings have been inconsistent (23). Although some older children were reported to have increased end diastolic pressure, cardiac output, stoke volume, and oxygen consumption are characteristically normal (24, 25).

Lack of standardization of measurements of the severity of the pectus deformity limits interpretation of these data. Although measuring the depth of the sternal defect may assess progression of the defect, it is not a good indicator of cardiopulmonary function. It is not known if subjective symptoms such as shortness of breath, difficulty exercising, or chest pain correlate with the severity of the defect. It has been reported that severe defects are associated with pulmonary function tests that are consistent with a restrictive pattern but that cardiorespiratory adaptations to exercise are normal (25). Others have noted that some young adults with pectus excavatum have exercise limitation because they experience increased O_2 uptakes at higher workloads due to decreased chest wall compliance and increased work of breathing (26, 27).

Although few data exist that address the natural history of pectus excavatum, clinical experience suggests that it is unusual for congenital pectus excavatum to progress from a mild case to a severe case unless significant airway obstruction is also present. Approximately 40% of pectus excavatum abnormalities that are present in young children improve over time (28). The more severely affected cases may stabilize but remain visible. It is not known if growth and development adversely affect a severe pectus deformity in a young child. At this time there are no good parameters that can predict accurately the natural course of a young child or adolescent with a pectus deformity.

Most clinicians agree that mild to moderate pectus excavatum calls for observation only. However, affected children (or their parents) may restrict physical activity because of concerns about potential dangers of exercise in a child whose chest wall looks so different.

In the past, a severe pectus excavatum associated with measurable abnormalities in pulmonary function and exercise tolerance was felt to be an indication for surgical repair. However, when available data are analyzed in detail, surgical correction has not been shown to improve definitively either lung function or exercise tolerance on a consistent basis. More data are needed in these children. An example of such a case is shown in Figure 41.6. It must be emphasized that because surgical repair does not guarantee significant improvement in cardiopulmonary function, it should not be considered routine treatment of this condition.

One group of patients who should be considered for surgery are those who have an asymmetric pectus that produces secondary thoracic scoliosis. If progression of the scoliosis is noted, correction of the pectus can result in a more horizontal alignment of the sternum and reduce the scoliosis.

Some children will undergo surgical repair of pectus excavatum for cosmetic reasons. These children are typically self-conscious about the defect (29) and are embarrassed to remove their shirts in public. These children should first be counseled to help them deal with their body image problems. However, even after counseling, some children, particularly adolescents, are willing to accept a surgical scar in place of their pectus excavatum.

A number of surgical approaches have been reported, including placing struts between the sternum and rib ends, chrondrotomy, osteotomy, sternal turnover, and insertion of synthetic plates. All of these methods are designed to reconfigure the sternum and, in general, to

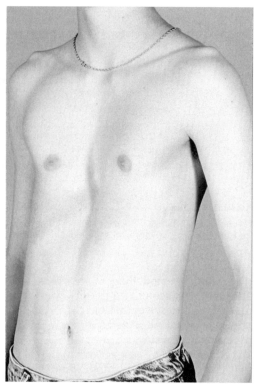

Figure 41.6. Fourteen-year-old male embarrassed by chest deformity was evaluated for surgery. Pulmonary function showed: total lung capacity = 89% predicted; vital capacity = 79% predicted; residual volume = 117% predicted; expiratory flows reduced in proportion to reduced vital capacity. Patient elected to undergo surgery.

reduce the degree of angulation of the sternum (30–34). An individual surgeon's preference dictates which procedure is selected. Some surgeons advocate surgical repair at an early age, according to a large retrospective series (35). There have not been prospective data to establish the most appropriate time for surgical intervention. Follow-up data suggest that surgical intervention may contribute to deterioration in pulmonary function (36).

In summary, available data show that, despite its appearance, pectus excavatum is a benign condition and that surgery is indicated only in select cases. Furthermore, these data also suggest that surgery can change the appearance of the thorax but appears to have little effect on cardiopulmonary function.

SCOLIOSIS

Although not a primary chest wall abnormality, scoliosis in children occurs as a complication of congenital vertebral body abnormalities and neuromuscular disease, and as an idiopathic condition that may affect chest wall function (37). Pediatric pulmonary physicians are frequently requested to evaluate patients with thoracic scoliosis who have developed chronic respiratory insufficiency, recurrent pneumonia, or atelectasis and to provide preoperative assessment prior to spinal and major thoracoabdominal surgery. An overview of the role of the pediatric pulmonologist in preoperative evaluation of patients with respiratory dysfunction is presented in Chapter 60.

Assessing patients with scoliosis calls for measuring the curvature of the spine on radiograph (38). It is essential to establish the nature of the underlying condition responsible for the development of the spinal curvature since that condition may influence the response to stress from surgery or infection more than the scoliosis itself. This is especially true in children with associated neuromuscular disease.

Ausculatation of the lungs of a patient with mild to moderate thoracic scoliosis is usually normal. With severe curves (> 90°) decreased breath sounds and/or crackles can be noted on the convex side of the curve. One possible explanation is inadequate clearance of secretions resulting in recurrent atelectasis and pneumonia on this side. The risk of these complications is increased in patients whose cough is impaired by muscular weakness. The examination is usually normal on the convex side (39).

Interpretation of a chest radiograph in a patient with severe scoliosis is complicated by displacement of the intrathoracic organs (Fig. 41.1). Despite these limitations, it is not uncommon to find evidence of volume loss on the convex side and recurrent chronic atelectasis.

Pulmonary function is usually affected adversely by severe scoliosis, particularly in the presence of underlying neuromuscular disease. Lung function is consistent with a restrictive pattern. Predicting normal values for lung volumes is difficult in patients with scoliosis because the relationship between standing height and lung volumes is discordant. Arm span has been used to predict height and, in turn (40), normal lung volumes, but this measurement is controversial because the

ratio of arm span to height is nearly 1:1 with curvature less than 46° (41). Nevertheless, for clinical purposes we suggest using arm span since it will remain relatively constant even as the scoliosis progresses. An increasing curvature of the spine may result in a decrease in height, either standing or sitting. This in turn reduces the predicted values, which may mask declining lung volume.

Pulmonary function abnormalities become detectable when the thoracic curve exceeds 50° (42). Several studies have demonstrated an inverse linear relationship between the angle of curvature and the vital capacity in patients with curves between 60° and 120° (43–45). Although total lung capacity (TLC) and functional residual capacity are also reduced, residual volume (RV) is preserved, resulting in an increased RV/TLC ratio. Increase in this ratio is not indicative of hyperinflation but, rather, a reflection of the effect of this disorder on vital capacity and TLC. Flow rates are decreased in proportion to the decrease in lung volume.

Compliance is decreased and work of breathing is increased. Exercise capacity may be diminished even in asymptomatic individuals (46). Hypoxia develops with progressive scoliosis. Despite limited data on the effects of sleep on ventilation in patients with scoliosis (47), there is concern that scoliosis, particularly in patients with underlying neuromuscular disease, may result in significant hypoventilation, particularly during rapid eye movement sleep. There is evidence that the risk of cardiorespiratory failure is increased in patients whose curve exceeds approximately 100° (48).

The management of thoracic scoliosis is based on early detection of respiratory compromise, aggressive control of respiratory infection, and prevention of progression of the spinal curvature. Patients with spinal curves > 60° should have routine serial assessment of lung function. Complaints of disturbed sleep, morning headaches, or development of polycythemia or cor pulmonale suggest hypoventilation during sleep. This is best evaluated with nocturnal polysomnography. Hypoxia without evidence of hypoventilation can be managed easily with supplemental oxygen. Children found to have significant nocturnal hypoventilation may be candidates for nocturnal ventilation. If the patient will tolerate a face mask this can be provided by nasal mask ventilation and a biphasic positive airway pressure device (49). Suspected infection should be treated aggressively with antibiotics and chest physical therapy.

Stabilization of the scoliosis is managed initially with bracing and eventually with spinal infusion. Bracing is not likely to help if thoracic lordosis is also present (50). For patients with a severe curve, a combination of the traditional posterior approach and an anterior intrathoracic approach is frequently used. This obviously increases the respiratory morbidity. Post-operative complications include atelectasis, pneumonia, and the need for prolonged assisted ventilation. Prediction of postoperative complications can be based on the degree and duration of pulmonary impairment, the nature of the underlying neuromuscular disease, and the need for an anterior as well as a posterior approach. Patients and parents should be advised of the risks of surgery and prepared for the possibility of chronic respiratory insufficiency. If lobar atelectasis develops and does not respond to chest physical therapy, fiberoptic bronchoscopy and bronchial lavage may be useful in removing mucus plugs.

REFERENCES

1. Harcke HT, Grissom LE, Lee MS, Mandell GA. Common congenital skeletal anomalies of the thorax. *J Thorac Imag* 1986; 1:1–6.
2. Argyle JC. Pulmonary hypoplasia in infants with giant abdominal wall defects. *Pediatr Pathol* 1989; 9:43–55.
3. Bowen A, Dominguez R. Sternal depression simulating mediastinal emphysema in neonates with respiratory distress. *Radiology* 1981; 139:599–601.
4. Pasterkamp, H. The history and physical examination. In Chernick V, ed. *Kendig's disorders of the respiratory tract in children.* Philadelphia, WB Saunders, 1990, pp 56–77.
5. Shamberger RC, Welch KJ. Surgical correction of pectus carinatum. *J Pediatr Surg* 1987; 22:48–53.
6. Urschel HC, Byrd HS, Sethi SM, Razzuk, MA. Poland's syndrome: Improved surgical management. *Ann Thorac Surg* 1984; 37:204–211.
7. Giorgi PL, Gabrielli O, Bonifazi V, Catassi C, Coppa GV. Mild form of Jeune syndrome in two sisters. *Am J Med Genet* 1990; 35:280–282.
8. Firmin RK, Fragomeni LS, Lennox SC. Complete cleft sternum. *Thorax* 1980; 35:303–306.
9. Kaplan LC, Matsuoka R, Gilbert EF, Opitz JM, Kurnit DM. Ectopia cordis and cleft sternum: Evidence for mechanical teratogenesis following rupture of the chorion or yolk sac. *Am J Med Genet* 1985; 21:187–202.
10. Mogilner J, Siplovich L, Bar-Ziv J, Mares AJ. Surgical management of the cleft sternum. *J Pediatr Surg* 1988; 23:889–891.
11. Teitelbaum SA, Fonkalsrud EW. Congenital bifid sternum. Report of an unusual case. *J Thorac Cardiovasc Surg* 1988; 96:162–165.
12. Arn PH, Scherer LR, Haller JA Jr, Pyeritz RE. Outcome of pectus excavatum in patients with Marfan syndrome and in the general population. *J Pediatr* 1989; 115:954–958.
13. Fan L, Murphy S. Pectus excavatum from chronic upper airway obstruction. *Am J Dis Child* 1981; 135:550–552.
14. Godfrey S. Association between pectus excavatum and sequential bronchomalacia. *J Pediatr* 1980; 96: 649–652.
15. Olsen KD, Kern EB, O'Connell EJ. Pectus excavatum: Resolution after surgical removal of upper airway obstruction. *Laryngoscope* 1980; 90:832–887.
16. Haller JA Jr, Kramer SS, Lietman S A. Use of CT scans in selection of patients for pectus excavatum surgery: A preliminary report. *J Pediatr Surg* 1987; 22:904–906.
17. Udoshi MB, Shah A, Fisher VJ, Dolgin M. Incidence of mitral valve prolapse in subjects with thoracic skeletal abnormalities: A prospective study. *Am Heart J* 1979; 97:303–311.
18. Saint-Mezard G, Duret J C, Chanudet X, et al. Prolapus valvulaire mitral et pectus excavatum. Association fortuite ou groupement syndromique? *Presse Med* 1986; 15:439.
19. Shamberger RC, Welch KJ, Sanders SP. Mitral valve prolapse associated with pectus excavatum. *J Pediatr* 1987; 111:404–407.
20. Gyllensward A, Irnell L, Michallsson M, Ovist O, Sahlstedt B. Pectus excavatum. A clinical study with long term postoperative follow-up. *Acta Pediatr Scand* 1975; 255:2–14.
21. Beiser GD, Epstein SE, Stampfer M, Goldstein RE, Noland SP, Levitsky S. Impairment of cardiac function in patients with pectus excavatum, with improvement after operative correction. *N Engl J Med* 1972; 287:267–272.
22. Peterson RJ, Young WG Jr, Godwin JD, Sabiston DC Jr, Jones RH. Noninvasive assessment of exercise cardiac function before and after pectus excavatum repair. *J Thorac Cardiovasc Surg* 1985; 90:251–260.
23. Diaz FU, Pelons AN, Valdis FG. Pectus excavatum: Hemodynamic and electrocardiographic considerations. *Am J Cardiol* 1968; 10:272–277.
24. Ghory MJ, James FW, Mays W. Cardiac performance in children with pectus excavatum. *J Pediatr Surg* 1989; 24:751–755.
25. Wynn SR, Driscoll DJ, Ostrom NK, Staats BA, O'Connell EJ, Mottram CD, Telander RL. Exercise cardiorespiratory function in adolescents with pectus excavatum. Observations before and after operation. *J Thorac Cardiovasc Surg* 1990; 99:44–47.
26. Castile RG, Staats BA, Westbrook PR. Symptomatic pectus deformities of the chest. *Am Rev Respir Dis* 1982; 126:564–568.
27. Mead J, Sly P, Le Souef P, Hibbert M, Phelan P. Rib cage mobility in pectus excavatum. *Am Rev Respir Dis* 1985; 132:1223–1228.
28. Humphreys GH, II, et al. Pectus excavatum. Late results with and without operation. *J Thorac Cardiovasc Surg* 1980; 80:686–695.
29. Ellis DG. Chest wall deformities in children. *Pediatr Ann* 1989; 18:161–165.

30. Nakahara K, Ohno K, Miyoshi S, Maeda H, Monden Y, Kawashima Y. An evaluation of operative outcome in patients with funnel chest diagnosed by means of the computed tomogram. *J Thorac Cardiovasc Surg* 1987; 93:577–582.

31. Hawkins JA, Ehrenhaft JL, Doty DB. Repair of pectus excavatum by sternal eversion. *Ann Thorac Surg* 1984; 38:368–373.

32. Shamberger RC, Welch KJ. Surgical repair of pectus excavatum. *J Pediatr Surg* 1985; 90:251–260.

33. Scherer LR, Arn PH, Dressel DA, Pyeritz RM, Haller JA Jr. Surgical management of children and young adults with Marfan syndrome and pectus excavatum. *J Pediatr Surg* 1988; 23:1169–1172.

34. Marks MW, Argenta LC, Lee DC. Silicone implant correction of pectus excavatum: Indications and refinement in technique. *Past Reconstr Surg* 1984; 74:52–58.

35. Watanabe Y, Iwa T. Surgical correction of pectus excavatum for adults and adolescents. *Jpn J Surg* 1984; 14:472–478.

36. Derveaux L, Ivanoff I, Rochette F, Demerits M. Mechanism of pulmonary function changes after surgical correction for funnel chest. *Eur Respir J* 1988; 1:823–825.

37. Bergofsky EH, Turino GM, Fishman AP. Cardiorespiratory failure in kyphoscoliosis. *Medicine* 1959; 38:263–317.

38. Cobb Jr. Outline for the study of scoliosis: Instructional course lecture. *Am Acad Orthop Surg* 1948; 5:261–275.

39. Canet E, Bureau MA. Chest Wall diseases and dysfunction in children. In Chernick V, ed. *Kendig's disorders of the respiratory tract in children*, 5th Ed. Philadelphia, WB Saunders, 1990, pp. 648–672.

40. Linderholm H, Lindgren V. Prediction of spirometric values in patients with scoliosis. *Acta Orthop Scand* 1978; 49:469–474.

41. Leech JA, Ernst P, Rogla EJ, Gurr J, Gordon I, Becklake MD. Cardiorespiratory status in relation to mild deformity in adolescent idiopathic scoliosis. *J Pediatr* 1985; 106:143–149.

42. Kafer ER. Idiopathic scoliosis: Mechanical properties of the respiratory system and the ventilatory response to carbon dioxide. *J Clin Invest* 1975; 55:1153–1163.

43. Weber B, Smith JP, Briscoe WA, Friedman SA, King TK. Pulmonary function in asymptomatic adolescents with idiopathic scoliosis. *Am Rev Respir Dis* 1975; 111:389–397.

44. Shneerson JM. The cardiorespiratory response to exercise in thoracic scoliosis. *Thorax* 1978; 33:457–463.

45. DiRocco PJ, Breed AI. Physical work capacity in adolescent patients with mild idiopathic scoliosis. *Arch Phys Med Rehabil* 1983; 64:476–478.

46. Smyth RJ, Chapman KR, Wright TA, Crawford JS, Rebuck AS. Ventilatory patterns during hypoxia, hypercapnia, and exercise in adolescents with mild scoliosis. *Am Rev Respir Dis* 1986; 77:692–697.

47. Sawicka EH, Branthwaite MA. Respiration during sleep in kyphoscoliosis. *Thorax* 1987; 42: 801–808.

48. Pehrsson K, Bake B, Larsson S, Nachemson A. Lung function in adult idiopathic scoliosis: A 20 year follow up. *Thorax* 1991; 46:474–478.

49. Padman R, Goodill J, Cicalo-Speiss T, VonNessen S. Use of independently adjusted inspiratory and exhalatory positive airway pressures via nasal mask in acute and chronic respiratory insufficiency in pediatric patients. *Am Rev Respir Dis* 1992; 145:A555.

50. Winter RB, Lovell WW, Moe JH. Excessive thoracic lordosis and loss of pulmonary function in patients with idiopathic scoliosis. *J Bone Joint Surg [AM]* 1975; 57:972–977.

42

Unusual Pulmonary Infections

GORDON E. SCHUTZE and RICHARD F. JACOBS

The majority of pulmonary infections in normal infants and children are treated with supportive measures and in many instances with standard antimicrobial agents. Occasionally, patients fail to improve with these regimens. When this occurs, unusual or less common etiologic agents should be considered (Table 42.1). The agents that should be considered vary according to the geographic location, presence of underlying disease, immune status, age, and exposure history of the patient. Being familiar with the early signs and symptoms of local pathogenic organisms and taking the time to obtain an adequate history will aid the clinician in establishing the diagnosis (Table 42.2).

MYCOTIC INFECTIONS

The incidence of mycotic pulmonary infections in children is on the rise. The improvements in diagnostic techniques is only part of the reason that infections with these organisms are increasing. Shifts in population from

Table 42.1.
Unusual Causes of Pneumonia in Children

Fungi

  Histoplasma capsulatum
  Blastomyces dermatitidis
  Coccidioides immitis
  Aspergillus fumigatus
  Paracoccidioides brasilensis

Bacteria

  Coxiella burnetii
  Legionella pneumophila
  Francisella tularensis
  Rickettsia rickettsii
  Ehrlichia chaffeensis
  Actinomyces
  Nocardia

large urban areas to rural regions have brought susceptible hosts into endemic areas. These nonimmune hosts become exposed and infected with the indigenous flora. Another important reason for the rise of these infections is the increasing population of immunosuppressed hosts. Whether the immunosuppression is due to a primary immunodeficiency, or to an acquired immunodeficiency, this population is growing rapidly. The discussion in this chapter will be limited to infants and children outside of the neonatal age without immunosuppressive disorders. Mycotic pulmonary infections of the neonate are quite rare but do occur (1). Infections in children who are immunosuppressed are discussed in Chapters 47 and 49.

HISTOPLASMOSIS

Histoplasma capsulatum is a fungus with nearly worldwide distribution. In the United States the organism is highly endemic along the Ohio and Mississippi river valleys. The organism is found in the soil and in areas contaminated with bird and bat dung. Infection occurs from inhalation of spores. Persons who work with or play with contaminated dirt or organic matter, raise roosting birds, or frequent caves are at risk for infection. Person-to-person transmission does not occur.

The major determinant of the clinical manifestations of disease is related to the inoculum size. About 1% of persons will develop symptomatic illness following exposure to a low inoculum of organisms. In contrast, 50–100% of individuals will develop symptoms with heavy exposure (2). The majority of individuals who develop symptoms will have an acute self-limited illness. Only about 1 in 2000

Table 42.2.
When to Suspect Infection with an Unusual Pathogen

- Residence or travel to endemic area
- Failure of pneumonia to respond to conventional anti-microbial therapy
- Atypical clinical presentation:
  Pneumonia with skin or bone lesions—blastomycosis
  Lobar infiltrate in a minimally symptomatic child or pneumonia, arthralgia, and erythema multiforme—coccidiomycosis
- Respiratory illness in a patient with a history of significant exposure:

Chicken or bird dropping	*Histoplasmosis*
Spelunking	*Cryptococcus*
Large scale excavation or landscaping activities	*Aspergillus* or *Histoplasmosis*
Exposure to sheep	Q fever
Tick exposures or ingestion of rabbit or deer meat	Tularemia

- Atypical radiograph for clinical illness (e.g., flu-like illness with nodules or hilar nodes on chest radiograph—*Histoplasmosis*)
- Persistent or poorly controlled symptoms despite adequate therapy (especially wheeze and productive cough with mucus plugs) in patients with asthma, CF, or bronchiectasis

infected individuals will develop a progressive or cavitary pulmonary infection.

In approximately 80% of the symptomatic patients the presenting complaints are of an influenza-like pulmonary infection. Symptoms include fever, chills, headache, myalgia, anorexia, nonproductive cough, and pleuritic chest pain. The physical examination is usually normal. Chest radiographs may be normal or may demonstrate pulmonary infiltrates, hilar nodules, or pulmonary nodules, as in Figure 42.1 (3). Disseminated histoplasmosis has become increasingly common because of the

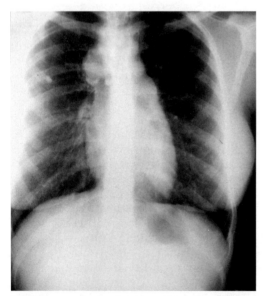

Figure 42.1. Chest radiograph demonstrating hilar adenopathy secondary to *Histoplasma capsulatum*.

increase of persons infected with the human immunodeficiency virus (HIV). This infection occurs uncommonly in hosts who are not immunosuppressed. When it does occur it should be viewed as a progression of the pulmonary infection with extrapulmonary spread. Chronic pulmonary histoplasmosis does not occur in children.

H. capsulatum is not present in the normal human flora, so its presence in body fluids is diagnostic. The isolation of the organism, therefore, is the most precise method of diagnosis. Specimens sent for culture should reflect the potentially infected site. A failure to isolate the organism, however, does not eliminate the possibility of histoplasmosis. A 1:500 dilution of the histoplasmin skin test placed intradermally may aid in the diagnosis. Induration of 5 mm or greater at 48 hours is considered a positive test. The positive skin test indicates that the patient has been infected with *H. capsulatum* some time in the past but does not discriminate an undiagnosed pulmonary infection as histoplasmosis. Although a valuable epidemiologic tool, the high frequency of positive skin tests in endemic regions invalidates this test in assessing individual patients (4).

Serologic assays may also be used but are sometimes negative early in the infection. These antibodies also clear very slowly, and positive test results may occur in patients with a past history of histoplasmosis. Assays that are currently available use complement fixation, immunodiffusion, latex agglutination, or radioimmunoassay for *H. capsulatum* antigen. False-positive tests may occur because of cross-reactivity in patients with blastomycosis, coccidioidomycosis, or other pulmonary mycoses. The most common serologic methods used are immunodiffusion and complement fixation. In the immunocompetent patient, the complement fixation test with the yeast-form antigen demonstrates greater sensitivity than the immunodiffusion method. Titers of 1:8–32 with either the yeast antigen or histoplasmin may be presumptive evidence of histoplasmosis. Many individuals in endemic regions, however, demonstrate such titers. Therefore, titers of > 1:32 or a demonstration of increasing titers offer better presumptive evidence of infection. Lack of a serologic response, however, does not exclude the diagnosis (5).

Patients with signs or symptoms of disseminated histoplasmosis may be diagnosed by the detection of *H. capsulatum* polysaccharide antigen. The antigen may be detected in one-half of serum specimens and in 90% of urine specimens in patients with disseminated histoplasmosis (6). This test offers an opportunity for early diagnosis of disseminated histoplasmosis but may be negative if dissemination has not occurred.

Most commonly, histoplasmosis presents as an acute, self-limited pulmonary infection. The decision to treat depends on the severity of clinical symptoms and the host defense status of the infected individual. Rarely does the immunocompetent host require therapy. In cases of severe or prolonged pulmonary disease, ketoconazole (400 mg/day) for 3–6 months or a short course of amphotericin B (2–4 weeks) has been shown to be effective. Intraconazole, a newer oral azole antifungal agent, may become quite useful in the future (7).

BLASTOMYCOSIS

Pulmonary infections due to *Blastomyces dermatitidis* occur through inhalation of the fungal spores. This organism is encountered most commonly in North America and especially in the Midwestern, Southeastern, and Appalachian states. The most common presenting clinical manifestation is a chronic pulmonary infiltrate. Patients who have signs or symptoms of dissemination may have skin or bony involvement. The different types of clinical

presentations of pulmonary infection include those patients with acute pneumonia, chronic pneumonia, or no pulmonary symptoms at all (8). Patients with acute pneumonia present with symptoms similar those of acute bacterial pneumonia. Fever, chills, and a productive cough are not uncommon. Although these patients will not respond to standard antimicrobial therapy, in many instances there will be some resolution of symptoms during the course of treatment, giving an appearance that the antimicrobial therapy was effective. However, fever, chest pain, shortness of breath, and productive cough may persist or return in association a chronic pneumonia. The duration of these symptoms in children is usually less than 6 months (9).

There are no diagnostic chest radiographic patterns in blastomycosis, and findings will vary depending on the chronicity of disease. Radiographic findings with an acute illness may mimic an acute bacterial pneumonia. Chronic disease may have findings consistent with neoplasms or tuberculosis, as in Figure 42.2 (10).

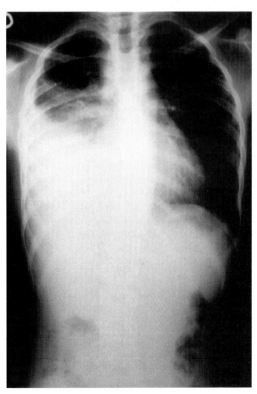

Figure 42.2.   Pulmonary infiltrate present for 6 months in a patient infected with *Blastomyces dermatitidis*.

The diagnosis should be considered in patients from endemic regions with chronic pulmonary infiltrates or in patients with pulmonary disease and skin or bone involvement. The diagnosis is confirmed by isolation of the organism from tissue or other body fluids. Examinations of fresh sputum may also be diagnostic since blastomycosis should not be part of the normal mouth flora and its presence is abnormal. Serologic tests for blastomycosis have improved but are mainly used for epidemiologic assessment and have little clinical utility (5). There are currently no skin-test antigens available for use in suspected blastomycosis.

Resolution of infection without therapy may occur, and an observation period of 1–2 weeks may be considered before therapy is started. If the patient's condition worsens, therapy should be started. Ketoconazole, 400–800 mg/day (6 mg/kg) for a total of 6 months, has been found to be effective (11). Intraconazole at a dose of 200 mg/day for 6 months has demonstrated good responses and may be the oral medication of choice in the future (7, 12). Relapses may occur with any therapy. Individuals with chronic pulmonary disease or those with signs and symptoms of disseminated disease warrant therapy with amphotericin B. A total of 2 g of drug or 30 mg/kg (total dose) has met with great success in these patients.

COCCIDIOIDOMYCOSIS

Coccidioides immitis is endemic in areas of North, Central, and South America. In the United States it is localized to the arid sections of the Southwest. Because of increased tourist activity in the endemic regions, infections with coccidioidomycosis are increasingly recognized outside of these regions. Primary pulmonary infections, disseminated infections, and primary cutaneous infections are the three types of involvement known to be caused by coccidioidomycosis. Disseminated coccidioidomycosis and primary cutaneous coccidioidomycosis are quite uncommon in children and will not be discussed in this section.

With primary pulmonary coccidioidomycosis, patients may be either symptomatic or asymptomatic. Only approximately 40% of patients will develop specific symptoms of an infection 1–3 weeks after exposure. The incubation period, duration, and severity of symptoms are related to the magnitude of the exposure. The symptoms, when present are usually related to the lower respiratory tract and may include cough, chest pain, fever, chills, night sweats, anorexia, weakness, and productive cough. Erythema nodosum or erythema multiforme may become part of the symptoms. "Acute valley fever" consists of erythema multiforme or nodosum in association with fever and diffuse arthralgias. This triad occurs in less than 25% of cases but may lead the clinician to suspect the diagnosis (13).

Chest radiographic manifestations of primary coccidioidomycosis are quite variable. Hilar adenopathy with an alveolar infiltrate, migratory infiltrates, and tissue excavation of an infiltrate leaving a thin-walled cavity are all consistent with coccidioidomycosis (14). Occasionally, pulmonary coccidioidomycosis may develop into a chronic, persistent pneumonia with pulmonary scarring and cavity formation.

The diagnosis can be established by culturing the organism from body fluids. Other methods include the use of skin testing. There are two skin test antigens used for diagnostic testing: coccidioidin, which is made from the mycelial phase, and spherulin (the tissue phase of the fungus). A 1:100 dilution of either preparation is used and evaluated at 48 hours, with a positive skin test demonstrating greater than 5 mm of induration (4). A positive skin test may occur 3 days to 3 weeks after the onset of symptoms but may be indicative of either prior or current infection. A recent conversion from a negative skin test to a positive skin test with appropriate symptoms is better evidence of infection. The performance of skin testing does not alter the results of serologic testing. A negative skin test, however, does not exclude the possibility of the diagnosis. Serodiagnostic tests for the presence of antibody are commercially available and are widely used for the diagnosis of coccidioidomycosis. Tests for antigenemia have not been developed sufficiently for diagnostic use in patients with early disease (15).

Primary pulmonary coccidioidomycosis is a self-limited disease that rarely requires therapy. Patients with severe pulmonary involvement, those with increasing titers, and those with fever, prostration, or worsening of pulmonary symptoms are all candidates for therapy. Those patients with disseminated disease or who are immunosuppressed should receive amphotericin B. The usual cumulative dose is 30 mg/kg. Ketoconazole, 6 mg/kg/day (maximum 400 mg) for 6 months, has been found to be effective in most instances of infiltrative pulmonary infection. Itraconazole therapy appears to have fewer side effects than does ketoconazole and may be the drug of the future (16).

ASPERGILLUS

Aspergillus fumigatus is the species of *Aspergillus* most commonly implicated in human disease. Other species such as *A. terreus, A. flavus, A. nidulans, A. oryzae,* and *A. niger* have been demonstrated occasionally to cause disease. The organism is ubiquitous and may be found in soil, decaying vegetation, bird droppings, and houses or buildings. The organism is obtained through inhalation, and pulmonary infections with *Aspergillus* may present in three forms. Invasive pulmonary infections will not be discussed since most are found in immunocompromised hosts. The remaining two forms are allergic bronchopulmonary aspergillosis and aspergillomas.

Allergic bronchopulmonary aspergillosis is generally thought to be due to a hypersensitivity reaction to antigens of *Aspergillus*. The majority of patients tend to be atopic and have a history of bronchial asthma (17). Patients with cystic fibrosis are known to be at risk as well (18). Patients usually present acutely with fever, wheezing, malaise, weight loss, chest pain, and a productive cough with blood-streaked sputum. Chest radiographs are variable but may demonstrate transient pulmonary infiltrates and signs of bronchiectasis.

The diagnosis of allergic bronchopulmonary aspergillosis should be entertained in individuals with chronic asthma and bronchiectasis who fail to respond to appropriate conventional therapy. Confirmatory examinations of the blood include a peripheral blood eosinophilia ($> 1000/mm^3$), immediate cutaneous reactivity to *A. fumigatus*, serum precipitins to *A. fumigatus*, elevated serum levels of total immunoglobulin E (IgE) (> 1000 ng/ml), and elevated serum levels of IgE and IgG to *A. fumigatus* (19).

Corticosteroid therapy is begun once the diagnosis of allergic bronchopulmonary aspergillosis is made. With the initiation of this therapy, pulmonary infiltrates should disappear and a decline in the total serum IgE of up to 35% may occur within the first 6 weeks of treatment. Prednisone, 0.5 mg/kg (maximum 40–60 mg) every day for 2 weeks, followed by 0.5 mg/kg every other day for 3 months after the infiltrates have cleared, is a standard regimen. Once this is completed, a tapering of the prednisone should be made over a 3-month period (20). A decreased and stable IgE level and a clearing of pulmonary infiltrates for at least 6 months should be seen with successful therapy. A rise in the serum IgE level and new pulmonary infiltrates should be considered a recrudescence of disease. The use of antifungal agents, cromolyn sodium, and topical inhaled steroids have been used but have not been found to be effective.

Aspergilloma may also arise when a patient has been infected with *Aspergillus*. The inhaled organisms gain access to a pre-existing lung space or cavity that has been devitalized. Once colonization has occurred in this devitalized region, necrosis continues and the growing mycelium gradually enlarges to form a mycetoma (fungus ball). These mycetomas tend to occur in the upper lobes at the site of previous lung damage due to such illnesses as tuberculosis, cysts, or neoplasms. Unless the patient develops a secondary infection or has hemoptysis, the condition is often asymptomatic. The diagnosis is usually established through chest radiography. Most aspergillomas found by chest radiograph tend to be distributed in the upper lobes and demonstrate a loose-appearing sphere in a large, thick-walled cavity (21). There is no standard accepted therapy for this disorder. Patients tend to have these removed surgically when the hemoptysis becomes severe (22). The role for medical therapy without surgery has not been established.

RARE PULMONARY MYCOSES

Paracoccidioides brasilensis (South American blastomycosis) is the predominant systemic mycosis in Latin America. The lungs are the site of primary infection but dissemination to the mucous membranes, skin, reticuloendothelial system, and adrenal glands is quite common. This disorder is only very rarely seen in children (23). Organisms such as *Cryptococcus neoformans*, mucormycosis, phycomycosis, and sporotrichosis are usually limited to immunosuppressed patients. The diagnosis in each is established with the isolation of one of these organisms from the sputum, bronchial washings, or lung tissue. The treatment and prognosis of these infections depends on the host, the organism isolated, and the extent of the infection.

BACTERIA

Coxiella burnetii is the etiologic agent of Q fever. This infectious disease has a worldwide distribution and is usually transmitted to children by inhalation of contaminated aerosols or consumption of unpasteurized milk products. Well-known reservoirs of this organism include cattle, sheep, and goats. These animals will shed the organisms in urine, feces, milk, and especially birth products. Humans are the only species known to regularly develop an illness with this organism (24).

Human pulmonary infections with this organism may present in different fashions. An incidental pulmonary infiltrate in a febrile patient is the most common finding. Patients may also present with atypical pneumonia or rapidly progressive pneumonia. The clinical signs associated with Q fever in children are not specific. Patients usually complain of influenza-like symptoms with sudden onset of fever, headache, malaise, myalgia, and photophobia (25). Chest radiographs in patients with Q fever show no features that might distinguish this disease from other types of pneumonia (26). The usual method of diagnosis is through the use of serologic testing with paired sera. Tests for detection of specific IgA, IgM, or IgG are available in research and reference laboratories.

The mainstay of therapy for Q fever is treatment with tetracyclines. Doxycycline appears to be the most active tetracycline preparation available and should be given for at least 3 days after the fever has subsided. Chloramphenicol or erythromycin appear to be alternative choices in the younger children with this disorder (27). Newer macrolide antimicrobial agents such as azithromycin may play a role in the future (28). In individuals suffering from chronic Q fever, multiple drugs may be used for prolonged periods in view of the risk of relapse (29).

Pulmonary infections with *Legionella pneumophila* may occur in immunocompetent children. The majority of these children have a history of chronic pulmonary disease. This organism can be cultured from water sources of all types; in adult epidemics the source of the infection is often linked to contaminated water sources. There is little information of this association concerning infections in children, but hospital water sources have often been implicated (30, 31).

Patients may have a nonspecific influenza-like prodrome but then usually become very acutely ill. They may have elevated temperatures (over 39.4° C), chills, nausea, vomiting, and a nonproductive or minimally productive cough. Lethargy, unsteadiness, slurring of speech, and confusion may also be present. As the disease progresses the pulmonary manifestations such as dyspnea and sputum production become evident (32). The chest radiograph demonstrates a patchy bronchopneumonia with poorly marginated rounded opacities, lobar consolidation, or perihilar densities. The abnormalities usually begin in one lobe and then rapidly progress to a lobar or multilobar consolidation. Pleural effusions in association with pulmonary infiltrates may also occur (30).

The diagnosis of *Legionella* pneumonia must be considered and actively pursued in children with pneumonia who do not respond to conventional antimicrobial therapy. Respiratory secretions can be cultured for the organism, or respiratory/lung tissue may be stained by direct fluorescent antibody to make the diagnosis. Positive direct fluorescent stains may only be helpful in about 60% of culture-proven cases. The use of serology may add valuable supportive evidence, but seroconversion may be difficult to document in the face of a rapidly progressive illness.

Since the diagnosis can be difficult to establish, empiric therapy should be instituted in those patients with the presumptive diagnosis of *Legionella* pneumonia. Erythromycin (50 mg/kg/day) is the drug of choice for treatment of infections caused by *Legionella*. Most patients will respond within 48 hours to the institution of therapy. The role of the newer antimicrobial agents such as clarithromycin and azithromycin is currently not known. The combination of erythromycin and rifampin has been used in the severely ill adults with good success. Treatment should continue for a minimum of 2 weeks (32).

Pulmonary involvement may be seen in children infected with *Francisella tularensis*.

Tularemia is a zoonotic disease transmitted through the bite of a tick or deer fly, the consumption of poorly cooked infected meats such as rabbit and deer, or inhalation of the organism. There are six clinical types of infections in tularemia: ulceroglandular, glandular, oculoglandular, typhoidal, pneumonic, and oropharyngeal. The ulceroglandular form is the most common clinical presentation. Pulmonary involvement may be seen with any of the forms but characteristically is seen in the typhoidal and pneumonic forms. Pneumonic tularemia has been increasing in children (33).

The diagnosis of tularemia should be entertained in those children with a history of tick exposure or bite, in those children with significant rabbit or deer exposure, and in those children who spend large amounts of time outdoors in endemic regions. The most common abnormality on chest radiograph in patients with tularemia is bronchopneumonia followed by hilar adenopathy and pleural effusion (34). The diagnosis can be established through the use of serologic testing. An acute titer of > 1:160 or a four-fold increase between acute and convalescent titers is diagnostic of tularemia. Streptomycin (30 mg/kg/day) twice daily or gentamicin (6 mg/kg/day) three times daily for 7–10 days is the current recommended therapy. The use of oral agents such as tetracycline has a high associated relapse rate.

Other tick-borne diseases that may have pulmonary involvement include Rocky Mountain spotted fever (*Rickettsia rickettsii*) and ehrlichiosis (*Ehrlichia chaffeensis*). Patients with Rocky Mountain spotted fever usually have a history of headache, fever, and rash. The rash starts on the extremities and progresses towards the body. Infections secondary to *E. chaffeensis* may present in a similar fashion, but patients may have pancytopenia with hepatitis or renal failure. A rash may be present but is rarely progressive.

Pulmonary infections with *Actinomyces* spp can be encountered. The infection is usually seen as a chronic fibrosing inflammatory process that spreads to adjacent tissue and contains small abscesses and purulent-filled sinus tracts. It is often difficult to diagnose since neither the clinical manifestations nor radiographic findings are specific for the disease (23). Simple recovery of *Actinomyces* from a sputum culture under anaerobic conditions does not establish the diagnosis since it can be indigenous to the oral flora. Tissue specimens containing the organisms or the classic sulphur granules may be considered diagnostic. High-dose penicillin therapy given intravenously for 2–6 weeks followed by oral penicillin for 3–12 months is an appropriate treatment for this pulmonary infection (35). Other antimicrobial agents have been used but with varying amounts of success.

The clinical manifestations of pulmonary infections with *Nocardia asteroides* include bronchopneumonia, lobar pneumonia, and necrotizing pneumonia with abscess. This occurs only very rarely in immunocompetent hosts. The diagnosis is established with isolation of the organism from pulmonary secretions. Treatment with trimethoprim-sulfamethoxazole has met with great success if given for prolonged periods.

CONCLUSIONS

Children with pulmonary infiltrates unresponsive to traditional therapy may have an unusual pathogen. Clinicians should be familiar not only with the clinical manifestations of the unusual pathogens in their area but be aware of others that may have been obtained with travel. Many times a history of animal exposure or tick bite is long forgotten, and the proper questions must be asked to elicit a response. Through the use of serology or respiratory secretion analysis the proper diagnosis can be made. The type and duration of therapy must be individualized to each patient.

REFERENCES

1. Miller MJ. Fungal infections. In Remington JS, Klein JO, eds. *Infectious diseases of the fetus and newborn infant*, 3rd ed. Philadelphia, WB Saunders, 1990, pp 475–515.
2. Wheat LJ. Histoplasmosis. *Infect Dis Clin North Am* 1988; 2:841–859.
3. Prechter GC, Prakash UBS. Bronchoscopy in the diagnosis of pulmonary histoplasmosis. *Chest* 1989; 95:1033–1036.
4. Sarosi GA, Catanzaro A, Daniel TM, Davies SF. Clinical usefulness of skin testing in histoplasmosis, coccidioidomycosis, and blastomycosis. *Am Rev Respir Dis* 1988; 138:1081–1082.
5. Kaufman L. Laboratory methods for the diagnosis and confirmation of systemic mycoses. *Clin Infect Dis* 1992; 14:S23–29.
6. Zimmerman SE, Stringfield PC, Wheat LJ, French MV, Kohler RB. Comparison of sandwich solid-phase radioimmunoassay and two enzyme-linked immunosorbent assays for detection of *Histoplasma*

capsulatum polysaccharide antigen. *J Infect Dis* 1989; 160:678–685.

7. Dismukes WE, Bradsher RW, Cloud GC, et al. Itraconazole therapy for blastomycosis and histoplasmosis. *Am J Med* 1992; 93:489–497.

8. Bradsher RW, Rice DC, Abernathy RS. Ketoconazole therapy of endemic blastomycosis. *Ann Intern Med* 1985; 103:872–879.

9. Yogev R, Davis AT. Blastomycosis in children: A review of the literature. *Mycopathologia* 1979; 68:139–143.

10. Bradsher RW. Blastomycosis. *Clin Infect Dis* 1992; 14:S82–90.

11. McManus EJ, Jones JM. The use of ketoconazole in the treatment of blastomycosis. *Am Rev Respir Dis* 1986; 133:141–143.

12. Bradsher RW. Itraconazole therapy of blastomycosis: Cure following progression or relapse after ketoconazole [Abstract no. 1351]. In *Program and Abstracts of the 27th Interscience Conference on Antimicrobial Agents and Chemotherapy*. Washington, DC, American Society for Microbiology, 1987.

13. Ampel NM, Wieden MA, Galgiani JN. Coccidioidomycosis: Clinical update. *Rev Infect Dis* 1989; 11:897–911.

14. Bayer AS. Fungal pneumonias; pulmonary coccidioidal syndromes (Part 1). Primary and progressive primary coccidioidal pneumonias—Diagnostic, therapeutic, and prognostic considerations. *Chest* 1981; 79:575–583.

15. Pappagianis D, Zimmer BL. Serology of coccidioidomycosis. *Clin Microbiol Rev* 1990; 89:282–290.

16. Graybill JR, Stevens DA, Galgiani JN, et al. Itraconazole treatment of coccidioidomycosis. *Am J Med* 1990; 89:282–290.

17. Slavin RG. Allergic bronchopulmonary aspergillosis. *Clin Rev Allergy* 1985; 3:167–182.

18. Maguire S, Moriarty P, Tempany E, Fitzgerald M. Unusual clustering of allergic bronchopulmonary aspergillosis in children with cystic fibrosis. *Pediatrics* 1988; 82:835–839.

19. Greenberger PA. Allergic bronchopulmonary aspergillosis and fungoses. *Clin Chest Med* 1988; 9:599–608.

20. Bierman CW, Pierson WE, Massie FS. Nonasthmatic allergic pulmonary disease. In Chernick V, Kendig EL, eds. *Disorders of the respiratory tract in children*, 5th ed. Philadelphia, WB Saunders, 1990, pp 608–614.

21. Singh P, Kumar P, Bhagi RP, Singla R. Pulmonary aspergilloma—Radiological observations. *Ind J Chest Dis Allied Sci* 1989; 31:177–185.

22. Stamatis G, Greschuchna D. Surgery for pulmonary aspergilloma and pleural aspergillosis. *Thorac Cardiovasc Surg* 1988; 36:356–360.

23. Medoff G, Kobayashi G. Pulmonary infections due to *Actinomyces* and *Nocardia*, and pulmonary mycoses. In Feigin RD, Cherry JD, eds. *Textbook of pediatric infectious diseases*, 2nd ed. Philadelphia, WB Saunders, 1987, pp 300–311.

24. Aitken ID, Bogel K, Cracea E, et al. Q fever in Europe: Current aspects of aetiology, epidemiology, human infection, diagnosis and therapy. *Infection* 1987; 15:323–327.

25. Richardus JH, Dumas AM, Huisman J, Schaap GJP. Q fever in infancy: A review of 18 cases. *Pediatr Infect Dis* 1985; 4:369–373.

26. Smith SL, Wellings R, Walker C, Ayres JG, Burge PS. The chest X-ray in Q fever: A report on 69 cases from the 1989 West Midland outbreak. *Br J Radiol* 1991; 64:1101–1108.

27. Perez-del-Molino A, Aguado JM, Riancho JA, Sampedro I, Matorras P, Gonzalez-Macias J. Erythromycin and the treatment of *Coxiella burnetii* pneumonia. *J Antimicrob Chemother* 1991; 28:455–459.

28. Schonwald S, Skerk V, Petricevic I, Car V, Majerus-Misic L, Gunjaca M. Comparison of three-day and five-day courses of azithromycin in the treatment of atypical pneumonia. *Eur J Clin Microbiol Infect Dis* 1991; 10:877–880.

29. Raoult D. Antibiotic treatment of rickettsiosis, recent advances and current concepts. *Eur J Epidemiol* 1991; 7:276–281.

30. Brady MT. Nosocomial legionnaires disease in a children's hospital. *J Pediatr* 1989; 115:46–50.

31. Carlson NC, Kuskie MR, Dobyns EL, Wheeler MC, Roe MH, Abzug MJ. Legionellosis in children: An expanding spectrum. *Pediatr Infect Dis* 1990; 9:133–137.

32. Swartz MN, Pasternack MS. Legionnaires' disease and other related pneumonias. In Chernick V, Kendig EL, eds. *Disorders of the respiratory tract in children*, 5th ed. Philadelphia, WB Saunders, 1990, pp 850–864.

33. Jacobs RF, Condrey YM, Yamauchi T. Tularemia in adults and children: A changing presentation. *Pediatrics* 1985; 76:818–822.

34. Rubin SA. Radiographic spectrum of pleuropulmonary tularemia. *Am J Roentgenol* 1978; 131:277–281.

35. Lerner PI. *Actinomyces* and *Arachnia* species. In Mandell GL, Douglas RG, Bennett JE, eds. *Principles and practice of infectious diseases*, 3rd ed. New York, Churchill Livingston, 1990, pp 1932–1942.

43

Sinusitis

BRUCE H. MATT

DEFINITIONS

Sinusitis is the inflammation of the mucosal lining of a paranasal airspace (sinus). Acute sinusitis lasts for 3 weeks or less, subacute for 3 weeks to 3 months, and chronic sinusitis inflammation for longer than 3 months, although the distinction between subacute and chronic is somewhat arbitrary (1).

ANATOMY AND DEVELOPMENT

The paranasal air sinuses develop as out-pouchings from the nasal cavity. The maxillary sinus begins at about 70 days in utero. The ethmoid and sphenoid buds begin at about 4 months of gestation. The frontal sinus is represented only by a furrow at birth (2).

The maxillary sinus is 7–8 mm (anterior to posterior) at birth. By age 1 year the lateral extension reaches the sagittal plane of the infraorbital nerve. Expansion of the sinus continues so that by age 9 years pneumatization has reached the zygomatic process (2) (Fig. 43.1).

Inferiorly the sinus expands as the maxillary permanent dentition erupts between ages 7 and 9 years. The floor of the maxillary sinus will generally reach the level of the floor of the nose between ages 8 and 12 years. By 15 years, the adult size (12–15 ml) is achieved, though pneumatization can continue, albeit slowly, in some persons (2, 3).

The ethmoid sinuses grow rapidly so by age 2 years the bone is filled from laterally (at the lamina papyracea) to medially (at the middle meatus) with tightly packed air cells. On each side are usually 3–15 cells, each with its own ostium. Pneumatization up to the floor of the cranial vault continues and all available bone,

often including the turbinates, sphenoid, and frontal bones, is invaded. The ethmoid sinuses tend to reach adult size between ages 12 and 14 years (3).

The sphenoid sinuses' growth is primarily posteriorly and laterally at first, thinning the bone around the optic nerve and first and second divisions of the trigeminal nerve. The growth rate is estimated at 0.25 mm per year posteriorly, accomplished in spurts. Adult size is reached in 50% of people by age 15 (2).

The frontal sinuses extend upward from the infundibulum (in the middle meatus) actually reaching the frontal bone by 20 months. The top of sinus is level with the nasion by age 3. It reaches the level of the orbital roof by age 8 in half the population. Growth is at 1.5 mm vertically per year on average, with slower growth under age 7 and more rapid growth thereafter. Adult size is generally seen by puberty, though slow growth can continue for life (2).

Given that the development of the sinuses starts antenatally, obviously even infants can have infection of their small sinuses. Additionally, surgical intervention in very small noses and sinuses is technically difficult and fortunately rarely needed. In fact 40% of sinusitis will resolve spontaneously without treatment (4, 5), and much of the rest will be able to be treated nonsurgically.

PATHOPHYSIOLOGY AND RISK FACTORS

The sinuses are lined by pseudostratified columnar ciliated epithelium incorporating goblet cells and submucosal glands. The cilia beat toward the sinus ostia, moving the secretions out of the sinus into the nose. These small openings from the sinus to the nose are

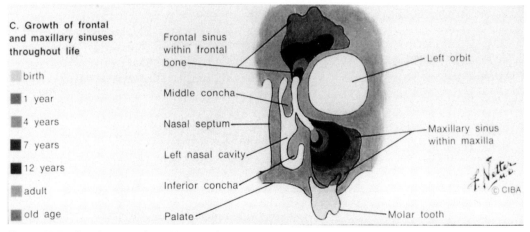

C. Growth of frontal
and maxillary sinuses
throughout life

birth

1 year

4 years

7 years

12 years

adult

old age

Frontal sinus
within frontal
bone

Middle concha

Nasal septum

Left nasal cavity

Inferior concha

Palate

Left orbit

Maxillary sinus
within maxilla

Molar tooth

Figure 43.1.   Development of maxillary and frontal sinuses (from CIBA symposium).

thought to be the choke point for sinusitis (6). If the ostium is blocked sinus secretions are trapped in the sinus space. Obstruction of the ostia contributes to the development of sinusitis. Because air cannot enter, the partial pressure of oxygen decreases and the partial pressure of carbon dioxide (Pco_2) increases, contributing to a low pH that impairs both ciliary movement and phagocytosis. A number of factors can contribute to the blockage of the sinus ostia (7). Hyperemia and edema resulting from an upper respiratory tract infection, allergy, or temperature changes are the most common cause. Most children have six to eight upper respiratory tract infections per year. Fortunately, only 5% or so of these children develop a sinusitis (8, 9).

Children with upper respiratory allergic symptoms seem to have an increased tendency for sinusitis (10). Thickened mucus from drugs (e.g., antihistamines) or systemic disorders (e.g., cystic fibrosis, hypothyroidism), vascular edema from cyanotic congenital heart disease (11), and barotrauma (e.g., diving) can produce injury and obstruction of the sinus ostia. Patients with cystic fibrosis often have radiographic abnormalities in their sinuses. Clinically only about 11% have symptoms of sinusitis; 6–9% of those under the age of 20 have polyps and 48% over the age of 20 have polyps in the nose. Obstruction leading to sinusitis can also occur from noxious agents (gases or foreign bodies), direct facial trauma, or the use of topical medications resulting in rhinitis medicamentosa. Nasal polyps, ade-

noiditis, tumors, or a deviated septum or turbinate can cause obstructed nasal airflow and block the sinus outflow tract (12).

Other conditions that predispose to sinusitis include dysmotile cilia syndromes (e.g., Kartagener syndrome), hypogammaglobulinemia, and defects in phagocytosis. Extension of the infection from the maxillary (upper) teeth to the sinuses also can occur (3, 11, 13, 14).

HISTORY

The symptoms of acute sinusitis are varied and change with age. Acute sinusitis is generally preceded by a viral upper respiratory tract infection. Sinus headaches are often localized over the involved sinus but may be projected to other parts of the head (15). Pain may be localized to the maxillary teeth, one eye, or a temple, or it can be projected to the occiput or vertex. The pain may be constant or intermittent but is clearly intensified when the head is placed in a dependent position. In acute sinusitis, patients may complain of dull ache that is most severe during the day. Pain is often associated with a purulent rhinorrhea. Cough, presumably from postnasal drip, is common (3). Children under 5 years usually have less specific symptoms. They often have purulent rhinorrhea with nasal congestion, a cough, and bad breath associated with sinusitis. Anecdotally, irritability, behavior change, and actions consistent with head pain (e.g., head holding or banging) can be seen even in young children (16).

Wald (4) suggests that acute sinusitis may have two types of presentation. The common form is a prolonged upper respiratory tract infection with cough and rhinorrhea lasting more than 10 days. Duration, not intensity, of symptoms is the concern. Less commonly, the "cold" is of unusual severity with a temperature above 39°C, pain, and pus discharging from the nose (17).

Some children will have painless swelling around the eyes, usually in the morning. Dental pain may also be reported by older children (4).

In chronic sinusitis the predominant symptoms are nasal obstruction, nasal discharge, cough, and persistent or recurrent "colds." Pain is often not present. Postnasal drip causes a sensation of dry throat and a throat-clearing cough. A history of recurrent pharyngitis is common. Nearly 50% of children with chronic sinusitis will have associated chronic otitis media, either bacterial or serous.

PHYSICAL EXAMINATION

Tenderness to palpation over the involved sinus is common in acute sinusitis, but is often not a finding in chronic sinusitis. The typical findings include copious nasal drainage, which is often thick purulent material, yellow or green in color, but can vary widely in these characteristics. Bright red and edematous mucosa suggests acute infection, whereas a pale or bosselated mucosa is often associated with allergy. Polyps suggest associated conditions such as allergy, asthma, aspirin sensitivity, or cystic fibrosis. Assessment of eye compressibility is important. Orbital extension of sinusitis can increase the pressure in the orbit and make the involved side more turgid. Evaluation of visual acuity and range of motion of the extraocular muscles is necessary to determine possible orbital involvement (3, 18, 19). Although it is quite rare in children, numbness in the distribution of the infra-orbital nerve (which passes through the roof of the maxillary sinus) or in other branches of the maxillary division of the trigeminal nerve (e.g., the teeth) suggests tumor as the cause of sinusitis.

Generally these patients do not have a problem with olfaction unless the mucosa is so swollen as to block air currents reaching the roof of the nose where olfactory receptors reside (cribriform plate) (3).

DIAGNOSIS

Chronic sinusitis is basically a persistent suppuration, manifested either grossly or by microabscess formation. Often one needs to search for the underlying causes such as allergies or polyps. Immune deficiencies and other problems with host defenses and offenses can obviously play a role here.

The differential diagnosis of "sinus" pain should be considered. Migraines (including histaminic cephalgia), temporomandibular joint (TMJ) syndrome, dental disease, and other problems can give similar symptoms. Purulent rhinitis is not pathognomonic for sinusitis because a foreign body in the nose, adenoid hypertrophy that obstructs the choanae, or isolated rhinitis without sinusitis can cause purulence and nasal drainage. Other obstructive problems including nasopharyngeal or sinus neoplasm and choanal atresia may lead to purulent rhinitis and must be considered during evaluation.

Transillumination of the sinuses is not helpful in children because of the thick bone in the anterior face of the maxilla and small size of the sinus. Even in adults it is only of limited value (20).

Anterior rhinoscopy in a patient with sinusitis will frequently reveal exudate in the middle or superior meatus. The discharge is usually creamy white but can be yellow or green. Topical vasoconstriction is useful to help identify the actual drainage site. Because most of the sinuses except for the sphenoid and posterior ethmoids drain into the middle meatus, one would expect most of the exudate there.

Imaging

If the history and physical examination are not characteristic for sinusitis, certain imaging studies may help localize the disease process. Sinus radiography is the simplest study, but its diagnostic sensitivity is questionable (21), especially in very young children whose sinuses may be poorly developed and aerated (22). The Waters view shows the maxillary sinuses, whereas a Caldwell view provides a look at the ethmoid and frontal sinuses (Table 43.2). The lateral view is particularly good for the sphenoid and frontal sinuses, whereas a submental vertex film often shows the sphenoid quite well, allowing one to differentiate right from left side. Obtaining a Waters view

Table 43.1.
Orbital Complications of Sinusitis

Periorbital cellulitis
Periorbital cellulitis with chemosis
Orbital cellulitis
Subperiosteal abscess
Orbital abscess
Cavernous sinus thrombosis

Adapted from Schramm VL Jr, Curtin HD, Kennerdell JS. Evaluation of orbital cellulitis and results of treatment. *Laryngoscope* 1982; 92:732–738.

Table 43.2.
Imaging in Sinusitis

Plain radiograph	
Waters view	Maxillary sinus
Caldwell view	Ethmoid and frontal sinuses
Lateral view	Sphenoid and ethmoid
Submental view	Sphenoids allowing differentiation of right from left air space
CT scan, coronal view	Gives good view of ostiomeatal complex and of structural defects or abnormalities
CT scan, axial view	Good view of relationship to deep structures (e.g., brain, optic nerve)

and a Caldwell view constitutes a minimum radiographic examination for children with acute sinusitis. Other views may be helpful (Table 43.1). The radiograph can be quite helpful in children over 1 year of age, and it correlates well with the presence of sinus disease. In patients under 1 year of age, sinus films are of no value because of the small size of the sinuses (22). The question of how crying effects the radiograph remains open (23). On the plain films, useful signs indicating sinus infection are a gas-liquid level, mucosal thickening, sinus opacity, and osteoblastic or osteoclastic changes. These last two changes take much longer to develop. In evaluating the radiographs, the size, symmetry, and shape of the abnormalities are useful clues (3, 24). In acute sinusitis, an air fluid level is classic, although often the sinus will be totally opacified. Osteolysis or mucosal thickening greater than 4 mm may be seen. In chronic sinusitis,

osteoblastic changes are often seen and mucosa is thickened (25, 26). In acute sinusitis approximately 88% of opaque sinuses will have pus when surgically aspirated. If only thickened mucoperiosteal membranes are seen on the radiograph, 50% may still have pus (22).

A computed tomography (CT) scan provides detailed anatomic information. Magnetic resonance imaging (MRI) offers little more information. The CT scan can also provide valuable information on sinus drainage passages.

Past history needs to be taken into account when evaluating the radiographs. If a procedure has been performed on a patient, changes such as blastic changes or mucosal thickening can be expected from that alone.

Transmaxillary ultrasonography in the A-mode has little or no place in evaluating children (27).

INFECTIOUS AGENTS

Streptococcus pneumoniae, Haemophilus influenzae, and *Moraxella catarrhalis* account for 60–75% of the organisms that cause acute bacterial sinusitis. Anaerobes make up less than 10% of the bacteriology of acute sinusitis (28, 29). However, in chronic sinusitis anaerobes predominate, with *Veillonella, Peptostreptococcus,* and *Corynebacterium acnes* being most common (30, 31).

Rarer still is fungal sinusitis, which can be caused by a number of organisms, including *Aspergillus, Mucor,* and *Alternaria* (3, 19, 32).

TREATMENT

In the pre-antibiotic era, treatment was based on the use of decongestants and/or nasal irrigation. If the condition was severe or not improving, aspiration of sinus secretions or sinus irrigation would be added. Modern treatment for acute sinusitis involves decongestants and antimicrobial agents. If a patient does not respond to appropriate treatment (see below), sinus cultures can be helpful in determining the adequacy of antibiotic coverage. Unfortunately, since no correlation exists between sinus cultures and nose or nasopharyngeal cultures, only direct sinus cultures are of benefit (32).

Patients with acute frontal or sphenoid sinusitis require hospitalization, since complications can occur. Additionally, if a complication of sinusitis has already occurred, the patient should be hospitalized (28).

For acute sinusitis, the first choice of antibiotic is amoxicillin, 40 mg/kg/day divided t.i.d. (5) (Table 43.3). For children who have received previous therapy with ampicillin, use of amoxicillin clavulanate, 40 mg/kg/day divided t.i.d, will overcome the problems with beta-lactamase resistance seen in 75% of *Moraxella catarrhalis* and 30% of *Haemophilus influenzae* (5). In any event, beta-lactamase coverage should be considered if the patient does not improve on initial treatment (3, 18).

Alternative initial choices include erythromycin-sulfisoxazole, 50 mg/150 mg/kg/day divided q.i.d., sulfamethoxazole/trimethoprim, 40 mg/8 mg/kg/day divided b.i.d., or cefaclor, 40 mg/kg/day divided t.i.d. Although no studies have evaluated duration of treatment, patients should be treated for at least 10–14 days, according to most authors (5).

Currently, the treatment for chronic sinusitis involves a minimum of 3 weeks of antibiotics. Chronic sinusitis is an infection not just of the mucosa but probably also of the bone itself. Decongestants and irrigations may also be required to allow for normalization of sinus function. If the medical treatment does not resolve the problem, surgical drainage may be required (3, 26, 28, 29).

Antihistamines should be avoided to prevent a drying and thickening of the mucus, which would tend to clog the outflow tracts (6, 18). Topical decongestants may be helpful but use for more than 4 days can result in rhinitis medicamentosa (18). Sodium cromolyn (Nasalcrom) and nasal steroids may be helpful in reducing mucosal edema and nasal obstruction in children with an allergic etiology. However, their use is controversial (33), and cooperation with nasal spray is often limited in young children.

In chronic sinusitis the first drug of choice would be amoxicillin clavulanate (Augmentin), 40 mg/kg/day divided t.i.d. or clindamycin, 40 mg/kg/day divided t.i.d., or in older children and adults, doxycycline, 5 mg/kg/day as a single dose (34). Fungal sinusitis may require amphotericin-B, ketoconazole, or 5-flucytosine in addition to surgical intervention (23, 32).

Patients for whom appropriate medical treatment, as outlined above, fails should be referred for possible surgical intervention (3). The first step in surgical intervention is aspiration and lavage if the maxillary sinuses are involved. Aspiration should be considered if maxillary sinusitis does not respond appropriately to medications within 5 days, symptoms recur after 10–14 days, or the patient is immunocompromised. Patients with severe discomfort would benefit from acute drainage of the infected maxillary sinus. Additionally, surgical intervention must be undertaken if complications exist (3, 9, 28).

A nasal antral window either through the middle or inferior meatus can be made to improve drainage of the maxillary sinus. Recent studies suggest that opening the natural ostium in the middle meatus is more important than opening an accessory window in the inferior meatus. Windows at the natural ostia allow for ciliary action to expel mucus from the sinus, whereas windows elsewhere do not take advantage of this surface-cleaning effect of the cilia. Additionally, windows at the natural ostia tend to stay open and reduce symptoms more than windows in the inferior meatus.

A more extensive procedure can be done to open the ostiomeatal complex to allow drainage. This can either be done externally (external ethmoidectomy with a Caldwell-Luc approach to the maxillary sinus) or internally using either macroscopic or endoscopic techniques.

Steps in management of sinusitis are listed in Table 43.4.

SINUS COMPLICATIONS

The most common complication of sinusitis occurs in the sinus itself in the form of a mucocele, a cyst of mucus trapped in one of the

Table 43.3.
Antibiotics for Sinusitis and Its Complications

Agent	Dosage
Oral	
Amoxicillin/Clavulanate (for older children only)	40 mg/kg/day give TID
Clindamycin	40 mg/kg/day give TID
Doxycycline	5 mg/kg/day q day
Intravenous	
Ampicillin	150–200 mg/kg/day
Cefuroxime	1500 mg/kg/day
Cefotaxime	50–100 mg/kg/day

Table 43.4.
Steps in Management of Sinusitis

Intervention	Drug Dose	Comment
Oral decongestant	Various (e.g., phenylpropanol-amine, ca. 2 mg/kg/d, divided BID to QID)	Pro—Decreases edema Con—Ciliary stasis; thickens secretions
Topical decongestant	Oxymetazoline 0.05% 1–2 puffs each side BID	Pro—Decreases edema Con—Ciliary stasis; rhinitis medicamentosa with prolonged used (>5 days)
Antiobiotic	Amoxicillin 40 mg/kg/day divided TID	Pro—Safe, effective Con—Continue for 10–14 days
Antihistamine	Various (e.g., chlorpheniramine maleate 0.2 mg/kg/d BID to QID)	Con—Controversial, may help allergy symptoms but thickens secretions
Mucolytic/expectorant	Guafenesin 10–20 mg/kg/day q 4–6 hrs; iodinated compounds	Pro—May thin secretions to allow clearance Con—Iodides can lead to goiter with prolonged use
Topical steroids	Beclomethasone flunisolide triamcinolone, 1–2 puffs each side QD to QID	Pro—Can help long term with nasal reactivity and allergic phenomena Con—Not well studied in sinusitis
Cromolyn nasal spray	Sodium cromolyn 1 puff each side, 4–6 times per day	Pro—Help underlying allergic responsiveness Con—Requires frequent dosing
Irrigation	Saline up to 1 L	Pro—Removes thickened infected mucus; allows topical treatments to reach mucosa more intimately; cheap Con—Difficult to use in young children; structural management
Surgical drainage	—	Con—Does not cure underlying systemic problem; risks of operation, anesthesia

sinuses (Fig. 43.2). These are usually slow growing, and found on the maxillary sinus radiograph. Mucoceles in the frontal or ethmoid sinuses are more likely to cause difficulties. Often the patient will have a frontal headache, and if the expansion of the cyst progresses long enough, the ocular globe may be pushed inferiorly or laterally, causing proptosis or diplopia. Plain x-ray films may show loss of scalloped edges in the frontal sinus, indicating bony destruction and osteosclerosis. If these are asymptomatic, observation is reasonable, since surgical excision is the treatment of choice.

Chronic sinusitis has also been implicated in the pathogenesis of difficult-to-control asthma (35). Aggressive therapy of sinusitis was associated with significant improvement in asthma symptoms and a decrease in bronchodilator therapy.

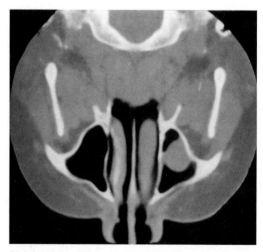

Figure 43.2.   CT scan: axial view of mucocele in right maxillary sinus.

ORBITAL COMPLICATION

Sinusitis may also progress to involve the orbit either by direct extension through the thin lamina papyracea (literally "paper layer") or by indirect extension as thrombophlebitis through ethmoidal veins. The stages of orbital sinusitis complications have recently been classified by Schramm et al. (36) (see Table 42.1).

Periorbital cellulitis without chemosis produces lid edema without limitation of extraocular mobility or disturbance of visual acuity. Periorbital cellulitis with chemosis is often due to bacteremic *Haemophilus influenzae* type B, which has a peak incidence in patients 6–18 months of age. Usually there is an antecedent upper respiratory tract infection. Subsequently the patient develops the high fever with rapid progression of findings. The eye will be swollen, discolored, and tender with induration surrounding the eye but without proptosis or ophthalmoplegia (3).

Treatment involves antibiotic therapy and close observation. If there is a progression or a lack of improvement for 24 hours, a CT scan is required. Patients with more severe symptoms require an immediate CT scan (37).

The third orbital complication, orbital cellulitis, results in diffuse edema in the orbit without discrete abscess. There may be ocular tenderness and some limitation of ocular mobility. An actual accumulation of pus in a subperiosteal abscess occurs if the condition remains untreated. The pus is between the bone and the periosteum and will tend to push the globe away; hence the eye will move down and laterally (Fig. 43.3). More serious is a collection of pus inside the orbital tissues themselves, deep to the orbital septum. Proptosis, chemosis, ophthalmoplegia, and decreased visual acuity occur. The most severe orbital complication is cavernous sinus thrombosis, which often spreads quickly to the opposite orbit, causing severe chemosis and ophthalmoplegia. Retinal vessels are massively engorged, fevers may be quite high (40°C), and the patient will appear "toxic." This complication carries a high mortality rate (10–27%), and is obviously a medical emergency (38, 39). The treatment involves treating the cause of abscess and orbital decompression if loss of visual acuity has occurred. Heparinization may be required to slow the progress of the thrombosis. In all these cases hospitalization for intravenous antibiotics is mandatory. Most will require a CT scan for evaluation and sinus drainage to remove the underlying cause. In children, the most common bacteria associated with orbital complications of sinusitis are *H. influenzae* and *Streptococcus pneumoniae*. This is somewhat different than in adults who have *S. pneumoniae*, and microaerophilic *Streptococcus*. Conjunctival cultures do not correlate with the bacteriology of the orbital complications and are not recommended. Treatment for these complications includes high doses of intravenous antibiotics that target the most common bacteria causing orbital complications (3, 18, 19, 34).

Intracranial complications are relatively rare, but 35–65% of subdural abscesses have been reported to come from sinusitis. The routes are direct spread either through the posterior wall of the frontal sinus through veins of Breschet or via the ophthalmic veins through the ethmoid system. Intracranial complications include epidural abscess, meningitis, subdural empyema or abscess, brain abscess, and cavernous sinus thrombosis. Again, the treatment involves hospitalization with medical as well as surgical treatment (3, 19, 40).

Localized complications such as osteomyelitis are seen occasionally. Osteomyelitis of the frontal bone with a subperiosteal abscess is also known as Pott's puffy tumor. Treatment involves intravenous antibiotics and surgical drainage of pus and removal of any irreversibly diseased bone. Long-term postoperative intravenous therapy of several weeks' duration followed by another 6 weeks of oral medica-

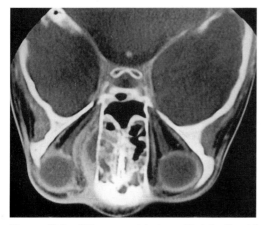

Figure 43.3. CT scan: axial view with left ethmoid sinusitis and subperiosteal orbital abscess causing proptosis.

tion is necessary. Fortunately, regeneration of the damaged bone generally occurs so that massive debridement is not required in most cases (19, 40).

The symptoms of malaise, headache, lethargy, and facial pain are certainly seen in sinusitis. Some patients may develop a secondary gain from continued complaints despite resolution of the initial sinusitis. A psychiatric disorder needs to be suspected if by history, physical examination, and laboratory testing and imaging no cause can be found to explain the complaints. Fortunately "psychosinusitis" is rare.

REFERENCES

1. Kern EB. Sinusitis. *J Allergy Clin Immunol* 1984; 73:25–31.
2. Fairbanks, DNF, Embryology and anatomy. In Bluestone CD, Stool SE, Scheetz MD, eds. *Pediatric otolaryngology*, 2nd ed. Philadelphia, WB Saunders, 1990, pp 605–631.
3. Wald ER. Rhinitis and acute and chronic sinusitis. In Bluestone CD, Stool SE, Scheetz MD, eds. *Pediatric otolaryngology*, 2nd ed. Philadelphia, WB Saunders, 1990, pp 729–744.
4. Wald ER. The diagnosis and management of sinusitis in children: Diagnostic considerations. *Pediatr Infect Dis* 1985; 4:S61–S62.
5. Wald ER. Medical management of sinusitis in pediatric patients. In Lusk RP, ed. *Pediatric sinusitis*. New York, Raven Press, 1992.
6. Reilly JS. The sinusitis cycle. *Otolaryngol Head Neck Surg* 1990; 103:856–862.
7. Rachelefsky GS, Katz RM, Siegel SC. Disease of paranasal sinuses in children. *Curr Probl Pediatr* 1982; 12:1–57.
8. Gwaltney JM Jr, Syndor A Jr, Sande MA. Etiology and antimicrobial treatment of acute sinusitis. *Ann Otol Rhinol Laryngol* 1981; 90:68–71.
9. Wald ER. Epidemiology, pathophysiology and etiology of sinusitis. *Pediatr Infect Dis* 1985; 4:S51–S54.
10. Slavin RG, Zilliox AP, Samuels LD. Is there a such an entity as allergic sinusitis? *J Allergy Clin Immunol* 1988; 81:284.
11. Slavin RG. Sinusitis in adults. *J Allergy Clin Immunol* 1988; 81:1028–1032.
12. Fujita A, Takahashi H, Honjo I. Etiological role of adenoids upon otitis media with effusion. *Acta Otolaryngol* 1988; 454(Suppl):210–213.
13. Chow AW, Roser SM, Brady FA. Orofacial odontogenic infections. *Ann Intern Med* 1978; 88:392–402.
14. Oxelius V, Laurell A, Lindquist B et al. IgG subclasses in selective IgA deficiency. *N Engl J Med* 1981; 304:1476–1477.
15. Greenfield HJ. Headache and facial pain associated with nasal and sinus disorders: A diagnostic and therapeutic challenge, Part 1. *Insights Otolaryngol* 1990; 5:1–8.
16. Parsons DS. Sinusitis: A pediatric perspective—Medical and surgical management. *Audiodigest Otolaryngol Head Neck Surg* 1992; 25(16).
17. Muntz HR, Lusk RP. Signs and symptoms of chronic sinusitis. In Lusk RP, ed. *Pediatric sinusitis*. New York, Raven Press, 1992.
18. Stafford, CT. The clinician's view of sinusitis. *Otolaryngol Head Neck Surg* 1990; 103:870–875.
19. Johnson JT. Infections. In Cummings CW, Fredrickson JM, Harker LA, Krause CJ, Schuller DE, eds. *Otolaryngology—Head and neck surgery*. St. Louis, CV Mosby, 1986, pp 887–900.
20. Wald ER, Chiponis D, Ledesma-Medina J. Comparative effectiveness of amoxicillin and amoxicillin-clavulanate potassium in acute paranasal sinus infections in children: A double-blind placebo-controlled trial. *Pediatrics* 1986; 77:795–800.
21. Lusk, RP, Lazar RH, Muntz HR. The diagnosis and treatment of recurrent and chronic sinusitis in children. *Pediatr Clin North Am* 1989; 36:1411–1421.
22. Glasier CM, Mallory GB Jr, Steele RW. Significance of opacification of the maxillary and ethmoid sinuses in infants. *J Pediatr* 1989; 114:45–50.
23. Hawkins DB. Advances in sinus disease in pediatrics. *Otolaryngol Clin North Am* 1989; 22:553–568.
24. Zinreich SJ. Paranasal sinus imaging. *Otolaryngol Head Neck Surg* 1990; 103:863–869.
25. Hamory BH, Sande MA, Syndor A Jr., Seale DL, Gwaltney JM Jr. Etiology and antimicrobial therapy of acute maxillary sinusitis. *J Infect Dis* 1979; 139:197–202.
26. Wald ER, Milmoe GJ, Bowen AD, Ledesma-Medina J, Salamon N, Bluestone CD. Acute maxillary sinusitis in children. *N Engl J Med* 1981; 1304:749–754.
27. Shapiro GG, Furukawa CT, Pierson WE, Gilbertson E, Bierman CW. Blinded comparison of maxillary sinus radiography and ultrasound for diagnosis of sinusitis. *J Allergy Clin Immunol* 1986; 77:59–64.
28. Wald ER, Pang D, Milmoe GJ, Schramm VL Jr. Sinusitis and its complications in the pediatric patient. *Pediatr Clin North Am* 1981; 28:777–796.
29. Wald ER, Byers C, Guerra N, Casselbrant M, Beste D. Subacute sinusitis in children. *J Pediatr* 1989; 115:28–32.
30. Brook I. Bacteriologic features of chronic sinusitis in children. *JAMA* 1981; 246:967–969.
31. Brook I. Bacteriology of chronic maxillary sinusitis in adults. *Ann Otol Rhinol Laryngol* 1989; 98:426–428.
32. Malow JB, Creticos CM. Nonsurgical management of sinusitis. *Otolaryngol Clin North Am* 1989; 22:809–818.
33. Druce HM. Adjuncts to medical management of sinusitis. *Otolaryngol Head Neck Surg* 1990; 103:880–883.
34. Fairbanks DNF. *Pocket guide to antimicrobial therapy in otolaryngology—Head and neck surgery*, 4th ed. Washington, DC, American Academy Otolaryngology—Head and Neck Surgery, 1987, pp 56–64.
35. Rachelsfsky GS, Katz RM, Siegel S. Chronic sinus disease with associated reactive airways disease in children. *Pediatrics* 1984; 73:526–529.
36. Schramm VL Jr, Curtin HD, Kennerdell JS. Evaluation of orbital cellulitis and results of treatment. *Laryngoscope* 1982; 92:732–738.
37. Lusk RP, Tyschen L, Park TS. Complications of sinusitis. In Lusk RP, ed. *Pediatric sinusitis*. New York, Raven Press, 1992.

38. Fearon B, Edmonds B, Bird R. Orbital facial complications of sinusitis in children. *Laryngoscope* 1979; 89:947–953.
39. Lew D, Southwick FS, Montgomery WW. Sphenoid sinusitis: A review of 30 cases. *N Engl J Med* 1983; 309:1149–1154.
40. Rabuzzi DD, Hengerer AS. Complications of nasal and sinus infections. In Bluestone CD, Stool SE, Scheetz MD, ed. *Pediatric otolaryngology*, 2nd ed. Philadelphia, WB Saunders, 1990, pp 745–751.

RESPIRATORY ASPECTS OF NONPULMONARY DISORDERS

the peristaltic wave (travelling at about 3 cm/second) reaches the LES (Fig. 44.1).

Pathophysiology and Symptoms

An older child or adolescent may describe difficulty swallowing. The infant or young child, on the other hand, must *demonstrate* the difficulty swallowing, sometimes quite dramatically (Table 44.2). An infant or child may choke, cough, gag, or become cyanotic during feedings. When these symptoms or signs occur during deglutition, the location of the disorder is usually oropharyngeal; following deglutition, coughing suggests a pharyngoesophageal disorder; and after the meal it may hint at reflux, or retention of material in a baggy esophagus enlarged by achalasia. If these symptoms are not attended to, the young child may begin to refuse to drink or eat, appearing hungry, but turning away from offered nutrition. Weight loss or lack of normal weight gain may ensue. Recurrent aspira-

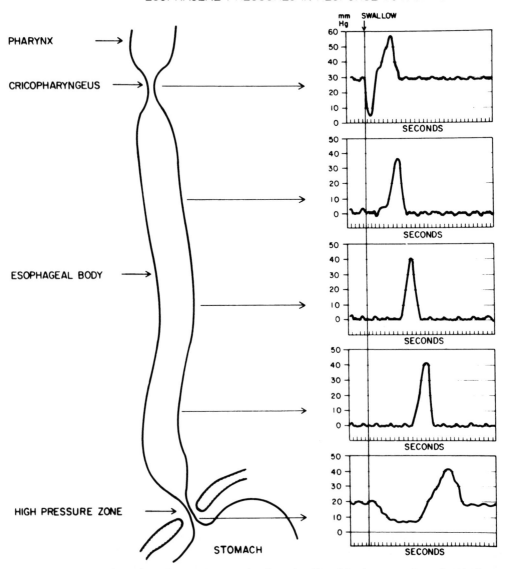

Figure 44.1. Tracing of esophageal pressure wave showing relaxation of the lower esophageal sphincter even before the peristaltic wave reaches that sphincter.

Table 44.2.
Symptoms Sometimes Associated with
Dysphagia

I.   Aspiration
     Cough, choke, gag
     Recurrent pneumonia
II. Nasopharyngeal regurgitation (sneezing)
III. Oral regurgitation (drooling if severe—unable to
     handle own secretions)
IV. Abnormalities of voice
     "Wet" voice—due to laryngeal soiling from
         dysfunctional swallowing
     Hoarse voice—due to laryngeal inflammation
     "Nasal" voice—due to velopharyngeal
         insufficiency and nasopharyngeal air escape
V.   Swallowing behavior
     Posturing of head and neck during swallowing
     Rapid or slow intake; multiple swallows;
         pocketing of food in cheeks

From Orenstein SR. Dysphagia and vomiting. In Wyllie R,
Hyams J, eds. *Pediatric gastrointestinal disease: Pathophysiology, diagnosis, management*. Philadelphia, WB Saunders,
1993.

tion pneumonia, initially seeming to be due to infection, may occur as a more subtle sequel of dysfunctional swallowing. Oral regurgitation during a meal is due to dysfunctional swallowing in some patients; nasal regurgitation during drinking may accompany severe disability of upper esophageal sphincter function; drooling because of inability to handle even oral secretions may befall some children with severe obstruction. Finally, symptoms of dysphagia may be accompanied by changes in voice quality, due to chronic laryngeal soiling and irritation by incompletely swallowed material. Dysphagia is usually perceived as discomfort rather than pain, and may be localized substernally or in the suprasternal notch. Older children may be able to distinguish dysphagia from other similar symptoms, such as odynophagia (painful swallowing) or heartburn, but these symptoms are often poorly distinguished, even by adults. A recent review of 1035 adults evaluated for "dysphagia" found that only 36% could be documented to have esophageal dysmotility, but 62% had increased esophageal acid exposure. Of the entire group with dysphagia, 74% also complained of heartburn (3). Particular forms of dysphagia have been separately identified: transfer dysphagia (dysphagia during the oropharyngeal phase of swallowing) and globus (the sensation that something is stuck in the upper esophagus).

Differential Diagnosis

When dysphagia for liquids is less than that for solids, a structural cause, such as a fixed esophageal narrowing, is likely. When dysphagia for liquids is the same as, or greater than, that for solids, dysmotility is suggested. A structural cause is also indicated by the need to regurgitate a bolus to gain relief, whereas movements of the neck or repeated swallowing will often permit material that is slowed by dysmotility to pass into the stomach. This differentiation between structural and functional basis for dysphagia is a basic step in the categorization of the causes for dysphagia (Table 44.3).

STRUCTURAL DISORDERS

Structural, fixed obstruction to forward movement of a swallowed bolus may result from intrinsic narrowing of the esophagus by congenital stenoses (Fig. 44.2), webs, acquired strictures (Fig. 44.3), or tumors. Extrinsic narrowing from compression of the esophagus also may present as dysphagia; the radiographic appearance aids in diagnosis of entities such as vascular rings.

FUNCTIONAL DISORDERS

Most nonstructural causes of dysphagia are due to dysmotility of the oropharynx and esophagus (Table 44.3). A host of neuromuscular disorders may affect normal swallowing. Cortical or brainstem disease may impair voluntary transfer of the bolus to the pharynx (i.e., the oral phase of swallowing); dysfunction of the brainstem or any of the six cranial nerves that participate in normal swallowing may affect initiation of the automatic, semireflexive portion of the swallow in the pharynx; and brainstem abnormalities, disorders of intrinsic esophageal neurons, or myopathies may hinder function of both the smooth muscle of the lower esophagus and the striated muscles of the oropharynx and upper esophagus (4).

In addition to being caused by systemic disease, dysmotility may result from isolated (primary) esophageal motility disorders, such as achalasia, diffuse esophageal spasm, and nonspecific esophageal motor disorders.

MISCELLANEOUS DISORDERS

Dysphagia may also be due to several common disorders that do not fit clearly into the struc-

Table 44.3.
Differential Diagnosis of Dysphagia

I. Structural causes (fixed narrowing)
  A. Intrinsic: stenosis, web, stricture, tumor, polyp
  B. Extrinsic: vascular ring, thyromegaly, exostosis, paraesophageal hernia, esophageal diverticula
II. Functional causes (dysmotility)
  A. Systemic neuromuscular disease
    1. Corticobulbar dysfunction
      a. Newborn transient pharyngeal weakness—"congenital flaccid bulbar palsy"
      b. Congenital malformations: Arnold-Chiari, syringobulbia
      c. Acquired disease: stroke (cortical, bulbar), tumor, trauma, bulbar polio
      d. Cerebral palsy, pseudobulbar palsy, bulbar palsy
    2. Neuropathy
      a. Metabolic: diabetic neuropathy
      b. Toxin: tetanus, lead poisoning, rabies
      c. Drug: nitrazepam
    3. Motor end plate: myasthenia gravis, botulism
    4. Myopathy
      a. Dystrophy : myotonic, oculopharyngeal
      b. Inflammatory
        1) Striated muscle: polymyositis, dermatomyositis
        2) Smooth muscle: systemic lupus erythematous
      c. Metabolic: hyperthyroid, hypothyroid
  B. Isolated esophageal dysmotility
    1. Diffuse esophageal spasm
    2. Nutcracker esophagus
    3. Achalasia
    4. Hypertensive lower esophageal sphincter
    5. Nonspecific esophageal motilty disorder
III. Miscellaneous causes
  A. Inflammatory
    a. Pharyngeal: pharyngitis, pharyngeal abscess
    b. Esophageal: esophagitis (reflux-associated, infectious, "pill-induced")
  B. Cicatricial: tracheostomy, other neck surgery
  C. Foreign body
  D. Psychogenic: globus
  E. Familial dysautonomia

From Orenstein SR. Dysphagia and vomiting. In Wyllie R, Hyams J, eds. *Pediatric gastrointestinal disease: Pathophysiology, diagnosis, management.* Philadelphia, WB Saunders, 1993.

tural-functional classification above. Inflammatory disease of the pharynx and esophagus (such as that due to gastroesophageal reflux) may produce nonspecific dysmotility, or may result in odynophagia (painful swallowing), which is difficult for the patient to distinguish from dysphagia. Similarly, a pharyngeal or esophageal foreign body may temporarily disturb motor function, may be partially obstructing, or may cause discomfort difficult to distinguish from dysphagia. The interactions of emotional state and esophageal function have been noted repeatedly, and may underlie some of the reported associations between dysphagia and psychiatric illness (5).

Several disorders of particular interest to the pulmonologist have been associated with difficulty swallowing. Scarring due to surgery in the neck, particularly tracheostomy, often impairs laryngeal elevation, which is necessary for normal cricopharyngeal opening, causing dysphagia (6). Anomalies such as "H-type" tracheoesophageal fistulas, laryngeal cleft, or unilateral vocal cord paralysis may also present as swallowing difficulties. Dysphagia is reported as an isolated manifestation of mealtime hypoxia in a young woman with severe pulmonary restriction caused by kyphoscoliosis (7). This confirms the clinical impression that other patients with borderline oxygenation may have more difficulty with meals if they do not use supplemental oxygen than if they do.

CRICOPHARYNGEAL DYSPHAGIA

Normal functioning of the upper esophageal sphincter (UES—largely the cricopharyngeus muscle) demands exquisite coordination

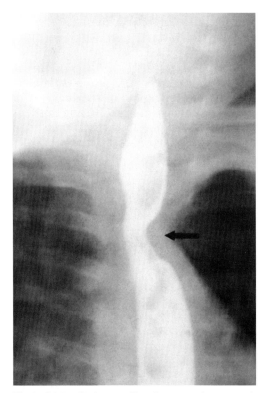

Figure 44.2.   Barium swallow demonstrating congenital esophageal stenosis.

between pharyngeal contraction and UES relaxation. In normal swallowing, pharyngeal contraction begins prior to UES relaxation, and ends before the UES resumes normal tone. The UES relaxes completely, and must be actively pulled open by the upward and forward movement of the larynx.

Abnormalities of several types have been identified in the function of this intricate unit. The pharyngeal contractions may be hypotensive. The UES may fail to relax or relax incompletely (cricopharyngeal achalasia). It may relax late or resume its tone early. Finally, the UES may fail to open completely because of inadequate elevation of the larynx. These abnormalities may be demonstrated by esophageal manometry and may be suggested radiographically. Because discrete treatable causes of cricopharyngeal dysphagia continue to be identified (8, 9) thorough investigation of children who have dysphagia is important before characterizing the symptom as idiopathic.

OROPHARYNGEAL DYSPHAGIA

Neurologic causes for oropharyngeal dysphagia interfere with bolus formation, causing

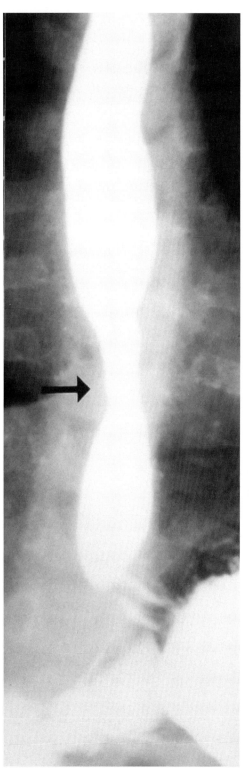

Figure 44.3.   Barium swallow demonstrating acquired esophageal stricture.

particular difficulty with thin liquids and grainy foods such as rice or crackers.

Diagnosis

RADIOLOGY

Diagnostic evaluation of children with dysphagia generally begins with radiographic evaluation (10). Structural abnormalities can be identified most readily; dysmotility of the oropharynx and esophagus can be seen; and sequelae such as laryngeal aspiration or nasopharyngeal regurgitation can be documented. Barium fluoroscopy provides particularly vivid demonstration of intrinsic (Figs. 44.2, 44.3) and extrinsic (Fig. 44.4) obstructive lesions of the esophagus. As with most diagnostic procedures, the yield of radiography depends on the interest and expertise of the person performing the study. Recording of motion per-

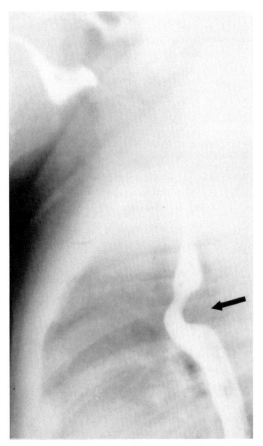

Figure 44.4. Barium swallow demonstrating extrinsic obstruction of the esophagus.

mits identification of functional disorders of swallowing (11).

MANOMETRY

Unless a clear structural lesion is demonstrated radiographically, most patients with dysphagia will benefit from manometric evaluation. Esophageal manometry examines the motility of the esophagus, including the lower and upper esophageal sphincters, and the pharynx. Resting tone of the upper and lower esophageal sphincters are measured and completeness and coordination of the relaxations of these sphincters are also noted (12).

ENDOSCOPY AND BIOPSY

Endoscopy is the optimal study for examination of mucosal detail, and also permits the sampling of tissue for histologic evaluation and some therapy during the same procedure. For dysphagia that has been shown radiographically to be due to intrinsic structural lesions, endoscopic biopsy provides information as to the presence of peptic esophagitis, and identifies the nature of inflammatory or neoplastic causes for dysphagia. Dilatation may be carried out at the same time (13, 14).

Therapy

The therapy of dysphagia is tailored to its cause (Table 44.4). Cricopharyngeal achalasia may be treated with neurosurgical decompression if it is due to Arnold-Chiari malformation (9) or with dilation if it is idiopathic, persistent, and associated with normal oropharyngeal function (15–18). Pharmacologic therapy is available for some primary disorders of esophageal motility (19, 20). For disorders without known definitive therapy, techniques to maintain nutrition while protecting the airway from aspiration are crucial. Attempts to maintain oral feedings, although laudable, must be based on the degree of dysphagia and associated symptoms. If symptoms are so severe that even oral secretions are not swallowed safely the swallowing mechanism must be bypassed to provide nutrition and prevent aspiration.

GASTROESOPHAGEAL REFLUX
Physiology

Gastroesophageal reflux, the retrograde movement of gastric contents into the esopha-

Table 44.4.
Therapy for Dysphagia

Treat primary disease if possible
  Esophageal structural abnormalities: dilatation or surgery
  Systemic neuromuscular disorders
    Neurosurgery (for brain tumor, Arnold-Chiari malformation, etc.)
    Pharmacologic treatment (for tetanus, polymyositis, hyperthyroidism, etc.)
  Esophageal dysmotility
    Dilatation or myotomy for hypertensive or nonrelaxing sphincters
    Pharmacologic treatment
      Calcium channel blocker: nifedipine, diltiazem
      Nitrates: isosorbide dinitrate
      Anticholinergic: propantheline bromide, valethamate bromide, L-hyoscyamine
      Adrenoceptor antagonists?
      Psychotropic medications (trazodone, etc.)?
Assure nutrition and airway protection
  Oral feeding: slow, careful: avoid distractions
    Nutrient characteristics
      Bolus volume and viscosity change timing of swallow components
      Semisolids and thick liquids generally easiest
    Head positions
      Neck flexion protects airway; neck extension speeds oral transit
      Head rotation directs bolus down opposite side; head tilt, down same side
    Maneuvers: supraglottic swallow. Mendelsohn maneuver
  Non-oral nutrition
    Nasogastric (beware reflux) or nasoduodenal feeds
    Gastrostomy (beware reflux) or intestinal feeds via gastrostomy
    Jejunostomy feeds
    Parenteral nutrition
  Laryngeal stents, etc., for patients unable to handle their secretions.

From Wylie R, Hyams JS. Gastrointestinal disease: Pathophysiology, diagnosis, management. Philadelphia, WB Saunders, 1993.

gus, is common in normal awake individuals following meals. Such physiologic reflux consists of infrequent, brief, and inconsequential return of small amounts of material into the esophagus. The buffering of gastric acid by ingested food contributes to the benign nature of physiologic postprandial reflux.

Reflux occurs most often during transient relaxations of the lower esophageal sphincter, unassociated with swallowing. Less often, reflux occurs in individuals with a hypotonic lower esophageal sphincter (LES), or during episodes of augmented intragastric pressure. The elevated intra-abdominal pressure that occurs with coughing or valsalva does not usually lead to reflux because contraction of the crural portion of the diaphragm bolsters the LES pressure, unless the LES is above the diaphragm, as with hiatal hernia.

Pathophysiology

Pathogenic reflux, that which causes untoward effects, may do so because of increased frequency or duration of the episodes, or because of the composition or fate of the refluxed

material. In addition to gastric acid, noxious components of refluxate may include pepsin, trypsin, and bile salts. The fate of refluxed material may be to remain in the esophagus for prolonged periods, or to enter the pharynx, whence it may be regurgitated, reswallowed, or, if the protective mechanisms fail, aspirated. Esophagitis results from prolonged residence of refluxate in the esophagus; failure to thrive results from regurgitation and/or chronic lung disease, and respiratory symptoms may result whether or not aspiration occurs. The remainder of this chapter will focus on respiratory problems associated with reflux.

The protections against reflux and against aspiration of refluxed material are listed in Table 44.5. Ways in which these protective mechanisms may fail, and thus predispose to reflux and respiratory sequelae, are also shown in Table 44.5.

Since protective mechanisms are apt to fail during sleep, it is fortunate that reflux rarely occurs during sleep in normal individuals (21). If it does occur during sleep, it is likely to be more acidic, more prolonged (because of the

Table 44.5.
Prevention of Respiratory Sequelae Due to Reflux

Structure	Protective Functions	Dysfunctions
Stomach	Antegrade emptying	Delayed gastric emptying
Esophagus		
Associated structures	Diaphragmatic hiatal tone	Hiatal hernia
Lower Esophageal sphincter (LES)	LES tone Distinction of gas vs. liquid	Hypotensive LES Transient LES relaxations to liquid
Body	Secondary peristalsis	Impaired esophageal clearance
Upper esophageal sphincter (UES)	UES tone Distinction of gas vs. liquid	Hypotensive UES Transient UES relaxations to liquid
Larynx, pharynx mouth	Swallow reflex Cord closure Arytenoid-epiglottic approximation	Impaired swallow reflex Impaired cord closure Impaired arytenoid epiglottic approximation

From Putnam PE, Ricker DH, Orenstein SR. Gastroesophageal reflux. In Beckerman RC, Brouillette RT, Hunt CE, eds. *Respiratory control disorders in infants and children.* Baltimore, Williams & Wilkins, 1992, p 323.

markedly reduced salivation, swallowing, and gravitational effects responsible for normal esophageal clearance), and more hazardous (because of impairment of protective mechanisms such as upper esophageal sphincter tone) (22, 23).

PATHOPHYSIOLOGY OF RESPIRATORY DYSFUNCTION CAUSED BY REFLUX

The effects of reflux on the upper and lower respiratory tract have several potential mechanisms (Fig. 44.5). We will discuss these mechanisms using the lower airway as a model, but similar mechanisms are likely in the upper airway, mediating such other reflux-associated respiratory findings as apnea, stridor, and hoarseness.

Lower airway narrowing manifested as wheezing or cough may occur as a result of airway obstruction by aspirated food particles, locally produced secretions, mucosal edema, or bronchial smooth muscle contraction (Fig. 44.6) (24). The latter three mechanisms may occur on the basis of aspiration (gross or microscopic), or may be initiated by a reflex response to acid stimulation of the esophagus. Although these mechanisms have been the subject of numerous studies in humans and animals, our understanding remains incomplete, largely because of the difficulties in documenting these effects and separating them from one another.

Direct Mechanical Effects from Macroaspiration

Aspiration of a large quantity of gastric material (macroaspiration) may lead to mechanical

obstruction of the airway lumen and chemical pneumonitis; the character of the refluxed material may influence the pulmonary reaction. Such aspiration may occur during dysfunctional swallowing or later, if swallowed material refluxes. Refluxed material may be more noxious than swallowed material, because it may be acidic, and contain pepsin, or even trypsin and bile salts (if there has also been duodenogastric reflux). In humans, aspiration of acidic material (pH <2.5) is associated with reflex airway closure, loss of surfactant, epithelial damage, pulmonary edema, and pulmonary hemorrhage, all resulting in severe hypoxia (25). Such blatant aspiration pneumonia is uncommon as a result of reflux, except in patients with depressed consciousness.

Indirect Effects: Neural Mediation from Airway

Macroaspiration has been generally considered the cause of all reflux-related respiratory morbidity (26). However, aspiration insufficient to cause radiographic changes may stimulate upper airway neural elements or the release of inflammatory mediators. Aspiration, noted by radionuclide scanning, occurs in 45% of normal adults following pharyngeal instillation of a radioactive tracer during sleep (27). Fifteen percent of normal subjects will be found to have lung contamination following a radiolabeled solid meal (28). Clearly, microaspiration does occur in spite of the fine neuromuscular control described above.

MECHANISMS FOR

REFLUX-ASSOCIATED RESPIRATORY DYSFUNCTION

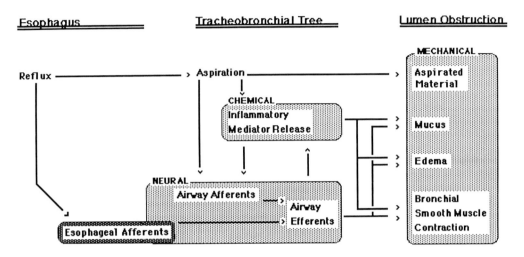

Figure 44.5. Mechanisms for reflux-associated respiratory dysfunction. Reflux may lead to direct pulmonary aspiration of refluxed material, producing mechanical obstruction of the airway lumen. Pulmonary aspiration also leads to release of chemical mediators of inflammation, which in return leads to obstruction of the lumen by mucus, by mucosal edema, and by bronchial smooth muscle contraction. Aspiration also stimulates airway neural afferents, which in turn influence airway efferents, which induce the release of chemical inflammatory mediators, and which also lead to mucus secretion, edema formation, and bronchial smooth muscle contraction. Finally, reflux can stimulate esophageal afferents, which also influence airway efferents.

FOUR POTENTIAL COMPONENTS OF
BRONCHIAL OBSTRUCTION

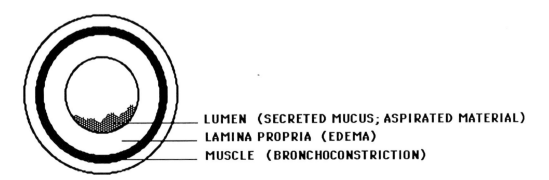

LUMEN (SECRETED MUCUS; ASPIRATED MATERIAL)
LAMINA PROPRIA (EDEMA)
MUSCLE (BRONCHOCONSTRICTION)

Figure 44.6. The four potential components of bronchial obstruction: (1) blockage of the lumen by secreted mucus and/or (2) aspirated material (not shown); (3) edema in the lamina propria; and (4) bronchial muscle constriction.

That irritation of upper airway mucosa may result in neurally mediated bronchoconstriction is suggested by work in animals (29). As little as 0.05 ml of 0.2 N HCl infused into a cat's trachea causes a four-fold increase in total lung resistance, whereas saline has no effect (30). The response to acid disappears within 1 minute after infusion, and may be abolished by bilateral vagotomy.

Indirect Effects: Neural Mediation from Esophagus

Instillation of 10 ml of the acid solution into the esophagus of cats also results in an increase in total lung resistance; the increase is smaller (1.5 times) but is sustained longer than after intratracheal acid. Intraesophageal saline infusion has no effect. Although this experiment suggests that microaspiration causes a greater degree of bronchospasm (via airway afferents), pulmonary effects also can result from stimulation of esophageal afferents.

Such vagal reflexes with gastroesophageal afferents were first postulated over 50 years ago as a mechanism of asthma attacks occurring after a heavy meal (31). Several studies in adults (32, 33) and children (34) have shown evidence of bronchoconstriction in patients with asthma during acid infusion into the esophagus but not during infusion of saline solution or antacid. This bronchoconstrictive response is eliminated in dogs by vagal blockade or section (35) and in humans by pretreatment with atropine (36, 37). Not all studies have demonstrated bronchoconstriction in response to acidification of the esophagus (38). One elegant investigation suggests an explanation: esophageal acid infusion decreases the threshold for bronchoconstriction in response to inhaled methacholine—that is, bronchial reactivity is increased, without the occurrence of bronchoconstriction (39).

Whether esophagitis is a prerequisite for reflex bronchoconstriction is unclear. Adult patients with asthma who complained of pyrosis during esophageal acid infusion (suggesting the presence of esophagitis) had a concomitant increase in respiratory system resistance, as compared to controls and to patients with asthma who did not develop pyrosis (32). However, no difference in lung resistance after esophageal acid infusion is observed in cats with and without esophagitis (30).

Indirect, Chemical, and Inflammatory Mediation

In addition to aspiration and neural reflexes, leukocyte-derived inflammatory mediators play an intermediary role in the production of bronchial obstruction (Fig. 44.5). Like neural reflexes, these mediators can narrow the bronchial lumen by inducing bronchial smooth muscle contraction, edema, and mucus secretion. The role of these mediators in producing reflux-associated bronchial obstruction is not clear.

PATHOPHYSIOLOGY OF REFLUX CAUSED BY RESPIRATORY DISORDERS

It is essential to note that just as reflux can cause a multitude of respiratory symptoms, the converse is also true, with various respiratory disorders aggravating reflux. Respiratory disorders may increase reflux by augmenting the gastroesophageal pressure gradient, or by causing transient inhibition of lower esophageal sphincter pressure.

Normally, the gastric pressure is positive relative to the esophagus, with the intra-abdominal lower esophageal sphincter providing a barrier to reflux. Abdominal pressure is made more positive by the forced expiration of coughing and wheezing, as is seen in asthma, bronchopulmonary dysplasia, and cystic fibrosis (40), but the increased pressure is transmitted to the lower esophageal sphincter, augmenting its anti-reflux function (41). This protection may be lost when the lower esophageal sphincter is above the diaphragm (i.e., hiatal hernia).

Intrapleural pressure with inspiration is more negative than normal during laryngospasm and bronchospasm, which may augment the gastroesophageal pressure gradient, favoring movement of gastric contents into the esophagus.

Lung inflation is followed by a transient inhibition of lower esophageal sphincter pressure in cats (42), which may occur in pulmonary diseases involving hyper-inflation.

PATHOPHYSIOLOGY OF REFLUX CAUSED BY RESPIRATORY THERAPIES

Pharmacologic

Pharmacologic agents used to treat asthma and other respiratory disorders may exacerbate reflux by relaxing the lower esophageal sphincter and increasing gastric acid secretion (43). Reflux should be considered in any patient with asthma whose symptoms worsen during theophylline use. A related situation may occur in premature infants treated with xanthines for apnea of prematurity: in one study of such infants, a subgroup treated unsuccessfully with xanthines, was found to have severe, unsuspected reflux (44). In a group of infants considered at risk for sudden infant death syndrome, pH probe monitoring documented increased reflux during treatment with theophylline and caffeine (45).

Some beta adrenergic agents (isoproterenol, carbuterol, terbutaline) decrease lower esophageal sphincter pressure (46), but this may not be associated with an increase in gastroesophageal reflux (47). In healthy adults, *inhaled* albuterol does not decrease lower esophageal sphincter tone; nor does it increase gastroesophageal reflux (48).

Nutritional Therapy

Tube feedings for the purpose of augmenting nutrition are frequently used in the care of malnourished or critically ill children. Nasogastric tubes predispose the child to reflux severe enough to cause esophagitis with strictures (49).

Surgical gastrostomy tube placement reduces lower esophageal sphincter pressure, and may impair the normally protective gastroesophageal relationship, and worsen reflux (50). Tube feeding has been used successfully to augment nutrition in children with reflux (51), but the effect of rapidly infused, high-pressure bolus feedings may instead provoke reflux.

The effects of percutaneous endoscopic gastrostomy (PEG) tubes has not been fully evaluated but it is felt to have less impact on LES function.

Mechanical Ventilation

Tracheal intubation impairs protective upper airway reflexes and may allow aspiration, prolonging the need for mechanical ventilation. Of 42 mechanically ventilated infants fed by nasogastric tube, six had sufficient lactose in the tracheal aspirates to suggest ongoing unrecognized aspiration (52).

Mechanically ventilated patients are often kept supine, a position that increases reflux (53) and slows gastric emptying (54). Keeping the patient in the prone position diminishes these problems and also improves gas exchange in preterm infants (55).

Reflux was provoked by routine chest percussion and postural drainage in 8 of 10 patients with cystic fibrosis (CF) (56), and was also found to occur significantly more frequently during chest physiotherapy than in control times in 63 infants with chronic vomiting (n = 28), acute respiratory disease (n = 8), or healthy controls (n = 21) (57), perhaps because of gravitational effects as well as altered thoracoabdominal pressure relationships.

Specific Respiratory Disorders

ASPIRATION PNEUMONIA

Pulmonary aspiration of refluxed gastric contents is a clear cause of some cases of pneumonia and has been long suspected as a cause of asthma-like symptoms (58). It may be difficult, however, to differentiate it from aspiration of oral contents during swallowing, or from neurally mediated reflex bronchoconstriction. Various diagnostic methods have implicated reflux with aspiration in some cases of pneumonia (59, 60), lung abscess (61), obliterative bronchiolitis (62), and apnea (59).

Major aspiration, as described here, occurs most often in patients with depressed consciousness, with its attendant suppression of protective mechanisms (Table 44.5) (27, 63). Even the partially depressed consciousness of physiologic sleep may be hazardous; although sleep markedly reduces reflux in normal individuals, it also decreases airway protection by decreasing upper esophageal sphincter tone (23). Increased risk for aspiration pneumonia has long been associated with general anesthesia, cardiopulmonary resuscitation, and neurologic disorders (58, 64, 65).

Through 24-hour pH measurements, pathogenic reflux was found in 65% of mentally retarded children, although no mention is made of pulmonary symptoms in this report (66). Two other studies of retarded children included those with recurrent aspiration pneumonia and found incidences of reflux as disparate as 11% and 86% (67, 68). Because of differences in diagnostic techniques, these figures are likely to be under- and over-estimated, respectively.

STRIDOR

Stridor can be caused by laryngospasm, which may be caused by reflux as suggested by the lessening of stridor (120, 121) with treatment of reflux in some infants. The association is further strengthened by the temporal relationship between episodes of reflux recorded by pH probe and stridor (Fig. 44.7) (122). In individual patients, episodes of stridor have been produced by esophageal acid perfusion (123). Reflex laryngospasm manifested as stridor may require the presence of esophagitis, laryngitis, or an abnormal upper respiratory tract. It is unclear why laryngospasm rather than bronchospasm occurs as a consequence of reflux in some younger children, but it may be related to the relatively small cross-sectional area of the upper airway, to a tendency towards greater laxity of upper airway structures, or to an immaturity of nervous control of the respiratory system.

HOARSENESS

Hoarseness has recently received attention as a possible consequence of gastroesophageal reflux in adults (124–126). The characteristics of the reflux, response to therapy, and postulated mechanisms have varied (124, 125). Laryngoscopic findings include normal anatomy (127); chronic arytenoid or vocal cord inflammation (edema, erythema), granulo-

mata, or "contact ulcers" (126); and scarring, stenosis, or cancer (125, 126). Postulated mechanisms include direct acid injury and an indirect path mediated by reflexive chronic coughing and throat-clearing in response to reflux (125). Hoarseness is associated with reflux in children, but no reports in the pediatric literature link the two (128). Reflux should be considered in the occasional patient with hoarseness and an otherwise negative evaluation.

COUGH

In some adults, cough has been identified as the sole manifestation of reflux, and has been responsive to anti-reflux therapy (129). Coughing is correlated with distal rather than proximal esophageal acidification. Coughing has also been associated with acid reflux in infants (107, 130). Coughing may occur as a consequence of bronchospasm, which may be precipitated by reflux.

HICCUPS

Hiccups have been shown to be temporally associated with spontaneous esophageal acidification (131), and have been provoked by esophageal acid perfusion in adults (132). A temporal association has been also demonstrated between hiccups and spontaneous reflux in two infants monitored simultane-

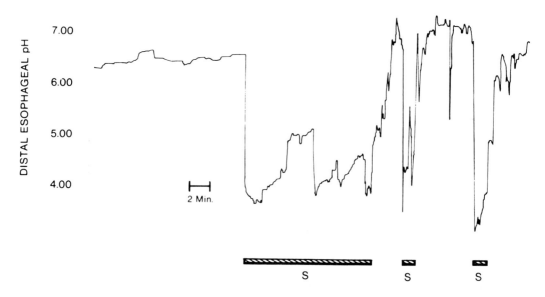

Figure 44.7. Esophageal pH record in an infant, showing ("S") stridor occurring only during episodes of reflux.

ously by video and pH probe (130). We have noted a history of excessive hiccups in some patients with severe reflux. Hiccups occurring with reflux may represent an involuntary reflex contraction of the diaphragm caused by esophagitis. Conversely, the increased gastroesophageal pressure gradient generated by the hiccups may produce the acid reflux.

Diagnosis of Reflux-Associated Respiratory Disease

EVALUATION FOR REFLUX

pH Probe

The pH in the esophagus drops when acidic gastric contents are refluxed, and returns to its normal range of 6–7 when peristalsis returns the refluxed material to the stomach and swallowed saliva neutralizes the residual.

The most reliable method of detecting acid reflux is by pH probe (133). Inserted through the nostril, the pH probe is left in the distal esophagus, where it monitors the pH of the surrounding fluid. A continuous tracing of the intra-esophageal pH is generated for subsequent interpretation.

By convention, a reflux episode is defined as the period during which the intraesophageal pH is < 4. Non-acid reflux is therefore not detected on pH probe studies, precluding the use of such studies in patients with achlorhydria, or those receiving antacids or H_2 blockers.

Detection of reflux may be impaired by the neutralization of gastric acid by food. To avoid this, apple juice (pH < 4) may be fed to subjects instead of milk or infant formula during pH probe studies.

Scintigraphy

Gastroesophageal reflux can be detected by nuclear imaging without regard to pH. Technetium-99m labeled sulfur colloid is mixed with milk (or formula) and given by mouth, nasogastric tube, or gastrostomy (134). The patient may be continuously monitored by gamma camera for an hour or so after the dose is given. Reflux is seen as return of radioactivity into the esophagus, and its frequency, duration, and volume are quantified. Aspiration may be documented by radioactivity appearing in the lung fields after swallowing or reflux

(135). Gastric emptying, which may be delayed in some patients with reflux (136), can be quantified.

This method suffers from insensitivity in detecting late postprandial reflux or aspiration, from poor resolution of anatomic structures (particularly proximal esophagus from trachea), and from the need to subject the patient to ionizing radiation, although only to a fraction of the radiation associated with fluoroscopic upper gastrointestinal examination (137).

Contrast Radiography

Barium studies are useful in evaluating infants and children with reflux. They allow observation of the contrast as it is affected by the mechanics of swallowing and the motility of the esophagus, stomach, and small intestine. They give a crude appreciation of the mucosa, and allow aspiration to be documented.

As a diagnostic tool for reflux, however, the upper gastrointestinal series must be considered inferior to pH probe and scintigraphy (138). The barium is nonphysiologic, and, although episodes of reflux can be seen, the periods of observation are too brief to allow conclusions about the frequency and duration of naturally occurring episodes.

One of the primary advantages of the upper gastrointestinal series in patients with suspected reflux is to exclude from consideration other abnormalities that result in persistent vomiting, such as gastric outlet obstruction, peptic ulcer disease, and malrotation of the intestine.

Endoscopy and Esophageal Biopsy

Although not routinely required for the evaluation of reflux, fiberoptic esophagogastroduodenoscopy with biopsy may be used as an adjunct to the evaluation of children with atypical chest pain. Pathogenic reflux is inferred from the presence of esophagitis, which may be seen grossly at endoscopy, but often is diagnosable only by histologic examination (139). Histologic esophagitis is present in the majority of infants and children with abnormal pH probe parameters (140).

Esophageal Manometry

Esophageal manometry has played an important role in the evolution of our understanding of gastroesophageal reflux by demonstrating the normal function of the esophagus and the changes that allow reflux to occur (141). Although currently used in selected patients with dysphagia, it is not required for routine evaluation of the patient with reflux.

EVALUATION FOR REFLUX-ASSOCIATED RESPIRATORY DISEASE

pH Probe with Observation

Documenting temporal association of occult reflux with other respiratory symptoms (cough, irritability, hiccups, stridor, wheezing) is best attempted by careful observation of the patient during a pH probe study. The onset of the symptom of interest must be noted exactly for correlation with intraesophageal pH; video recording may be useful in this regard.

Unfortunately, pH probe data may be difficult to interpret when obtained during acute respiratory illnesses that include frequent coughing or persistent wheezing and are best performed after the acute illness has abated (141a).

pH Probe with Polysomnography

Patients in whom there is concern about the contribution of reflux to apnea or ALTE should be evaluated by concurrent pH probe and multichannel sleep study. Patient monitoring includes simultaneous intraesophageal pH probe, chest wall impedance, electrocardiogram, pulse oximetry, and nasal thermistor or end-tidal CO_2 to identify obstructive apnea. Thus, apneic events can be examined in temporal relation to changes in intra-esophageal pH (112).

One must keep in mind that this type of study answers only questions about the temporal relationship between a reflux episode and another symptom, but does not prove causation.

Esophageal Acid Infusion (Modified Bernstein Test)

Many respiratory symptoms are episodic and infrequent, and may not occur during a pH probe study. Furthermore, the prolonged intensive observation required to link spontaneous esophageal acidification with respiratory symptoms may not be feasible.

The Bernstein test is a provocative test that attempts to reproduce a patient's symptoms by infusing 0.1 N HCl into the esophagus, mimicking prolonged reflux episode (142). Normal saline is infused to clear the acid, and as a "control" solution. Irritability, wheezing, apnea, coughing, choking, stridor, or changes in oxygen saturation can be seen and correlated with the solution being infused (34, 123). In the older child, spirometry may be performed during acid and saline infusion (36). However, there is always uncertainty as to whether the infused acid produced respiratory symptoms by entering the airway, or solely by stimulating the esophagus.

EVALUATION FOR ASPIRATION

Documenting reflux, even reflux into the proximal esophagus, is not sufficient for the diagnosis of aspiration. Although aspiration of refluxed material may be difficult to prove, the patient's clinical condition and the chest radiograph may provide clues. The right lung is involved more often than the left, and various segments may be affected, depending on body position at the time of aspiration, and the volume aspirated. Fluid obtained by bronchoalveolar lavage or endotracheal tube suctioning can be examined for lipid-laden macrophages (143, 144), lactose (52), or dye (145). The invasive nature and possible false-positive results (146) limit the clinical usefulness of these techniques. Imaging studies used to diagnose aspiration are contrast radiography (59, 147) and the more sensitive radionuclide scintigraphy (59, 148–150).

INDICATIONS FOR EVALUATION

Patients with reflux manifested as recurrent effortless regurgitation or with symptoms of esophagitis should need only an upper gastrointestinal series to exclude obstruction before instituting therapy.

In patients without overt reflux and regurgitation, the contribution of reflux to respiratory disease is often uncertain. It remains difficult to determine which individuals with respiratory disease fall into a subgroup that should be evaluated for reflux. The following are general guidelines for the evaluation of such patients.

Bronchospasm and Asthma

Patients with asthma and unsatisfactory response to conventional bronchodilator therapy may benefit from pH probe monitoring to document increased reflux, and to correlate reflux with the respiratory symptoms. This is especially useful in patients with severe symptoms at night.

If pH probe data do not allow one to associate reflux and wheezing definitively, a modified Bernstein test can be done during an asymptomatic period to attempt to elicit the respiratory symptoms by esophageal acidification. Pulmonary function testing following both esophageal acid infusion and neutralization is a useful adjunct to such testing (36).

Apnea and ALTE

Because of the serious consequences of apnea, and the desire to prevent further episodes, any infant with otherwise unexplained apnea or ALTE should undergo simultaneous pH probe and polysomnograph to document the type of apnea present and to correlate reflux with the event and any associated physiologic sequelae such as decreased oxygen saturation. Unfortunately, such correlation is not possible when a single event, witnessed at home, does not recur during the study interval. In that case, the detection of abnormal quantities of reflux (by pH probe), or of pathologic effects of reflux (by esophageal biopsy) may suggest the association and justify a trial of anti-reflux therapy.

Other Recurrent or Persistent Respiratory Disorders

Patients with chronic cough, stridor, hoarseness, or recurrent pneumonia, whose routine evaluation fails to disclose an underlying etiology, or whose response to treatment is unsatisfactory, should be evaluated for reflux. For intermittent symptoms such as cough or stridor, standard pH probe testing should be supplemented by careful documentation of the association between reflux and the symptom. If aspiration is suspected, scintigraphy may be helpful, although the sensitivity is low. Endoscopic procedures to evaluate both the esophagus and airway are useful in many of these situations as well. As in bronchospastic conditions, the modified Bernstein test may be used as a provocative test if no relationship with reflux can be demonstrated by pH probe despite strong clinical suspicion.

In any of the clinical situations cited above, esophageal histology consistent with esophagitis provides evidence for pathogenic reflux, whether or not reflux is held responsible for the respiratory symptoms. Esophagitis should be treated, even in the absence of its symptoms, to prevent esophageal (stricture or Barrett esophagus) or respiratory sequelae.

Follow-Up Studies

Intra-esophageal pH monitoring with the patient receiving anti-reflux treatment is occasionally valuable, though not routinely required. Patients with vomiting have an easily observable symptom, the reduction of which usually reflects the adequacy of treatment. Improvement in respiratory symptoms during treatment for reflux is indicative of the effectiveness of anti-reflux therapy in those patients with reflux-associated respiratory disease. Patients without overt reflux who have a positive pH probe study and persistence of respiratory symptoms during anti-reflux measures may benefit from a second study to establish the effectiveness of the anti-reflux treatment, and to reconsider the correlation of reflux with the symptom of interest.

Therapy for Reflux-Associated Respiratory Disease

NONPHARMACOLOGIC

Gastroesophageal reflux can be treated in a variety of ways depending on the needs of the patient. Conservative, nonpharmacologic measures including thickening of infants's formula and appropriate body positioning may be effective for patients with repeated emesis in the absence of esophagitis or respiratory symptoms. Several other dietary measures have been recommended (151) and make good sense, but lack rigorous scientific backing. These measures include small and frequent feedings (based on the theory that increased gastric volume increases reflux), fasting for several hours before bedtime in the older child, weight reduction in the obese child, avoiding tight clothing, and avoiding foods known to have a detrimental effect on gastric acidity and/or lower esophageal sphincter tone (fatty foods, acid foods, coffee, and alcohol). The likelihood of excellent compliance with these recommendations is low.

Thickening

One tablespoon of rice cereal may be added to each ounce of formula to increase the caloric density (152). Patients with reflux and failure to thrive may benefit most from this approach. The use of this therapy in infants with respiratory symptoms requires further study, since it may increase coughing (152).

Positioning

Body position influences gastroesophageal reflux (53, 54, 153). Because the gastroesophageal junction is posterior to the stomach, the semi-reclining seated position or the supine position cause it to be below the air-fluid interface when the stomach is full (Fig. 44.8)

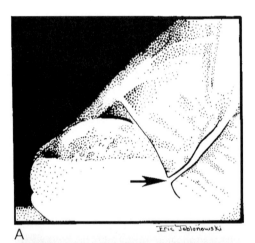

A

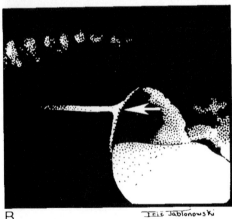

B

Figure 44.8. Drawing taken from barium swallow with infant seated in the semi-reclining position, showing the gastroesophageal junction to below the air-fluid level *(A)* and in contrast, with the infant prone, showing the gastroesophageal junction to be above the air-fluid level *(B)*.

(154). In this position, transient lower esophageal sphincter relaxations are more likely to result in gastroesophageal reflux than when the gastroesophageal junction is "above water" with the infant in other positions. Therefore, infants with significant reflux and respiratory disease should be positioned prone in the *post-prandial period*, when reflux is most likely. Elevation of the head in the prone position provides little benefit beyond that found in flat-prone positioning (155).

These conservative measures should be continued in patients with more severe reflux or its complications, even when pharmacologic agents are required.

PHARMACOLOGIC TREATMENT

Prokinetic Agents

Several medications are available that decrease reflux.

Metoclopramide. A dopamine antagonist, metoclopramide stimulates gastric motility and increases the pressure of the lower esophageal sphincter (156). Infants and older children are treated with 0.1 mg/kg/dose, given four times a day (one-half hour before meals and at bedtime). Side effects at this dose are infrequent, but include irritability and extrapyramidal effects. Dosing errors must be assiduously avoided because of troublesome extrapyramidal symptoms at higher doses; when such symptoms occur acutely, they may be treated with diphenhydramine if necessary.

Bethanechol. Bethanechol, a cholinergic agonist that promotes gastric motility, has been reported to be variably successful in patients with reflux (157–159). However, it may provoke bronchospasm (160) and is best avoided as initial therapy in patients with wheezing. It may be useful in infants who do not respond to metoclopramide therapy but it should be started under close supervision.

Other prokinetic agents are available abroad and include cisapride and domperidone. Their use in this country is currently investigational.

Anti-Acid Agents

Antacids. Although useful for the acute amelioration of discomfort due to esophagitis, antacid solutions (e.g., magnesium hydroxide, aluminum hydroxide, calcium carbonate) are seldom indicated for long-term treatment of esophagitis. At conventional dosing intervals, the acid-neutralizing capacity of antacids is overwhelmed by ongoing gastric acid secretion (161). Excessive use of antacids may lead to metabolic alkalosis.

H₂ Receptor Blockers. Type 2 histamine receptor antagonists (H_2 blockers) are commonly employed in children to reduce gastric acid output, thereby resulting in gastric contents with less potential to damage the esophageal mucosa, although digestive enzymes or bile may still cause injury (162, 163). Combined with metoclopramide to decrease reflux, cimetidine has become a mainstay in treatment of esophagitis in children. Its dose is 5–10 mg/kg/dose four times a day, given on the same schedule as for metoclopramide. Treatment should be continued for 2 months, or until reflux resolves clinically.

Ranitidine, famotidine, and nizatidine are newer alternatives to cimetidine; their advantages include less frequent administration, but their use in infants is as yet incompletely evaluated.

Sucralfate

The aluminum salt of sucrose sulfate, sucralfate binds to mucosal proteins and has emerged as an effective agent in the treatment of peptic ulcer disease, but evidence to support its use in the treatment of esophagitis in children is limited. In a comparative study, children with endoscopic evidence of esophagitis were treated with cimetidine, sucralfate tablets, or sucralfate suspension, with no statistically significant difference in outcome among the groups (164). However, there was no histologic assessment of the esophageal mucosa in these patients, without which the true prevalence of esophagitis is likely underestimated (139).

Other Agents

Omeprazole, a hydrogen-potassium adenosine triphosphatase inhibitor, may be the most effective treatment for severe esophagitis in adults (165), but it has not been adequately studied in children.

SURGICAL TREATMENT

Spontaneous resolution of reflux is anticipated in approximately 90% of otherwise normal infants within the first year of life, and in many of the remainder in the second year (166). Spontaneous resolution is less frequent in children who become symptomatic after infancy. Surgical treatment should be reserved for patients unlikely to have spontaneous resolution (such as those with neurologic impairment) (167, 168), and for patients with persistent sequelae of reflux (such as growth failure, esophagitis, and bronchopulmonary disease) despite maximal medical management (73). Nissen fundoplication is the surgical procedure of choice in most situations (73), but situations such as esophageal atresia, with disordered esophageal motility, make a loose wrap advisable.

SPECIAL CONSIDERATIONS IN PATIENTS WITH CONCOMITANT RESPIRATORY DISEASE

In general, the treatment of reflux in children with respiratory disorders is the same as for other children. However, some infants who present with apnea or recurrent pulmonary symptoms have comparatively little overt reflux, and only mildly increased reflux on pH probe. Although one might choose conservative (nonpharmacologic, nonsurgical) management of the reflux in the absence of the other symptoms, the more serious respiratory complications suggest the need for more aggressive anti-reflux therapy. These patients can be treated with metoclopramide, and cimetidine can be added if esophagitis is present on biopsy.

Consideration should also be given to modifying respiratory therapies, including drugs, that provoke reflux. There are some children with difficult-to-control "asthma" who are found to have reflux, and whose symptoms resolve entirely when all their medications are discontinued. Presumably, their bronchodilators caused or worsened reflux, and reflux caused increased bronchial reactivity. Chest physiotherapy in the head-down position should be performed before, rather than after, meals. Patients who are intubated, mechanically ventilated, and receiving boluses of enteral feed by nasogastric tube should be positioned on their right side, perhaps with the head of the bed elevated, following meals. In these patients, the supine position should be avoided in the postprandial period when possible.

Exposure to tobacco smoke should be avoided by all, particularly by those patients with reflux and respiratory symptoms. Nicotine, perhaps with concomitant adrenergic stimulation, decreases lower esophageal sphincter tone, thereby increasing the frequency of reflux (169–171). The additional respiratory effects are obvious. To date, the effects of passive smoking on reflux are undefined, but it may be of clinical importance and should be avoided.

ACKNOWLEDGEMENT

This chapter contains material adapted from Putnam PE, Ricker DH, Orenstein SR. Gastroesophageal reflux. In Beckerman RC, Brouilette R, Hunt C, eds. *Respiratory control disorders in infants and children.* Baltimore, Williams & Wilkins, 1993; and Orenstein SR. Dysphagia and vomiting. In Wyllie R, Hyams JS, eds. *Pediatric gastrointestinal disease: Pathophysiology, diagnosis, management.* Philadelphia, WB Saunders, 1993. The authors were supported in part by NIH grant R01HL35334 to D. Orenstein, NIH grant HD21445 to S. Orenstein, and the Cystic Fibrosis Foundation.

REFERENCES

1. Lear C, Flanagan J, Moorrees C. The frequency of deglutition in man. *Arch Oral Biol* 1965; 10:83–99.
2. Koenig J, Davies A, Thach B. Coordination of breathing, sucking, and swallowing during bottle feedings in human infants. *J Appl Physiol* 1990; 69:1623–1629.
3. Decktor D, Allen M, Robinson M. Esophageal motility, heartburn, and gastroesophageal reflux: Variations in clinical presentation of esophageal dysphagia. *Dysphagia* 1990; 5:211–215.
4. Buchholtz D. Neurologic causes of dysphagia. *Dysphagia* 1987; 1:152–156.
5. Clouse R, Lustman P. Psychiatric illness and contraction abnormalities of the esophagus. *N Engl J Med* 1983; 309:1337–1342.
6. Rosnagle R, Yanagisawa E. Aerophagia: An unrecognized complication of tracheotomy. *Arch Otolaryngol* 1968; 89:537.
7. Chapman K, Rebuck A. Dysphagia as a manifestation of occult hypoxemia. The role of oximetry during meal times. *Chest* 1991; 99:1030–1032.
8. Wyllie E, Wyllie R, Cruse R, Rothner A, Erenberg E. The mechanism of nitrazepam-induced drooling and aspiration. *N Engl J Med* 1986; 314:35–38.
9. Putnam P, Orenstein S, Pang D, Proujansky R, Kocoshis S. Cricopharyngeal achalasia associated with Arnold-Chiari malformation (ACM). *Pediatr Res* 1990; 27:113A.
10. Jones B, Donner M. Examination of the patient with dysphagia. *Radiology* 1988; 167:319–326.
11. Ott D, Gelfand D, Wu W, Chen Y. Radiological evaluation of dysphagia. *JAMA* 1986; 256:2718–2721.
12. Davidson G, Dent J, Willing J. Monitoring of upper oesophageal sphincter pressure in children. *Gut* 1991; 32:607–611.
13. Lindor K, Ott B, Hughes R Jr. Balloon dilation of upper digestive tract strictures. *Gastroenterology* 1985; 89:545–548.
14. Bourgeois N, Coffernils M, Buset M, Gelin M, Deltenre M, Panzer JM, Cremer M. Management of dysphagia in suspected esophageal motor disorders. *Dig Dis Sci* 1991; 36:268–273.
15. Dinari G, Danziger Y, Mimouni M, Rosenbach Y, Zahavi I, Grunebaum M. Cricopharyngeal dysfunction in childhood: Treatment by dilatations. *J Pediatr Gastroenterol Nutr* 1987; 6:212–216.
16. Frank M, Gatewood O. Transient pharyngeal incoordination in the newborn. *Am J Dis Child* 1966; 111:1966.
17. Bluestone C, Stool S, Sieber W, Sieber A. Congenital cricopharyngeal achalasia. *Ann Otol* 1977; 86:603–610.
18. Berg H, Jacobs J, Persky M, Cohen N. Cricopharyngeal myotomy: A review of surgical result in patients with cricopharyngeal achalasia of neurogenic origin. *Laryngoscope* 1985; 95:1337–1340.
19. Clouse R, Lustman P, Eckert T, Ferney D, Griffith L. Low-dose trazodone for symptomatic patients with esophageal contraction abnormalities. *Gastroenterology* 1987; 92:1027–1036.
20. Traube M, McCallum R. Primary oesophageal motility disorders: Current therapeutic concepts. *Drugs* 1985; 30:66–77.
21. Joley S, Johnson D, Herbst J, Pena A, Garnier R. An assessment of gastroesophageal reflux in children by extended monitoring of the distal esophagus. *Surgery* 1978; 84:16–22.
22. Paton J, MacFadyen U, Simpson H. Sleep phase and gastroesophageal reflux in infants at possible risk of SIDS. *Arch Dis Child* 1989; 64:264–269.
23. Kahrilas P, Dodds W, Dent J, Haeberle B, Hogan W, Arndorfer R. Effect of sleep, spontaneous gastroesophageal reflux, and a meal on upper esophageal sphincter pressure in normal human volunteers. *Gastroenterology* 1987; 92:466–471.
24. Barnes P. Neural control of human airways in health and disease. *Am Rev Respir Dis* 1986; 134:1289–1314.
25. Wynne J, Modell J. Respiratory aspiration of stomach contents. *Ann Intern Med* 1977; 87:466–474.
26. Pellegrini C, DeMeester T, Johnson L, Skinner D. Gastroesophageal reflux and pulmonary aspiration: Incidence, functional abnormality, and results of surgical therapy. *Surgery* 1979; 86:110–119.
27. Huxley E, Viroslav J, Gray W, Pierce A. Pharyngeal aspiration in normal adults and patients with depressed consciousness. *Am J Med* 1978; 64:564–568.
28. Crausaz F, Favez G. Aspiration of solid food particles into lungs of patients with gastroesophageal reflux and chronic bronchial disease. *Chest* 1988; 93:376–378.
29. Widdicombe J. Respiratory reflexes from the trachea and bronchi of the cat. *J Physiol* 1954; 123:55–70.

30. Tuchman D, Boyle J, Pack A, et al. Comparison of airway responses following tracheal or esophageal acidification in the cat. *Gastroenterology* 1984; 87:872–881.

31. Bray G. Recent advances in the treatment of asthma and hay fever. *Practitioner* 1934; 133:368–379.

32. Spaulding H, Mansfield L, Stein M, Sellner J, Gremillion D. Further investigation of the association between gastroesophageal reflux and bronchoconstriction. *J Allergy Clin Immunol* 1982; 69:516–521.

33. Mansfield L, Stein M. Gastroesophageal reflux and asthma: A possible reflex mechanism. *Ann Allergy* 1978; 41:224–226.

34. Davis R, Larsen G, Grunstein M. Respiratory response to intraesophageal acid infusion in asthmatic children during sleep. *J Allergy Clin Immunology* 1983; 72:393–398.

35. Mansfield L, Hameister H, Spaulding H, Smith N, Glab N. The role of the vagus nerve in airway narrowing caused by intraesophageal hydrochloric acid provocation and esophageal distention. *Ann Allergy* 1981; 47:431–434.

36. Andersen L, Schmidt A, Bundgaard A. Pulmonary function and acid application in the esophagus. *Chest* 1986; 90:358–363.

37. Denjean A, Herve P, Simonneau G, Lockhart A, Duroux P. Effects of acid infusion into the esophagus on airflow obstruction and bronchial hyperreactivity in adult asthmatic patients. *Chest* 1985; 5(Suppl):210S–202S.

38. Ekstrom T, Tibbling L. Gastroesophageal reflux and triggering of bronchial asthma: A negative report. *Eur J Respir Dis* 1987; 71:177–180.

39. Herve P, Denjean A, Jian R, Simonneau G, Duroux P. Intraesophageal perfusion of acid increases the bronchomotor response to methacholine and to isocapnic hyperventilation in asthmatic subjects. *Am Rev Respir Dis* 1986; 134:986–989.

40. Orenstein S, Orenstein D. Gastroesophageal reflux and respiratory disease in children. *J Pediatr* 1988; 112:847–858.

41. Mittal R, Rochester D, McCallum R. Sphincteric action of the diaphragm during a relaxed lower esophageal sphincter in humans. *Am J Physiol* 1989; 256:G139–G144.

42. Boyle J, Altschuler S, Patterson B, Pack A, Cohen S. Reflex inhibition of the lower esophageal sphincter (LES) following stimulation of pulmonary vagal afferent receptors [Abstract]. *Gastroenterology* 1986; 90:1353.

43. Johannesson N, Andersson K, Joelsson B, Persson C. Relaxation of the lower esophageal sphincter and stimulation of gastric secretion and diuresis by antiasthmatic xanthines. *Am Rev Respir Dis* 1985; 131:26–31.

44. Newell S, Booth I, Morgan M, McNeish A. Gastroesophageal reflux in the pre-term infant. *Pediatr Res* 1987; 22:104.

45. Vandenplas Y, De WD, Sacre L. Influence of xanthines on gastroesophageal reflux in infants at risk for sudden infant death syndrome. *Pediatrics* 1986; 77:807–810.

46. DiMarino A, Cohen S. Effect of an oral beta2-adrenergic agonist on lower esophageal sphincter pressure

47. in normals and in patients with achalasia. *Dig Dis Sci* 1982; 27:1063–1066.

47. Berquist WE, Rachelefsky GS, Rowshan N, Siegel S, Katz R, Welch M. Quantitative gastroesophageal reflux and pulmonary function in asthmatic children and normal adults receiving placebo, theophylline and metaproterenol sulfate therapy. *J Allergy Clin Immunol* 1984; 73:253–8.

48. Schindlbeck N, Heinrich C, RM H, Mueller–Lissner S. Effects of albuterol (salbutamol) on esophageal motility and gastroesophageal reflux in healthy volunteers. *JAMA* 1988; 260:3156–3158.

49. Spiliopoulos A, Megevand R. Oesophagite peptique stenosante apres sondage oeso-gastrique. *Helv Chir Acta* 1980; 47:527–532.

50. Berezin S, Schwarz S, Halata MS, Newman LJ. Gastroesophageal reflux secondary to gastrostomy tube placement. *Am J Dis Child* 1986; 140:699–701.

51. Ferry GD, Selby M, Pietro TJ. Clinical response to short-term nasogastric feeding in infants with gastroesophageal reflux and growth failure. *J Pediatr Gastroenterol Nutr* 1983; 2:57–61.

52. Hopper A, LK K, Stevenson D, et al. Detection of gastric contents in tracheal fluid of infants by lactose assay. *J Pediatr* 1983; 102:415–418.

53. Meyers WF, Herbst JJ. Effectiveness of positioning therapy for gastroesophageal reflux. *Pediatrics* 1982 69:768–772.

54. Yu V. Effect of body position on gastric emptying in the neonate. *Arch Dis Child* 1975; 500:500–504.

55. Martin R, Herrel N, Rubin D, Fanaroff A. Effect of supine and prone positions on arterial oxygen tension in the preterm infant. *Pediatrics* 1979; 63:528–531.

56. Foster A, Voyles J, Murphy S. Twenty-four-hour pH monitoring in children with cystic fibrosis: Association of chest physical therapy to gastroesophageal reflux. *Pediatr Res* 1983; 17:118A.

57. Vandenplas Y, Diericx A, Blecker U, Lanciers S, Deneyer M. Esophageal pH monitoring data during chest physiotherapy. *J Pediatr Gastroenterol Nutr* 1991; 13:23–26.

58. Mendelson C. The aspiration of stomach contents into the lungs during obstetric anesthesia. *Am J Obstet Gynecol* 1946; 52:191–205.

59. McVeagh P, Howman–Giles R, Kemp A. Pulmonary aspiration studied by radionuclide milk scanning and barium swallow roentgenography. *Am J Dis Child* 1987; 141:917–921.

60. Christie D, O'Grady L, Mack D. Incompetent lower esophageal sphincter and gastroesophageal reflux in recurrent acute pulmonary disease of infancy and childhood. *J Pediatr* 1978; 93:23–27.

61. Perlman L, Lerner E, D'Esopo N. Clinical classification and analysis of 97 cases of lung abscess. *Am Rev Respir Dis* 1969; 99:390–398.

62. Hardy K, Schidlow D, Zaeri N. Obliterative bronchiolitis in children. *Chest* 1988; 93:460–466.

63. Epstein P. Aspiration diseases of the lungs. In Fishman A, ed. *Pulmonary diseases and disorders.* New York, McGraw-Hill, 1988, pp 877–892.

64. Bannister W, Sattilaro A. Vomiting and aspiration during anesthesia. *Anesthesiology* 1962; 23:251–264.

65. Arms R, Dines D, Tinstman T. Aspiration pneumonia. *Chest* 1974; 65:136–139.

66. Mollitt DL, Golladay ES, Seibert JJ. Symptomatic gastroesophageal reflux following gastrostomy in neurologically impaired patients. *Pediatrics* 1985; 75:1124–6.

67. Sondheimer J, Morris B. Gastroesophageal reflux among severely retarded children. *J Pediatr* 1979; 94:710–714.

68. Wesley J, Coran A, Sarahan T, Klein M, White S. The need for evaluation of gastroesophageal reflux in brain-damaged children referred for feeding gastrostomy. *J Pediatr Surg* 1981; 16:866–870.

69. Hoyoux C, Forget P, Lambrechts L, Geubelle F. Chronic bronchopulmonary disease and gastro-esophageal reflux and the premature infant. *Pediatr Pulmonol* 1985; 1:149–153.

70. Martin M, Grunstein M, Larsen G. The relationship of gastroesophageal reflux to nocturnal wheezing in children with asthma. *Ann Allergy* 1982; 49:318–322.

71. Shapiro G, Christie D. Gastroesophageal reflux in steroid-dependent asthmatic youths. *Pediatrics* 1979; 63:207–212.

72. Berquist WE, Rachelefsky GS, Kadden M, Siegel SC, Katz RM, Mickey MR, Ament ME. Effect of theophylline on gastroesophageal reflux in normal adults. *J Allergy Clin Immunol* 1981; 67:407–11.

73. Andze G, Brandt M, St. Vil D, Bensoussan A, Blanchard H. Diagnosis and treatment of gastro-esophageal reflux in 500 children with respiratory symptoms: The value of pH monitoring. *J Pediatr Surg* 1991; 26:295–3000.

74. Jeffrey H, Rahilly P, Read D. Multiple causes of asphyxia in infants at high risk for sudden infant death. *Arch Dis Child* 1983; 58:92–100.

75. Henderson-Smart D, Read D. Reduced lung volume during behavioral active sleep in the newborn. *J Appl Physiol* 1979; 46:1081–1085.

76. Henderson-Smart D, Read D. Depression of intercostal and abdominal muscle activity and vulnerability to asphyxia during active sleep in the newborn. In Guilleminault C, Dement W, eds. *Sleep apnea syndromes: Proceedings of the Kroc Symposium 1977.* New York, AR Liss, 1978, pp 93–117.

77. Gustafsson P, Kjellman N, Tibbling L. Oesophageal function and symptoms in moderate and severe asthma. *Acta Paediatr Scand* 1986; 75:729–736.

78. Allen J, Wohl M. Pulmonary function in older children and young adults with gastroesophageal reflux. *Clin Pediatr* 1986; 25:541–546.

79. Hughes D, Spier S, Rivlin J, Levison H. Gastro-esophageal reflux during sleep in asthmatic patients. *J Pediatr* 1983; 102:666–672.

80. Lew C, Keens T, O'Neal M, et al. Gastroesophageal reflux recovery from bronchopulmonary dysplasia. *Clin Res* 1981; 29:149A.

81. Sindel B, Maisels M, Ballantine T. Gastroesophageal reflux to the proximal esophagus in infants with bronchopulmonary dysplasia. *Am J Dis Child* 1989; 143:1103–1106.

82. Hrabovsky EE, Mullett MD. Gastroesophageal reflux and the premature infant. *J Pediatr Surg* 1986; 21:583–587.

83. Sindel B, Maisels M, Ballantine T, Karl S. The effect of a Nissen fundoplication on infants with chronic lung disease. *Pediatr Res* 1985; 19:365A.

84. Motoyama E, Fort M, Klesh K, Mutich R, Guthrie R. Early onset of airway reactivity in premature infants with bronchopulmonary dysplasia. *Am Rev Respir Dis* 1987; 136:50–57.

85. Hazinski T. Bronchopulmonary dysplasia. In Chernick V, Kendig E, eds. *Disorders of the respiratory tract in children.* Philadelphia, WB Saunders, 1990, pp 300–320.

86. Bendig DW, Seilheimer DK, Wagner ML, Ferry GD, Barrison GM. Complications of gastroesophageal reflux in patients with cystic fibrosis. *J Pediatr* 1982; 100:536–540.

87. Scott RB, OLoughlin EV, Gall DG. Gastroesophageal reflux in patients with cystic fibrosis. *J Pediatr* 1985; 106:223–227.

88. Dab I, Malfroot A. Gastroesophageal reflux: A primary defect in cystic fibrosis? *Scand J Gastroenterol* 1988; 23(Suppl 143):125–131.

89. Stringer D, Sprigg A, Juodis E, Corey M, Daneman A, Levison H, Durie P. The association of cystic fibrosis, gastroesophageal reflux and reduced pulmonary function. *Can Assoc Radiol* 1988; 39:100–102.

90. Vinocur CD, Marmon L, Schidlow DV, Weintraub WH. Gastroesophageal reflux in the infant with cystic fibrosis. *Am J Surg* 1985; 149:182–6.

91. Cucchiara S, Santamaria F, Andreotti M, et al. Mechanisms of gastro-esophageal reflux in cystic fibrosis. *Arch Dis Child* 1991; 66:617–622.

92. Dudgeon D, Colombani P, Beaver B. Tracheo-esophageal fistula and esophageal atresia. In Rudolph A, Hoffman J, eds. *Pediatrics.* Norwalk, CT, Appleton & Lange, 1987, pp 909–911.

93. Dudley N, Phelan P. Respiratory complications in long-term survivors of oesophageal atresia. *Arch Dis Child* 1976; 51:279–282.

94. Desjardins J, Stephens C, Moes C. Results of surgical treatment of congenital tracheo-esophageal fistula, with a note on cine-fluorographic findings. *Ann Surg* 1964; 160:141–145.

95. Whitington P, Shermeta D, Seto D, Jones L, Hendrix T. Role of lower esophageal sphincter incompetence in recurrent pneumonia after repair of esophageal atresia. *J Pediatr* 1977; 91:550–554.

96. Parker A, Christie D, Cahill J. Incidence and significance of gastroesophageal reflux following repair of esophageal atresia and tracheoesophageal fistula and the need for anti-reflux procedures. *J Pediatr Surg* 1979; 14:5–8.

97. Laks H, Wilkinson R, Schuster S. Long-term results following correction of esophageal atresia with tracheoesophageal fistula: A clinical and cinefluorographic study. *J Pediatr Surg* 1972; 7:591–597.

98. Chrispin A, Friedland G, Waterston D. Aspiration pneumonia and dysphagia after technically successful repair of oesophageal atresia. *Thorax* 1966; 21:104–110.

99. Shepard R, Fenn S, Sieber W. Evaluation of esophageal function in postoperative esophageal atresia and tracheoesophageal fistula. *Surgery* 1966; 59:608–617.

100. Emery J, Haddadin A. Squamous epithelium in respiratory tract of children with tracheo-oesophageal fistula. *Arch Dis Child* 1971; 46:236–242.

101. Nakazato Y, Wells T, Landing B. Abnormal tracheal innervation in patients with esophageal atresia and

tracheo-esophageal fistula: Study of the intrinsic tracheal nerve plexuses by a microdissection technique. *J Pediatr Surg* 1986; 21:838–844.

102. Menon A, Schefft G, Thach B. Frequency and significance of swallowing during prolonged apnea in infants. *Am Rev Respir Dis* 1984; 130:969–973.

103. Herbst J, Book L, Bray P. Gastroesophageal reflux in the "near miss" sudden infant death syndrome. *J Pediatr* 1978; 92:73–75.

104. Herbst J, Minton S, Book L. Gastroesophageal reflux causing respiratory distress and apnea in newborn infants. *J Pediatr* 1979; 95:763–768.

105. Menon A, Schefft G, Thach B. Apnea associated with regurgitation in infants. *J Pediatr* 1985; 106:625–629.

106. MacFadyen U, Hendry G, Simpson H. Gastro-oesophageal reflux in near-miss sudden infant death syndrome or suspected recurrent aspiration. *Arch Dis Child* 1983; 58:87–91.

107. Berquist W, Ament M. Upper GI function in sleeping infants. *Am Rev Respir Dis* 1985; 131(Suppl):S29–S32.

108. Spitzer A, Boyle J, Tuchman D, Fox W. Awake apnea associated with gastroesophageal reflux: A specific clinical syndrome. *J Pediatr* 1984; 104:200–205.

109. Perkett E, Vaughan R. Evidence for laryngeal chemoreflex in some human preterm infants. *Acta Paediatr Scand* 1982; 71:969–972.

110. Downing S, Lee J. Laryngeal chemosensitivity: A possible mechanism for sudden infant death. *Pediatrics* 1975; 55:640–649.

111. Harned H Jr., Myracle J, Ferreiro J. Respiratory suppression and swallowing from introduction of fluids into the laryngeal region of the lamb. *Pediatr Res* 1978; 12:1003–1009.

112. Walsh J, Farrell M, Keenen W, Lucas M, Kramer M. Gastroesophageal reflux in infants: Relation to apnea. *J Pediatr* 1981; 99:197–201.

113. Ariagno R, Guilleminault C, Baldwin R, Owen-Boeddiker M. Movement and gastroesophageal reflux in awake term infants with "near miss" SIDS, unrelated to apnea. *J Pediatr* 1982; 100:894–897.

114. Sacre L, Vandenplas Y. Gastroesophageal reflux associated with respiratory abnormalities during sleep. *J Pediatr Gastroenterol Nutr* 1989; 9:28–33.

115. Rosen C, Frost J, Harrison G. Infant polygraphic studies and follow-up monitoring. *Pediatrics* 1983; 71:731–736.

116. Leape L, Holder T, Franklin J, Amoury R, Ashcraft K. Respiratory arrest in infants secondary to gastroesophageal reflux. *Pediatrics* 1977; 60:924–928.

117. Ramenofsky M, Leape L. Continuous upper esophageal pH monitoring in infants and children with gastroesophageal reflux, pneumonia and apneic spells. *J Pediatr Surg* 1981; 16:374–378.

118. See C, Newman L, Berezin S., Glassman M, Meadow M, Dozor A, Schwartz S. Gastroesophageal reflux-induced hypoxemia in infants with apparent life-threatening event(s). *Am J Dis Child* 1989; 143:951–954.

119. Veereman-Wauters G, Bochner A, Van Caillie-Bertrand M. Gastroesophageal reflux in infants with a history of near–miss sudden infant death. *J Pediatr Gastroenterol Nutr* 1991; 12:319–323.

120. Henry R, Mellis C. Resolution of inspiratory stridor after fundoplication: Case report. *Aust Paediatr J* 1982; 18:126–127.

121. Nielson D, Heldt G, Tooley W. Stridor and gastroesophageal reflux in infants. *Pediatrics* 1990; 85:1034–1039.

122. Orenstein S, Orenstein D, Whitington PF. Gastroesophageal reflux causing stridor. *Chest* 1983; 84:301–302.

123. Orenstein S, Kocoshis S, Orenstein D, Proujansky R. Stridor and gastroesophageal reflux: diagnostic use of intraluminal esophageal acid perfusion (Bernstein Test). *Pediatr Pulmonol* 1987; 3:420–424.

124. Katz P. Ambulatory esophageal and hypopharyngeal pH monitoring in patients with hoarseness. *Am J Gastroenterol* 1990; 85:35–40.

125. Wiener G, Koufman J, Wu W, Cooper J, Richter J, Castell D. Chronic hoarseness secondary to gastroesophageal reflux disease: Documentation with 24-hour ambulatory pH monitoring. *Am J Gastroenterol* 1989; 84:1503–1508.

126. Wilson J, White A, vonHaacke N, Maran A, Heading R, Pryde A, Piris J. Gastroesophageal reflux and posterior laryngitis. *Ann Otol Rhinol* 1989; 98:405–510.

127. Hallewell J, Cole T. Isolated head and neck symptoms due to hiatus hernia. *Arch Otolaryngol* 1970; 92:499–501.

128. Putnam P, Orenstein S. Hoarseness in a child with gastroesophageal reflux. *Acta Paediatr Scand* 1992; 81:635–636.

129. Irwin R, Zawacki J, Curley F, French C, Hoffman P. Chronic cough as the sole presenting manifestation of gastroesophageal reflux. *Am Rev Respir Dis* 1989; 140:1294–1300.

130. Feranchak A, Orenstein S, Cohn J. Behaviors associated with gastroesophageal reflux episodes in infants: A study using pH probe and split-screen video. *Pediatr Res* 1990; 27:9A.

131. Shay S, Myers R, Johnson L. Hiccups associated with reflux esophagitis. *Gastroenterology* 1984; 87:201–207.

132. Gluck M, Pope C II. Chronic hiccups and gastroesophageal reflux disease: the acid perfusion test as a provocative maneuver. *Ann Intern Med* 1986; 105:219–220.

133. Sondheimer J. Continuous monitoring of distal esophageal pH: A diagnostic test for gastroesophageal reflux in infants. *J Pediatr* 1980; 96:804–807.

134. Heyman S, Kirkpatrick J, Winter H, Treves S. An improved radionuclide method for the diagnosis of gastroesophageal reflux and aspiration in children (milk scan). *Radiology* 1979; 131:479–482.

135. Heyman S, Respondek M. Detection of pulmonary aspiration in children by radionuclide "salivagram". *J Nucl Med* 1989; 30:697–699.

136. Hillemeier A, Lange R, McCallum R, et al. Delayed gastric emptying in infants with gastroesophageal reflux. *J Pediatr* 1981; 98:190–193.

137. Fawcett H, Hayden C, Adams J, Swischuk L. How useful is gastroesophageal reflux scintigraphy in suspected childhood aspiration. *Pediatr Radiol* 1988; 18:311–313.

138. Leonidas J. Gastroesophageal reflux in infants: Role of the upper gastrointestinal series. *AJR* 1984; 143:1350–1351.

139. Biller J, Winter H, Grand R, Allred E. Are endoscopic changes predictive of histologic esophagitis in children. *J Pediatr* 1983; 103:215–218.

140. Hyams J, Ricci A Jr, Leightner A. Clinical and laboratory correlates of esophagitis in young children. *J Pediatr Gastroenterol Nutr* 1988; 7:52–56.

141. Werlin S, Dodds W, Hogan W, et al. Mechanisms of gastroesophageal reflux in children. *J Pediatr* 1980; 97:244–249.

141a. Orenstein S, Orenstein D. Gastroesophageal reflux and respiratory disease in childen. *J Pediatr* 1988; 112:847–858.

142. Bernstein L, Baker L. A clinical test for esophagitis. *Gastroenterology* 1958; 34:760–780.

143. Williams H, Freeman M. Milk inhalation pneumonia: The significance of fat filled macrophages in tracheal secretions. *Aust Paediatr J* 1973; 9:286–288.

144. Colombo J, Hallberg T. Recurrent aspiration in children: lipid-laden alveolar macrophage quantitation. *Pediatr Pulmonol* 1987; 3:86–89.

145. Brand J, Brodsky N, Hurt H. No evidence of aspiration in intubated infants fed by orogastric (OG) or oroduodenal (OD) routes. *Pediatr Res* 1986; 20:405A.

146. Stagus R, Martin A, Binns G, Steven I. The significance of fat-filled macrophages in the diagnosis of aspiration associated with gastro-oesophageal reflux. *Aust Paediatr J* 1985; 21:275–277.

147. McCauley R, Darling D, Leonidas J, Schwartz A. Gastroesophageal reflux in children: A useful classification and reliable physiologic technique for its demonstration. *Am J Roentgenol* 1978; 130:47–50.

148. Chernow B, Johnson L, Janowitz W, Castell D. Pulmonary aspiration as a consequence of gastroesophageal reflux: A diagnostic approach. *Dig Dis Sci* 1979; 24:839–844.

149. Fisher R, Malmud L, Roberts G, Lobis I. Gastroesophageal (GE) scintiscanning to detect and quantitate GE reflux. *Gastroenterology* 1976; 70:301–308.

150. Stein M, Ghaed N. An isotope study of pulmonary aspiration of gastric contents in asthmatics with gastroesophageal reflux (GER). *Am Rev Respir Dis* 1978; 117:82.

151. Orenstein S. Gastroesophageal reflux. *Curr Prob Pediatr* 1991; 21:193–241.

152. Orenstein S, Magill H, Brooks P. Thickening of infant feedings for therapy of gastroesophageal reflux. *J Pediatr* 1987; 110(2):181–186.

153. Orenstein S, Whitington PF. Positioning for prevention of infant gastroesophageal reflux. *J Pediatr* 1983; 103:534–537.

154. Orenstein S, Whitington P, Orenstein DM. The infant seat as treatment for gastroesophageal reflux. *N Engl J Med* 1983; 309:760–763.

155. Orenstein S. Prone positioning in infant gastroesophageal reflux: Is elevation of the head worth the trouble? *J Pediatr* 1990; 117:184–187.

156. Hyams J, Leichtner A, Zamett L, Walters J. Effect of metoclopramide on prolonged intraesophageal pH testing in infants with gastroesophageal reflux. *J Pediatr Gastroenterol Nutr* 1986; 5:716–720.

157. Strickland AD, Chang JH. Results of treatment of gastroesophageal reflux with bethanechol. *J Pediatr* 1983; 103(2):311–5.

158. Sondheimer J, Mintz H, Michaels M. Bethanechol treatment of gastroesophageal reflux in infants: Effect on continuous esophageal pH records. *J Pediatr* 1984; 104:128–131.

159. Orenstein S, Lofton S, Orenstein D. Bethanechol for pediatric gastroesophageal reflux: A prospective, blind, controlled study. *J Pediatr Gastroenterol Nutr* 1986; 5:549–555.

160. Taylor P. Cholinergic agonists. In Gilman A, Goodman L, Rall T, Murad F, eds. *The pharmacological basis of therapeutics*. New York, MacMillan, 1985, pp 100–109.

161. Cucchiara S, Staiano A, Romaniello G, Capobianco S, Auricchio S. Antacids and cimetidine treatment for gastro-oesophageal reflux and peptic oesophagitis. *Arch Dis Child* 1984; 59:842–847.

162. Fiasse R, Hanin C, Lepot A, Descamps C, Lamy Dive D. Controlled trial of cimetidine in reflux esophagitis. *Dig Dis Sci* 1980; 25:750–755.

163. Cucchiara S, Gobio–Casali L, Balli F, et al. Cimetidine treatment of reflux esophagitis in children: An Italian multicentric study. *J Pediatr Gastroenterol Nutr* 1989; 8:150–156.

164. Arguelles-Martin F, Gonzalez-Fernande F, MG G. Sucralfate versus cimetidine in the treatment of reflux esophagitis in children. *Am J Med* 1989; 86(Suppl 6A):73–76.

165. Hetzel D, Dent J, Reed W, et al. Healing and relapse of severe peptic esophagitis after treatment with omeprazole. *Gastroenterology* 1988; 95:903–912.

166. Carre I. The natural history of the partial thoracic stomach (hiatus hernia) in children. *Arch Dis Child* 1959; 34:344–353.

167. Wilkinson J, Dudgeon D, Sondheimer J. A comparison of medical and surgical treatment of gastroesophageal reflux in severely retarded children. *J Pediatr* 1981; 99:201–205.

168. Byrne WJ, Euler AR, Ashcraft E, Nash DG, Seibert JJ, Golladay ES. Gastroesophageal reflux in the severely retarded who vomit: Criteria for and results of surgical intervention in twenty-two patients. *Surgery* 1982; 91:95–8.

169. Dennish G. Castell D. Inhibitory effect of smoking on the lower esophageal sphincter. *N Engl J Med* 1971; 284:1136–1137.

170. Stanciu C, Bennett J. Smoking and gastro-oesophageal reflux. *Br Med J* 1972; 3:793–795.

171. Cryer P, Haymond M, Santiago J, Shah S. Norepinephrine and epinephrine release and adrenergic mediation of smoking-associated hemodynamic and metabolic events. *N Engl J Med* 1976; 295:573–577.

45

Neuromuscular Disease

DEBORAH C. GIVAN

Respiratory failure is a well known sequela of the respiratory muscle weakness associated with neuromuscular disease. The importance of respiratory muscle function in chronic airway disease in adult disease has only recently been acknowledged. The unique properties and configuration of the infant chest—"the respiratory pump"—makes muscle failure a major factor in any respiratory disease affecting this age group. A better understanding of muscle mechanics, then, is essential to understanding pulmonary disease in pediatric patients.

This chapter will address the following aspects of respiratory muscle function: (a) functional anatomy, (b) structural organization of the muscles, (c) assessment of respiratory muscle function, (d) diseases that adversely affect respiratory muscle performance, and (e) treatment of respiratory muscle failure. Aspects unique to pediatrics will be included whenever data are available.

The mechanics of respiration deal with the respiratory muscle forces required to overcome both the elastic recoil of the lung and the resistance to flow through the airways. This and the fact that they are the only skeletal muscles whose repetitive and continuous function are essential for life differentiate them from other skeletal muscles whose major function is to overcome inertia. The three basic functions of the respiratory muscles are to support breathing, perform expulsive efforts (cough, vomiting, defecation), and to stabilize the thorax during physical labor. This chapter will discuss those aspects of respiratory muscle function related to breathing.

FUNCTIONAL ANATOMY

The diaphragm is the primary muscle of inspiration. The sole motor supply to the dia- phragm is the phrenic nerve (C5-C7). The function of the diaphragm in adults has been recently reviewed and only a brief overview will be given here (1). The function of the diaphragm can best be understood if the diaphragm is conceived as a collapsible cylinder topped by a dome (Fig. 45.1). The part of the diaphragm adjacent and parallel to the rib cage (the cylinder portion) is the zone of apposition. Inspiration occurs by two different mechanical actions. The *appositional component* begins when muscle contraction decreases muscle fiber length along the zone of apposition, resulting in a piston-like descent of the dome (Fig. 45.1). The concomitant rise in intra-abdominal pressure expands the lower rib cage. These combined motions increase the depth and width of the chest. The *insertional action* occurs as the costal fibers of the diaphragm contract and shorten. For this phase, the abdominal viscera and muscles

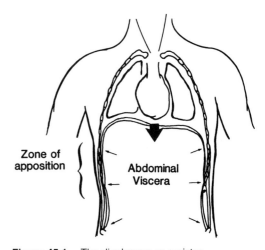

Figure 45.1. The diaphragm as a piston.

maintain the cranial orientation of the costal muscles and act as a fulcrum for the diaphragm to lift the lower ribs and rotate them outward.

Respiration in the infant requires great energy expenditure. The infant chest is circular rather than elliptic, and the diaphragm inserts horizontally. This decreases the zone of apposition, thus decreasing the distance of diaphragm descent. The infant's compliant chest wall also distorts when the diaphragm contracts. The infant is most compromised during rapid eye movement (REM) sleep when contraction of the intercostal muscles is inhibited, thus depriving the chest wall of muscular support (2).

The remaining chest wall muscles are considered accessory muscles of respiration. The internal intercostals consist of a parasternal portion, which contracts during inspiration, rotating the chondrosternal junctions and elevating the lower ribs, and an interosseous portion, which contracts during expiration. The function of the external intercostals, which also contract during inspiration, is unclear, but it is probable that together with the interosseous intercostals they participate in the rotation of the trunk (3). The scalenes appear to contract synchronously with the diaphragm; the parasternals expand the upper rib cage as do the sternocleidomastoid, hyoid muscles, and platysma (1).

Although primarily muscles of expiration, the abdominal muscles contract tonically during inspiration, lengthening the diaphragm and preventing excessive shortening. Just prior to inspiration these muscles relax, allowing lung volume to increase.

The primary function of the abdominal muscles is to perform expulsive maneuvers (i.e., coughing) or to exhale in the presence of obstructive airway disease. These maneuvers are accomplished by displacing the diaphragm upward and pulling lower ribs down and outward.

STRUCTURAL ORGANIZATION OF THE MUSCLES

Respiratory muscles are striated, and the motor units can be classified into two muscle fiber groups based on their histochemical staining for glycogen stores and their contractile properties. Fibers with low glycogen stores are high in oxidative capacity and have excellent endurance. These fibers are *slow twitch*. Fibers with low oxidative activity are *fast twitch*—they are stronger but with poor endurance. The fast twitch fiber can be divided into fatigue resistant, fatigue intermediate, and fatigable categories by the tendency of the fiber to fatigue during repetitive activity (4). The respiratory muscle fiber composition changes markedly from the fetus to early childhood. Although premature infants have less than 10% high-oxidative, slow twitch fibers in the diaphragm, the newborn infant has 25% (5). The adult diaphragm contains approximately 30% slow twitch fibers, 4% fast fatigue resistant, 25% fast fatigue intermediate, and 42% fast fatiguable (4). Fiber type is an important determinant of respiratory muscle endurance, as will be discussed later.

ASSESSMENT OF RESPIRATORY MUSCLE FUNCTION

Muscle performance is assessed by its strength, endurance, and ability to resist fatigue. Although some of these properties can be measured and extrapolated in limb muscle and animal models, these parameters cannot be assessed directly in human respiratory muscles. Some of these parameters can be measured indirectly by evaluating aspects of lung function dependent on the actions of these muscles.

Muscle Strength

Respiratory muscle strength (RMS) is determined by a patient's age, sex, and general muscle development, and on these muscle properties: the length-tension relationship, the force-velocity relationship, the force-frequency relationship, and the integrity of the contractile apparatus. The length-tension relationship proposes that a muscle generates its greatest force when it is at its resting (optimal) length. Muscle tension decreases as the muscle shortens or is stretched (Fig. 45.2). The force-velocity relationship proposes that the force of muscle contraction decreases with increasing speed of muscle contraction if stimulus frequency remains unchanged (Fig. 45.3). The force-frequency relationship states that the force of muscle contraction increases as the stimulation frequency increases and emphasizes the role of neural drive in determining muscle contractile force (Fig. 45.4).

Using a pressure gauge to occlude the airway, one can measure RMS by obtaining

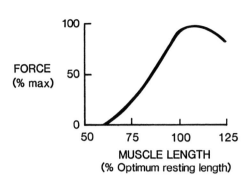

Figure 45.2. The length tension curve of a normal diaphragm. Force (tension) is the percentage of maximum tension developed during isometric contraction. Length is percentage of the optimum resting length. (From Rochester DF, Braun NMT. The respiratory muscles. *Basics RD* 1978; 6:1.)

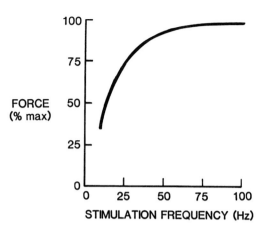

Figure 45.4. The force frequency curve of a normal diaphragm where force is the percentage of maximum force attained during isometric contraction and stimulation frequency is the rate of a supramaximal stimulus to the phrenic nerve. (From Rochester DF, Arora NS. The respiratory muscles in asthma. In Lavietes MH, Reichman LB, eds. *Diagnostic aspects and management of asthma.* Norwalk, CT, Purdue Frederick, 1981.)

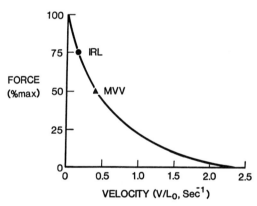

Figure 45.3. The force-velocity curve of a normal diaphragm. Force is the percent maximum force attained during isometric contraction. Velocity is the ratio of the actual velocity (V) to the optimum muscle resting length (L_o). The triangle describes the force velocity relationship during maximum voluntary ventilation (MVV); the circle during inspiratory resistive loading (IRL). (From Rochester DF. Fatigue of the diaphragm. In Fishman AP, ed. *Pulmonary diseases and disorders update.* New York, McGraw-Hill, 1982.)

inspiratory (P_I max) and expiratory (P_E max) static pressures at the mouth. P_I max is measured after expiration to residual volume (RV), and P_E max is measured at total lung capacity (TLC) (Fig. 45.5). These parameters can be adversely affected by intrinsic pulmonary disease, neuromuscular disease, and poor effort. Inspiratory muscle strength can also be assessed by measuring the transdiaphragmatic pressure (P_{di}). This measurement is obtained by inserting a balloon catheter into the esoph-

agus to measure esophageal pressure (P_{es}), which approximates pleural pressure, and into the stomach to measure gastric pressure (P_{ga}). The P_{di} is the difference between P_{es} and P_{ga} and is measured during a maximal inspiratory effort against a closed glottis (Mueller maneuver). Although technically valuable it is not usually practical in children.

Pulmonary function tests may be helpful in evaluating RMS, usually showing a restrictive pattern when RMS is decreased. The RV is usually increased with expiratory muscle weakness, resulting in a decreased forced vital capacity. TLC is decreased when inspiratory muscle weakness is present.

Muscle Endurance

Respiratory muscle endurance (the capacity to sustain high levels of ventilation) is a function of muscle fiber type, adequacy of blood supply, integrity of contractile elements, and the pattern of contraction. It is quantified by relating the level of ventilation to the time it can be sustained. The endurance can be measured by calculating the *tension-time index* of the diaphragm (TTI_{di}) (6). This is done by multiplying the contractile force by the transdiaphragmatic pressure measured during a breath (P_{di} breath), then dividing by the maximum transdiaphragmatic pressure (P_{di} max) and the time

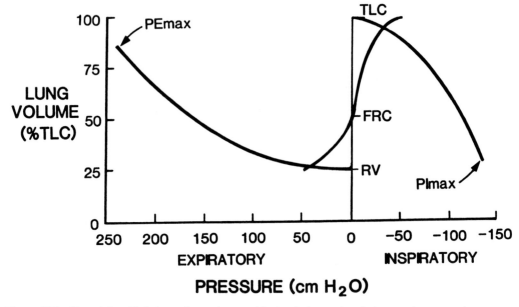

Figure 45.5.   The relationship between lung volume and the inspiratory and expiratory maximum muscle pressures. Pressures are expressed as a percentage of maximum, and lung volumes are expressed as a percentage of TLC. (From Rochester DF, Braun NMT. The respiratory muscles. *Basics RD* 1978; 6:1.)

of inspiration (measured as a fraction of the duration of the respiratory cycle.)

A less invasive but less reproducible way of determining respiratory muscle endurance is the maximum voluntary ventilation (MVV), which is measured by having the patient breathe as quickly and deeply as possible for 10–12 seconds, then extrapolating this ventilatory volume to 1 minute. The maximal sustainable ventilatory capacity (MSVC) is the level of ventilation that can be sustained for 15 minutes or longer and is approximately 60–80% of MVV in normal patients, usually calculated rather than directly measured. Both the absolute and relative levels of MSVC may be increased by endurance training, to be discussed later.

Muscle Fatigue

Muscle fatigue is the reversible decrease in muscle strength or force as a result of exertion (7). Mechanisms of muscle fatigue may be one or all of three reversible types (8):

1. *Central fatigue.* Decrease in central drive caused by muscle overuse, either motivational or nonmotivational.
2. *Transmission fatigue.* Impairment or blockage of neural impulse transmission at the axonal

branch, neuromuscular junction, or muscle membrane level (9).

3. *Contractile fatigue.* Failure of muscle contraction after neural stimulation. High-frequency fatigue, the failure to respond to high stimulation frequency of 50–100 Hz, recovers quickly and may be caused by accumulation of toxic metabolic products, altered calcium or electrolyte balance, or decreased energy supplies. In low-frequency fatigue, the failure to respond to low stimulation of 10–20 Hz, recovery takes 24 hours or longer and may be caused by minor muscle injury (7).

Respiratory muscle fatigue can be measured by direct tests such as determining the P_i max or P_{di} max before and after fatiguing efforts or measuring the length of time a maximum voluntary effort can be performed. These two tests are unable to differentiate among the types of fatigue and depend on patient effort. Electrical stimulation of the phrenic nerve with measurement of the conduction time or measurement of the P_{di} at increasing stimulation frequencies differentiates the cause of fatigue, but this technique is painful, and it is very difficult to confirm maximal stimulation of the nerve in humans.

Clinical evaluation of muscle fatigue is a helpful but poorly sensitive technique. Thoracic cage inspection may show chest wall movements that are out of phase with the abdomen (paradoxical breathing). This type of breathing, as well as use of accessory muscles of respiration, increases with approaching fatigue. Paradoxical breathing, however, may be normal in the infant and may more commonly reflect an increased respiratory load in the older child or adult. Inductive plethysmography can be used to measure dimensional changes of the rib cage and abdomen and help quantitate and confirm clinical observations. Pulmonary function tests may show a decreased TLC and RV, indirectly reflecting muscle fatigue. Using the tension-time index, one can identify the contractile pattern and use this to determine if a fatiguing pattern is present. Fatigue usually occurs when the TTI_{di} exceeds 0.15 (6). Although sensitive, this technique is invasive, as noted earlier, and requires multiple calculations.

Another indirect measure is based on the observation that the diaphragm relaxes more slowly as the muscle fatigues. This inspiratory relaxation rate (IRR) can be calculated by obtaining the first derivative of pressure with respect to time from maximum contraction to relaxation (dP/dt) and then dividing by the peak pressure (P). The measurement is taken from pressure tracings derived either from a voluntary sniff or phrenic nerve stimulation (10). Measuring the time constant of relaxation (Tr) is an alternative way to determine IRR.

Measurement of the electromyographic spectrum of the diaphragm is the most commonly used method for determining a fatiguing pattern, especially in human research. The frequency content of the diaphragm is normally 20–250 Hz (11). During fatigue, high-frequency power (or amplitude) falls and low-frequency power increases. Both the centroid frequency (point at which half the power lies above and half the power lies below) and Hi/Lo ratio (the ratio of the power in high-frequency bands to low-frequency bands) fall with fatigue (6).

RESPIRATORY DISEASE AND MUSCLE FUNCTION

Respiratory muscle failure occurs either when pulmonary or thoracic disease increase the work of breathing or when the muscles become so weak they can not sustain the work

of normal breathing. Factors that can compromise respiratory muscle function include certain metabolic states, nutritional deficiencies, and disease processes that affect the airway, lung, chest wall, or muscles.

Metabolic and Nutritional Factors

Metabolic derangements such as hypoxia, hypercapnia, hypophosphatemia, hypocalcemia, hypomagnesemia, and hypokalemia all adversely affect pulmonary function by decreasing neural drive or impairing muscle performance. These problems frequently accompany thoracopulmonary disorders and compound the disability. Malnutrition has also been associated with impaired respiratory muscle function. Undernourished patients with chronic obstructive pulmonary disease (COPD) require more frequent hospitalization, are more likely to develop cor pulmonale, and have overall increased mortality (12). In COPD patients with a progressive weight loss the life expectancy is less than 3 years (13, 14).

Studies in malnourished rats show decreased diaphragm muscle mass and strength (15). In a necropsy study, subjects whose mean weight was 71% of ideal body weight showed significant loss of diaphragm muscle mass and impairment of respiratory muscle performance as measured by MVV and P_i max (16).

Disease States

Diseases can cause respiratory muscle fatigue through airway obstruction (increasing the work of breathing), restricting chest wall motion (increasing inertia and therefore muscle work), or compromising neuromuscular integrity. Examples from each group will be used to illustrate how these diseases adversely affect respiratory muscle function.

AIRWAY OBSTRUCTION

COPD has been extensively studied, and many aspects of this disease relate directly to childhood respiratory problems such as cystic fibrosis and bronchopulmonary dysplasia. COPD adversely affects respiratory muscle function in at least three ways: (a) by increasing energy demands, (b) by hyperinflation, and (c) by affecting respiratory muscle strength and endurance (17).

Even at rest, the patient with COPD may have increased work of breathing and energy demands. Minute ventilation may be increased by 30–50% (18) and oxygen cost of breathing may account for 15% of the total oxygen consumption in patients with COPD, compared to 1–2% in the normal subject (19). Ventilatory reserve is diminished so that resting ventilation may be as high as 40% of the maximal ventilatory capacity, compared to 5% in the normal patient (20).

Hyperinflation has a marked effect on the lungs. Flattening of the diaphragm creates an unfavorable length-tension curve that cannot efficiently convert tension into transdiaphragmatic pressure changes. Diaphragm flattening also results in a decreased zone of apposition, which makes the "piston" less effective, and when the appositional fibers contract, their medial orientation causes the rib cage to move inward. When the functional residual capacity (FRC) is increased, thoracic recoil is directed inward instead of outward and the muscles have to work against the recoil of both the thoracic cage and the lung. The inspiratory intercostal muscles are also placed at a mechanical disadvantage and cannot lift the ribs. Both external and internal intercostals have an expiratory action as lung volumes approach TLC (3). Muscle weakness has been documented in COPD (21, 22). The decreased P_I max in COPD can be partially attributed to hyper-inflation and decreased diaphragm length. The cause of decreased P_E max can only be speculated on, but may be due to changes in muscle morphology (caused by steroids), decreased fuel supply (caused by undernutrition or impaired blood supply), or an abnormal metabolic milieu as in hypoxia, hypercapnia, and abnormal electrolytes (16).

THORACIC RESTRICTIVE DISEASE

Of all the thoracic restrictive disorders, kyphoscoliosis has been most widely studied. Respiratory dysfunction becomes detectable when the angle between the upper and lower limbs of the spinal curve is greater than 70° (23), with the severity of pulmonary abnormalities correlating with the angle of curvature (24). The risk of complications is greater in patients whose scoliosis is present before age 5 (25). All muscles, including the diaphragm, may be at a mechanical disadvantage because of the misshapen thoracic cage. The increased work and high oxygen cost of breathing in these patients increases markedly for only small increases in tidal ventilation. RMS in patients with severe scoliosis is reduced at least 50% from normal, and correlates inversely with carbon dioxide retention, suggesting that decreased RMS plays a role in muscle failure (26). Kyphoscoliosis may be seen as an isolated condition but is also commonly seen in conditions associated with muscle weakness and often compounds the respiratory problems.

NEUROMUSCULAR DISEASE

Clinical problems associated in general with neuromuscular disease and resultant respiratory muscle weakness include shallow restricted chest wall motion with inadequate alveolar ventilation, weak abdominal and glottic musculature associated with poor cough and secretion clearance, reduced mobility often resulting in atelectasis, and swallowing dysfunction causing poor nutrition and occasionally aspiration. Some forms of neuromuscular disease (NMD) have pulmonary problems peculiar to the disease.

Quadriplegic patients suffer from pulmonary complications primarily because of the impaired ability to cough and breathe deeply. The lower the level of spinal cord dysfunction, the more respiratory function is spared. Approximately 40% of adult patients with lesions at C3, 14% with lesions at C4, and 11% with lesions at C5 become ventilator dependent (27). Adults with lower levels of damage are rarely ventilator dependent but have mild to moderate impairment of expiratory muscle strength (28). The lower resting position of the diaphragm that occurs when the patient is seated decreases diaphragm excursion. Activation of the diaphragm causes the abdominal contents to fall forward, removing the fulcrum that normally supports the diaphragm and stabilizes the lower rib cage. Because of this, relatively small increases in breathing resistance can produce diaphragm fatigue.

Some myopathies have distinctive characteristics that require special consideration. Duchenne muscular dystrophy patients may have associated cardiomyopathies that may cause arrhythmias and precipitate cardiac failure. The muscles of expiration, especially abdominal muscles, exhibit the greatest weakness, and the diaphragm is spared until late in the disease. The beginning of pulmonary function impairment is usually associated with a functional Class V (before the child is wheelchair bound) (29). The myotonic dystrophy patient may present with apnea either in the newborn period or post anesthesia. Patients with this disease commonly have gastroesophageal reflux and are prone to aspiration, especially in the postoperative period. Infants of affected mothers may develop respiratory failure at birth. This problem can improve with age if adequate respiratory support is provided, but chronic respiratory failure to some degree often persists. Chronic sleep hypoventilation is extremely common in these patients who are also at risk for cardiac arrhythmias. Certain congenital myopathies and those caused by mitochondrial defects may have diaphragm weakness out of proportion to skeletal muscle weakness, with respiratory failure occurring in patients with otherwise minimal disability. Any neuromuscular disease associated with diaphragmatic involvement has a high risk of respiratory failure, manifested initially as sleep hypoventilation or exercise intolerance.

MANAGEMENT OF PULMONARY PROBLEMS IN NEUROMUSCULAR DISEASE

Despite advancements in understanding the mechanisms and genetics of NMD, with few exceptions, these diseases are irreversible and often progressive. Management is directed at stabilizing lung function.

When respiratory involvement becomes apparent by either a decrease in vital capacity, evidence of diaphragm weakness, or recurrent or chronic pneumonia, specific measures to decrease muscle fatigue and improve secretion clearance should be instituted. Chest percussion and postural drainage *with assisted cough* is an effective method for mobilizing secretions in this group of patients. IPPB may be helpful in patients with kyphoscoliosis (30, 31), but its effect in patients with NMD remains questionable. It does not appear to improve either lung or total respiratory system compliance immediately following a treatment in adult patients with muscular dystrophy or quadriplegia (32, 33). No studies have evaluated the effectiveness of the long-term use of this modality. The use of IPPB in the

treatment of children with NMD has not been studied, though theoretically it may have more value in children since they have less intrinsic lung disease and a more compliant chest wall.

Children with neuromuscular disease should have serial measurements of lung function including spirometry, inspiratory and expiratory force measurements, and measurement of their maximum voluntary ventilation. A plateau in the vital capacity often precedes the final decline in pulmonary function in Duchenne, and an early plateau at low lung volumes is predictive of early respiratory failure (34). Respiratory insufficiency occurs predictably in patients with Duchenne once vital capacity drops below 500 ml and daytime arterial CO_2 exceeds 45 mm Hg (35). Measurement of the inspiratory force is especially helpful in assessing the degree of diaphragmatic involvement in an otherwise seemingly stable patient with NMD.

Correction of scoliosis should be strongly considered before the vital capacity drops below 50% predicted. Correction of curvature before pulmonary function deteriorates results in a better prognosis, since morbidity increases significantly if the vital capacity is 30% or less (37). New correction techniques such as the Luque rod and Cotrel Dubousset technique have decreased the morbidity of the procedure and improved the outcome (38, 39).

Pneumonia is a frequent complication. Routine immunizations should be obtained, and yearly vaccination against influenza should be given.

Polysomnography provides a tool for early detection of respiratory failure and should be performed in patients with symptoms of hypoventilation, to screen patients with diaphragm involvement, and in patients with NMD prior to scoliosis surgery. An overnight study is necessary since abnormalities are most likely to occur during REM sleep (36). Early identification of hypoventilation will allow appropriate counseling and ventilation, if elected, prior to onset of acute respiratory failure. It may also identify upper airway obstruction, a commonly occurring and potentially reversible cause of respiratory compromise in NMD patients.

Pharmacotherapy

Theophylline, caffeine, dopamine, isoproterenol, and digoxin have all been shown to modify muscle performance. Therapeutic levels of caffeine have been shown to increase normal diaphragm contractility by 40% (40). Theophylline decreases diaphragm fatigue and increases diaphragm strength in normal patients (41) and paralyzed patients (42), but conflicting effects have been reported in patients with COPD (43). The therapeutic effects of caffeine and theophylline in asthma and apnea of prematurity may be due in part to their effect on diaphragm contractility (44). The human diaphragm has numerous beta receptor sites and theoretically would respond to beta agonists (45). Animal studies using isoproterenol, fenoterol, and terbutaline showed increased contractile force in the fatigued diaphragm (46–48). Human studies using albuterol have failed to show a similar response (49).

Digitalis, a cardiac inotropic drug, has an inotropic effect on the diaphragm in patients with COPD (50). The effectiveness and usefulness of these drugs in infants and children with NMD has not yet been explored, and the routine use of these medications to modify muscle performance in children with NMD is not recommended. However, treatment with theophylline or beta agonists is indicated in the patient with concomitant asthma.

Training

Training has been shown to enhance respiratory muscle contractility by increasing strength and endurance in a selected group of patients, namely those with chronic obstructive lung disease, cystic fibrosis, and spinal cord injury. Effective training requires adherence to three basic principles: (a) *overload:* muscle fibers must be pushed beyond a certain level of work to improve their function, (b) *specificity:* the training must be performed in the same type of exercise in which the enhanced performance is desired; and (c) *reversibility:* the effects of training begin to reverse once training is stopped (51).

People can be trained to increase respiratory muscle strength or endurance. For RMS training, small amounts of intense stimuli create muscle fiber hypertrophy. Endurance training uses repetitive low-intensity stimuli to increase oxidative enzymes, mitochondria, and capillary density (51).

Studies suggest that RMS training can improve RMS in normal humans and those with COPD, cystic fibrosis (CF), and quadriplegia (52, 53). Training techniques consist of repetition of maximal forced inspiratory respiration maneuvers or inspiratory resistive loading. Low work loads and subject adaptive responses can produce an inconsistent response, making study results difficult to reproduce.

Respiratory muscle endurance training has been achieved in patients with CF and normal patients by nonspecific programs (total body exercise) (54, 55). Specific programs that enhance respiratory muscle endurance are of three types:

1. *Voluntary isocapnic hyperpnea.* Individuals maintain high target levels of ventilation up to 15 minutes. Improvement is measured as a change in the MSVC. Positive effects on respiratory muscle endurance have been reported in COPD, CF, and normal controls (52, 56).
2. *Inspiratory resistance load.* Devices are prescribed that apply a resistive load for 5–15 minutes. The response expected is an increase in maximum load tolerance or maximum time tolerance. Positive effects have been reported in COPD, CF, and normal individuals (53, 57, 58). Positive results have also been reported for patients with quadriplegia, muscular dystrophy, and myopathy (59–61). Patients can adapt to this type of training by developing different breathing strategies, an issue not addressed by most studies (51).
3. *Inspiratory threshold loading.* A weighted inspiratory pressure load is applied to the inspiratory port of a one-way valve. The response is assessed by the length of time a subject can breathe against a certain load. Positive results have been reported for COPD (58).

No studies of the long-term effect of respiratory muscle training are available. Good programs are expensive, labor-intensive, and time-consuming, and questions continue as to what constitutes an optimal program and when intervention should begin. Training in the patient with advanced NMD may precipitate respiratory failure by depleting muscle energy stores or by increasing the work of breathing. Training appears to most benefit those patients with static NMD (i.e., spinal cord injury patients). Its use in patients with progressive NMD is potentially hazardous, and unless further studies demonstrate its usefulness, should be avoided.

Respiratory Muscle Rest Therapy (RMR)

Rest is the most important treatment available to restore respiratory muscle contractility. Devices used to effect respiratory muscle rest therapy and thus decrease respiratory muscle energy expenditure include the mechanical rocking bed, the pneumobelt, negative pressure ventilators, and positive pressure ventilators.

GENERAL DEVICES

The mechanical rocking bed produces diaphragm motion by shifting intra-abdominal contents toward and away from the diaphragm. This motion may assist a weak diaphragm and place the diaphragm in a more functional position for breathing. It has only limited usefulness in the treatment of respiratory compromise, but has been advocated as an adjunct to treating patients with diaphragm weakness or paralysis following heart surgery (62).

The pneumobelt can be used in the seated patient. An air bladder strapped to the abdomen inflates, pushing up on the diaphragm and assisting expiration, and then deflates, allowing the diaphragm to descend, causing inspiration. At least part of the benefit derived from this device is secondary to abdominal support.

NEGATIVE PRESSURE DEVICES

The cuirass or turtle shell respirator covers the chest and upper abdomen. The device attaches by a hose to a negative pressure generator that cycles at a prescribed frequency. The negative pressure elevates the anterior chest wall, assisting inspiration. Expiration occurs passively when the unit cycles off. This can be custom made to fit small or unusually shaped chests. The major drawbacks to this device are its inability to move a poorly compliant chest wall (i.e., the hyper-expanded or kyphoscoliotic chest) and the difficulty in achieving a good fit in patients with deformed chest walls. Since the patient must be supine, movement is somewhat hampered. This is especially problematic in the child.

The poncho-type ventilator uses a metal or plastic grid that lies over the patient's chest and rests on a backplate. An airtight suit encloses the patient's body. The ventilator attaches to the suit with a hose and generates a vacuum between the grid and chest wall, which causes the chest wall to rise. Expiration occurs passively when the ventilator cycles off. The major difficulties with this respirator include the need to maintain the patient supine during ventilation and problems with discomfort caused from heat trapping. The heat trapping can be controlled somewhat by changing the air temperature around the intake chamber of the ventilator. Some of the newer materials have less tendency to cause this problem.

The tank respirator, or Iron Lung, is one of the oldest forms of respiratory support (Fig. 45.6). It was first used during the 1950 poliomyelitis epidemic. Cyclic movement of a diaphragm (up to 40 times a minute) allows the tank to generate negative pressure (maximum of 60 cm). The chest wall expands and inspiration occurs. Expiration occurs passively but may be facilitated by the addition of positive pressure, generated by a hand-operated flap. The machine is sturdy, as evidenced by the fact that many of the early models are still in operation. It is simple to use and inexpensive to maintain. Three sizes were made—the adult, intermediate, and infant (fitted to children less than 30 inches tall). A lightweight, portable version (Portalung) is also available. The chief drawbacks of the tank respirator are its size and weight, poor patient accessibility for treatment, and the need of the patient to remain supine. Many adult patients experience some initial claustrophobia when placed in the tank; this is less of a problem with children.

One major complication associated with negative pressure ventilation is the tendency to aggravate upper airway obstruction. Since the patient does not initiate respiration, stimulation of the upper airway muscles may not occur synchronously with respiration. Cardiovascular complications are theoretically possible since negative pressure ventilation has been shown to decrease cardiac output by decreasing venous return in animal models (63).

POSITIVE PRESSURE VENTILATORS

Positive pressure ventilation with a tracheostomy is an alternative mode of therapy. Indications for its use would be total ventilator dependence, severe intrinsic lung disease,

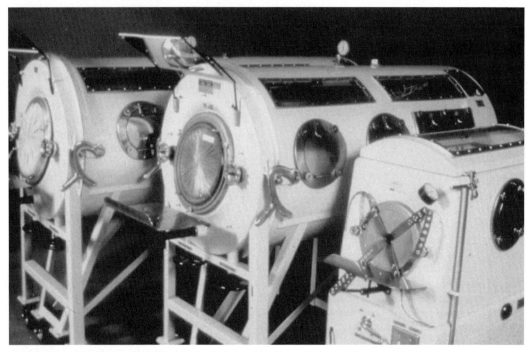

Figure 45.6. The three sizes of the tank respirator. (Courtesy of Lifecare Services, Inc.)

upper airway obstruction, severe cervical deformity, and chronic aspiration. Drawbacks for this type of ventilation include the need for a tracheostomy with its attendant morbidity. Recently, investigators have described successful application of ventilation through a nasal mask as used for nasal continuous positive airway pressure (CPAP) (64, 65).

Recent data suggesting that RM weakness plays a role in ventilatory failure associated with COPD has caused some centers to evaluate the use of mechanical ventilation in COPD.

Braun and Marino evaluated patients with COPD repeatedly hospitalized with episodes of respiratory failure. RMR was instituted in 18 patients (4 with positive pressure ventilation via tracheostomy and 14 with a poncho-type ventilator) (66). RMR was continued for 4–10 hours per night at home, resulting in improved respiratory muscle strength and vital capacity. Work by Cropp and Dimarco using negative pressure ventilation showed similar findings, and improvement was documented as soon as 3 days after initiation of therapy (67).

Frates et al. described their experience with home mechanical ventilation for neuromuscular disease using negative pressure devices in 21 children and positive pressure devices in 33 children (68). The children's ages ranged from 4 months to 18 years. Over 20 years, there were 17 deaths, including 3 from ventilator disconnection. Using life table analysis they predicted a 1-year survival rate of 84% and a 5-year survival rate of 64%. Other benefits included decreased cost (homecare was 6% of the cost for in-hospital care) and improved ability to function as measured by return to school and increased daytime activities. Similar reports have come from other investigators.

RMR is an effective form of therapy for stabilizing lung function in patients with progressive neuromuscular disease. Nocturnal ventilation is viewed positively by many families, rarely hampers the patient, and often improves the patient's psychologic and physical functioning (67–69, 71). The form of ventilation chosen should be individualized with either negative pressure ventilation or nasal positive pressure ventilation preferred to allow for oral communication. Tracheostomy and positive pressure ventilation should be reserved for those patients with swallowing or secretion difficulties, those requiring continuous ventilator support, or those patients unable to tolerate the other modalities.

ETHICAL ISSUES

The effectiveness of artificial ventilation in prolonging life for children with neuromuscular disease has been well documented (35, 68–70). Functional existence, even professional and social success, has been achieved by persons on chronic ventilation (68, 69, 71). There is no general consensus as to whether patients with progressive neurologic disease should be offered mechanical ventilation, largely because of concerns about the quality of life for ventilator-dependent patients and their families (69, 71). A recent report, however, showed that ventilator-dependent individuals had an overall positive affect and that ventilator assistance was perceived as less a disability than the inability to use upper arms (71). In addition, health care professionals significantly underestimated the degree of life satisfaction experienced by these patients (71).

The current medical practice necessitates that patients and their families participate in medical decisions affecting them. Quality of life is a subjective and by nature a personal experience. The physician's responsibility is to communicate factual information to the patient regarding the disease, its prognosis and complications, and treatment options in a sympathetic and supportive setting. Clinical parameters can be obtained that allow the physician to reasonably predict when respiratory failure is imminent (35). Discussions regarding care issues should be held when the patient is not in crisis. By presenting all options nonjudgementally, the patients and their families are able to make decisions regarding care based on their own religious, ethical, and personal values (69). Medical and psychosocial support should remain available to all families, no matter what decision is made.

CONCLUSIONS

Respiratory muscle dysfunction is a major factor not only in neuromuscular disease but also in illnesses that affect the lung itself. Infants and children are at the greatest risk for such problems. Evaluation of respiratory muscle function primarily depends on measuring indirect parameters of pulmonary function, with some new techniques on the horizon.

Treatment modalities are supportive and aimed at correcting metabolic disturbances, improving nutritional parameters, and decreasing respiratory muscle work. The utility of pharmacologic interventions and muscle training programs are areas still being explored. Mechanical ventilation has allowed patients to live longer lives. The physician's responsibilities now include frank, unbiased discussions with patients and their families about life-sustaining equipment.

REFERENCES

1. DeTroyer A, Estenne M. Functional anatomy of the respiratory muscles. *Clin Chest Med* 1988; 9:175–193.
2. Muller N, Bryan AC. Chest wall mechanics and respiratory muscles in infants. *Pediatr Clin North Am* 1979; 26:503–516.
3. DeTroyer A, Kelly S, Macklem PT, Walter AZ. Mechanics of intercostal space and actions of external and internal intercostal muscles. *J Clin Invest* 1985; 75:850–857.
4. Sieck, G. Diaphragm muscle: Structural and functional organization. *Clin Chest Med* 1988; 9:195–210.
5. Keens TG, Bryan AC, Levison H, Ianuzzo CD. Developmental pattern of muscle fiber types in human ventilatory muscles. *J Appl Physiol* 1978; 44:909–913.
6. Bellemare F, Grassino A. Effect of pressure and timing of contraction on human diaphragm fatigue. *J Appl Physiol* 1982; 53:1190–1195.
7. Aldrich TK. Respiratory muscle fatigue. *Clin Chest Med* 1988; 225–236.
8. Asmussen E. Muscle fatigue. *Med Sci Sports* 1979; 11:313–321.
9. Aldrich TK. Transmission fatigue of the rabbit diaphragm. *Respir Physiol* 1987; 69:307–319.
10. Rochester DF. Tests of respiratory muscle function. *Clin Chest Med* 1988; 9:249–261.
11. Schweitzer TW, Fitzgerald JW, Bowden JA, Lynne-Davies P. Spectral analysis of human inspiratory diaphragmatic electromyogram. *J Appl Physiol* 1979; 46:152.
12. Braun SR, Dixon RM, Keim NL, Luby MS, Anderegg A, Shrago ES. Predictive clinical value of nutritional assessment factors in COPD. *Chest* 1984; 85:353–357.
13. Vandenbergh E, Van de Woestijne KP, Billier L, et al. Evaluation et propoistic de la bronchite chronique au stade de la retention de CO2. *Bull Eur Physiopathol Respir* 1965; 1:260.
14. Driver AG, McAlevy MTR, Smith JL. Nutritional assessment of patients with chronic obstructive pulmonary disease and acute respiratory failure. *Chest* 1982; 82:568–571.
15. Lewis MI, Sieck GC, Fournier M, Belman MJ. The effect of nutritional deprivation on diaphragm contractility and muscle fiber size. *Appl Physiol* 1986; 60:596–603.
16. Arora NS, Rochester DF. Respiratory muscle strength and maximal ventilation in undernourished patients. *Am Rev Respir Dis* 1982; 126:5–8.

17. Tobin MJ. Respiratory muscles in disease. *Clin Chest Med* 1988; 9:263–286.
18. Tobin MJ. Breathing patterns, diseased subjects. *Chest* 1983; 84:286–294.
19. Cherniack RM. The oxygen consumption and efficiency of the respiratory muscles in health and emphysema. *J Clin Invest* 1959; 38:494–499.
20. Clark THJ, Freedman S, Campbell EJM, Winn RR. The ventilatory capacity of patients with chronic airways obstruction. *Clin Sci* 1969; 36:307–316.
21. Byrd RB, Hyatt RE. Maximal respiratory pressure in chronic obstructive lung disease. *Am Rev Respir Dis* 1968; 98:848–856.
22. Rochester DF, Braun NMT. Determinants of maximal inspiratory pressure in chronic obstructive pulmonary disease. *Am Rev Respir Dis* 1985; 132:42–47.
23. Bergofsky EH. Thoracic deformities. In Roussos C, Macklin PT, eds. *The thorax (Part B)*. New York, Marcel Dekker, 1985, pp 941–978.
24. Kafer ET. Idiopathic scoliosis: Mechanical problems of the respiratory system and the ventilatory response to carbon dioxide. *J Clin Invest* 1975; 55:1153–1163.
25. Branthwaite MA. Cardiorespiratory consequences of unfused idiopathic scoliosis. *Br J Dis Chest* 1986; 80:360–368.
26. Lisboa C, Moreno R, Fava M, Ferretti R, Edgardo C. Inspiratory muscle function in patients with severe kyphoscoliosis. *Am Rev Respir Dis* 1985; 132:48–52.
27. Wicks AB, Menter RR. Long-term outlook in quadriplegic patients with initial ventilator dependency. *Chest* 1986; 90:406–410.
28. Arora NS, Suratt PM, Rochester DF. Respiratory muscle and ventilatory function in spinal cord injury [Abstract]. *Clin Res* 1978; 26:443A.
29. Inkley SR, Oldenburg FC, Viguos PJ. Pulmonary function in Duchenne muscular dystrophy related to stage of disease. *Am J Med* 1974; 56:297–306.
30. Sinha R, Bergofsky EH. Prolonged alteration of lung mechanics in kyphoscoliosis by positive pressure hyperinflation. *Am Rev Respir Dis* 1972; 106:47–57.
31. George, RB, O'Donohue WJ, Brooks JG, et al. Intermittent positive pressure breathing (IPPB). *Clin Notes Resp Dis* Winter, 1979.
32. DeTroyer A, Deisser P. The effects of intermittent positive pressure breathing on patients with respiratory muscle weakness. *Am Rev Respir Dis* 1981; 124:132–137.
33. McCool FD, Mayewski RF, Shayne DS, Gibson, CJ, Griggs RC, Hyde RW. Ret al. Intermittent positive pressure breathing in patients with respiratory muscle weakness. *Chest* 1986; 90:546–552.
34. Rideau Y, Jankowski LW, Grellet J. Respiratory function in the muscular dystrophies. *Muscle Nerve* 1981; 4:155–164.
35. Baydur A, Gilgoff I, Prentice W. Guidelines for assisted ventilation in Duchenne's muscular dystrophy. *Am Rev Respir Dis* 1985; 131(Suppl):A268.
36. Smith PEM, Calverley PMA, Edwards RHT. Hypoxemia during sleep in Duchenne muscular dystrophy. *Am Rev Respir Dis* 1988; 137:884–888.
37. Jenkins, JG, Bohn D, Edmonds JF, Levison H, Barker GA. Evaluation of pulmonary function in muscular dystrophy patients requiring spinal surgery. *Crit Care Med* 1982; 10:645–649.
38. Luque ER. The correction of postural curves of the spine. *Spine* 1982; 7:270–275.
39. Farcy JP, Weidenbaum M, Roye D. Correction of thoracic scoliosis using the Cotrel–Dubousset technique. *Surg Rounds Orthop* 1987; May, 11–19.
40. Supinski GS, Deal EC, Kelson SG. Comparison of the effects of aminophylline and caffeine on diaphragmatic contractility in man. *Am Rev Respir Dis* 1984; 130:429–433.
41. Aubier M, DeTroyer A, Sampson M, Macklem PT, Roussos C. Aminophylline improves diaphragm contractility. *N Engl J Med* 1981; 305:249–252.
42. Chevrolet JC, Reverdin A, Suter PM, Tshopp JM, Junod AF. Ventilatory dysfunction resulting from bilateral anterolateral high cervical cordotomy: Dual beneficial effect of aminophylline. *Chest* 1983; 84:112–115.
43. Aubier M. Pharmacotherapy of respiratory muscles. *Clin Chest Med* 1988; 9:311–324.
44. Nichols DG. Respiratory muscle performance in infants and children. *J Pediatr* 1991; 118:493–502.
45. Bowman WC, Roper C. The effects of adrenergic and other drugs affecting carbohydrate metabolism and contractions of the diaphragm. *Br J Pharmocol* 1984; 23:184–200.
46. Howell S, Roussos CS. Isoproterenol and aminophylline improve contractility of fatigued canine diaphragm. *Am Rev Respir Dis* 1984; 129:118–124.
47. Suzuki S, Numata H, Sano F, Yoshiike Y, Miyashita A, Okubot. Effects and mechanism of fenoteral on fatigued canine diaphragm. *Am Rev Respir Dis* 1988; 137:1048–1054.
48. Aubier M, Viires N, Murciano D, Medrano G, Lecocguic Y, Pariente R. Effects and mechanisms of action of terbutaline on diaphragmatic contractility and fatigue. *J Appl Physiol* 1984; 56:922–929.
49. Javaheri S, Smith JT, Thomas JP, Guilfoile TD, Donovan EF. Albuterol has no effect on diaphragmatic fatigue in humans. *Am Rev Respir Dis* 1988; 137:197–201.
50. Aubier M, Murciano D, Viires N, Lebargy F, Curran Y, Jean-Phillipe S, Pariente R. Effects of digoxin on diaphragmatic strength generation in patients with chronic obstructive pulmonary disease during acute respiratory failure. *Am Rev Respir Dis* 1987; 135:544–548.
51. Pardy RL, Reid WD, Belman MJ. Respiratory muscle training. *Chest Clin North Am* 1988; 9:287–296.
52. Belman MJ, Thomas SF, Lewis MI. Resistive breathing training in patients with chronic obstructive pulmonary disease. *Chest* 1986; 90:663–670.
53. Asher MI, Pardy RL, Coates AL. The effects of inspiratory muscle training in patients with cystic fibrosis. *Am Rev Respir Dis* 1982; 126:855–859.
54. Orenstein DM, Franklin BA, Doerschuk CF, Hellerstein HK, Germann KJ, Horowitz JG, Stern RC. Exercise conditioning and cardiopulmonary fitness in cystic fibrosis. *Chest* 1981; 80: 392–398.
55. Robinson EP, Kjeldgaard JM. Improvement in ventilatory muscle function with running. *J Appl Physiol* 1982; 52:1400–1406.
56. Keens TG, Krastins IRB, Wanamaker EM, Levison H, Crozier DN, Bryan AC. Ventilatory muscle endurance training in normal subjects and patients with cystic fibrosis. *Am Rev Respir Dis* 1977; 116:853–860.
57. Pardy RL, Rivington RN, Despas PJ, Macklem PT. The effects of inspiratory muscle training on exercise

performance in chronic airflow limitation. *Am Rev Respir Dis* 1981; 123:426–433.

58. Clanton TL, Dixon G, Drake J, Gadek JE. Inspiratory muscle conditioning using a threshold loading device. *Chest* 1985; 87:62–66.

59. Gross D, Ladd HW, Riley EJ, Macklem PT, Grassino A. The effect of training on strength and endurance of the diaphragm in quadriplegia. *Am J Med* 1980; 68:27–35.

60. DiMarco AF, Kelling J, Sajovic M et al. Respiratory muscle training in muscular dystrophy. *Clin Res* 1982; 30:427A.

61. Martin RJ, Sufit RL, Ringel SP, Hudgel DW, Hill PL. Respiratory improvement by muscle training in adult onset acid maltase deficiency. *Muscle Nerve* 1983; 6:201–203.

62. Abd AG, Braun NMT, Baskin MI, O'Sullivan MM, Alkaitis DA. Diaphragmatic dysfunction after open heart surgery: Treatment with a rocking bed. *Ann Intern Med* 1989; 111:881–886.

63. Maloney JV, Whittenberger JL. Clinical implications of pressure used in the body respirator. *Am J Med Sci* 1951; 221:425.

64. Ellis E, Bye PT, Bruderer JW, Sullivan CE. Treatment of respiratory failure during sleep in patients with neuromuscular disease: Positive pressure ventilation through a nose mask. *Am Rev Respir Dis* 1987; 135:738–740.

65. Kerby GR, Mayer LS, Pingleton SK. Nocturnal positive pressure ventilation via nasal mask. *Am Rev Respir Dis* 1987; 135:739–740.

66. Braun NMT, Marino WD. Effect of daily intermittent rest of respiratory muscles in patients with severe chronic airflow limitation (CAL). *Chest* 1984; 85:595.

67. Cropp A, DiMarco AF. Effects of intermittent negative pressure ventilation on respiratory muscle function in patients with severe chronic obstructive pulmonary disease. *Am Rev Respir Dis* 1987; 135:1056–1061.

68. Frates RC, Splaingard ML, Smith EO and Harrison GM. Outcome of home mechanical ventilation in children. *J Pediatr* 1985; 106:850–856.

69. Gilgoff IS, Kahlstrom E, MacLaughlin E, Keens TG. Long-term ventilatory support in spinal muscle atrophy. *J Pediatr* 1989; 115:904–909.

70. Heckmatt JZ, Loh L, Dubowitz V. Nocturnal hypoventilation in children with nonprogressive neuromuscular disease. *Pediatrics* 1989; 83:250–255.

71. Bach, JR, Campagnolo DI, Hoeman S. Life satisfaction of individuals with Duchenne muscular dystrophy using long-term ventilatory support. *Am J Phys Med Rehabil* 1991; 70:129–135.

72. Rochester DF, Braun NMT. The respiratory muscles. *Basics RD* 1978; 6:1.

73. Rochester DF. Fatigue of the diaphragm. In Fishman, AP, ed. *Pulmonary diseases and disorders update.* New York, McGraw-Hill, 1982.

74. Rochester DF, Arora NS. The respiratory muscles in asthma. In Lavietes MH, Reichman LB, eds. *Diagnostic aspects and management of asthma.* Norwalk, CT, Purdue Frederick, 1981.

46

Congenital Heart Disease

GEORGE LISTER and J. JULIO PEREZ FONTAN

In the healthy subject there is usually close linkage between the functions of the cardiac and respiratory systems such that changes in the metabolic demands of the body are rapidly followed by proportional changes in both cardiac output and minute ventilation. As a result, oxygen (O_2) is transported to the tissues at a rate commensurate with metabolic need, and O_2 and carbon dioxide (CO_2) tensions and pH are maintained within narrow limits in arterial and venous blood. However, in the presence of congenital anomalies of the circulation this linkage is almost always broken. Under such circumstances, the ability of the heart to increase systemic blood flow is often limited, arterial Po_2 may be decreased, and therefore O_2 delivery cannot keep pace with the demands of the tissues. Not infrequently the circulatory derangement also places stress on the respiratory system itself, causing signs and symptoms that mimic primary respiratory disease. Because congenital defects of the circulation are so common (approximately 7 infants per 1000 live births are affected) and the alterations in respiratory function are often so profound, it is essential that the physician interested in respiratory diseases be well acquainted with the spectrum of congenital heart disease and the ways in which it is manifested in the infant and child.

Accordingly, it is our aim in this chapter to provide an overview of the common types of congenital cardiac defects by grouping the lesions according to their major functional effect. We will try to convey the current understanding of the pathogeneiss of respiratory dysfunction caused by these defects. In the process we will call particular attention to developmental factors that render the immature and young subject particularly susceptible to respiratory compromise. For the purposes of our discussion we have grouped cardiac defects into two categories based on the predominant pathophysiologic alteration in respiratory function.

LESIONS IN WHICH THE WORK OF BREATHING IS INCREASED

In general, three types of problems cause disturbances in mechanical function of the lungs and increase the work of breathing. These include large-volume left-to-right shunts, inflow or outflow obstruction of the systemic ventricle, and vascular anomalies that obstruct the airways.

Large Volume Left-to-Right Shunt

Lesions that permit communication between the systemic and pulmonary circulations and cause a large left-to-right shunt are the most frequent congenital cardiac anomalies. These include common problems such as ventricular septal defect or patent ductus arteriosus as well as defects with similar physiologic consequences but more complex anatomy, such as single ventricle, aortopulmonary window, or truncus arteriosus. These lesions are characterized by the recirculation of oxygenated blood through the lungs and pulmonary vascular congestion. The shunt produces excessive pulmonary blood flow and increased return of pulmonary venous blood to the left side of the heart (except when the output of the systemic ventricle is substantially decreased). In addition, when the abnormal communication is large and occurs at the level of the ventricles or great vessels, the high pressure of the left side of the heart is transmitted to the pulmonary circulation, causing pulmo-

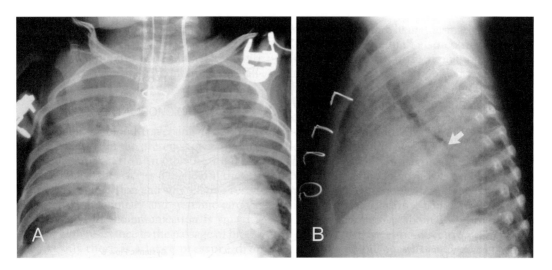

Figure 46.2. Anteroposterior (*A*) and lateral (*B*) chest radiographs of a 1-year-old infant with severe mitral valve regurgitation. The regurgitation places a large volume load on the left ventricle and markedly increases left atrial volume and pressure. There is cardiomegaly, pulmonary edema, and left lower lobe collapse (loss of shadow of left hemidiaphragm), which are easily appreciated on the anteroposterior view, and compression and elevation of the left mainstem bronchus (*arrow*) by the left atrium, which can be seen best in the lateral projection.

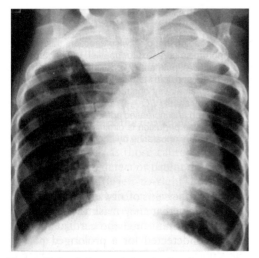

Figure 46.3. Anteroposterior chest radiograph of an infant with a large left-to-right ventricular and atrial shunt. This infant was initially treated for presumed asthma because of the prominent wheezing and retractions. The radiograph called attention to the cardiomegaly in addition to the significant air trapping and collapse of the upper lobes.

shunt) both minimize the effects of intrapulmonary right-to-left shunting on arterial O_2 saturation. Thus, arterial Po_2 and Pco_2 are usually near normal unless there is respiratory fatigue.

The excessive left-to-right shunt may also reduce systemic blood flow and, in response, increase adrenergic tone in the systemic circulation (9). Increase catecholamine stimulation and release of other vasoactive hormones (e.g., angiotensin II, aldosterone, and antidiuretic hormone) redistribute systemic blood flow to the organs and tissues whose needs are most important. In addition, these vasoconstricting hormones maintain blood pressure and increase peripheral O_2 extraction (10). However, favorable for the survival of the whole organism, these adaptive responses always reduce perfusion (and O_2 transport) to some organs, possibly impairing their function. For example, reduced renal perfusion decreased glomerular filtration rate, often resulting in an elevation in serum creatinine concentration. Similarly, reduced gastrointestinal perfusion may cause intolerance to feeding. Furthermore, when systemic flow is markedly decreased, the respiratory muscles may not receive sufficient perfusion to sustain their function, particularly in the face of the greater metabolic demands imposed by the abnormalities in the mechanical function of the lungs (11). In addition, as the hemoglobin concentration declines postnatally, O_2 transport to systemic tissues decreases even further. The "physiologic anemia" of infancy increased the left-to-right shunt and raises the demand for systemic blood flow, but the ability to respond to such a demand is limited by the left-to-right shunt and the large volume load already imposed on the left ventricle (3). Thus, events that we consider part of normal postnatal development (such as the decrease in pulmonary vascular resistance and in hemoglobin concentration) promote the emergence of congestive circulatory failure and create a marked mismatch between the metabolic supply and demand of the systemic tissues.

Inflow or Outflow Obstruction of the Systemic Ventricle

Anomalies that commonly cause left-sided (systemic ventricular) obstruction include coarctation of the aorta, interruption of the aortic arch, aortic stenosis or atresia, mitral stenosis or atresia, and obstruction to pulmonary venous return. These anomalies are generally characterized by decreased systemic perfusion and pulmonary venous congestion. Although the nature of the respiratory abnormalities may be similar with left heart obstruction and with large volume left-to-right shunts, infants with obstruction of the left heart usually develop signs and symptoms at an earlier postnatal age and have more severe respiratory compromise (12). This is because closure of the ductus arteriosus, which usually occurs within the first few days after birth, may substantially reduce blood flow through the aorta and decrease systemic perfusion (13). Alternatively, when the pulmonary artery pressure is suprasystemic (e.g., with total anomalous pulmonary venous return and obstruction), ductus closure eliminates a mechanism for amelioration of the pulmonary hypertension via right-to-left shunting. Thus, the pulmonary and systemic venous congestion can occur precipitously.

DEVELOPMENTAL CONSIDERATIONS

The time at which signs become apparent with severe left heart obstruction depends on both the site and severity of the obstruction. With complete outflow obstruction, such as in aortic atresia, the infant will develop cardiogenic shock as soon as the ductus arteriosus closes. With aortic stenosis or coarctation, the onset of signs of poor perfusion can be delayed until after the ductus closes if the left ventricle can eject a sufficient volume of blood through the narrowing (14). The clinical presentation of partial left ventricular obstruction is therefore quite variable; some infants develop failure abruptly within the first postnatal week, whereas others tolerate the obstruction for an extended period before they come to medical attention. In some patients with outflow obstruction the signs of low systemic perfusion predominate, whereas in other infants the leading manifestations are usually respiratory. The elevated pulmonary venous pressure causes severe pulmonary edema and invariably results in respiratory distress. But even then, an occasional infant may tolerate one of these severe obstructive lesions for a while before having respiratory failure, possibly because the left atrium is decompressed through an imcompetent foramen ovale or, more rarely, through an alternative route, such as a persistent levoatrial cardinal vein (15).

When there is significant obstruction to pulmonary venous return as with total anomalous pulmonary venous return below the diaphragm or pulmonary venous stenosis respiratory distress invariably occurs very soon after birth. Under such circumstances there will be severe pulmonary edema hypoxia and respiratory insufficiency. Similar findings may occur with cor triatriatum, a membrane within the left atrium that obstructs pulmonary venous return. Infants with each of these problems have pulmonary edema usually with a normal or small heart. Accordingly, venous obstruction should be considered in the differential diagnosis of respiratory distress of the newborn, particularly the full-term infant.

PATHOPHYSIOLOGY

The problems occurring with left heart obstruction arise from its effects on systemic blood flow, ventricular loading, and pulmonary function. For a clearer understanding of the pathophysiology of left ventricular obstruction, it is helpful to separate the lesions into inflow and outflow obstruction. Outflow obstruction produces an increased afterload on the left ventricle, which will be tolerated very poorly if the obstruction is severe or if it occurs abruptly. The hemodynamic consequences of outflow obstruction are increased ventricular end-diastolic, left atrial, and pulmonary venous and pulmonary arterial pressures that cause variable degrees of pulmonary venous congestion and pulmonary edema (interstitial and alveolar) and obstruction of both large and small airways, just as with the large left-to-right shunt. As mentioned above the left atrial pressure is often increased enough to distend the foramen ovale and create a left-to-right atrial shunt. This may help relieve some of the pulmonary venous congestion but it further diminishes systemic perfusion. In response to these effects on ventricular function, systemic blood flow may be markedly reduced and redistributed, as previously described for the left-to-right shunt. In the most severe of forms of obstruction, usually found in the neonate, there are always signs of poor systemic perfusion (increased capillary refill time, decreased or absent peripheral pulses, cool extremities) accompanied by lactic acidosis.

In contrast, left ventricular inflow obstruction (e.g., mitral atresia or stenosis) impedes left ventricular filling and raises the afterload on the right ventricle. The preload on the right ventricle also becomes increased by the excess flow entering the right ventricle from the portion of the pulmonary venous return, which is shunted from the left to the right atrium through the foramen ovale. The impairment of systemic perfusion depends on the amount of anterograde flow from the systemic ventricle and the right-to-left flow, if any, through the ductus arteriosus. Thus, when there is atresia of the mitral or aortic valve, the left-to-right atrial shunt represents the only means for blood to reach the systemic circulation (via the right ventricle and through the ductus arteriosus to the descending aorta).

The frequent association of pulmonary venous obstruction with anomalous pulmonary venous return also increases markedly the afterload on the right ventricle. However, rather than left-to-right atrial shunting, there is right-to-left intra-atrial shunting, which provides the only source for left ventricular filling because pulmonary venous blood returns to the heart via some communication with the systemic veins. When total venous return is anomalous but not obstructed, respiratory signs may be absent or minimal for a long time. Pulmonary veins may drain anomalously above the diaphragm without obstruction; under these circumstances there may be mild hypoxia signs of a left-to-right shunt, and a mediastinal mass corresponding to the anomalous venous connections noted on chest radiograph.

With most of these lesions, particularly those with obstruction of pulmonary veins or inflow to the left heart, there is such severe pulmonary edema that not only the mechanical function of the lungs but also the gas exchange function is disrupted. Mild hypoxia is common with left ventricular outflow obstruction, whreas more severe hypoxia is expected with inflow or pulmonary venous obstruction. These disturbances in gas exchange are caused both by extrapulmonary right-to-left shunting and by areas within the lung that, owing to pulmonary edema and alveolar collapse, are perfused but not ventilated. In addition, when the excessive respiratory work overwhelms the respiratory muscles (see below), hypercarbia also develops.

Vascular Anomalies that Obstruct Airways

Compression of the trachea and bronchi can be caused by developmental abnormalities of both the pulmonary vessels or the major arterial branches of the aorta. These lesions, which generally arise from failure of abnormal regression of one or more segments of the early fetal paired aortic arch system, can produce substantial distortion of the trachea and large bronchi (16). The most common types involve either complete encirclement of the trachea by vascular structures (vascular rings) or compression of the trachea or bronchi by vessels that follow an anomalous trajectory. Examples of the latter include the pulmonary artery sling and anomalous origin of the innominate arteries. In addition pulmonary regurgitation owing to congenital absence of the pulmonary valve can result in massive enlargement of the pulmonary arteries and severe compression of the large intrathoracic airways (17). As a group, vascular anomalies obstruct the intrathoracic airways exclusively. Consequently their mainfestations are predominantly expiratory, and include expiratory prolongation, wheezing, and pulmonary hyper-inflation. When the compression is severe, inspiratory stridor is also seen, indicating the relatively fixed nature of the obstruction. Surgical correction does not usually eliminate all the respiratory signs immediately (if ever) because the alterations in both the geometry of the airways and the stiffness of the airway cartilage tend to persist for months.

In fact, in some cases it is unclear whether the airway ever becomes normal.

Although the clinical manifestations are usually the same, the possible combinations of vascular abnormalities that can cause respiratory difficulty from airway compression is virtually unlimited. In years past, the first approach to diagnosis was the use of a radiograph taken in frontal and lateral projections with barium in the esophagus (18). Although there is little doubt that magnetic resonance imaging will supplant this approach in the future, the barium esophagogram still has an important role in the initial assessment of infants and children suspected of having airway compression by an anomalous vessel, and merits some discussion.

The esophagogram usually falls into one of several patterns in most anomalies that cause airway obstruction (Fig. 46.4). One of the patterns consists of a large posterior indentation in the esophagus in association with an anterior notch in the tracheal air column. This pattern is usually caused by complete vascular rings (double aortic arch and the complex of right aortic arch, a left ductus arteriosus. and an abberant left subclavian artery) encircling the esophagus and trachea. In these cases, the degree of respiratory difficulty depends on the severity of the compression, but the clinical manifestations tend to occur very early in infancy and require surgical intervention. It is also important to recognize that a complete vascular ring can be associated with intracardiac defects such as a ventricular septal defect, which can complicate the diagnosis by diverting attention from the extracardiac anomalies. Even at the time of cardiac catheterization, aortic arch anomalies are difficult to diagnose unless there is a high index of suspicion.

Another radiographic finding is the presence of an isolated anterior tracheal indentation with compression of the esophagus. This pattern occurs when there is an anomalous innominate artery or common bracheocephalic trunk (incorporating the innominate and left carotid arteries) that arises too far from its normal original and has to cross the midline in front of the trachea. Unlike the complete vascular rings, antcrior tracheal compression may appear as an incidental observation and produce few or no symptoms. The onset of signs and need for surgical intervention depends on the severity of the clinical manifestations in each specific case.

Finally, an unusual radiographic finding is an anterior identation of the esophagus associated with a posterior impression on the tracheal air column. This combination is seen when the left pulmonary artery originates from the right pulmonary artery (pulmonary vascular sling). The anomalous left pulmonary artery must find its way to the left lung anterior to the esophagus and posterior to the trachea. In the process, it passes over the right mainstem bronchus, behind the trachea, and down over the left mainstem bronchus, and may compress any of these structures, frequently causing air trapping or collapse of either lung.

Although the embryogenesis is quite different from the previous anomalies, congenital absence of the pulmonary valve is an important cause of airway obstruction. This lesion usually occurs in association with tetralogy of Fallot, and accordingly it is accompanied by a ventricular septal defect with either left-to-right or bidirectional shunting. The aortic arch is on the right. Regurgitation of blood through the pulmonary outflow tract results in extremely enlarged pulmonary arteries (17). These compress the trachea and mainstem bronchi, causing lobar collapse or lobar emphysema and severe respiratory distress. Airway compression can be bilateral or, if the pulmonary artery enlargement is asymmetric, predominantly unilateral. The more severe the obstruction, the earlier the problem presents. Some patients are symptomatic at or shortly after birth, but in other infants the signs may not emerge for a few weeks. Frequently, the respiratory difficulty occurs as the pulmonary artery becomes gradually dilated when the postnatal decrease in pulmonary vascular resistance increases left-to-right shunting and pulmonary regurgitation. Surgical repair of the cardiac anomaly and placement of an artificial pulmonary valve are invariably necessary. However, the timing of the surgery very much depends on the significance of the respiratory distress. As a result of the residual severe tracheobronchomalacia there is, in many patients, a need for mechanical ventilation for weeks or months following surgical repair even if the hemodynamic function is near normal and there is no regurgitation (Fig. 46.5).

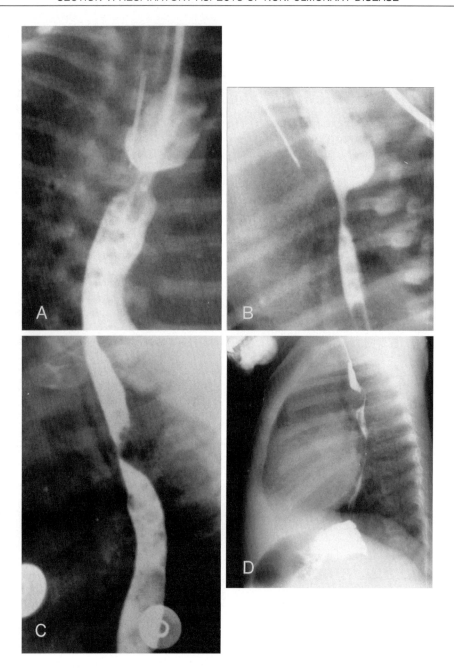

Figure 46.4. Esophagograms of vascular lesions causing airway obstruction. Panels *A* and *B* show anteroposterior and lateral projections of a child with a double aortic arch. Note how tightly the esophagus is constricted (*A*) by the ring formed by the double arch. There is also substantial compression of the esophagus posteriorly (*B*) and obliteration of the tracheal air column by the vascular ring immediately below the tip of the endotracheal tube. Panel *C* shows the lateral projection of a child with an abnormal aortic arch causing posterior compression of the esophagus (see oblique indentation) and compression of the trachea anteriorly. This child had a right aortic arch that descended in the left hemithorax. The first branch of the aorta was a left carotid artery that arose from the anterior part of the arch; it then coursed horizontally and leftward, anterior to the trachea. The second arch vessel was the right carotid artery, and the third vessel was a right subclavian artery. The posterior indentation was caused by the aortic arch crossing from the right to the left side. Panel *D* shows a lateral projection of a child with a pulmonary artery sling. Note the anterior esophageal compression and mass of tissue between the esophagus and trachea.

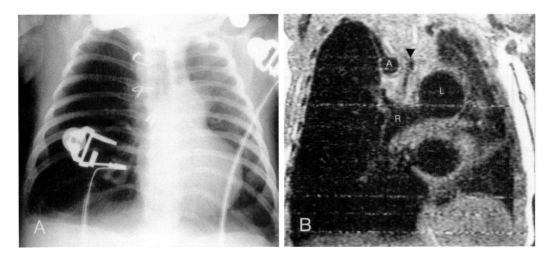

Figure 46.5. Anteroposterior chest radiograph (*A*) and magnetic resonance image (*B*) of a 2-month-old infant with severe dilatation of the pulmonary arteries caused by tetralogy and absent pulmonary valve. This child developed respiratory failure shortly after birth and required ventilatory support. Her ventricular septal defect was closed and an artificial valve was placed in the pulmonary outflow tract at 2 weeks after birth. The radiograph, taken at 2 months, demonstrates persistent hyper-inflation of the lungs, especially on the right. The magnetic resonance image shows how dilated the pulmonary arteries are and how narrow the trachea (*arrowhead*) and right mainstem bronchus are even though they are no longer directly compressed. To appreciate the mammoth size of the left (*L*) and right (*R*) pulmonary arteries, compare them to the caliber of the ascending aorta (*A*). The image also demonstrates the hyper-inflation of the right lung.

Pathophysiology of Respiratory Manifestations

From a clinical point of view, all the cardiovascular anomalies we have discussed until now are characterized by the severity of their respiratory manifestations. Regardless of the exact nature of the anomaly, these manifestations always include an increase in the amount of work that the respiratory system must do in order to maintain adequate ventilation. The increased work taxes further the limited energy reserves of most patients and often leads to the development of respiratory failure as the first indication of the anomaly's existence.

The mechanisms responsible for the increase in work of breathing, however, vary depending on the mechanical alterations produced by each cardiovascular anomaly (Fig. 46.6). A careful analysis of the patient's signs and symptoms usually provides the clinician with helpful clues to unravel these mechanisms, thereby facilitating a better understanding of the disease. For instance, most patients with a large left-to-right shunt or a left ventricular obstruction will develop pulmonary edema. As a result, their alveoli become unstable and collapse, causing an increase in the amount of force that the respiratory muscles have to generate to overcome the elastic recoil of the lungs (19). Under these circumstances, intercostal and subcostal retractions develop and the respiratory pattern tends to become rapid and shallow. Moreover, the patient frequently tries to preserve lung volume by closing the glottis at the end of expiration, producing a grunt. A group of similar patients can develop airway obstruction as their predominant respiratory abnormality. Where it is caused by direct compression of the trachea and large bronchi by enlarged vessels or heart chambers or by narrowing of the small airways by edema, the obstruction is almost always intrathoracic and as such is exacerbated during expiration (6, 7). In these children, respiration tends to be slower and deeper, and the physical examination shows gas trapping, wheezing, and expiratory prolongation.

The increase in the work of breathing represents a challenge for patients who are usually in a poor state of nutrition and whose respiratory muscles may have a reduced ability to increase their blood flow because of reduced

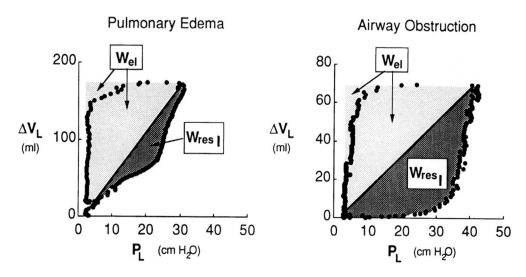

Figure 46.6. Volume-pressure relationships of the respiratory system in the two patients whose chest radiographs are shown in Figures 46.2 and 46.5. ΔV_L and P_L represent the change in the volume of the lungs and the transpulmonary pressure during a breath delivered by a positive pressure ventilatory. The stippled areas indicate the resistive (W_{resl}) and elastic (W_{el}) work that the respiratory muscles would have had to perform on the lungs in order to generate a similar breath during spontaneous ventilation. Note that, as expected, the patient with airway obstruction, on the right, must perform more work against resistive forces than the patient with pulmonary edema. Note also that both patients have to do an increased amount of elastic work. This increased work is caused by alveolar collapse and the presence of interstitial and alveolar fluid in the patient with pulmonary edema, and from lung overdistention in the patient with airway obstruction.

systemic perfusion. In addition, the mechanical abnormalities produced by the disease itself tend to decrease the efficiency with which the respiratory system uses its limited resources (Fig. 46.7). The development of severe retractions, for example, creates an undue burden on the diaphragm, which, for the same amount of work done on the lungs, has to consume more energy to deform the rib cage (20, 21). Similarly, flattening of the diaphragm in the presence of airway obstruction causes the muscle to generate less volume displacement for the same degree of fiber shortening and diminishes its area of apposition to the rib cage (22). Under such conditions, it is not surprising that the energy cost of breathing becomes extraordinary. Although there are very little data in infants and children, some adults with heart disease may devote 50% or more of the O_2 consumption to breathing alone (23). It is obvious that such demands cannot always be fully met, particularly in situations, such as when the patient develops fever or agitation or receives metabolic-stimulating catecholamines, in which the respiratory muscles must compete with

other energy hungry activities. It is then that respiratory failure develops.

Medical Therapy

Although corrective or palliative surgery is the ultimate therapy of each of the defects discussed in this section initial medical management can be invaluable for stabilizing a infant with critical congenital heart disease. Many of these infants are in severe circulatory and respiratory failure at the time of presentation and require interventions that provide the opportunity for and reduce the risks of surgery. Here we will briefly outline the initial approach and rationale for such medical therapy.

For the infant with a large left-to right shunt, treatment has traditionally focused on improving myocardial function, removing excess fluid accumulated in the lungs, and, in some patients, providing assisted respiration. In the acutely decompensated infant, an intravenous inotropic medication such as dopamine, dobutamine, or isoproterenol is most useful. These drugs have rapid onset and metabolism and have few risks even when

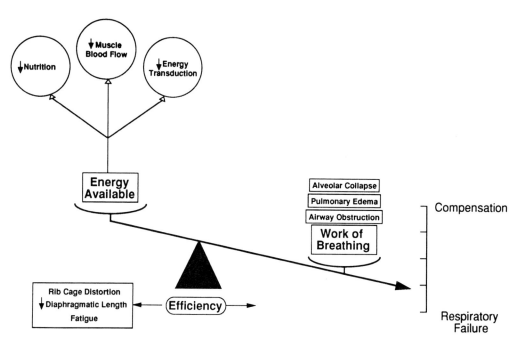

Figure 46.7. Schematic representation of the balance between the energy available to the respiratory muscles and the work that these muscles do during breathing in the presence of a mechanical alteration. Whether the balance tips toward compensation or respiratory failure depends not only on the relative magnitudes of the energy available to the muscles and the increased work load (represented by the weights on both sides of the balance), but also on the efficiency with which the energy is transformed into work (represented by the position of the fulcrum). In the presence of heart disease, alveolar collapse, pulmonary edema, and airway obstruction can increase the work load; poor nutrition, decreased blood flow, and, in general, the inability of the muscle's contractile machinery to transduce energy into work can decrease the energy available. Under such circumstances, decreased efficiency caused by rib cage distortion (retractions), a flattened diaphragm, or muscle fatigue can easily displace the fulcrum to the left, precipitating respiratory failure.

renal function and serum electrolyte concentrations are abnormal. For chronic use, a medication that can be given enterally, such as digoxin, is more appropriate. It is important to note that although most patients with large left-to-right shunts seem to benefit from the use of inotropic drugs, the rationale for their use has been questioned because many of these patients also have normal or increased systolic ventricular function (24). It has been suggested in response to such objections that digoxin may have effects other than augmentation of ventricular function that ameliorate circulatory failure (25). In particular, digoxin might reduce peripheral metabolic demands, which are increased in many infants with large left-to-right shunts. Regardless of the controversy, inotropic suspport is still a mainstay of therapy for the infant with a large-volume left-to-right shunt and circulatory failure.

Diuretics can improve respiratory function by controlling the accumulation of pulmonary edema. In particular, the combination of diuretics and inotropic drugs can decrease filling pressure in the left atrium and reduce pulmonary microvascular pressure, thereby attenuating edema formation. Thus, both the restrictive and obstructive complications of a left-to-right shunt can be controlled by diuretics. However, diuretics also have the risk of disrupting electrolyte homeostasis or compromising systemic blood flow by decreasing intravascular volume, so close monitoring is warranted.

The use of "systemic" vasodilators has been often proposed to decrease the left-to-right shunt. However, these drugs are not selective for the systemic circulation in their vasodilating properties, and therefore do not have predictable effects on the shunt.

For the decompensated infant positive pressure ventilation may be necessary; this can reduce the excessive work devoted to breathing and improve perfusion to non-respiratory tissue (11, 26). It also improves gas exchange by increasing functional residual capacity and overall ventilation-perfusion ratio. Positive airway pressure usually decreases total pulmonary blood flow and, under such conditions, can be expected to diminish transvascular fluid flux in the lung (27). However, if measures are used to maintain pulmonary perfusion, the effect of positive pressure breathing on fluid flux in the lung is less predictable. Although the tendency is often to ventilate patients with supplemental O_2, a high inspired O_2 concentration can reduce pulmonary vascular resistance and increase the left-to-right shunt. For this reason it is important to keep the inspired O_2 concentration as close as possible to room air as long as arterial O_2 saturation is in a clinically acceptable range.

It is quite common for infants with a left-to-right shunt to present with circulatory failure near the nadir of their postnatal anemia, and increasing the hematocrit (usually to the range of 45%) is another approach that can reduce the shunt (3). Although transfusion of blood has obvious infectious risks, it may be valuable as a short-term measure to control pulmonary blood flow, reduce demands on the left ventricle, and maintain systemic O_2 transport.

With some exceptions, the same strategies outlined above—inotropic support, diuretics, and ventilatory assistance—are also used to stabilize the infant with obstruction to inflow or outflow of the left heart. The use of prostaglandin E_1 (PGE_1) is an essential component of the initial therapy for the infant who depends on a patent ductus for systemic perfusion (28). This includes the baby with aortic or mitral atresia, critical aortic or mitral stenosis, or juxtaductal coarctation of the aorta. Infusion of PGE_1 can dramatically improve systemic perfusion, reverse systemic acidosis, and sustain an infant with left heart obstruction for an extended period. Augmentation of the hematocrit, however, has no specific value unless there is significant anemia, which in itself could compromise systemic oxygenation.

There is no specific medical therapy for management of infants with obstruction of the airways except for support of respiration when there is impending fatigue. Because the obstruction is relatively close to the carina or it involves the bronchi, bypassing the lesion with an endotracheal tube is impractical. These infants have usually been stressed by excessive work of breathing so that positive pressure ventilation is usually necessary. The infants with absent pulmonary valve represent a particularly formidable challenge because they have such severe air trapping.

LESIONS IN WHICH THE PREDOMINANT DISTURBANCE IS INCREASED VENOUS ADMIXTURE

Physiologic Classification

Cardiac lesions that cause some of the systemic venous blood to be diverted into the systemic circulation before passing through the lungs result in increased venous admixture and some degree of arterial hypoxia. These congenital anomalies of the heart can be grouped into four general categories (Fig. 46.8): (a) The coexistence of an obstruction of pulmonary blood flow and a communication between the right and the left heart forces blood to flow from the right to the left side of the heart, bypassing the lungs. Examples of this type of right-to-left shunt include those cases in which severe pulmonary stenosis is associated with a ventricular septal defect (as in tetralogy of Fallot) or with a simple patent foramen ovale. In these conditions there is diminished pulmonary blood flow. (b) Anomalous connections of the major vessels with the ventricles can direct a large portion of the systemic venous blood into the aorta and a similar volume of the pulmonary venous blood into the pulmonary artery. This effectively prevents oxygenation of the arterial blood even if pulmonary blood flow is normal or, as is commonly the case, increased. Obviously there must be some mixing between the two circulations, but the magnitude of this mixing, which is the major determinant of arterial oxygenation, varies widely. The most common example of this second group of lesions is the transposition of the great arteries, but a double-outlet right ventricle with preferential streaming of left ventricular blood through a ventricular septal defect into the pulmonary artery (Taussig-Bing anomaly) can produce a similar pattern of blood flow. (c) Cardiac anomalies that produce complete mixing of

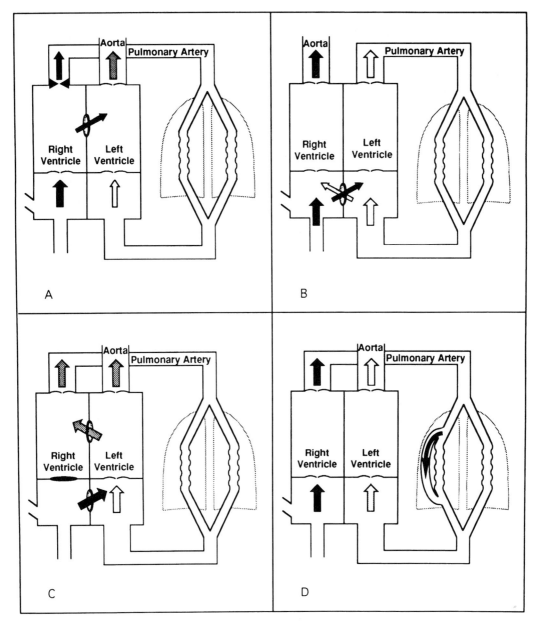

Figure 46.8.   Four mechanisms by with cardiocirculatory anomalies can cause arterial hypoxia. These are described in detail in the text. Panel *A* shows obstruction to pulmonary blood flow and diversion of desaturated systemic venous blood (*dark arrow*), which mixes with well-oxygenated pulmonary venous blood (*light arrow*). The net effect is arterial hypoxia (*shadow arrow*). Panel *B* shows aortopulmonary transposition. Desaturated systemic venous blood mixes with the small amount of oxygenated pulmonary venous blood, which passes through an interartrial connection and returns to the systemic circulation. The resultant arterial hypoxia depends on how much mixing there is between the two circulations. Panel *C* shows tricuspid atresia and a ventricular septal defect. Here all systemic and pulmonary venous blood mix and then this mixture is distributed to both the aorta and the pulmonary artery. The degree of hypoxia depends on the relative flows through the pulmonary and systemic circulations. Panel *D* demonstrates the effect of pulmonary arteriovenous fistulae. Here are some pulmonary arterial blood bypasses ventilated alveoli, causing systemic venous blood to enter the left side of the circulation and producing arterial hypoxia.

systemic and pulmonary venous blood within the heart or great vessels necessarily cause the arterial blood to have a lower than normal O_2 saturation. This occurs whenever there is atresia of one of the cardiac valves because blood must be diverted to the other side of the heart. It also happens if the blood returning from the systemic and pulmonary veins converge into a single chamber or major vessel, as in patients with a single ventricle or truncus arteriosus. Under such conditions pulmonary blood flow may be diminished, normal, or increased; it is the ratio of pulmonary to systemic blood flow that dictates the level of arterial oxygenation. (d) On rare occasions an anomalous vascular channel is formed between a branch of the pulmonary arteries and a pulmonary vein. These pulmonary arteriovenous malformations can allow considerable flow of deoxygenated venous blood to reach the arterial circulation, and therefore they are manifested by cyanosis, which is sometimes positional. Additional signs may include a bruit audible in one lung field or the presence of a mass on chest radiograph. The diagnosis is usually confirmed by angiography, but frequently a contrast echocardiogram with injection of aerated saline into the venous circulation will provide the diagnosis by demonstrating a rapid appearance of bubbles in the left side of the heart in the absence of intracardiac anomalies.

Pathophysiology of Venous Admixture

Although each of the types of cardiac anomalies described above causes venous admixture, the arterial O_2 saturation varies widely depending on the quantity of *mixed systemic venous blood* that effectively traverses the lungs and passes into the systemic circulation. As a general rule for lesions that produce a pure right-to-left shunt or for lesions with complete mixing, the greater the pulmonary blood flow (or pulmonary-to-systemic blood flow ratio), the higher the arterial O_2 saturation. In contrast, when there is transposition (or an analogous circulatory abnormality), pulmonary blood flow can be quite high and the ratio of pulmonary to systemic flow does not determine arterial oxygenation. Rather, it is the small amount of blood that mixes between the systemic and pulmonary circulations that dictates arterial oxygenation. In simple transposition of the great vessels, this mixing can

occur at the atrial level, through a patent ductus arteriosus or, not infrequently, through an associated ventricular septal defect. The blood flow that passes from the right side of the circulation to the left side of the circulation in transposition is really the flow that effectively takes up O_2 and relinquishes it to the systemic tissues. This is because whatever volume of blood passes from the right side of the circulation to the left must, over a period, be balanced by an equal volume of blood passing in the other direction (i.e., that the blood volume in each of the two circulations remains constant.

DEVELOPMENTAL CONSIDERATIONS

Not only the degree of the hypoxia but also its onset varies with each of these lesions. In infants with a right-to-left shunt, hypoxia may not be apparent immediately after birth if the degree of right ventricular outflow obstruction is not severe. An example of these is the tetralogy of Fallot in which the obstruction frequently progresses over infancy. There may even be predominant left-to-right shunting initially. If there is complete obstruction to right ventricular outflow, however, hypoxia is usually apparent shortly after birth, particularly if pulmonary blood flow is low and decreases further as the ductus arteriosus begins to constrict. Alternatively, if pulmonary blood is relatively high, as with tricuspid atresia and a large ventricular septal defect, there may be little hypoxia in the neonatal period. This situation may persist if pulmonary blood flow remains relatively high; however, hypoxia will occur if pulmonary blood flow is progressively curtailed as the ventricular septal defect gets smaller. Finally, with transposition of the great vessels or similar lesions, the hypoxia is usually marked soon after birth.

Physiologic Response to Hypoxia

Hypoxia provokes important adaptive responses that serve to sustain O_2 transport near normal, particularly during infancy when the metabolic demands are high. Cardiac output is usually increased because of an expanded blood volume (29) that augments venous return, and increased sympathetic stimulation that enhances contractility and heart rate (30). Hypoxia also stimulates an increase in hemoglobin synthesis. As with normal infants, subjects with cyanosis caused by congenital cardiac disease experience a postnatal decrease in hemoglobin concentration during the first few weeks, even though in the most hypoxic infants the decline in hemoglobin concentration is blunted and subsequently there is progressive polycythemia (31). In the older child the level of polycythemia is inversely related to the arterial hemoglobin saturation so that arterial O_2 content is near normal despite the hypoxia (32). These circulatory and hematologic adjustments are similar to those observed when healthy subjects ascend to high altitude for a sustained period. They permit restoration of O_2 transport toward normal and help maintain early postnatal growth in many infants despite the severe hypoxia. However, for a variety of reasons many of the infants with significant hypoxia will eventually fail to thrive. In some children, the polycythermia may restrict blood flow in the systemic circulation, thus ablating the benefits derived from this critical adaptation (33). In other infants the hypoxia progresses rapidly to the point where no compensation is sufficient. Still other infants suffer complications of their shunts such as a cerebral stroke; this appears to be particularly likely when the right-to-left shunting is coupled with iron deficiency, which reduces red cell deformability and predisposes to vascular occlusion (34). Another response to chronic hypoxia is the development of bronchial vessels that arise from the aorta and proliferate within the lung parenchyma. These vessels increase pulmonary blood flow and can improve arterial oxygenation. However, with time bronchial blood flow can be excessive enough to produce a volume load on the systemic ventricle. In addition, bronchial vessels rupture easily and become the site of pulmonary hemorrhage, often a life-threatening complication in later years.

Pathophysiology of Respiratory Manifestations

Hypoxia stimulates the peripheral chemoreceptors causing an increase in minute ventilation. However, it is important to note that, for the same arterial Po_2, the increase in minute ventilation in subjects with cyanotic congenital heart disease is less than that in subjects with acute alveolar hypoxia (35). One possible reason for this discrepancy is that with cyanotic heart disease, alveolar oxygen tension is normal and an increase in minute ventilation has minimal effect on both pulmonary venous and arterial Po_2. In contrast, with alveolar hypoxia, an increase in minute ventilation can increase pulmonary venous and arterial Po_2 substantially. Even if the reason is clear, the mechanism for the blunted response to hypoxia of patients with cyanotic heart disease is unknown; re-establishment of normal arterial oxygenation following repair of a cardiac lesion usually results in a return to a normal response (36). However, the clinician must remember that before the repair an infant who has cyanotic heart disease with superimposed factors may have an inappropriate ventilatory response in the presence of *added* alveolar hypoxia, such as that produced by conditions such as parenchymal pulmonary disease, ascent to high altitude, or flight in a poorly pressurized airplane.

When mechanical function of the lungs is relatively normal, as may be anticipated in most lesions that reduce pulmonary blood flow, minute ventilation is raised by an increase in tidal volume and a small increase in respiratory rate (hyperpnea) (37). This usually results in a reduced alveolar and pulmonary venous Pco_2 and high alveolar and pulmonary venous Po_2, consistent with having higher than normal ventilation-perfusion ratio and physiologic dead space. Therapeutic interventions, such as positive pressure ventilation, which further disturb pulmonary blood flow and its distribution, can on occasions interfere further with CO_2 elimination by derecruiting pulmonary capillaries and increasing alveolar (i.e., physiologic) dead space (38).

Although the pathophysiologic changes associated with increased pulmonary blood flow and hypoxia have not been studied in detail in infants, certain problems can be anticipated. If there is significant engorgement of the pulmonary circulation and pulmonary edema, then the disturbances in pulmonary gas exchange might be quite similar to those seen in infants with left-to-right shunts or with left heart obstruction. For example, in infants with transposition and a ventricular septal defect, pulmonary blood flow can be sufficiently high to cause pulmonary venous oxygen desaturation through the development of interstitial or alveolar pulmonary edema, alveolar collapse, and low ventilation-perfu-

47

Hematologic and Oncologic Disorders

WAYNE R. RACKOFF and ROBERT M. WEETMAN

Children with blood disorders and cancer may have pulmonary problems related directly to the disease process, as is the case with acute chest syndrome in sickle cell disease, or may have problems associated with treatment for the underlying disease process, as is the case with interstitial pneumonitis in the immuno-compromised host. In this chapter, the most commonly seen diseases and associated pulmonary problems will be described. Acute chest syndrome and chronic lung changes in sickle cell disease and pulmonary problems associated with homozygous beta-thalassemia will be described first. The discussion of problems in oncology patients is divided into two sections. The first describes problems directly related to oncologic disease or seen during treatment for oncologic disease; the second describes problems encountered as late effects of cancer therapy.

HEMATOLOGIC DISEASES

Sickle Cell Disease

ACUTE CHEST SYNDROME

Now that the risk of infection has been decreased by the use of penicillin prophylaxis, and pneumococcal and *Haemophilus influenzae B* vaccines, acute chest syndrome has become a leading cause of morbidity and mortality among children with sickle cell disease (1, 2). Acute chest syndrome refers to a common set of signs and symptoms that are found in patients with a number of pathologic processes in the lung. Patients with acute chest syndrome present with fever, cough, tachypnea, chest pain, shortness of breath, hypoxia, and a new infiltrate on chest radiograph

(Fig. 47.1) (3). Although adults often present to the clinic or emergency department with these symptoms, children often develop symptoms during the course of treatment for vaso-occlusive pain, or other complications of their disease.

The etiology and pathogenesis of acute chest syndrome have been the subject of much

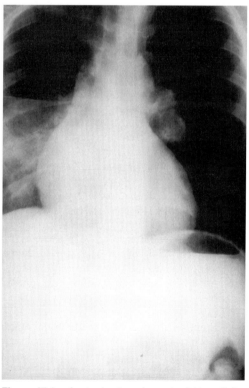

Figure 47.1. Acute chest syndrome in sickle cell disease. PA chest radiograph shows right lower lobe infiltrate that developed on the third day of an admission for vaso-occlusive pain. (Courtesy of Dr. Mervyn Cohen, Riley Hospital for Children.)

debate, but few studies have adequately addressed these questions. Prior to the advent of control measures, bacterial pneumonia was found to account for most cases of acute chest syndrome in children, whereas pulmonary infarction due to sickling and subsequent vaso-occlusion was thought to cause the majority of cases in adults (3–5). In a prospective study of 102 episodes of acute chest syndrome in children who were receiving penicillin prophylaxis, and most of whom had received pneumococcal vaccine, a bacterial etiology could be identified in only 12% of the episodes. Only 3% were secondary to *Streptococcus pneumoniae* (6). The remaining episodes were associated with viral pneumonia (8%) or *Mycoplasma* pneumonia (16%), or were of undetermined etiology. Most were presumed to be due to pulmonary infarction, atelectasis, or missed infections. The patients with bacterial pneumonia had higher temperatures at presentation, were febrile for more days, and had longer hospitalizations than those without a known bacterial etiology. The low incidence of bacterial pneumonia found in this study was presumed to be a result of adequate prophylaxis for and vaccination against *Streptococcus pneumoniae*. The relatively high incidence of *Mycoplasma* infection found in this study, and the finding of unusually severe *Mycoplasma* pneumonia in children with sickle cell disease (7), has resulted in the recommendation to treat for *Mycoplasma* infection in children with acute chest syndrome.

Rib infarction, with secondary soft tissue reaction, pleural effusion, splinting, hypoventilation, and resultant pulmonary infarction, has been proposed as a cause of acute chest syndrome (8). This process may explain the onset of acute chest syndrome in patients hospitalized for painful vaso-occlusion in the ribs or sternum. The use of appropriate analgesia and incentive spirometry may help prevent acute chest syndrome in patients with pain in the bony thorax.

Fat embolism to the lung after bone infarction has also been proposed as a cause of acute chest syndrome (9). Patients may have stainable fat in the urine and may have the classic syndrome of fever and neurologic, respiratory, and renal complications. Whether the hypoxia associated with acute chest syndrome is the cause or result of fat embolism is still under investigation.

Differentiation among the various conditions that result in acute chest syndrome is difficult. Currently, most episodes are treated as though bacterial or *Mycoplasma* pneumonia is present. Initial therapy with a second-generation cephalosporin (e.g., cefuroxime) and oral erythromycin is given to cover the most common treatable microbiologic agents. Intravenous fluid should be used judiciously, with the goal of maintaining intraerythrocyte hydration using hypotonic saline solutions at a maintenance rate. The fluid rate may need to be adjusted downward if pulmonary edema or pleural effusion develops.

Arterial oxygenation should be monitored with continuous pulse oximetry, periodic arterial blood gas measurements, or both. Initial values should be obtained prior to giving supplemental oxygen. The goal is to maintain the PaO_2 at greater than 70 mm Hg and the hemoglobin oxygen saturation above 95%. Pulse oximetry has been demonstrated to be accurate in patients with sickle cell disease (10, 11). However, the limitations of pulse oximetry—poor accuracy below 70% hemoglobin oxygen saturation and poor reflection of oxygen delivery in the severely anemic patient (12)—and the rightward shift of the hemoglobin oxygen dissociation curve in patients with sickle cell disease must be considered in the interpretation of values obtained using this technique (10, 11).

Supplemental oxygen is indicated in patients with hypoxia due to acute chest syndrome, but not indicated for patients with uncomplicated vaso-occlusive pain episodes. In a prospective, randomized trial of children with vaso-occlusive pain, supplemental oxygen had no beneficial effect on pain relief or the duration of hospitalization (13). In fact, continuous inhalation of oxygen may have a detrimental effect in the absence of hypoxia. Continuous oxygen inhalation for 5 days in three otherwise well sickle cell patients resulted in lower erythropoietin levels, and a fall in irreversibly sickled cells. All three patients had rapid reversal of the process after cessation of oxygen therapy, resulting in acute painful episodes that were thought to have been caused by rebound erythropoiesis in two patients (14).

The role of red blood cell transfusion in the treatment of acute chest syndrome has not been thoroughly investigated. Reports of small numbers of patients show dramatic reversal of acute chest syndrome using either partial exchange transfusion (15) or simple transfusion (16), suggesting that vaso-occlusion plays a significant role in the pathogenesis of acute chest syndrome. A reasonable approach to patients with acute chest syndrome is to give simple transfusion to those patients with moderate hypoxia on supplemental oxygen (PaO_2 greater than 70 mm Hg), reserving partial exchange transfusion for patients with moderate to severe hypoxia (PaO_2 less than 70 mm Hg) despite supplemental oxygen therapy, and those who have a worsening chest radiograph despite other supportive measures.

A significant drop in the hemoglobin is characteristic of acute chest syndrome (17). Therefore, significant lowering of the hemoglobin S percentage may be accomplished by simple transfusion in patients who are severely anemic. However, the hematocrit should not be raised above 30–35% in order to avoid too rapid an increase in blood viscosity that may contribute to vaso-occlusion or congestive heart failure from volume overload.

After recovery from acute chest syndrome, new baseline pulmonary function tests, including flow volume loops pre- and post-bronchodilators, diffusion capacity of the lung for carbon monoxide (DLCO), and lung volumes when possible, and pulse oximetry should be done. This will facilitate more appropriate interpretation of such tests at the time of subsequent evaluations for acute or chronic pulmonary problems.

CHRONIC LUNG DISEASE

In adults, sickle cell chronic lung disease is characterized by reduction in total lung capacity, forced vital capacity, forced expiratory volume, and hemoglobin oxygen desaturation (5, 8). The DLCO may be decreased in patients with sickle cell disease, but is often normal when corrected for anemia (19). However, diffusion across the alveolar membrane is frequently decreased in hemoglobin SS disease, with the lowest values observed in patients with a history of pulmonary complications (20). Progressive pulmonary vascular disease, and the complications of pulmonary hypertension, are the cause of significant morbidity and mortality in older patients with sickle cell disease (21).

There is increasing evidence that the development of sickle cell chronic lung disease in adults is associated with episodes of acute chest syndrome (20, 22). Thus, chronic lung disease may have its origins in childhood. In a study of 108 children with sickle cell disease, those with hemoglobin SS disease and a history of acute chest syndrome had lower transcutaneous hemoglobin oxygen saturation (mean = 94%) than those without a history of acute chest syndrome (mean = 98%) (11). The difference is not seen in children with hemoglobin SC disease, all of whom had transcutaneous hemoglobin oxygen saturation in the normal range. In Hb SS patients, a similar difference was seen when those 5 years old or younger were compared with those 6 years old and older, suggesting that the changes occur at an early age.

In contrast to these findings, studies of pulmonary function using spirometry have not shown an association between a history of acute chest syndrome and pulmonary function abnormalities in children with sickle cell disease. A comparison of 12 children with sickle cell disease and 12 race-, sex-, and height-matched control subjects showed no significant difference in lung volumes or expiratory flow rates between the groups (23). However, children with sickle cell disease had mild hypoxia and abnormal increases in calculated shunt. A similar study of 37 children with sickle cell disease and 22 matched control subjects showed that the FVC and FEV_1 were significantly less for sickle cell disease patients than for control subjects (24). The FEV_1/FVC ratio was normal. Total lung capacity in Hb SS patients was lower than in control subjects, but the ratio of residual volume to total lung capacity was normal. No differences were found between the patients with acute chest syndrome episodes and other patients with sickle cell disease. Exercise testing of some of the same patients showed an increased ventilatory response caused in part by anemia and increased physiologic dead space (V_D/V_T) (25).

The apparent discrepancy between studies based on spirometry and the study using pulse oximetry may be explained by the inclusion in the spirometry studies of children who are already likely to have had clinically unrecognized acute chest syndrome that occurs by age 6 years, the age at which children are usually able to be studied with spirometry. The oximetry study included many patients less than 6 years of age, and so would have a comparison group with less chest disease.

Whether it is associated with multiple episodes of acute chest syndrome or not, chronic lung disease, with hypoxia and cor pulmonale, is seen in children after severe episodes of acute chest syndrome and as a more insidious process in older patients. Unfortunately, there are no controlled trials of the treatment of sickle cell chronic lung disease. Chronic transfusion has been proposed, but not subjected to rigorous study (22). The use of supplemental oxygen is usually limited to the most severely affected. It is not yet known whether agents that increase hemoglobin F percentage will have a beneficial effect on chronic pulmonary pathology.

Homozygous Beta-Thalassemia

Homozygous beta-thalassemia is an inherited disorder of globin synthesis. A lack of beta globin production results in a severe, microcytic anemia due to hemolysis of red blood cells containing aggregates of insoluble alpha globin. Patients usually become dependent on red blood cell transfusion during the first 2 years of life. Chronic transfusion therapy results in the accumulation of excess iron unless adequate chelation therapy is undertaken.

Pulmonary function studies in patients with homozygous beta-thalassemia have shown varying results. One study of 19 patients with homozygous beta-thalassemia showed increased residual volume, ratio of residual volume to total lung capacity, and airway resistance (26). These results indicate mild to moderate small airway obstruction. None of the patients had normal pulmonary function testing. Transfusion history and the degree of iron accumulation did not influence the results of pulmonary function testing in this study. A similar study of 28 Chinese patients with homozygous beta-thalassemia showed decreases in forced vital capacity and FEV_1, indicative of mild restrictive lung disease (27).

Patients with homozygous beta-thalassemia have iron deposition in the lungs at postmortem examination (28). Presumably, iron deposition contributes to small airway obstruction or fibrosis and restriction. Yet, in one study (26), there was no difference between the group with a high mean ferritin value, a marker of tissue iron deposition, and the group with a low mean ferritin value. This finding suggests that iron deposition does not make a major contribution to the lung abnormalities seen in these patients. Thus, no good explanation exists to explain the various abnormalities in lung function found in patients with homozygous beta-thalassemia.

Although iron deposition and chelation therapy with deferoxamine may not contribute to the abnormalities found in otherwise well patients with homozygous beta-thalassemia, a syndrome of acute pulmonary interstitial disease has been described in four patients receiving continuous, high-dose infusions of the drug (29). Patients suffered the acute onset of cough, tachypnea, and hypoxia associated with new interstitial infiltrates on chest radiograph. Infectious agents were not identified. Lung biopsy was normal in one patient; in a second patient, the biopsy showed diffuse alveolar damage, obliteration of alveolar spaces, interstitial fibrosis, and an inflammatory response. The infiltration of eosinophils and mast cells with surface IgE suggested that sensitization to deferoximine may have occurred. Although one of the patients had life-threatening respiratory failure, all recovered. We have treated a patient with this syndrome who died of respiratory failure. Postmortem examination revealed lung pathology similar to that seen in adult respiratory distress syndrome (ARDS). A cause-and-effect relationship has not been proven, but the risk of this syndrome must be considered when high-dose intravenous deferoximine is administered.

ONCOLOGIC DISEASES

Disease- and Acute Treatment-Related Complications

Chest findings in children with cancer are varied. Knowledge of the distribution of chest lesions in children by site of origin can help in the differential diagnosis of the underlying oncologic problem (30, 31). Table 47.1 lists categories of pediatric oncologic diagnoses by their more common sites of origin within the chest. Specifically, the differential diagnosis can be divided into those lesions arising in the anterior, middle, and posterior mediastinum, and those arising in the chest wall. Primary

Table 47.1.
Malignant and Benign Chest Lesions In Children

Affected region	Malignant	Benign
Anterior mediastinum	Lymphoma Germ cell tumor	Normal thymus Teratoma Lymphangioma Bronchogenic cyst Cystic hygroma

Middle mediastinum	Lymphoma
	Germ cell tumor
		Teratoma
		Pericardial cyst
		Granulomatous disease
		  (histoplasmosis, tuberculosis)
		Esophageal duplication and
		  enteric cyst
		Bronchial cyst

Posterior mediastinum	Neuroblastoma Ganglioneuroblastoma Lymphoma	Ganglioneuroma Bronchiogenic cyst Thoracic meningocele Cystic hygroma Neurofibroma
Chest wall origin	Ewing sarcoma PNET[a] Rhabdomyosarcoma	Lipoma Hemangioma Osteochondroma Neurofibroma
Pulmonary nodules	Wilms tumor Ewing sarcoma PNET[a] Rhabdomyosarcoma Osteosarcoma Hepatoblastoma Hepatocellular carcinoma Hodgkin disease	Granulomatous disease (histoplasmosis; tuberculosis) Round pneumonia Inflammatory pseudotumor Hamartoma
Diffuse pulmonary infiltrates	Langerhans cell histiocytosis Leukemia Non-Hodgkin lymphoma	Radiation pneumonitis Opportunistic infection

[a]Primitive neuroectodermal tumor.

pulmonary neoplasms are extremely rare in children. Pleural effusions occasionally accompany mediastinal masses in children, and usually signify the presence of non-Hodgkin lymphoma or leukemia-lymphoma syndrome (Fig. 47.2). Rarely, pleural effusions are associated with other oncologic diagnoses.

PULMONARY METASTATIC LESIONS IN CHILDREN WITH CANCER

The accurate diagnosis of pulmonary metastatic lesions in children with known cancer can be difficult. When multiple pulmonary nodules are present in the child known to have a cancer with a natural history of metastasis to the lung, the diagnosis of pulmonary metastases may often be assumed. However, in the child with a single pulmonary nodule, the diagnosis of pulmonary metastasis cannot be assumed. In a study of 39 pulmonary nodules in 37 children with known malignant tumors, 33% were benign lesions and required no further intervention or change in antineoplastic therapy (32). In this study, the etiology of the benign nodules included histoplasmosis, round pneumonia, round atelectasis, inflammatory pseudotumor, hamartoma, and radiation pneumonitis.

The evaluation of the child with cancer for suspected pulmonary metastatic disease depends on the clinical presentation. In children with posterior-anterior (PA) and lateral chest radiographs that revealed no abnormalities, whole lung tomography detected a new lesion in only 1% of studies, provided new information in only 8% of studies, and when performed for routine screening, yielded new information in only 2.7% of studies (33).

ance to the lung, sometimes progressing to bullae formation (52, 53, 58). Spontaneous pneumothorax, particularly if recurrent, in the presence of chronic interstitial lung disease should suggest the diagnosis of pulmonary histiocytosis. This complication is reported to occur in 10–20% of patients (52, 53, 55). Hilar or mediastinal adenopathy in the presence of histiocytic pulmonary infiltrates is more likely to be present in the young child with multi-organ system disease than in the adolescent or young adult with isolated pulmonary histiocytosis. In the absence of generalized adenopathy, or multi-organ system disease, the presence of hilar or mediastinal adenopathy should suggest the possibility of another disease (55, 59).

The pulmonary function abnormalities in LCH involving the lung depend to a certain degree on the extent of disease. A decrease in the oxygen diffusion capacity, hypoxia, and decreased lung compliance with a restrictive pattern may result from histiocytic infiltration and fibrosis of the lung. With the formation of blebs, and bullae, air trapping occasionally occurs, resulting in an obstructive abnormality (52, 53, 58). High-resolution chest CT appears to be superior to the plain chest radiograph for the assessment of pulmonary disease in LCH (60, 61). Lung biopsy should be used to establish a definite diagnosis of pulmonary histiocytosis because of the similarity of the clinical picture with other diseases and the lack of a definitive, non-invasive diagnostic technique.

There is ongoing controversy about the treatment of LCH. Generally, young infants and children with multi-organ system disease and pulmonary dysfunction require chemotherapy. Commonly used drugs are vinblastine, 6-mercaptopurine, etoposide, and corticosteroids in some combination. However, pulmonary involvement with LCH has been reported to respond to corticosteroids alone (55). In one series, pulmonary LCH was not felt to worsen the prognosis in a group of patients with multi-organ system involvement (53). In young adults, isolated or primary LCH frequently is related to cigarette smoking. The process may regress spontaneously after cessation of smoking or with corticosteroid therapy (56, 62, 63). Isolated pulmonary histiocytosis in the young adult occasionally may progress to chronic debilitating lung dis-

ease (63). In isolated or primary LCH of the lung, the radiographic findings secondary to fibrosis, honeycomb appearance, and bullae formation typically are more prominent in the upper lung fields and peri-hilar areas, with the costophrenic areas less involved (55, 63). Bronchogenic carcinoma has been reported following primary pulmonary histiocytosis in the young adult population and may relate to the prominent history of tobacco abuse in this population (64). Pulmonary histiocytosis has also been reported following the treatment of Hodgkin disease (65).

TRACHEAL COMPRESSION AND SUPERIOR VENA CAVA SYNDROME

Large tumors in the anterior mediastinum can cause tracheal compression, superior vena cava syndrome, or both. The most common tumors in this area are Hodgkin and non-Hodgkin lymphomas (see Table 47.1). Tracheal compression may cause cough, stridor, dyspnea, or orthopnea. However, tracheal compression is not always obvious from the physical examination or chest radiograph. It may become apparent only when a patient is forced from a position of comfort for an examination or diagnostic study. Compression of the superior vena cava may cause headache, dyspnea, orthopnea, syncope, or cardiovascular collapse due to decreased venous return. Together, these findings are known as superior vena cava syndrome (Fig. 47.3). Physical examination may be unremarkable or may show venous distension, plethora, cyanosis, and edema of the head, neck, thorax, or upper extremities (41).

Children with tracheal compression or superior vena cava syndrome are often anxious and diaphoretic. They resist efforts to be placed in the supine position and should not be forced to do so. Efforts to assess airway patency with CT or flexible bronchoscopy are often ill advised, because patients do not tolerate procedures well and may be very difficult to resuscitate if they suffer cardiorespiratory collapse (66, 67). Narcotic analgesia, sedation, and any drug that interferes with venous return should be avoided, or if required, should be used with great care. Intravenous infusions administered in the affected extremity may cause respiratory distress, thrombosis, or phlebitis.

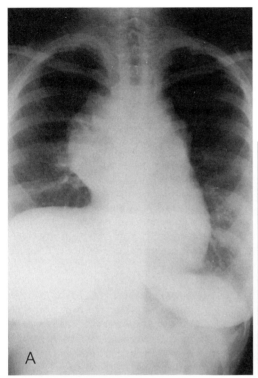
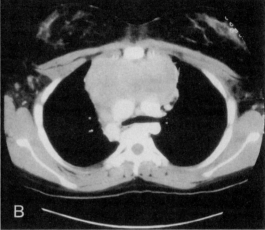

Figure 47.3. Superior vena cava syndrome and tracheal compression. *A,* PA chest radiograph shows large anterior mediastinal mass. *B,* Chest CT with contrast shows compression of the trachea at the level of the carina and filling of the azygous vein due to occlusion of the superior vena cava. The azygous vein is not usually visualized on contrast CT in the absence of superior vena cava obstruction. (Courtesy of Dr. Mervyn Cohen, Riley Hospital for Children.)

In a child, tracheal compression and superior vena cava syndrome are almost always caused by Hodgkin's disease or non-Hodgkin's lymphoma. Often, the diagnosis can be made from bone marrow or peripheral lymph node biopsy. If the diagnosis cannot be made from tissue outside of the mediastinum, therapy should be based on the impression of the treating oncologist. Studies of histologic specimens made after the initiation of emergent therapy show that the impression of the treating oncologist is usually correct (68). Therapy with radiation (50–100 cGy to the midplane for 2–3 days) or corticosteroids (hydrocortisone 2 mg/kg every 6 hours), or both, usually will alleviate symptoms (69).

INTERSTITIAL PNEUMONITIS

Interstitial pneumonitis in oncology patients may be seen in a number of clinical settings and may be caused by a wide array of infectious agents or may be due to the effects of chemo-therapy or radiation therapy (see the sections on pulmonary metastatic lesions in children and pulmonary late effects of cancer therapy). Patients present with cough, fever, hypoxia, and an interstitial, reticular pattern on the chest radiograph. Often, the initial physical findings belie the degree of hypoxia and underlying lung pathology. Patients may be at the depth of a neutrophil nadir or have normal leukocyte counts at the time of onset.

Prior to the use of prophylaxis with trimethoprim-sulfamethoxazole (TMP-SMZ), pneumonia due to *Pneumocystis carinii* (PCP) was a frequent cause of interstitial pneumonitis and death in patients with acute lymphoblastic leukemia (ALL) in remission (39). PCP has been virtually eliminated from this group of patients since the advent of effective prophylaxis, but is still seen in those who are unable to take TMP-SMZ due to hypersensitivity phenomena or drug-induced myelosuppression. Patients who have had lung irradiation or who are taking high-dose corticosteroids are also at risk of PCP if they are not on TMP-SMZ prophylaxis.

Other than PCP, causative organisms in interstitial pneumonitis include the following: viruses—cytomegalovirus (CMV), varicella (VZV), Epstein-Barr virus (EBV), herpes simplex virus (HSV), respiratory syncytial virus (RSV), and influenza species; bacteria, especially viridans streptococci; atypical bacteria—*Mycoplasma* and *Legionella* species; and fungi, especially *Candida* and *Aspergillus* species. PCP should be suspected in patients at risk who are not receiving adequate prophylaxis. *Mycoplasma* or viral infection often presents in a patient with a history of upper respiratory tract infection, with or without wheezing. *Aspergillus* infection may present as a diffuse interstitial pneumonia in the patient with neutropenia. Pleuritic chest pain is sometimes present and probably is due to the presence of pleural-based lesions. A fungus ball is usually not seen until the patient has an adequate neutrophil count (69). Often, the chest radiograph does not show the extent of disease seen on CT (Fig. 47.4) (70). A cluster of *Aspergillus* pneumonia has been reported in the setting of poor maintenance of the air handling system of an oncology unit (71).

Interstitial pneumonitis may be a manifestation of bacterial pneumonia in the severely neutropenic patient. It may also follow septicemia by 1–3 days and be a harbinger of ARDS. Viridans streptococcal infection is particularly prone to cause pulmonary complications (72, 73). This organism should not be considered a contaminant in cultures from an oncology patient.

Initial evaluation and treatment of an oncology patient with interstitial pneumonitis should be directed toward the identification and treatment of bacterial infection. Blood culture, and sputum culture when feasible, should be obtained. Varicella or herpetic pneumonia are rare in the absence of skin lesions. When skin lesions are present, scrapings should be obtained from the base of the lesion and submitted for Tzanck preparation, viral culture, and rapid immunologic detection tests.

The role of flexible bronchoscopy was examined in 60 consecutive procedures for pulmonary infiltrate of unknown cause in pediatric oncology patients (74). Fifty of these patients had broncho-alveolar lavage (BAL). A specific diagnosis was identified in 27% of patients, with the largest proportion from the group that had BAL. *Aspergillus* infection was the most commonly missed diagnosis: only four of eight patients who were proven to have the infection were diagnosed with bronchoscopy.

Based on these findings, a reasonable approach to the oncology patient with interstitial pneumonitis would be to perform flexible bronchoscopy with BAL if no diagnosis is evident within 24 hours after the onset of signs or symptoms. If a diagnosis is not evident 24–36 hours after bronchoscopy, open lung biopsy is indicated. In some institutions, open lung biopsy is the initial diagnostic procedure of choice.

Initial treatment of the neutropenic oncology patient with interstitial pneumonitis should be with broad-spectrum antibiotics. The choice of drugs should be guided by the flora seen in the treating institution, but should include coverage for *Pseudomonas* species and gram-positive organisms. Additional treatment should be directed toward the most likely organism. TMP-SMZ (20 mg/kg/day of TMP) should be given for suspected PCP. Acyclovir is given for suspected HSV (250 mg/m^2/day divided every 8 hours) or VZV (1500 mg/m^2/day divided every 8 hours). Ganciclovir (2–5 mg/kg every 8 hours) and intravenous gamma globulin are used for proven CMV infection or when CMV is highly suspected, as would be the case in a patient with interstitial pneumonitis 1–3 months after bone marrow transplantation. Erythromycin is used to cover atypical bacteria, and is rarely contraindicated. Therapy with amphotericin B or other anti-fungal agents should be instituted if fungal infection is suspected (75, 76).

Supplemental oxygen is used as indicated. Mechanical ventilation should be used except when precluded by prior discussions with the patient or family. Most patients who are being treated with chemotherapy will have some degree of anemia. Packed red blood cell transfusion is indicated to increase oxygen-carrying capacity in the hypoxic patient.

Pulmonary Late Effects of Cancer Therapy

With modern pediatric oncologic therapy, 60–70% of childhood cancer patients survive

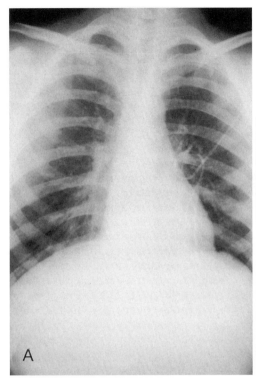
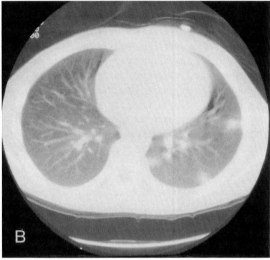

Figure 47.4. Pulmonary aspergillosis in a patient with acute myeloid leukemia. *A,* PA chest radiograph does not show distinct infiltrates. *B,* Chest CT shows multiple wedge-shaped pleural-based lesions typical of pulmonary aspergillosis. (Courtesy of Dr. Mervyn Cohen, Riley Hospital for Children.)

their disease. It is estimated that by the year 2000, 1 in 900 young adults in the age range 15–45 years will be a survivor of childhood cancer (77). This section will briefly review the pulmonary late effects of cancer therapy. A number of recent articles are available for more in-depth review of the subject (78–84).

PULMONARY LATE EFFECTS OF RADIATION THERAPY

Therapeutic radiation that encompasses normal pulmonary tissue can lead to acute and chronic reactions (82). Acute radiation pneumonitis usually occurs 1–6 months after the start of radiation therapy (82, 85). Chronic pulmonary fibrosis usually requires months to years to develop with most changes being apparent by 1–2 years post radiation exposure (82, 85). Irradiation of type I and II pneumocytes, endothelial cells, macrophages, and fibroblasts may lead to interference with lung growth and alveolar multiplication, changes in compliance and airway resistance, volume loss with a decrease in total lung capacity and

vital capacity, chronic pulmonary fibrosis, and a decrease in the diffusion capacity (79, 82). The effect of therapeutic radiation on the growth of normal muscle, cartilage, and bone of the thorax of the young child may also contribute to chronic pulmonary dysfunction (79, 82). Pulmonary function testing after radiation injury may reveal restrictive changes, pulmonary volume loss, and arterial hypoxia secondary to decreased diffusion capacity, with a potential for more chronic problems, including dyspnea, orthopnea, cyanosis, and cor pulmonale (82). However, many patients remain asymptomatic after radiation therapy to the lungs.

The risk of radiation damage to normal pulmonary tissue is enhanced by the concomitant administration of chemotherapeutic agents with radiomimetic effects (anthracyclines and actinomycin-D) or the potential for primary pulmonary damage secondary to the chemotherapeutic agent itself (85). In the absence of chemotherapy, fractionated whole lung radiation tolerance in children is in the range of

1800–2000 cGy, whereas in the presence of chemotherapy, whole lung tolerance is in the range of 1500–1800 cGy. There is a 5–10% incidence of toxicity at this level (85, 86). When less than 30% of one lung is irradiated in the absence of chemotherapy, pulmonary tolerance is in the 2500–3000 cGy range with a less than 5–10% incidence of toxicity. However, when partial lung radiation is given with chemotherapy, tolerance is reduced to less than 2000 cGy (85, 86).

Certain chemotherapy agents (anthracyclines and actinomycin-D), when administered shortly following therapeutic radiation, can result in the reactivation of radiation injury to the lung, a process termed "radiation recall." Anthracyclines and actinomycin-D must be given at a reduced dosage when used shortly after radiation therapy (88, 89). Other chemotherapy agents reported to cause radiation recall reactions include bleomycin, etoposide, hydroxyurea, methotrexate, trimetrexate, and vinblastine (90).

Although post-irradiation pneumonitis is usually a self-limited phenomena, corticosteroids may be effective in ameliorating symptoms and shortening the course (85). The corticosteroid dose should be tapered cautiously in order not to precipitate an exacerbation of the radiation pneumonitis (91). It has been postulated that radiation pneumonitis represents a lymphocyte-mediated hypersensitivity reaction, and exacerbation of radiation pneumonitis following withdrawal of corticosteroids, an immunosuppressive agent, further supports this theory (92, 93).

PULMONARY LATE EFFECTS OF CHEMOTHERAPY

A number of chemotherapeutic agents have been reported to have pulmonary toxicity, and an extensive review of the pulmonary toxicity of antineoplastic agents recently has been published (87). Agents with pulmonary toxicity that currently are in use in the field of pediatric oncology include bleomycin, BCNU, CCNU, busulfan, cyclophosphamide, melphalan, methotrexate, cytosine arabinoside, 5-azacitidine, vinblastine, etoposide, and procarbazine. In addition, the immunotherapeutic agent interleukin-2 has been associated with a life-threatening syndrome characterized by hypotension, respiratory distress (which often requires mechanical ventilation),

and both pulmonary and peripheral edema (94). Bleomycin, cyclophosphamide, and BCNU are the chemotherapy agents commonly used in the pediatric age group with pulmonary toxicity that may be enhanced by concomitant administration of oxygen (95–101). The most common injury pattern is that of alveolar damage, with the development of pulmonary fibrosis and restrictive disease, and decreased diffusion capacity (87). Bleomycin, procarbazine, and methotrexate may also produce pulmonary injury through a hypersensitivity mechanism (102–104).

In the pediatric age group, the agents most commonly associated with pulmonary toxicity are bleomycin, BCNU, busulfan, and cyclophosphamide. Most of the information known about bleomycin comes from the adult literature, with little information primarily in pediatric patients (87, 97). This agent produces direct injury to the pulmonary capillary endothelium and pneumocytes, resulting in pulmonary fibrosis. Pulmonary injury is felt to be mediated through an oxygen free-radical mechanism, and may be potentiated by an FiO_2 of greater than 25% (Fig. 47.5) (95–97). Although a cumulative dose of 400 units of bleomycin in adults increases the risk of pulmonary toxicity, toxicity in children may occur at a much lower cumulative dose (78, 97). Radiation to the lung concomitant with bleomycin therapy increases the risk of pulmonary toxicity. Clinically, this has been manifested primarily in patients with Hodgkin disease receiving combination chemotherapy and radiation for mediastinal disease. Bleomycin is excreted by the kidneys. Therefore, administration of bleomycin with cisplatin, or other agents that produce renal dysfunction, increases the risk of bleomycin toxicity (105–110). An acute and often fatal hypersensitivity reaction associated with hypotension and cardiorespiratory collapse may be initiated by bleomycin. During bleomycin therapy, pulmonary function tests should be followed. If the diagnosis of bleomycin pulmonary toxicity is established, this agent should be discontinued and corticosteroids should be administered (87, 97, 111).

BCNU, a nitrosourea compound commonly used for the treatment of brain tumors in children, also produces pulmonary fibrosis, restrictive lung disease, hypoxia, and decreased diffusion capacity. A total cumula-

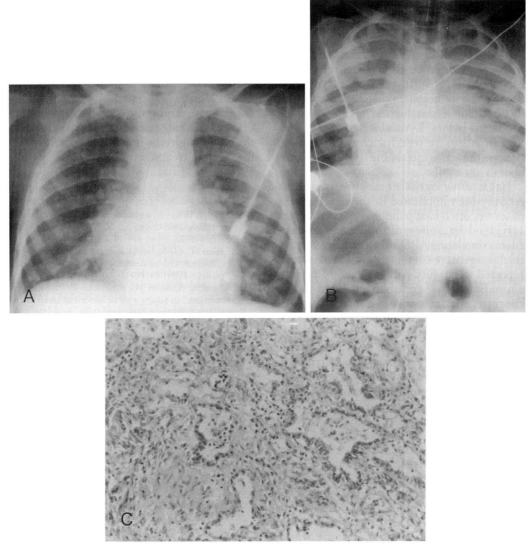

Figure 47.5. Bleomycin-induced pulmonary injury. *A,* PA chest radiograph shows diffuse reticulonodular densities. *B,* PA chest radiograph of the same patient shows worsening after the administration of supplemental oxygen. *C,* Histologic findings of interstitial fibrosis and hyperplastic pneumocytes at the time of autopsy in the same patient. (Courtesy of Drs. Mervyn Cohen and Phillip Faught, Riley Hospital for Children.)

tive BCNU dose of 1000 mg/m^2 has been associated with an increased risk of pulmonary toxicity, but toxic effects have been reported to occur at lower doses (87, 112–114). Pulmonary fibrosis frequently occurs within 3 years of the start of BCNU therapy, but may be delayed for many years following completion of therapy (112). Patients receiving BCNU should have periodic pulmonary function tests for surveillance of pulmonary toxicity. In one study, corticosteroid administration did not prevent BCNU-induced pulmonary toxicity

(114). Other nitrosourea compounds (CCNU and methyl-CCNU) are less likely to produce pulmonary fibrosis than BCNU. However when combined with spinal irradiation for the treatment of childhood brain tumors, the incidence of pulmonary toxicity has been reported to be higher than with CCNU alone, suggesting that spinal irradiation contributes to the development of pulmonary toxicity (115).

The alkylating agents cyclophosphamide and busulfan cause pulmonary toxicity that may be augmented by concomitant radiation

manifestations of a single nosologic entity. *Arch Pathol* 1953; 56:84–102.

51. Chu T, D'Angio GJ, Favara B, Ladisch S, Nesbit M, Pritchard J. Histiocytosis syndromes in children. *Lancet* 1987; 1:208–209.

52. Berry DH, Becton DL. Natural history of histiocytosis X. *Hematol Oncol Clin North Am* 1987; 1:23–34.

53. Ha SY, Helms P, Fletcher M, Broadbent V, Pritchard J. Lung involvement in Langerhans' cell histiocytosis: Prevalence, clinical features, and outcome. *Pediatrics* 1992; 89:466–469.

54. Carlson RA, Hattery RR, O'Connell EJ, Fontana RS. Pulmonary involvement in histiocytosis X in the pediatric age group. *Mayo Clin Proc* 1976; 51:542–547.

55. Nondahl SR, Finlay JL, Farrell PM, Warner TF, Hong R. A case report and literature review of "primary" pulmonary histiocytosis of childhood. *Med Pediatr Oncol* 1986; 14:57–62.

56. McDowell HP, MacFarlane PI, Martin J. Isolated pulmonary histiocytosis. *Arch Dis Child* 1988; 63:423–426.

57. Basset F, Corrin B, Spencer H, Lacronique J, Roth C, Soler P, Battesti J, Georges R, Chretien J. Pulmonary histiocytosis X. *Am Rev Respir Dis* 1978; 118:811–819.

58. Marcy TW, Reynolds HY. Pulmonary histiocytosis X. *Lung* 1985; 163:129–150.

59. Brambilla E, Fontaine E, Pison CM, Coulomb M, Paramelle B, Barmbilla C. Pulmonary histiocytosis X with mediastinal lymph node involvement. *Am Rev Respir Dis* 1990; 142:1216–1218.

60. Grenier P, Valeyre D, Cluzel P, Brauner MW, Lenoir S, Chastang C. Chronic diffuse interstitial lung disease: Diagnostic value of chest radiography and high resolution CT. *Radiology* 1991; 179:123–132.

61. Lee WA, Hruban RH, Kuhlman JE, Fishman EK, Wheeler PS, Hutchins GM. High resolution computed tomography of inflation-fixed lungs: Pathology-radiologic correlation of pulmonary lesions in patients with leukemia, lymphoma or other hematopoietic proliferative disorders. *Clin Imag* 1992; 16:15–24.

62. Von Essen S, West W, SItiorius M, Rennard SI. Complete resolution of roentgenographic changes in a patient with pulmonary histiocytosis X. *Chest* 1990; 98:765–767.

63. Friedman PJ, Liebow AA, Sokoloff J. Eosinophilic granuloma of lung: Clinical aspects of primary histiocytosis in the adult. *Medicine* 1981; 60:385–396.

64. Sadoun D, Vaylet F, Valeyre D, et al. Bronchogenic carcinoma in patients with pulmonary Histiocytosis X. *Chest* 1992; 101:1610–1613.

65. Shanley DJ, Lerud KS, Leutkehans TJ. Development of pulmonary histiocytosis X after chemotherapy of Hodgkin's Disease. *Am J Roentgenol* 1990; 155:741–742.

66. Keon TC. Death on induction of anesthesia for cervical node biopsy. *Anesthesiology* 1981: 55:471–472.

67. Halpern S, Chatten J, Meadows AT, et al. Anterior mediastinal masses: Anesthesia hazards and other problems. *J Pediatr* 1983; 102:402–410.

68. Loeffler JS, Leopold KA, Recht A, et al. Emergency pre-biopsy radiation for mediastinal masses: Impact on subsequent pathologic diagnosis and outcome. *J Clin Oncol* 1986; 417:716–721.

69. Gefter WB, Albelda SM, Talbot GH, Gerson SL, Cassileth PA, Miller WT. Invasive pulmonary aspergillosis and acute leukemia: Limitations in the diagnostic utility of the air crescent sign. *Radiology* 1985; 157:605–610.

70. Scullier JP, Feld R. Superior vena cava obstruction syndrome: Recommendation for management. *Cancer Treat Rev* 1985; 12:209–218.

71. Kramer SS, Jakacki RI, Rackoff WR, Glass TS. Invasive pulmonary aspergillosis in immune compromised children [Abstract]. Presented at the European Society of Radiology, May, 1990.

72. Ruutu P, Valtonen V, Tiitanen L, et al. An outbreak of invasive aspergillosis in a haematologic unit. *Scand J Infect Dis* 1987; 19:347–351.

73. Sotiropoulos SV, Jackson MA, Woods GM, Hicks RA, Cullen J, Freeman AI. Alpha-streptococcal septicemia in leukemic children treated with continuous or large dosage intermittent cytosine arabinoside. *Pediatr Infect Dis J* 1989; 8:755–758.

74. Weisman SJ, Scoopo FJ, Johnson GM, Altman AJ, Quinn JJ. Septicemia in pediatric oncology patients: The significance of viridans streptococcal infections. *J Clin Oncol* 1990; 8:453–459.

75. Stokes DC, Shenep JL, Parham D, Bozeman PM, Marienchek W, Mackert P. Role of flexible bronchoscopy in the diagnosis of pulmonary infiltrates in pediatric patients with cancer. *J Pediatr* 1989; 115:561–567.

76. Pizzo PA, Rubin M, Friedfeld A, Walsh TJ. The child with cancer and infection. I. Empiric therapy for fever and neutropenia, and preventive strategies. *J Pediatr* 1991; 119:679–694.

77. Pizzo PA, Rubin M, Friedfeld A, Walsh TJ. The child with cancer and infection. II. Nonbacterial infections. *J Pediatr* 1991; 119:845–857.

78. Bleyer WA. The impact of childhood cancer on the United States and the world. *CA* 1990; 40:355–367.

79. Blatt J, Copeland DR, Bleyer WA. Late effects of childhood cancer and its treatment. In Pizzo PA, Poplack DG, eds. *Principles and practice of pediatric oncology*, 2nd ed. Philadelphia, JB Lippincott, 1993, pp 1091–1114.

80. De Latt CA, Lampkin BC. Long-term survivors of childhood cancer: Evaluation and identification of sequelae of treatment. *CA* 1992; 42:263–282.

81. Meadows AT, Silber J. Delayed consequences of therapy for childhood cancer, *CA* 1985; 35:271–286.

82. Neglia JP. Late effects of treatment of children with cancer. *Semin Pediatr Surg* 1993; 2:29–36.

83. Constine LS. Late effects of radiation therapy. *Pediatrician* 1991; 18:37–48.

84. Miller RW, Fusner JE, Fink RJ, et al. Pulmonary function abnormalities in long-term survivors of childhood cancer. *Med Pediatr Oncol* 1986; 14:202–207.

85. Shaw NJ, Tweeddale PM, Eden OB. Pulmonary function in childhood leukemia survivors. *Med Pediatr Oncol* 1989; 17:149–154.

86. Kun LE, Moulder JE. General principals of radiation therapy. In Pizzo PA, Poplack DG, eds. *Principles and practice of pediatric oncology*, 2nd edition. Philadelphia, JB Lippincott, 1993, pp 273–302.

87. Emami B, Lyman J, Brown A, et al. Tolerance of normal tissue to therapeutic irradiation. *Int J Radiat Oncol Biol Phys* 1991; 21:109–122.

88. Kreisman H, Wolkove N. Pulmonary toxicity of antineoplastic therapy. In Perry MC, ed. *The chemotherapy source book*. Baltimore, Williams & Wilkins, 1992, pp 598–619.

89. McInerney DP, Bullimore J. Reactivation of radiation pneumonitis by Adriamycin. *Br J Radiol* 1977; 50:224–227.

90. Wara WM, Phillips TL, Margolis LW, et al. Radiation pneumonitis: A new approach to the derivation of time-dose factors. *Cancer* 1973; 32:547–552.

91. Patterson W, Perry MC. Chemotherapeutic toxicities: A comprehensive overview. *Contemp Oncol* 1993; 3:56–64.

92. Castellino RA, Glatstein E, Turbow MM, et al. Latent radiation injury of lungs or heart activated by steroid withdrawal. *Ann Intern Med* 1974; 80:593–599.

93. Gibson PG, Bryant DH, Morgan GW, et al. Radiation induced lung injury: A hypersensitivity pneumonitis? *Ann Intern Med* 1988; 109:288–291.

94. Roberts CM, Foulcher E, Zaunders JJ, et al. Radiation pneumonitis: A possible lymphocyte-mediated hypersensitivity reaction. *Ann Intern Med* 1993; 118:696–700.

95. Lee RE, Lotze MT, Skibber JM, et al. Cardiorespiratory effects of immunotherapy with interleukin-2. *J Clin Oncol* 1989; 7:7–20.

96. Goldiner PL, Carlon GC, Cvitkovic E, Schweizer O, Howland WS. Factors influencing postoperative morbidity and mortality in patients treated with bleomycin. *Br Med J* 1978; 1:1664–1667.

97. Goldiner PL, Schweizer O. The hazards of anesthesia and surgery in bleomycin-treated patients. *Semin Oncol* 1979; 6:121–124.

98. Eigen H, Wyszomierski D. Bleomycin lung injury in children, pathophysiology and guidelines for management. *Am J Pediatr Hematol Oncol* 1985; 7:71–78.

99. Ingrassia TS, Ryu JH, Trastek VF, Rosenow EC. Oxygen-exacerbated bleomycin pulmonary toxicity. *Mayo Clin Proc* 1991; 66:173–178.

100. Kehrer JP, Kacew S. Systemically applied chemicals that damage lung tissue. *Toxicology* 1985; 35:251–293.

101. Hakkinen PJ, Whiteley JW, Witschi HR. Hyperoxia, but not thoracic x-irradiation, potentiates bleomycin and cyclophosphamide-induced lung damage in mice. *Am Rev Respir Dis* 1982; 126:281–285.

102. Kehrer JP, Paraidathathu T. Enhanced oxygen toxicity following treatment with 1,3-bis (2-chloroethyl)-1-nitrosourea. *Fund Appl Toxicol* 1984; 4:760–767.

103. Holoye PY, Luna MA, Mackay B, Bedrossian CWM. Bleomycin hypersensitivity pneumonitis. *Ann Intern Med* 1978; 88:47–49.

104. Sostman HD, Matthay RA, Putman CE, Smith GJW. Methotrexate-induced pneumonitis. *Medicine* 1976: 55:371–388.

105. Garbes ID, Henderson ES, Gomez GA, Bakshi SP, Parthasarathy KL, Castillo NB. Procarbazine induced interstitial pneumonitis with a normal chest x-ray: A case report. *Med Pediatr Oncol* 1986; 14:238–241.

106. Dalgleish AG, Woods RL, Levi JA. Bleomycin pulmonary toxicity: Its relationship to renal dysfunction. *Med Pediatr Oncol* 1984; 12:313–317.

107. Yee GC, Crom WR, Champion JE, Brodeur GM, Evans WE. Cisplatinum induced changes in bleomycin elimination. *Cancer Treat Rep* 1983; 67:587–589.

108. Rabinowits M, Souhami L, Gill RA, Andrade CAV, Paiva HC. Increased pulmonary toxicity with bleomycin and cisplatinum chemotherapy combinations. *Am J Clin Oncol* 1990; 13:132–138.

109. Perry DJ, Weiss RB, Taylor HG. Enhanced bleomycin toxicity during acute renal failure. *Cancer Treat Rep* 1982; 66:592–593.

110. Bennett WM, Pastore L, Houghton DC. Fatal pulmonary bleomycin toxicity in cisplatinum-induced renal failure. *Cancer Treat Rep* 1980; 64:921–924.

111. McLeod BF, Lawrence HJ, Smith DW, Vogt PJ, Gandara DR. Fatal bleomycin toxicity from a low cumulative dose in a patient with renal insufficiency. *Cancer* 1987; 60:2617–2620.

112. Cooper AD, White DA, Matthay RA. State of the art: Drug induced pulmonary disease. *Am Rev Respir Dis* 1986; 133:321–340.

113. O'Driscoll PR, Hasleton PS, Taylor PM, Poulter LW, Gattamaneni HR, Woodcock AA. Acute lung fibrosis up to 17 years after chemotherapy with carmustine (BCNU) in childhood. *N Engl J Med* 1990; 323:378–382.

114. Limper AH, DcDonald IA. Delayed pulmonary fibrosis after nitrosourea therapy. *N Engl J Med* 1990; 323:407–409.

115. Aronin PA, Mahaley MS, Rudnick SA, et al. Prediction of BCNU pulmonary toxicity in patients with malignant gliomas: An assessment of risk factors. *N Engl J Med* 1980; 303:183–188.

116. Jakacki R, Schramm C, Haas F, Allen J. Restrictive lung disease in survivors of childhood brain tumors [Abstract]. *Proc Am Soc Clin Oncol* 1992; 11:150.

117. Baker WJ, Fistel SJ, Jones RV, Weiss RB. Interstitial pneumonitis associated with Ifosfamide therapy. *Cancer* 1990; 65:2217–2221.

118. Mäakipernaa A, Heino M, Laitinen LA, Siimes MA. Lung function following treatment of malignant tumors with surgery, radiotherapy, or cyclophosphamide in childhood: A follow-up study after 11 to 27 years. *Cancer* 1989; 63:625–630.

119. Andersson BS, Luna MA, Yee C, Hui KK, Keating MJ, McCredie KB. Fatal pulmonary failure complicating high-dose cytosine arabinoside therapy in acute leukemia. *Cancer* 1990; 65:1079–1084.

120. Weitman SD, Buchanan GR, Kamen BA. Pulmonary toxicity of deferoxamine in children with advanced cancer. *J Natl Cancer Inst* 1991; 83:1834–1835.

121. Hudson MM, Greenwald C, Thompson E, et al. Efficacy and toxicity of multiagent chemotherapy and low-dose involved field radiotherapy in children and adolescents with Hodgkin's disease. *J Clin Oncol* 1993; 11:100–108.

122. Mefferd JM, Donaldson SS, Link MP. Pediatric Hodgkin's disease: pulmonary, cardiac, and thyroid function following combined modality therapy. *Int J Radiat Oncol Biol Phys* 1989; 16:679–685.

123. Tarbell NJ, Thompson L, Mauch P. Thoracic irradiation in Hodgkin's disease: Disease control and

long-term complications. *Int J Radiat Oncol Biol Phys* 1990; 18:275–281.

124. Green DM, Finklestein JZ, Tefft ME, Norkool P. Diffuse interstitial pneumonitis after pulmonary irradiation for metastatic Wilms' tumor, a report from the National Wilms' Tumor Study. *Cancer* 1989; 63:450–453.

125. Shaw NJ, Eden OB, Jenney MEM, Stevens RF, Morris-Jones PH, Craft AW, Castillo L. Pulmonary function in survivors of Wilms' tumor. *Pediatr Hematol Oncol* 1991; 8:131–137.

126. Thomas PRM, Griffith KD, Fineberg BB, Perez CA, Land VJ. Late effects of treatment for Wilms' tumor. *Int J Radiat Oncol Biol Phys* 1983; 9:651–657.

127. Benoist MR, Lemerle J, Jean R, Rufin P, Scheinmann P, Paupe J. Effects on pulmonary function of whole lung irradiation for Wilms' tumor in children. *Thorax* 1982; 37:175–180.

128. Steinherz LJ, Steinherz PG, Tan CTC, Heller G, Murphy ML. Cardiac toxicity 4 to 20 years after completing anthracycline therapy. *JAMA* 1991; 266:1672–1677.

129. Lipshultz SE, Colan SD, Gelber RD, Perez-Atayde AR, Sallan SE, Sanders SP. Late cardiac effects of Doxorubicin therapy for acute lymphoblastic leukemia in childhood. *N Engl J Med* 1991; 324:808–815.

130. Jakacki RI, Goldwein JW, Larsen RL, Barber S, Silber JH. Cardiac dysfunction following spinal irradiation during childhood. *J Clin Oncol* 1993; 11:1033–1038.

48

Pulmonary Hypertension

GREGORY J. REDDING

Pulmonary hypertension results from alterations in the pulmonary vascular bed or heart that lead to an increase in pulmonary vascular resistance and impedance. Pulmonary hypertension resulting only from lung disease in infants and children will be the focus of this chapter. The consequence of severe or sustained pulmonary hypertension due to respiratory disease is cor pulmonale and, when extreme, right heart failure. The disorders that produce pulmonary hypertension may affect primarily either lung vessels (e.g., vasculitis) or various lung compartments (e.g., central or peripheral airways, interstitial tissue). They may also include extrapulmonary processes adversely affecting respiratory function, such as sickle-cell thrombosis, and central hypoventilation syndromes.

The prevalence of pulmonary hypertension in childhood is unknown because of a lack of systematic screening and a sensitive, inexpensive, non-invasive means of detection. Screening electrocardiogram and echocardiograms have been used in particular patient populations with chronic pulmonary conditions such as cystic fibrosis, interstitial fibrosis, and bronchopulmonary dysplasia (1–3). In these studies, the children with severe disease and hypoxia are most likely to have cor pulmonale. In addition, conditions such as sleep-associated airway obstruction predispose children to pulmonary hypertension and cor pulmonale (4, 5), but no epidemiologic studies have been conducted to determine the prevalence of pulmonary vascular disease in children who snore or develop oxyhemoglobin desaturation at night. Pulmonary diseases of childhood that can lead to pulmonary hypertension and/or cor pulmonale are listed in Table 48.1.

Table 48.1.
Pulmonary Etiologies for Pulmonary Hypertension in Children

Airway Disease
Cystic Fibrosis
Bronchopulmonary dysplasia
Upper airway obstruction
Chronic aspiration syndromes

Pulmonary vascular disorders
Primary pulmonary hypertension
Thromboembolic diseases
Pulmonary vasculitides
Veno-occlusive disease
Atresia/hypoplasia of pulmonary vessels

Others
Interstitial lung disease
Bronchiolitis obliterans/bronchiectasis
Respiratory muscle weakness
Restrictive chest wall disorders
Central hypoventilation syndromes

Cor pulmonale often occurs as an expected consequence of chronic or progressive respiratory abnormalities in a child with known pulmonary disease. Its presence serves as a marker of disease severity that can be monitored in conjunction with other indices of lung function. Cor pulmonale also contributes to the morbidity of chronic lung disease, such as exercise intolerance and syncope, and contributes to mortality when right heart failure occurs. Alternatively, cor pulmonale occurs in conjunction with right heart failure as the initial presenting feature in an apparently normal child. In the child with unexplained right heart failure, the underlying mechanism(s) producing pulmonary hypertension must be identified. Such mechanisms include pulmonary vasoconstriction, vaso-occlusion, vascular injury, and vascular remodeling. In order to produce pulmonary hypertension, these mechanisms must affect a large proportion of pulmonary vessels (6). In addition, cardiac reasons for pulmonary hypertension, such as left heart failure or left-to-right shunts resulting from congenital cardiac disease, must be confirmed or ruled out.

MECHANISMS

The majority of pulmonary diseases affecting children result in alveolar hypoxia, which in turn produces pulmonary vasoconstriction. The degree to which a level of alveolar hypoxia produces pulmonary vasoconstriction varies among individuals (7). Nonetheless, the relationship between hypoxia and pulmonary vascular resistance, depicted in Figure 48.1 for neonatal animals (8), is believed to apply to humans of all ages. The relationship is influenced mostly by alveolar oxygen tensions and much less by mixed venous oxygen tensions (9). It is also influenced by acid-base status rather than by carbon dioxide per se, with less vigorous vasoconstriction occurring under conditions of alkalosis and more vigorous constriction by acidosis. Regional hypoxic pulmonary vasoconstriction due to localized lung disease improves ventilation-perfusion matching by redistributing pulmonary blood flow to better ventilated areas without great changes in pulmonary artery pressure (10). However, diffuse vasoconstriction associated with diffuse alveolar hypoxia leads to pulmonary hypertension and increased afterload to the right ventricle. Resolution of acute hypoxia leads to resolution of acute pulmonary vasoconstriction; this is one basis for oxygen therapy in children with lung disease and hypoxia. Vasoconstriction can be caused by other constrictors such as angiotensin, catecholamines, eicosanoids, endothelins, and cytokines, but the pathogenic role of these circulating mediators in most clinical diseases remains undefined.

More importantly, repeated episodes and persistent exposure to alveolar hypoxia lead to structural alterations in pulmonary vessels known as "remodeling." The site of the remodeling associated with hypoxic pulmonary hypertension is primarily in small arterioles, which are believed to be the major but not exclusive site of active pulmonary vasoconstriction. The features of remodeled arterioles include increased medial muscle wall thickness due to proliferation and hypertrophy of smooth muscle cells and significant enlargement of the adventitial tissue surrounding the vessel, made up of fibroblasts and deposition of collagen and elastin (11). Examples of normal and remodeled pulmonary arterioles are illustrated in Figure 48.2. In addition, there is extension of smooth muscle into smaller, usually partially or non-muscularized precapillary arterioles. Structural alterations in the surface appearance of the endothelial cells have also been described (12). The net effect of these changes is a vessel with a narrowed lumen that is no longer distensible. Whether a remodeled pulmonary arteriole vasoconstricts more intensely and at higher oxygen tensions compared to normal pulmonary vessels remains controversial (13). It may also be less able to relax because of lower production of vasodilator mediators within the vessel (14). With progressive narrowing of the lumen, intravascular thrombosis occurs, leading to complete occlusion and vessel obliteration. When this process occurs diffusely within the lung, there is a loss of cross-sectional surface area, which contributes to irreversibly increased pulmonary vascular resistance.

It is unclear if repeated pulmonary vasoconstriction per se leads to vascular remodeling or whether hypoxia is also a mitogenic stimulus for cellular proliferation within and around vessel walls. It is important to note that recurrent episodic vasoconstriction, as occurs with hypoventilation and airway obstruction during sleep, also produces pulmonary hypertension and cor pulmonale despite normal oxygenation during wakefulness (4). The rate at which this process occurs may depend on the frequency of hypoxic events, their duration, and the degree of hypoxia during each event. It also depends on the vasoconstrictive response to hypoxia and remodeling tendencies of the host. The duration of time necessary to produce remodeled pulmonary vessels and pulmonary hypertension in rats is several weeks (15); the correlate in humans has not been described. In newborns, however, it is likely that postnatal alveolar hypoxia, as occurs in many neonatal lung diseases, may retard the natural regression of pulmonary arterial muscularization found in the fetus and newborn, resulting in an earlier tendency for pul-

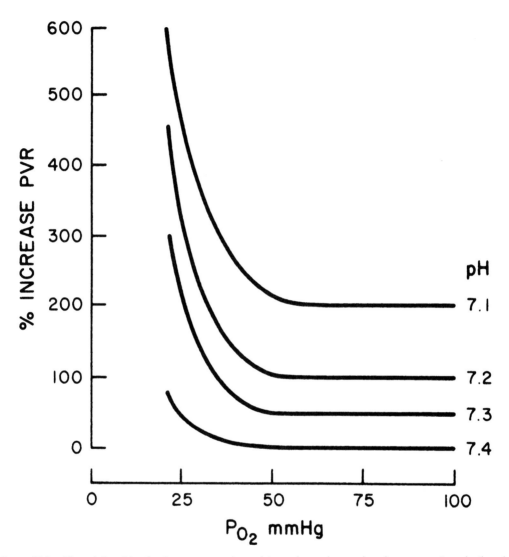

Figure 48.1. The relationship of pulmonary vascular resistance in newborn calves in response to reductions in inspired oxygen concentration and variations in arterial blood pH. (From Rudolph AM, Yuen S. Response of the pulmonary vasculature to hypoxia and H+ ion concentration changes. *J Clin Invest* 1966; 45:399–411.)

monary hypertension in neonates than in infants and older children.

There are few studies describing the resolution of features associated with hypoxia-induced vascular remodeling after hypoxia has been treated. In rats, the thickened medial smooth muscle diminishes as does the fibroblast number within the adventitia. However, the deposition of collagen and elastin remains increased (16). These features may explain why only a minority of patients on long-term oxygen therapy will experience an incomplete return of pulmonary hemodynamics to normal levels. The rate at which remodeled pulmonary vessels revert toward normal appearance in humans is not known. However, the resolution of pulmonary hypertension in children has occurred within 3 months following tonsillectomy an adcnoidectomy for sleep-related hypoxia (17).

Most of the other mechanisms for pulmonary hypertension due to lung disease affect

hypoxia is due to reduced mixed venous oxygen tension as a result of increased tissue extraction in the presence of low cardiac output resulting from poor right ventricular function. Hypoxia worsens during exercise because of additional tissue needs for oxygen which cannot be met by the failing right ventricle. As a result of restrictive lung mechanics and hypoxia, tachypnea and hypocapnia are frequent clinical findings in patients with pulmonary hypertension. These are produced in part by the increase in physiologic dead space, which occurs as pulmonary vessels are obliterated and capillary surface area diminishes. In these circumstances, the loss of pulmonary vasculature also leads to a reduction in volume-corrected diffusion capacity of the lung (35).

In children who have severe lung disease and associated pulmonary hypertension and cor pulmonale, the contributions of the abnormal vasculature to poor lung function are far outweighed by the impact of the underlying lung disease itself. In patients with cystic fibrosis and bronchopulmonary dysplasia, the lung disease produces abnormal lung mechanics, gas exchange abnormalities, and exercise intolerance. The contribution of the remodeled pulmonary vessels to these functional abnormalities in any particular case may be additive but difficult to measure.

CLINICAL FEATURES

The clinical features of pulmonary hypertension per se are often obscured by signs and symptoms of the lung disease producing pulmonary hypertension. Among patients with primary pulmonary hypertension, the most common initial symptoms are dyspnea and fatigue (35). This is manifested earliest during exercise or equivalent activities that require effort. These symptoms occur at rest when pulmonary hypertension is severe. The remainder of symptoms found in patients with primary pulmonary hypertension are listed in Table 48.2. Physical findings specific for pulmonary hypertension are most evident when cor pulmonale has already developed. They reflect the early compensatory changes and the later ineffective compensation for progressively increasing right heart work. The earliest findings are a narrowing of the normal split in the second heart sound heard with rapid closure of the pulmonic valve as right ventric-

Table 48.2.
Signs and Symptoms Associated with Primary Pulmonary Hypertension

Symptoms	Signs
Dyspnea	Tachypnea
Fatigue	Tachycardia
Exercise intolerance	Diaphoresis
Failure to thrive in infancy	Increased P2 heart sound
Excessive napping	Narrowed splitting of S2
Chest pain	S3 or S4 heart sounds
Syncope	Tricuspid or pulmonic insufficiency murmur
Palpitations	Hepatic enlargement and pain
	Pedal edema
	Jugular venous distension

ular pressure falls at the end of systole (36). With progressive right ventricular dilation to maintain stroke volume, pulmonic valve incompetency and high pulmonary artery diastolic pressures lead to an audible diastolic flow murmur of pulmonic regurgitation. This occurs much more often than the holosystolic murmur heard with tricuspid regurgitation, which results from right ventricular dilation, loss of ventricular compliance, and increased ventricular diastolic pressures. Giant "a" waves and S4 extra heart sounds reflect atrial compensation for the poorly compliant right ventricle. With right heart failure, central venous and hepatic engorgement occur, as does edema of peripheral dependent tissue. The radiographic features of pulmonary hypertension, unobscured by underlying lung disease, depend on whether precapillary or postcapillary vessels are primarily involved. When pulmonary arteries are involved, as with primary pulmonary hypertension, central pulmonary vessels in the hilum are enlarged but peripheral vascular markings taper quickly (35). Lung parenchyma appears underperfused. In contrast, pulmonary venous obstruction increases pulmonary extravasation of intravascular fluid, producing diffuse parenchymal densities in ground-glass or nodular interstitial patterns (37). In addition, right heart enlargement may be seen, reflecting both atrial and ventricular dilation. Regardless of the type of pulmonary hypertension, its severity and functional consequences may be substantial without notable radiographic findings.

Other radiographic techniques, such as pulmonary wedge angiography, have been used to define the vascular appearance more clearly (38); however, they are not commonly used in children. The exception to this is the ventilation-perfusion scan used to detect localized pulmonary obstruction caused by thrombosis or emboli. As in adults, this technique is most helpful in detecting localized or patchy pulmonary vascular obstruction when the patient's chest film is normal and perfusion scan defects are identified in the absence of ventilation defects (39).

ASSESSMENT OF PULMONARY VASCULAR AND RIGHT HEART FUNCTION

The most direct way to diagnose and manage pulmonary hypertension is to measure pulmonary vascular and cardiac function. Unlike the clinical examination, which reflects the likelihood of pulmonary hypertension, measurement of pulmonary artery pressure as well as structure and function of the right heart directly quantitates the degree of pulmonary vascular disease and cardiac compensation. The methods to do this include electrocardiography, echocardiography, and cardiac catheterization. Of these methods, electrocardiography measures exclusively cardiac changes. The echocardiogram and pulmonary catheterization measure pulmonary hemodynamics, right heart function, and their interrelationship.

The electrocardiogram (EKG) is less sensitive in assessing right heart function than vectorcardiography or echocardiography (40–43). Reduced right ventricular ejection fraction may exist in the presence of pulmonary hypertension without diagnostic electrocardiographic abnormalities. However, the characteristic EKG changes of right ventricular hypertrophy, right atrial hypertrophy, and right bundle branch block are very suggestive of cor pulmonale in the presence of chronic lung disease (44). Such findings should prompt further documentation of right heart structural and functional changes using echocardiography. In patients without apparent lung disease, such electrocardiographic features mandate a search for pulmonary hypertension and structural heart disease. The usefulness of the electrocardiogram lies in its widespread availability and ease of use by most physicians, and it should be considered a screening tool to identify patients with moderate pulmonary hypertension. In patients with cor pulmonale, the EKG is less useful than the echocardiogram to follow resolution of pulmonary hypertension, since EKG features of cor pulmonale will regress much more slowly than the functional and structural echocardiographic abnormalities.

Echocardiographic characteristics of cor pulmonale include increased right ventricular wall thickness, paradoxical interventricular septal motion, and both increased regurgitation through and abnormal movement of the tricuspid and pulmonary valves (45). In addition, right-to-left shunts through the foramen ovale, indicative of increased right atrial pressures, suggest poor right ventricular function in the presence of pulmonary hypertension. The foramen ovale is probe-patent in 50% of children less than 5 years old, and remains so in 25% of adults (46). There are several ways to quantitate mean, diastolic, and systolic pulmonary artery pressures using M-mode and Doppler echocardiographic techniques. These include measurements of the isovolumic right ventricular relaxation time, time of peak velocity of the pulmonary artery pressure wave divided by rate-corrected ejection time, and velocity of regurgitant blood flow across the tricuspid and pulmonic valves. All of these techniques correlate well with concurrent direct measurements of pulmonary artery pressures (45). They are most useful when the techniques are used together to confirm one another. It is important to note that echocardiographic findings reflect both long-standing features, such as hypertrophy, and the current hemodynamic function at the time of the measurement. This makes the technique helpful as a diagnostic tool as well as the optimal way to monitor severity of disease non-invasively and to evaluate immediate responses to therapy. The major limitation of echocardiography is the technical difficulty in obtaining a satisfactory view of the heart in patients with pulmonary hyper-inflation.

The most precise method to assess pulmonary hypertension and right heart function is right heart catheterization. The normal mean pulmonary artery pressure in infants and older children is 10–16 mm Hg, and pulmonary hypertension is diagnosed when it exceeds 20 mm Hg or pulmonary artery systolic pressure exceeds 30 mm Hg (47). Pulmonary hypertension also exists when calculated pulmonary vascular resistance, normalized by dividing pulmonary driving pressure (Ppa-Pcw) by cardiac index, exceeds 3 units per square meter. The severity of pulmonary hypertension is also estimated by comparing mean pulmonary artery pressure to systemic artery pressure. In normal individuals, pulmonary artery pressure is 20–25% of systemic pressure. Such norms are not applicable in neonates, who have higher pulmonary artery pressures until at about 8 weeks of age (48).

In addition to pulmonary artery measurements, right ventricular end-diastolic volumes and pressures, indices of contractility, and stroke volume can all be measured to determine the degree of right heart compensation in the presence of pulmonary hypertension. Measurements of cardiac output using indicator dilution techniques are particularly helpful pre- and post-therapy since improvement in cardiac reserve despite the persistence of pulmonary hypertension is a common outcome of treatment (49).

The pulmonary vascular response to vasodilators has been used to design long-term treatment regimens and also to make prognoses about life expectancy. The assumption made with vasodilator trials is that pulmonary vasoconstriction is a variable but important component of pulmonary hypertension in an individual patient and that reversal of this component will reduce the severity of the hypertension, reduce cardiac work, and prevent or forestall progression of pulmonary vascular disease. In a review of multiple acute pulmonary vasodilator trials in adults with pulmonary hypertension, 45% of patients were found to experience a $\geq$ 30% reduction in pulmonary vascular resistance (50). The majority of patients with this degree of vasorelaxation improved clinically on treatment over the ensuing 6 months, in contrast to only 6% of patients with < 30% fall in PVR acutely. This study has been confirmed more recently by a report that compared the course of responders to acute and chronic vasodilator therapy over 3 years to nonresponders with similar degrees of pulmonary hypertension prior to treatment (51) (Fig. 48.3). The prediction of an individual patient's clinical course based on his acute hemodynamic response to a pulmonary vasodilator is more difficult. Some individuals with a static pulmonary disease such as interstitial fibrosis may have fixed unresponsive pulmonary hypertension from vascular remodeling that does not progress. In contrast, patients with primary pulmonary hypertension can have a significant response to vasodilator agents on initial catheterization but lose the response on subsequent catheterizations as the vascular disease progresses (52).

The hemodynamic response to pulmonary vasodilators depends on the agent and route of administration. There are currently no selective pulmonary vasodilators that can be administered orally or intravenously. All agents delivered by these routes produce systemic vasodilation as well. In contrast, oxygen, and more recently, nitric oxide, are inhaled agents that reduce pulmonary vasoconstriction acutely without adverse systemic effects (53, 54). Intravenous pulmonary vasodilators also can produce arterial hypoxia due to ventilation-perfusion mismatching by reducing regional hypoxic pulmonary vasoconstriction and increasing blood flow to poorly ventilated regions of lung (55). This adverse effect is more common in patients with parenchymal lung disease and airway disease than in patients with primary pulmonary vascular disease (49).

The goal of both acute and chronic pulmonary vasodilator therapy is to reduce right heart afterload, thereby increasing right heart function and functional reserve, and to increase oxygen delivery to tissues without producing systemic hypotension. The most common acute hemodynamic response to parenteral vasodilator trials reported from the NIH Registry of Primary Pulmonary Hypertension was an increased cardiac output, a decreased systemic artery pressure, and little or no change in mean pulmonary artery and right atrial pressure (49). This results in a calculated reduction in both pulmonary and systemic vascular resistance. There is no single accepted definition of a "positive" vasodilator response. Those suggested in the Registry report are either (a) a $\geq$ 10% increase in cardiac output associated with a $\geq$ 5 mm Hg decrease in mean pulmonary artery pressure, or (b) a 20% or greater reduction in calculated pulmonary vascular resistance (49). These hemodynamic responses have been associated with an improvement in symptoms (i.e., dyspnea and exercise intolerance) when chronic

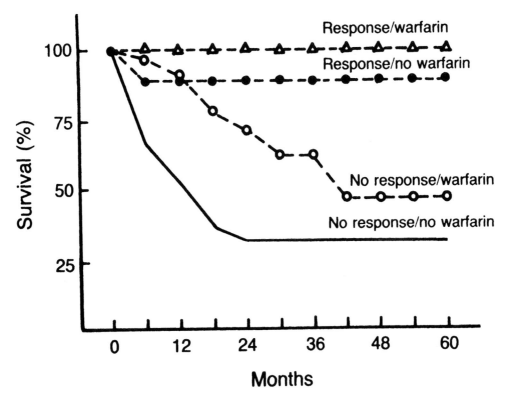

Figure 48.3. Kaplan-Meier estimates of 50-year survival of adult patients with primary pulmonary hypertension stratified according to acute responses to intravenous vasodilators (responders vs nonresponders) and according to treatment or no treatment with the anticoagulant warfarin. (From Rich S, Kaufmann E, Levy PS. The effect of high doses of calcium-channel blockers on survival in primary pulmonary hypertension. *N Engl J Med* 1992; 327:76–81.)

vasodilator therapy is instituted (56). An adverse hemodynamic response also encountered during cardiac catheterization is a greater drop in systemic artery pressure than in pulmonary artery pressure, due to an unresponsive pulmonary vascular bed and a right heart that cannot increase cardiac output in response to systemic vasodilation. Acute vasodilator trials in patients with pulmonary hypertension have produced sudden death (49, 55). For this reason, short-acting or readily reversible vasodilator agents are used within the intensive care unit, and chronic vasodilator therapy is not instituted prior to a vasodilator trial during cardiac catheterization.

The vasodilators used most often in the NIH Registry are listed in Table 48.3 (49). Of these agents, prostacyclin and nifedipine are most likely to produce significant reductions in pulmonary vascular resistance. Data

from adults undergoing catheterizations suggest that most individuals who respond to one parenteral vasodilator will respond similarly to others (57).

DIAGNOSTIC APPROACH TO PULMONARY HYPERTENSION OF UNKNOWN ETIOLOGY

In addition to assessment of the functional severity of pulmonary hypertension, the child with unexplained right heart failure requires an assessment as to the etiology of the condition. Most often, such a child will have undiagnosed lung, heart, or systemic disease. Less often, the patient may have primary pulmonary vascular disease. The algorithm in Figure 48.4 outlines an efficient way to identify most categories of diseases producing unanticipated right heart failure. Evaluation of the structure and function of the left and right heart can be accomplished with an echocardiogram.

Table 48.3.
Times for Vasodilator Half-life and Peak Effect*

Drug	Route	Half-life (published range)	Peak Effect Window (time in min)
Diltiazem	PO	3.2 h (1.9–4.5)	180–240
	IV	3.1 h (2.1–4.1)	0–246
Hydralazine	PO	3.1 h (2.2–4)	48–132
	IV	3.1 h (2.2–4)	10–80
Isoproterenol	IV	3.8 min (2.5–5)	0–5
Ketanserin	PO	10.0 h	96–600
	IV	12.8 h (8–17.6)	12–1056
Nifedipine	PO	3.4 h (3–3.8)	20–45
	SL	2.0 h	20–30
Nitrendipine	PO	2.8 h (0.7–4.9)	96–294
Nitroglycerine	IV	2.7 min (1–4.4)	0–4.4
	SL	2.7 min (1–4.4)	1–5
	TD	2.7 min (1–4.4)	60–120
Nitroprusside	IV	3.5 min (3–4)	0–4
Prostaglandin E_1	IV	Not known	0–2
Prostacyclin	IV	3.0 min	0–3
Phentolamine	PO	Not known	192–288
	IV	Not known	0–2
CGS 13080	PO	1 h (0.74–1.2)	30–60
(Thromboxane synthetase inhibitor Transdermal patch			

*The available published data are given for each of the vasodilators used in at least three patients. From Weir EK, Rubin LJ, Ayres SM, et al. The acute administration of vasodilators in primary pulmonary hypertension. Experience for the National Institutes of Health Registry on Primary Pulmonary Hypertension. *Am Rev Respir Dis* 1989; 140:1623–1630.

Screening blood gas analysis, spirometry, and chest radiography will characterize lung disease previously unsuspected. If cor pulmonale is present but blood gas tensions and chest evaluations are normal, focus should be directed on sleep-related disorders of breathing, autoimmune disease, and tendencies for thrombosis or embolus. As yet, there are no definitive criteria (i.e., degree, frequency, or duration of oxyhemoglobin desaturation or hypercapnia) that demonstrate a causal relationship between sleep-related disorders of breathing and pulmonary hypertension. However, multiple or "severe" abnormalities (e.g., SaO_2 <80% during sleep) merit a trial of treatment to ameliorate both the sleep-related abnormalities and the severity of pulmonary hypertension. If vascular obstruction is seriously considered, a ventilation-perfusion scan will prove useful. Right heart catheterization and measurement of multiple capillary occlusion pressures will determine if regional or diffuse pulmonary venous obstruction is present. The final diagnostic maneuver, the open lung biopsy, will provide histologic data that may be diagnostic (e.g., granulomatous vasculitis) or nonspecific because of advanced remodeling.

THERAPY

Therapy for pulmonary hypertension due to lung disease is primarily treatment directed toward the pulmonary process (e.g., antibiotics for children with endobronchial infection due to cystic fibrosis) or toward the consequences of the lung disease (e.g., supplemental oxygen for alveolar hypoxia). Additional treatments are designed to reverse underlying pathologic mechanisms of a specific vascular disease (e.g., warfarin for recurrent pulmonary emboli and steroids for pulmonary vasculitis). Treatment strategies differ when reversing pulmonary hypertension and right heart failure acutely, rather than in chronic supportive care. In either case, the response to treatment will vary depending on the reversibility of the underlying vascular pathophysiology (i.e., vasoconstriction vs. remodeling).

Acute Therapy

Ideally, immediate treatment of right heart failure due to pulmonary hypertension will

DIAGNOSTIC APPROACH TO UNEXPLAINED RIGHT HEART FAILURE

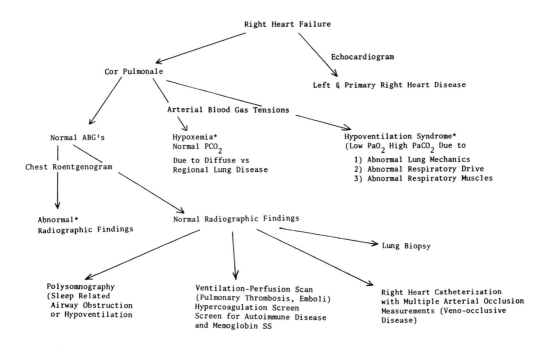

Figure 48.4. An algorithm used to investigate the etiology of unexplained right heart failure in children.

reduce right ventricular afterload, improve cardiac output, maintain coronary perfusion to both ventricles, and maintain adequate oxygen delivery to tissues. Supplemental oxygen sufficient to keep oxyhemoglobin saturations at 90–92% will avoid CO_2 narcosis in chronically hypercapnic patients while reducing hypoxic pulmonary vasoconstriction (58, 59). If CO_2 retention is not a concern, there is no reason to maintain SaO_2 values below 96%, since the level of alveolar hypoxia that elicits pulmonary vasoconstriction in an individual patient is unknown. If signs of inadequate cardiac output, such as metabolic acidosis and hypotension, are present, close cardiopulmonary monitoring to quantitate systemic and pulmonary artery pressures as well as cardiac output will provide immediate feedback as to the effects of fluid administration, diuretics, digoxin, vasopressors, and vasodilators. Fluid therapy may increase preload to the heart, thus improving cardiac output (60). However, it can also exacerbate the function of a dilated, poorly compensated right ventricle and pro-

mote further peripheral edema and discomfort. Diuretics may improve right heart dimensions along the Starling curve, thereby improving contractility and function. Alternatively, diuretics may reduce preload sufficiently to compromise cardiac output. Recurrent trials of diuretics or intravenous fluids are contraindicated without quantitative hemodynamic monitoring. Agents producing systemic vasoconstriction will raise aortic and hence coronary perfusion pressures, thereby maintaining right ventricular perfusion, but may also produce pulmonary vasoconstriction, aggravating poor right heart function (61). In the absence of systemic hypotension, pulmonary vasodilators (Table 48.3) have been used to treat pulmonary hypertensive crises.

In contrast to intravenous pulmonary vasodilators, inhaled nitric oxide (NO) has recently been used successfully to treat acutely severe pulmonary hypertension in both adults and newborns (53, 62, 63). Nitric oxide appears to be endothelium-derived relaxant factor

(EDRF), a substance that is produced by pulmonary endothelial cells on an ongoing basis. It is derived from L-arginine by the action of several nitric oxide synthase enzymes (64). Nitric oxide then diffuses to adjacent vascular smooth muscle where it increases cyclic GMP, thereby causing active vasorelaxation. Its therapeutic potential is great because excessive nitric oxide combines with hemoglobin and is inactivated as a vasodilator (64). Inhaled nitric oxide is therefore a *selective* pulmonary vasodilator that neither worsens gas exchange nor produces systemic hypotension. NO therapy at high doses (greater than 50 parts per million) may produce methemoglobinemia (65). In addition, nitric oxide can interact with water in the airways to produce nitrous oxide, which has the potential to injure the lung (66). Preliminary evidence indicates that these are not problems when nitric oxide is administered for hours or days. Its potential as a long-term pulmonary vasodilator and its effects on remodeled vessels are under study.

Chronic Therapy

The major modalities for treatment of chronic pulmonary hypertension include oxygen, vasodilators, anticoagulants, and lung transplantation. Oxygen and oral vasodilators are used to minimize pulmonary vasoconstriction, which may not only compromise cardiac function but also may promote further vascular remodeling by increasing vessel wall tension and endothelial cell shear stress. It is unclear to what extent pulmonary vasoconstriction contributes to abnormal hemodynamic function in an individual child with remodeled pulmonary vessels due to chronic lung disease, but most groups of children with alveolar hypoxia (e.g., from bronchopulmonary dysplasia or cystic fibrosis) demonstrate some reduction in pulmonary vascular resistance when supplemental oxygen is administered (41, 54). In animal studies, long-term oxygen administration has actually reduced medial smooth muscle hypertrophy characteristic of pulmonary vascular remodeling, suggesting that vessels are capable of structural reversal toward normal when factors promoting remodeling are eliminated (67). Thus, the beneficial effects of oxygen may not be apparent simply from immediate hemodynamic responses during pulmonary catheterization studies; therapeutic trials of supplemental oxygen lasting a

month or more may be necessary before improvement is apparent.

According to the results of two studies conducted in the United States and Great Britain, oxygen therapy for patients with moderately severe chronic lung disease and pulmonary hypertension improves survival (68, 69). The results of the British Medical Research Council (MRC) and the NIH-sponsored Nocturnal Oxygen Therapy Trial (NOTT) are summarized in Figure 48.5. Patients in the MRC study who received no oxygen therapy experienced a 67% mortality rate over a 5-year period. Patients receiving 12–15 hours of supplemental oxygen in the MRC and NOTT studies sufficient to maintain Pao_2 values at > 55 mm Hg experienced a 41–45% mortality rate. In contrast, only 22% of the group (NOTT study) receiving 19–24 hours of oxygen treatment per day died after 2 years of therapy. In both the MRC and NOTT studies, pulmonary artery pressure and vascular resistance measurements were not substantially improved in the treatment groups who lived longer. The results suggest that improved oxygen delivery to tissues may explain the improvement in survival of chronically hypoxemic patients. A similar improvement in survival with long-term oxygen therapy has been demonstrated in children with Eisenmenger syndrome (70).

To determine the amount of oxygen an individual patient requires, arterial oxygenation is monitored as an indirect estimation of alveolar hypoxia. Using oximetry, it is apparent that oxygen requirements will often increase with exercise, feeding, sleep, and the onset of superimposed minor respiratory infections (5, 71). Strategies that increase inspired oxygen concentrations during such periods reduce the episodes of hypoxia that cause recurrent pulmonary vasoconstriction, a response that perpetuates or worsens pulmonary hypertension. Studies in animals made hypoxic for 30-minute intervals several times each night demonstrate that intermittent hypoxic events can produce pulmonary hypertension and cor pulmonale (72). In order to reverse pulmonary hypertension, oxygen therapy must be individualized to meet the varying needs of each patient for oxygen depending on daily activities and sleep patterns. Measuring oxyhemoglobin during all phases of daily activity and sleep is necessary to devise an

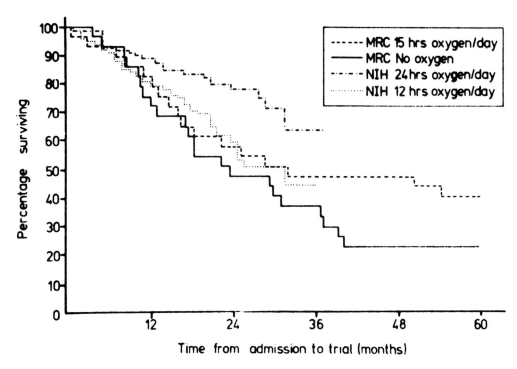

Figure 48.5. Survival rates in two trials (MRC and NIH-NOTT) of long-term oxygen therapy for adults with COPD and cor pulmonale. Follow-up in the NIH study was for 36 months and in the MRC study was 60 months. Survival was greatest among patients using oxygen 24 hours/day. (From MRC Working Party. Long-term domiciliary oxygen therapy in chronic hypoxic cor pulmonale complicating chronic bronchitis and emphysema: A clinical trial. *Lancet* 1981; 1:681–685; and from Nocturnal Oxygen Therapy Trial Group. Continuous or nocturnal oxygen therapy in hypoxia chronic obstructive lung disease: A clinical trial. Ann Intern Med 1980; 93:391–398.)

effective plan of treatment. In children with progressive pulmonary disease, such as cystic fibrosis or interstitial lung disease, significant hypoxia may first manifest itself as poor sleep quality and frequent arousals (73). Initial use of oxygen at night is often sufficient to forestall the progression of pulmonary hypertension until the underlying lung disease progresses to the stage that both night and daytime oxygen therapy is necessary.

There are no data available to know the minimal duration, strength, and frequency of pulmonary vasoconstriction that promotes or perpetuates pulmonary hypertension and cor pulmonale; nor is an individual's threshold of pulmonary vasoconstriction in response to alveolar hypoxia routinely measured in a serial fashion to see if it changes as lung disease improves or worsens. Consequently, most practitioners opt to use oxygen liberally and maintain SaO_2 values at $> 94\%$ in patients

with cor pulmonale in order to minimize the likelihood of intermittent hypoxic events.

The use of chronic pulmonary vasodilators occurs more commonly in patients with primary pulmonary vascular disease than in patients with chronic lung disease. The latter respond readily to oxygen and therefore require oral vasodilator agents less frequently. The most commonly used agents for chronic management of pulmonary hypertension are oral calcium-channel blockers, hydralazine, and more recently, chronic continuous infusions of prostacyclin (74). Several short-term drug trials have demonstrated the relative efficacy of these agents in patients with COPD, cystic fibrosis, and primary pulmonary hypertension (75–77). Outcome indices vary with each study, but improvements have included reduced pulmonary vascular resistance, improved cardiac index, improved oxygen tissue delivery, and improved exercise tolerance. In contrast, there are few long-term clinical trials of vasodilator therapy to demonstrate improvements in survival. In one report (51), patients with primary pulmonary hypertension who responded during initial catheterization studies to nifedipine and diltiazem continued to do so for up to 5 years of continuous vasodilator therapy (Fig. 48.6). Such "responders" also enjoyed a 94% survival rate compared to the 55% survival rate among patients who did not respond initially to these agents. It remains unclear if these results reflect differences among patients with inherently more reversible and hence responsive vascular disease or whether chronic vasodilator therapy improves survival in patients who would otherwise worsen over time.

It is important to note that in this study, high doses of calcium channel blockers were used and were based on hemodynamic

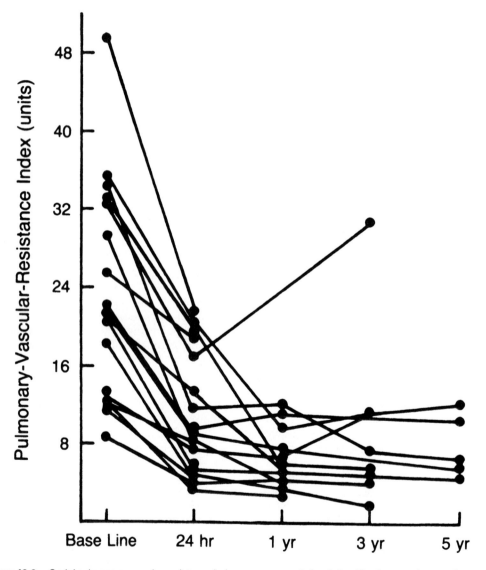

Figure 48.6. Serial pulmonary vascular resistance index measurements in adults with primary pulmonary hypertension who initially responded to pulmonary vasodilators over a 3–5 year follow-up period. (From Rich S, Kaufmann E, Levy PS. The effect of high doses of calcium-channel blockers on survival in primary pulmonary hypertension. *N Engl J Med* 1992; 327:76–81.)

responses to progressive increments in vasodilator dose during the initial evaluations. Such protocols have demonstrated that doses of vasodilators must be individualized and may be greater than anticipated in order to produce hemodynamic improvement (78). Because vasodilators may worsen ventilation-perfusion matching in patients with chronic lung disease, supplemental oxygen therapy is often used in conjunction with long-term vasodilator therapy. Systemic hypotension due to nonspecific vasodilation remains an additional complication limiting the use and dose of vasodilators to treat pulmonary hypertension. Minor but distressing side effects reported with vasodilator therapy include headache, nausea, vomiting, and abdominal cramps (49).

Anticoagulant therapy is now recognized as an important adjunct therapy for patients with severe, end-stage pulmonary hypertension. As vascular remodeling progresses and vessel lumens narrow, thrombosis occurs locally. This is reflected by a patchy distribution of perfusion defects noted on perfusion scans of patients with primary pulmonary hypertension (51, 79). Warfarin has been used to treat not only primary thromboembolic pulmonary disease but also primary pulmonary vascular disease. Rich and colleagues demonstrated significant improvement in survival of adults with primary pulmonary hypertension, particularly among those patients who did not respond to vasodilator therapy (51). Survival within the first year of treatment was 91% in patients treated with warfarin and 52% in those who did not receive anticoagulant therapy (Fig. 48.3). This work confirms earlier findings at the Mayo Clinic where survival rates were almost twice as great for patients with pulmonary hypertension who received anticoagulation therapy compared to those who did not (80). The role of platelet inhibitors such as dipyridamole as an alternative means of reducing spontaneous clotting of pulmonary vessels is less clear, according to clinical trials in patients with pulmonary hypertension (81). The study of anticoagulants has been limited to adults and to patients with primary pulmonary vascular disease rather than children with chronic lung disease. Its efficacy in the pediatric age group remains to be determined.

Lung and heart-lung transplantation have been performed on children in multiple centers to treat pulmonary hypertension secondary to heart and lung diseases. The age of recipients has ranged from 4 months to 18 years in the 23 children reported on from 1989 to 1992 (82–85). Postoperative complications mirror those encountered in adults, including recurrent lung rejection, infections, and late bronchiolitis obliterans. Long-term survivors have experienced substantial improvement in function and reduction in symptoms. However, the number of centers performing lung transplantation remains limited as does the availability of donors (86). Currently, this represents a treatment option for very few children with pulmonary hypertension.

Current clinical treatment of pulmonary hypertension has had limited impact on the outcome of the disease because it neither corrects the underlying lung disease nor directly modifies the process of vascular remodeling. Active research to understand the regulators of cell growth and proliferation within pulmonary vessels under normal and adverse conditions will ideally lead to novel treatment modalities with greater efficacy. In the meantime, treatment for this disorder will remain primarily supportive for most children.

REFERENCES

1. Allen H, Taussig LM, Gaines JA. Echocardiograph profiles of the long-term cardiac changes in cystic fibrosis. Chest 1979; 75:428–433.
2. Goodman G, Perkin RM, Anas NG, Sperling DR, Hicks DA, Rowen M. Pulmonary hypertension in infants with bronchopulmonary dysplasia. J Pediatr 1988; 112:67–72.
3. Stack HR, Choo-Kang YF, Heard BC. The prognosis of cryptogenic fibrosing alveolitis. Thorax 1972; 27:535–542.
4. Flenley DC. Sleep in chronic obstructive lung disease. Clin Chest Med 1985; 6:651–661.
5. Krieger J. Breathing during sleep in normal subjects. Clin Chest Med 1985; 6:577–594.
6. Brandfonbrener M, Turino G, Himmelstein A, Fishman A. Effects of occlusion of one pulmonary artery on pulmonary circulation in man. Fed Proc 1958; 17:19.
7. Ahmed T, Oliver WJ, Wanner A. Variability of hypoxic pulmonary vasoconstriction in sheep. Role of prostaglandins. Am Rev Respir Dis 1985; 127:59–62.
8. Rudolph AM, Yuen S. Response of the pulmonary vasculature to hypoxia and H+ ion concentration changes. J Clin Invest 1966; 45:399–411.
9. Benumof JL, Pirlo AF, Johanson I, Trousdale FR. Interaction of PVO_2 with PAO_2 on hypoxic pulmonary vasoconstriction. J Appl Physiol 1981; 51:871–874.
10. Marshall BE. Importance of hypoxic pulmonary vasoconstriction with atelectasis. Adv Shock Res 1982; 8:1–12.

tion in infants, children, and adolescents. *J Pediatr Surg* 1991; 26:434–438.

84. Vouh'e PR, Le Bidois J, Dartevelle P, et al. Heart- and heart-lung transplantation in children. *Eur J Cardiothorac Surg* 1989; 3:191–195.

85. Smyth RL, Higenbottam TW, Scott JP, et al. Early experience of heart-lung transplantation. *Arch Dis Child* 1989; 64:1225–1229.

86. Kaiser LR, Cooper JD. The current status of lung transplantation. *Adv Surg* 1992; 25:259–307.

87. Stenmark KR, Fasules J, Hyde DM, et al. Severe pulmonary hypertension and arterial adventitial changes in newborn calves at 4,300 m. *J Appl Physiol* 1987; 62:821–830.

49

AIDS and Other Immune Deficiency States

MEYER KATTAN

The respiratory tract is the organ system most commonly involved in a wide variety of immunodeficiency disorders. These disorders encompass a diverse group of illnesses resulting from one or more abnormalities of the immune system. The immunodeficiencies can be primary or, much more commonly, secondary to chronic or acute disorders (Table 49.1). The immune system dysfunction results in recurrent or chronic sinopulmonary infections, which in turn can lead to chronic lung disease, fibrosis, and bronchiectasis.

Immunodeficiency states are increasingly common in pediatrics because of the growing number of children infected with the human immunodeficiency virus (HIV). In addition, there are many more children requiring immunosuppresive therapy for organ transplants and for a wide variety of other chronic conditions.

The clinical history is helpful in distinguishing the immunodeficient child from the normal child with "frequent respiratory infections" or allergies. Six to eight upper respiratory tract infections per year are common, especially in those in day-care settings or nursery schools. A positive family history of allergies, absence of fever, normal growth patterns, and chronic clear nasal discharge suggest allergies.

PRIMARY IMMUNODEFICIENCIES

Defects in the immune system can affect four components: the B lymphocyte (antibody) system, the T lymphocyte (cell-mediated immune) system; the phagocytic system; and the complement system. The World Health Organization (WHO) classification of the primary immunodeficiencies is shown in Table 49.2 (1). The organisms that are most frequently encountered in the respiratory system in B and T cell deficiencies are presented in Table 49.3. Although most of the primary immunodeficiencies can result in recurrent pneumonias, there are many other sites of infection and problems that are life-threatening. The conditions discussed in this section are limited to those in which chronic respiratory problems are prominent features.

IgA Deficiency

IgA deficiency is the most common primary immunodeficiency. The incidence varies in different population groups. The relative frequency is approximately one in every 600–700 individuals in North America and Europe, and

Table 49.1.
Factors Associated with Secondary Immunodeficiencies

1. Prematurity
2. Hereditary and metabolic disorders (e.g., diabetes mellitus, sickle cell disease, malnutrition)
3. Infections (e.g., measles, HIV, Epstein-Barr virus)
4. Immunosuppressive agents (e.g., radiation, immunosuppressive drugs)
5. Malignancies (e.g., leukemia, lymphoma)
6. Miscellaneous (e.g., burns, splenectomy)

Table 49.2.
World Health Organization (WHO) Classification of Primary Immunodeficiencies

I. Predominantly antibody defects
II. Combined immunodeficiencies
III. Immunodeficiencies with other major defects
IV. Complement deficiencies
V. Defects of phagocytic function

657

Table 49.3.
Frequent Organisms in B Cell and T Cell Immunodeficiency States

Immunodeficiency	Organisms Isolated
B cell	Encapsulated bacteria
	Pseudomonas aeruginosa
	Pnemocystis carinii
	Ureaplasma urealyticum
	Mycoplasma pneumoniae
T cell	Encapsulated bacteria
	Mycobacterium tuberculosis
	Escherichia coli
	Pseudomonas aeruginosa
	Klebsiella spp
	Serratia marcesans
	Nocardia spp
	Viruses
	Pneumocystis carinii
	Fungi

approximately one in 18,000 in Japan (2–5). African-Americans are reported to have a lower incidence of IgA deficiency compared to whites (6). Serum IgA is usually undetectable at birth and reaches the adult level around the time of puberty. IgA accounts for about 10–20% of serum immunoglobulin normally, but is the most prevalent immunoglobulin in secretions, including the nasal and bronchial secretions. Mucosal IgA is synthesized by local plasma cells, and serum IgA is derived mainly from plasma cells in the bone marrow. There are two subtypes of IgA, IgA_1 and IgA_2. Both isotypes are reduced in IgA deficiency, but the degree of reduction of each is highly variable. In this deficiency, serum levels of IgA are usually 5 mg/dl or less.

An important biologic function of IgA antibodies is to protect the host from organisms invading the respiratory mucosal surface. Secretory IgA antibodies may inhibit adherence of pathogens to epithelial cells, neutralize virus infectivity, and regulate the absorption of antigens.

The clinical consequences of IgA deficiency are variable. It is often not associated with clinical illness, but IgA-deficient individuals are more prone to recurrent respiratory tract illnesses and allergies in addition to autoimmune diseases, gastrointestinal disorders, and malignancies. Recurrent upper respiratory infections are most common, although a few IgA-deficient patients have recurrent pneumonias and bronchiectasis (7–9). IgA deficiency appears to predispose to allergic conjunctivitis, rhinitis, urticaria, atopic eczema, and asthma.

Selective IgA deficiency requires no treatment, and those individuals with sinopulmonary disease or asthma should be treated in the same manner as patients with normal IgA concentrations. Care should be taken in administering immunoglobulins in IgA-deficient patients because of the risk of severe anaphylactic reactions as a result of production of IgA antibodies.

Other cellular and humoral defects may be associated with IgA deficiency. Approximately 20% of patients have an associated IgG subclass deficiency (10). IgA deficiency is frequent in ataxia telangectasia, an autosomal recessive disorder characterized by thymic hypoplasia, progressive ataxia, oculocutaneous telangectasia, and recurrent sinopulmonary infections. There have been case reports of IgA deficiency in association with alpha-1 antitrypsin deficiency and chronic granulomatous disease (11, 12).

IgG Subclass Deficiencies

IgG subclass deficiency is an antibody deficiency of one or two subclasses but with normal or increased levels of other subclasses. IgG_1 deficiency is usually associated with other IgG subclass deficiencies. These patients often present with recurrent lung disease (13).

IgG_2 deficiency has been associated with recurrent and chronic pulmonary disease (13). IgA-deficient patients are more likely to have respiratory symptoms when they have an associated IgG_2 subclass deficiency (10). IgG_3 deficiency can be isolated or found in combination with other subclass deficiencies. This deficiency has been associated with lung disease (14). IgG_4 is present in low concentration in serum and requires sensitive methods for detection. Beck and Heiner reported that selective IgG_4 deficiency increases the risk for recurrent pulmonary infections (15). Treatment of IgG subclass deficiency has been successful with immunoglobulin infusions.

Common Variable Immune Deficiency (CVID)

CVID is a primary immunodeficiency in which B lymphocytes produce little or no antibody, resulting in reduced levels of immunoglobulins. About half the patients also have associated T cell defects. The IgG levels are generally less than 500 mg/dl (normal range 800–1800), IgA levels are less than 90 (normal range 90–450), and IgM levels are less than 100 (normal range 80–350). Patients with this disorder often have recurrent infections of the sinopulmonary tract. Chronic lung disease, particularly bronchiectasis, and cor pulmonale may develop. In one reported series, the majority of patients had pneumonia at least once, and 7% developed chronic pulmonary complications before the age of 20 years (16). Both obstructive and restrictive changes on pulmonary function testing have been described (17). Over the years, patients have been diagnosed earlier, possibly reflecting an increased awareness of the disease. Respiratory failure, infections, and malignant lymphoma are the major causes of death. Treatment consists of intravenous immunoglobulin infusions.

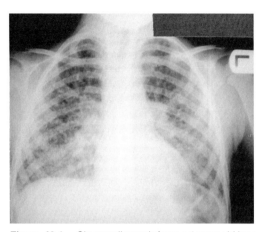

Figure 49.1. Chest radiograph from a 4-year-old boy with CGD. There is a reticulonodular pattern throughout the lung fields representing granulomas. Hilar adenopathy is present.

Chronic Granulomatous Disease (CGD)

CGD is an inherited disorder characterized by recurrent pyogenic infections. It can be either an X-linked recessive disorder (approximately 55% of patients) or an autosomal recessive one. Pulmonary infections occur in nearly all patients. CGD granulocytes ingest microorganisms normally, but killing is deficient because the phagocytes fail to produce superoxide, an ion, and related microbicidal oxygen intermediates. This results from an NADPH oxidase deficiency. The patients usually present with infections beginning in the first few months of life. The pulmonary manifestations include hilar adenopathy, pneumonia, empyema, and lung abcesses. Infections result from catalase-producing organisms. *Staphlococcus aureus, Serratia marcescens,* and *Aspergillus* spp are common organisms. Pulmonary infiltrates persist for weeks or months as granulomas form in response to infection. The chest radiograph can show reticulonodular densities representing the granulomas (Figs. 49.1, 49.2). Treatment consists of antibiotics aimed at the organism. Blood and sputum cultures are often negative because of the ability of the phagocytes to ingest the organisms. Lung biopsy is usually needed for identification of the infecting agent. Continuous prophylaxis with trimethoprim-sulfamethoxazole (TMP-SMX) is used,

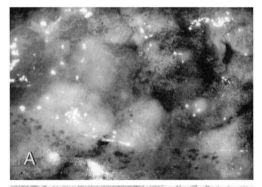

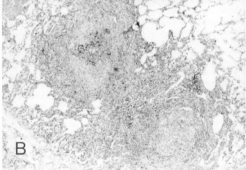

Figure 49.2 Lung biopsy specimen, same patient as in Figure 49.1. *A,* Cut surface of pulmonary parenchyma displaying numerous ill-defined pale firm nodules with necrotic centers. *B,* Section of lung showing focally confluent granulomata with histiocytes, multinucleated giant cells, and central abscess pockets. (Magnification: × 20.)

because this antibiotic penetrates granulocytes (18). In a recent double-blind controlled clinical trial, interferon-gamma (50, $\mu g/m^2$ of body surface area) reduced the frequency of serious infections and was well tolerated (19).

IMMUNODEFICIENCY SECONDARY TO IMMUNOSUPPRESSIVE AGENTS

Advances in the field of transplantation have led to a rapid rise in the number of organ transplants in children. Renal, liver, heart, lung, and bone marrow transplants are increasing, and with this comes an increase in pulmonary problems related to immunosuppressive agents. The most common chemical agents presently used to control rejection are steroids, cyclosporine A, FK506, and OKT3.

The effects of steroids include the suppression of the accumulation of leukocytes at the site of inflammation, blocking of reticuloendothelial cell clearance, decreasing helper T lymphocytes, and reduction of bacterial and fungicidal activity of monocytes. Cyclosporine A has a selective effect on T cells by inhibiting DNA translation and the expression of interleukin-2 receptors as well as the release of interleukin-1 and -2. FK506 has more powerful immunosuppressive activity than does cyclosporine (20). This agent also inhibits interleukin-2 synthesis and release. OKT3 is a monoclonal antibody directed against the OKT3 antigen in mature human T cells (21).

In studies of solid organ and bone marrow transplants, the risk of pulmonary complications has been related to the immunosuppressive regimens and to host factors. A major risk factor for CMV pneumonitis is a seropositive donor, especially when coupled with a seronegative recipient (22, 23). Steroids, OKT3, and the use of antilymphocyte globulins also increase the risk of CMV infection (24, 25). High-dose steroids in neutropenic patients increase the susceptibility to invasive aspergillosis (26).

Many conditions present with fever tachypnea and infiltrates on chest radiograph; a precise diagnosis is difficult on clinical grounds alone. Bronchoalveolar lavage and open lung biopsy are often required to establish a diagnosis. Lavage has some limitations in that CMV or *Aspergillus* in lavage fluid may not be indicative of invasive infection.

LIVER TRANSPLANTATION

Bacterial, CMV, fungal, and *Pneumocystis carinii* pneumonia (PCP) are infectious complications arising after orthotopic liver transplant. CMV is the most common infection in this population, especially if the donor is seropositive (23). Pneumonia most commonly occurs during the second month after liver transplant. Onset of CMV appears to be related to increased immunosuppression and particularly OKT3 therapy (27). CMV pneumonitis is often preceded by prolonged fever and hepatitis. Gancyclovir is an effective treatment of CMV pneumonia, especially if started early in the course of infection (28). CMV hyperimmune globulin and CMV-negative blood have been used for prevention of CMV disease (29).

Fungal pneumonia usually occur within the first month after transplantation. *Candida* and *Aspergillus* are the most common agents (30). PCP occurs several months after transplantation (30). Prophylaxis with trimethoprim-sulfamethoxazole is usually given to children after transplant, although there have been no controlled studies to determine the effectiveness of this practice.

Lymphoproliferative disease resulting from long-term immunosuppression has been reported on long-term follow-up of children with liver transplants (31). Patients can have asymptomatic hilar adenopathy, mild upper airway obstruction from tonsillar hypertrophy, or systemic symptoms with respiratory distress.

RENAL TRANSPLANTATION

Infectious pulmonary complications of renal transplantation are similar to those seen after liver transplantation, but in addition, mycobacterial pneumonia has been reported (32). CMV is the most common complication (33). Symptoms usually appear in the first 2 months. Fever is present in the majority of cases. Gancyclovir is an effective treatment (34). CMV hyperimmune globulin may also be effective in the treatment of CMV pneumonitis in renal transplant recipients (35). In adults, oral administration of acyclovir prophylactically has reduced the rate of CMV pneumonia (36).

Introduction of cyclosporine in renal transplant recipients has been associated with increased incidence of PCP (37). PCP usually presents with acute respiratory distress and fever occurring 2–4 months after transplantation. TMP-SMX is the preferred treatment and is also used for prophylaxis.

Aspergillus is the most common fungal infection in this population and usually occurs within the first 4 months after transplantation (38).

Symptoms with mycobacterial infection may be nonspecific with little respiratory compromise. The only pulmonary manifestation may be an abnormal chest radiograph.

BONE MARROW TRANSPLANTATION

The goal of immunosuppression in marrow transplantation is the complete eradication of the immune system. The lung is affected by infectious and non-infectious processes that result from the major alterations in the immune system and the degree of immunosuppression. Chemotherapeutic agents and irradiation can also directly damage the lung.

Graft versus host disease (GVHD) occurs as a result of immunocompetent donor cells destroying host tissues. Acute GVHD occurs 20–100 days after transplantation. Infections are common during this phase. Chronic GVHD occurs more than 3 months after transplantation. Bacterial and viral pneumonias are common, and severe airway obstruction and bronchitis obliterans may occur (39).

Interstitial pneumonitis is observed in bone marrow transplant recipients. Bacterial and fungal etiologies have been identified. More commonly, CMV or no etiology is found (40, 41). The clinical picture is nonspecific with dyspnea, fever, hypoxia, and diffuse interstitial infiltrates.

CMV pneumonitis occurs about 2 months after transplantation. It is much more common after allogeneic transplantation than autologous graft recipients. Mortality with this infection is high. Prophylaxis with high-dose intravenous acyclovir has been successful in reducing the incidence of pneumonias (42). Herpesvirus pneumonia and RSV pneumonia are less common than CMV (43).

Bone marrow transplant patients are at risk for invasive fungal infections, which usually occur within the first month after transplantation. Invasive aspergillosis is the most common fungal infection (44).

Bacterial pneumonia occurs but most commonly in those with GVHD. Gram-negative organisms predominate. PCP is a less common finding in marrow transplantation because of the use of prophylaxis with TMP-SMX. It usually occurs around 2 months after transplantation.

HEART AND LUNG TRANSPLANTATION

Pulmonary infections are common after heart transplantation, usually occuring within the first 3 months (45). Pneumonia, mediastinitis, and emphysema can occur. Bacterial pneumonias occur within the first few weeks after transplantation, usually secondary to gram-negative organisms. *Legionella* pneumonia, *Nocardia*, and mycobacterial infections have been reported in adults after cardiac transplant (46, 47).

CMV pneumonia is the most common viral infection, although this appears to be less of a problem with cyclosporine-based regimens. Gancyclovir is an effective treatment. Fungal pneumonia has been observed, with *Aspergillus* as the leading agent. PCP can occur, although prophylaxis with trimethoprin-sulfamethoxazole has reduced its occurence. There is little experience in heart-lung or lung transplants in children, but infections reported in adults are similar to those observed in heart transplants.

ACQUIRED IMMUNODEFICIENCY SYNDROME

In 1982, a year after the initial description of the acquired immunodeficiency syndrome (AIDS) in adults, cases were described in infants and children (48–51). Over the past decade, this disease has emerged as a major problem in pediatrics worldwide. HIV was established as the cause of the syndrome. The incubation period of the virus is variable, ranging from months to years. HIV affects multiple organ systems. The primary target cell of HIV is the CD4 helper-inducer lymphocyte. The identifiable risk factors associated with HIV infection in children include parental intravenous drug abuse, bisexual fathers, and transfusion of blood or blood products to the mother or directly to the child. Although approximately 20% of AIDS cases are presently transfusion-related, screening of blood for infection has reduced this risk.

A major public health problem is now perinatally acquired infection. The HIV seroprevalence rate in childbearing women was estimated to be 0.15% in the United States in 1989, with rates as high as 1.63% in areas in New York City and 1.2% in Connecticut (52). Studies in the United States and Europe suggest maternal-to-infant transmission rates between 13 and 35% (53–56). Prospective studies have so far not been able to identify the mode of delivery (vaginal vs. caesarean section) as a risk factor for transmission.

There are a growing number of cases among adolescents. As in the adult population, male homosexuals and intravenous drug abusers are at highest risk. The female-to-male ratio of infection in adolescents in higher than in adults, suggesting a greater role of heterosexual transmission.

Definition

HIV infection results in a disease spectrum ranging from asymptomatic infection to symptomatic cases meeting the Centers for Disease Control (CDC) case definition for AIDS (57). Asymptomatic children under 15 months of age who are HIV antibody positive are considered to be indeterminate (P-0), CDC classification). Maternal HIV antibodies persist for a median of 10 months but usually are not present after 15 months. Criteria for early diagnosis of HIV infection will need to be established as other methods of detection become more routinely available. Infected patients, greater than 15 months of age, who are asymptomatic are classified as CDC stage P-1. Asymptomatic patients can have defects in helper T cell function. Symptomatic patients are classified as CDC state P-2. P-2 patients require specific illnesses or opportunistic infections to meet the CDC surveillance definition for AIDS (Table 49.4) (58).

A screening assay (ELISA) detects specific antibody to the virus. Serum is incubated with HIV antigen and treated to detect a spectrophotometric color change. The color change correlates with the amount of antibody in the test sample. This test has a sensitivity and specificity of 99% (59). The test is confirmed using an immunoblot analysis (Western blot). In this assay, HIV antigens are electrophoretically separated into bands. Antibodies to HIV can be identified when bound to specific antigenic bands. Infection can be detected by more sophisticated testing such as culture of peripheral blood lymphocytes for HIV, detec-

Table 49.4.
Centers for Disease Control (CDC) Surveillance Definition for AIDS-Diagnosis Indicative of AIDS

Candidiasis of the esophagus[a,b]
Candidiasis of the trachea, bronchi, or lungs[a]
Coccidioidomycosis, disseminated or extrapulmonary[c]
Cryptococcosis, extrapulmonary[a]
Cryptosporidiosis, chronic intestinal[a]
Cytomegalovirus disease (other than liver, spleen, nodes) onset at >1 month of age[a]
Cytomegalovirus retinitis (with loss of vision)[a,b]
Herpes simplex ulcer, chronic (>1 month's duration) or pneumonitis or esophagitis, onset at >1 month of age[a]
HIV encephalopathy[c]
Histoplasmosis, disseminated or extrapulmonary[c]
Isosporiasis, chronic intestinal (>1 month's duration)
Karposi sarcoma[a,b]
Lymphoid interstitial pneumonitis[a,b]
Lymphoma, primary brain[a]
Lymphoma (Burkitt, or immunoblastic sarcoma)[c]
Multiple or recurrent bacterial infections[c]
Mycobacterium avium complex or *M. kansasii*, disseminated or extrapulmonary[a]
M. tuberculosis or acid-fast infection (species not identified), disseminated or extrapulmonary[c]
Pneumocystis carinii pneumonia[a,b]
Progressive multifocal leukoencephalopathy[a]
Toxoplasmosis of brain, onset at >1 month of age[a,b]
Wasting syndrome due to HIV[c]

[a]If indicator disease is diagnosed definitively (e.g., biopsy or culture) and there is no other cause of immunodeficiency, laboratory documentation of HIV infection is not required.
[b]Presumptive diagnosis of indicator disease is accepted, if there is laboratory evidence of HIV infection.
[c]Requires laboratory evidence of HIV infection.

tion of circulating viral antigens such as the p24 viral core protein, or the polymerase chain reaction, which enables the detection of viral genomes.

Clinical Manifestations

The initial signs and symptoms of HIV infection include pulmonary disease, lymphadenopathy, hepatosplenomegaly, chronic diarrhea, failure to thrive, recurrent sepsis, and encephalopathy. Infectious and noninfectious pulmonary diseases are major complications of HIV infection (Table 49.5). A pulmonary problem is the first symptom of infection in more than half of the cases (60).

PNEUMOCYSTIS CARINII PNEUMONIA

Pneumocystis carinii pneumonia (PCP) was the most common opportunistic infection with HIV infection before the use of prophylaxis.

Table 49.5.
Pulmonary Complications of HIV Infection

Infections
Viruses:
  Cytomegalovirus
  Respiratory syncytial virus
  Herpes simplex virus
  Parainfluenza virus
  Influenza virus
  Adenovirus

Bacteria:
  Encapsulated organisms (e.g., *Streptococcus
    pneumoniae, Haemophilus influenzae,
    Staphylococcus aureus*)
  Gram-negative organisms (e.g., *Escherichia coli,
    Klebsiella, Pseudomonas aeruginosa*)
  Mycobacterium tuberculosis
  Mycobacterium avium intracellulare

Fungi:
  Pneumocystis carinii
  Candida albicans
  Histoplasma capsulatum
  Cryptococcus neoformans
  Aspergillus spp
  Coccidioides immitis

Malignancies
Kaposi sarcoma
Lymphoma

Interstitial pneumonia
Lymphoid interstitial pneumonia
Pulmonary lymphoid hyperplasia
Desquamative interstitial pneumonia

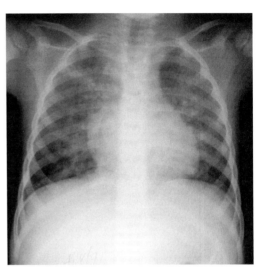

Figure 49.3. Chest radiograph in a 3-month-old boy with *Pneumocystis carinii* pneumonia. There is a diffuse interstitial pattern.

PCP was diagnosed in more than one-third of HIV-infected children (61, 62). It can be the initial presentation of HIV infection. The organism primarily affects the lung and attaches to the type II cells of the alveolar epithelium. The median age at presentation of PCP is 5 months (60, 61). Children with this infection present with acute or progressive fever, tachypnea, and retractions. Decreased breath sounds or crackles may be present on auscultation. The patients are commonly markedly hypoxic and have an elevation of serum lactic dehydrogenase levels (60, 64). The majority of cases of PCP progress to respiratory failure necessitating intubation and mechanical ventilation (65, 66). Co-infection with bacteria, CMV, and *Mycobacterium avium* intracellulare has been reported.

Chest radiographs commonly show a diffuse, reticulonodular infiltrate, but focal infiltrates or pneumatoceles can also be seen (Fig. 49.3). Radionuclide scans with intravenous gallium-67 citrate or aerosolized technetium-99m diethylenetriamine pentaacetate (^{99m}Tc-

DTPA) have been used to study the lungs of patients with HIV infection. Because of the low specificity of these tests, they have added little to the chest radiograph and arterial blood gas in the diagnosis of PCP. Studies are presently being conducted to determine if ^{99m}Tc-DTPA can be helpful in the earlier detection of lung disease in HIV-infected children.

The diagnosis of PCP relies on identification of the organism obtained from bronchial washings or lung tissue. The common stains used for identification are Gomori methenamine silver stain, Giemsa stain, and toluidine blue stain. Bronchoalveolar lavage with fiberoptic bronchoscopy is a reliable method for establishing the diagnosis of PCP (65, 67). In intubated patients, installation of 2–3 aliquots of 5–10 ml of saline into the endotracheal tube followed by suctioning also provides a high yield in isolating PCP. However, there are cases in which a lavage is negative for PCP but open lung biopsy is positive.

Trimethoprin-sulfamethoxazole is the drug of choice for the treatment of PCP, usually for 3 weeks, and is initially given intravenously. A clinical response to therapy is usually noted by 5–7, days and the drug should not be discontinued if there is deterioration in the patient's condition in the first few days. Adverse reactions to TMP-SMX include rashes and thrombocytopenia, but these are not as frequent as they are in adult patients with

AIDS. Pentamidine administered intravenously or intramuscularly is also effctive in PCP and can be used if TMP-SMX is not well tolerated. Pentamidine is nephrotoxic and can also cause hypoglycemia and thrombocytopenia. Corticosteroids have been advocated as an adjunct to therapy in the treatment of PCP in some HIV-infected adults based on studies showing improved survival and a decreased incidence of respiratory failure (68). The use of corticosteroids in children with PCP has not been studied. Extrapolation from adult studies to children is limited by the fact that the immune system is still developing and that the pathogenesis of PCP may be a *primary* infection, rather than reactivation. Clinical trials regarding steroid use in PCP have been recommended.

The prognosis is poor, with a mortality rate in excess of 50%. There does not appear to be a correlation between survival and LDH or CD4 cell count. Some survivors of PCP are oxygen-dependent, and approximately one-half die within a year of infection (65, 66). Recurrence of PCP has occurred and is associated with a high mortality rate. The prognosis of children with PCP is worse than in adults, and may be related to the likelihood that infection is primary rather than reactivation, combined with severe immunodeficiency.

Typically, the CD4 cell count decreases as HIV infection progresses. Studies in both adults and children have shown a greater likelihood of developing PCP with lower CD4 cell counts. In HIV-infected adults, CD4 lymphocyte counts less than 200 cells/μl are associated with a high risk of PCP (69). However, CD4 cell counts are higher in healthy children than in healthy adults and decline with age (70). Therefore, it is not surprising that infants with PCP and CD4 cell counts over 1000 cells/μl have been reported (71, 72). Because of the high mortality of PCP, the CDC has published guidelines for prophylaxis of HIV-infected children (73). Prophylaxis should be initiated if the CD4 counts are: 1500 cells/mm^3 for children 1–11 months; 750 cells/mm^3 for children 12–23 months; 500 cells/mm^3 for children 24 months through 5 years; and 200 cells/mm^3 for children 6 years and older. Prophylaxis is also recommended for if the percentage of CD4 cells is less than 20, regardless of the absolute count. Trimethoprim-sulfamethoxazole is currently the preferred drug for prophylaxis. Alternatives include aerosolized pentamidine and dapsone, but there is limited experience with these agents in children.

LYMPHPOID INTERSTITIAL PNEUMONIA/ PULMONARY LYMPHOID HYPERPLASIA

LIP/PLH is a common pulmonary complication of children with HIV infection (64). The association of LIP/PLH in children with HIV infection is so striking that histologically confirmed LIP without any other cause of immunodeficiency in an HIV-seropositive child less than 13 years satisfies the CDC surveillance definition for AIDS. The pathology consists of a diffuse infiltration of lymphocytes in the interstitium and scattered nodules of mononuclear cells 0.5 mm in diameter. These mononuclear cells are lymphocytes, plasma cells, and immunoblasts, and are mainly B cells. In LIP the infiltration is diffuse throughout the parenchyma, and in PLH the infiltration is primarily associated with the bronchial and bronchiolar walls. The etiology of LIP/PLH is unknown but this condition has been observed in other immunodeficiency states (74). Epstein-Barr viral DNA has been found in lung biopsies of children with LIP (75, 76). HIV RNA has been identified in the lung of an infant with LIP (77). However, the relationship between EBV, HIV infection, and LIP/PLH remains to be elucidated.

The onset of LIP/PLH is insiduous and may be associated with cough and tachypnea. It usually becomes apparent after the first year of life at a median age of 2.5–3.0 years (60, 78). Patients usually hae generalized lymphadenopathy, and may have hepatosplenomegaly, clubbing, and parotid gland enlargement. Auscultation of the chest is often normal, but crackles and wheezes may be present. Patients should be monitored for pulmonary infections that may co-exist with LIP/PLH. The disease is slowly progressive.

Some patients develop hypoxia although this is usually mild. Elevated immunoglobulin levels are associated with LIP/PLH. The radiograph typically shows a diffuse interstitial nodular pattern with or without hilar adenopathy (Fig. 49.4). The gallium scan is positive but is not specific (79).

Lung biopsy definitively establishes the diagnosis of LIP/PLH. A presumptive diag-

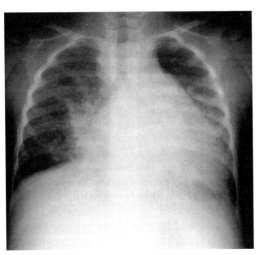

Figure 49.4. Chest radiograph in a child with lymphocytic interstitial pneumonia. There is a reticulonodular pattern with hilar adenopathy.

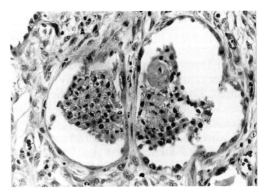

Figure 49.5. High-power microscopic photograph of lung with diffuse alveolar damage in an infant with HIV infection. This shows desquamated alveolar lining cells and histiocytes within alveolar spaces, hyperplasia of type II pneumocytes lining alveolar spaces, and fibroplasia of intra-alveolar septa. (Magnification: × 200.)

nosis can be made in the HIV-infected child based on the clinical findings and the typical radiographic pattern lasting more than 2 months without another documented cause.

There is no specific therapy for LIP/PLH. Oxygen is administered for hypoxia. Although treatment of LIP/PLH with corticosteroids has been reported to result in clinical improvement in a small number of patients, clinical trials have not been done (80).

DIFFUSE ALVEOLAR DAMAGE (DAD)

DAD is a nonspecific pattern of acute lung injury associated with a variety of clinical conditions. It has been reported in patients with HIV infection (81). Possible etiologies in these patients are *P. carinii* infection, adult respiratory distress syndrome, and oxygen toxicity. DAD has an exudative phase developing over 2 or 3 days and is characterized by interstitial edema and hyaline membranes. This progresses to a proliferative phase after 1 week. There is hyperplasia of alveolar lining cells, thickening of the interstitium, and chronic inflammation (Fig. 49.5).

This entity should be suspected if there is persistent hypoxia following acute respiratory failure from PCP or other opportunistic infections. Recurrent episodes of respiratory failure may represent viral infections superimposed on a lung with DAD.

VIRAL INFECTION

Viral pneumonia with common pathogens, such as respiratory syncytial virus (RSV), parainfluenza, influenza, and adenovirus, has occurred in HIV-infected patients (60, 67). Measles virus and varicella-zoster virus can cause severe pulmonary disease in this group of patients (82). CMV and herpes simplex virus have been isolated from bronchial washings, but do not necessarily indicate the presence of pneumonia. Documentation of infection requires histopathologic evidence of tissue invasion with the virus and recovery of the virus on culture. In a recent review, Murray and Mills proposed criteria for a tentative clinical diagnosis, which included (a) CMV recovered on culture, (b) CMV inclusions in bronchoalveolar lavage cells or from biopsy specimens, (c) no other pathogens, and (d) progressive pneumonitis (83).

The clinical symptoms with viral pneumonia are variable. A history of exposure associated with cough or tachypnea suggests a viral etiology. Mild hypoxia is common. The chest radiograph can reveal diffuse interstitial or alveolar infiltrate. Since the clinical picture is nonspecific and infection may occur with other pulmonary disease such as LIP/PLH, further workup may be necessary. A nasopharyngeal specimen for rapid viral diagnosis and culture is helpful. If the patient with a presumed viral infection is deteriorating, bronchoalveolar lavage or lung biopsy is warranted to rule out other infections.

19. The International Chronic Granulomatous Disease Cooperative Study Group. A controlled trial of interferon gamma to prevent infection in chronic granulomatous disease. *N Engl J Med* 1991; 324:509–516.

20. Anon. FK 506-An investigational immunosuppressant. *Med Lett* 1991; 33:94.

21. Chatenoud L, Jonker M, Villemain F, Goldstein G, Bach JF. The human immune response to OKT3 monoclonal antibody is oligoclonal. *Science* 1986; 232:1406–1408.

22. Chou S. Acquisition of donor strain of cytomegalovirus by renal-transplant recipients. *N Engl J Med* 1986; 314:1418–1423.

23. King SM, Petric M, Superin R, Graham N, Roberts EA. Cytomegalovirus infections in pediatric liver transplantation. *Am J Dis Child* 1990; 144:1307–1310.

24. Velasco N, Catto RD, Edward N, et al. The effect of the dosage of steroids on the incidence of cytomegalovirus infections in renal transplant recipients. *J Infect* 1984; 9:69–78.

25. Pass RF, Whitley RJ, Deithelm AG, et al. Cytomegalovirus infections in patients with renal transplants: Potentiation by antithymocytic globulin and an incompatible graft. *J Infect Dis* 1980; 142:9–17.

26. Gerson SL, Talbot GH, Hurwitz S, Strom BL, Lusk EJ, Cassileth PA. Prolonged granulocytopenia: The major risk factor for invasive pulmonary aspergillosis in patients with acute leukemia. *Ann Intern Med* 1984; 100:345–351.

27. Singh N, Dummer JS, Kusne S, et al. Infections with cytomegalovirus and other herpesviruses in 121 liver transplant recipients: Transmission by donated organs and the effect of OKT3 antibodies. *J Infect Dis* 1988; 158:124–131.

28. Gudnason T, Belani KK, Balfour HH. Gancyclovir treatment of cytomegalovirus disease in immunocompromised children. *Pediatr Infect Dis J* 1989; 8:436–440.

29. Saliba F, Arulnaden JL, Gugenheim J, et al. CMV hyperimmune globulin prophylaxis after liver transplantation: A prospective randomized controlled study. *Transplant Proc* 1989; 21:2260–2262.

30. Kusne S, Dummer JS, Singh N, et al. Infections after liver transplantation: An analysis of 101 consecutive cases. *Medicine* 1988; 63:131–143.

31. Malatack JJ, Gartner JC, Urbach AH, Zitelli BJ. Orthotopic liver transplantation, Epstein-Barr virus, cyclosporine and lymphoproliferative disease: A growing concern. *J Pediatr* 1991; 118:667–675.

32. Lloveras J, Peterson PK, Simmons RL, Najarian JS. Mycobacterial infections in renal transplant recipients. *Arch Intern Med* 1982; 142:888–892.

33. Glenn J. Cytomegalovirus infections following renal transplantation. *Rev Infect Dis* 1981; 3:1151–1178.

34. Hecht DN, Syndman DR, Crumpacker CS, Weiner B, Heinz-Lacey B. Gancyclovir for treatment of renal transplant-associated primary cytomegalovirus pneumonia. *J Infect Dis* 1988; 157:187–190.

35. Lautenschlager I, Ahonen J, Eklund B, et al. Hyperimmune globulin therapy of clinical cytomegalovirus infection in renal allograft recipients. *Scand J Infect Dis* 1989; 21:139–143.

36. Balfour HH, Chace BA, Stapleton JT, Simmons RL, Fryd DS. Randomized placebo controlled trial of oral acyclovir for the prevention of cytomegalovirus disease in recipients of renal allografts. *N Engl J Med* 1989; 320:1381–1387.

37. Talseth T, Holdaas H, Albrechtsen D, et al. Increasing incidence of *Pneumocystis carinii* pneumonia in renal transplant patients. *Transplant Proc* 1988; 20:400–401.

38. Weiland D, Ferguson RM, Peterson PK, Snover DC, Simmons RL, Najarian JS. Aspergillosis in 25 renal transplant patients. *Ann Surg* 1983; 198:622–629.

39. Clark JG, Schwartz DA, Flournoy N, Sullivan KM, Crawford SW, Thomas ED. Risk factors for airflow obstruction in recipients of bone marrow transplants. *Ann Intern Med* 1987; 107:648–656.

40. Meyers JD, Flournoy N, Thomas ED. Risk factors for cytomegalovirus infection after human marrow transplantation. *J Infect Dis* 1986; 153:478–488.

41. Stein R, Hummel D, Bohn D, Levison H, Roifman C. Lymphocytic pneumonitis following bone marrow transplantation in severe combined immunodeficiency. *Am Rev Respir Dis* 1991; 143:1406–1408.

42. Meyers JD, Reed EC, Shepp DH, et al. Acyclovir prophylaxis for prevention of cytomegalovirus infection and disease after allogenic marrow transplantation. *N Engl J Med* 1988; 318:70–75.

43. Meyers JD, Flournoy N, Thomas ED. Non-bacterial pneumonia after allogeneic marrow transplantation: A review of ten years' experience. *Rev Infect Dis* 1982; 4:1119–1132.

44. Peterson PK, McGlare C, Ramsay NKC, et al. A prospective study of infectious diseases following bone marrow transplantation: Emergence of aspergillus and cytomegalovirus as the major causes of mortality. *Infect Control* 1983; 4:81–89.

45. Green M, Wald E, Fricker FJ, et al. Infections in pediatric orthotopic heart transplant recipients. *Pediatr Infect Dis J* 1989; 8:87–93.

46. Redd SC, Schuster DM, Quan J, Plikaytis BD, Spika JS, Cohen ML. Legionellosis in cardiac transplant recipients: Results of a nationwide survey. *J Infect Dis* 1988; 158:651–652.

47. Krick JA, Stinson EB, Eqger MJ, Remington JS. Noncardia infections in heart transplant patients. *Ann Intern Med* 1975; 82:18–26.

48. Centers for Disease Control. Unexplained immunodeficiency and opportunistic infections in infants: New York, New Jersey, California. *MMWR* 1982; 31:665–667.

49. Oleske J, Minnefor A, Cooper R, et al. Immune deficiency in children. *JAMA* 1983; 249:2345–2349.

50. Rubinstein A, Sicklick M, Gupta A, et al. Acquired immunodeficiency with reversed T4/T8 ratios in infants born to promiscuous and drug addicted mothers. *JAMA* 1983; 249:2350–2356.

51. Scott AB, Buck BE, Letterman JG, Bloom FL, Parks WP. Acquired immunodeficiency syndrome in infants. *N Engl J Med* 1984; 310:76–81.

52. Gwinn M, Pappaioanou M, George R, et al. Prevalence of HIV infection in childbearing women in the United States: Surveillance using newborn blood samples. *JAMA* 1991; 265:1704–1708.

53. Blanche S, Rouzioux C, Guiherd Moscato ML, et al. A prospective study of infants born to women seropositive for human immunodeficiency virus type 1. *N Engl J Med* 1989; 320:1643–1648.

54. European Collaborative Study. Mother to child transmission of HIV infection. *Lancet* 1988; 2:1039–1042.

55. European Collaborative Study. Children born to women with HIV-1 infection: Natural history and risk of transmission. *Lancet* 1991; 337:253–260.

56. Andiman WA, Simpson J, Olsen B, Dember L, Silva TJ, Miller G. Rate of transmission of human immunodeficiency virus Type I infection from mother to child and short-term outcome of neonatal infection. *Am J Dis Child* 1990; 144:758–766.

57. Classification for human immunodeficiency virus (HIV) infection in children under 13 years of age. *MMWR* 1987; 36:225–230, 235–236.

58. Serologic testing in diagnosing AIDS based on case definition. *MMWR* 1987; 36:1S–14S.

59. Weiss SH, Goedert JJ, Sarngadharan MG, Bodner AJ, Gallo RC, Blattner WA. Screening test for HTLV-III (AIDS agent) antibodies: Specificity, sensitivity and application. *JAMA* 1985; 253:221–225.

60. Marolda J, Pace B, Bonforte RJ, Kotin NM, Rabinowitz J, Kattan M. Pulmonary manifestation of HIV infection in children. *Pediatr Pulmonol* 1991; 10:231–235.

6.1 Oxtoby MJ. Perinatally acquired human immunodeficiency virus infection. *Pediatr Infect Dis J* 1990; 9:609–619.

62. AIDS Surveillance Update. Albany, NY, New York State Department of Health, Dec. 26, 1990.

63. Scott, GB, Hutto C, Makuch RW, et al. Survival in children with prenatally acquired human immunodeficiency virus type 1 infection. *N Engl J Med* 1989; 321:1791–1796.

64. Rubinstein A, Moreski R, Silverman B, et al. Pulmonary disease in children with acquired immune deficiency syndrome and AIDS-related complex. *J Pediatr* 1986; 108:498–503.

65. Marolda J, Pace B, Bonforte RJ, Kotin N, Kattan M. Outcome of mechanical ventilation in children with acquired immunodeficiency syndrome. *Pediatr Pulmonol* 1989; 7:230–234.

66. Bernstein LJ, Bye MR, Rubenstein A. Prognostic factors and life expectancy in children with acquired immunodeficiency syndrome and *Pneumocystis carinii* pneumonia. *Am J Dis Child* 1989; 143:775–778.

67. Bye MR, Bernstein LJ, Shah K, Ellaune M, Rubinstein A. Diagnostic lavage in children with AIDS. *Pediatr Pulmonol* 1987; 3:425–428.

68. National Institutes of Health. Consensus statement on the use of corticosteroids as adjunctive therapy for pneumocystis pneumonia in the acquired immunodeficiency syndrome. *N Engl J Med* 1990; 523:1500–1504.

69. Masur H, Ognibene F, Yarchoan R, et al. CD4 counts as predictors of opportunistic pneumonias in human immunodeficiency virus infection. *Ann Intern Med* 1989; 111:223–231.

70. Denny TN, Niven P, Skuza C, et al. Age related changes of lymphocyte phenotypes in healthy children [Abstract]. *Pediatr Res* 1990; 27:155A.

71. Leibovitz E, Regaud M, Pollack H, et al. *Pneumocystis carinii* pneumonia in infants infected with the human immunodeficiency virus with more than 450 CD4+ lymphocytes per cubic millimeter. *N Engl J Med* 1990; 323:531–533.

72. Kovacs A, Fredrick T, Church J, Eller A, Oxtoby M, Mascola L. CD4 T-Lymphocyte counts and *Pneumocystis carinii* pneumonia in pediatric HIV infection. *JAMA* 1991; 265:1698–1703.

73. Guidelines for prophylaxis against *Pneumocystis carinii* pneumonia for children infected with human immunodeficiency virus. *MMWR* 1991; 40(No. RR2):1–3.

74. Church JA, Isaacs H, Saxon A, Keens TG, Richards W. Lymphocytic interstitial pneumonitis and hypogammaglobulinemia in children. *Am Rev Respir Dis* 1981; 124:491–496.

75. Fackler JC, Nagel JE, Adler WH, Mildvan PT, Ambinder RF. Epstein-Barr virus infection in a child with acquired immunodeficiency syndrome. *Am J Dis Child* 1985; 139:1000–1004.

76. Andiman WA, Eastman R, Martin K, et al. Opportunistic lymphoproliferations associated with Epstein-Barr viral DNA in infants and children with AIDS. *Lancet* 1985; 2:1390–1393.

77. Chayt KJ, Harper ME, Marselle LM, et al. Detection of HTLV-III RNA in lungs of patients with AIDS and pulmonary involvement. *JAMA* 1986; 256:2356–2359.

78. Blanche S, Tardieu M, Duliege A-M, et al. Longitudinal study of 94 symptomatic infants with perinatally acquired human immunodeficiency virus infection: Evidence for a bimodal expression of clinical and biological symptoms. *Am J Dis Child* 1990; 144:1210–1215.

79. Schiff RA, Kabat L, Kamani N. Gallium scanning in lymphoid interstitial pneumonitis of children with AIDS. *J Nucl Med* 1987; 28:1915–1919.

80. Rubinstein A, Bernstein L, Charytan M, et al. Corticosteroids treatment for pulmonary lymphoid hyperplasia in children with acquired immune deficiency syndrome. *Pediatr Pulmonol* 1988; 4:13–17.

81. Welch K, Finkbeiner W, Alpers CE, et al. Autopsy findings in the acquired immune deficiency syndrome. *JAMA* 1984; 252:1152–1159.

82. Pahwa S, Bison K, Lim W, et al. Continuous varicella-zoster infection associated with acyclovir resistance in a child with AIDS. *JAMA* 1988; 290:2879–2882.

83. Murray JF, Mills J. Pulmonary infectious complications of human immunodeficiency virus infection. *Am Rev Respir Dis* 1990; 141:1356–1372.

84. Jacobson MA, Mills J. Serious cytomegalovirus disease in the acquired immunodeficiency syndrome (AIDS): Clinical findings, diagnosis and treatment. *Ann Intern Med* 1988; 108:585–594.

85. Schwyn PA, Hartel D, Lewis VA, et al. A prospective study of the risk of tuberculosis among intravenous drug users with human immunodeficiency virus infection. *N Engl J Med* 1989; 320:545–550.

86. Grant IH, Armstrong D. Fungal infection in AIDS: Cryptococcosis. *Infect Dis Clin North Am* 1988; 2:457–464.

87. Johnson PC, Haml RJ, Sarvosi GA. Clinical review: Progressive disseminated histoplasmosis in the AIDS patient. *Semin Respir Infect* 1989; 4:139–146.

88. Pervez NK, Kleinerman J, Kattan M, et al. Pseudomembranous necrotizing bronchial aspergillosis in a patient with hemophilia and acquired immune deficiency syndrome. *Am Rev Respir Dis* 1985; 131:961–963.

89. Asnis DI, Chitkara RK, Jacobson M, Goldstein JA. Invasive aspergillosis: An unusual manifestation of AIDS. *N Y State J Med* 1988; 88:653–655.

50

Collagen Vascular Diseases in Childhood

DEREK A. UCHIDA, J. ROGER HOLLISTER, and GARY L. LARSEN

The child with a collagen vascular disorder who presents with pulmonary symptoms can pose difficult and challenging questions for the principle care providers. They must discern whether the lung disease is directly a result of the underlying collagen vascular disease or perhaps is due to infection, drug therapy, or an unrelated process. In addition, although many of the pulmonary complications of collagen vascular disorders are well characterized in pediatrics, child care providers must often rely on the experience gained from adult patients for disease processes that are rare in childhood. A complete history and physical examination combined with a careful selection of laboratory tests, pulmonary function tests, and proper imaging techniques (including some of the newly available technologies described in Section II) may provide important clues to the etiology of the lung disease. However, more invasive procedures such as flexible or rigid bronchoscopy, bronchoalveolar lavage, thoracentesis, and/or lung biopsy may be required to elucidate the true diagnosis. The following discussion provides an overview of the pulmonary complications associated with childhood collagen vascular diseases, beginning with the processes most likely to lead to pulmonary symptoms.

SYSTEMIC LUPUS ERYTHEMATOSUS (SLE)

Systemic lupus erythematosus is a disease that can affect multiple organ systems, including the respiratory system. Of the collagen vascular diseases, SLE is the one most likely to involve the respiratory system (1). Virtually every element of the respiratory system can be affected including the pleura and pleural space, interstitium, alveolar space, airways, pulmonary vasculature, and diaphragm.

Pleural disease in SLE can be manifested as pleuritis with or without effusion. "Dry" pleuritis may have no findings on chest radiographs, with the only clinical manifestation being pleuritic pain. Pleural effusions in childhood SLE are relatively common (Fig. 50.1). In one series of childhood onset SLE, 7 of 22 patients were noted to have evidence of pleural effusions on chest radiographs or ultrasonography (2). The typically small volume effusions may be either unilateral or bilateral;

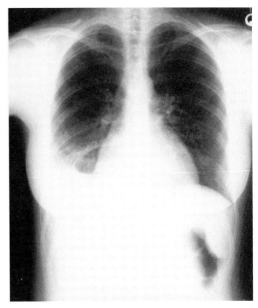

Figure 50.1. Systemic lupus erythematosis: Pleural effusion. PA chest radiograph of a female patient with SLE. A right pleural effusion is present. These findings persisted over a period of several years despite corticosteroid treatment. Heart size is slightly enlarged, which is suggestive but not diagnostic of a pericardial effusion.

large volume effusions have also been described (3). Patients with effusions secondary to SLE often have dyspnea, cough, and fever in addition to pleuritic pain (4), making the differentiation between empyema and lupus effusion difficult without sampling the fluid. The pleural fluid of SLE is typically exudative in nature, and leukocyte counts vary (5). The presence of antinuclear antibodies in the pleural fluid (and absence of findings typical of infection—e.g., negative Gram stain) may be of help in distinguishing lupus effusion from other causes of pleural effusion (4). Once the diagnosis of lupus effusion is made, treatment usually consists of corticosteroid administration (3, 5, 6), which is effective in alleviating the chest discomfort, pain, and fever associated with the pleuritis. Pleural effusions may be slower to respond to corticosteroid treatment, and rarely the effusion may be so large and refractory to medical therapy that pleural sclerosis or pleurectomy is required (5). Nonsteroidal anti-inflammatory medications may be effective in relieving the pleuritic pain of dry pleuritis.

Acute lupus pneumonitis, frequently encountered in adult SLE, occurs in pediatric patients as well (2, 7). Respiratory distress, fever, cough, and a need for oxygen supplementation are the usual clinical manifestations. Chest radiographs often show bilateral hazy alveolar infiltrates in the bases. The diagnosis of lupus pneumonitis is one of exclusion because infection, a common cause of lung infiltrates in SLE, must be ruled out. Corticosteroids are the first-line therapy in uncomplicated lupus pneumonitis. Immunosuppressive agents or plasmapheresis are of benefit in some patients refractory to corticosteroid treatment (3, 5, 6, 8).

Alveolar hemorrhage occurs in children with SLE (9) and can present in much the same way as lupus pneumonitis. In this instance, acute bleeding into the acinar portion of the lung results in ventilation-perfusion mismatching and hypoxia. Even extensive bleeding may result in only minimal or no hemoptysis, making the clinical and radiographic distinction from lupus pneumonitis difficult. An abrupt fall in hemoglobin concentration unexplained by hemolysis and an increase in the diffusing capacity for carbon monoxide (10, 11) may provide clues that bleeding into the acini has occurred.

Chronic interstitial lung disease (ILD) is uncommonly seen in the adult SLE population, with a reported incidence of less than 3%. Reliable estimates for childhood SLE are not available. In one pediatric series, 4 out of 8 children with SLE who presented with pulmonary symptoms had evidence of ILD (7). A postmortem study of the lungs in 26 cases of childhood onset SLE found chronic interstitial pneumonitis in all 26 (severe in 5) (12), suggesting that ILD, though present, does not manifest itself clinically. Rarely, diffuse interstitial infiltrates may be the presenting feature of SLE in a child (13). Clinical signs such as dyspnea (exacerbated by exertion), cough, and chest discomfort need not be present. Chest radiographs may be normal in the early stages of ILD, but in later stages a persistent granular, reticular, or reticulonodular infiltrate may be seen. Other associated findings include pleural changes (with or without small effusions), unilateral elevated diaphragm, reduced lung fields, and plate-like atelectasis, usually in the lower lobes just above the diaphragms (14). Pulmonary function testing may show a restrictive process and an abnormal diffusing capacity (15). Histologically, there can be a wide range of findings from mild fibrous thickening, mononuclear cell infiltrates, intra-alveolar cellularity, and focal type II epithelial hyperplasia to gross honeycombing within the lung (14). The treatment of ILD associated with SLE usually consists of corticosteroids (and immunosuppressive agents in those unresponsive to corticosteroids) (5, 15), although large clinical trials in pediatric patients are lacking. The histologic changes in the lung may predict response to therapy, in that those with active inflammation may respond more favorably than those with fibrosis (5, 15).

Abnormal function of the diaphragm, associated with a loss of lung volume (the so-called "shrinking lung" of SLE) was first recognized in adult patients (16, 17) and may also occur in the pediatric patient (2, 4, 7). Myopathy of the diaphragm, with or without pleural adhesions and atelectasis, is thought to contribute to this process (2, 3). This entity tends not to be disabling or progressive in nature (2, 7, 16).

Perhaps the most insidious pulmonary complication of SLE is the development of pulmonary hypertension (PHTN). Little is known about the prevalence of PHTN in children with SLE. Although severe PHTN is rare in the adult SLE population, a recent report suggests that mild PHTN is common (18). In adults, PHTN is associated with the lupus anticoagulant, rheumatoid factor, and ribonucleoprotein (RNP) positivity (19). The pathogenesis of PHTN in SLE is unknown, although various theories for its origin have been put forth including pulmonary vasculitis, loss of pulmonary capillary units associated with interstitial lung disease, pulmonary arteriole thrombosis, and increased pulmonary vasoreactivity (18). Clinical signs may be as nonspecific as chronic dyspnea or dyspnea on exertion. Chest radiographs may be normal, show an enlarged pulmonary artery, or show cardiomegaly (Fig. 50.2). The development of more sophisticated echocardiographic techniques to assess pulmonary artery pressure has helped the clinician screen for PHTN without the need for cardiac catheterization (18).

The airways are rarely affected in SLE. Airflow obstruction due to small airways disease is uncommon and not often of clinical significance (5). Upper airway obstruction secondary to laryngeal involvement has also been reported (20) but is rare.

Infection as a cause of pulmonary disease in the child with SLE plays a major role in SLE. Various factors including immune dysfunction, the use of immunosuppressive medications, and SLE-induced changes in parenchyma, pleura, or respiratory muscular function contribute to the increased susceptibility to pulmonary infections. The organisms that cause disease in the normal pediatric host as well as opportunistic organisms should be sought in the child with SLE and lung disease. Acute bronchopneumonia was found in over 50% of 21 children who had postmortem assessment of their lungs (21). In that series, a variety of organisms including *Klebsiella*, *Aerobacter*, *Escherichia coli*, cytomegalovirus, and *Pneumocystis carinii* were isolated or identified histologically. Another postmortem study found acute pneumonia present in 20 of 26 childhood SLE cases (mild in 13, moderate in 2, and severe in 5) (12). Nocardiosis, tuberculosis, and Legionnaire disease have been reported in adults (5). Clinically, it may be difficult or impossible to distinguish between an infectious process and a noninfectious complication of SLE. Flexible bronchoscopy with bronchoalveolar lavage may be of benefit in

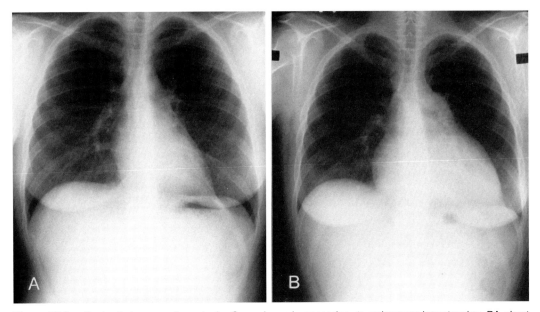

Figure 50.2. *Systemic lupus erythematosis: Cor pulmonale secondary to pulmonary hypertension.* PA chest radiographs of a female patient with SLE; the radiograph shown in *A* was obtained three years prior to *B*. This patient rapidly developed cor pulmonale due to pulmonary hypertension, as reflected by the increase in heart size. Cardiomegaly may also be due to a cardiomyopathy or pericardial effusion. Echocardiography would be helpful in distinguishing between these entities.

isolating an organism from the lungs of immune-deficient hosts. Other more invasive methods of establishing an infectious etiology (e.g., transbronchial lung biopsy, endobronchial brush biopsy, percutaneous needle biopsy, and open lung biopsy) may be necessary (21).

PROGRESSIVE SYSTEMIC SCLEROSIS (PSS)

Progressive systemic sclerosis is a rare disorder that is characterized by thickening, induration, and tightness of the skin (so called "sclerodermatous" changes) and involvement of the visceral organs. Pulmonary manifestations of PSS are common, and along with cardiac abnormalities are the chief causes of childhood deaths from this disease (23). Indeed, histologic evidence of lung involvement can occur without clinical symptoms or radiographic changes (24). The primary pulmonary manifestations of PSS are interstitial lung disease and pulmonary vasculitis.

Interstitial lung disease occurs in 50–90% of adult patients with PSS (25), and is a frequent cause of death in these patients (26). Early in the development of pulmonary fibrosis, the patient may be asymptomatic. The classic symptoms of cough, dyspnea, and breathlessness may not appear until late in the course of illness (26). Bilateral rales (often basilar in distribution) are commonly discovered upon chest auscultation (8, 24, 26). Typical chest radiographic findings in PSS include diffuse reticulonodular interstitial densities with primarily a bibasilar distribution (3, 24). Cystic changes occur late in the course of the disease (24) with rupture of the cysts resulting in pneumothorax (27). Honeycombing is also seen, but only occasionally. As noted above, the most common histologic finding is interstitial fibrosis (5, 28).

Pulmonary hypertension is another common complication of PSS reported in children (29). The appearance of pulmonary hypertension can be sudden and result in rapid development of cor pulmonale with lethal consequences (26). Cor pulmonale may also develop more insidiously with the loss of pulmonary capillary units as pulmonary fibrosis progresses (30). Patients with the CREST syndrome (calcinosis, Raynaud phenomenon, esophageal dysfunction, sclerodactyly, telangiectasias) may be predisposed to developing

pulmonary vascular changes in the absence of interstitial fibrosis (31). Physical examination may reveal a prominent P2 or a widened or fixed split between A2 and P2. An enlarged pulmonary artery with or without cardiomegaly may be noted on chest radiographs. Routine cardiac evaluations are important in the care of children with PSS because the heart may be the primary target of the underlying disease (arrhythmias, myocardial fibrosis, pericardial effusions) or may be secondarily involved because of pulmonary hypertension.

Pulmonary function testing (PFT) is helpful in the evaluation of the patient with PSS (25). The most common findings in the 70% of patients (25) with abnormal PFTs are restrictive lung disease and a decrease in the diffusing capacity for carbon monoxide (DLCO) (5, 32, 33). The early detection of pulmonary function abnormalities does not predict future progression of lung disease in these patients (33, 34).

There is no definitive treatment for PSS-related lung disease at the present time. Glucocorticoids alone, colchicine, para-aminobenzoic acid, and chlorambucil seem not to be of benefit (5, 25, 26). Treatment with D-penicillamine has been associated with an improvement in DLCO, although forced vital capacity (FVC) was unchanged by therapy (35, 36). In preliminary studies, treatment with cyclophosphamide and low-dose prednisone resulted in improvement in dyspnea, DLCO, and FVC in patients with alveolitis detected by bronchoalveolar lavage (BAL) (37). The use of BAL to identify "at risk" patients so that early, aggressive treatment can be instituted during the inflammatory phase and prior to the fibrotic phase may hold some promise (24–26). Treatment options for pulmonary hypertension are even more limited. The minimal reversibility of the pulmonary hypertension may be due to the role of medial and intimal changes in the production of increased pulmonary vascular pressures (25). There are advocates for the use of a calcium channel blocker along with an anti-hypertensive agent that does not selectively decrease renal blood flow (e.g., hydralazine, captopril, or enalapril) (26). Mixed success has been noted with a 6- to 12-week trial of daily prednisone. For now pediatric patients must be treated on the basis of information obtained in adults.

DERMATOMYOSITIS (DM)/ POLYMYOSITIS (PM)

The childhood form of dermatomyositis is a myopathy characterized by chronic inflammation with vasculitis involving the skin and muscles. A diagnosis of DM is made if certain criteria are met including the characteristic skin rash, symmetrical proximal muscle weakness, elevated serum levels of enzymes derived from muscle tissue, muscle biopsy showing histologic features of inflammation or degeneration, and an electromyogram showing changes consistent with the disease (38). It appears that the childhood form of DM differs from the adult disease in that a diffuse, systemic angiopathy is present in children (39). The disease is termed polymyositis if a rash is absent from the constellation of findings. Interstitial lung disease, aspiration-induced pulmonary abnormalities, and ventilatory insufficiency are the pulmonary complications most commonly associated with DM (40, 41).

In the adults with DM, 5–9% of patients will have evidence of interstitial pneumonitis (42, 43). These patients have been placed into three groups according to their pattern of presentation (41, 42). The first is characterized by an acute onset of fever, dyspnea, and dry cough; the second involves the more insidious, gradual progression of dyspnea; the third is the asymptomatic group with evidence of lung involvement on chest radiograph or pulmonary function testing. The few case reports of biopsy-proven interstitial lung disease in childhood DM have been either acute and rapidly progressive or insidious in presentation (44, 45). Chest radiographs may show diffuse interstitial infiltrates consistent with pulmonary fibrosis. Of note, pneumothoraces have been described as part of childhood dermatomyositis (44, 45). Pulmonary function studies may show abnormalities consistent with a restrictive process (i.e., decreased FVC, TLC, RV, and DLCO). Upon histologic examination of the lungs, fibrosis of varying degrees as well as interstitial accumulations of mononuclear cells, polymorphonuclear leukocytes, and plasma cells are described (3, 46). In adults with PM and DM, three groups are identified using major histologic patterns: (a) bronchiolitis obliterans organizing pneumonia (BOOP), (b) usual interstitial pneumonia (UIP), and (c) diffuse alveolar damage (DAD).

Prognosis is best for patients with BOOP; patients with UIP do somewhat more poorly, and those with DAD have an extremely poor outlook (47). Whether these findings may extend to the pediatric population is presently unclear. Lung biopsy results were presented in two of the pediatric case reports previously mentioned. Findings included thickening of the alveolar septa, pleural fibrosis, irregular patterns of aeration, and focal bronchiolitis obliterans (44, 45).

Approximately one-half of adult patients with interstitial lung disease associated with DM/PM respond favorably to corticosteroid therapy (5). Although it appears that responders are generally those with active inflammatory disease on lung biopsy rather than those having more mature ILD with fibrosis (5, 41), this distinction is not necessarily clear (47). Drawing on the experience in treating adults, a trial of corticosteroids seems to be an appropriate first step in therapy when ILD complicates childhood DM/PM (8, 21). Early intervention may be a way of forestalling the progression from inflammation to irreversible fibrosis.

Palatorespiratory inefficiency is a major cause of death in children with DM (48); caregivers must be vigilant for these complications. Pharyngeal dysfunction caused by weakness of the muscles of the soft palate, pharynx, and esophagus can lead to aspiration (41). Other abnormalities including impaired cough mechanisms, esophageal lesions, and inability to use airway protective movements such as turning and bending when vomiting or coughing may contribute to the tendency to aspirate food and secretions (3, 41). Weakness of the respiratory muscles may also complicate DM/PM and may progress to the point of respiratory failure (49). Chest radiographs in patients with respiratory muscle weakness may reveal small lung volumes, elevated diaphragms, and basilar plate-like densities, probably representing atelectasis (50). Maximal inspiratory and expiratory pressures are helpful in following the degree of ventilatory insufficiency and can be measured at the bedside; VC measurements may also be of benefit (41). As in other neuromuscular diseases, care must be taken to provide adequate pulmonary toilet and, if necessary, assist ventilation.

JUVENILE RHEUMATOID ARTHRITIS (JRA)

Clinically apparent pulmonary involvement in patients with JRA is uncommon. This is unlike the situation with rheumatoid arthritis in adults, in whom pulmonary manifestations are frequently encountered. In the largest series in the literature consisting of 191 patients with JRA, eight children had symptoms referable to the lungs (52). Seventy-five percent of those with JRA and lung involvement had the febrile, systemic form of the disease. Common symptoms included cough, dyspnea, tachypnea, and chest pain. The patients with chest pain all had pleural effusions, the most common pulmonary manifestation in this series. Pericarditis was commonly found in those with pleural effusions. Interstitial parenchymal disease occurs in JRA and is associated with a decreased vital capacity in those tested (52). Other pulmonary abnormalities that are rarely seen include restrictive lung disease secondary to chest wall deformity (21), pulmonary hemosiderosis (52, 53), and bronchiolitis obliterans (Fig. 50.3).

Although clinically apparent lung disease may be rare in JRA, a relatively high incidence of pulmonary function abnormalities has been

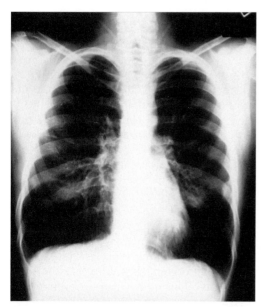

Figure 50.3. Juvenile rheumatoid arthritis: Bronchiolitis obliterans. AP chest radiograph of a female with JRA. Hyper-inflation is present, consistent with bronchiolitis obliterans. This diagnosis was confirmed with open lung biopsy.

reported (54). The abnormalities included reduced lung volumes and airflows, decreased DLCO, and oxygen desaturation during exercise most likely due to ventilation/perfusion mismatching. Longitudinal studies of pulmonary function in children with JRA have not been performed.

JUVENILE ANKYLOSING SPONDYLITIS (JAS)

Ankylosing spondylitis (AS) is an inflammatory disease that involves the sacroiliac joints and spine. Pulmonary involvement in children with JAS has not been reported. In adults with AS, one review of 2080 patients found the incidence of pleuropulmonary involvement to be only 1.3%, and a high percentage of those affected were either smokers or ex-smokers (55). Upper lobe fibrobullous disease and pulmonary restriction caused by limitation of chest wall expansion are the primary pulmonary abnormalities found in adults with AS. The fibrobullous involvement of the upper lobes has been reported to be asymptomatic, unless a secondary infection occurs; pulmonary aspergilloma was a major cause of morbidity in patients with pre-existing bullae (55). The chest wall restriction is due to inflammation or ankylosis of sternocostal and costovertebral joints and adjacent synchondroses in affected patients (56). A study of pulmonary function in 32 patients with AS and without symptoms of lung disease and normal chest radiographs found reduced VC and TLC with normal FRC and RV (56). Maximal elastic recoil pressure, static compliance, and diffusion capacity were normal, suggesting that pulmonary fibrosis was not a major contributor to the restrictive pattern of lung function observed in this study (56). Increased diaphragmatic excursion compensates for the chest wall restriction in many patients, thus minimizing the clinical symptoms (5).

MIXED CONNECTIVE TISSUE DISEASE (MCTD)

In 1972, a clinical syndrome with some features each of SLE, dermatomyositis-polymyositis, and scleroderma was described. This entity, termed "mixed connective tissue disease," was associated with a circulating hemagglutinating antibody specific for the ribonucleoprotein component of extractable nuclear antigen (57). Pulmonary disease is a common finding in children and adults with MCTD. Singsen et al. reported that 6 of 14 children with MCTD had pulmonary involvement that included pulmonary hypertension, pleural effusions, and restrictive lung disease manifested by pulmonary function abnormalities (58). The incidence of pulmonary involvement in adults with MCTD ranges from 25% (59) to 80% (60). Pleuropulmonary involvement in adults includes the childhood manifestations of MCTD plus massive pulmonary hemorrhage (61) and aspiration pneumonitis (59). Pulmonary disease including pulmonary hypertension was the most serious clinical problem noted in a prospective study of 34 adult patients with MCTD (60). Pulmonary involvement is common but often clinically inapparent until relatively far advanced, and then is not always responsive to corticosteroids or immunosuppressive agents (60). The pulmonary disease can be severe and rapidly progressive, with either disabling interstitial lung disease (Fig. 50.4) or severe pulmonary hypertension (62). Although corticosteroid therapy has been ineffective, early use of cytotoxic agents may be of benefit (62).

SJÖGREN SYNDROME (SS)

Sjögren syndrome is a chronic autoimmune disease characterized by lymphocytic inflammation and infiltration of exocrine glandular tissue. This leads to the classic symptoms of the disease: keratoconjunctivitis sicca (dry eyes) and xerostomia (dry mouth). Although SS may occur as a solitary disease process (primary SS), there is frequently an association with other connective tissue diseases including rheumatoid arthritis, SLE, PSS, and DM/PM. Although SS has been documented to occur in the pediatric population (63), information on pulmonary involvement in children with SS is scant. The incidence of pulmonary manifestations in adults with SS was reported to be 9% in one series of 343 patients (63). Lung disease can manifest early in primary SS, and progression may occur over a relatively short period (64). The pulmonary abnormalities associated with primary SS include pleurisy, pleural effusion, discoid atelectasis, pulmonary fibrosis, lymphocytic interstitial pneumonitis, and an increased incidence of respiratory infections (3, 65). "Xerotrachea," or a dryness of the larynx, trachea, and

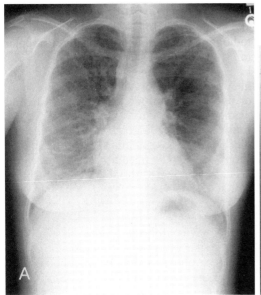
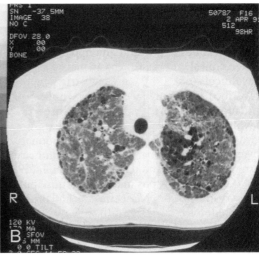

Figure 50.4. Mixed connective tissue disease: Interstitial and cystic lung disease. *A,* PA chest radiograph of a female patient with MCTD. Patchy groundglass and reticulonodular infiltrates are present throughout both lungs. The pulmonary vessels are prominent, suggesting pulmonary hypertension. *B,* High-resolution CT scan of this patient's chest. Extensive peripheral and intraparenchymal cystic changes as well as patchy interlobular septal thickening are present, consistent with pulmonary fibrosis. Diffuse groundglass opacities are also present, possibly representing ongoing alveolitis.

of deaths due to alveolar hemorrhage (87, 88). For pulmonary complications associated with other vasculitides, the reader is referred to review articles on this subject (71, 89).

ACUTE RHEUMATIC FEVER (ARF) AND RHEUMATIC PNEUMONIA

Rheumatic pneumonia is a well described complication of acute rheumatic fever and may be the initial manifestation of ARF, may occur during the polycyclic course of rheumatic fever, or may be subclinical (90). Rheumatic pneumonia should be suspected in a patient with rheumatic fever who has marked diffuse and extensive pulmonary consolidation, tachypnea, and lack of a response to antibiotic and/or steroid therapy (91). Diagnosis can be difficult since many other disease processes of the lungs and heart can mimic the symptoms of rheumatic pneumonia. Typical histologic findings include alveolar hemorrhage, fibrinous edema, interstitial inflammatory exudates, and globular tufts of intra-alveolar fibrous tissue (Masson bodies). Septal necrosis may also be seen, but is almost always associated with bronchopneumonia. Unfortunately, these findings are not pathognomonic for rheumatic pneumonia (92). Prognosis is generally guarded (91), although the disease may also be mild (93). Data on drug therapy for rheumatic pneumonia is very scant. Case reports in the literature have described patients who have recovered with (94) or without (93) the use of corticosteroids. The vast majority of reported cases have been unresponsive to steroids, and fatalities have been common. One report suggested the use of immunosuppressive agents in biopsy-proven rheumatic pneumonia, but no data exist on the efficacy of such treatment (95).

PULMONARY COMPLICATIONS SECONDARY TO DRUG THERAPY OF COLLAGEN VASCULAR DISEASES

When one is faced with a child being treated for a collagen vascular disease who develops pulmonary symptoms, the possibility of drug-induced lung disease should be entertained. Because this topic is too large for an extensive review, the reader is directed to two articles for detailed discussions on this topic (96, 97). What follows is a brief overview of the lung complications seen with drugs more commonly used in the treatment of pediatric collagen vascular diseases.

Penicillamine

Penicillamine is used in the treatment of JRA and scleroderma. There have been reports of hypersensitivity pneumonitis, bronchiolitis obliterans, alveolar and/or interstitial fibrosis, and pulmonary hemorrhage in association with penicillamine use (98, 99). Bronchiolitis obliterans due to penicillamine is well documented in patients with rheumatoid arthritis, but this complication is rare in scleroderma patients (5). A pulmonary-renal syndrome much like Goodpasture syndrome has also been described after treatment with penicillamine (100).

Gold

Hypersensitivity pneumonitis is the most common pulmonary complication of gold therapy (101). As with penicillamine, bronchiolitis obliterans has also been reported (102).

Methotrexate

Pneumonitis with symptoms of cough, shortness of breath, fever, and rales has been described with methotrexate use (103). Pulmonary fibrosis can also be a complication of methotrexate therapy (96, 97). There is a report of a teenage girl who died of noncardiogenic pulmonary edema after an oral dose of methotrexate for acute lymphocytic leukemia (104). A previous dose of intrathecal methotrexate is believed to have caused sensitization.

Salicylates

Salicylates can cause bronchoconstriction in sensitive individuals. The classic triad of rhinitis with nasal polyps, asthma, and aspirin sensitivity (105) has been modified by some to include sinusitis and to withdraw the absolute requirement for nasal polyps (106). The asthma is chronic and severe in greater than 60% of sensitive individuals (106). Because individuals sensitive to aspirin can be susceptible to having bronchospasm with other nonsteroidal anti-inflammatory medications, care must be taken that all use of these medications is avoided (including eyedrops) (107).

Noncardiogenic pulmonary edema has been described with salicylate ingestion; most cases are associated with intentional or nonintentional overdoses (97). The pathogenesis is unknown, although increased permeability of the pulmonary vascular bed has been implicated (108).

Nonsteroidal Anti-Inflammatory Drugs (NSAIDs)

Bronchoconstriction, noncardiogenic pulmonary edema, and hypersensitivity pneumonitis have been described in association with NSAID use (96, 97). A systemic reaction to ibuprofen consisting of aseptic meningitis, rash, abdominal pain, and pulmonary infiltrates has also been reported in patients with SLE and MCTD (109).

REFERENCES

1. Turner-Stokes L, Turner-Warwick M. Intrathoracic manifestations of SLE. *Clin Rheum Dis* 1982; 8:229–242.
2. Delgado EA, Malleson PN, Pirie GE, Petty RE. The pulmonary manifestations of childhood onset systemic lupus erythematosus. *Semin Arth Rheum* 1990; 19:285–293.
3. Hunninghake GW, Fauci AS. Pulmonary involvement in the collagen vascular diseases. *Am Rev Respir Dis* 1979; 119:471–503.
4. Good JT, King TE, Antony VB, Sahn SA. Lupus pleuritis: Clinical factors and pleural fluid characteristics with special reference to pleural fluid antinuclear antibodies. *Chest* 1983; 84:714–718.
5. Wiedeman HP, Matthay RA. Pulmonary manifestations of the collagen vascular diseases. *Clin Chest Med* 1989; 10:677–722.
6. Boulware DW, Weissman DN, Doll NJ. Pulmonary manifestations of the rheumatic diseases. *Clin Rev Allergy* 1985; 3:249–267.
7. De Jongste JC, Neijens HJ, Duiverman EJ, Bogaard JM, Kerrebijn KF. Respiratory tract disease in systemic lupus erythematosus. *Arch Dis Child* 1986; 61:478–483.
8. Hepburn B. Interstitial lung disease in childhood rheumatic disorders. In Laraya-Cuasay LR, Hughs WT, eds. *Interstitial lung diseases in children*, vol III. Boca Raton, FL, CRC Press, 1988, pp 105–119.
9. Miller RW, Salcedo JR, Fink RJ, Murphy TM, Magilavy DB. Pulmonary hemorrhage in pediatric patients with systemic lupus erythematosus. *J Pediatr* 1986; 108:576–579.
10. Ewan PW, Jones HA, Rhodes CG, Hughes JM. Detection of intrapulmonary hemorrhage with carbon monoxide uptake. Application in Goodpasture's syndrome. *N Engl J Med* 1976; 295:1391–1396.
11. Greening AP, Hughs JMB. Serial estimations of carbon monoxide diffusing capacity in intrapulmonary haemorrhage. *Clin Sci* 1981; 60:507–512.
12. Nadorra RL, Landing BH. Pulmonary lesions in childhood onset systemic lupus erythematosis: Analysis of 26 cases, and summary of the literature. *Pediatr Pathol* 1987; 7:1–18.

13. Pohlgeers AP, Eid NS, Schikler KN, Shearer LT. Systemic lupus erythematosus: Pulmonary presentation in childhood. *South Med J* 1990; 83:712–714.
14. Eisenberg H, Dubois EL, Sherwin RP, Balchum OJ. Diffuse interstitial lung disease in systemic lupus erythematosis. *Ann Intern Med* 1973; 37–45.
15. Eisenberg H. The interstitial lung diseases associated with the collagen vascular disorders. *Clin Chest Med* 1982; 3:565–578.
16. Gibson GJ, Edminds JP, Hughs GRV. Diaphragm function and lung involvement in systemic lupus erythematosis. *Am J Med* 1977; 63:926–932.
17. Hoffbrand BI, Beck ER. "Unexplained" dyspnea and shrinking lungs in systemic lupus erythematosis. *Br Med J* 1965; 1:1273–1277.
18. Simonson JS, Schiller NB, Petri M, Hellman DB. Pulmonary hypertension in systemic lupus erythematosus. *J Rheumatol* 1989; 16:918–925.
19. Asherson RA, Oakley CM. Pulmonary hypertension and systemic lupus erythematosus. *J Rheumatol* 1986; 13:1–5.
20. Smith GA, Ward PH. Laryngeal involvement in systemic lupus erythematosis. *Trans Am Acad Ophthalmol Otolaryngol* 1977; 84:124–128.
21. Singsen BH, Platzker ACG. Pulmonary involvement in the rheumatic disorders of childhood. In Chernick V, Kendig EL, eds. *Disorders of the respiratory tract in children*. Philadelphia, WB Saunders, 1990, pp 890–916.
22. Wagener JS. Fatality following fiberoptic bronchoscopy in a two-year old child. *Pediatr Pulmonol* 1987; 3:197–199.
23. Cassidy JT, Petty RE. *Textbook of pediatric rheumatology*. New York, Edinburgh, London, Melbourne, Churchill Livingstone, 1990.
24. McCarthy DS, Baragar FD, Dhingra S, et al. The lungs in systemic sclerosis (scleroderma): A review and new information. *Semin Arth Rheum* 1988; 17:271–283.
25. Silver RM, Miller KS. Lung involvement in systemic sclerosis. *Rheum Dis Clin North Am* 1990; 16:199–216.
26. Leroy EC, Lomeo R. The spectrum of scleroderma (II). *Hosp Pract* 1989; 24:65–84.
27. Israel MS, Harley BJS. Spontaneous pneumothorax in scleroderma. *Thorax* 1956; 11:113–118.
28. D'Angelo WA, Fries JF, Masi AT, Shulman LE. Pathologic observations in systemic sclerosis (scleroderma). A study of fifty-eight autopsy cases and fifty-eight matched controls. *Am J Med* 1969; 46:428–440.
29. Bulkley BH, Ridolfi RL, Salyer WR, Hutchins GM. Myocardial lesions of progressive systemic sclerosis. A cause of cardiac dysfunction. *Circulation* 1976; 53:483–490.
30. Trell E, Lindstrom C. Pulmonary hypertension in systemic sclerosis. *Ann Rheum Dis* 1971; 30:390–400.
31. Ungerer RG, Tashkin DP, Furst D, et al. Prevalence and clinical correlates of pulmonary arterial hypertension in progressive systemic sclerosis. *Am J Med* 1983; 75:65–74.
32. Steen VD, Owens GR, Fino GJ, Rodnan GP, Medsger TAJ. Pulmonary involvement in systemic sclerosis (scleroderma). *Arthritis Rheum* 1985; 28:759–767.

33. Bagg LR, Hughes DT. Serial pulmonary function tests in progressive systemic sclerosis. *Thorax* 1979; 34:224–228.

34. Greenwald GI, Tashkin DP, Gong H. Longitudinal changes in lung function and respiratory symptoms in progressive systemic sclerosis. Prospective study. *Am J Med* 1987; 83:83–92.

35. Steen VD, Owens GR, Redmond C, et al. The effect of D-penicillamine on pulmonary findings in systemic sclerosis. *Arthritis Rheum* 1985; 28:882–888.

36. de Clerck LS, Dequeker J, Francx L, Demedts M. D–Penicillamine therapy and interstitial lung disease in scleroderma. A long-term follow up study. *Arthritis Rheum* 1987; 3:643–650.

37. Silver RM, Miller KS, Kinsella MB, Smith EA, Schabel SI. Evaluation and management of scleroderma lung disease using bronchoalveolar lavage. *Am J Med* 1990; 88:470–476.

38. Pachman LM. Juvenile dermatomyositis. *Pediatr Clin North Am* 1986; 33:1097–1117.

39. Banker BO, Victor M. Dermatomyositis (systemic angiopathy) of childhood. *Medicine* 1966; 45:261–289.

40. Hepper NG, Ferguson RH, Howard FM. Three types of pulmonary involvement in polymyositis. *Med Clin North Am* 1964; 48:1031–1042.

41. Dickey BF, Myers AR. Pulmonary disease in polymyositis/dermatomyositis. *Semin Arthritis Rheum* 1984; 14:60–76.

42. Frazier RA, Miller RD. Interstitial pneumonitis in association with polymyositis and dermatomyositis. *Chest* 1974; 65:403–408.

43. Salmeron G, Greenberg SD, Lidsky MD. Polymyositis and diffuse interstitial lung disease: A review of the pulmonary histopathologic findings. *Arch Intern Med* 1981; 141:1005–1010.

44. Park S, Nyhan WL. Fatal pulmonary involvement in dermatomyositis. *Am J Dis Child* 1975; 129:723–726.

45. Singsen BH, Tedford JC, Platzker ACG, Hanson V. Spontaneous pneumothorax: A complication of juvenile dermatomyositis. *J Pediatr* 1978; 92:771–774.

46. Duncan PE, Griffin JP, Garcia A, Kaplan SB. Fibrosing alveolitis in polymyositis: A review of histologically confirmed cases. *Am J Med* 1974; 57:621–626.

47. Tazelaar HD, Viggiano RW, Pickersgill J, Colby TV. Interstitial lung disease in polymyositis and dermatomyositis. Clinical features and prognosis as correlated with histologic findings. *Am Rev Respir Dis* 1990; 141:727–733.

48. Bitnum S, Daeschner CWJ, Travis LB, Dodge WF, Hopps HC. Dermatomyositis. *J Pediatr* 1964; 64:101–131.

49. DeVere R, Bradley WG. Polymyositis: Its presentation, morbidity and mortality. *Brain* 1975; 98:637–666.

50. Fraser RG, Paré JAP, Paré PD, Fraser RS, Genereux GP. *Diagnosis of diseases of the chest*, vol 2, 3rd ed. Philadelphia, WB Saunders, 1989.

51. Samuels MP, Warner JO. Pulmonary alveolar lipoproteinosis complicating juvenile dermatomyositis. *Thorax* 1988; 43:939–940.

52. Athreya BH, Doughty RA, Bookspan M, Schumacher HR, Sewell EM, Chatten J. Pulmonary

53. Smith BS. Idiopathic pulmonary haemosiderosis and rheumatoid arthritis. *Br Med J* 1966; 1:1403–1404.

54. Wagener JS, Taussig LM, DeBenedetti C, Lemen RJ, Loughlin GM. Pulmonary function in juvenile rheumatoid arthritis. *J Pediatr* 1981; 99:108–110.

55. Rosenow EC, Strimlan CV, Muhm JR, Ferguson RH. Pleuropulmonary manifestations of ankylosing spondylitis. *Mayo Clin Proc* 1977; 52:641–649.

56. Feltelius N, Hedenström H, Hillerdal G, Hällgren R. Pulmonary involvement in ankylosing spondylitis. *Ann Rheum Dis* 1986; 45:736–40.

57. Sharp GC, Irvin WS, Tan EM, Gould RG, Holman HR. Mixed connective tissue disease: An apparently distinct rheumatic disease syndrome associated with a specific antibody to an extractable nuclear antigen (ENA). *Am J Med* 1972; 52:148–159.

58. Singsen BH, Bernstein BH, Kornreich HK, King KK, Hanson V, Tan EM. Mixed connective tissue disease in childhood. *J Pediatr* 1977; 90:893–900.

59. Prakesh UBS, Luthra HS, Divertie MB. Intrathoracic manifestations of mixed connective tissue disease. *Mayo Clin Proc* 1985; 60:813–821.

60. Sullivan WD, Hurst DJ, Harmon CE, et al. A prospective evaluation emphasizing pulmonary involvement in patients with mixed connective tissue disease. *Medicine* 1984; 63:92–107.

61. Sanchez-Guerrero J, Cesarman G, Alarcón-Segovia D. Massive pulmonary hemorrhage in mixed connective tissue disease. *J Rheumatol* 1989; 16:1132–1134.

62. Wiener–Kronish JP, Solinger AM, Warnock ML, Churg A, Ordonez N, Golden JA. Severe pulmonary involvement in mixed connective tissue disease. *Am Rev Respir Dis* 1981; 124:499–503.

63. Athreya BH, Norman ME, Myers AR, South MA. Sjögren's syndrome in children. *Pediatrics* 1977; 59:931–938.

64. Kelly C, Gardiner P, Pal B, Griffiths I. Lung function in primary Sjögrens syndrome: A cross sectional and longitudinal study. *Thorax* 1991; 46:180–183.

65. Strimlan CV, Rosenow EC, Divertie MD, et al. Pulmonary manifestations of Sjögren's syndrome. *Chest* 1976; 70:354–361.

66. Hatron PY, Wallaert B, Gosset D, et al. Subclinical lung inflammation in primary Sjögrens syndrome. Relationship beween bronchoalveolar lavage cellular analysis findings and characteristics of the disease. *Arthritis Rheum* 1987; 30:1226–1231.

67. Anderson LG, Talal N. The spectrum of benign to malignant lymphoproliferation in Sjögren's syndrome. *Clin Exp Immunol* 1972; 10:199–221.

68. Ammann AJ, Johnson A, Fyfe GA, Leonards R, Wara DW, Cowan M. Behçet syndrome. *J Pediatr* 1985; 107:41–43.

69. Cadman EC, Lundberg WB, Mitchell MS. Pulmonary manifestations in Behçet's syndrome. *Arch Intern Med* 1976; 136:944–947.

70. Raz I, Okon E, Chajek–Shaul T. Pulmonary manifestations in Behçet's syndrome. *Chest* 1989; 95:585–589.

71. Leavitt RY, Fauci AS. Pulmonary vasculitis. *Am Rev Respir Dis* 1986; 134:149–166.

manifestations of juvenile rheumatoid arthritis. A report of eight cases and review. *Clin Chest Med* 1980; 1:361–374.

72. McCombs RP. Diseases due to immunologic reactions in the lung (two parts). *N Engl J Med* 1972; 286:1186–1194, 1245–1252.

73. Hunder GG, Arend WP, Bloch DA, et al. The American College of Rheumatology 1990 criteria for the classification of vasculitis. *Arthritis Rheum* 1990; 33:1065–1067.

74. Wolff SM, Fauci AS, Horn RG, Dale DC. Wegener's granulomatosis. *Ann Intern Med* 1974; 81:513–525.

75. Hall SL, Miller LC, Duggan E, Mauer SM, Beatty EC, Hellerstein S. Wegener granulomatosis in pediatric patients. *J Pediatr* 1985; 106:739–744.

76. Landman S, Burgener F. Pulmonary manifestations in Wegener's granulomatosis. *Am J Roentgenol Radium Ther Nucl Med* 1974; 122:750–757.

77. Cohen Tervaert JW, van der Woude FJ, Fauci AS, et al. Association between active Wegener's granulomatosis and anticytoplasmic antibodies. *Arch Intern Med* 1989; 149:2461–2464.

78. Specks U, Wheatley CL, McDonald TJ, Rohrbach MS, DeRemee RA. Anticytoplasmic antibodies in the diagnosis and follow–up of Wegener's granulomatosis. *Mayo Clin Proc* 1989; 64:28–36.

79. Weiss MA, Crissman JD. Segmental necrotizing glomerulonephritis: Diagnostic, prognostic, and therapeutic significance. *Am J Kidney Dis* 1985; 6:199–211.

80. Fauci AS, Haynes B, Katz P, Wolff S. Wegener's granulomatosis: Prospective clinical and therapeutic experience with 85 patients for 21 years. *Ann Intern Med* 1983; 98:76–85.

81. Lanham JC, Elkon KB, Pusey CD, Hughes GR. Systemic vasculitis with asthma and eosinophilia: A clinical approach to Churg-Strauss syndrome. *Medicine* 1984; 63:65–81.

82. Buschman DL, Waldron JA, King TE. Churg-Strauss pulmonary vasculitis. High-resolution computed tomography scanning and pathologic findings. *Am Rev Respir Dis* 1990; 142:458–461.

83. Koss MN, Antonovych T, Hochholzer L. Allergic granulomatosis (Churg-Strauss syndrome): Pulmonary and renal morphologic findings. *Am J Surg Pathol* 1981; 5:21–28.

84. Meade III RH, Brandt L. Manifestations of Kawasaki disease in New England outbreak of 1980. *J Pediatr* 1982; 100:558–562.

85. Byard RW, Edmonds JF, Silverman E, Silver MM. Respiratory distress and fever in a 2-month-old child. *J Pediatr* 1991; 118:306–313.

86. Umezawa T, Saji T, Matsuo N, Odagiri K. Chest x-ray findings in the acute phase of Kawasaki disease. *Pediatr Radiol* 1989; 20:48–51.

87. Weiss VF, Naidu S. Fatal pulmonary hemorrhage in Henoch-Schonlein purpura. *Cutis* 1979; 23:687–688.

88. Kathuria S, Cheifec G. Fatal pulmonary Henoch-Schonlein syndrome. *Chest* 1982; 82:654–656.

89. Chandler DB, Fulmer JD. Pulmonary vasculitis. *Lung* 1985; 163:257–273.

90. Griffith GC, Phillips AW, Asher C. Pneumonitis occuring in rheumatic fever. *Am J Med Sci* 1946; 212:22.

91. Massumi RA, Legier JR. Rheumatic pneumonitis. *Circulation* 1972; 33:417–427.

92. Grunow WA, Esterly JR. Rheumatic pneumonitis. *Chest* 1972; 61:298–301.

93. Yamamoto LG, Seto DSY, Reddy V. Pneumonia associated with acute rheumatic fever. *Clin Pediatr* 1987; 26:198–200.

94. Raz I, Fisher J, Israeli A, Gottehrer N, Chisin R, Kleinman Y. An unusual case of rheumatic pneumonia. *Arch Intern Med* 1985; 145:1130–1131.

95. Serlin SP, Rimsza ME, Gay JH. Rheumatic pneumonia: The need for a new approach. *Pediatrics* 1975; 56:1075–1078.

96. Cannon GW. Pulmonary complications of antirheumatic drug therapy. *Semin Arthritis Rheum* 1990; 19:353–364.

97. Zitnik RJ, Cooper Jr. JAD. Pulmonary disease due to antirheumatic agents. *Clin Chest Med* 1990; 11:139–150.

98. Stein HB, Patterson AC, Offer RC, Atkins CJ, Teufel A, Robinson HS. Adverse effects of D-penicillamine in rheumatoid arthritis. *Ann Intern Med* 1980; 92:24–29.

99. Howard-Lock HE, Lock CJL, Meura A, et al. D-penicillamine: Chemistry and clinical use in rheumatic disease. *Semin Arthritis Rheum* 1986; 15:261–281.

100. Peces R, Riera JR, Arboleya LR, et al. Goodpasture's syndrome in a patient receiving penicillamine and carbimazole. *Nephron* 1987; 45:316–320.

101. Evans RB, Ettensohn DB, Fawaz-Estrup F, et al. Gold lung: Recent developments in pathogenesis, diagnosis, and therapy. *Semin Arthritis Rheum* 1987; 16:196–205.

102. O'Duffy JD, Luthra HS, Unni KK, Hyatt RE. Bronchiolitis in a rheumatoid arthritis patient receiving auranofin. *Arthritis Rheum* 1986; 29:556–559.

103. Carson CW, Cannon GW, Egger MJ, Ward JR, Clegg DO. Pulmonary disease during the treatment of rheumatoid arthritis with low dose pulse methotrexate. *Semin Arthritis Rheum* 1987; 16:186–195.

104. Lascari AD, Strano AJ, Johnson WW, Collins JG. Methotrexate-induced sudden fatal pulmonary reaction. *Cancer* 1977; 1393–1397.

105. Samter M, Beers Jr. RF. Intolerance to aspirin. *Ann Intern Med* 1968; 68:975–983.

106. Stevenson DD, Simon RA. Aspirin sensitivity: Respiratory and cutaneous manifestations. In Middleton E Jr, Reed CE, Ellis EF, Adkinson NF Jr, Yunginger JW, eds. *Allergy. Principles and practice.* St. Louis, CV Mosby, 1988, pp 1537–1554.

107. Sheehan GJ, Kutzner MR, Chin WD. Acute asthma attack due to opthalmic indomethacin. *Ann Intern Med* 1989; 3:337–338.

108. Hormaechea E, Carlson RW, Rogoue H, et al. Hypovolemia, pulmonary edema and protein changes in severe salicylate poisoning. *Am J Med* 1979; 66:1046–1050.

109. Ruppert GB, Barth WF. Ibuprofen hypersensitivity in systemic lupus erythematosus. *South Med J* 1981; 74:241–243.

51

Indoor Pollution

GERALD M. LOUGHLIN

GENERAL PRINCIPLES

The history of indoor pollution dates back to the days of the caveman and the discovery of fire. Over the centuries, advances in the technology used to prepare our meals and heat our homes have reduced the indoor pollution burden substantially for most homes in western society (1). Despite these advances, the effort to make our homes more energy-efficient in order to reduce the costs of heating and cooling has resulted in a dramatic reduction in the exchange rate of the air within our homes with the outside air (1). In the past, the average exchange rate was approximately 1 exchange/hour. Many modern energy efficient homes have dropped this rate to less than 0.5 exchanges/hour (2). The net result of this efficiency is that whatever pollutant is produced in the indoor environment is likely to be around for quite some time (2). Although we may have cleaned up the smoke, we have added other and perhaps more toxic substances to the indoor environment and we have eliminated the pathway by which these substances can escape. The following relationship can be used to determine the concentration of a pollutant in the environment (3):

$$C_{(room)} = C_{(outside)} + \frac{G - E}{Q}$$

C = concentration of the pollutant
G = rate of generation of the pollutant
E = rate of elimination through reaction
Q = rate of air exchange with outside

This equation indicates that the level of indoor pollution can be effected by a variety of factors in addition to simple rate of production within a closed environment.

Another aspect of studying the effects of pollution lies in determining what constitutes an adverse health effect (5). A committee of the American Thoracic Society defined an adverse health effect as a "medically significant physiologic or pathologic change evidence by one or more of the following: (1) interference with the normal activity of the affected person or persons, (2) episodic respiratory illness, (3) incapacitating illness, (4) permanent respiratory injury, and/or (5) progressive respiratory dysfunction." Although no one would argue that increased asthma symptoms and increased otitis media are adverse health affects, eye irritation and chronic nasal congestion, symptoms often found in children exposed to cigarette smoke, are more difficult to label as a significant adverse health effect. In addition, in children, the adverse effect may not be detected for quite some time after the exposure, such as might occur with the increased risk of lung cancer seen in nonsmoking spouses of smokers.

Children are particularly vulnerable to the effects of indoor pollution since they, especially the very young, are in essence captives of the indoor environment. The average housewife (mother and child) spends approximately 20 hours a day indoors (4). Furthermore, the immaturity of the child's lung defense systems and the fact that their lungs are involved in a vigorous process of growth and development adds to their vulnerability. Their increased minute ventilation relative to their size ensures that they will experience a significant exposure to whatever pollutes the ambient air.

SOURCES AND TYPES OF INDOOR POLLUTANTS

The nature and adverse health effects of indoor air pollution have been the subject of extensive review, and the reader is referred to these reviews for detailed discussion of the topic (2, 5). This chapter will focus on pollutants that are encountered commonly in dealing with children with lung disease. Table 51.1 summarizes some of the sources and types of indoor pollutants found in the home. Each of these has been implicated in producing respiratory symptoms (Table 51.2). This chapter will also review ways to clean up the indoor environment with particular emphasis on the commercially available home air filtration systems, since physicians are frequently asked by families if they should purchase one of these systems for the home.

Involuntary Exposure to Tobacco Combustion Products

A custom loathsome to the eye, hateful to the nose, harmful to the brain, dangerous to the lungs, and in the black, stinking fume thereof, nearest resembling the horrible Stygian smoke of the pit that is bottomless.

—King James I of England, 1604 (6)

Nearly four centuries later, the Surgeon General's office heeded this royal admonition and issued a series of statements warning of the dangers of cigarette smoke (7, 8). This was followed in 1993 by a warning issued by the Environmental Protection Agency that identified environmental tobacco smoke as a Class 1 carcinogen (9). Passive smoking describes the involuntary exposure of nonsmokers to the combustion products of tobacco in the indoor environment. When tobacco is smoked it produces two types of smoke:

Mainstream smoke, which arises after being drawn through the cigarette filtered by the lung and exhaled
Sidestream smoke, which arises from the burning end of the cigarette

The components of mainstream and sidestream smoke are different, with the more potentially toxic agents contained in the sidestream smoke (Table 51.3). Sidestream smoke contributes to approximately 85% of the smoke in a room. Although these constituents are diluted by the air in the room, the fact that significant exposure occurs has been confirmed by studies measuring carboxyhemoglobin and cotinine levels in nonsmokers (4, 10). Elevation of carboxyhemoglobin levels reflects acute exposure since the half-life of carboxyhemoglobin in a person breathing room air is about 4 hours. Cotinine, on the other hand, confirms long-term exposure (10).

Since the initial report by the Surgeon General warning of the dangers of active smoking, there has been increased attention also focused on the adverse healths effects on children of parental smoking. These findings are summarized in a review by Weiss and coworkers and by and official statement by the American Thoracic Society (10, 11). The body

Table 51.1.
Sources and Types of Indoor Pollutants

Source	Type
Cigarette smoke	Respirable particles, CO, volatile organic substances
Gas stoves	NO_2, CO
Wood stoves	Respirable particles, CO, polycyclicaromatic hydrocarbons
Kerosene heaters	NO_2, CO_2, SO_2
Building materials	Formaldehyde, radon, asbestos
Miscellaneous	Dust, allergens, cleaning solvents

Adapted from Samet JM, Marburg MC, Spangler JD. Health effects and sources of indoor air pollution. Part 1. *Am Rev Respir Dis* 1987; 136:1486–1508.

Table 51.2.
Potential Health Effects of Indoor Pollution

Pollutant	Adverse Effect
CO	Tissue hypoxia
NO_2	Increased respiratory infections
SO_2	Bronchospasm
CO_2	Hypoxia, discomfort
Formaldehyde	Mucous membrane irritation, ? bronchospasm
Radon	Cancer
Suspended particles	Increased respiratory illness, bronchospasm
Asbestos	Cancer, restrictive lung disease
Aeroallergens	Rhinitis, conjunctivitis, asthma

Table 51.3.
Selected Constituents of Cigarette Smoke—Ratio of Constituents in Sidestream Smoke (SS) to Mainstream Smoke (MS)

Gas Phase Constituents	MS	SS/MS Ratio	Particulate Phase Constituents	MS	SS/MS
Carbon dioxide	20–60 mg	8.1	Tar	1–40 mg	1.3
Carbon monoxide	10–20 mg	2.5	Water	1–4 mg	2.4
Methane	1.3 mg	3.1	Toluene	108 μg	5.6
Acetylene	27 μg	0.8	Phenol	20–150 μg	2.6
Ammonia	80 μg	73.0	Methylnaphthalene	2.2 μg	28.0
Hydrogen cyanide	430 μg	0.25	Pyrene	50–200 μg	3.6
Methyifuran	20 μg	3.4	Benzo(a)pyrene	20–40 μg	3.4
Acetonitrile	120 μg	3.9	Aniline	360 mg	30.0
Pyridine	32 μg	10.0	Nicotine	1.0–2.5 mg	2.7
Dimethyinitrosamine	10–65 μg	52.0	2-Napthylamine	2 mg	39.0

From Weiss ST, Tager IB, Schenker M, Speizer FE. The health effects of involuntary smoking. *Am Rev Respir Dis* 1983; 128:933–942.

of evidence that chronic exposure to smoke from parents is dangerous continues to accumulate. The negative impact on the health of both the child and his parents of parental smoking is staggering (Table 51.4).

The adverse effects of involuntary exposure to tobacco smoke begin in utero and extend certainly through childhood and probably for life. Maternal smoking during pregnancy increases the risk of fetal loss and compromises the growth and overall well-being of the baby (11–13). Recent data have implicated maternal smoking during pregnancy as a major risk factor for sudden infant death syndrome (SIDS) (14, 15). After birth, the adverse effects of involuntary smoking escalate. Children whose parents smoke have increased rate of otitis media (16), adenotonsillectomy (16), bronchitis, and other lower respiratory tract illnesses (4, 10, 18, 19). Although some studies have demonstrated no effect on acute wheezing (20), others have shown an affect both on pulmonary function and asthma symptoms in patients with asthma (21–23). The effects of exposure to cigarette smoke on asthma go beyond simply increasing wheezing. As a known bronchial irritant, cigarette smoke adds to the inflammation in the lung, a major factor in increasing the severity of asthma in children and adults. Our clinical experience in a large pulmonary practice confirms this effect, as we have seen a dramatic reduction in wheezing and other respiratory symptoms simply by removing the child, especially infants from smoke filled rooms. Parental

Table 51.4.
Adverse Effects of Passive Smoking on Children

Fetal

Decreased fetal weight
Increased incidence of
　Placenta previa
　Abruptio placenta
　Antepartum hemorrhage
　Preterm delivery
　Stillbirths

Neonatal

Increased deaths from
　Respiratory distress syndrome
　Neonatal asphyxia
　Pneumonia

Infants and children

Reduces lung size and function
Increases risk for
　SIDS
　Recurrent otitis media
　Recurrent tonsillopharyngitis
　Adenotonsillectomy
Increases incidence of lower respiratory tract illness
Increases symptoms in children with asthma
Probable similar role in infants with CF, BPD, etc.

Older children and adolescents

Role model for smoking
Increases risk that the child will start smoking (most adult smokers start prior to age 18)
Increases risk of premature disability in parents
May increase the risk of lung cancer (unproven for children but has been shown for nonsmoking spouses)

smoking has also been shown to cause small but consistent changes in lung function and on subsequent lung growth in children exposed both in utero and in early life (4, 10, 11, 24, 25). Even though these changes are small, available evidence strongly suggests that they should not be ignored (26).

There are also data that suggest an increased risk of developing lung cancer in nonsmoking spouses of smokers (27–29). From a pediatric perspective, we must also be concerned about a similar increased risk of developing lung or other cancers in children who are exposed to cigarette smoke from infancy. Are these children more susceptible to lung cancer as adults and is this effect magnified if they start smoking themselves as teenagers and young adults?

Approximately two-thirds of adults who smoke started smoking as adolescents, most before the age of 16 (10). Parental smoking provides a poor role model for children and undermines the anti-smoking campaigns of the school, government, and voluntary health agencies.

RECOMMENDATION

A detailed history of smoking in the home should be obtained in all children referred for evaluation of chronic respiratory symptoms. Counseling parents about the dangers of smoking should be included as an essential component of well child care by the primary pediatrician (30, 31). The pulmonary consultant should re-enforce the particular importance of a smoke-free environment to a child with respiratory disease. All pregnant women should stop smoking before attempting to get pregnant or as soon as possible after they are aware of the pregnancy. This is quite simply part of the responsibility of parenthood. The defense that the parents or adults in the home "don't smoke around the child" should not be accepted at face value. Parents who smoke should be encouraged to stop smoking in the home and the car. Ideally, the home should be completely smoke-free. A first step involves moving all smoking to the outdoors. However, smoking cessation should be the goal rather than shifting the smoking outside, since as soon as the weather turns bad, human nature brings smokers back indoors. The phone numbers of the various smoking cessation programs in the community should be provided

to the parents. It is also useful to refer the parents who smoke to an internist to discuss the use of one of the nicotine patch smoking cessation programs.

Other Combustion Products

Although cigarette smoke constitutes the major source of indoor pollution, the use of gas cooking, kerosene heaters, and wood burning stoves also contributes to increased respiratory symptoms in children. Gas cooking produces CO, CO_2, and a variety of nitrogen oxides (NO and NO_2). Kerosene heaters produce similar compounds with the addition of SO_2. Exposure to NO_2 has received the most attention. Initial studies implicated a role for NO_2 in increasing the risk of chronic respiratory disease in children living in homes dependent on gas cooking (2, 4). This association seemed to affect females more, possibly reflecting the amount of time mothers and daughters spend together. However, the results of subsequent studies have been somewhat equivocal, and at the present time it would appear that exposure to NO_2 at concentrations encountered in the average American home does not place the occupants at increased risk of developing respiratory illness (4). However, more data are needed in certain populations, especially the urban poor who use gas not only to cook but also to heat their apartments. In this setting, the concentrations of NO_2 may be considerably higher and thus may be a contributing factor to the increased respiratory illness seen in this population. A similar conclusion can be reached regarding low-level exposure to CO, another byproduct of gas combustion (4).

As a part of the effort to reduce heating costs and dependence on oil, many homes have switched to alternative sources of heat, such as fireplaces, wood-burning stoves, and kerosene space heaters. The regular use of fireplaces and non-airtight wood-burning stoves can result in substantial levels of pollutants such as polyaromatic hydrocarbons, CO, and respirable particles (2, 4). These substances can be reduced dramatically by the use of the newer airtight stoves that operate under negative pressure conditions in order to minimize leaks. Another advance is the addition of catalytic convertors. In less developed countries, indoor combustion of wood products has been implicated as a risk factor for lung disease. However, this exposure is often in the form of open fires in a hut with poor ventilation, which is several orders of magnitude more intense than that encountered in developed countries.

There are limited data on the effects of wood-burning stoves in causing respiratory disease in children. Honicky et al. reported an increase in moderate to severe respiratory symptoms in children from homes using wood-burning stoves (32). This finding was confirmed in a study of American Indians (33). However, a similar study from Massachusetts could not confirm these effects (34). Additional data are needed that are carefully controlled for the duration of exposure, the type of stove used, and some quantification of the magnitude of the exposure.

RECOMMENDATION

At the present time, the available data on the adverse health effects of exposure to gas combustion in the home do not warrant abandoning use of gas to heat homes and prepare food. Use of a pilotless ignition system can help reduce some of burden in the home. Space heaters should be used in uninhabited areas, and adequate ventilation of the home should be guaranteed in order to reduce the concentration of these byproducts in the living space.

More data are needed before a policy geared toward the use of wood-burning stoves can be developed. Nonetheless, families who are interested in heating their home with a wood-burning stove should be strongly encouraged to purchase state-of-the-art equipment in order to minimize the indoor pollution burden. Families should also be instructed to have the stove checked for leaks and efficiency regularly. Electrostatic filters may also be helpful. If a wood-burning stove or fireplace is used regularly in the home of a child who continues with chronic respiratory symptoms despite appropriate medical management, the family should be requested to use an alternative heat source for several weeks in order to determine if wood burning is the culprit. Families should also be cautioned about what to burn. Peters and co-workers reported a family that experienced chronic arsenic poisoning from burning treated plywood in their stove (35).

Formaldehyde

Modern home construction and insulation techniques have resulted in increased use of formaldehyde-containing materials in homes. Formaldehyde is a volatile gas with an easily recognizable odor. It is a water-soluble gas that is highly irritating to the mucous membranes of the upper respiratory tract (2, 4). The first reports of problems arising from formaldehyde were seen following widespread use of urea formaldehyde foam insulation (UFFI) (36, 37). Although this compound has been removed from the market, formaldehyde-containing products (e.g., particle board, paper products, carpets, adhesives) are still widely used, and the potential risk of side effects is still present. This risk is a particular problem for those living in new mobile homes. Table 51.5 summarizes the relationship between concentrations of formaldehyde and symptoms. Comparable levels have been reported in a number of studies investigating homes and offices thought to be the source of the patient's complaints. Acute effects include eye and nasal mucosa irritation and vague neuropsychologic complaints (headache, memory lapse, fatigue, and difficulty sleeping). The major pulmonary symptom of concern is formaldehyde-induced wheezing. However, the data on domestic exposure to formaldehyde and exacerbation of asthma symptoms are equivocal (4). Unfortunately, a number of studies that either claimed an effect or did not

Table 51.5.
Acute Human Health Effects of Formaldehyde at Various Concentrations

Reported Effects	Formaldehyde Concentration (ppm)
None reported	0.0–0.5
Neurophysiologic effects[a]	0.05–1.5
Odor threshold	0.05–1.0
Eye irritation[b]	0.01–2.0
Upper airway irritation	0.10–25
Lower airway and pulmonary effects	5–30
Pulmonary edema, inflammation, pneumonia	50–100
Death	> 100

[a]As measured by determination of optical chronaxy, electroencephalography, and sensitivity of dark-adapted eyes to light.
[b]The low concentration (0.01 ppm) was observed in the presence of other pollutants that may have been acting synergistically.
Adapted from Samet JM, Marburg MC, Spangler JD. Health effects and sources of indoor air pollution. Parts 1 and 2. *Am Rev Respir Dis* Pt 1 1987; 136:1486–1508. Pt 2 1988; 137:221–242.

reveal any problem did not measure formalde-hyde levels in the home (38, 39). When a number of patients thought to be suffering from formaldehyde-induced asthma under-went bronchoprovocation testing with form-aldehyde, the majority were found to be non-responders (40), raising doubt about its role in the pathogenesis of asthma.

RECOMMENDATION

Current data do not support formaldehyde as a major cause of respiratory symptoms. If there is concern that formaldehyde may be playing a role in causing persistent asthma symptoms, several steps should be taken. First, an environmental history should be obtained with specific emphasis on living conditions and any changes or additions to the home environment associated with onset of symp-toms. Next, a thorough inspection of the home environment should be undertaken with specific measurement of formaldehyde levels. Kits are available that can be used to measure the indoor formaldehyde levels (Table 51.6). If the patient is old enough to undergo pulmo-nary function testing, a formaldehyde inhala-tion challenge study should be performed before a diagnosis can be made (4, 40).

Aeroallergens

A number of allergens have been identified that may be found in significant concentra-tions in the home and that may be a source of chronic respiratory symptoms. These include house dust mite and cockroach droppings (a particular problem for inner city and other disadvantaged populations), animal skin scales, and molds. House dust mites have received considerable attention as the most common cause of indoor environmental allergy. Mites thrive in environments of high relative humidity and temperatures around 23°C. An allergic environmental cause should be suspected in a child with a personal or family history of atopy whose symptoms include cough, wheeze, or chronic rhinitis/conjunctivitis that either are worse in the home or are improved when the child is out of the home for an extended period and then recur shortly after the child returns.

RECOMMENDATION

As with other indoor pollutants, a thorough environmental history and, with the child with difficult-to-control asthma symptoms, a home visit by an individual trained to look for poten-tial environmental allergens should be obtained. Common sense dictates that in any child with chronic asthma or other respiratory illness that the parents be strongly encouraged to reduce the risks of environmental aeroaller-gen exposure. This should at a minimum include removal of stuffed animals and carpet from the child's room. The mattress and pil-low should be covered with hypoallergenic covers to reduce exposure to dust mites. If carpet cannot be removed, it should be cleaned regularly using appropriate solutions to reduce the burden of mites in the carpeting. Steps should be taken to reduce dampness in the home since this fosters growth not only of mites but also of molds (41). Household pets, especially cats, should be removed or restricted to the outdoors. If the family does not already have a pet they should be strongly discouraged from introducing one into the home. When the house is being cleaned, the infant or child should be in another room to reduce exposure to dust churned up by clean-ing. An evaluation by an allergist in the hopes of identifying a specific allergen should be considered in children whose symptoms per-sist despite these simple environmental pre-cautions.

Radon

Experience with miners who were exposed to radon decay products has demonstrated that these workers are at increased risk of develop-ing lung cancer (2, 4, 42). However, the risk to the general population from exposure to radon and radon daughters in the home has only recently come under study and become a source of concern. Uranium and radium are present in varying concentrations in all rocks and soil. Radium decays to radon, an inert, colorless, odorless, water-soluble gas that, because it is inert, easily diffuses out of source material into the atmosphere or dissolves in water. Radon decays into a number of daugh-ters, two of which (Polonium-214 and Poloni-um-218) emit alpha energy that is injurious to the respiratory epithelium. This exposure to ionizing radiation is thought to cause the tissue injury that eventually leads to malig-nancy.

The soil beneath the home is the major source of radon gas. It diffuses out of the soil

Table 51.6.
Commercially Available Sampling Equipment for Indoor Air Pollutants Other than Particulates

Pollutant Sampler	Manufacturing Company	Sensitivity and Integrating Time	Approximate Cost
Radon: track etch detector	Terradex Corporation 460 N. Wiget Lane Walnut Creek, CA 94598 (415) 938-2545	1- to 3-month exposure 1–4 pCi/L	$20–$60 depending on sensitivity desired
Radon: charcoal canister detector	RTCA 12 West Main Street Elmsford, NY 10523 (914) 347-5010	4 days 0.1 pCi/L	$35/canister; includes shipment and analysis costs
Organic vapors	Industrial Scientific Corporation 355 Steubenville Pike Oakdale, PA 15071 (412) 758-4353		
Organic vapors: Hydrocarbon chemical reaction tubes	National Draeger Inc. P.O. Box 120 Pittsburgh, PA 15230 (412) 787-8383	100–3000 ppm for 4–8 hours	$3/tube, $900 for pump and accessories
Organic vapors: charcoal badges	3M Corporation Technical Service Department 3M Center St. Paul, MN 55144 (612) 733-1110	Depends on vapors and sampling times; minimum level, 10/mg	$10 badge; $50–$300 analysis by GC or GC/MS
Formaldehyde: diffusion tube	Air Quality Research, Inc. 901 Grayson Street Berkeley, CA 94710 (415) 644-2097	5–7 days	$48 kit, includes two monitors, analysis, and report
Formaldehyde: Pro-tek adsorption badge	E.I. Dupont Company Applied Technical Division P.O. Box 110 Kennett Square, PA 19348 1(800) 344-4900	1.6–54 ppm/hour up to 7 days or 0.2 to 6.75 ppm/8 hour TWA	$20/badge; $25–$80 for analysis
Formaldehyde: diffusion monitor	3M Corporation Technical Service Department 3M Center St. Paul, MN 55144 (612) 733-1110	0.1 ppm for 8 hours	$37/monitor and analysis
NO$_2$: personal and alarm	*MDA Scientific 405 Barclay Blvd. Lincolnshire, IL 60069 1(800) 323-2000*	*2–3 ppm; 1/3 TLV electrochemical cell based 15 minutes to 8 hours TWA*	*$800/detector; $100/output: $2075/dosimeter; $1045/ readout unit*
NO$_2$: diffusion tubes	Environmental Sciences and Physiology Harvard School of Public Health 665 Huntington Avenue Boston, MA 02115 (617) 732-1000	50 ppb/hour integrated	$10/tube, research only
NO$_2$: diffusion badge	Environmental Sciences and Physiology Harvard School of Public Health 665 Huntington Avenue Boston, MA 02115 (617) 732-1000	50 ppb/hour	$15/badge, research only
CO: passive badge	Lab Safety Supply Co. P.O. Box 1368 Janesville, WI 53547 (608) 754-2345	50 ppm for 8 hours produces color change	$3/holder: $12.75/10 indicating papers
CO: detector tube integrated	National Draeger Inc. P.O. Box 120 Pittsburgh, PA 15230 (412) 787-8383	2.5 ppm for 8 hours	$255 pump and accessories; $3/tube
CO: detector tube grab	Sensidyne Inc. 12345 Sparkey Road Suite E Largo, FL 33543 (813) 530-3602	5 ppm/minute	$130 pump; $2/tube

From Samet JM, Marburg MC, Spangler JD. Health effects and sources of indoor air pollution. Parts 1 and 2. *Am Rev Respir Dis* Pt 1 1987; 136:1486–1508. Pt 2 1988; 137:221–242.

into the basement or crawl space beneath the house. The concentration of radon varies widely. It is increased in certain areas because of the geologic formations beneath the home. One example of this is the Reading prong, a geologic formation extending from eastern Pennsylvania through Maryland and into New Jersey. Homes along this prong have been shown to have radon concentrations greater than 20 pCi/L, which is dramatically higher than the average domestic levels in the United States, which range from 0.01 to 4 pCi/L. It can also be increased inadvertently if high-radium-containing building materials are used in constructing the foundation for the home. It has been estimated that over 1 million homes in the United States may have concentrations that exceed 8 pCi/L, a level that is well above the EPA action standard of 4 pCi/L. At the present time, it is not known what level of domestic exposure constitutes significant health risk. Unfortunately, the data obtained from the mining experience are not strictly applicable to a domestic exposure. Mines are generally dustier, the ventilation of this space is different than that in the average home, and the dose delivered to the lung is considerably greater for miners whose minute ventilation is increased from manual labor. Furthermore, active smoking, a behavior common among the miners, is a confounding variable. The risk of developing lung cancer in this population is enhanced by this double exposure. Another difficulty relates to the fact that infants are exposed from birth, and it is unclear what difference injury from ionizing radiation will have in a growing and developing organism.

Although the exact role residential exposure to radon plays in increasing the risk of lung cancer, it has been estimated that domestic radon exposure at a rate of 0.5 pCi/L contributes approximately 10% of lung cancer deaths in nonsmokers. Assuming the model holds, this figure rises to 30% at a background exposure of 1.5 pCi/L. The risk figure is even higher in active smokers. It is not known how radon exposure interacts with exposure to environmental tobacco smoke.

RECOMMENDATION

As with a number of other environmental pollutants, even though the data defining a risk are incomplete, public awareness of the prob-

lem has generated considerable concern among home owners. Anxiety has been heightened by a vigorous advertising campaign. Radon testing kits can be found routinely in local supermarkets or hardware stores, creating a perception of risk among the general population. However, for most American homes the radon levels are not increased and the actual danger to children is simply unknown. With this in mind, who should have their homes tested and what test should be used? The answer to the first question is relatively simple. If your patient resides in an area known to have elevated background concentrations of radon in the soil such as the area along the Reading Prong, the home should be tested, if for no other reason than to give the family peace of mind. Information on high-risk areas can be obtained from many local American Lung Association chapters or from the Environmental Protection Agency (EPA). The EPA has developed a information pamphlet on radon entitled *A Citizen's Guide to Radon: What Is It and What to Do About It* (43).

Two types of testing kits are currently available. The short-term kit consists of a charcoal canister, whereas longer-term measurements can be made with an etched track detector or its equivalent. The longer-term techniques have less variability and are more accurate. Regardless of the test used, the results should be obtained from a laboratory accredited by the EPA's Radon Measurement Proficiency Program. The EPA's action level is 4 pCi/L. If the level is high, one should not panic. Often these measurements are obtained in a basement or crawl space. If high levels are found in these areas, it is worthwhile to repeat the test, perhaps including measurements in actual living spaces, and to consider some inexpensive options. Abatement techniques are based on mitigation and ventilation. Mitigation can be accomplished by placing a vapor barrier around the foundation; sealing cracks and holes in basement floor, traps, and drains; installing a charcoal water-scrubber for well water; and reducing dampness in basements or crawl space. Ventilation should be improved in the crawl space, the sump hole, and bathrooms; the laundry room should be ventilated to the outside, and the subslab area should be depressurized. Unfortunately, these techniques may get expensive for the homeowner, and the solution should be based on the severity of the problem.

IMPROVING INDOOR AIR QUALITY

Physicians are frequently asked about ways to clean up the indoor air in the home of a child with significant respiratory disease. The first step involves identifying the pollutant and its concentration in the home. Table 51.6 lists commercially available kits for measuring common sources of pollution (4). Once identified, some approaches to reducing pollution in the home, which are listed in Table 51.7, can be considered (4). For many indoor pollutants such as combustion products, however, the best way to clean the air is to stop the production of the pollutant in the home. Simple smoking cessation is the cheapest way to clean the air in the home of a smoker. Opening a window to increase the exchange rate for a tight home is also effective in improving indoor air quality. However, this is a less appealing solution when one is dealing with extremes of temperature outdoors.

Alternative approaches have included the use of room and whole-house filtering systems. Societal concerns about purifying the environment has spawned the birth of the home air purification business. There are many machines on the market, many of which do not live up to the manufacturers' claims (43). These machines are based on the use of filters, electrical attraction, and ozonation. The most efficient filters are the high-efficiency particulate arresting (HEPA) filters. which capture approximately 99% of particles 0.3 μm or greater in size. These can be supplemented with activated charcoal or carbon filters, which facilitate trapping gas molecules. The pleated filter variant is slightly less effective (95%), but both are considerably better than a room air-conditioner filter, which removes only about 30% of particles greater than 10 μm. There are three types of electrical attraction filters. Electrostatic precipitating cleaners operate by passing air drawn into the system by a fan over a high-voltage wire. These charged particles are then attracted to precipitating cells of the opposite charge. An electret filter employs statically charged fibers to trap particulate matter. The third system is a negative ion generator that uses electronically charged needles and wires to trap ionized particles. They are not as efficient, and these ionized particles may accumulate on furnishings or the walls of the room. None of these systems removes gas molecules. The final and generally not recommended system is the ozone generator. In this system a high-voltage charge is used to convert oxygen to ozone. At high concentrations ozone destroys gas molecules and microorganisms but has no effect on particles. These machines may also foul the air by the excess production of ozone in an enclosed space.

Choice of a particular machine should be based on what pollutant one wants to remove and the documented performance characteristics of the machine in question (43). In general, even the best available equipment can handle only a single room. Thus, if the family wants to purchase a filtering system, they will need to purchase a portable machine or place it in the room where the child spends the most time. This is usually the bedroom. Whole house systems are available but they are expensive to purchase and operate. The better systems require instillation by a professional. Unless an auxiliary fan is installed, they depend on the heating or cooling being on for them to filter the air. They also add to the heating and cooling costs.

This is a changing field, and thus a physician should advise families to consult the various consumer guides before making an investment. After the family has made a choice, it is helpful to review the choice to see if the characteristics of the machine suit the intended purpose.

REFERENCES

1. Frank R, Lebowitz MD. The risk of staying in. *Am Rev Respir Dis* 1981; 124:521–522.
2. Angle CR. Indoor air pollutants. *Adv Pediatr* 1988; 35:239–280.
3. Witek TJ, Schachter EN, Leaderer BP. Indoor air pollution and respiratory health. *Respir Care* 1984; 29:147–154.
4. Samet JM, Marburg MC, Spangler JD. Health effects and sources of indoor air pollution. Part 1 and 2. *Am Rev Respir Dis* Pt 1 1987; 136:1486–1508. Pt 2 1988; 137:221–242.
5. Guidelines as to what constitutes an adverse respiratory health effect, with special reference to epidemiologic studies of air pollution. *Am Rev Respir Dis* 1985; 131:666–668.
6. *Oxford dictionary of quotations*, 3rd ed. Oxford, Oxford University Press, 1979, p 271.
7. US Department of Health, Education and Welfare, Public Health Service, Office on Smoking and Health. Report of the advisory committee to the sur-

Table 51.7.
Control Measures for Pollutants

Pollutant	Control Measures	
	Equipment and Materials	Ventilation and Design
Respirable particles	High-efficiency filters Tight sealing doors and grates Properly drafting chimney Electrostatic precipitators	Zone and Ventilate for smoking Supply outside combustion air to heater and fireplace Relocate air intakes Maintain filter system
NO, NO_2	Remove gasoline engine Pilotless ignition	Effective hood vent over source Isolate garage from indoor space
CO	Pilotless ignition Restrict heater use to uninhabited space Use Catalytic converter Replace indoor gaslone engines with electric	Supply outside combustion air Vent emission outside Kitchen/hood vent Relocate vents Provide smoking zones Isolate garage from indoor space
CO_2	Check static pressure in return air ducts to make sure return is not over-riding fresh air intake	Isolate garage from indoor space
Agents from biologic sources	Insulate to prevent condensation Damp-proof foundation, ducts Proper drainage of drip pans under condenser coils Add bacteriocides to steam and water for humidifiers and cooling towers Proper maintenance of filters and ducts Routine cleaning Discard water-damaged floor coverings Do not use cool-mist humidifiers and vaporizers	Maintain inside relative humditiy of 35–50% Exhaust bath and kitchen Vent crawl spaces
Formaldehyde	Substitute products such as phenolic resin plywood Seal sources Removal of materials	Increase air exchange to house or office
Radon and radon daughters	Vapor barrier around foundation Damp-proof basement and crawl space Seal cracks and holes in floor, traps and drains Install charcoal water-scrubber for well water Complete seal foundation	Vent crawl space Vent sumphole to exterior Subslab depressurization Vent bathroom and laundry to exterior
Volatile organic compounds	Substitute products Isolate storage area Apply only according to specifications Do not locate transformers indoors	Use only with adequate ventilation Ventilate laundry, shop Provide separate ventilation to storage area
Asbestos	Removal Injection sealant Wrap pipes with plastic and duct tape	Ventilation does not provide adequate protection

From Samet JM, Marburg MC, Spangler JD. Health effects and sources of indoor air pollution. Parts 1 and 2. *Am Rev Respir Dis* Pt 1 1987; 136:1486–1508. Pt 2 1988; 137:221–242.

geon general. PHS Publication No. 1103. Washington, DC, US Government Printing Office, 1964.

8. US Department of Health, Education and Welfare, Public Health Service, Office on Smoking and Health. *The health consequences of involuntary smoking. A report of the surgeon general.* Washington DC, US Government Printing Office, 1986.

9. Respiratory health effects of passive smoking: *Lung cancer and other disorders.* Environmental Protection Agency, EPA/600/6–90/006F, December, 1992.

10. Weiss ST, Tager IB, Schenker M, Speizer FE. The health effects of involuntary smoking. *Am Rev Respir Dis* 1983; 128:933–942.

11. Health effects of smoking on children: official ATS statement. *Am Rev Respir Dis* 1985; 132:1137–1138.

12. Abel EL. Smoking during pregnancy: A review of effects on growth and development of offspring. *Hum Biol* 1980; 52:593–625.

13. Holsclaw DS, Topham AL. The effects of smoking on fetal, neonatal, and childhood development. *Pediatr Ann* 1978; 7:105–136.

14. Haglund B, Cnattinguis S. Cigarette smoking as a risk factor for sudden infant death syndrome: A population-based study. *Am J Pub Health* 1990; 80:29–32.

15. Lewak N, van den Berg BJ, Beckwith JB. Sudden infant death syndrome risk factors. *Clin Pediatr* 1979; 18:404–411.

16. Pukander J, Luotonen J, Timonen M, Karmer P. Risk factors effecting the occurrence of acute otitis media among 2–3 year old urban children. *Acta Otolaryngol* 1985; 100:260–265.

17. Said G, Zalokar J, Lellouch J, Patois E. Parental smoking related to adenoidectomy and tonsillectomy in children. *J Epidemiol Commun Health* 1978; 32:97–101.

18. Harlap S, Davies AM. Infant admissions to hospital and maternal smoking. *Lancet* 1974; 1:529–532.

19. Fergussen DM, Horwood LJ, Shannon FT, et al. Parental smoking and lower respiratory illness in the first three years of life. *J Epidemiol Commun Health* 1981; 35:180–184.

20. Wiedemann HP, Mahler DA, Loke J, et al. Acute effects of passive smoking on lung function and airway reactivity in asthmatic subjects. *Chest* 1986; 89:180–185.

21. Martinez FD, Antognoni G, Macri F, et al. Parental smoking enhances bronchial responsiveness in nine year old children. *Am Rev Respir Dis* 1988; 138:518–523.

22. Gortmaker SL, Walker DK, Jacobs FH, Ruch–Ross H. Parental smoking and the risk of childhood asthma. *Am J Pub Health* 1982; 72:574–579.

23. Cogswell JJ, Mitchell EB, Alexander J. Parental smoking, breast feeding, and respiratory infections in development of allergic disease. *Arch Dis Child* 1987; 62:338–344.

24. Burchfiel CM, Higgins MW, Keller JB, et al. Passive smoking in childhood; respiratory conditions and pulmonary function in Techumseh, Michigan. *Am Rev Respir Dis* 1986; 133:966–973.

25. Berkey CS, Ware JH, Dockery DW, et al. Indoor air pollution and pulmonary function growth in preadolescent children. *Am J Epidemiol* 1986; 123:250–260.

26. Tager IB. Passive smoking and respiratory health in children—Sophistry or cause for concern? *Am Rev Respir Dis* 1986; 133:959–961.

27. Trichopoulos D, Kalandidi A, Sparros L, MacMahon BB. Lung cancer and passive smoking. *Int J Cancer* 1981; 27:1–4.

28. Hirayama T. Non-smoking wives of heavy smokers have a higher risk of lung cancer: A study from Japan. *Br Med J* 1981; 282:183–185.

29. Dalager NA, Pickle LW, Mason TJ, et al. The relation of passive smoking to lung cancer. *Cancer Res* 1986; 46:4808–4811.

30. Koop CE. The pediatrician's obligation in smoking education. *Am J Dis Child* 1985; 139:973.

31. Involuntary smoking – a hazard to children. *Pediatrics* 1986; 77:755–757.

32. Honicky RE, Osborne JS, Akpom CA. Symptoms of respiratory illness in young children and the use of wood-burning stoves for indoor heating. *Pediatrics* 1985; 75:587–593.

33. Morris K, Morganlander M, Coulehan JL, et al. Wood-burning stoves and lower respiratory tract infection in American Indian children. *Am J Dis Child* 1990; 144:105–108.

34. Tuthill RW. Woodstoves, formaldehyde, and respiratory disease. *Am J Epidemiol* 1984; 120:952–955.

35. Peters HA, Croft WA, Wooson EA, et al. Seasonal arsenic exposure from burning chromium-copper-arsenate treated wood. *JAMA* 1984; 251:2392–2396.

36. Dally K, Hannahan L, Woodburg M, Kanarek M. Formaldehyde exposure in non-occupational environments. *Arch Environ Health* 1981; 36:277–284.

37. Sardinas AV, Guilretti MA, Most RS, Honchar P. Health effects associated with urea-formaldehyde foam insulation in Connecticut. *J Environ Health* 1979; 41:270–272.

38. Thun MJ, Lakat MF, Altman R. Symptoms survey of residents of homes insulated with urea-formaldehyde foam. *Environ Res* 1982; 29:320–324.

39. Norman GR, Pengelly LD, Kerigan AT, et al. Respiratory function of children in homes insulated with urea formaldehyde foam insulation. *Can Med Assoc J* 1986; 134:1135–1138.

40. Frigas E, Filley WV, Reed CE. Asthma induced by dust from urea-formaldehyde foam insulation material. *Chest* 1981; 79:706–707.

41. Bun ML, Dean BV, Merrett TG, et al. Effects of anti-mite measures on children with mite sensitive asthma: A controlled trial. *Thorax* 1980; 35:506–512.

42. Samet JM, Nero AV. Indoor radon and lung cancer. *N Engl J Med* 1989; 320:591–594.

43. Household air cleaners. *Consumer Reports* October, 1992, pp 657–662.

52

Central Hypoventilation and Hyperventilation Syndromes

CAROLE L. MARCUS and JOHN L. CARROLL

CENTRAL HYPOVENTILATION

Central alveolar hypoventilation is defined as a persistently elevated arterial carbon dioxide tension (> 45 mm Hg) due to a decrease in central nervous system ventilatory drive. It is usually associated with hypoxia. Patients with central hypoventilation fail to breathe normally despite the presence of normal lungs, upper airway, and chest wall.

Etiology

Central hypoventilation may be congenital or acquired, and primary or secondary. Causes of central hypoventilation are listed in Table 1.

History and Physical Examination

Patients with congenital central hypoventilation usually present at birth or soon thereafter with cyanosis, apnea, respiratory depression, or hypoxic seizures. The infant may be misdiagnosed as having perinatal asphyxia. Some patients present in infancy with apparent life-threatening events (ALTEs). A few children with congenital central hypoventilation present later in childhood with nonspecific symptoms (lethargy, poor sleep, irritability, morning headaches), cor pulmonale, seizures, or respiratory failure precipitated by sedation or a respiratory tract infection. Usually, these older children have symptoms dating back to infancy. A high index of suspicion is required for early diagnosis, and it is not unusual for patients to be diagnosed only following catastrophic events.

Patients with central hypoventilation have been described as having "happy hypoxia."

They appear oblivious to cyanosis or respiratory failure, and do not manifest respiratory distress or increased respiratory effort in response to hypoxia or hypercapnia. This is in marked contrast to patients with respiratory failure secondary to pulmonary mechanical abnormalities or ventilatory muscle weakness. The physical examination in children with central hypoventilation is usually normal, especially when the child is awake. Cyanosis, shallow breathing, bradypnea, or central apnea may be noticeable during sleep. In the severely affected child, these respiratory abnormalities may be noticeable during wakefulness as well. Children with central hypoventilation may be able to take normal breaths on command, but the effort is transient. Growth failure or signs of pulmonary hypertension are frequently present in the untreated patient. In children with secondary central hypoventilation, the underlying condition or associated neurologic abnormalities are usually evident.

Specific Disease Conditions

CONGENITAL CENTRAL HYPOVENTILATION SYNDROME

Patients with congenital central hypoventilation syndrome (CCHS, Ondine's curse) have intact voluntary control of ventilation, but lack automatic control. The name "Ondine's curse" was derived from a German fable. Ondine was a mermaid who married a mortal man. When he abandoned her for another woman, a curse was cast upon him, depriving him of automatic control of his bodily func-

Table 52.1.
Causes of Central Hypoventilation

Primary

Congenital central hypoventilation syndrome (CCHS)
Central hypoventilation syndromes associated with
  endocrine dysfunction (e.g., hypothyroidism and
  diabetes insipidus)

Secondary

Obesity hypoventilation syndrome

Increased intracranial pressure

  Arnold-Chiari malformation type I
  Arnold-Chiari malformation type II
  Ventriculoperitoneal shunt malfunction
  Achondroplasia (106–109)
  Other causes of increased intracranial pressure

Brainstem lesions

  Hypoxic-ischemic encephalopathy
  Trauma
  Hemorrhage
  Tumor
  Congenital anomalies (60)
  Moebius syndrome (110)
  Meningoencephalitis
  Poliomyelitis (64)

Neurologic syndromes

  Autonomic neuropathies (familial dysautonomia)
  Subacute necrotizing encephalomyelopathy (Leigh
    disease)
  Mitochondrial defects
  Neurodegenerative syndromes

Miscellaneous

  Depressant drugs
  Hyperthermia (111)
  Hypothyroidism
  Metabolic dysfunction, inborn errors of metabolism

tions. He died when he forgot to breathe (1). The name "Ondine's curse" is no longer used because of its negative connotations. CCHS has been considered extremely rare. However, increased recognition of the syndrome and improved methods of ventilatory support have resulted in an increasing number of children diagnosed with CCHS. It is possible that some infants dying from the sudden infant death syndrome (SIDS), or from unexplained cardiac failure (2), may actually have had CCHS.

Classically, children with CCHS were described as having normal breathing during wakefulness, but severe hypoventilation during sleep. However, it is now apparent that CCHS consists of a spectrum of severity. The most severely affected patients hypoventilate during both wakefulness and sleep (3, 4). Some patients maintain adequate ventilation during wakefulness from birth. In others, sleep/wake discrimination develops as the child grows older, usually by 6 months of age (3, 5). Even the mildly affected patients do not exhibit the normal increase in ventilation in response to exercise (6–8) and tend to develop respiratory failure during infections.

Patients with CCHS may have associated abnormalities. Subtle autonomic dysfunction, such as lack of heart rate variability (9–11), is present in most patients. Episodes of severe bradycardia or hypotension may occur unrelated to hypoxia or hypoventilation (3). Swallowing dysfunction is frequently present (3, 9, 12, 13) and is a predisposing factor for aspiration. It improves with age. A few patients have been reported to have stridor (3, 14, 15). This may be due to lack of central augmentation of upper airway tone in response to hypoxia or hypercapnia (16). Other associated medical conditions include Hirschsprung disease (9, 14, 17–21), neural tumors (ganglioneuromas [22], neuroblastomas [20], and ganglioneuroblastomas [9, 23]), and minor ocular abnormalities (4).

The literature from the previous decade described a high rate of morbidity and mortality in children with CCHS (9, 14, 23, 24). Death usually resulted from cor pulmonale, aspiration, or sepsis. Recent reports from centers experienced with CCHS describe prolonged survival, with a good quality of life (3–5). Our oldest patient is currently 16 years of age. However, children continue to need ventilatory support, and do not "outgrow" their disease. In the three centers reporting long-term outcome in patients with CCHS, mortality was 0% (of 6 patients) (5), 7.7% (1 of 13 patients) (3), and 31% (10 of 32 patients) (4), respectively. Cor pulmonale, the commonest cause of death, can be prevented by providing adequate ventilatory support. Reversible episodes of pulmonary hypertension occur with infections or with hypoventilation due to inadequate ventilatory support (3, 5). Intelligence is usually in the normal or low-normal range, although some children are retarded; a few children are of above average intelligence (3, 5, 25). Hypoxemic episodes result in seizures or permanent neurologic damage (3, 5, 9, 12, 14, 19, 23). Early diagnosis of CCHS, with vigilant detection and correction of intermittent hypoxia, will help prevent neurologic sequelae.

The etiology of CCHS is not known. One theory is that it is due to a defect in neural crest migration (14, 20); hence the association with autonomic dysfunction, Hirschsprung disease, and neural tumors. An alternative hypothesis is that it is due to a defect in serotonin metabolism (9). CCHS has occasionally occurred in siblings and twins (9, 13, 18), although most cases do not appear to be genetic in origin (26, 27). No teratogens or perinatal risk factors have been determined; most infants with CCHS are born at term, following an uneventful pregnancy (3, 4).

Children with CCHS have decreased or absent ventilatory chemosensitivity in response to progressive hypoxia and hypercapnia during wakefulness and sleep (5, 9, 14, 23, 28–32). However, they do respond to acute hypoxia, hypercapnia, and hyperoxia (9, 14, 23, 29, 30, 33). They also arouse in response to progressive hyperoxic hypercapnia (34). Therefore, the primary physiologic defect in CCHS may be in the area of the brainstem where afferent impulses from the central and peripheral chemoreceptors are integrated. Pathologic and radiologic studies have not shown specific abnormalities (19, 35). Brainstem auditory evoked potentials have been reported to be normal in 16 of 17 children in one series (4), and to be mildly abnormal in 4 of 4 infants in another series (36).

OBESITY HYPOVENTILATION SYNDROME

The obesity hypoventilation syndrome (Pickwickian syndrome) occurs in morbidly obese children and adolescents (37). Its manifestations are similar to those described in adults. The syndrome can occur in patients with either primary obesity or obesity secondary to such conditions as hypothalamic disease or Prader Willi syndrome. Hypoventilation may be severe enough to result in cor pulmonale or respiratory failure (37, 38). In addition, morbidly obese patients are predisposed to other pulmonary problems, such as obstructive sleep apnea syndrome and restrictive lung disease (39). Patients with the obesity hypoventilation syndrome have decreased hypoxic and hypercapnic ventilatory drives. It is hypothesized that they have chronic hypoxia and hypercapnia due to mechanical limitation of ventilation, and therefore develop secondary blunting of their ventilatory drive (40–42). The ventilatory drive normalizes with weight loss. The amount of weight loss required for resolution of the obesity hypoventilation syndrome has not been established; however the level of hypercapnia has been shown to decline in proportion to the degree of weight loss (40).

ARNOLD-CHIARI MALFORMATION

Central hypoventilation occurs in association with both type I (43) and type II Arnold-Chiari malformations, as well as with hydrocephalus from other causes. The type I Arnold-Chiari malformation consists of caudal herniation of the cerebellar tonsils through the foramen magnum. The type II malformation consists of caudal displacement of the cerebellar vermis, brainstem, and fourth ventricle, and is associated with brainstem compression and/or dysplasia. It is present in the vast majority of patients with myelodysplasia. Patients with Arnold-Chiari malformations can have abnormalities ranging from subclinical abnormalities on pneumograms (44) to central apnea, cyanotic spells, and respiratory failure. Sudden, unexpected death during sleep may occur (45–47).

Children with Arnold-Chiari malformation have decreased ventilatory and arousal responses to hypercapnia (47, 48), suggesting an abnormality of central chemoreceptor function or of brainstem processing of central chemoreceptor signals. The hypoxic ventilatory response is usually intact (48), although it may be decreased in patients with glossopharyngeal nerve dysfunction and resultant carotid chemoreceptor dysfunction (49).

The incidence of clinical ventilatory control abnormalities or stridor has been reported to be between 6 and 13% (45, 46). However, even asymptomatic infants have subtle abnormalities of ventilatory control (47), and these abnormalities persist through adolescence (48). Although children with myelodysplasia may present with apnea soon after birth, they frequently do not become symptomatic until a later age. Severe breath-holding spells are common (50, 51), and are possibly secondary to vagal dysfunction or abnormal behavioral control of ventilation. The presence of ventilatory control abnormalities in patients with the Arnold-Chiari malformation are not necessarily associated with cognitive impairment (45, 46). Many patients with severe ventilatory control dysfunction have normal intellectual function, and can lead fulfilling lives once appropriate treatment is provided.

Children with myelodysplasia are predisposed to other pulmonary problems, such as restrictive lung disease, secondary to ventilatory muscle weakness or scoliosis. Bilateral vocal cord paralysis can occur as a result of traction on the vagal nerve roots, and can result in stridor, airway obstruction, and aspiration (51). Concomitant pharyngeal abnormalities can occur secondary to bulbar paralysis (52). These factors, combined with the central hypoventilation, place them at risk for aspiration, atelectasis, and pneumonia.

An increase in apnea or stridor frequently heralds an increase in intracranial pressure. If the child has a ventriculoperitoneal shunt in place, the functional status of the shunt should be assessed. "Croup" in children with myelomeningocele should always be regarded as a sign of increased intracranial pressure until proven otherwise. Previous studies have shown a high mortality rate in children with myelodysplasia and ventilatory control abnormalities (45). Wider recognition of the relationship between respiratory symptoms and increased intracranial pressure, and earlier treatment of respiratory complications, should lead to improved survival.

DYSAUTONOMIA

Patients with familial dysautonomia have abnormal control of ventilation (53, 54). Central hypoventilation has also been reported in a child with acquired dysautonomia secondary to a ganglioneuroma (55). During sleep, breathing is irregular (56, 57). In children with dysautonomia, hypercapnic ventilatory responses are moderately decreased, and hypoxic ventilatory responses are markedly decreased (53, 54). In addition, the normal cardiovascular response to hypoxia is absent. It has been postulated that the decreased ventilatory response to hypoxia is due to central hypoxic ventilatory depression resulting from diminished cerebral blood flow, rather than to abnormal chemoreceptor function (53). Hypoxia results in hypotension and relative bradycardia, and may be accompanied by seizures or syncope (54). Patients with dysautonomia are usually asymptomatic, but decompensate in the face of stress, such as a respiratory infection or a hypoxic environment. Deaths from hypoxia have been reported in patients who held their breath while swimming underwater (54).

MISCELLANEOUS CAUSES OF CENTRAL HYPOVENTILATION

Central hypoventilation can result from any congenital or acquired central nervous system lesion affecting the brainstem (58–64). Hypoventilation from these causes may occur during sleep only, or during both wakefulness and sleep. Central hypoventilation has been reported in conjunction with endocrine abnormalities, such as diabetes insipidus and hypothyroidism (65, 66). Presumably this is due to a hypothalamic defect that has not been localized.

Hypoventilation can also result from severe, diffuse central nervous system (60) or metabolic (67, 68) disease. Sedative drugs, especially narcotics, can cause temporary respiratory depression. Central hypoventilation occurs in patients with mitochondrial disorders (69–71). It may be a presenting sign in patients with Leigh disease, prior to the development of other gross neurologic abnormalities (personal experience, 72).

Diagnosis

The presence of hypoventilation can be established by arterial blood gas analysis, or noninvasively by polysomnography. Gas exchange should be assessed during both wakefulness and sleep. The hypoventilation can be assumed to be central in origin if tests of pulmonary function and ventilatory muscle strength are normal. Ventilatory responses to hypoxia and hypercapnia are abnormal in patients with central hypoventilation, but will also be abnormal in patients with mechanical limitation of ventilation. Techniques for ventilatory control testing are discussed in Chapter 11. Potential diagnostic tests are shown in Table 52.2; the choice of tests must be individualized for each patient. Magnetic resonance imaging of the brainstem and evaluation of diaphragmatic function are recommended for all patients with central hypoventilation of undetermined etiology. The diagnosis of CCHS is made primarily by exclusion, according to the following criteria: (a) persistent hypoventilation during sleep (PCO_2 consistently > 60 mm Hg), (b) onset of symptoms from birth or early infancy, and (c) absence

Table 52.2.
Diagnostic Evaluation of Suspected
Hypoventilation

Documenting hypoventilation
Arterial blood gas
Polysomnography

Establishing the etiology
Chest radiograph
Pulmonary function tests
Ventilatory responses to hypoxia and hypercapnia
Diaphragm fluoroscopy
Ventilatory muscle strength evaluation
   (transdiaphragmatic muscle strength, maximal and
   sustained inspiratory pressure measurement)
Fiberoptic laryngoscopy
Magnetic resonance imaging of brainstem
Brainstem auditory evoked potentials
Endocrine evaluation
Serum glucose, ammonia, pyruvate, lactate
Serum and urinary amino acids, organic acids

Assessing the severity
Hematocrit/hemoglobin
Serum bicarbonate
EKG, echocardiogram

of primary pulmonary, cardiac, neurologic, neuromuscular, or metabolic dysfunction (5, 28).

Treatment

Treatment depends on the severity of hypoventilation and the overall prognosis of the underlying condition. In the few patients with mild hypoventilation (mild hypercarbia, no pulmonary hypertension, normal growth, and good cognitive function), observation with close follow-up may be sufficient.

SPECIFIC THERAPY

Whenever possible, the primary cause of the hypoventilation should be treated. Patients with Arnold-Chiari malformation frequently improve following the relief of elevated intracranial pressure by ventriculoperitoneal shunting or posterior fossa decompression (43, 46, 51, 73). However, some patients with chronic or severe abnormalities may have irreversible dysplastic changes or necrosis of the brainstem (46, 51). Patients with airway compromise secondary to vocal cord paralysis should undergo tracheostomy if decompression procedures are unsuccessful. In patients with hypoventilation secondary to severe central nervous system dysfunction, palliative

treatment (e.g., supplemental oxygen) or no treatment may be preferable to invasive measures that will prolong life without enhancing the quality of life. However, supplemental oxygen alone should be administered with caution, since it may suppress the hypoxic ventilatory drive and therefore worsen hypoventilation. Obese patients will improve with weight loss, but this may be extraordinarily difficult to achieve. Hospital admission for supervised weight loss is justifiable in children with life-threatening hypoventilation.

PHARMACOLOGIC MANAGEMENT

A variety of drugs have been used in patients with central hypoventilation. Very few systematic studies have been performed, and it is difficult to derive recommendations based on isolated case reports. Oren et al. reported that two children with myelodysplasia, central apnea, and breath-holding spells responded to atropine (50). Hesz and Wolraich reported that children with myelodysplasia and breath-holding respond to acetazolamide, although details are not provided in the report (51). Progesterone has been used as a respiratory stimulant in adults with the obesity-hypoventilation syndrome (74). It was reported to be successful in the treatment of one child with this condition (38). Milerad et al. (75) demonstrated an improvement in two children with CCHS treated with progesterone. However, the children did not attain normal P_{O_2} or P_{CO_2} values, and long-term results were not reported. In other cases of CCHS, progesterone has been unsuccessful (9, 21). Drugs that have been tried in children with CCHS include doxapram, almitrine bimesylate, L-dopa, theophylline, caffeine, methylphenidate, dexedrine, pemoline, imipramine, progesterone, ACTH, naloxone, and acetazolamide; none has resulted in sustained improvement (9, 12–14, 18, 20, 21, 23, 24, 32, 76, 77). Thus, at this time, no drug has been shown to be effective in the treatment of central hypoventilation in children.

VENTILATORY SUPPORT

The mainstay of treatment for patients with CCHS, or those in whom the primary cause of hypoventilation cannot be successfully treated, is ventilatory support. Modern techniques for home ventilation enable these children and their families to lead fulfilling lives. Ventilatory support may be provided by positive pressure ventilation via tracheostomy or nasal mask, diaphragm pacing, or negative pressure cuirass ventilation. At this time, our preference is to initially stabilize infants using positive pressure ventilation via tracheostomy. At a later stage, the child can be considered for other modalities of ventilatory support. A tracheostomy is usually necessary in conjunction with diaphragm pacing or negative pressure ventilation, in order to prevent the occurrence of obstructive apnea (due to lack of synchronous activation of the upper airway and diaphragmatic muscles). Portable diaphragm pacers are especially useful for ambulatory children who require ventilatory support during wakefulness (3, 78). However, diaphragm pacers require bilateral thoracotomies for insertion, must be replaced as the child grows, cannot currently be used in children 24 hours a day with conventional techniques, and should be used only in a center with expertise in this technique. Positive pressure ventilation via nasal mask is a promising new technique that has been used successfully in children with central hypoventilation during sleep (79, 80).

It is our practice to hyperventilate children slightly during sleep, maintaining P_{CO_2} at 30–35 mm Hg and arterial oxygen saturation at > 95% (3, 81). This is to compensate for hypoventilation during wakefulness, and to provide physiologic leeway during respiratory infections. In addition, because children are more active at home than in the hospital, and because tracheostomy care and chest physical therapy are unlikely to be administered as thoroughly at home as in the hospital, it is likely that P_{CO_2} measurements obtained when the child is hospitalized are lower than the child's baseline at home. As ventilatory requirements change with age and growth, gas exchange and ventilatory support should be re-evaluated every 6–12 months or whenever there is a change in clinical status.

SUPPORTIVE CARE

Supportive care includes the prevention and treatment of atelectasis and pneumonia with chest physical therapy, bronchodilators, antibiotics, and influenza immunization. Good nutrition is essential. If persistent aspiration is present, gastrostomy feedings may be necessary. Sedative medications or anesthetic agents should not be administered unless appropriate monitoring and ventilatory support are available (66, 69–71). Parents should be warned of the potential dangers of hypoxic environments, such as underwater swimming (54) or high altitude. Patients should have an electrocardiogram and echocardiogram every 6–12 months, or whenever there is a deterioration in clinical status, in order to detect pulmonary hypertension.

Children with central hypoventilation frequently decompensate during minor illnesses, and develop insidious respiratory or cardiac failure. Parents and physicians should be alert for the presence of such subtle signs as pallor, lethargy, puffiness, or duskiness. However, as the children grow older, they tend to become more stable medically, and their parents became more familiar with their care, resulting in fewer hospitalizations.

VENTILATORY CONTROL AND CHRONIC LUNG DISEASE

Ventilatory drive varies widely in the normal population. It is largely determined by genetic factors (82–86). An individual with a congenitally low ventilatory drive may remain asymptomatic as long as the respiratory system is not stressed. However, if an asymptomatic individual with a congenitally low ventilatory drive develops lung disease, ventilation may not be increased in response to the stress. This can result in disproportionate hypoxia and/or hypercarbia (87–90). Patients with chronic lung disease and hypercapnia, such as patients with bronchopulmonary dysplasia or cystic fibrosis, may develop secondary blunting of their hypercapnic ventilatory drive.

CENTRAL HYPERVENTILATION

Hyperventilation usually occurs in response to a physiologic stimulus, such as hypoxia, metabolic acidosis, hypotension, or hyperthermia. Uncommonly, hyperventilation may be central in origin. Causes of central hyperventilation are listed in Table 52.3. Psychogenic hyperventilation will not be discussed in this section.

Hyperventilation Secondary to Neurologic Dysfunction

True central hyperventilation is rare. It is defined as hyperventilation associated with

Table 52.3.
Causes of Central Hyperventilation

Pain, anxiety, fear
Psychogenic hyperventilation
Salicylate toxicity
Brainstem tumor
Central nervous system lymphoma
Rett syndrome

normal or high P_{O_2}, low P_{CO_2}, and high pH, which persists during sleep (91). In adults, it has been reported most commonly secondary to central nervous system lymphomas (92). Most cases in children are secondary to brainstem tumors (91, 93–95). Central hyperventilation has been postulated to be due to direct mechanical effects on the respiratory centers, or possibly the production of a respiratory stimulant by the tumor. The hyperventilation may be extreme, with $P_{CO_2} < 10$ mm Hg (91, 94, 95). Narcotics have been used as palliative therapy (94, 96–98).

DISORDERED BREATHING

Disordered, irregular patterns of breathing may be seen in children with profound neurologic damage that is either diffuse or localized to the brainstem. The patient may have an erratic breathing pattern, central apnea, or Cheyne-Stokes ventilation. As with other ventilatory control disorders, these abnormalities may be more pronounced during sleep. Central causes of disordered breathing are listed in Table 52.4. No specific treatment is available. Supportive measures, such as cardiorespiratory monitoring, supplemental oxygen, or tracheostomy, may be indicated in selected cases.

There are a few rare disorders in which alternating bouts of tachypnea and central apnea occur (99, 100). These have been studied most extensively in Rett syndrome.

Table 52.4.
Causes of Disordered Breathing

Diffuse central nervous system damage from any cause

Syndromes with Tachypnea-apnea

Rett syndrome
Joubert syndrome (agenesis of the cerebellar vermis) (99, 100)
Mohr syndrome (99)
Dandy-Walker syndrome (99)

Rett Syndrome

Rett syndrome is a degenerative encephalopathy associated with autistic mannerisms, occurring in girls. The etiology is unknown. Typically, patients have cycles of hyperventilation, with resultant hypocapnia and central apnea (101–105). Severe hypoxia may ensue before spontaneous ventilation is resumed. It has been postulated that the abnormal ventilatory pattern is due to either (a) excessive stimulation of the brainstem respiratory center or (b) lack of cortical inhibition of ventilation, as an obsessive type of behavior or due to a physiologic defect (105). Breathing during sleep is normal, suggesting that the second explanation is the most likely. No treatment is currently available.

REFERENCES

1. Sugar O. In search of Ondine's curse. *JAMA* 1978; 240:236–237.
2. Rosenberg HS, Williams RL. Ondine's curse: A pathogenetic mechanism in pulmonary hypertension. *Arch Dis Child* 1975; 50:667A.
3. Marcus CL, Jansen MT, Poulsen MK, Keens SE, Nield TA, Lipsker LE, Keens TG. Medical and psychosocial outcome of children with congenital central hypoventilation syndrome. *J Pediatr* 1991; 119:888–895.
4. Weese-Mayer DE, Silvestri JM, Menzies LJ, Morrow-Kenny AS, Hunt CE, Hauptman SA. Congenital central hypoventilation syndrome: Diagnosis, management, and long-term outcome in thirty–two children. *J Pediatr* 1992; 120:381–387.
5. Oren J, Kelly DH, Shannon DC. Long-term follow-up of children with congenital central hypoventilation syndrome. *Pediatrics* 1987; 80:375–380.
6. Paton JY, Swaminathan S, Sargent CW, Hawksworth A, Keens TG. Ventilatory response to exercise in children with congenital central hypoventilation syndrome. *Am Rev Respir Dis* 1993; 147:1185–1191.
7. Shea SA, Andres LP, Banzett RB, Guz A, Shannon DC. The ventilatory response to exercise in the absence of CO_2 sensitivity. *Am Rev Respir Dis* 1991; 143:A194.
8. Weese-Mayer DE, Silvestri JM, Morrow AS, Conway LP, Barkov GA. Ventilatory recovery from exercise in children with congenital central hypoventilation syndrome. *Am Rev Respir Dis* 1991; 143:A799.
9. Haddad GG, Mazza NM, Defendini R, Blanc WA, Driscoll JM, Epstein MF, Epstein RA, Mellins RB. Congenital failure of automatic control of ventilation, gastrointestinal motility and heart rate. *Medicine* 1978; 57:517–526.
10. Woo MS, Woo MA, Gozal D, Jansen MT, Keens TG, Harper RM. Heart rate variability in congenital central hypoventilation syndrome. *Pediatr Res* 1992; 31:291–296.

respiratory failure. *Semin Respir Med* 1990; 11:269–281.

82. Beral V, Read DJC. Insensitivity of respiratory centre to carbon dioxide in the Enga people of New Guinea. *Lancet* 1971; 2:1290–1294.

83. Scoggin CH, Doekel RD, Kryger MH, Zwillich CW, Weil JV. Familial aspects of decreased hypoxic ventilatory response in endurance runners. *J Appl Physiol* 1978; 44:464–468.

84. Saunders NA, Leeder SR, Rebuck AS. Ventilatory response to carbon dioxide in young athletes: A family study. *Am Rev Respir Dis* 1976; 113:497–502.

85. Collins DD, Scoggin CH, Zwillich CW, Weil JV. Hereditary aspects of decreased hypoxic response. *J Clin Invest* 1978; 62:105–110.

86. Arkinstall WW, Nirmel K, Klissouras V, Milic-Emili J. Genetic differences in the ventilatory response to inhaled CO_2. *J Appl Physiol* 1974; 36:6–11.

87. Bayadi SE, Millman RP, Tishler PV, Rosenberg C, Saliski W, Boucher MA, Redline S. A family study of sleep apnea. *Chest* 1990; 98:554–559.

88. Mountain R, Zwillich C, Weil J. Hypoventilation in obstructive lung disease. *N Engl J Med* 1978; 298:521–525.

89. Hudgel DW, Weil JV. Asthma associated with decreased hypoxic ventilatory drive. *Ann Intern Med* 1974; 80:622–625.

90. Moore GC, Zwillich CW, Battaglia JD, Cotton EK, Weil JV. Respiratory failure associated with familial depression of ventilatory response to hypoxia and hypercapnia. *N Engl J Med* 1976; 295:861–865.

91. Plum F. Mechanisms of "central" hyperventilation. *Ann Neurol* 1982; 11:636–637.

92. Pauzner R, Mouallem M, Sadeh M, Tadmor R, Farfel Z. High incidence of primary cerebral lymphoma in tumor-induced central neurogenic hyperventilation. *Arch Neurol* 1989; 46:510–512.

93. Tinaztepe B, Tinaztepe K, Yalaz K, Aysun S. Microgliomatosis presenting as sustained hyperventilation. *Turk J Pediatr* 1981; 23:269–275.

94. Tobias JD, Heideman RL. Primary central hyperventilation in a child with a brainstem glioma: Management with continuous intravenous fentanyl. *Pediatrics* 1991; 88:818–820.

95. Suzuki M, Kawakatsu T, Komoshita S, et al. A case of pontine tumor associated with repeated episodes of hyperventilation and ketosis. *Paediatr Univ Tokyo* 1964; 10:58.

96. North JB, Jennett S. Abnormal breathing patterns associated with acute brain damage. *Arch Neurol* 1974; 31:338–344.

97. Jaeckle KA, Digre KB, Jones CR, Bailey PL, McMahill PC. Central neurogenic hyperventilation. *Neurology* 1990; 40:1715–1720.

98. Rodriguez M, Baele PL, Marsh HM, Okazaki H. Central neurogenic hyperventilation in an awake patient with brainstem astrocytoma. *Ann Neurol* 1982; 11:625–628.

99. Boltshauser E, Lange B, Dumermuth G. Differential diagnosis of syndromes with abnormal respiration (tachypnea-apnea). *Brain Dev* 1987; 9:462–465.

100. Friede RL, Boltshauser E. Uncommon syndromes of cerebellar vermis aplasia. *Dev Med Child Neurol* 1978; 20:758–763.

101. Glaze DG, Frost JD, Zoghbi HY, Percy AK. Rett's syndrome: Characterization of respiratory patterns and sleep. *Ann Neurol* 1987; 21:377–382.

102. Cirignotta F, Lugaresi E, Montagna P. Breathing impairment in Rett syndrome. *Am J Med Genet* 1986; 24:167–173.

103. Kerr A, Southall D, Amos P, et al. Correlation of electroencephalogram, respiration and movement in the Rett syndrome. *Brain Dev* 1990; 12:61–68.

104. Elian M, Rudolf N. EEG and respiration in Rett syndrome. *Acta Neurol Scand* 1991; 83:123–128.

105. Southall DP, Kerr AM, Tirosh E, Amos P, Lang MH, Stephenson JBP. Hyperventilation in the awake state: Potentially treatable component of Rett syndrome. *Arch Dis Child* 1988; 63:1039–1048.

106. Mador MJ, Tobin MJ. Apneustic breathing. A characteristic feature of brainstem compression in achondroplasia? *Chest* 1990; 97:877–883.

107. Nelson WF, Hecht JT, Horton WA, Butler IJ, Goldie WD, Miner M. Neurological basis of respiratory complications in achondroplasia. *Ann Neurol* 1988; 24:89–93.

108. Reid CS, Pyeritz RE, Kopits SE, et al. Cervicomedullary compression in young patients with achondroplasia. *J Pediatr* 1987; 110:522–530.

109. Stokes DC, Phillips JA, Leonard CO, et al. Respiratory complications of achondroplasia. *J Pediatr* 1983; 102:534–541.

110. Sudarshan A, Goldie WD. The spectrum of congenital facial diplegia (Moebius syndrome). *Pediatr Neurol* 1985; 1:180–184.

111. Gozal D, Colin AA, Daskalovic YI, Jaffe M. Environmental overheating as a cause of transient respiratory chemoreceptor dysfunction in an infant. *Pediatrics* 1988; 82:738–740.

53

Chest Trauma

DAVID F. WESTENKIRCHNER

Approximately 22,000 deaths per year in children less than 19 years of age are because of trauma (1). The great majority of trauma deaths are related to the severity of head injury, although other associated injuries such as thoracic and abdominal trauma contribute to the morbidity and mortality of trauma (Table 53.1). Chest trauma is less common in children than in adults. Children sustain thoracic trauma in a variety of ways including motor vehicle accidents, child abuse, falls, and less commonly violent trauma from a stab or gunshot wound. Mechanisms of thoracic trauma are differentiated as either blunt or penetrating, with blunt thoracic trauma related either to rapid deceleration or a direct blow to the chest. Although mechanisms of injury for thoracic trauma may be similar in adults and children, there are some physiologic differences that have bearing on management of thoracic trauma. Particularly in children less than 1 year of age the thorax is amazingly compliant, and injury to thoracic

contents may occur from compression without fracture of the bony thorax. The mediastinum in children can move freely within the thorax but is relatively fixed in adults, and therefore dislocation, compression, or angulation of structures within the mediastinum occurs more often in children, with pronounced cardiopulmonary consequences. Children sustain isolated thoracic trauma infrequently and usually have concurrent head injuries or abdominal injuries. Children tend to be free of pre-existing multisystem disease as compared to their adult counterparts. This review will concentrate on a discussion of blunt thoracic trauma as it occurs in children and will not review penetrating injuries, since they are not usually in the provence of the pediatric pulmonologist.

Blunt trauma commonly is categorized according to the following scheme for intrathoracic injury: (a) rib fractures with or without flail chest, (b) pulmonary contusion/laceration, (c) pneumothorax/hemothorax, (d) tracheobronchial disruption, and (e) diaphragmatic rupture (Table 53.2). Injuries to the heart and great vessels are not discussed in this review.

Table 53.1.
Thoracic Trauma: Diagnosis and Therapy

Sucking wounds: Seal at end expiration
Airway obstruction: Clear mechanically—intubate patient—
(be certain of stability of cervical spine)
Tension pneumothorax:
  Signs: Cyanosis, poor air entry, Shock
  Action: Needle aspiration, *then* chest tube
Pneumothorax: Chest tube
Hemothorax: Chest tube
Flail chest with/without pulmonary contusion: Intubation, ventilation, possibly PEEP
Ruptured bronchus:
  Signs: Fracture of 1st rib; mediastinal emphysema, poor expansion despite thoracostomy drainage
  Action: Increase drainage
       Surgical consultation

Table 53.2.
Types of Chest Trauma (94 Children)

Type	Percentage
Pulmonary contusion	62%
Pulmonary laceration	7%
Pneumo/hemothorax	16%
Fractured ribs (sole injury)	10%
Ruptured airway	6%

From Guyer B, Ellers B. Childhood injuries in the United States, mortality, morbidity and cost. *Am J Dis Child* 1990; 144: 649–652.

RIB FRACTURES

Rib fractures are a very common accompaniment of major thoracic injury. When present, they usually involve the posterolateral area of the ribs and are usually multiple. Multiple rib fractures most commonly involve the 7th–10th ribs. In younger children, significant thoracic compression may occur without accompanying rib fractures. The pain and the reflex muscle spasm associated with rib fractures can worsen hypoventilation and lead to retained secretions and subsequently pulmonary atelectasis. Adequate pain control is important in maintaining ventilation and stability of alveolar volume. The incidence of serious complications with injury to underlying structures increases with the number of ribs fractured. The greater the number of ribs fractured the greater the amount of force that has been applied to the thorax.

FLAIL CHEST

When multiple sequential ribs are fractured, each in two locations, the result can be a chest wall segment that is unstable and may move independently of the remaining thorax. Flail chest refers to the paradoxical expiratory expansion and inspiratory retraction of this unstable chest wall segment. With flail chest, mortality may be as high as 50% (2). Because of the pliability of the thorax, flail chest is much less common in the pediatric trauma patient, although the exact incidence is unknown. On physical examination the patient may demonstrate subcutaneous emphysema; in addition, there will be a palpable rib fracture and paradoxical motion of the involved segment with protrusion of the segment during expiration and retraction of the segment during inspiration. Therapy for flail chest may range from simple chest wall external stabilization and adequate analgesia and bronchial hygiene to elective intubation and controlled mechanical ventilation if respiratory failure exists. Pulmonary contusion of the parenchyma underlying the flail segment is a more serious component of the injury; in fact, some authors think that the pathophysiology of flail segment is related to the underlying contusion, rather than to the flail segment itself (3).

PULMONARY CONTUSION

Pulmonary contusion may occur to underlying pulmonary parenchyma without rib fractures or flail segment. The energy imparted to the chest wall and underlying pulmonary parenchyma by increasing intra-alveolar pressure can result in rupture of the alveolar-capillary interface and result in an intra-alveolar hemorrhage and alveolar pulmonary edema (4). This reduces ventilation to the affected lung parenchyma, and the resultant ventilation-perfusion inequality leads to arterial hypoxia. Pulmonary contusion may be more prevalent in the pediatric age group, wherein the pliable chest wall may allow greater transmission of energy to the underlying pulmonary parenchyma rather than being dissipated by fracturing the thoracic ribs. The region of the lung affected usually is localized to that area underneath the area of impact, but bilateral pulmonary contusions can occur in crush injuries. Chest radiographs will delineate the localized area of hazy density that is consistent with the hemorrhage, edema, or fluid-filled alveolar spaces. Therapy for pulmonary contusion is largely supportive. Because there has been disruption of the alveolar-capillary interface, aggressive fluid resuscitation may worsen edema formation in the injured lung. Fluid administration *should be guided by objective measurements of fluid balance* such as central venous pressure (CVP) or pulmonary capillary wedge pressure (PCWP) measurement (4). The degree of respiratory support should be dictated by the degree of respiratory insufficiency. This may range from supplemental oxygen for hypoxia to mechanical ventilation in patients who progress to respiratory failure. The application of positive end expiratory distending pressure may be helpful in reversing the hypoxia. In addition, pain control, particularly for the rib fractures, may improve lung mechanics and assist in clearance of retained secretions by allowing an improved cough. Widespread intraalveolar edema may develop in the noncontused lung. This may be associated with fluid overload from aggressive fluid resuscitation of the traumatized patient. In addition, the trauma patient is predisposed to adult respiratory distress syndrome and a host of factors, including leukocyte aggregation within the lung, vasoactive mediators, and immunomodulators, that may be involved in the development of widespread lung injury. The development of adult respiratory distress syndrome associated with trauma has been reviewed elsewhere.

PNEUMOTHORAX

The development of a simple pneumothorax is the most common injury noted in pediatric thoracic trauma (5). A pneumothorax occurs when air enters into the pleural space from the pulmonary parenchyma or airways. This can result from disruption of the lung parenchyma, a tear within the tracheobronchial tree, an esophageal rupture, or chest wall penetration. On physical examination there will be ipsilateral reduction of intensity of breath sounds with a shift of the trachea to the contralateral side. The ipsilateral chest is typically hyper-resonant to percussion and there may be associated subcutaneous emphysema. A chest radiograph should confirm the diagnosis. In an emergency, evacuation of the air may be necessary without obtaining a chest radiograph. When air progressively enters into the pleural space but cannot escape, intrapleural pressure will increase, creating a tension pneumothorax. As the tension increases, there is progressive mediastinal shift to the contralateral side and subsequent reduction of cardiac output. When a tension pneumothorax exists there is need for rapid evacuation of the retained air, either by immediate needle aspiration or chest tube insertion. Prompt aspiration of air is indicated for a pneumothorax that exceeds 25% even in the absence of tension pneumothorax (6).

HEMOTHORAX

Blood may be introduced into the pleural space from the pulmonary parenchyma, the chest wall, the great vessels, or the heart, creating a hemothorax. Physical examination findings consistent with a hemothorax include diminished ipsilateral breath sounds associated with a flat percussion note. If a large hemothorax has occurred, the findings will include those of systemic blood loss as well as respiratory distress. An upright chest radiograph will demonstrate blunting of the costophrenic angle or, if there is a hemopneumothorax, an air-fluid interface. A supine chest radiograph may demonstrate apical "capping" of fluid surrounding the superior pole of the lung or there may be a lateral extrapulmonary density consistent with fluid in the pleural space. If the hemothorax is so large that findings of systemic blood loss and hypovolemia are evident, therapy consists of aggressive fluid

resuscitation. Removal of the hemothorax should be by insertion of a thoracotomy tube. Removal of blood from the pleural space should allow expansion of the underlying lung and should not instigate further bleeding (4). Thoracotomy for direct control of bleeding may be necessary if bleeding and hypotension persist despite aggressive fluid resuscitative measures.

TRACHEOBRONCHIAL DISRUPTION

Rupture of the trachea or a bronchus in children as well as adults is rare, but appears to be increasing in incidence over the last 20 years (7). In addition, there may be more common recognition of this complication of thoracic trauma. For this injury to occur there usually must have been a severe compression injury of the chest or a very sharp blow to the anterior part of the neck. There have been reports of disruption of the tracheobronchial tree at all levels, although the majority of tears are within 2.5 cm of the carina (8). Rupture or tear within the tracheobronchial tree may occur by one of the following mechanisms. There may be a sudden forceful external posterior compression of the airway with a simultaneous expansion of the lungs; this may cause traction on the pericarinal structures with subsequent rupture or tearing. Secondly, there may be a reflex glottic closure at the moment of chest impact with a sudden increase in intrabronchial pressure with the resultant rupture. Lastly, there may be shearing forces that are produced at points of fixation of the airways because of a rapid deceleration injury (4). Ten percent of patients with tracheobronchial disruption are asymptomatic. The majority of patients will demonstrate some symptoms or findings typical of tracheobronchial disruption including subcutaneous emphysema, cutaneous hemorrhages noted about the face and chest, hemoptysis, dyspnea, and cough. Two distinct clinical forms of tracheobronchial disruption have been identified, according to whether or not there is free communication of the airway with the mediastinal pleura. When free communication exists a pneumothorax results; however, a chest tube insertion fails to reexpand the affected lung. In the absence of such free communication there is no pneumothorax or perhaps only a small pneumothorax, which will resolve with chest tube insertion. On rare occasion, chest radiographs allow visualization of disruptions within the normally smooth tracheobronchial walls. However, this is uncommon and the diagnosis usually is made on the basis of a persistent pneumothorax and a bronchoscopic demonstration of the disruption of the tracheobronchial tree. Acute, severe injury with a major disruption requires immediate surgical management for maintenance of a patent airway and evacuation of pleural air (7). Often the diagnosis is not suspected initially because the rupture is of a smaller airway or does not communicate freely with the mediastinal pleural. A diagnosis of tracheobronchial disruption should be entertained if the patient develops recurrent pneumonitis or atelectasis. These complication usually occur in an area distal to development of a stricture associated with a tracheobronchial tear.

REFERENCES

1. Guyer B, Ellers B. Childhood injuries in the United States, mortality, morbidity and cost. *Am J Dis Child* 1990; 144:649–52.
2. Pate JW. Chest wall injuries. *Surg Clin North Am* 1989; 69:59–70.
3. Craven KD, Oppenheimer L, Wood LDH. Effects of contusion and flail chest on pulmonary perfusion and oxygen exchange. *J Appl Physiol* 1979; 47:729–737.
4. Jackson J. Management of thoraco abdominal injuries. In Capan LM, Miller SM, Turndorf H, eds. *Trauma: Anesthesia and intensive care*. Philadelphia, JB Lippincott, 1991, pp 481–510.
5. Eichelberger MR, Randolph JG. *Thoracic trauma in children. Surg Clin North Am* 1981; 61:1181–1197.
6. Salzberg AM, Brooks JW, Krummel TM. Disorders of the respiratory tract due to trauma. In Chernick VC, Kendig EL, eds. *Disorders of the respiratory tract in children*. Philadelphia, WB Saunders, 1990, pp 976–991.
7. Pate JW. Tracheobronchial and esophageal injuries. *Surg Clin North Am* 1989; 69:111–123.
8. Kirsh MM, Orringer MB, Behrendt DM, Sloan H. Management of tracheobronchial disruption secondary to nonpenetrating trauma. *Ann Thorac Surg* 1976; 22:93–101.

PRINCIPLES OF THERAPY

54

Evaluating Clinical Trials

EDWARD N. PATTISHALL and J. HEYWARD HULL

One of the first randomized clinical trials reported in the literature was by the pulmonologist J.B. Amberson, Jr and colleagues in 1931 (1). After randomizing treatment groups by the flip of a coin, they found intravenous sanocrysin to be no more effective than intravenous distilled water for therapy of pulmonary tuberculosis. These negative results were important in guiding later research toward streptomycin in the treatment of tuberculosis, which was proven effective in a subsequent randomized trial (2). The subsequent streptomycin trial was one of the first investigations with design features reflective of modern scientific methods for evaluation of medical therapy. Along with sanocrysin, many other anecdotal therapies, such as mist tent therapy for patients with cystic fibrosis and tonsillectomy for patients with asthma, have succumbed to the objectivity of clinical trials.

Initially used to evaluate pharmaceutical products, clinical trial methodology was slowly accepted for use in trials of therapy for cancer and cardiovascular diseases in the 1950s and 1960s (3). Today, the randomized clinical trial is a prerequisite for the acceptance of most therapies. Unfortunately, despite these gains in experimental design, many pediatric pulmonologists continue to let anecdotal therapy determine clinical practice. In some instances, the lack of adequate data makes anecdotal therapy unavoidable; no level of understanding of scientific methods will solve the absence of data. For example, several modes of ventilation are available, but in almost all instances, no randomized clinical trials have been conducted to evaluate the efficacy of these different methods of ventilation.

A second, often more frustrating problem occurs when clinical trials exist, but may be inadequate, and interpretation of the findings is problematic. In this setting, greater knowledge of scientific methods can be extremely helpful to the clinician in understanding the strengths and limitations of published clinical studies. Accordingly, the purpose of this chapter is to discuss the appropriate evaluation of clinical trials to determine if the data are adequate and should be applied in clinical practice.

COMPONENTS OF CLINICAL TRIALS

Given the importance of sound clinical trial methodology, it is important to recognize the strengths and limitations of particular experimental methods to satisfy oneself that the conclusions from an article are warranted. Spilker has reviewed a number of guidelines published to help evaluate clinical trials in the medical literature (4). Some guidelines are rather extensive; however, several key components are common and are discussed below.

Purpose of the Study (Objective)

Every study should have a major research question (primary objective) clearly defined and stated in advance. If the question is not relevant to the reader, then no further evaluation of the study may be necessary. If the question is relevant, the study should be designed to efficiently answer that question. The structure and the size of the trial should be determined by the primary objective.

Study design

METHODOLOGY AND MEASUREMENTS

In the pure sense, the study design includes all experimental elements of a trial. Randomization is the first (and cornerstone) of two essential features of well-designed studies. The second is inclusion of a concurrent control group to permit an objective comparison. Studies without a control group and without random allocation to treatment groups often have fatal biases. These trials are not only difficult to interpret, they may actually steer the reader to an incorrect therapeutic regimen.

When study measurements are subjective (e.g., signs and symptoms), the patient treatment assignment should be masked (blinded) for both the investigator and the patient. This limits the potential for accidental or deliberate bias in interpretation of response to treatment and ensures that each patient is managed during the trial in a uniform manner. For some objective measurements (e.g., death, blood chemistry values, antibody titers) open or unblinded trials may be acceptable, although not ideal. When treatment is unblinded, the patient must be enrolled in the study before the assigned treatment group is known, to prevent selection bias by the investigator. In addition, both groups should undergo the same study procedures and be handled similarly, other than the specific therapy being studied, to ensure that subsequent response differences seen in the study can be attributed to the test treatment. The study outcome measures used should be appropriate to the research question and need to be well defined in advance, including how the data will be statistically analyzed. The measures should be objective whenever possible and accurate (or at least precise).

TREATMENT STRUCTURE

In addition to experimental elements, the term "study design" is often used to refer to the treatment structure or architecture of the study. The most common treatment structure used in trials today has two or more groups of patients who are assigned and remain in separate treatment groups (parallel group design) (5). Because all groups are treated equally and at the same time, this design is considered to be the most scientifically valid. The major disadvantage of this design is that large patient-to-patient variability often necessitates a large sample size and stratification of patients. An example of this design would be a study comparing the response to inhaled steroids versus placebo in two groups

of asthmatic patients, one of whom receives only inhaled steroids and the other group received only placebo (Fig. 54.1A).

In other studies, the treatment assignment is switched during the course of the study so that the patient receives each of the treatments being compared in the trial (crossover design) (6). Because the patient serves as his own control, study efficiency is increased and a smaller sample size is required. This design should not be used when the disease is episodic in nature or varies in severity, or if it is likely that patients will drop out of the study. An example of this approach would be a study comparing the effectiveness of two antihistamines in perennial allergic rhinitis, in which the patient is administered one antihistamine for half the period in the study and another antihistamine for the second half of the trial (Fig. 54.1B).

A third design used more frequently in the past is the self-controlled (before-and-after) design (6). With this design, a patient serves as his own control, and changes in measurements taken before and after therapy are considered the treatment effect. Because there is no concurrent control, and blinding is not feasible, this design is considered less acceptable and

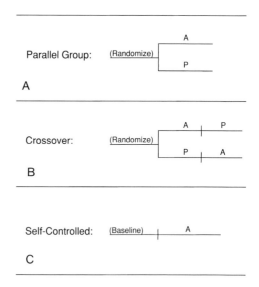

Figure 54.1. Schematic diagrams of three common study designs (treatment structures) used in clinical trials: *A,* Parallel. *B,* Cross-over. *C,* Self-controlled. In these examples, treatment A = active drug, and treatment P = placebo.

thus, is used less today. Dose-response and dose-titration studies of inhaled bronchodilators often use this design, with comparisons made to baseline or the response to the previous dose (Fig. 54.1C). Pivotal trials for drug efficacy usually do not use a before-and-after design.

The self-controlled design should not be confused with a parallel-group design wherein before and after measurements are performed, but there is a concurrent control group. This study design is used often in studies of patients with cystic fibrosis or other diseases in which there is large variability of outcome measures between patients. This is a well-accepted, rigorous design that allows comparisons of within-in-patient changes, which are often less variable than the values obtained before and after treatment.

Subjects

The subjects should be from a representative (appropriate and well-defined) population. Recruitment methods (and if practical, the patients not enrolled in the trial) should be discussed to help the reader appreciate the generalizability of study findings to a particular clinical setting. Both treatment groups should be selected during the same period and at the same location. How well the results of the study apply to broader patient populations (generalizability) depends on how similar the original population is to the general population, and how the subjects were selected. As an obvious example, if a study was conducted in severe, refractory patients with asthma in an intensive care unit of a teaching institution, the results may not be applicable to patients with milder disease in the setting of a small community hospital.

Bias

Bias is a systematic error (distortion) incorporated in either the design or the analysis of a trial. Systematic bias can fatally flaw a trial. Some instances of bias can be determined by common sense, whereas others are hard to recognize, especially from the limited data available in publications. Systematic bias should not be confused with chance (random) error such as occurs when two treatment groups differ in one or more baseline variables despite randomization, although in the litera-

ture this is sometimes called bias. Current statistical methods can usually adjust for bias due to chance imbalance of a known prognostic factor, but usually cannot adjust for systematic bias.

Sackett has described 57 examples of bias in the medical literature (7). The most common systematic errors occur because of preferential selection of patients (selection bias), preferential execution of therapy between groups (treatment bias), and consistently distorted measurements of outcome (measurement bias). The situation in an unblinded trial where the investigator might preferentially assign sicker patients to the active treatment would be an example of selection bias. If one treatment group had their drugs administered by the study nurse and the other group by the physician investigator, there would be a significant potential for treatment bias. Finally, if different scales were used to record weights of patients in the two treatment groups, there would be a potential for measurement bias.

Randomization into treatment groups that are unknown (blinded) to the patient and the investigators is essential for helping to eliminate selection and measurement bias. Treating the groups in a similar fashion helps to control treatment bias. Although randomization, blinding, and similar treatment of groups may be stated in the methodology of the study, compliance with the protocol should also be assessed to evaluate the possibility of bias.

Statistical Issues

There are numerous articles and books that describe appropriate statistical evaluations for different situations, and these will not be discussed here. However, some common issues or problems involving statistics are mentioned.

SAMPLE SIZE

A sample size calculation should be included in the experimental methods of the study with a definition of the magnitude of treatment effects to be detected (i.e., considered clinically meaningful or important). With many published trials, the actual probability of detecting a difference between therapies, assuming a true difference exists (the power of the study), is often small. For studies with negative findings, power calculations should be presented to enable the reader to interpret fairly the strength of the evidence being presented. Treatment effects that are not statistically different may not be statistically the same, or, as noted by Sackett, "... absence of proof, is not proof of absence" (8). For example, vigorous cough and chest physiotherapy were found to result in similar increases in maximal expiratory flows in a study of nine patients with cystic fibrosis (9). The authors concluded, "Because there was no clear-cut benefit of chest physiotherapy over cough alone ... cough is an attractive alternate method of treatment." Even with each subject serving as his or her own comparison, the small sample size gives only a 55% chance (slightly more than the odds in a coin flip) of detecting a difference of one standard deviation of the test. In this example, one standard deviation for change in FEV_1 from baseline was 17%. Thus, there was only a 55% chance of detecting a difference if one group had a 17% greater change in FEV_1 than the other group.

A nomogram relating power, total study size, standardized difference, and significance level for comparisons of continuous variables is shown in Figure 54.2. The standardized difference is the change one wants to detect

divided by the estimated standard deviation. For example, if the investigator wishes to detect a 10% change of FEV_1 where the mean FEV_1 is 2.0 (i.e., 0.2 L) and the standard deviation is 1.0 L, the standardized difference would be 0.2 (0.2 L divided by 1.0 L). Using the nomogram, a study with the power to detect such a difference 90% of the time (power of 0.9) would require about 1000 patients using a significance level of 0.05.

MULTIPLE COMPARISONS

The more comparisons made between groups, the higher the probability that one of the comparisons will yield a statistically significant result. It is not uncommon to see many variables compared between groups. When this is done using t-tests, a multiple comparison technique should be employed, such as the bonferonni correction or Tukey HSD test (10). A more subtle form of multiplicity occurs when the accumulating data from a trial are repeatedly analyzed, without adjusting for this in the analysis. Thus, if interim analyses are performed, the significance level used for the final analysis should be adjusted (11).

REGRESSION TOWARD THE MEAN

Just by random chance, some values from an assessment will be higher or lower than the rest of the group. If patients with extreme values are selected as a subgroup to evaluate a second time, repeated measurements in these patients will tend to have values more toward the mean of the original population (12). This may incorrectly be construed as a treatment effect. For example, if patients are selected because their FEV_1 is below 80% of predicted, some of those values will be decreased (at that particular time) because of random variation rather than disease. Subsequent tests in these patients will have a mathematical tendency to be closer to normal, which may incorrectly be interpreted as clinical improvement. This phenomenon is a particular problem when self-controlled designs are used, because of the lack of a concurrent control group.

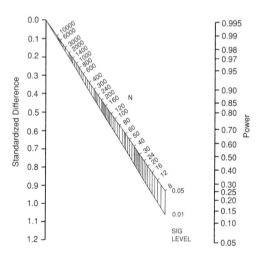

Figure 54.2. Nomogram for a two-sample comparison of a continuous variable, relating power, total study size, the standardized difference, and significance level. (From Altman DG. Statistics and ethics in medical research. III. How large a sample? *Br Med J* 1980; 281:1336–1338.)

CAUSALITY VS. ASSOCIATION

Although two factors must be associated to be causal, not all associations are causal. Although it is the intent of investigators to prove causality by associating a result with a treatment, bad study design may identify associations not directly related to the treatment. Unfortunately, associations can be the result of bias, or can occur indirectly through another factor (confounding). The association is more plausible when there are consistent results between studies, dose-response relationships, or when the association is very strong. However, some of the biases may persist between studies, and the randomized clinical trial is only one piece of supporting evidence of causality that should also be examined for biologic plausibility. The issue of potential confounding is particularly difficult, since there are often a number of factors associated with the true cause, and therefore associated with the outcome, and thus appear to be causal.

APPLYING PREDICTIVE MODELS DERIVED FROM ONE POPULATION TO OTHER POPULATIONS

It is common to see mathematical models derived from a study that accurately predict an outcome for patients in that study. The clinically relevant question is how well these equations predict outcome when applied to another group with the same disease. For example, a study in patients with adult respiratory distress syndrome (ARDS) found that discriminate analysis correctly identified 95% of survivors and 95% of nonsurvivors using five physiologic and laboratory parameters (13). But, when applied to a second group of ARDS patients, the mortality in predicted nonsurvivors was 81% and survival in predicted survivors was 60%. Thus, the results of a mathematical model derived from a population always need to be validated in another group of patients to evaluate its true utility and should be expected to do less well in its reliability.

CONCLUSIONS AND LIMITATIONS OF CLINICAL TRIALS

After the experimental design of the trial and the quality of the data is evaluated, the next issue to consider is whether the conclusions can be accepted or rejected. Were the interpretations and conclusions of the study justified? Often some of the conclusions can be accepted while others are rejected. Were the

patients and methods evaluated similar to patients and methods applicable in other settings—that is, are the results generalizable to other patients? In order to answer specific questions, clinical trials often use specific methodology or equipment that may not be practical for many clinicians. For example, a particular nebulizer used in a study may not be readily available to patients. Another example is a study comparing an intravenous and oral therapy in patients with COPD, where both groups are hospitalized to avoid bias. However, the oral therapy will normally be used in outpatients, and the results may differ in that setting.

A common error in interpreting the results of a clinical trial is to confuse statistical significance with clinical significance. Statistical tests address the question concerning the probability that findings in a study are real, not whether they are important. There is an inverse relationship of the number of subjects in a study and the magnitude of change (treatment effect) that is statistically significant. Thus, a very large study may find small, clinically unimpressive changes to be statistically significant. For example, a study with a large number of patients may find that a therapy improves FEV_1 by 3%, but clinically such a change, although a real effect, would be unimportant.

No clinical trial is perfect, and studies should not be totally discredited because of some limitations of the study. The limitations must be weighed against how the results may have been influenced. A potential bias may not be important enough to influence the outcome of the study. And in some cases, biases inherent in the study are acknowledged, but technically or ethically cannot be overcome. For example, a treatment requiring a surgical procedure may not be appropriate for a placebo group. In this instance, the study design should minimize known potential biases by randomization to treatment groups and using objective outcome measures, which should be influenced less in an unblinded study. In other instances, the study may have limitations, but may offer the only data available. In this case, the data need to be interpreted intelligently, but with caution. An example of this situation is a five-patient crossover study conducted in patients with systemic mastocytosis, a rare disease, that demonstrated the efficacy of oral disodium cromoglycate (14).

Not all clinically important questions can be answered by clinical trials (15). Some example situations include trials that are cost-prohibitive, require too long a follow-up period (e.g., studies of effects of treatment to offspring), unethical (e.g., trials in pregnant women to study the teratogenicity of drugs), or diseases in which there may be too few patients with a particular disease to study (e.g., idiopathic pulmonary alveolar microlithiasis or pulmonary alveolar proteinosis). Despite these limitations, the randomized clinical trial is here to stay and the experimental design of clinical trials continues to evolve and improve. Even if the clinician has no plans to serve as a study investigator for future trials, clinicians need to understand the strengths and limitations of data provided by clinical trials to maximally utilize the literature.

REFERENCES

1. Amberson JB Jr, McMahon BT, Pinner M. A clinical trial of sanocrysin in pulmonary tuberculosis. *Am Rev Tuberc* 1931; 24:401–435.
2. Streptomycin in Tuberculosis Trials Committee, Medical Research Council. Streptomycin treatment of pulmonary tuberculosis: A Medical Research Council investigation. *Br Med J* 1948; 2:767–782.
3. *The impact of randomized clinical trials on health policy and medical practice: Background paper.* Washington, DC, US Congress, Office of Technology Assessment, OTA-BP-H-22, August 1983.
4. Spilker B. Systems of evaluating published data. In Spilker B, ed. *Guide to clinical interpretation of data.* New York, Raven Press, 1986, pp 301–325.
5. Lavori PW, Louis TA, Bailar JC, Polansky M. Designs for experiments—Parallel comparisons of treatment. *N Engl J Med* 1983; 309:1291–1299.
6. Louis TA, Lavori PW, Bailar JC, Polansky M. Designs for experiments—Parallel comparisons of treatment. *N Engl J Med* 1984; 310:24–31.
7. Sackett DL: Bias in analytical research. *J Chronic Dis* 1979; 32:51–63.
8. Sackett DL. The competing objectives of randomized trials. *N Engl J Med* 1980; 303:1059–1060.
9. De Boeck C, Zinman R: Cough versus chest physiotherapy. A comparison of the acute effects on pulmonary function in patients with cystic fibrosis. *Am Rev Respir Dis* 1984; 129:182–184.
10. Wallenstein S, Zucker CL, Fleiss JL. Some statistical methods useful in Circulation Research. *Circ Res* 1980; 47:1–9.
11. McPherson K. Statistics: The problem of examining accumulating data more than once. *N Engl J Med* 1974; 290:501–502.
12. Oldham PD. A note on the analysis of repeated measurements of the same subjects. *J Chron Dis* 1962; 15:969–977.
13. Gottlieb JE, McKee L, Kubis JM, Burns JR, Machiedo G, Gee M, Fish J. Individual patient outcome in adult respiratory distress syndrome (ARDS): Prediction and validation by discriminant analysis from a multicenter registry. *Am Rev Respir Dis* 1991; 143:A676.
14. Soter NA, Austen KF, Wasserman SI. Oral disodium cromoglycate in the treatment of systemic mastocytosis. *N Engl J Med* 1979; 301:465–469.
15. Feinstein AR. An additional basic science for clinical medicine: II. The limitations of randomized trials. *Ann Intern Med* 1983; 99:544–550.

Appendix 54.1
Sample Size Calculations

Total sample size required when using the t-test to compare means of continuous outcome variables:

$$\text{Total sample size} = \frac{4(Z_\alpha + Z_\beta)^2 \, (\text{Std. Dev.})^2}{\text{Absolute Difference}}$$

Where

Z_α = 1.96 for a two-tailed α = 0.05 or a one-tailed α = 0.025
Z_β = 0.842 for β = 0.2, Z_β = 1.282 for β = 0.1
Std. Dev. = standard deviation of the control sample
Absolute Difference = smallest absolute difference between the two study groups thought important to detect.

Total sample size required when using the z statistic to compare proportions of dichotomous outcome variables:

$$\text{Total sample size} = \frac{\left[Z_\alpha \sqrt{4P(1-P)} + Z_\beta \sqrt{2P_1(1-P_1) + 2P_2(1-P_2)}\right]^2}{(P_1 - P_2)^2}$$

Where n, Z_α, and Z_β are as defined above, and

$$P = \frac{(P_1 + P_2)}{2}$$

P_1 = the smallest proportion developing the disease in the exposed study group that one considers important to detect.
P_2 = the proportion expected to develop the disease in the unexposed control group.

55

Aerosol Delivery Systems

BETH L. LAUBE

In recent years, aerosol therapy for respiratory diseases has gained acceptance as an alternative to oral or parenteral therapy because of the ability to administer smaller doses of drug, with a more rapid onset of action and a lower incidence of systemic side effects. These advantages derive from drug being deposited directly in the lung. Systemic absorption of drugs via the oropharynx or airways and their subsequent redistribution to the lungs via the circulation plays only a minor role in the effect of inhaled drugs (1–3).

To achieve a full therapeutic effect, an adequate amount of the inhaled drug must be deposited in the lungs. However, the precision of delivering aerosolized drug to the lungs is limited by physical parameters of the aerosol particle, breathing maneuvers, and airway patency. Knowledge of how these factors affect deposition of inhaled particles in adults has been obtained from aerosol deposition experiments, but ethnical issues have limited the number of such studies in children and adolescents. Therefore, much of our knowledge concerning aerosol deposition in children is extrapolated from studies in adults or from predictive models of aerosol behavior within the growing human lung.

DETERMINANTS OF AEROSOL DEPOSITION IN THE HUMAN RESPIRATORY TRACT

It is often assumed that dose delivered to the lungs is determined primarily by the output of the aerosol generator. Although it is true that output may vary considerably between generators, particularly nebulizer generators (4–5), and this variability affects the dose of aerosol available for inhalation, other factors are more important determinants of dose

delivered. Aerosol particle size, aerosol velocity, and inspiratory flow rate determine how much of the inhaled dose penetrates beyond the nasopharynx (or oropharynx if mouth-breathing), whereas breathholding and the degree of airway patency combine with these factors to determine the site of deposition within the lungs.

Aerosol Particle Size

The particles of a given therapeutic aerosol are heterodisperse, which means they vary in size. The mass median aerodynamic diameter (MMAD) is used to describe the particle size distribution of heterodisperse aerosols. MMAD is the size such that 50% of the mass of the aerosol is contained within larger particles and 50% within smaller particles. According to a standard model of aerosol deposition, particles < 5 μm deposit predominantly in the tracheobronchial and pulmonary zones of the lung, whereas particles > 5 μm have their peak deposition in the nasopharynx (or oropharynx if mouth-breathing) (6). Particles < 5 μm are therefore defined as within the respirable range. Figures 55.1 and 55.2 show the effect of particle size on the fraction of aerosol deposited in the lungs of two adult subjects. When an aerosol consisting of 10 μm particles was inhaled, only 4% of the deposited fraction was in the lower airways (below the larynx) (Fig. 55.1). The remainder deposited in the oropharynx. In contrast, approximately 85% of the deposited fraction of an aerosol consisting of smaller particles (MMAD = 1.12 μm) was deposited in the lungs (Fig. 55.2). Although aerodynamic diameter is a useful parameter for predicting deposition site within the human respiratory tract, the particle size distribution of therapeutic aerosols is

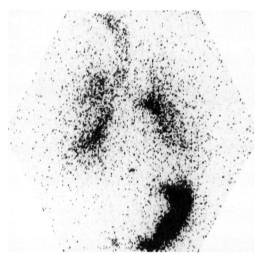

Figure 55.1. Anterior gamma camera scan of the lungs of a normal subject following inhalation of an aerosol consisting of 10-μm monodisperse particles, generated by a spinning top generator from a technetium-labeled saline solution. (From Bowes SM, Laube BL, Links JM, Frank R. Regional deposition of inhaled fog droplets: Preliminary observations. *Environ Health Perspect* 1989; 79:151–157.

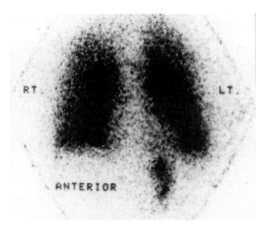

Figure 55.2. Anterior gamma camera scan of the lungs of an asymptomatic asthma patient following inhalation of a heterodisperse aerosol (MMAD = 1.12 μm), generated by a raindrop nebulizer (Puritan Bennett) from a technetium-labeled saline solution. Forced expiratory volume in one second (FEV_1 at the time of aerosol inhalation was 83% of predicted. (From Labue BL, Swift DL, Wagner HN, Norman PS, Adams GK III. The effect of bronchial obstruction on central airway deposition of a saline aerosol in patients with asthma. *Am Rev Respir Dis* 1986; 133:740–743.

dynamic. Size characteristics may be altered after leaving the generator or may change upon entering the airways. Therefore, it is best to estimate size distribution during simulations of inspiration.

Aerosol Velocity and Inspiratory Flow Rate

Particles > 1 μm deposit by inertial impaction in regions of the respiratory tract where airflow velocity is high and changes direction rapidly. For this reason, inertial impaction of aerosol particles occurs predominantly in the nasopharynx (or oropharynx if mouth breathing) and at bifurcations in the larger, central airways. When jet nebulizers and metered dose inhalers (MDIs) are placed directly in the mouth, a significant fraction of the inertial impaction of particles in the oropharynx is due to high aerosol velocities at the mouthpiece (7, 8). The use of a spacer device in conjunction with an MDI or nebulizer (see spacers below) reduces aerosol velocity and oropharyngeal impaction. Inspiratory flow rates < 60 L/min also reduce impaction at these sites and improve deeper penetration into the smaller airways (9–13).

Breathholding

Particles > 0.5 μm that penetrate to the smaller airways deposit by sedimentation as the result of gravity. Breathholding for up to 10 seconds enhances the residence time, and so increases deposition (14). Particles less than 0.5 μm in size deposit primarily by diffusion beyond the terminal bronchioles.

Airway Patency

Impaction of aerosol particles is enhanced in airways that have become narrowed as the result of bronchoconstriction, edema, or increased mucus because airflow velocity has increased. (13,15). In patients with mucus plugs, aerosol particles may not penetrate beyond the obstruction. Figure 55.3 shows the effect of bronchial obstruction on aerosol deposition within the lungs. In this severely obstructed asthma patient, the distribution of aerosol (MMAD = 1.12 μm) is extremely uneven, with greater deposition in the larger, central airways and little penetration to the lung periphery. Contrast this distribution with the homogeneous deposition pattern for the

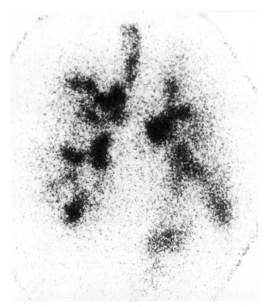

Figure 55.3. Anterior gamma camera scan of the lungs of a severely obstructed asthma patient following inhalation of a heterodisperse aerosol (MMAD = 1.12μm), generated by a raindrop nebulizer (Puritan Bennett) from a technetium-labeled saline solution. FEV_1 at the time of aerosol inhalation was 36% of predicted. (From Laube BL, Swift DL, Wagner HN, Norman PS, Adams GK III. The effect of bronchial obstruction on central airway deposition of a saline aerosol in patients with asthma. *Am Rev Respir Dis* 1986; 133:740–743.

patient with normal pulmonary function shown in Figure 55.2. In some cases, inhalation of a bronchodilator may decrease airway narrowing and thereby improve subsequent aerosol distribution beyond sites of obstruction.

Age

Equations based on the structural components of the lung and ventilation conditions as a function of age have been derived to predict aerosol deposition in the developing lung. Knight and associates (16) calculated deposition of aerosolized ribavirin using equations from Hofmann et al. (17) and Yu and Xu (18) and found that total and regional dosage was higher for infants and children than for adults. Recent in-vivo studies also indicate a tendency for greater deposition in children compared to adults (19). Becquemin et al. (19) found that this tendency was significant for 1- and 2-μm aerosol particles in children younger than 8 years, and Schiller et al. (20) reported similar findings for children aged 7–16 years.

With some nebulizers, the concentration of aerosolized drug per unit volume of inspired air can be greater in very young children (< 6 months) compared to older children (21). This is because older children inspire at higher flow rates, resulting in greater entrainment of room air through the nebulizer and consequent dilution of the aerosol. Because deposition fraction and drug concentration may be greater in children, adult doses of aerosolized drugs should be given to children on an adjusted basis, perhaps as a function of body weight (21).

AEROSOL GENERATION AND DELIVERY EQUIPMENT

MDIs

MDIs are small, pressurized canisters that contain drug either in suspension or in solution with propellants. Hiller et al. (22) and Kim et al. (23) report MMAD between 2.8–4.3 and 4.9–5.5 μm, respectively, for various MDIs after "aging" of aerosol under conditions of ambient humidity. These data suggest that MDI aerosol particles are within the respirable range. However, incomplete evaporation of the propellants that coat the drug particle or the presence of nonvolatile surfactants may result in significantly larger suspension droplets (24). Slowly evaporating ethanol (a co-solvent) may also result in larger solution droplets (24). The large effective size of the particles and the high velocity of the aerosol spray as it leaves the canister (may exceed 50 m/second) combine to deliver, on average, approximately 10% of the aerosol dose to the lungs (25–28). Approximately 10% of the dose remains on the actuator, and 80% is deposited in the oropharynx and swallowed (24).

There are currently two techniques recommended to achieve optimal delivery of aerosol by MDI. These techniques were derived from experiments that determined the inhalation manuevers that maximized bronchodilator response (29) or aerosol dose to the lungs (28). First, the cap is removed and the canister shaken thoroughly. The canister should be upright. According to Newman et al. (29), the patient should breathe out fully, place the canister between the lips, and fire the inhaler slowly and deeply. A 10-second breathhold should follow. Patients with respiratory disorders who are not able to hold their breath for that long should be encouraged to hold their breath for as long as possible. At least 1 minute should pass before taking a second dose. Dolovich et al. (28) recommends placing the canister 3–4 cm in front of the open mouth and firing the inhaler while inhaling from functional residual capacity (FRC) for 3–5 seconds. The time of the breathhold and the time between doses is similar to that recommended by Newman et al. (29). Some studies have demonstrated that bronchodilatation and deposition in the lungs are significantly higher with the open-mouth technique (30–32). However, the open-mouth technique requires accurate alignment of the MDI in front of the mouth, which may be difficult for children. Poor aim on the part of the child could result in drug deposited on the face or in the eyes.

Although an MDI appears simple to use, simultaneous coordination of inhalation and actuation of the aerosol, which may be difficult for many young patients, is essential for effective drug delivery. Newman et al. (33) showed that this coordination is necessary for the therapuetic effect of inhaled bronchodilators, and it is likely an important determinant of the treatment outcome for other aerosolized medications. Nevertheless, a significant percentage of patients (especially children) are incapable of this coordinated effort, are never instructed as to proper inhaler technique, misunderstand the directions, or forget the instructions. Common mistakes that patients make when instruction has been omitted in the use of an MDI device are failure to take the cap off of the inhaler before use, holding the inhaler upside down, failure to shake the canister before use, and failure to synchronize aerosol release with inhalation (34–36). In a recent study (37), only 32% of a group of 25 children (ages 7.5–18 years) who had received formal instruction in the use of their inhaler inhaled slowly and deeply. Only 48% activated the inhaler and inhaled simultaneously, and only 44% held their breath for 10 seconds. Approximately half of the children had not been observed using their inhalers after the initial education process. Other studies have reported that only 46% and 57%, respectively, of children use their inhalers correctly (38, 39). To achieve the maximum benefit from aerosolized medications, it is clear that children should be carefully instructed in the use of an MDI and should be checked periodically for inhaler technique.

Spacers

In an attempt to overcome the problems associated with coordination of inhalation and aerosol release, spacer devices (also known as holding chambers and extension tubes) have been developed. A spacer allows the discharge of aerosol from an MDI into a chamber where particles are suspended for a few seconds. Then, the patient inhales, with no coordination necessary. During the time in the chamber, large particles sediment from the mist and propellant evaporates. This leads to an overall reduction in aerosol particle size. Spacers also add distance between the actuator and the patient's mouth, which allows the aerosol particles to slow down before reaching the mouth. A reduction in aerosol particle size and aerosol velocity results in decreased oropharyngeal deposition (40–42). Kim et al. (43) have demonstrated that various spacer devices reduce oropharyngeal deposition to 6% or less.

Reducing oropharyngeal deposition is particularly important for minimizing oral candidiasis in patients who inhale high doses of steroids (44). With high doses, following the standard instruction of rinsing out the mouth with water after each MDI adminisration may not be adequate to decrease the amount of retained drug to levels that prevent the occurrence of oral candidiasis. For this reason, Toogood recommends the use of a spacer for those patients who need more than 800 µg of inhaled steroid a day (45).

The use of a spacer is also recommended for the delivery of bronchodilators in pediatric patients who have difficulty using MDIs correctly. A recent study compared the efficacy of a bronchodilator administered with and without a spacer in preventing exercise asthma in children with good versus unsatisfactory MDI inhaler technique (46). The authors found that children who use good technique did not benefit from the addition of a spacer, whereas all the children with poor technique required a spacer to achieve the full therapeutic benefit. Other studies have shown that the use of a spacer enhances the effective delivery of bronchodilators, even in very young children (47–49). Simple instructions for the use of an MDI with and without a spacer are shown in Figure 55.4.

Spacers that are currently available in the United States include Aerochamber (rigid

Correct Use of a Metered-Dose Inhaler *

Steps for checking how much medicine is in the canister

1. If the canister is new, it is full.

2. If the canister has been used repeatedly, it might be empty. (Check product label to see how many inhalations should be in each canister.)

   To check how much medicine is left in the canister, put the canister (not the mouthpiece) in a cup of water.
   —If the canister sinks to the bottom, it is full.
   —If the canister floats sideways on the surface, it is empty.

Steps for using the inhaler

1. Remove the cap and hold inhaler upright.

2. Shake the inhaler.

3. Tilt the head back slightly and breathe out.

4. Position the inhaler in one of the following ways (A is optimal, but C is acceptable for those who have difficulty with A or B):

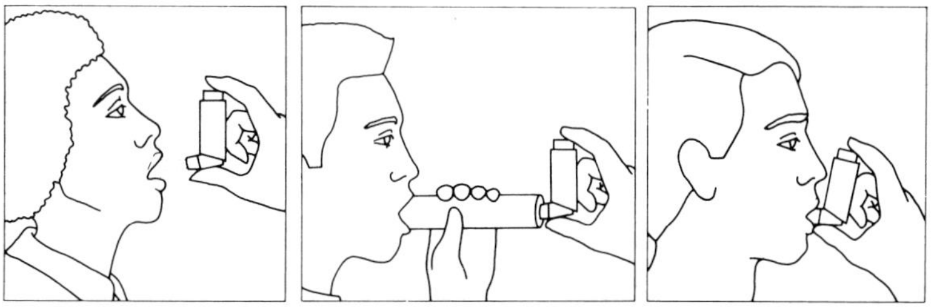

A. Open mouth with inhaler 1-2 inches away.

B. Use spacer (this is recommended especially for young children).

C. In the mouth.

5. Press down on inhaler to release medication as you start to breathe in slowly.

6. Breathe in *slowly* (3-5 seconds).

7. *Hold* breath for 10 seconds to allow medicine to reach deeply into lungs.

8. Repeat puffs as directed. Waiting 1 minute between puffs may permit second puff to penetrate the lungs better.

9. Spacers are useful for all patients. They are particularly recommended for young children and older adults and for use with inhaled steroids.

Note: Inhaled dry powder capsules require a different inhalation technique. To use a dry powder inhaler, it is important to close the mouth tightly around the mouthpiece of the inhaler and to inhale rapidly.

Figure 55.4. Correct use of a metered dose inhaler with and without a spacer. (Courtesy NIH.)

tube: 145 ml), Azmacort Extender (rigid tube: 90 ml), Brethancer (retractable tube: 80 ml), InhalAid (rigid chamber: 700 ml), and InspirEase (collapsible bag: 700 ml). A high percentage of aerosol that is actuated from the MDI is retained in these various spacer devices. However, the dose that penetrates beyond the oropharynx and deposits in the lungs is only marginally affected by a spacer when compared to MDI alone (50). The dose to the lung varies slightly according to the volume of the spacer. In two studies, the dose was similar, whether using an MDI optimally or a spacer device with a 145-ml volume (51, 52). The dose was slightly enhanced for devices with volumes of 750 ml (43). The simplest tube spacer reduces oropharyngeal deposition by allowing the velocity of the aerosol

particles to diminish before entering the mouth. Other devices have features that provide for control of inspiratory flow rate at the time of inhalation. However, these features may not be suitable for young patients since they either require coordination of inspiration at a specific rate during inhalation using visual cues (InhalAid) or rely on a noise to inform the patient that they are inhaling too fast (InspirEase, Aerochamber). Children may prefer to hear the whistle.

Experience with an MDI in conjunction with a spacer in infants is limited. Salmon et al. (53) found that delivery of sodium cromoglycate aerosol by either nebulizer/face mask or MDI with a spacer/face mask resulted in low deposition fractions in a group of infants between 9 and 36 months of age. Only 0.76%

of a 20-mg dose was delivered by a jet nebulizer during tidal breathing and only 0.30% was delivered by a metered dose inhaler into a spacer deposited within the lungs. The majority of the aerosol was deposited in the spacer, on the face, or in the nasopharynx. These low doses may be inadequate to treat some children successfully with cromolyn aerosol. However, this low deposition fraction may be sufficient for a therapeutic bronchodilator response, since albuterol delivered by an MDI/spacer and a face mask resulted in significantly greater bronchodilatation than placebo aerosol in infants aged 1.6–25.2 months (54).

Dry Powder Inhalers

These devices do not use freon propellants, but depend on a rapid inspiration ($\geq$ 60 L/minute) to deliver a dry powder form of drug. Children who have poor MDI technique may benefit from these inhalers because they eliminate the need for coordinating aerosol actuation and inhalation. In the case of bronchodilators, at least one type of device has been shown to produce the same effect as the pressurized aerosol (55). Nonetheless, there are several disadvantages to dry powder inhalers. First, particles of drug form nonrespirable agglomerates with large carrier particles (30–70 μm), and very little (5–10%) of the dry powder penetrates to the lower airways (56, 57). Secondly, the inhalation of the powder itself may cause irritation. Finally, the necessary high inspiratory flow rate may be difficult for patients who are severely obstructed (56, 57). When prescribing the use of a dry powder inhaler, it is important to emphasize to the patient that a rapid inspiration is required. This is opposite to the instructions for an MDI.

Jet Nebulizers

Nebulized aerosols are useful in treating young children who may be unable to coordinate the actuation and inhalation necessary for MDI delivery, or may be unable to generate high inspiratory flow rates for the inhalation of dry powder aerosols. There are two types of nebulizer devices: jet and ultrasonic. In the jet nebulizer, compressed air passes over a tube that resides in the liquid to be aerosolized. The resulting pressure drop causes liquid

to be drawn up the tube where it is entrained in the airstream and broken into droplets of various sizes by baffles that are incorporated within the internal structure of the nebulizer. Large particles impact on these baffles and return to the nebulizer solution for re-aerosolization. A small fraction of the aerosol leaves the nebulizer as fine particles. Mercer reported that the mass median diameter for aerosols generated by various jet nebulizers ranged between 1.2 and 6.9 μm (58).

High compressed gas flow rates (6–8 L/minute) maximize jet nebulizer output and decrease aerosol particle size (59). For example, Williams et al. (60) reported an output rate of 0.07 ml/minute at a flow rate of 4 L/minute, whereas output increased to 0.25 ml/minute at 8 L/minute. Increased rate of output will decrease nebulization time and, thereby, enhance patient compliance. In the hospital, jet nebulizers utilize compressed air or oxygen sources that are regulated by a flow meter that can be adjusted as high as 10 L/minute. If nebulizer treatment occurs at home, gas flow from portable sources should be checked to be sure that is is between 6 and 8 L/minute. Warming the nebulizer in the hand before nebulization will minimize the reduction in aerosol output that occurs as the result of a temperature drop during aerosolization (59). Most drug manufacturers recommend that nebulizers be filled with a 2 ml solution reservoir. However, some volume of the solution (usually 0.5–1.0 ml) remains on the internal structures of the nebulizer and is not aerosolized. In order to reduce the percentage of "dead" volume, Clay et al. (59) suggest increasing the reservoir to 4–6 ml.

Jet nebulization combined with intermittent positive-pressure breathing (IPPB) has been used to treat children with various respiratory disorders. IPPB increases the pressure differential during inspiration, which is thought to increase the flow and penetration of an aerosol into the lungs. Nevertheless, it appears that IPPB does not improve drug delivery to the lungs or drug efficacy, since it has been shown that 32% less aerosol is delivered to the lungs with IPPB compared to quiet breathing, and aerosol tends to impact in the larger, central airways, presumably because of an increase in ventilation rate (61).

Jet nebulizers are also used in conjunction with pressure-limited, time-cycled ventilators to treat infants with respiratory distress syndrome or bronchopulmonary dysplasia. Dahlback et al. (62) recently reported that when an aerosol was nebulized during the last 25% of the respiratory cycle, the amount of drug delivered to the tip of a tracheal cannula was significantly less than when nebulization took place during the last 50% of the cycle. Drug delivery was also diminished when the volume of tubing between the nebulizer and the cannula was less than tidal volume or ventilation frequency was increased from 20 to 60/minute. Ahrens et al. (63) have shown that small diameter tubing in the breathing circuit will also reduce the yield of aerosol.

Only 1.2–2.9% of the administered dose of a radioactively labeled aerosol generated by jet nebulizer was deposited in the lungs of adult patients during mechanical ventilation (64, 65). Percentage of deposition could be increased to 5.6% by substituting an MDI plus spacer for the nebulizer (64). The observed differences in delivered dose may be due to variations in aerosol particle size, drug solubility, or absorption of drug on the ventilator tubing, but probably is not due to differences in the positioning of the aerosol generators (66). The efficacy of using an MDI and spacer to deliver aerosolized drugs to infants and children who are receiving mechanical ventilation is not known, although it appears to be a more efficient method in adults.

Ultrasonic Nebulizers

An ultrasonic nebulizer generates particles by focusing vibrations from a piezoelectric transducer on the surface of the liquid to be aerosolized. The liquid surface becomes unstable, producing an aerosol fountain. Continuous aerosolization requires 10 ml of liquid in the reservoir (67). Although nebulizer output is higher than with the jet nebulizer, ultrasonic nebulizers also produce larger aerosol droplets, in the range of 3.7–10.5 μm MMAD (58). Droplet size varies inversely with the oscillating frequency of the piezoelectric transducer (24), which is usually fixed by the manufacturer.

Of the dose of aerosol that is generated by a jet or ultrasonic nebulizer, it is generally agreed that an average of 10% is deposited in the lungs (24). Estimates range from 2–11% (68), to 3–23% (69), to 7–32% (70), depending on nebulizer design, operating conditions,

breathing patterns, and subject propulation. There are a few disadvantages to the administration of aerosolized medications by either jet or ultrasonic nebulizer. The time for treatment with a nebulizer averages 10–15 minutes. A compressor or electrical power source is necessary. In the hospital, treatment requires specialized personnel, which adds to the expense. When aerosol is administered through a mouthpiece or face mask, a large percentage of the dose is deposited on the accessory apparatus. During continuous breathing, significant losses will occur as the result of a diversion of incoming aerosol to the expired air.

CONCLUSIONS

Ideally, treatment with aerosolized medications will be optimal when the relationship between drug dose and distribution within the lungs and drug effect are well understood. We have discussed the major factors that determine how much of an aerosolized drug is deposited in the lungs and described operational information for a variety of aerosol generating equipment and their recommended use in order to improve that understanding. With aerosol therapy, the selection of an appropriate device for aerosol generation, according to patient age and/or capability, to acuate and inhale effectively is crucial. Once the device is selected, the second most important step is for the patient to receive proper instruction in its use with periodic observations of technique to ensure that the patient is getting the dose that is required.

REFERENCES

1. Davies DS. Pharmacokinetics of inhaled substances. *Postgrad Med J* 1975; 51 (Suppl 7):69–76.
2. Ruffin RE, Montgomery JM, Newhouse MT. Site of beta-adrenergic receptors in the respiratory tract. *Chest* 1978; 74:256–260.
3. Martin AJ, Erben A, Landau LT, Phelan PD. Recent advances in aerosol therapy. In Baran D, ed. First Belgium Symposium on Aerosols in Medicine, Brussels, 1979, pp 113–116.
4. Newman SP, Pellow PGD, Clay MM. Nebulisation of gentamicin solution. In Lawson D, ed. *Cystic fibrosis: Horizons.* Chichester, John Wiley, 1984, p 270.
5. Dahlback M, Nerbrink O, Arborelius M, Hansson HC. Output characteristics from three medical nebulisers. *J Aer Sci* 1986; 17:563–564.
6. Bates DV. Deposition and retention models for internal dosimetry of the human respiratory tract: Task Group on Lung Dynamics. *Health Phys* 1966; 12:173–207.

7. Laube BL, Swift DL, Adams, GK III. Single-breath deposition of jet-nebulized saline aerosol. *Aer Sci Tech* 1984; 3:97–102.

8. Rance RW. Studies of the factors controlling the action of hair sprays—III. The influence of particle velocity and diameter on the capture of particles by arrays of hair fibres. *J Soc Cosmet Chem* 1974;25:545–561.

9. Newhouse MT, Dolovich MB. Control of asthma by aerosols. *N Engl J Med* 1986; 315:870–874.

10. Newman SP, Clarke SW. Therapeutic aerosols: Physical and practical considerations. *Thorax* 1983; 38:881–886.

11. Inhalation therapy in the management of airway obstruction. Proceedings of a Symposium in Lund, Sweden. *Eur J Respir Dis* 1982; 63(Suppl 119):1–125.

12. Lippmann M, Albert RE. The effect of particle size on the regional deposition of inhaled aerosols in the human respiratory tract. *Am Ind Hyg Assoc J* 1969; 30:257–275.

13. Pavia D, Thomson ML, Clarke SW, Shannon HS. Effect of lung function and mode of inhalation on penetration of aerosol into the human lung. *Thorax* 1977; 32:194–197.

14. Palmes ED. Measurement of pulmonary air spaces using aerosols. *Arch Intern Med* 1973; 131:76–79.

15. Dolovich MB, Sanchis J, Rossman C, Newhouse MT. Aerosol penetrance: A sensitive index of peripheral airway obstruction. *J Appl Physiol* 1976; 40:468–471.

16. Knight V, Yu CP, Gilbert BE, Divine GW. Estimating the dosage of ribavirin aerosol according to age and other variables. *J Infect Dis* 1988; 158:443–448.

17. Hofmann W. Mathematical model for the postnatal growth of the human lung. *Respir Physiol* 1982; 49:115–129.

18. Yu CP, Xu GB. Predicted deposition of diesel particles in young humans. *J Aer Sci* 1987; 18:419–429.

19. Becquemin MH, Roy M, Bouchikhi A, Teillac A. Deposition of inhaled particles in children. In Hofmann W ed. *Deposition and clearance of aerosols in the human respiratory tract.* Vienna, Facultas, 1987, pp 22–27.

20. Schiller-Scotland CF, Hlawa R, Gebhart J, Wonne R, Heyder J. Particle deposition in the respiratory tract of children during spontaneous and controlled mouth-breathing. Seventh International Symposium on Inhaled Particles, British Occupational Hygiene Society, 1991.

21. Collis GG, Cole CH, LeSouef PN. Dilution of nebulised aerosols by air entrainment in children. *Lancet* 1990; 336:341–343.

22. Hiller FC, Mazumder MK, Wilson JD, Bone RC. Aerodynamic size distribution of metered-dose bronchodilator aerosols. *Am Rev Respir Dis* 1978; 118:311–317.

23. Kim CS, Trujillo D, Berkley BB. Aerodynamic size distribution of metered dose aerosols in low and high humidity conditions. *Am Rev Respir Dis* 1981; 123(Suppl):110.

24. Newman SP, Pavia D. Aerosol deposition in man. In Moren F, Newhouse MT, Dolovich MB, eds. *Aerosols in medicine, principles, diagnosis and therapy.* Amsterdam, Elsevier Science, 1985, pp 193–217.

25. Davies DS. Pharmacokinetic studies with inhaled drugs. *Eur J Respir Dis* 1982; 63(Suppl 119):67–72.

26. Short MD, Singh CA, Few FD, Studdy PT, Heaf PJD, Spiro SG. *Chest* 1981; 80(Suppl):918–921.

27. Newman SP, Pavia D, Moren F, Sheahan NF, Clarke SW. Deposition of pressurized aerosols in the human respiratory tract. *Thorax* 1981; 36:52–55.

28. Dolovich MB, Ruffin RE, Roberts R, Newhouse MT. Optimal delivery of aerosols from metered/dose inhalers. *Chest* 1981; 80(Suppl):911–915.

29. Newman SP, Pavia D, Clarke SW. Simple instructions for using pressurized aerosol bronchodilators. *J Roy Soc Med* 1980; 73:776–779.

30. Thomas P, Williams T, Reilly P. Bradley D. Modifying delivery technique of fenoterol from a metered dose inhaler. *Ann Allergy* 1984; 52:279–281.

31. Connolly CK. Method of using pressurized aerosols. *Br Med J* 1975; 5:21.

32. Dolovich M, Ruffin RE, Roberts R, Newhouse MT. Optimal delivery of aerosols from metered dose inhalers. *Chest* 1981; 80:911–915.

33. Newman SP, Pavia D, Clarke SW. How should a pressurized β-adrenergic bronchodilator be inhaled? *Eur J Respir Dis* 1981; 62:3–21.

34. Epstein SW, Manning CPR, Ashley MJ, Corey PN. Survey of the clinical use of pressurized aerosol inhalers. *Can Med Assoc J* 1979; 120:813–816.

35. Crompton GK. Problems patients have using pressurized aerosol inhalers. *Eur J Respir Dis* 1982; 119(Suppl):101–104.

36. Coady TJ, Stewart CJ, Davies HJ. Synchronization of bronchodilator release. *Practitioner* 1976; 217:273–275.

37. Baciewicz AM, Kyllonen, KS. Aerosol inhaler technique in children with asthma. *Am J Hosp Pharm* 1989; 46:2510–2511.

38. Pedersen S, Frost L, Arnfred T. Errors in inhalation technique and efficiency in inhaler use by asthmatic children. *Allergy* 1986; 41:118–124.

39. Lee HS. Proper aerosol inhalation technique for delivery of asthmatic medications. *Clin Pediatr* 1983; 22:440–443.

40. Corr D, Dolovich M, McCormack D, Ruffin RE, Obminski G, Newhouse M. The aerochamber: A new demand-inhalation device for delivery of aerosolized drugs. *Am Rev Respir Dis* 1980; 121(Suppl):123.

41. Moren F. Drug deposition of pressurized inhalation aerosols. I. Influence of actuator tube design. *Int J Pharm* 1978; 1:205.

42. Newman SP, Moren F, Pavia D, Little F, Clarke SW. Deposition of pressurized suspension aerosols inhaled through extension devices. *Am Rev Respir Dis* 1981; 124:317–320.

43. Kim CS, Eldridge MA, Sackner MA. Oropharyngeal deposition and delivery aspects of metered-dose inhaler aerosols. *Am Rev Respir Dis* 1987; 135:157–164.

44. Toogood J, Jennings B, Baskerville J, Lefcoe N, Newhouse M. Assessment of a device for reducing oropharyngeal complications during beclomethasone of asthma. *Am Rev Respir Dis* 1981; 123(Suppl):113.

45. Toogood JH. Are spacers of any use in the treatment of asthma? [Letter]. *Pediatr Pulmonol* 1986; 2:250.

46. Heno N, Kivity S, Greif J, Greif Z, Freundlich E, Topilsky M. The use of spacers in the prevention of exercise-induced asthma. *Pediatr Asthma Allergy Immunol* 1989; 3:135–139.

47. Sly RM, Barbera JM, Middleton HB, Eby DM. Delivery of albuterol aerosol by Aerochamber to young children. *Ann Allergy* 1988; 60:403–406.
48. Conner WT, Dolovich MB, Frame RA, Newhouse MT. Reliable salbutamol administration in 6- to 36-month-old children by means of a metered-dose inhaler and Aerochamber with mask. *Pediatr Pulmonol* 1989; 6:263–267.
49. Konig P, Gayer D, Kantak A, Kruetz C, Douglass B, Hordvik NL. A trial of metaproterenol by means of metered-dose inhaler and two spacers in preschool asthmatics. *Pediatr Pulmonol* 1988; 5:247–251.
50. Clark AR, Rachelefsky G, Mason PL, Goldenhersh MJ, Hollingworth A. The use of reservoir devices for the simultaneous delivery of two metered-dose aerosols. *J Allergy Clin Immunol* 1990; 85:75–79.
51. Newman SP, Moren F, Pavia D, Little F, Clarke SW. Deposition of pressurized suspension aerosols inhaled through extension devices. *Am Rev Respir Dis* 1981; 121:317–320.
52. Dolovich M, Ruffin R, Corr D, Newhouse M. Clinical evaluation of a simple demand inhalation MDI aerosol delivery device. *Chest* 1983; 84:36–44.
53. Salmon B, Wilson NM, Silverman M. How much aerosol reaches the lungs of wheezy infants and toddlers? *Arch Dis Child* 1990;65:401–403.
54. Kraemer R, Frey U, Sommer CW, Russi E. Short-term effect of albuterol, delivered via a new auxiliary device, in wheezy infants. *Am Rev Respir Dis* 1991; 144:347–351.
55. Svedmyr N, Lofdahl CG, Svedmyr K. The effect of powder aerosol compared to pressurized aerosol. *Eur J Respir Dis* 1982; 119(Suppl):81–88.
56. Smith G, Hiller C, Mazumder M, Bone R. Aerodynamic size distribution of cromolyn sodium at ambient and airway humidity. *Am Rev Respir Dis* 1980; 121:513–517.
57. Walker SR, Evans ME, Richards AJ, Paterson JW. The fate of (^{14}C) sodium cromoglycate in man. *J Pharm Pharmacol* 1972; 24:525.
58. Mercer TT. Production of therapeutic aerosols: Principles and techniques. *Chest* 1981; 80(Suppl):813–818.
59. Clay MM, Pavia D, Newman SP, Lennard-Jones T, Clarke SW. Assessment of jet nebulizers for lung aerosol therapy. *Lancet* 1983; 2:592–594.
60. Williams PE, Renowden SA, Ward MJ, Audit of nebuliser use. *Postgrad Med J* 1985; 61:1055–1056.
61. Dolovich MB, Killian D, Wolff RK, Obminski G, Newhouse MT. Pulmonary aerosol deposition in chronic bronchitis: Intermittent positive pressure breathing versus quiet breathing. *Am Rev Respir Dis* 1977; 115:397–402.
62. Dahlback M, Wollmer P, Drefeldt B, Jonson B. Controlled aerosol delivery during mechanical ventilation. *J Aer Med* 1989; 2:339–347.
63. Ahrens RC, Ries RA, Popendorf W, Wiese JA. The delivery of therapeutic aerosols through endotrachel tubes. *Pediatr Pulmonol* 1986; 2:19–26.
64. Fuller HD, Dolovich MB, Posmituck G, Pack, WW, Newhouse MT. Pressurized aerosol versus jet aerosol delivery to mechanically ventilated patients. *Am Rev Respir Dis* 1990; 141:440–444.
65. MacIntyre NR, Silver RM, Miller CW, Schuler F, Coleman RE. Aerosol delivery in intubated, mechanically ventilated patients. *Crit Care Med* 1985; 13:81–84.
66. Hughes J, Saez J. Effects of nebulized mode and position in a mechanical venilator circuit on dose efficiency. *Respir Care* 1987; 32:1131–1135.
67. Swift DL. Aerosol characterization and generation. In Moren F, Newhouse MT, Dolovich MB, eds. *Aerosols in medicine, principles, diagnosis and therapy*. Amstedam, Elsevier, 1985, pp 53–75.
68. Ruffin RE, Obminski G, Newhouse MT. Aerosol salbutanol administration by IPPB: Lowest effective dose. *Thorax* 1978; 33:689–693.
69. Wasnich RD. A high frequency ultrasonic nebulizer system for radioaerosol delivery. *J Nucl Med* 1976; 17:707–710.
70. Lin MS, Hayes TM, Goodwin DA, Kruse SL. Distal penetration in radioaerosol inhalation with an ultrasonic nebulizer. *Radiology* 1974; 112:443–447.
71. Bowes SM, Laube BL, Links JM, Frank R. Regional deposition of inhaled fog droplets: Preliminary observations. *Environ Health Perspect* 1989; 79:151–157.
72. Laube BL, Swift DL, Wagner HN, Norman PS, Adams GK III. The effect of bronchial obstruction on central airway deposition of a saline aerosol in patients with asthma. *Am Rev Respir Dis* 1986; 133:740–743.

56

Oxygen Therapy

RAEZELLE ZINMAN

This chapter will consider oxygen therapy from a pediatric perspective. The chapter begins with a review of the principles underlying oxygen delivery. These provide the basis for evaluation of a patient's oxygenation status. The causes for hypoxia will then be discussed. This is followed by a section on the treatment of acute hypoxia and complications of oxygen therapy. The chapter closes with a review of long-term home oxygen therapy that focuses on patient selection and techniques. There are issues related to maturation and size that make oxygen therapy different in an infant or child as compared to an adult.

OXYGEN DELIVERY

Oxygen is carried in the blood in two ways. The amount dissolved in blood (0.3 ml O_2/100 ml plasma/100 mm Hg PaO_2) is only a small proportion of the total. The greater proportion is bound to hemoglobin, which when fully saturated can bind 1.34 ml O_2/g hemoglobin at 38° C. The extent to which hemoglobin is saturated is described by the oxyhemoglobin dissociation curve (Fig. 56.1). The P_{50} (the point where hemoglobin is 50% saturated) is about 26 mm Hg. The steep portion of the curve, up to a PaO_2 of 50 mm Hg, accounts for the release of large amounts of oxygen for small changes in PaO_2 in the peripheral tissues. On the relatively flat portion of the curve, above a PaO_2 of 60 mm Hg, there is little change in oxygen content despite a considerable change in PaO_2. The curve is shifted to the right (i.e., the P_{50} is increased) in the presence of a decrease in pH, or an elevation of CO_2, temperature, and D-2, 3-diphosphoglycerate (2,3-DPG). The curve is shifted to the left with an increase in pH, or decrease in CO_2, temperature, or 2,3-DPG.

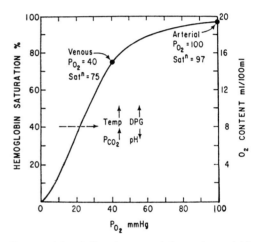

Figure 56.1. Salient features of the oxyhemoglobin dissociation curve. The oxygen content scale is based on a hemoglobin concentration of 14.5 g/100 ml. (From West JB. *Pulmonary pathophysiology—The essentials.* Baltimore, Williams & Wilkins, 1977.)

The fetal oxyhemoglobin dissociation curve is shifted to the left in comparison to the adult curve. This occurs because 2,3-DPG binds less well to the gamma chain of hemoglobin found in fetal cells than to the beta chain in adult cells. Fetal blood thus contains more oxygen than adult blood at low PaO_2, which is in keeping with fetal needs in the intrauterine environment, where PaO_2 is 30 mm Hg.

Oxygen delivery, the product of blood oxygen content and cardiac output (CO), can be summarized by equation (a):

(a) O_2 delivery = [(0.003 ml/mm Hg/100 ml) (PaO_2) + (1.34 ml/g.Hb) (Hb g/100 ml) SaO_2%] CO

In a patient with a hemoglobin of 15 g, the oxygen content of arterial blood, 98% saturated, will be 20 ml O_2/100 ml of blood, whereas the content of venous blood, 75% saturated, will be 15 ml O_2/100 ml of blood. Thus 5 ml of oxygen will be delivered to the tissues for each 100 ml of cardiac output. If hemoglobin is reduced to 10 g, oxygen delivery is 3 ml for each 100 ml of cardiac output. Thus for an anemic patient to maintain oxygen delivery to the tissues, cardiac output must increase.

EVALUATION OF OXYGENATION

The clinical signs of hypoxia are initially an increase in respiratory rate and heart rate, and decrease in exercise tolerance. The older patient may become irritable or show a reduction in mental capacity, especially with acute hypoxia. In infants and especially premature neonates, hypoxia can lead to apnea and bradycardia. Cyanosis is a notoriously poor indicator of hypoxia. Cyanosis depends on the presence of a sufficient quantity of unsaturated hemoglobin ($\geq$ 5 g%), which occurs at a hemoglobin saturation of 75% in an infant with normal hemoglobin concentration. It follows that an anemic patient will not appear cyanotic until PaO_2 falls even further.

The laboratory evaluation gold standard is the arterial blood gas, but this requires an invasive procedure to procure the sample and is limited to a moment in time. Capillary blood gases are frequently obtained in the pediatric setting, since this is technically easier than arterial blood gas sampling. Examination of the oxyhemoglobin dissociation curve makes it apparent that slight contamination of the sample with venous blood will substantially lower the oxygen content and resultant $P_{cap}O_2$. This is difficult to circumvent even when care is taken to "arterialize" the sample by prewarming the sampling site. Transcutaneous PO_2 is routinely measured in neonates, but its use is limited to this population. Its slow response time to changes in PaO_2 and the risk of burns have further limited its usefulness. Pulse oximetry is used to measure hemoglobin saturation on a continuous basis (see Chapter 13). Since this is based on physical rather than chemical principles, it is very stable and internally calibrated. Its accuracy is reported to be ± 2%. The response time is 15 seconds although 95% of a step change in SaO_2 is displayed within 8 seconds. This makes the oximeter an excellent device for continuous monitoring. Its major drawback is that it cannot be used to assess hyperoxia, which is especially important in the premature infant, and is subject to artifacts from ambient light and motion. Pulse oximetry cannot differentiate carboxyhemoglobin from oxygenated hemoglobin. Methemoglobin drives the reading towards 85%. The accuracy of the device in the presence of poor peripheral perfusion has been enhanced by newer units that compensate by increasing the light source and gain. Pulse detection and problems related to movement artefact have also been overcome by use of the electrocardiogram to lock into the pulse signal.

Oxygen delivery may be adequate in the presence of marked cyanosis and decreased SaO_2 as illustrated by children with cyanotic congenital heart disease. Alternatively, oxygen delivery may be inadequate in the presence of a normal PaO_2, as in the child with carbon monoxide poisoning. When oxygen delivery is inadequate, oxygen extraction at the tissue level will increase prior to the development of acidemia. This will result in a fall in the mixed venous PO_2 and saturation.

CAUSES OF HYPOXIA

There are four main causes of arterial hypoxia in patients, and in many patients more than one cause may be operative at a time. *Ventilation-perfusion mismatching*, in which areas of the lung are perfused but relatively underventilated, is the most common reason for hypoxia. This is the mechanism underlying hypoxia in asthma, pneumonia, atelectasis, pulmonary edema, and respiratory distress syndrome.

In the presence of *hypoventilation* the alveolar PO_2 ($PalvO_2$) drops as the $PaCO_2$ increases as described by the abbreviated alveolar gas equation (b):

(b) $PalvO_2 = P_IO_2 - (PalvCO_2/0.8)$

where the inspired PO_2 (P_IO_2) is equal to 760 mm Hg at sea level minus 47 mm Hg of water vapor times the percentage of inspired oxygen, the alveolar PCO_2 ($PalvCO_2$) is estimated by the arterial PCO_2, and 0.8 is the respiratory exchange ratio of CO_2 production to O_2 consumption. The more common causes of hypoventilation in children are categorized in Table 56.1.

Table 56.1.
Causes of Hypoventilation

Respiratory center depression
  Drugs
  Anesthesia

Respiratory center disease
  Congenital hypoventilation syndrome
  Encephalitis
  Hemorrhage
  Neoplasm

Spinal cord lesion
  Trauma
  Syringomyelia
  Arnold-Chiari malformation

Anterior horn cell disease
  Poliomyelitis
  Spinal muscular atrophy

Neuropathy and neuromuscular junction disorder
  Guillain-Barré syndrome
  Botulism
  Myasthenia gravis

Myopathies
  Nemaline myopathy
  Duchenne muscular dystrophy
  Congenital myotonic dystrophy

Chest wall abnormalities
  Flail chest
  Kyphoscoliosis
  Asphyxiating thoracic dystrophy

Upper airway obstruction
  Epiglottitis
  Croup
  Subglottic stenosis

In the presence of a true right-to-left *shunt*, blood passes from the systemic venous circulation directly to the systemic arterial circulation without coming into contact with ventilated portions of the lung. Persistent pulmonary hypertension syndrome in the newborn and tetralogy of Fallot are classic examples in which right-to-left shunt occurs predominantly via atrial and ventricular septal defects, respectively.

Diffusion can present a barrier to adequate oxygenation of blood during its passage through the lung. In pediatrics pure diffusion block is relatively uncommon, but it occurs in the presence of severe lung hypoplasia, because the surface area available for diffusion is limited. This results in a shorter transit time for blood through the lung, which can critically lessen the time for diffusion. By supplying an increased concentration of inspired oxygen, the concentration gradient is enhanced and the time needed for diffusion is decreased and oxygenation improved.

ACUTE OXYGEN THERAPY

The approach to the management of acute hypoxia in part depends on recognition of the cause. Many of the techniques used in the intensive care setting to improve oxygenation are aimed at improving ventilation/perfusion mismatching and involve increasing mean airway pressure. This can be accomplished by adding positive end expiratory pressure, increasing or even inverting the inspiratory to expiratory time ratio, or developing a pressure plateau earlier in inspiration. One must balance the negative impact that increases in mean airway pressure will have on systemic venous return and pulmonary vascular resistance, and in turn cardiac output, with the improvement that can be achieved in oxygenation. In fact the goal must be to maximize oxygen delivery to the tissues, not just Pao_2. Returning to equation (a), which defines oxygen delivery, it is evident that if the price for increasing Sao_2 is a decrease in cardiac output, there may be no improvement or even a decline in oxygen delivery. Equation (a) also highlights the importance of maintaining an appropriate oxygen-carrying capacity, which means that anemic patients can be improved by transfusion. Pharmacologic intervention to improve cardiac output may also be beneficial in the acute care setting.

If a patient is hypoventilating, the most effective intervention is to reestablish adequate minute ventilation, although oxygenation can be improved by increasing the concentration of inspired oxygen.

The methods of delivering an increased inspired oxygen concentration are numerous and varied. An underlying principle is that unless the rate of oxygen delivery exceeds the peak inspiratory flow rate, there will be entrainment of room air and the inspired oxygen concentration will be less than the concentration at the oxygen source.

Nasal Cannula (Prongs)

The most convenient means of oxygen delivery is by nasal prongs. The use of nasal prongs can be difficult in infants since the prongs often need to be taped in place. Using special short prongs for infants or cutting the prongs off completely can be helpful but they may be easily dislodged and oxygen delivery may be compromised. When prongs need to be taped in place for long-term use, stomadhesive placed on the cheeks allows anchoring of the nasal cannula without chronic irritation of the baby's face.

Nasal cannulae do not need to be removed for feedings and are less likely than a face mask to be displaced during sleep. Flows up to 2 L/m can be tolerated by infants and 4 L/m by older patients. High flows can be drying and irritating and are better tolerated when inspired humidity is kept high. The delivered oxygen concentration depends on the amount of room air entrained around the nasal prongs and the patient's breathing pattern. There is no accurate way to equate a given liter flow with a delivered FiO_2, and so adjustments are best made by adjusting oxygen flow to achieve a desired oxygen saturation. It has been nicely demonstrated that the FiO_2 achieved with a flow rate of 1 L/m is substantially greater in a premature infant than in a 3.5-kg baby (Fig. 56.2) (2). In premature infants it is not uncommon to find that oxygen flow rates are adjusted in 0.125-L/m increments. The real issue however is not the FiO_2, but rather the SaO_2 that

can be achieved. If the SaO_2 is inadequate, then the use of a face mask can be considered.

Face mask

Face masks can deliver higher oxygen concentrations, approaching 100% under ideal circumstances. Of course it is essential that the mask be worn covering the nose and mouth and not over one ear. This isn't easy in a 2-year-old who is constantly moving.

Face masks with air entrainment devices (the so-called "Venturi masks") are designed to deliver a fixed FiO_2 by mixing a precise quantity of air with oxygen. The larger the air intake port, the lower the final FiO_2. These require a relatively leakproof fit on the face to deliver the stated FiO_2. In practice we usually use a soft plastic mask to deliver oxygen. We attach large bore corrugated tubing to the mask and run it off an oxygen blender to achieve the desired oxygen concentration. The blended gas is passed through a high-efficiency humidifier (such as a Fisher-Pykell MR-6000) and then to the patient. This provides high humidity gas at the desired FiO_2

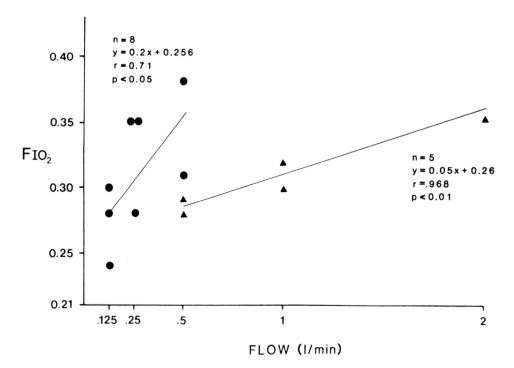

Figure 56.2. FiO_2 delivered at specific flow rates by nasal cannula in infants weighing < 3500 g (•) and > 3500 g (▲). (From Fan LL, Voyles JB. Determination of inspired oxygen delivered by nasal cannula in infants with chronic lung disease. *J Pediatr* 103:924, 1983.)

and requires only an adjustment to the oxygen blender to change concentrations. Oxygen saturation should be monitored in patients on high concentrations of mask oxygen. Delivery of well humidified gas in these patients is very important and should not be confused with delivery of particulate water in the gas stream. The use of "bubblers" and cool mist devices as a source of moisture is to be avoided. They are inefficient and the water particles can serve as an irritant, causing bronchospasm in children with hyper-reactive airways.

The flow to the face mask should be such that it prevents entrainment of room air and prevents rebreathing of carbon dioxide. This flow will be at least three times the minute ventilation of the patient.

When high oxygen concentrations are needed or when young patients won't tolerate a face mask, a head hood, canopy, or head box can be used. Attention needs to be paid to proper humidification and to sufficient gas flow to prevent rebreathing. If a small infant is placed in a large tent, temperature control can be a problem, and the baby should be monitored carefully to be sure he does not get chilled or overheated. The old style "croup tents" that produced large quantities of cold mist are not desirable for supplying oxygen.

The physician should be certain that patients in oxygen tents can be observed clearly and that mist or condensation does not reduce the nursing staff's ability to observe the child's color or respiratory effort. Wiping the inside of the tent with liquid soap is an easy way to prevent condensation.

COMPLICATIONS

The risk of oxygen therapy is the development of pulmonary oxygen toxicity. During hyperoxia free radicals are produced that promote oxidation reactions with cell components, including enzymes containing sulfhydryl groups, membrane lipids, and nucleic acids. These products are produced in excess of the capacity of antioxidant enzymes and other scavengers to detoxify them. Ultimately this results in cell death and lysis, and microvascular and alveolar cell injury. Initially this manifests as a worsening in ventilation-perfusion relationships, decreased lung compliance, and small airways dysfunction, which can progress to pulmonary fibrosis and pulmonary hypertension. Frank pulmonary edema occurs after 48–72 hours of exposure to a FiO_2 greater than 0.50 at 1 atmosphere pressure. However, there is no clear dose-response relationship between oxygen dose and toxic manifestations, since this depends on oxygen delivery and intracellular PO_2 as well as the antioxidant capabilities of the individual(6).

There is also a phenomenon that has been described as the "oxygen paradox"; an explosion of tissue damage that occurs during reoxygenation of hypoxic tissue. During reoxygenation the accumulated hypoxanthine is washed out into the circulation and metabolized by xanthine oxidase, and in the process oxygen-free radicals are produced (12). This type of reoxygenation damage has been proposed as a common mechanism for the development of retrolental fibroplasia, necrotizing enterocolitis, and bronchopulmonary dysplasia.

There are other risks involved in oxygen therapy that should be considered. In a chronically hypoxemic patient with compensated respiratory acidosis, correction of the hypoxia may depress minute ventilation by removing the hypoxic drive to breathe. This is well documented in adult patients with chronic obstructive pulmonary disease (COPD) and has been noted in some patients with cystic fibrosis, but appears to be less of a problem in infants. However, it would be prudent in this setting to monitor arterial PO_2 and PCO_2 as well as SaO_2. In a patient in whom ventilation is compromised to a portion of the lung, the risk of atelectasis is increased when high concentrations of oxygen are inspired.

LONG-TERM OXYGEN THERAPY

Patient Selection

The use of long-term home oxygen therapy has been best established in COPD. The landmark studies on which present recommendations are based for COPD patients were the Nocturnal Oxygen Therapy Trial and Medical Research Council studies (9, 10). It is now accepted that oxygen therapy improves survival in hypoxemic COPD patients (Fig. 56.3) (7–10). In the pediatric population home oxygen therapy is commonly prescribed for patients with bronchopulmonary dysplasia (BPD) and cystic fibrosis (CF) (13), and on an individual basis for those with pulmonary hypertension associated with congenital heart

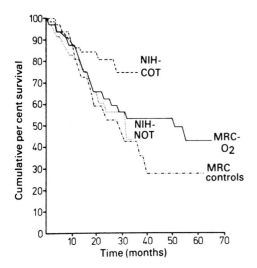

Figure 56.3. Comparison of survival curves from the National Institute of Health and the Britisih Medical Research Council studies in COPD patients. NIH-COT: continuous oxygen therapy of 19 hours or more per day; NIH-NOT: nocturnal oxygen therapy of 12 hours per day; MRC-O₂: oxygen for 15 hours per day including sleep time; MRC controls: no oxygen therapy. (From Flenley DC. *Respir Care* 28:881, 1983.)

disease, metastatic lung diseases, and advanced interstitial lung disease.

Long-Term Oxygen in BPD

The pulmonary vascular bed in BPD is responsive to oxygen; pulmonary artery pressures fall when hypoxia is relieved, though not necessarily to normal (1). This relates to the fact that there is an increase in smooth muscle of the pulmonary vasculature. It has been postulated that remodeling of the pulmonary vasculature may be normalized by maintaining adequate oxygenation (1). Supplemental oxygen therapy, therefore, has become a cornerstone in the long-term management of these patients in an effort to prevent cor pulmonale (17). Continuous SaO_2 monitoring indicates that in BPD, oxygenation can decrease with feedings as well as with sleep (4, 22). There is also evidence to suggest that home oxygen therapy promotes weight gain in infants with BPD (5). In order to prescribe oxygen optimally, children requiring oxygen supplementation should be evaluated with the goal of maintaining $SaO_2 \geq 90\%$ during all periods of the day. Awake oxygen supplementation requirements can be assessed by increasing nasal cannula flows in increments of 0.25 lpm in infants, or 0.5 lpm in older children, until the SaO_2 reaches 90%. Oxygen requirements during sleep can be assessed with continuous oximetry and a program that records trends for the night and highlights periods of desaturation.

Oxygen desaturation during sleep occurs in infants with BPD (4, 22), as it does in other COPD patients (3, 14). In BPD patients, 6 of 14 patients with an acceptable awake SaO_2 between 90 and 92% in room air dropped their asleep SaO_2 to < 88%, whereas only 1 of 25 patients with an awake $SaO_2 \geq 92\%$ on room air dropped their asleep SaO_2 to < 88%. It was not possible to discriminate which patients on supplemental oxygen would desaturate to a critical extent based on their awake SaO_2. A prospective study is required to define the natural history of sleep desaturation in BPD patients and determine whether there are simple predictors that discriminate patients at risk for sleep desaturation. In the interim, it seems prudent to take into account sleep desaturation when formulating guidelines for oxygen supplementation in infants with BPD, so we have proposed the following: (a) obtain sleep studies to regulate oxygen administration during sleep for all patients requiring awake oxygen supplementation and (b) continue oxygen supplementation during sleep until the quiet awake SaO_2 in room air is equal to or exceeds 92%. The first recommendation is aimed at preventing repeated desaturation in a population still at risk for developing cor pulmonale, and the second at preventing the need for repeated sleep studies.

Long-Term Oxygen in Cystic Fibrosis

It is tempting to extrapolate from COPD to cystic fibrosis (CF) that oxygen therapy in hypoxemic patients will improve survival, especially since the prognostic implications of right-sided heart failure seem ominous in both (15, 18). However, as compared to COPD patients, CF patients are younger and have not had a prolonged history of smoking, both of which could affect the response of the right ventricle to increased pulmonary artery pressures. This led us to undertake a double-blind randomized study of the effect of nocturnal oxygen therapy on mortality, morbidity, and disease progression in 28 patients with advanced CF (21). Patients were selected on the basis of an awake stable PaO_2 < 65 mm Hg. Oxygen was prescribed to achieve an awake PaO_2 ≥ 70 mm Hg. Two groups were randomly assigned to receive either humidified oxygen or room air from modified concentrators. There were four deaths in each group. The progression of disease, as ascertained from nutritional status, pulmonary function, exercise ability, and right ventricular response to exercise was not improved by oxygen therapy. However, school or work attendance was maintained in the oxygen group, whereas it deteriorated in the air group. We speculated that this could reflect improvement in quality of sleep. We concluded that oxygen therapy in CF should be reserved for symptomatic relief and not be instituted early in an effort to retard the progression of disease. Symptoms in this context should be defined as clinical signs of cor pulmonale, such as abdominal tenderness in the right upper quadrant or peripheral edema, and/or evidence of decreased attendance at school or work.

Oxygen Delivery Systems for the Home

Oxygen therapy has been provided by transporting large cylinders of compressed gas to the home, a process that is cumbersome, costly, and potentially dangerous. This has been supplanted by the use of electrically powered oxygen concentrators and enrichers that work by passing room air through a molecular sieve bed that absorbs gases other than oxygen. There are many models available but most achieve concentrations of approximately 95% at flow rates as high as 3 lpm with slightly lower concentrations at higher flow rates. This is the least expensive means of oxygen delivery but does not provide for patient mobility. A supplemental portable system is available that uses tanks weighing 7–10 lbs that can deliver 2 lpm of oxygen for 8 hours. These are refilled in the home from larger liquid oxygen reservoirs. Liquid oxygen is subject to large amounts of waste from evaporation losses which, in small infants requiring low flow, can even exceed the actual consumption. However, it remains the most practical portable delivery method, although it is the most expensive because of the need for home delivery of liquid oxygen on a regular basis.

In-home oxygen delivery is usually by low-flow system using high concentrations (e.g., 0.5 lpm of 100% oxygen) rather than with high-flow blended systems, as used in hospitals. Adaptors that fit over tracheostomies have also been designed to facilitate the administration of low-flow oxygen (19).

In infants with BPD, the use of nasal cannula or tracheal low-flow oxygen during the day permits freedom of movement and interaction with the environment, which is important to promote childhood development. The concern that the cannula might be displaced during the night led to the development of an alternative means for night time oxygen administration (20), the "inverted tent." The sides, ends, and floor of the crib are lined with plastic and a partial canopy is placed over half the length of the crib (Fig. 56.4). The concentrator is run at 3 lpm and an air entrainment device is placed in the oxygen line coming from the concentrator. This line is introduced at the mattress level of the crib. The FiO_2 delivered into the crib is adjusted by the setting on the air entrainment device. At an FiO_2 setting of 0.50, a mattress level FiO_2 of 0.40 is achieved within 5 minutes and 0.46 within 20 minutes. A major advantage of the system is that it does not depend on secure fixation of

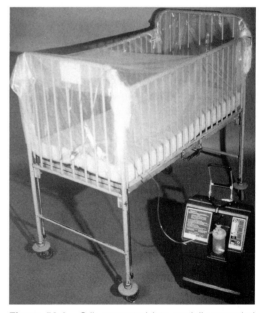

Figure 56.4. Crib converted into partially canopied "inverted tent" for oxygen delivery. The oxygen concentrator is connected to an air entrainment device at the head of the crib just before the oxygen line enters the tent. (From Zinman R, Franco I, Pizzuti-Daechsel R. Home oxygen delivery system for infants. *Pediatr Pulmonol* 1:326, 1985.)

the nasal cannula, which can be troublesome, especially in older infants. The air entrainment device allows the system to run off a concentrator at relatively low oxygen flow and assures a consistent FiO_2.

For adult patients different devices have been designed to conserve oxygen (11). This is of particular importance with respect to patient mobility, because small portable tanks will last longer if the flow requirements are less. The first such device was based on a reservoir system built into the nasal cannula. The reservoir was shaped like a moustache; it filled during expiration and provided a small bolus of oxygen in early inspiration. Because the moustache was unsightly, the design was modified, and the reservoir was placed in a pendant positioned over the chest. However, this required stiff tubing and was uncomfortable. More recently a technique of transtracheal oxygen flow has been used in some patients. This consists of a catheter placed through the skin and into the trachea. The fact that the catheter can be completely hidden from view makes it an attractive alternative to many patients; however, it requires more care than a nasal cannula, and is difficult to use in patients who produce large amounts of sputum. There is some limited experience in its use in patients with cystic fibrosis. Another approach to conserving oxygen is to limit flow just to the inspiratory phase of the respiratory cycle so that it is not wasted during expiration. Such devices are now available to be used with liquid reservoirs or compressed gas cylinders but have not been modified for infant use.

Home Care Planning

Pediatric expertise with respect to delivery systems and laboratory evaluation is essential, but is only one component of effective discharge planning. For best care of these patients, a team is required that includes a physician, nurse, respiratory therapist, and social worker, and the parents need to become actively involved in the care of their child in hospital (see Chapter 58). Parents need to acquire the necessary nursing and respiratory care skills to recognize if their child is in difficulty, and need to know how to intervene successfully. Home care also requires organization to procure and pay for the equipment that will be needed at home. Emergency services have to be notified, such as the electric

and telephone companies, as well as ambulance and local health care services. Not least of all there must be built into the home care plan some form of respite for the primary care giver.

REFERENCES

1. Abman SH, Wolfe RR, Accurso FJ, Koops BL, Bowman M, Wiggins JW Jr. Pulmonary vascular response to oxygen in infants with severe bronchopulmonary dysplasia. *Pediatrics* 1985; 75:80–84.
2. Fan LL, Voyles JB. Determination of inspired oxygen delivered by nasal cannula in infants with chronic lung disease. *J Pediatr* 1983; 103:923–925.
3. Flenley DC. Sleep in chronic obstructive lung disease. *Clin Chest Med* 1985; 6:651–661.
4. Garg M, Kurzner SI, Bautista DB, Keen TG. Clinically unsuspected hypoxia during sleep and feeding in infants with bronchopulmonary dysplasia. *Pediatrics* 1988; 81:635–642.
5. Groothuis JR, Rosenberg AA. Home oxygen promotes weight gain in infants with bronchopulmonary dysplasia. *Am J Dis Child* 1987; 141:992–995.
6. Jackson RM. Molecular, pharmacologic, and clinical aspects of oxygen-induced lung injury. *Clin Chest Med* 1990; 11:73–86.
7. Levi Valensi P, Aubry P, Donner CF, Robert D, Ruhle KH, Weitzenblum E, Wurtemburger R. Recommendations for long-term oxygen therapy (LTOT). *Eur Respir J* 1989; 2:160–164.
8. Levin DC, Neff TA, O'Donohue WJ Jr, Person DJ, Petty TL, Snider GL. Further recommendations for prescribing and supplying long-term oxygen therapy (Summary of the second conference on long-term oxygen therapy held in Denver, Colorado, Dec 11–12, 1987). *Am Rev Respir Dis* 1988; 138:745–747.
9. Medical Research Council Working Party. Long-term domiciliary oxygen therapy in chronic hypoxic cor pulmonale complicating bronchitis and emphysema. *Lancet* 1981; 1:681–686.
10. Nocturnal Oxygen Therapy Trial Group. Continuous or nocturnal oxygen therapy in hypoxemic chronic obstructive lung disease. A clinical trial. *Ann Intern Med* 1980; 93:391–398.
11. O'Donohue WJ Jr. Oxygen conserving devices. *Respir Care* 1987; 32:37–42.
12. Saugstad OD. Oxygen radicals and pulmonary damage. *Pediatr Pulmonol* 1985; 1:167–175.
13. Sewell EM, Holsclaw D, Schidlaw D, McGrady S, Berger B, Kolb S. The use of oxygen for children in their homes. *Pediatr Pulmonol* 1986; 2:72–74.
14. Spier S, Rivlin J, Hughes D, Levison H. The effect of oxygen on sleep, blood gases and ventilation in cystic fibrosis. *Am Rev Respir Dis* 1984; 129:712–718.
15. Stern RC, Borkat G, Hirschfield SS, Boat TF, Matthews LW, Liebman J, Doershuk CF. Heart failure in cystic fibrosis. Treatment and prognosis of cor pulmonale with failure of the right side of the heart. *Am J Dis Child* 1980; 134:267–272.
16. Suter PM, Fairley B, Isenberg MD. Optimum end-expiratory airway pressure in patients with acute pulmonary failure. *N Engl J Med* 1975; 292:284–289.
17. Taussig LM. Long-term management and pulmonary prognosis in bronchopulmonary dysplasia. In Farrell PM, Taussig LM eds. *Bronchopulmonary dys-*

plasia and related chronic respiratory disorders, Report of the ninetieth Ross conference in pediatric research. Columbus, OH, Ross Laboratories, 1986, pp 126–134.

18. Traver GA, Cline MG, Burrows B. Predictors of mortality in chronic obstructive pulmonary disease. *Am Rev Respir Dis* 1979; 119:895–902.

19. Whipple TJ, Lusk R. A device for administering low-flow oxygen to patients with tracheostomies. *Respir Care* 1985; 30:266–267.

20. Zinman R, Franco I, Pizzuti-Daechsel R. Home oxygen delivery system for infants. *Pediatr Pulmonol* 1985; 1:325–327.

21. Zinman R, Corey M, Coates AL, Canny GJ, Connolly J, Levison H, Beaudry PH. Nocturnal home oxygen in the treatment of hypoxemic cystic fibrosis patients. *J Pediatr* 1989; 114:368–377.

22. Zinman R, Blanchard PW, Vachon F. Oxygen saturation during sleep in patients with bronchopulmonary dysplasia. *Biol Neonate* 1992; 61:69–75.

57

Pharmacotherapy

ELIZABETH FARRINGTON

The previous chapters have reviewed the various respiratory diseases and made recommendations on treatment. The purpose of this chapter is to review the pharmacokinetics and pharmacodynamics of drugs used to treat various respiratory disorders and aid the physician with dosing strategies and the development of safe patient monitoring parameters.

A basic knowledge of pharmacokinetic principles is needed to order and interpret serum medication concentrations properly and calculate dosage regimens. These will be reviewed prior to discussing drug dosing (82), starting with theophylline.

The therapeutic range for a given drug is defined as the plasma concentrations that are both effective and safe; that is, within this range the desired effects of the drug are most likely to outweigh the side effects. Below this range, the therapeutic benefits are not realized; above it, toxicity is more likely to occur. There are no absolute boundaries for a given drug that separate subtherapeutic, therapeutic, and toxic drug concentrations. Individual differences in drug metabolism, elimination, and absorption will affect the therapeutic response.

PLASMA CONCENTRATIONS

Unless otherwise noted, the plasma concentration (Cp) of a drug is the total amount of drug (i.e., drug bound to plasma proteins and that unbound or free) in plasma. Since only the unbound portion is pharmacologically active, Cp may be only an indirect reflection of the concentration of active drug available.

Two major plasma proteins are responsible for approximately 95% of all drug binding: albumin (acidic drugs) and alpha-1 acid glycoprotein (basic drugs). Some disease states are associated with decreases in plasma proteins (renal failure, hepatic dysfunction, burns, malnutrition, and stress/trauma) or with decreased binding to plasma proteins (hyperbilirubinemia, hyper-uremia,). Changes in the binding characteristics of a drug may affect pharmacologic response to the drug, or the development of side effects.

VOLUME OF DISTRIBUTION

The volume of distribution (Vd) does not necessarily refer to an identifiable physiologic volume but to the fluid volume that would be needed to account for all the drug in the body. A small Vd implies that the drug is largely retained within the vascular compartment, whereas a large Vd implies distribution throughout the total body water or sequestration in certain tissues (see Table 57.5).

Loading Dose

Since the Vd relates the amount of drug in the body to the plasma drug concentration (Cp), it may be used to estimate the loading dose (LD) necessary to achieve a desired Cp (see Table 57.5).

Equation 2 in Table 57.5 can also be used to calculate the LD that will be required to achieve a higher CP than the present measured Cp. To calculate the new LD, one replaces Cp in equation 2 with (Cp [desired]—Cp [measured]), an expression that represents the increment in Cp that is desired (see Table 57.5).

HALF-LIFE AND STEADY STATE

The elimination half-life ($t_{1/2}$) of a drug is the time required for a 50% decrease in the Cp.

One pharmacokinetic relationship that is directly related to $t_{1/2}$ is steady state. When drugs are administered chronically, they accumulate in the body until the amount administered in a given time period (maintenance dose) is equal to the rate of elimination. When this occurs, Cp will plateau and will have reached "steady state." The time required for Cp to reach steady state is determined by the drug's half-life ($t_{1/2}$). After one $t_{1/2}$, 50% of steady state is achieved; after two, 75%; after three, 87.5%; after four; 93.75%; and after five, 97%. In most clinical situations, the attainment of steady state can be assumed after three to five half-lives. Whenever there is a change in either dose or interval, one must wait another three to five half-lives before a new steady state is attained *irrespective of the dosing interval.* The administration of a loading dose achieves a higher Cp, but does not shorten the time to reach steady state.

METHYLXANTHINES

Theophylline

ASTHMA

Theophylline, 1-dimethyl-xanthine, is used as a bronchodilator for the treatment of acute and chronic asthma. It is used for the treatment of apnea because of its central stimulation of respiration, and may be useful in weaning patients from mechanical ventilation.

MECHANISM OF ACTION

The mechanism of action of theophylline as a bronchial smooth muscle relaxant remains undefined. Historically, theophylline has been described as a potent inhibitor of phosphodiesterase, the enzyme that degrades cyclic 3'5' adenosine monophosphate (cAMP). However, in therapeutic concentrations theophylline does not inhibit this enzyme, and other phosphodiesterase inhibitors are not bronchodilators.

Theophylline binds to adenosine receptors at therapeutic concentrations and functions pharmacologically as an adenosine antagonist in lung tissue in vitro (5). However, in vitro, adenosine receptors are not antagonized by enprofylline, a xanthine derivative that is a more potent bronchodilator than theophylline (6). Furthermore, enprofylline has less

central nervous system (CNS) and cardiac toxicity than theophylline, suggesting that adenosine antagonism may account for some of the side effects of methylxanthines but not their bronchodilator effect (7). Other postulated mechanisms of action of theophylline include action as a prostaglandin antagonist (2), or as an agent that changes intracellular concentration of free calcium (3, 8). In addition to its effects on the lungs, theophylline produces a transient diuresis, stimulates the CNS, causes cerebral vasoconstriction, and inhibits uterine contractions. The drug also increases the acidity and volume of gastric contents. At therapeutic levels, theophylline reduces experimentally induced fatigue of diaphragmatic muscles, stimulates hypoxic ventilatory response, and enhances mucociliary clearance (8).

ABSORPTION

The absorption of theophylline (liquid and uncoated tablets) from the gastrointestinal tract is generally rapid and complete (9–11). The time to peak serum concentration of rapidly released formulations is from 30 minutes to 2 hours. Neither the presence of alcohol in solutions (12) nor micronized crystals in tablets (e.g., Theolair) or capsule formulations (e.g., Bronkodyl) speeds up absorption to a clinically important degree (13, 14). Delayed gastric emptying caused by the presence of food in the stomach (15) or magnesium-containing antacids (16, 17) slows the rate but not the extent of absorption of rapid-release theophylline preparations.

The slow-release dosage forms of oral theophylline are formulated using either a slowly dissolving tablet matrix or coated theophylline beads. With most preparations, the peak serum concentration occurs from 4–5 hours. Theo-Dur Sprinkle has good bioavailability when sprinkled on food (18, 19). However, significantly delayed absorption and reduced bioavailability occur when Theo-Dur Sprinkle is administered with meals (18, 20–22). Food has no clinically important effect on Theo-Dur tablets (23–26), Theo-Bid (26), Somophyllin-CRT (22, 27, 28) or Slo-Bid (29). In contrast, food results in dumping of potentially toxic amounts of theophylline from once-daily preparations (30–33). A study showed that in children, food significantly delayed theophylline absorption and resulted in approximately 50% greater peak concentrations compared to the fasting state (32).

Antacids increase the rate of theophylline absorption from Theolair-SR but not from Theo-Dur tablets (35) or Slophylline gyrocaps (36). The rate of absorption from a slow-released product with pH-dependent dissolution might be altered in the presence of antacids, H_2 histamine antagonists, or other factors that affect gastric pH.

Knowledge of the in-vivo absorption characteristics that exhibit delayed or slow dissolution is needed for safe and effective oral theophylline therapy. Products least affected by food and other factors such as pH should be considered for routine clinical use (Table 57.1).

Rectal theophylline solution is absorbed rapidly and completely (37, 38), and may be an acceptable alternative in the presence of vomiting or when fasting before surgery. Commercially available rectal suppositories are absorbed slowly and erratically (38), and are unreliable for chronic theophylline dosing.

DISTRIBUTION

Once theophylline enters the systemic circulation, it is rapidly distributed throughout extracellular fluids and body tissues, with peak serum levels occurring 1 hour after an IV loading dose (40). Theophylline protein binding ranges from 36% in neonates to 50–60% in the older child and adult (41). The drug readily crosses the placenta (42, 43) and is distributed into breast milk in concentrations about 70% those in serum (44, 45). The apparent Vd of theophylline ranges from 0.3 to 1.03 L/kg in premature infants (46) to 0.3–0.7 L/kg in children (47, 48) and adults (average 0.45 L/kg) (49).

METABOLISM AND ELIMINATION

Ten to fifteen percent of theophylline is eliminated by the kidneys unchanged (50); the remainder is metabolized exclusively by the liver microsomal system via oxidation and demethylation (51). In the premature neonate about 10% of the dose is metabolized to caffeine, but serum caffeine levels may be 30–50% of serum theophylline levels (52) because of delayed excretion of caffeine in this age group. Measurement of caffeine serum levels is only necessary when adverse effects appear.

Renal clearance of theophylline depends on urine flow rate (54), but dosage adjustments are not required in the presence of renal dysfunction.

There are differences in theophylline concentrations in asthmatic patients after daytime and nighttime oral dosing (55–57) that appear to be due to differences in nocturnal absorption. In healthy subjects, there is no evidence of time-dependent variation in theophylline biotransformation.

The half-life of theophylline varies with age (Table 57.2). In adult smokers there is induc-

---

Table 57.1.
Effect of Administration with Food on Selected Sustained-Release Theophylline (SRT) Products

SRT Product	Significant Effect	Clinical Significance
Theo-24 capsules	Yes	Dose-dumping reported with potentially toxic STCs
Uniphyllin tablets	Yes	Dose-dumping reported with potentially toxic STCs
Uniphyl tablets	Yes	Significant increased C_{max} and bioavailability—faster T_{max}
Theo-Dur sprinkles	Yes	Significantly decreased C_{max} and bioavailability
Theolair-SR tablets	No	Decreased C_{max} and bioavailability; clinical significance likely
Theo-Dur tablets	No	None likely
Slo-Bid gyrocaps	No	None likely
Slo-Phyllin gyrocaps	No	No effect with soft food; not tested with full meal
Somophyllin-CRT capsules	No	None likely, only effect is delay in absorption

Table 57.2.
Theophylline Half-Life and Clearance Values from Various Patient Populations

Patient Population	Age (years) Mean ± 50	Total Body Clearance Mean ± 50 (ml/kg/min)	Half-Life (hours)
Premature neonates	7.5 ± 4.4 days	0.29 ± 0.1	30 ± 6.5
	41 ± 12 days	0.64 ± 0.3	20 ± 5.3
Term infants	12 ± 4 weeks	Incomplete data	14 ± 4
(<6 months)	18 ± 2 weeks	0.8 ± 0.1	6.9 ± 1
6–11 months	34 ± 10 weeks	2.0 ± 0.5	4.6 ± 1
Young children	2.5 ± 0.9	1.7 ± 0.6	3.4 ± 1.1
(1–4 years)			
Older children	9.4 ± 3	1.6 ± 0.4	Not measured
(4–12 years)			
(6–17 years)	10.7 ± 0.6	14 ± 0.6	3.7 ± 1.1
(13–15 years)	14 ± 0.8	0.9 ± 0.2	Not measured
Adults (otherwise healthy	31 ± 10	0.65 ± 0.19	6.1 − 12.8
nonsmoking asthmatics)			(8.2)
Healthy nonsmoking volunteers	22-3 g	0.86 ± 0.35	8.1 ± 2.4
Heavy cigarette smokers	33	—	4.1 ± 1
	22–31 (27)	1.05 ± 0.3	5.4 ± 1
Marijuana alone	20–25	1.2 ± 0.5	4.3 ± 1
Marijuana + cigarettes	19–27	1.5 ± 0.4	4.3 ± 1

Adapted from Hendeles L, et al. Theophylline. In Evans WE, Schentag JJ, Jasko WJ, eds. *Applied pharmacokinetics.* San Francisco, Applied Therapeutics, 1986, pp 1105–1188.

tion of the metabolizing enzymes in the liver resulting in a half life of 4–5 hours (60, 61).

Variability of dosage requirements (Table 57.3) among individuals occurs as a result of variable rates of elimination. Theophylline clearance and therefore dosage requirements are markedly reduced in neonates (46, 62) and increase during the first year of life (59). Thereafter, they remain constant for the first 9 years and gradually decline to adult mean values by age 16 (63).

EFFECTS OF DISEASE AND ALTERED PHYSIOLOGY

Theophylline clearance is reduced during febrile (T > 102°F) viral illnesses (64), but it is not clear if this is due to the fever or the viral infection. Regardless of the mechanism, a temporary dosage reduction of 50% is recommended during the acute febrile period. The decrease in theophylline clearance associated with hepatic cirrhosis (65, 66), acute hepatitis (67), cardiac decompensation (68, 69), and cor pulmonale (as in bronchopulmonary dysplasia, or BPD) (70) can be quite large and require a significant dosage decrease to prevent toxicity. Theophylline clearance in patients with cholestasis (67) does not appear to be reduced. Enhanced theophylline clear-

ance occurs in adolescents with cystic fibrosis (71) and in patients with hyperthyroidism (72).

DRUG INTERACTIONS

Many drugs have been found to either inhibit or enhance theophylline clearance (73, 74). Co-administration of intravenous terbutaline or isoproterenol increases theophylline clearance, resulting in a shortened half-life of theophylline. Other drugs induce or inhibit hepatic metabolizing enzymes. Erythromycin and troleandomycin inhibit theophylline metabolism by way of competitive metabolism in the liver.

Theophylline may exhibit synergistic toxicity with ephedrine and other sympathomimetics. When administered concurrently, these agents increase the frequency of headache, insomnia, nervousness, and nausea disproportionate to that seen with either drug alone (75). Concomitant administration of intravenous beta-adrenergic agonist (e.g., isoproterenol, terbutaline) and theophylline may produce increased cardiotoxic effects. Cardiac arrhythmias have been reported in adolescents and adults receiving these combinations (76, 77).

Phenytoin levels appear to be decreased when it is taken with theophylline (78), and

Table 57.3.
Aminophylline/theophylline Dosing in Infants and Children

Patient Population	Age (years)	Theophylline (aminophylline) infusion rate (mg/kg/hour)	Oral maintenance therapy mg/kg/24 hours[a]
Premature neonates	Up to 40 weeks postconception	1 mg/kg q 12h	
	Postnatal age (weeks) 1–4	1–2 mg/kg q 12h	(0.2) (age in weeks ± 5)
	4–8	1–2 mg/kg q 8h	
	>8 weeks	1–3 mg/kg q 6h	
Infants	6–52 weeks old	mg/kg/hour − (0.008) (age in weeks) + 0.21	(0.3) (age in weeks + 8.0)
Young children	1–9	0.8 (1.0)	24
Older children	9–12	0.7 (0.9)	20
Adolescents (cigarette or marijuana smokers)	12–16	0.7 (0.9)	—
Adolescents (nonsmokers)	12–16	0.5 (0.6)	18
Adults (otherwise healthy cigarette or marijuana smoker)	16–50	0.7 (0.9)	—
Adults (otherwise healthy nonsmokers)	>16 (including the elderly)	0.4 (0.5)	13 (up to 900 mg/day)
Cardiac decompensation; hepatic dysfunction	>16	0.2 (0.25)	—

[a]Median dose necessary to achieve a serum concentration within the therapeutic range.

theophylline increases renal excretion of lithium, which may decrease its therapeutic effectiveness (79).

Recommendations of dosage adjustment when adding an interfering drug to a patient currently on theophylline are summarized in Table 57.4.

ADVERSE EFFECTS/TOXICITY

The adverse effects of theophylline are extensions of its pharmacologic properties and most likely occur when serum concentrations exceed 20 μg/ml. Low serum protein levels and altered protein binding may cause patients, especially neonates, to experience toxicity within the therapeutic range. These may occur as subtle symptoms such as failure to gain weight, sleeplessness, irritability, and tachycardia.

Theophylline side effects are manifested clinically by symptoms in three organ systems: the gastrointestinal (GI) tract, the central nervous system (CNS), and the heart (58). Theophylline produces GI irritation and CNS stimulation following administration by any route. The GI symptoms occur primarily as a result of a central effect on the medulla rather than a local irritative effect on the stomach. The most common adverse GI effects include nausea, vomiting, gastric irritation, and intestinal bleeding. Adverse CNS effects, which are often more severe in children than in adults, include headache, irritability, restlessness, nervousness, insomnia, and seizures. Cardiovascular effects include palpitations, tachycardia, and flushing.

Symptoms of frank toxicity are more pronounced manifestations of the effects mentioned above. Nausea and vomiting may be more pronounced and accompanied by abdominal tenderness, epigastric pain, hematemesis, and diarrhea. Hyper-reflexia, fasciculations, and generalized seizures can occur. Cardiovascular effects include palpitations and tachycardia. Hypertension is seen initially, but volume and vasopressor-resistant hypotension develops. Arrhythmias such as paroxysmal supraventricular tachycardia have also been documented (80).

Respiratory symptoms include tachypnea, which leads to respiratory alkalosis and respiratory arrest. Less frequently seen are hypophosphatemia, hypo-magnesemia, hypocalcemia, hypo-kalemia, and hyper-glycemia.

Table 57.4.
Recommendations of Dosage Adjustment When Adding an Interfering Drug to a Theophylline Regimen

Drug	Interaction	Suggested Adjustment
	Enhanced theophylline metabolism	
Carbamazepine	Increases elimination by average of 60%	Measure theophylline serum level to guide final dosage during concurrent therapy
Phenobarbital	Increases elimination by average of 25%	Measure theophylline serum level after 1 month of concurrent therapy and adjust dose if indicated
Phenytoin	Increases elimination by average of 75% (additionally theophylline appears to inhibit absorption of phenytoin)	Measure both phenytoin and theophylline serum levels at 5-day intervals to adjust the dose of each drug
Rifampin	Increases elimination by 50–80%	If rifampin is used for more than a few days measure theophylline serum level to guide final dose during concurrent therapy.
	Unknown	
Isoproterenol (IV)	Increases elimination by average of 20%	Measure theophylline serum level within 4–6 hours after adding isoproterenol or terbutaline and adjust theophylline dose accordingly
Terbutaline (IV)	Increases elimination by average of 20%	
	Inhibition of Theophylline Metabolism	
Allopurinol (high dose)	Decreases elimination by average of 25%	Reduce dose by 25% when >600 mg/24 hours allopurinol are required; pediatric high dose not established
Cimetidine	Decreases elimination by average of 40%. The interaction begins with 24 hours after initiation of therapy and is gone 3 days after discontinuing it	Use ranitidine, famotidine nizatidine, or antacids in place of cimetidine
Ciprofloxacin	Decreases elimination by average of 30%	Measure theophylline serum level to guide final dosage during concurrent therapy
Contraceptive pills	Decreases elimination by average of 30% (may be less with lower doses of estrogen)	Reduce theophylline by 30% and measure serum level 5 days later to make final adjustment
Propranolol	Decreases elimination by average of 20%	Measure theophylline serum level to guide final dosing during concurrent therapy
Erythromycin	Decreases elimination by average of 25% after 5 days of concurrent therapy	Reduce theophylline dose by 25% *or* measure serum theophylline level if erythromycin therapy is continued ≥ 5 days and serum concentration was ≥ 13
Troleandomycin	Decreases elimination by average of 50%	Reduce theophylline dose by 50% *and* measure serum theophylline in 5 days
	Unknown	
Interferon (recombinant interferon alpha)	Decreases elimination by average of 50%	Measure theophylline serum level to guide final dosage during concurrent therapy
Methotrexate	Decreases elimination by average of 20%	Measure theophylline serum level to guide final dosage during concurrent therapy
Mexiletin	Decreases elimination by average of 40%	Measure theophylline serum level to guide final dosage during concurrent therapy
Thiabendazole	Decreases elimination by average of 65%	Measure theophylline serum level to guide final dosage during concurrent therapy

Adapted from reference 7.

The clinical presentations of acute and chronic toxicity differ significantly (81). Acute toxicity generally presents with many, if not all, of the above symptoms in an orderly progression; seizures may be the only presenting symptom of chronic toxicity.

DRUG DOSING AND THERAPEUTIC MONITORING

Acute Bronchodilation

Inhaled and parenteral sympathomimetic therapies have demonstrated superiority over theophylline in the treatment of acute asthma (83, 84); however, when response to these agents is inadequate, theophylline may provide additional bronchodilation (85, 86). The optimal bronchodilatory effect of theophylline is achieved with serum concentrations of 10–20 μg/ml.

To obtain a therapeutic serum concentration as rapidly as possible one uses an intravenous loading dose. The serum concentration (C) obtained from an initial dose (D) is related to the volume of distribution (Vd); therefore, assuming an average volume of distribution of about 0.5 kg (range 0.3–0.7 L/kg), each milligram per kilogram of theophylline will raise the serum concentration 2 μg/ml. Aminophylline is 80% theophylline; therefore 1 mg of theophylline equals 1.25 mg aminophylline. Because of its limited distribution into fat, the loading dose of theophylline in obese individuals should be based on *effective body weight* (EBW), which is ideal body weight (IBW) plus 60% of the difference between actual (ACW) and IBW (87) (Table 57.5, equation 4).

For an acutely ill patient who has not had theophylline in the past 24 hours, the loading dose is calculated on the basis of ideal body weight and an assumed volume of distribution of 0.5 L/kg, and a desired serum level of 15 μg/ml (7.5 mg/kg). Because of the variation in volume of distribution among patients the serum level may fall between 11 and 26 μg/ml. In less acutely ill patients, a loading dose of theophylline to produce a serum theophylline concentration (STC) of 10 μg/ml (5 mg/kg) may be sufficient to eliminate the signs and symptoms of bronchospasm with a reduced risk of theophylline toxicity (expected serum level range 7–17 μg/ml.)

Table 57.5.
Pharmacokinetic Calculations

1. Volume of distribution (Vd)
   $$VD\ (L) = D\ (mg)\ Cp\ (mg/L)$$
   D = drug dose
   Cp = plasma concentrations

2. Loading dose (LD)
   $$LD = Vd \times Cp$$

3. Incremental loading dose
   $$LD - Vd \times [Cp(desired) - Cp(present)]$$

4. Effective body weight (EBW)
   $$EBW = [IBW + 0.6\ (ABW\text{-}IBW)$$
   ABW = actual body weight
   IBW = ideal body weight

5. $$Cl = \frac{2R}{(C_1 + C_2)} + \frac{2\ Vd^*\ (C_1 - C_2)}{(C_1 + C_2)(t_2 - t_1)}$$
   Cl = clearance (L/hour)
   R = infusion rate (mg/hour)
   C_1 = serum concentrations at time 1(t_1)
   C_2 = serum concentrations at time 2(t_2)

6. $$R = Cl \times Cp$$
   R = fusion rate
   Cp = desired plasma concentration

If a patient has a known but subtherapeutic STC, the loading dose of theophylline to produce a higher serum concentration can be calculated assuming 1 mg/kg of theophylline will raise the serum level 2 μg/ml. The desired serum level should be conservative (e.g., 10–15 μg/ml) to allow for the variability in volume of distribution. If the clinical situation requires prompt intervention, it is usually safe to administer a 2.5 mg/kg bolus of theophylline (i.e., raise the CP by 5 μg/ml) as long as the patient does not already have signs of theophylline toxicity.

The loading dose should be administered IV over 20 minutes to avoid adverse effects and should be followed immediately by a continuous infusion at a rate consistent with the child's clearance (Table 57.3). To monitor effectively the serum concentration of theophylline in patients on infusions, one must know whether the loading dose achieved the desired therapeutic concentration, and if the maintenance dose is keeping the concentration in the desired range. A serum level obtained 30 minutes after the completion of the intravenous loading dose when distribution is complete can be used to assess the need for and the size of subsequent loading doses. A second serum level is obtained one half-life (usually

4–6 hours) after starting the continuous infusion to determine if the serum concentration is accumulating or declining from the post-loading dose level. At this point, if the level is lower, a second bolus dose is indicated, but one should not increase the maintenance infusion rate until a steady-state STC is obtained. An additional sample, obtained 12–24 hours later, will help guide adjustments in the maintenance infusion. STC is obtained at 24-hour intervals to adjust for changes in clearance as they occur.

A simple equation may be used to compute the infusion rate necessary to achieve the desired serum concentration (88). This requires two serum levels obtained on the *same maintenance infusion rate*, but attainment of steady state (five half-lives) is not required. The time interval between the two levels should be at least one half-life, as estimated for age, to enhance the reliability of the method (Table 57.5, equation 5).

Once the clearance (Cl) is known, the rate of infusion can be adjusted to obtain the desired serum concentration using equation 6 of Table 57.5. This method is most accurate if the desired concentration is between the two measured values. The farther the desired concentration is outside this range, the greater the chance for error. In general, infusion rates should not be increased by more than 25% regardless of the calculated increment. Another method for adjusting continuous theophylline infusions is summarized in Table 57.6. A summary of pharmacokinetic equations is found in Table 57.5.

When the patient is sufficiently improved, therapy can be continued with an oral formulation by changing the continuous aminophylline infusion rate that produced a therapeutic steady state concentration to divided oral dosing appropriate for the age of the patient. Remember aminophylline is 80% theophylline; therefore,

Aminophylline (mg/hour) (24 hours) (0.80) =
   Total daily dose of theophylline (mg)

When the first dose of a slow-release oral formulation is administered, the intravenous infusion can be discontinued. A list of commercially available theophylline/aminophylline products can be found in Tables 57.7 and 57.8.

DOSAGE FOR TREATMENT OF CHRONIC ASTHMA

The recommended initial oral doses for theophylline (Table 57.3) can be associated with mild side effects such as nausea, headache, nervousness, and insomnia. These symptoms can be minimized by beginning with low doses (e.g., 12–14 mg/kg/24 hours (maximum 300 mg/24 hours) for children beyond 1 year old and adults. In infants the initial dose should not exceed the results of the following formula: mg/kg/24 hours = (0.2)(age in weeks) + 5. Increases in dose can be made, in 25% increments, every 3 days until the calculated daily dosage or a therapeutic theophylline level is obtained.

Blood samples obtained for assessment of long-term therapy should be collected during steady-state conditions, at least three half-lives after the last dose adjustment. In addition the patient should not have missed doses in the last 48 hours, taken additional doses, or changed his usual routine for theophylline dosing. Dosage adjustments (Table 57.6) should be guided by an estimation of the peak serum concentration that occurs.

Differences in theophylline concentrations occur depending on whether the dose is given in daytime or night-time (55–57). These result from differences in absorption of theophylline, which is slower at night, and not diurnal variation in theophylline metabolism. Therefore, in some patients information obtained around daytime dosing may not predict serum concentrations achieved at night.

Dosage adjustments should be guided by measuring peak and not trough serum concentrations, since a trough level under 10 μg/ml can be associated with a peak near 20 μg/ml, and an increase in dose could result in peak concentrations that exceed 20 μg/ml. Measurement of trough theophylline concentrations may be helpful if asthma symptoms occur repeatedly at the end of the dosage interval even though the peak is within the therapeutic range.

Once the appropriate dosage regimen is established, serum concentrations should be monitored every 4–6 months in children, depending on growth. This will allow for adjustment in the patient's theophylline regimen prior to "outgrowing" his or her theophylline dose. In adults, measurements can be

Table 57.6.
Dosage Adjustment After Serum Theophylline Measurement

Peak Serum Concentrations	Directions
<7.5 µg/ml	Increase dose by about 25%.[a] Recheck serum theophylline concentration for guidance in further dosage adjustment (another increase will probably be needed, but this provides a safety check).
7.5–10.0 µg/ml	Increase dose by about 25%.[a] Recheck serum theophylline concentration in 3 days, then at 6–12 month intervals.[b]
10–20 µg/ml	Maintain dosage if tolerated. Recheck serum theophylline concentrations at 6–12 month intervals.[b]
20–25 µg/ml	Decrease dose by about 10%. Recheck serum theophylline concentration after 3 days, then at 6–12 month intervals.[b]
25–30 µg/ml	Skip next dose and decrease subsequent doses by about 25%. Recheck serum theophylline.
>30 µg/ml	Skip next two doses and decrease subsequent doses by 50%. Recheck serum theophylline.

[a]Dividing the daily dose into three doses administered at 8-hour intervals may be indicated if symptoms occur repeatedly at the end of the dosing interval.
[b]Finer dosage adjustments may be needed for some patients.
From Weinberger M, Hendeles L. A practical guide to using theophylline. *J Respir Dis* 1981; 212–227.

obtained yearly. Changes in concurrent drug therapy (the addition or deletion of an interfering drug), the presence of sustained fever, or changes in cardiac or hepatic function may alter drug elimination and warrant more frequent measurement of serum theophylline levels. A list of available theophylline/aminophylline preparations can be found in Tables 57.7 and 57.8.

APNEA

Theophylline serum concentrations considered therapeutic for the treatment of apnea are 5–12 µg/ml (89). An initial loading dose of 5 mg/kg should be administered, followed by a maintenance dose; higher doses are suggested by some for premature neonates (91). Since the half-life of theophylline in newborns is generally greater than 20 hours, there is no need to administer the maintenance dose more often than every 12 hours. However, the theophylline clearance increases with age, resulting in increased dosage requirements. Dosage recommendations are summarized in Table 57.3, but must be guided by careful monitoring of serum theophylline concentrations.

Caffeine

The methylxanthine caffeine has been demonstrated to decrease the frequency of neonatal apnea.

MECHANISM OF ACTION

The mechanism by which methylxanthines affect apnea is not known. However, several actions seem to be beneficial, and it may be a combination of these effects that decrease the frequency of neonatal apnea. The proposed mechanisms include (a) increased sensitivity of the medullary respiratory center to CO_2 (92, 93), (b) increased vagal activity (94), improving both the contractibility of respiratory muscles and their recovery from fatigue (95–97), (c) improved metabolic homeostasis (98), (d) competitive inhibition of adenosine receptors (99–101), and (e) increased circulating catecholamine levels (101).

CAFFEINE VERSUS THEOPHYLLINE

The advantages of caffeine over theophylline include a higher therapeutic index, once-daily administration with smaller fluctuation in plasma concentrations, no active metabolites to confuse the interpretation of the serum concentration measurement, and fewer adverse drug effects (99).

ABSORPTION AND DISTRIBUTION

Caffeine is rapidly and completely absorbed from the gastrointestinal tract with peak serum concentrations reached in 30–120 minutes (102). Caffeine is rapidly distributed into body tissues, readily crossing the blood-

103). Caffeine toxicity is not common if serum levels are less than 40 μg/ml (99). Therapy is initiated with a 10 mg/kg loading dose of caffeine base, followed 24 hours later by a maintenance regimen of 2.5 mg/kg/24 hours of caffeine base, as a single daily dose (106). Caffeine citrate is about 50% caffeine base. Neonates failing to respond to this dosage regimen should receive incremental increases with monitoring of plasma concentrations. Steady-state plasma concentrations reflective of a dosage change will not occur for three to five half-lives (approximately 2 weeks in neonates and 1 week in infants). A trough plasma concentration is recommended for monitoring therapy.

Doxapram

Doxapram hydrochloride has been used in treating apnea of prematurity refractory to methylxanthine therapy (107–110). Doxapram hydrochloride stimulates all levels of the CNS, augmenting descending CNS impulses. It transiently increases the volume, and to a lesser extent, the rate of respiration by stimulating the medullary respiratory centers. In addition to the treatment of apnea, doxapram has been used to control central hypoventilation syndromes and narcotic-induced respiratory depression.

Doxapram is administered as a continuous intravenous infusion of 1.0–2.5 mg/kg/hour. After approximately 6 hours of therapy (non–steady-state doxapram concentrations of 3.7 ± 1.8 μg/ml), a significant decrease in the frequency of apnea has been reported (107). With control of apnea, the infusion rate should be decreased to 0.5–0.8 mg/kg/hour to avoid significant adverse effects. An alternative dosing scheme (109) is to administer a 3 mg/kg loading dose over 15 minutes, followed by an infusion rate of 1 mg/kg/hour.

Adverse drug effects are associated with infusion rates greater than 3 mg/kg/hour and serum doxapram concentrations greater than 5 μg/ml (107). These include CNS stimulation, seizures, hypertension, hypothermia, salivation, abdominal distension, vomiting, hyperglycemia, and glycosuria.

The use of the drug is limited by its availability only in parenteral form. Doxapram should be considered a second-line pharmacologic agent for infants who fail to respond to methylxanthines. In the United States, doxapram is available only in a preparation that contains benzyl alcohol 0.9% as a preservative. The recommended doxapram dosage of 0.5–2.5 mg/kg/hour would deliver 5.4–32.4 mg/kg/24 hours benzyl alcohol. Although this quantity is below the dose (94–245 mg/kg/24 hours) reported to cause "gasping syndrome" (112), it has been recommended that low-birth-weight infants receive no fluids or drugs containing benzyl alcohol as a preservative (112).

Beta-Adrenergic Agonists

The beta-2 agonists have become first-line agents for the treatment of asthma because of their ease of administration, rapid onset of action, and relatively uncommon side effects.

MECHANISM OF ACTION/PHARMACOLOGY

The beta-adrenergic drugs dilate bronchial smooth muscle exclusively by stimulating beta-adrenergic receptors. Beta-1 receptors do not appear to play a role in the modulation of bronchial tone in humans (113). Phenylethylamine derivatives (i.e., ephedrine) dilate the bronchi indirectly, by stimulating the release of catecholamines from nerve endings.

Stimulation of the beta adrenoreceptors causes activation of adenylate cyclase, which increases production of adenosine 3', 5'-cyclic phosphate (cAMP). The accumulation of cAMP blunts the phosphorylation of myosin light-chain kinase, and therefore prevents the interaction of actin with light-chain phosphorylated myosin; thus, the muscle contraction is blocked. The result is smooth muscle relaxation (114).

In addition, cAMP appears to disinhibit protein kinase, which leads to increases in calcium binding to the endoplasmic reticulum and cell membrane. This results in a lowering of the intracellular calcium concentration and in smooth muscle relaxation (115). Beta-adrenergic agonists may also induce increased mucociliary transport of respiratory secretions. Stimulation of beta-2 receptors in mast cells inhibits the release of histamine and leukotrienes, but does not alter release of mediators from granulocytes. Therefore, the beta-agonists reverse and prevent the early asthmatic response but do not inhibit either the late response to allergens or the subsequent bronchial hyper-responsiveness (117).

Distinctions between beta-adrenergic agonists are based on differences in chemistry and selectivity for the beta-2 receptor over the beta-1 receptor (Table 57.9) (118).

PHARMACOKINETICS

Few pharmacokinetic data are available on beta-adrenergic agonists owing to the very low serum levels of drug that are achieved after dosing, particularly following inhalation. Only metaproterenol, terbutaline, and albuterol are available orally. Other beta-2 agonists are rapidly conjugated and inactivated in the mucosa of the gastrointestinal tract (119). The oral administration of these drugs is followed by blood concentration–dependent bronchodilation; peak drug concentration in blood is achieved in 1–2 hours.

With aerosol drug delivery, a high percentage of each drug dose is trapped in the upper airways or is swallowed; only 13% of a dose from a metered dose inhaler and 1–5% of a dose administered by nebulization reach the lower respiratory tract (120). For all inhaled catecholamine beta-adrenergic agonists (except bitolterol), peak effects occur 5–15 minutes after administration and persist for 1–3 hours. Bitolterol's actions are maximal at 0.5–2 hours after administration and continue for up to 6 hours (121).

Metaproterenol has a slower onset of action (30 minutes), peak effects in 1 hour, and a duration of action (DOA) of 3–5 hours. Albuterol, of the saligen class, has a rapid onset of 5–15 minutes, with peak effects in 0.5–2 hours and a DOA of 3–6 hours. Salmeterol, a saligen agent, has an onset of action of 10–20 minutes, with peak effects in 3–4 hours and a DOA of at least 12 hours. The resorcinol agents terbutaline and fenoterol have similar pharmacokinetic profiles: onset of action 5–15 minutes; peak effects 1–2 hours; effects last for as long as 6 hours.

SIDE EFFECTS

The side effects of the beta-adrenergic agonists are extensions of their pharmacologic effects; the majority are transient or disappear promptly after the drug is withdrawn (120, 121). Skeletal muscle tremor, tachycardia, palpitations, and nervousness are the most common adverse effects reported (122). The cardiac effects can be either direct beta-1 reception stimulation or reflex tachycardia through beta-2 mediated peripheral vasodilation (123).

Other beta-mediated side effects occurring after relatively high doses are headache, dizziness, nausea, weakness, sweating, and a worsening of ventilation-perfusion (V/Q) ratio. Metabolic effects observed after intravenous administration of beta agonists are a 10–25% increase in blood glucose, lactate, pyruvate, ketone bodies, and non-esterified fatty acids, with minor decreases in serum potassium, magnesium, calcium, and phosphate. The

Table 57.9.
Beta-Adrenergic Agents

Drug	Route of Administration			Duration of Action (hours)	Receptor		
	Injection	Inhaled	Oral		β_2	β_1	α
Catecholamines							
Bitolterol	No	Yes	No	4–6	+ +	+	−
Ephedrine	Yes	No	Yes	2–3	+	+	+
Epinephrine	Yes	Yes	No	1–2	+	+	+
Isoetharine	No	Yes	No	2–3	+ +	+	−
Isoproterenol	Yes	Yes	No	2–3	+	+	+
Resorcinols							
Fenoterol[a]	No	Yes	No	4–6	+ +	+	−
Metaproterenol	No	Yes	Yes	3–5	+ +	+	−
Terbutaline	Yes	Yes[b]	Yes	4–6	+ +	+	−
Saligen							
Albuterol	No	Yes	Yes	4–6	+ +	±	−
Pirbuterol	No	Yes	No	5	+ +	+	−
Salmeterol[c]	No	Yes	No	12	+ + +	−	−

[a]Not available in the United States.
[b]Not FDA-approved for this indication.
[c]Awaiting FDA approval in the United States.

alteration in serum potassium is an initial rise, resulting from potassium efflux from the liver as a result of glycogenolysis, followed by a more pronounced fall as the potassium enters muscle cells. There is concern that these potassium shifts may contribute to the development of cardiac arrhythmias, particularly in patients whose potassium stores are depleted; therefore beta agonists should be used cautiously in patients with heart disease and hypokalemia (123). The frequency of adverse effects with the beta agonists depends on their route of administration. Adverse effects are least frequently associated with drug inhalation since the drug is delivered directly to the lungs. Oral and injectable administration are more often associated with adverse effects (121). In general, the adverse effects of beta agonists are dose-dependent, regardless of the route of administration.

Tolerance

Tolerance does develop to the nonbronchial effects of beta agonists in both animals and humans within approximately 1 month of initiating therapy. These include reduced effects on tremor, heart rate, and nervousness. In-vitro studies have demonstrated that beta-adrenergic receptors may become desensitized (tolerant) to stimulation by beta agonists. This may occur because of down-regulation of the receptors (receptors are removed from the cell surface and stored within the cell) or from phosphorylation of the receptors, which makes them unable to activate adenyl cyclase (124).

Numerous studies have attempted to determine if tachyphylaxis to the bronchodilatory effects of beta-2 agonists develops after long-term use. Although the results have been conflicting, most evidence indicates that prolonged use of oral or inhaled beta agonists results in a shortening of the duration of effect, not a lessening of effect; thus, tolerance may influence the dosage interval in some patients (114).

ADMINISTRATION

Table 57.10 summarizes the currently available formulations of beta-adrenergic drugs. Beta-adrenergic drugs can be administered by inhalation using five different methods: (a) metered dose inhalers (MDIs), (b) MDIs with auxiliary delivery systems, (c) nebulizers driven by compressed air or ultrasonic crystals, (d) intermittent positive pressure breathing (IPPB), and (e) powder aerosols. These methods differ in ease of use, portability, and convenience. However, if good technique is performed, there is probably no difference between them in terms of efficacy (125).

There are two main advantages to inhalation therapy over oral, subcutaneous, or intravenous administration that make it the preferred initial route of administration. First, the drug is delivered directly to the respiratory tract, necessitating substantially smaller quantities of drug to achieve the desired therapeutic effect; consequently, the blood level achieved and the corresponding systemic side effects are less. Second, the onset of action is immediate (5–15 minutes), much shorter than after oral administration (1–2 hours) and comparable with the onset after intravenous dosing (5 minutes).

The reliability of any specific method of administration depends on the ability of the patient to coordinate breathing with activation of the device. The nebulizer is the most reliable drug delivery system, especially in an acutely ill or dyspneic patient, because it requires only tidal breathing. With the exception of infants, spacer devices simplify MDI use and reduce oropharyngeal deposition, therefore increasing the amount of drug that reaches the lungs (126–128). The devices probably do not add benefit in patients with good MDI technique (129, 130).

In choosing among the spacers available in the United State, the practitioner must consider the reservoir size, the inclusion of and type of incentive device in the design, and the cost (Table 57.11).

Albuterol powder can be administered using a dry powder inhaler (DPI), Rotahaler. This is as effective as administration via MDI, with both dosage forms producing a comparably low frequency of adverse effects (131, 132).

The DPI offers the convenience of MDI use, but eliminates the need for hand-breath coordination. Two limitations of DPI devices available in the United States are the need for high inspiratory flow rates and the cumbersome loading procedure. Inspiratory flow rates below 50 L/minute are associated with a significant reduction in clinical response using the Rotahaler device (133). During acute epi-

Table 57.10.
Beta Agonist Dosages

Medication	Form	Pediatric	Adult
Subcutaneous			
Epinephrine	1:1000 (1 mg/ml)	0.01 mg/kg up to 0.5 mg/kg every 20 min for 3 doses	0.3–0.5 mg every 20 min for 3 doses
Sustained-action epinephrine (susphrine)	1:200 (5 mg/ml)	0.005–0.01 mg/kg every 6–10 hours PRN	0.5–0.75 (0.10 to 0.15 ml) mg every 6–10 hours PRN
Terbutaline	1 mg/ml	0.01 mg/kg q 20 min × 3 doses, then q 2–6 hours PRN	0.25–0.5 mg q 20 min × 3 doses, then q 2–6 hours PRN
Nebulizer solution			
Albuterol	5 mg/ml	0.05–0.15 mg/kg 8–20 min × 3 doses, then q 2–4 hours PRN (continuous aerosol 0.30 mg/kg/hour	2.5–5 mg every 20 min × 3 doses, then q 2–4 hours PRN
Fenoterol	5 mg/ml[b]	Same as albuterol	Same as albuterol
Isoproterenol	1:400 (2.5 mg/ml) 1:200 (5 mg/ml) 1:100 (10 mg/ml)	0.05–0.1 mg/kg q 20 min × 3 doses, then q 2–4 hours PRN	3.5–7 mg q 20 min × 3 doses, then q 2–4 hours PRN
Isoetharine	0.1–1%	0.1–0.2 mg/kg q 20 min × 3 doses then q 2–4 hours PRN	3–10 mg q 20 min × 3 doses, then q 2–4 hours PRN
Metaproterenol	50 mg/ml	0.25–0.5 mg/kg q 2–4 hours PRN; maximum: 15 mg	15 mg (.3 ml) in 3–4 ml NS q 2–4 hours PRN
Terbutaline	Injection: 1 mg/ml[a] nebulizer solution: 10 mg/ml[b]	0.1–0.3 mg/kg q 20 min × 3 does then q 2–4 hours PRN	5–10 mg undiluted ? q 20 min × 3 doses then q 2–4 hours PRN
Epinephrine racemic	2.25%	0.03 ml/kg q 1–2 hours PRN (min: 0.25 ml; max: 125 ml)	1.25 ml q 1–2 hours PRN
Metered dose inhaler			
Albuterol	MDI: 90 μg/puff	1–2 puffs q 4–6 hours and prior to exercise	1–2 puffs q 4–6 hours and prior to exercise
	Powder inhaler 200 μg Rotacaps	1–2 caps q 4–6 hours PRN	1–2 caps q 4–6 hours PRN
Bitolterol	MDI: 370 μg/puff	1–2 puffs q 4–6 hours PRN	1–3 puffs q 4–6 hours PRN
Epinephrine	MDI: 300 μg/puff MDI: 270 μg/puff MDI: 200 μg/puff	1–2 puffs q 4 hours PRN	1–2 puffs q 4 hours PRO
Fenoterol	MDI: 160 μg/puff	1–2 puffs q 4–6 hours PRN	1–2 puffs q 4–6 hours PRN
Isoetharine	MDI: 340 μg/puff	1–2 puffs q 4–6 hours	1–2 puffs q 4–6 hours
Isoproterenol[b]	MDI: 131 μg/puff	1–2 puffs q 4–6 hours	1–2 puffs q 2–4 hours
Metaproterenol	MDI: 65 μg/puff	1–2 puffs q 4–6 hours and before exercise	2–3 puffs q 4–6 hours and before exercise
Pirbuterol	MDI: 200 μg/puff	2 puffs q 4–6 hours PRN	2 puffs q 4–6 hours
Salmeterol[b]	MDI: 25 μg/puff	2 puffs q 12 hours	2 puffs q 12 hours
Terbutaline	MDI: 200 μg/puff	1–2 puffs q 4–6 hours and before exercise	1–2 puffs q 4–6 hours and before exercise

Table 57.10.
Beta Agonist Dosages, *continued*

Medication	Form	Pediatric	Adult
Oral formulations			
Albuterol	Tablets: 2,4 mg	2–6 years: 0.1 mg/kg/ dose, maximum 0.2 mg/dose (4 mg) TID	Regular release: 2–4 mg TID–QID
	Extended release: 4,8 mg	6–12 years: 2 mg/dose qd–qid, maximum 24 mg/24 hours QID	Extended release: 4–8 mg q 12 hours, maximum 32 mg/24 hours
	Syrup: 2 mg/5 ml		
Ephedrine	Capsules: 25, 50 mg Syrup: 11 mg/5 ml; 20 mg/5 ml	3 mg/kg/24 hours q 4–6 hours	
Fenoterol[b]	Tablet: 2.5, 5 mg	0.1–0.2 mg/kg q 6–8 hours	2.5–5 mg q 6–8 hours
Metaproterenol	Tablets: 10, 20 mg Syrup: 10 mg/5 ml	Children <12 years: 0.3–0.5 mg/kg/dose	10–20 mg/dose q 6–8 hours
Terbutaline	Tablets: 2.5, 5 mg	< 12 years initial: 0.05 mg/kg/dose TID; maximum 0.15 mg/kg/ dose TID–QID	25–50 mg/dose q 6–8 hours

[a]Not FDA-approved for this use.
[b]Not available in the United States.

Table 57.11.
Spacer Devices

Brand Name	Manufacturer	Volume	Description
Aerochamber	Monaghan Medical Co.	—	Cylinder with *one-way valve* that traps aerosol until inhaled by subject. Available with flowsignal and with a mask.
Brethancer	Geigy Pharmaceuticals	—	10-cm open-ended telescopic tube *(no valve).*
Inhal-Aid	Key Pharmaceuticals	700 ml	Plastic spherical chamber with a flowmeter and *one-way valves* for directed airflow.
Inspirease	Key Pharmaceuticals	700 ml	A collapsible bag with a flow indicator whistle.
Nebuhaler	A.B. Dracho[a]	750 ml	Conical spacer with a *one-way valve* at the mouth piece.
Optihaler	HealthScan Products, Inc.		10-cm open-ended telescopic tube *(no valve).*
Ace (aerosol cloud enhancer)	Diemolding Health Care Division	150 ml	Frustoconical spacer with a *one-way valve* at the mouthpiece and a flow indicator whistle.
Ellipse Compact Spacer	Allen Hanburys	172 ml	Eliptically shaped hollow cylinder; 12 cm, *(no valve).*

[a]Not available in the United States.

sodes, children may have peak inspiratory flow rates below this level, and it is recommended that another form of aerosol delivery be used. The need for high flow rates does not appear to be present with the terbutaline-dry-powder multiple dose inhaler, available in the United Kingdom and Europe (but not the United States) as the Turbohaler and Turbuhaler, respectively. Children as young as 3 years can use this device with good results (133).

MDIs are portable and have a short preparation and administration time compared to nebulizers. However, it is often difficult for children to use inhalers correctly (130, 134).

MDI use may be complicated further by the lack of knowledge among health care professionals on proper use (135). Thirty to seventy percent of asthmatics use MDIs *incorrectly* (136).

It is important to check each child's technique periodically to ensure that no bad habits develop. Lee and Evans found that 30% of children who previously demonstrated correct MDI technique were later unable to perform the technique correctly.

ORAL ADMINISTRATION

If adequate doses of an aerosol preparation can be taken, there is no compelling reason to use an oral preparation. There are two instances, however, wherein oral administration may be indicated. Oral sustained-release beta-2 agonists are useful in the treatment of nocturnal asthma (137, 138), and oral beta-2 agonists may be used in infants and small children when the severity of the disease does not warrant purchase of nebulizer equipment.

SUBCUTANEOUS/INTRAVENOUS ADMINISTRATION

Prior to the development of beta-2 selective aerosolized bronchodilators, subcutaneous administration of epinephrine was the standard of care for the emergency management of status asthmaticus. Subcutaneous administration of beta-2 agonists may still be required, if for any reason an aerosolized beta-2 agonists cannot be administered immediately, or if the child cannot tolerate or will not cooperate with a nebulizer treatment. Subcutaneously administered beta agonists (epinephrine or terbutaline) are well established as effective therapy for acute exacerbations of asthma. Terbutaline, however, may have a therapeutic advantage because of its longer duration of action and beta-2 selectivity (139).

Intravenous administration of beta-2 agonists may be attempted in order to avoid endotracheal intubation in a patient with status asthmaticus or to treat a patient in respiratory failure. This therapeutic intervention must be performed only in a pediatric intensive care unit, where continuous cardiac monitoring is available, because of the risk of arrhythmias and or myocardial ischemia. Isoproterenol, terbutaline, and albuterol have been used in

this way (139–142) (Table 57.12). Isoproterenol may cause dysrhythmia, sudden deaths, EKG changes consistent with myocardial ischemia, and cardiac enzyme elevations (77). The reported patients were adolescents or adults who were also receiving theophylline. Intravenous terbutaline has also demonstrated arrhythmogenic potential when combined with theophylline (76). Isoproterenol, terbutaline, and albuterol may initially worsen ventilation-perfusion mismatch; thus, an increase in oxygen requirement should be anticipated. Hypokalemia and a 10–25% increase in serum glucose level may occur with intravenous beta agonist therapy. Lastly, all three agents are efficacious in treating respiratory failure, although terbutaline and albuterol have a potential for a lower incidence of cardiovascular adverse effects (141, 142). Terbutaline does not have a Food and Drug Administration (FDA) indication for the treatment of status asthmaticus, and intravenous albuterol is not available in the United States.

Corticosteroids

ASTHMA

Corticosteroids have been used in the management of asthma for years, but the recent focus on the inflammatory nature of asthma has shifted their role to one of primary therapy (Table 57.13) (143).

Table 57.12.
Intravenous Dosing of Beta Agonists in Asthma

Isoproterenol	*Continuous infusion:* 0.1 μg/kg/min Increment: 0.1 μg/kg/min every 15 minutes *Maximum:* 1.5 μg/kg/min or HR>200
Terbutaline[a]	*Load:* 2 μg/kg given over 2 minutes *Continuous infusion:* 0.05–0.1 μg/kg/min Increment: 0.1 μg/kg/min every 15 minutes *Maximum:* 1.0 μg/kg/min or HR>200
Albuterol[b]	*Load:* 10 μg/kg given over 10 minutes *Continuous infusion:* 0.2 μg/kg/min Increment: 0.1 μg/kg/min every 15 minutes *Maximum:* 4 μg/kg/min

[a]Not FDA-approved for this use.
[b]Not available in the United States.

Table 57.13.
Factors Associated with Corticosteroid Side Effects

Factor	Effect
Duration of treatment	At least 2 weeks of therapy is required for suppression of the normal adrenal response to stress.
Time of dose	Single oral morning doses, in patients requiring chronic CCS administration, will mimic the normal pituitary diurnal rhythm, thereby resulting in the least suppression of the HPA-axis.
Preparation	Because of the constant stimulation of the peripheral tissue receptors, due to their longer plasma half-lives, the longer-acting corticosteroids are more likely to produce cushingoid side effects and induce suppression of the HPA-axis.
Route of administration	The less drug systemically absorbed, the less suppression of the HPA-axis, therefor inhalation < oral < intravenous.
Dose	The higher the dose, the greater risk of CCS adverse effects. Doses should be compared using the equivalent anti-inflammatory dose found in Table 57.17.
Dosage interval	Alternate-day CCS causes fewer adverse effects than daily dosing or q6–12 hour dosing.

MECHANISM OF ACTION

Corticosteroids (CCSs) pass through cell membranes and bind to cytoplasmic receptors. The interaction of the steroid and the receptor produces a complex that is taken up by the nucleus to interact with nuclear DNA, initiating the synthesis of messenger RNA, which in turn leads to the production of specific proteins (144–146). These proteins include the beta-adrenergic receptor. It appears that CCSs may facilitate beta-adrenergic receptor numbers and their coupling to adenylate cyclase. In addition, CCSs restore and prevent tolerance induced with chronic administration of beta-adrenergics.

Other actions of CCSs helpful in treating asthma include reduction of mucus production and hyper-secretion and inhibition of the inflammatory response at all levels. CCSs constrict the microvasculature, inhibiting fluid and protein influx and inhibit migration of neutrophils and eosinophils into tissues as well as inhibiting their function. CCSs also induce the production of lipocortin, a protein that inhibits the synthesis of phospholipase A_2 and thus leads to a decrease in the synthesis of leukotrienes, platelet activating factor, and release of arachidonic acid from membrane phospholipids. Lastly, CCSs inhibit the synthesis but not the release of histamine from most cells. Corticosteroids initially exert their primary effect on the late asthmatic response, and only after extended administration do these agents decrease bronchial hyper-activity (147).

TIME COURSE OF RESPONSE

CCSs act through production of lipocortin; therefore, the time required to see a particular effect depends on the time required for lipocortin synthesis, decreased formation of the particular mediator, and resolution of the response (148). Generally the cellular and biochemical effects are immediate, but longer time is required to produce a clinical response. Beta receptor density increases within 4 hours of glucocorticoid administration (148), although improved responsiveness to beta agonists may not occur until 12 hours (149). In acute severe asthma (status asthmaticus), 12–36 (average 24) hours may be required until any clinical response is noted. Reversal of seasonal increased bronchial hyper-reactivity requires at least 1 week of therapy (148). Reactivity to exercise decreases after 4 weeks of therapy (150). CCS therapy continued for 1 week will partially block the immediate asthmatic response to antigen challenge (151).

TOXICITY

The frequency of adverse effects with CCSs depends on the factors listed in Table 57.14.

Adverse effects have mostly been associated with continuing long-term therapy. The greatest risk of long-term CCS therapy is suppression of the hypothalamic-pituitary-adrenal axis (HPA-axis). Adrenal-CCS insufficiency after chronic CCS administration may be life-threatening. It appears that at least 2 weeks of therapy is required for suppression of the normal adrenal response to stress (152). Recovery of normal adrenal response after long-term therapy may take up to 1 year (153).

Table 57.14.
Complications Associated with Corticosteroids

Site	Unpleasant Effects	Significant Effects
Skin	Acne, hirsutism, striae, flushing, facial erythema, increased perspiration hypopigmentation, burning, folliculitis	Loss of subcutaneous tissue, poor wound healing
Vascular	Petechiae, bruising	Thromboemboli or fat embolism, vasculitis, periarteritis nodosa, thrombophlebitis
Appearance	Fat deposition (facial mooning, buffalo hump, truncal obesity, etc.)	Stunting of growth in children
Central nervous system	Insomnia, restlessness, agitation, headache, vertigo	Altered personality, psychosis (euphoria, mania, depression, confusion) pseudotumor cerebri, seizures, neuritis/paresthesias
Cardiovascular	Edema (due to Na retension)	Hypertension, heart failure, arrhythmias, myocardial infarction
Metabolic	Sodium and fluid retention hypokalemia, alkalosis hypocalcemia, negative nitrogen balance, hyperlipidemia	Deceased carbohydrate tolerance, hyperglycemia, glycosuria (diabetogenic effect), hyperosmolar ketotic coma
Musculoskeletal	Weakness (due to myopathy, hypokalemia, and wasting), osteoporosis, leg cramps	Vertebral and other fractures, aseptic bone necrosis of femoral and humeral heads, tendon rupture, growth suppression, abnormal teeth
Endocrine	Menstrual disorders, menopausal symptoms, impotence, delayed sexual maturation, decreased number and mobility of spermatozoa	HPA-axis suppression
Gastrointestinal	Nausea vomiting, fatty liver, increased appetite, with excessive weight gain	Increased risk of peptic ulceration, pancreatitis, perforation of the bowel, peritonitis, gastric hemorrhage esophagitis
Ocular	Exophthalmos, posterior subcapsular cataract, 6th-nerve palsies (diplopia)	Papilledema, increased Iop, glaucoma, increased risk of fungal and viral keratitis
Immunologic	Oral candidiasis, suppression of skin test reaction, increased susceptibility to infections	Masking infections, latent infections becoming active, opportunistic infection, decreased serum IgG levels
Renal system	Incresed urinary frequency and nocturia	Nephrosclerosis, nephrolithiasis, uncosuria
Hematopoietic	Leukocytosis, monocytopenia, lymphopenia, eosinopenia	Agranulocytosis, disturbances in coagulation
Fetus		Risk of teratogenicity in first trimester, possible adrenal insufficiency in newborn infant

The side effects of long-term CCS therapy are listed in Table 57.14. There are minimal risks of serious toxicity with short-term ($<$ 2 weeks) use of daily oral or injected CCS (153). However, four or more short-term courses of corticosteroids per year may place some patients at greater risk for HPA-axis suppression. The risks of long-term use or oral CCS can be minimized by administering shorter-acting agents (e.g., prednisone, prednisolone, or methylprednisolone) and an alternate-day schedule. However, when one uses large doses for extended periods, alternate-day therapy can still lead to the serious side effects discussed above (154, 155).

Systemic side effects can be reduced but not avoided using inhaled corticosteroids. Both HPA-axis suppression and growth suppression have been reported (156–160). Still other investigators have noted normal height and HPA-axis function in children receiving inhaled CCS. These effects are dose-dependent.

Other adverse effects unique to treatment with inhaled CCS include dry or sore throat, dysphonia, and esophageal candidiasis (153).

These effects rarely lead to discontinuation of therapy and can be minimized by using a spacing device or by rinsing the mouth after dosage administration.

CHOICE OF DRUG

When choosing a CCS agent, the goal is to minimize the potential for adverse effects. This is accomplished by using an agent with potent glucocorticoid activity, minimal mineralocorticoid activity, and a short to intermediate duration of action (Table 57.15). Oral CCSs that fit these criteria are prednisone, prednisolone, and methylprednisolone. Prednisone is equally effective and is less expensive than prednisolone or methylprednisolone. Liquid preparations of prednisone and prednisolone are available.

When injectable CCSs are indicated, methylprednisolone or hydrocortisone is recommended. Methylprednisolone has fewer mineralocorticoid effects than hydrocortisone, but in the majority of patients, this is unlikely to be clinically important.

PHARMACOKINETICS

CCSs are readily absorbed when taken orally and rapidly distributed when given intravenously. Systemic bioavailability percentages of aerosol CCSs are summarized in Table 57.16. More than 90% of circulating CCSs are bound to albumin or corticosteroid binding globulin (163). The plasma half-life of the CCSs in serum is relatively short compared to their biologic half-life (Table 57.15). CCSs are eliminated by conjugation with sulfate or glucuronic acid to form water-soluble complexes that are excreted (161). Conjugation occurs primarily in the liver, although the kidney participates to a small degree.

DRUG INTERACTIONS

A number of drugs may have a significant clinical effect on CCS synthesis and metabolism. Phenytoin, barbiturates and rifampin have all been reported to cause an increase in CCS metabolism, leading to diminished patient response to CCSs. In contrast, estrogens in oral contraceptives cause an increase in the total and unbound concentrations of prednisolone because of lower clearance rates and decreased affinity for protein binding sites. Concurrent administration of CCS with aspirin decreases plasma salicylate levels. Accordingly, caution should be exercised when decreasing CCS dosages that avoid salicylate intoxication. Macrolide antibiotics, specifically troleandomycin, cause a significant decrease in methylprednisolone clearance. This interaction has been utilized to decrease the methylprednisolone dose.

DOSAGE AND ADMINISTRATION

Status Asthmaticus/Acute Exacerbations

The indication for the use of CCS in acute asthma is the loss of bronchodilator response. Although CCS do not provide immediate benefit, recent studies of CCS therapy in acute asthma document a significantly higher Pao_2 following 24 hours of therapy (160) and accelerated recovery of forced expiratory flow (FEF) 15–75% to normal. A short course of CCS has been shown to reduce the duration

Table 57.15.
Corticosteroid Comparison Chart (Oral/Intravenous)

Preparation	Equivalent Anti-inflammatory Dose	Relative Anti-inflammatory Potency	Relative Mineralocorticoid Activity	Increased Appetite	Muscle Myopathy	Plasma Half-Life (hours)	Biologic Half-Life (hours)
Short-acting							
Cortisone	25	0.8	0.8	2+	1+	0.5	8–12
Hydrocortisone	20	1.0	1.0	2+	1+	1.5	8–12
Intermediate-acting							
Prednisone	4	5	0.5	3+	1+	3.3	18–36
Prednisolone	5	4	0.8	3+	1+	3.0	18–36
Methylprednisolone	5	4	0.8	2+	1+	3.6	18–36
Triamcinolone	4	5	0	0	3+	3.3	24–48
Long-acting							
Betamethasone	0.6	25	0	4+	2+	5	36–54
Dexamethasone	0.75	30	0	4+	2+	5	36–54

Table 57.16.
Inhaled Aerosol Corticosteroid Comparison Chart

Drug	Relative Topical Potency	Systemic Bioavailability (percentage)	Plasma Half-Life (hours)
Beclomethasone dipropionate	500	<5	15
Dexamethasone sodium phosphate	0.8	80	5
Flunisolide	>100	20	1.6
Triamcinolone Acetonide	100	Unknown	0.5–1
Budesonide	1000	10	1–2.8

and severity of severe bronchospasm, with very early use preventing hospitalization (162, 163).

Empirically determined doses of prednisone used for the treatment of acute symptoms are 10 mg q12h for infants under 1 year of age, 20 mg q12 h for toddlers 1–3 years, 30 mg q12h for children 3–13 years, and 40 mg q12h for adolescents and adults (Table 57.17).

This therapy is referred to as "burst" steroids, is continued for 5–7 days, then discontinued without tapering. The dosages of prednisone used for burst therapy are at the upper end of the commonly recommended dosage range for children, approximately 2 mg/kg/24 hours. Hospitalized patients with more serious dyspnea may need injectable therapy with methylprednisolone or hydrocortisone.

Table 57.17.
Corticosteroid Dosing

Drug	Dosage Form	Dosage
Hydrocortisone	Injection	10 mg/kg (up to 300 mg) once, then 10 mg/kg/24 hours q6 hours
Methylprednisolone	Injection	2 mg/kg (up to 125 mg) once, then 2 mg/kg/24 hours q6 hours
Prednisone	Oral tablets 1, 2.5, 5, 10, 20, 50 mg Oral solution (Roxane) 5 mg/5 ml Itensol concentrate (Roxane) 5 mg/ml Liquid Pred (Muro) syrup 5 mg/5 ml	*Burst therapy:* <1 year 10 mg q12 hours 1–3 years 20 mg q12 hours 3–13 years 30 mg q12 hours >13 years 40 mg q12 hours *Long-term therapy:* <1 year 10 mg QOD 1–3 years 20 mg QOD 3–13 years 30 mg QOD >13 years 40 mg QOD
Prednisolone	Tablets 5 mg Prelone syrup (Muro) 15 mg/5 μl	Same as prednisone
Beclomethasone diproprionate	MDI-42 μ/spray Beclovent (Allen & Hanburys) Vanceril (Schering)	*Child:* 1–2 inhalations 3–4 times daily; max 10 *Adult:* 2 inhalations 3–4 times daily; max 20
Dexamethasone sodium phosphate	MDI-84 μ/spray Decadron phosphate respihaler (MSD)	*Child:* 2 inhalations 3–4 times daily; max 8 *Adult:* 3 inhalations 3–4 times daily; max 12
Flunisolide	MDI-250 μ/spray Aerobicl (Forest)	*Child:* 2 inhalations q12 hours; max 4 *Adult:* 2 inhalations q 12 hours; max 8
Triamcinolone acetonide	MDI-100 μ/spray Azmacort (Rhone-Poulence-Rorer)	*Child:* 1–2 inhalations 3–4 times daily; max 12 *Adult:* 2 inhalations q6–12 hours; max 16

Doses equivalent to prednisone therapy are used, but the frequency of administration is every 4–6 hours. In addition, a loading dose equivalent to a 24-hour dose is administered. Dosing for hydrocortisone would be 10 mg/kg load (maximum 300 mg/dose) followed by 10 mg/kg/24 hours q6h and methylprednisone 2 mg/kg load (maximum 125 mg/dose), followed by 2 mg/kg/24 hours (Table 57.17).

Once acute symptoms have been relieved, daily CCS can be discontinued. Tapering is not necessary for treatment less than 14 days, but for courses > 14 days tapering over 2 weeks is recommended. If withdrawal symptoms occur, the dose should be increased to the previous dose and a more gradual tapering process implemented. Withdrawal symptoms are summarized in Table 57.18.

LONG-TERM THERAPY

Pediatric patients with chronic asthma who are inadequately controlled by bronchodilators or cromolyn and who require frequent hospitalizations or frequently miss school or work, or patients whose symptoms recur following the discontinuation of a short course of (burst) therapy, should be considered for chronic corticosteroids. Long-term administration of CCSs may be accomplished by inhalation or alternate-day oral therapy; frequency of adverse effects from both methods is comparably low (164, 165). The concomitant use of inhaled and oral CCSs may lead to increased adrenal suppression and other adverse effects (164, 165). The initial dosage should be high (e.g., for a 12-year-old child, 30 mg every other day for prednisone or two inhalations three to four times daily for inhaled beclomethasone diproprionate) (Table 57.17). Information comparing the available inhaled CCS can be found in Table

Table 57.18.
Corticosteroid Withdrawal Syndrome

Emotional "letdown," depression
Malaise, headache, fatigue, lethergy, weakness
Orthostatic hypotension, dizziness and fainting
Anorexia, nausea
Hypoglycemia
Weight loss
Conjunctivitis, rhinitis
Pseudorheumatism (arthralgias, myalgias, stiffness)
Desquamation of the skin
Exacerbation of primary disease

57.16. The lowest amount of drug that maintains adequate control of asthmatic symptoms can then be determined by cautious reduction in dosage (e.g., 5 mg for prednisone and 42 µg per dose for the inhaled beclomethasone dipropionate) at intervals no shorter than 1–2 weeks. If asthmatic symptoms increase, the dose should be increased to the previous dose that kept the patient relatively free of symptoms, and further tapering should be postponed. Once the airway obstruction is cleared, a slower wean may be attempted. A drop in post bronchodilator pulmonary function may be useful in identifying early signs of inadequate control from a decrease in CCS dosage. Theophylline or cromolyn should remain at optimal doses to minimize CCS requirements.

CROUP

The use of CCSs in croup has been controversial for years. Most of the studies have been either poorly designed or poorly controlled (166). More recently, Super et al. published a prospective, randomized, double-blind study that showed that the use of 0.6 mg/kg of dexamethasone intravenously decreases the severity of moderate to severe disease during the first 24 hours after intravenous administration (167). Dexamethasone should not be used in place of standard treatments for moderate to severe croup, but considering the relatively low toxicity of a single dose of dexamethasone, an empiric trial of dexamethasone should be considered.

ALLERGIC RHINITIS

Intranasal CCSs are effective in controlling symptoms or seasonal or perennial rhinitis when effectiveness or tolerance to conventional treatment is unsatisfactory. Available products and dosage recommendations are summarized in Table 57.19. Improvement in symptoms in patients with seasonal rhinitis usually becomes apparent within a few days, although in some patients relief may not occur until 3 weeks of treatment. Do not continue beyond 3 weeks in absence of significant symptomatic improvement. Patients suffering from perennial rhinitis may require 8 weeks to see a response. After desired clinical effect is obtained, one should attempt to reduce the maintenance dose to the smallest amount necessary to control symptoms (168).

Table 57.19.
Intranasal Corticosteroid Dosing

Drug	Form	Dose
Beclomethasone dipropionate	Aerosol: 42 μm/spray Beconase (Allen & Hanburys) Vancenase Nasal (Schering) Spray: 0.042% Beconase AQ/Vancenase AQ	*Child: 6–12* 1 inhalation in each nostril 3 times a day *Adult:* 1 inhalation in each nostril 2–4 times a day
Dexamethasone sodium phosphate	Aerosol: 84 μm/spray Decadron Phosphate Turbinaire (MSD)	*Child:* 1–2 sprays in each nostril 2 times a day; max 8 *Adult:* 2 sprays in each nostril 2–3 times a day; max 8
Flunisolide	Spray: 25 μm/spray Nasalide (syntex)	*Child:* 1 spray in each nostril 3 times daily or 2 sprays in each nostril 2 times daily; max 8 *Adult:* 2 sprays in each nostril 2 times daily. May increase to 2 sprays in each nostril 3 times daily; max 16
Triamcinolone acetonide	Spray: 55 μm/spray Nasacort (Rhone-Poulence Rorer)	*Adult:* 2 sprays in each nostril once daily. May increase to 2 sprays twice a day or one spray four times a day; max 8

In the presence of excessive nasal mucosa secretions or edema of the nasal mucosa, the drug may fail to reach the site of intended action. In such cases, use a nasal vasoconstrictor during the first 2–3 days of therapy.

The most common adverse effects observed following administration of intranasal CCSs are mild nasopharyngeal irritation, nasal irritation, burning, stinging, dryness, and headache. Other reported adverse effects include lightheadedness, nausea, transient epistaxis or bloody mucus, rebound congestion, sneezing attacks, throat discomfort, and loss of sense of taste.

Cromolyn Sodium

ASTHMA

Cromolyn, known as cromolyn sodium or disodium cromoglycate, was serendipitously discovered during the testing of new bronchodilators. Cromolyn was extracted from a Mediterranean plant, ammi visnaga (Umbelliferae), and was marketed in England in 1968 and in the United States in 1975.

Mechanism of Action

Cromolyn sodium's precise mechanism of action remains unknown. Cromolyn prevents the release of the chemical mediators of the type I (IgE-related) hyper-sensitivity reactions, including histamine and slow-reacting substance of anaphylaxis (SRS-A), from sensitized mast cells after the antigen-antibody union has taken place (169). The drug does not inhibit the binding of IgE to the mast cells or the antigen-antibody interactions, nor does it oppose the action of the mediators once they are released. Instead, the mast cells simply do not degranulate. The cellular mechanism for mast cell stabilization is still unclear, but investigators have proposed that cromolyn interferes with calcium transport across the mast cell membrane, thereby interfering with mediator release (170). Cromolyn prevents the release of mediators from mast cells induced by both immunologic (171) and non-immunologic (171, 172) stimulation. Cromolyn also blocks both the early and late asthmatic responses (173).

Pharmacokinetics

Cromolyn is poorly absorbed from the gastro-intestinal tract, with < 1% of an oral dose being absorbed (174). When administered by inhalation using a turbo-inhaler (Spinhaler) for powder insufflation, about 75% of the dose is delivered. Of the delivered dose, only

5–10% (7.5%) reaches the site of action in the peripheral airways, where it is rapidly absorbed into the systemic circulation. Following inhalation, absorption of the drug is highest following administration of the powder via the Spinhaler and lowest following administration of solution via a nebulizer. Absorption from the metered dose inhaler is intermediate to the Spinhaler and nebulizer. Less than 7% of an intranasal dose of cromolyn as a solution is absorbed systemically.

The absorbed fraction of an inhaled dose of cromolyn is rapidly excreted unchanged in the urine and bile with a biologic half-life of 46–99 minutes. No biotransformation occurs. The remainder of the dose is swallowed and excreted in the feces.

Toxicity

Cromolyn is the least toxic of all medications used for asthma, regardless of route of administration (175, 176). No clinically important adverse effects have been reported from large multicenter studies evaluating cromolyn's long-term safety.

With cromolyn sodium powder for oral inhalation, the most common adverse effects are irritation of the throat and trachea, cough, and bronchospasm caused by inhalation of the dry drug powder. These effects were also reported following inhalation of the lactulose vehicle. Bronchospasm may be avoided by concurrent administration of an inhaled beta agonist, whereas the dryness and cough may be avoided by drinking water before and after inhalation.

The most frequent adverse effects occurring in patients using other forms of cromolyn sodium are (when using aerosol inhalation) irritation and dryness of the throat, bad taste, cough, wheezing, and nausea; (when using MDI) nasal congestion, cough, sneezing, wheezing, and nausea; and (following intranasal administration) a sensation of nasal burning and stinging, nasal irritations, and sneezing. Sneezing occurs in about 10% of patients. Although most side effects are mild, there are rare case reports of more severe cromolyn-associated reactions, including anaphylaxis (177).

Administration

Three dosage forms of cromolyn sodium for inhalation are available in the United States:

20 mg powdered capsule delivered via Spinhaler apparatus, 1% solution containing cromolyn sodium 20 mg in 2 ml distilled water delivered by nebulizer, and a pressurized MDI that delivers 800 μg per activation.

Spinhaler. The Spinhaler delivery system can be used by any patient older than 4 years of age. It requires little coordination because it is a breath-activated system. No spacer devices are necessary and there are no fluorocarbons. The starting dose is one 20 mg capsule four times a day. When symptoms are under control, usually after 1–2 months, the schedule can be reduced to three times a day and then twice daily. Some patients may require higher doses to control symptoms. The maximum recommended dose is six capsules in 24 hours. A full trial on the drug should be a least 6 weeks, although improvement may be seen after 1 or 2 weeks of therapy.

Nebulizer Solution. The dosing of cromolyn with the nebulizer solution is the same as for the Spinhaler capsules. For young children who cannot use the Spinhaler or those who cannot tolerate the irritant effects from the inhaled powder, the nebulizer solution is a safe and effective alternative. In addition, the cromolyn sodium nebulizer solution has been shown to be physically and chemically compatible for up to 60 minutes with the bronchodilator and mucolytic drugs listed in Table 57.20. Cromolyn sodium did not adversely affect the stability of the individual drugs in the admixtures. Therefore, it is possible to make a mixture of medications that can be simultaneously nebulized to the patient. This provides an advantage for the more severely ill patients who benefit from both drugs.

Metered Dose Inhaler. The recommended dosage is two inhalations (1.6 mg) four times a day. To prevent acute bronchospasm following exercise or exposure to cold dry air or

Table 57.20.
Drugs Physically and Chemically Compatible with Cromolyn Sodium Nebulizer Solution

Albuterol nebulizer solution
Atropine sterile aqueous solution
20% acetylcysteine solution
Epinephrine hydrochloride solution
Isoetharine hydrochloride 0.25% inhalation solution
Isoproterenol hydrochloride solution
Metaproterenol sulfate solution
Terbutaline sulfate sterile aqueous solution

environmental agents, the recommended dosage is two inhalations 10–15 minutes, but no more than 60 minutes, before exposure to the precipitating factor.

ALLERGIC RHINITIS

Cromolyn sodium nasal solution is used for the symptomatic prevention and treatment of seasonal or perennial allergic rhinitis. Intranasal administration of cromolyn generally provides symptomatic relief of rhinorrhea, nasal congestion, sneezing, and postnasal drip. For optimal symptomatic relief in patients with perennial allergic rhinitis, up to 2–4 weeks of therapy may be required. Supplemental therapy with topical nasal decongestants and/or oral antihistamines may be necessary until acceptable clinical response is achieved. Intranasal cromolyn therapy typically does not provide symptomatic relief or eye or throat irritation associated with allergic rhinitis. Intranasal cromolyn is ineffective in patients with nonallergic rhinitis.

The nasal inhaler (Nasalcrom) delivers 5.2 mg of cromolyn sodium per metered spray. The usual initial dose of intranasal cromolyn sodium in adults and children 6 years of age and older is one spray in each nostril three or four times daily. For patients with seasonal rhinitis, therapy should be continued throughout the period of exposure. When necessary, the dosage may be increased to one spray in each nostril six times daily.

Nedocromil Sodium

ASTHMA

Nedocromil sodium is a disodium salt of a pyranoquinolone dicarboxylic acid. Its chemical structure differs significantly from that of cromolyn sodium. As reported for cromolyn sodium, the exact mechanism of action of nedocromil sodium is unknown. However, the in-vitro inhibitory effect of nedocromil sodium has been examined on the activation of, and mediator release from, a variety of inflammatory cells that have been implicated in the pathogenesis of asthma (179). Nedocromil appears to inhibit both the immediate and late phase bronchial obstruction and decreases hyper-responsiveness (12). It blocks mediators other than histamine and has a greater spectrum of activity compared with cromolyn.

Pharmacokinetics

After inhalation, approximately 90% of the dosage is deposited in the throat and swallowed, but the portion of the dose reaching the lungs is completely absorbed. Oral absorption is low, approximately 3% of the amount swallowed. Nedocromil has an elimination half-life of approximately 90 minutes. Elimination is predominately via the kidney.

Toxicology

No toxicity was observed in long-term studies of up to 24 months in various animal species. In human trials the main side effects reported include distinctive bitter taste (14%), headache (5%), and nausea (4%) (181).

Nedocromil sodium is a drug that (a) exhibits a good safety profile, (b) is able to prevent bronchospasm induced by a variety of stimuli, (c) can inhibit late reaction after antigen inhalation and reduces bronchial hyper-reactivity, both generally related to the inflammatory process, and (d) is effective in asthma therapy irrespective of age or association with allergic factors.

A full evaluation of the mechanism of action of nedocromil sodium and its effectiveness in treating various forms of asthma is needed, but overall the preliminary clinical data indicate that nedocromil sodium will have an important place in the treatment of reversible airway disease.

Anticholinergic Agents

The major neural control of the airways is through the parasympathetic system, with impulses mediated through vagal pathways. Parasympathetic nerve endings release acetylcholine, which binds to cholinergic receptors and stimulates the enzyme guanyl cyclase to produce cyclic 3',5'-monophosphate (cGMP). Increased concentrations of cGMP appear to favor bronchoconstriction.

MECHANISM OF ACTION

Anticholinergic drugs act in asthma by antagonizing the effect of acetylcholine on muscarinic cholinergic receptors through inhibition of release of intracellular cGMP (182). In addition, the anticholinergic drugs may inhibit the release of mast-cell derived mediators by competitive antagonism of acetylcholine at the postganglionic neuromuscular junction (183). In contrast to beta sympathomimetic drugs, which act on both the large and small airways, anticholinergic agents act primarily on the large airways (184, 185).

The effect of anticholinergic drugs on respiratory secretions varies. Atropine has been shown to block the production of respiratory secretions in response to cholinergic stimulation. However, atropine also reduces mucociliary clearance and decreases ciliary beat frequency, which is the reason cited to avoid its use in asthma. Ipratropium bromide does not affect ciliary beat frequency or mucociliary clearance, even after chronic high-dose therapy (186).

PHARMACOKINETICS

Atropine is well absorbed from the GI tract, and following oral inhalation atropine appears in the serum within 15 minutes and peak concentrations are achieved within 1.5–4 hours. Atropine is metabolized in the liver (50–70%), and 30–50% is excreted in the urine unchanged. The elimination half-life of atropine is about 2–3 hours.

Ipratropium bromide has poor systemic absorption after oral and inhaled administration. Most of an inhaled dose is swallowed and excreted unchanged in the stool. The small portion that is systemically absorbed is rapidly metabolized to inactive metabolites. The elimination half-life of ipratropium bromide is about 3 hours.

TOXICITY/SIDE EFFECTS

Atropine delivered via nebulization greatly reduces the incidence of side effects. Many patients will develop some dryness of the mouth, although this is usually minor. Blurred vision, urinary retention, and other side effects associated with systemic therapy are rare, but flushing, lightheadedness, and slight tachycardia may occur.

Ipratropium bromide is remarkably free of unwanted side effects as a result of its minimal systemic absorption. Side effects reported by study volunteers and patients throughout the literature are relatively mild and infrequent. Adverse effects reported by the manufacturer include cough (5.9%), nervousness (3.1%), nausea (2.8%), dizziness, headache, GI distress and dry mouth (2.4%), and irritation from the aerosol (1.6%).

DOSAGE AND ADMINISTRATION

Table 57.21 summarizes the currently available formulations of anticholinergic drugs. The pediatric dose of aerosolized atropine sulfate is 0.05–0.075 mg/kg (187). There is generally a measurable bronchodilator response within 15 minutes of giving the aerosol; in contrast, most sympathomimetic bronchodilators produce a response in 5 minutes. The maximum response to an atropine aerosol may be found by 30 minutes, or may take as long as 3 hours. Significant bronchodilation may last for only 2–3 hours (187), but most commonly persists for 3–5 hours. Therefore repeat dosing is every 4–6 hours.

Ipratropium bromide is available in the United States in an MDI and is dosed two inhalations (36 μm) four times a day (maximum 12 inhalations in 24 hours). In Europe, ipratropium bromide is available on an investigational basis as a respiratory solution for aerosol use in a concentration of 0.25 mg/ml. The suggested dose for children 3–15 years is 0.25 mg (187). Although substantial bronchodilation is seen rapidly following inhalation (50% of the eventual maximum in the first 3–5 minutes and 80% within 30 minutes), the maximum effect occurs relatively slowly (1.5–2 hours) (187); therefore ipratropium bromide appears to be most appropriate for prophylaxis of asthma rather than for treating acute symptoms.

Glycopyrrolate is used orally to control gastric acid output and is a more effective antisialagogue than atropine. Intravenous administration has been shown to cause bronchodilation; more recently, aerosolization of 100–200 μg of the drug was found to produce prolonged bronchodilation lasting 6–12 hours (188–190). No significant side effects were reported. Thus, the aerosol may prove useful in the treatment of asthma.

Miscellaneous Anti-Asthma Drugs

CALCIUM-CHANNEL BLOCKERS

Calcium ions participate in the pathogenesis of asthma. Increased cellular concentrations of Ca^{++} trigger smooth muscle contraction, mast cell mediator release, mucous gland secretion, vagal nerve activity, and the movement of inflammatory cells into the walls of the airways. Calcium-channel blockers, vera-

Table 57.21.
Anticholinergic Dosages

Drug	Availability	Dosage	
		Pediatric	Adult
Aerosol			
Atropine SO_4	0.2% (1 mg) injectable solution[a] 0.5% (2.5 mg)	0.05–0.075 mg/kg q 4–6 hours PRN	0.025 mg/kg or 2.5–5 mg q 4–6 hours PRN
Ipratropium bromide[a]	0.25 mg/ml	0.25 mg q 4–6 hours PRN	0.50 mg q 4–6 hours PRN
Glycopyrrolate[b]	0.2 mg/ml injectable solution	0.025–0.05 mg/kg nebulized q 6 hours	2 mg nebulized q 6 hours
MDI			
Ipratropium bromide	Atrovent 18 μm/ puff	2 inhalations 4 times a day Max: 12	2 inhalations 4 times a day Max: 12

[a]Not available in the United States.
[b]Not FDA-approved for this use.

pamil and nifedipine, inhibit airway smooth muscle contraction and mast cell and basophil mediator release. Other experiments indicate that verapamil and nifedipine may interfere with exercise-induced asthma and broncho-constriction caused by cold air and methacholine. However, studies do not confirm their usefulness as bronchodilators on a long-term basis (191). It is possible that more specific calcium antagonists will be developed and find use in the treatment of asthma.

H_1 RECEPTOR ANTAGONIST

The development of nonsedating H_1 antihistamines has generated interest in the possible value of these medications in the treatment of asthma. Examples of antihistamines showing possible value in asthma include terfenadine (192, 193), loratidine (196), and astemizole (194), as well as drugs not available in the United States, including cetirizine (195) and azelastine (196). Potent H_1-receptor blockers antagonize histamine-induced bronchoconstriction and require further study in seasonal asthma.

KETOTIFEN

Ketotifen, an orally administered drug with antihistamine and cromolyn-like activity, has been investigated as a possible alternative to cromolyn because of its long-acting oral properties. Clinical studies indicate ketotifen to be less effective than cromolyn and to possess marked antihistamine-like side effects (sedation and weight gain) (197, 198).

OTHER ANTI-INFLAMMATORY DRUGS

Methotrexate

Methotrexate (MTX), an antimetabolite that inhibits the enzyme dihydrofolate reductase,

has been used in high doses to treat cancers and leukemias since 1947 (199). In lower doses, it has been used as an anti-inflammatory agent to treat a variety of chronic inflammatory diseases. The initial observation of the use of MTX in asthma involved a 63-year-old woman with severe psoriasis, erosive psoriatic arthritis, and steroid-dependent asthma. MTX was started to treat the patient's psoriasis, and it was incidently noted that she also had a significant improvement in her asthma control, with deceased dependence on CCS. A pilot study was then done with CCS-dependent asthmatics; seven of eight patients were able to reduce their CCS requirements significantly while on MTX (200). A double-blind study of the use of MTX in CCS-dependent asthmatics confirmed this observation (201). MTX, used 18–22 months, appears to remain effective with minor side effects (202). Patients with steroid-dependent asthma are generally started on 15 mg of MTX per week; the dose is increased to 25 mg if there is no improvement in steroid requirements in 3–4 months (203). MTX is metabolized more rapidly by children than by adults; therefore children may require or tolerate higher doses. The most common minor toxicity is GI intolerance, reported in 3–74% of patients taking oral MTX. Nausea is reported in less than 5% of patients receiving intramuscular therapy. Transient elevations of liver enzymes up to two times normal are reported in all studies and generally resolve without changing the dose of methotrexate. Side effects reported in rheumatoid arthritis patients receiving long-term MTX include mild hepatic fibrosis (25–50%) and pulmonary fibrosis (< 5%) (203).

Because the long-term side effects of MTX reported in rheumatoid arthritis include pulmonary fibrosis and hepatic damage, such therapy should be reserved for patients with severe CCS-dependent asthma. Many questions remain unanswered with regard to the use of MTX in asthma, including the optimal dose and route of administration. The need to continue MTX therapy in asthmatics after CCS have been discontinued needs to be assessed. Observed toxicity in asthmatic patients treated with MTX seems to be minor, but this needs to be confirmed with larger numbers of patients. Whether other immunomodulator drugs, such as azathioprine or cyclosporine, are useful has not been determined.

Gold

Like MTX, gold salts have anti-inflammatory properties and have been used to treat rheumatoid arthritis. In Japan, gold injections (chrysotherapy) have been used to treat asthma (204). Studies suggest that they reduce the need for orally administered CCS and in some patients reduced bronchodilator use (205).

Twenty-nine percent of parenteral gold-treated patients are forced to discontinue therapy because of drug-related side effects. Auranofin, an oral gold preparation, has less toxicity than reported with parenteral gold therapy. Bernstein et al. (205) evaluated auranofin in 20 steroid-dependent patients in a 20-week open label trial. The auranofin dose was 3 mg twice daily. The results of the study were encouraging in that patients exhibited clinical improvement in their asthmatic symptoms during treatment with auranofin, and CCS requirements were reduced in 72% of patients. A surprising finding was a decrease of methacholine-induced bronchial hyperresponsiveness in 50% of the auranofin-treated group. GI symptoms were the most frequently reported adverse effects during auranofin therapy. Loose stools or diarrhea were reported within the first month of therapy and either resolved spontaneously or diminished with a reduction in the auranofin dose. No patient discontinued therapy because of side effects, but the high incidence indicates that patients receiving auranofin will require close surveillance until more extensive safety data become available. The use of oral gold should only be considered for patients who require moderate to high doses of daily steroids for long-term control of their disease.

COMMON COLD

The common cold is probably the most common disease entity in the pediatric age group. About half of our total population gets at least one cold during the winter months every year. In fact, 15% of the population have colds in any given week during the winter months. During the summer, about 20% of the population contract a cold, often progressing among children to otitis media.

Treatment

There are no clinically available antiviral agents that are effective against the viruses that cause the common cold. No therapy is indicated in the majority of cases. Over-the-counter cough and cold preparations may be used for symptomatic treatment of specific complaints. Individual therapy directed at controlling specific symptoms is better than all-inclusive cold remedies.

ANTIPYRETICS

Many people feel miserable with malaise when they have a cold, and in those cases an analgesic is often useful. Acetaminophen 10–15 mg/kg/dose q4–6h is generally preferred over aspirin since recent studies have implicated aspirin as an etiologic factor in Reye syndrome. Ibuprofen may be administered 5–10 mg/kg/dose q6–8h. Caution should be used in treating a fever in infants less than 6 months of age, as fever may be the only indicator of a more severe infection.

DECONGESTANTS

Relief of nasal obstruction is the most important therapeutic intervention in young children. Locally applied (Table 57.22) or orally administered (Tables 57.23, 57.24), systemically active decongestants may be used. It is clear that excessive use of sprays and drops with vasoactive drugs (phenylephrine, ephedrine) for more than 3–5 consecutive days causes "rebound phenomenon," producing copious nasal secretions. This may prolong the illness. If congestion persists, normal saline nose drops may be substituted for the

Table 57.22.
Locally Applied Decongestants

Drug	Age	Concentration	Dose	
Phenylephrine	Infants	0.125–0.2%	1 drop ea. nostril q2–4 hours	
	Children >6	0.25%	1–2 sprays ea. nostril q3–4 hours	
Oxymetazoline	Children 2–5	0.025%	2–3 drops ea. nostril q12 hours	
	Children >6	0.05%	2–3 sprays or 2–4 drops ea. nostril q12 hours	
Xylometazoline	Children 2–12	0.05%	2–3 drops ea. nostril q8–10 hours	

Phenylephrine

Neosynephrine St. Joseph's measured dose		Solution 0.125%	Drops: 30 ml 15 ml	Winthrop Consumer Plough
Alconefrin 12		Solution 0.16%	Drops: 30 ml	Webcon
Rhinall-10		Solution 0.2%	Drops: 30 ml	Scherer
Alconefrin 25		Solution 0.25%	Drops: 30 ml Spray: 30 ml	Webcon
Doktors			Drops: 30 ml Spray: 30 ml	Scherer
NeoSynephrine			Drops: 15 ml Spray: 15 ml	Winthrop Consumer
Nostril			Spray: 15 ml	Boehinger-Ingelheim
Rhinall			Drops: 30 ml Spray: 30 ml	Scherer

Oxymetazoline

Afrin Children's Nose Drops		Solution 0.025%	Drops: 20 ml	Schering
Afrin		Solution 0.05%	Drops: 20 ml Spray: 15, 30 ml Spray: 15 ml (menthol)	Schering
Allerest-12 Hour Nasal			Spray: 15 ml	Pharmacraft
Coricidin Nasal Mist			Spray: 20 ml	Schering
Dristan Long Lasting			Spray: 15, 30 ml Spray: 15 ml (menthol)	Whitehall
Duramist Plus			Spray: 15 ml	Pfeiffer
Duration			Spray: 15, 30 ml	Plough
4-Way Long Acting Nasal			Spray: 15 ml	Bristol-Myers
NeoSynephrine-12 Hour			Drops: 30 ml Spray: 15 ml Spray: 15 ml (menthol)	Winthrop Consumer
Nostrilla			Spray: 15 ml	Boehinger-Ingelheim
NTZ Long Acting Nasal			Drops: 15 ml Spray: 15 ml	Winthrop Consumer
Sinarest 12-Hour			Spray: 15 ml	Pharmacraft
Sinex Long Acting			Spray: 15, 30 ml	Vicks Health Care

Xylometazoline

Otrivin Pediatric Nasal Drops		Solution 0.05%	Drops: 20 ml	Ciba Consumer
Otrivin		Solution 0.1%	Drops: 20 ml Spray: 15 ml	Ciba Consumer

Table 57.24
Pediatric Decongestant Combinations, *continued*

	Decongestant-Antihistamine Liquids (content given per 5 ml liquid or 1 ml drops)		
Product	Decongestant	Antihistamine	Manufacturer
R-Tannamine Pediatric Suspension	5 mg phenylephrine tannate	2 mg chlorpheniramine tannate 12.5 mg pyrilamine tannate	Qualitest
Rynatan Pediatric Suspension	5 mg phenylephrine tannate	2 mg chlorpheniramine tannate 12.5 mg pyrilamine tannate	Wallace
Triotann Pediatric Suspension	5 mg phenylephrine tannate	2 mg chlorpheniramine tannate 12.5 mg pyrilamine tannate	Duramed
Tri-Tannate Pediatric Suspension	5 mg phenylephrine tannate	2 mg chlorpheniramine tannate 12.5 mg pyrilamine tannate	Rugby
Triaminic oral infant drops	20 mg phenylpropanolamine	10 mg pyrilamine maleate 2 mg phenyltoloxamine citrate	Sandoz
Naldecon Pediatric Syrup	5 mg phenylpropanolamine HCl 1.25 mg phenylephrine HCl	0.5 mg chlorpheniramine maleate 2 mg phenyltoloxamine citrate	Bristol Labs
Naldecon Pediatric Drops	5 mg phenylpropanolamine HCl 1.25 mg phenylephrine HCl	0.5 mg chlorpheniramine maleate 2 mg phenyltoloxamine citrate	Bristol Labs
Nalgest Pediatric Syrup	5 mg phenylpropanolamine HCl 1.25 mg phenylephrine HCl	0.5 mg chlorpheniramine maleate 2 mg phenyltoloxamine citrate	Major
Nalgest Pediatric Drops	5 mg phenylpropanolamine HCl 1.25 mg phenylephrine HCl	0.5 mg chlorpheniramine maleate 2 mg phenyltoloxamine citrate	Major
Drixoral Syrup[a]	30 mg pseudoephedrine sulfate	2 mg brompheniramine maleate	Schering-Plough
Dimetane Decongestant Elixir (2.3% Alcohol)	5 mg phenylephrine HCl	2 mg brompheniramine maleate	Robins
Benelyn Decongestant Liquid (5% Alcohol)	30 mg pseudoephedrine HCl	12.5 mg diphenhydramine	Parke-Davis
Benadryl Decongestant Elixir (5% Alcohol)	30 mg pseudoephedrine HCl	12.5 mg diphenhydramine	Parke-Davis
Children's NyQuil Nighttime Head Cold Allergy Formula[a]	10 mg pseudoephedrine HCl	0.67 mg chlorpheniramine maleate	Richardson-Vicks
Actifed Syrup[a]	30 mg pseudoephedrine HCl	1.25 mg triprolidine HCl	Burroughs Wellcome
Pedia Care Cold Formula[a]	15 mg pseudoephedrine HCl	1 mg chlorpheniramine maleate	McNeil
Dorcol Pediatric Cold Formula Liquid	15 mg pseudoephedrine HCl	1 mg chlorpheniramine maleate	Sandoz

[a]Alcohol-free.

effects include tremor, nervousness, insomnia, dizziness, headache, hallucinations, and rarely, convulsions. Nausea and sleepiness may also occur. Cardiovascular effects include tachycardia, palpitations, exacerbation of hypertension, and arrhythmias. Therefore, the drugs should be used with caution in patients with underlying congenital heart disease, hypertension, or cardiac arrhythmias. Oral decongestants should also be used with caution in patients with hyperthyroidism and diabetes mellitus. The side effects associated with topical use include initial burning or stinging sensations in the nose and subsequent dryness of the mucosa. Rebound congestion may occur with overuse.

ANTIHISTAMINES

Antihistamines have historically been used in over-the-counter cough and cold preparations. Naclerio and co-workers studied the response of inflammatory mediators to induced viral infections (207). All variables except histamine grew stronger in direct relationship with the symptoms as the cold increased in severity. This indicates that antihistamines are not likely to have effect on shortening the duration of symptoms. They may be helpful to treat the "cold-like" symptoms of allergic rhinitis.

Antihistamines competitively antagonize histamine at the H_1 receptor site, but do not bind with histamine to inactivate it. Terfenadine and astemizole, the most specific H_1 antagonists available, bind preferentially to peripheral rather than central H_1 receptors. Antihistamines do not block histamine release, antibody production, or antigen-antibody interactions. They antagonize the pharmacologic effects of histamine. They also have anticholinergic, antipruritic, and sedative effects; terfenadine and astemizole have little or no anticholinergic or sedative effects.

If a patient becomes refractory to the effects of a particular antihistaminic agent, it is necessary to switch from one class of antihistamines to another (Table 57.24) to restore responsiveness. In general, antihistamines should be used with caution in patients with lower respiratory tract symptoms, including asthma, since their anticholinergic effects may cause thickening of secretions and impair expectoration.

CNS depression is common with the usual dosage of antihistamines, except terfenadine and astemizole (Table 57.25). Sedation, ranging from drowsiness to deep sleep, occurs most frequently. Dizziness, lassitude, disturbed coordination, and muscular weakness may also occur. In some patients, the sedative effects disappear spontaneously after the antihistamine has been administered for 2–3 days. Children may experience paradoxical excitement characterized by restlessness, insomnia, tremors, euphoria, nervousness, delirium, palpitations, and even seizures. Antihistamines may also precipitate epileptiform seizures in patients with focal lesions of the cerebral cortex, and therefore should be used with caution in patients with a focal seizure disorder. Although the mechanism has not been determined, respiratory depression, sleep apnea, and sudden infant death syndrome (SIDS) have occurred in young infants. Therefore, antihistamines should be used with special caution in these patients.

MUCOKINETIC AGENTS

Guaifenesin is the most commonly prescribed oral mucolytic agent in the United States. Its action is to reduce the surface tension and viscosity of the mucus, thereby making thick mucous secretions into thin secretions, which increases the ease of expectoration. However, studies on the efficacy of guaifenesin have failed to demonstrate either improved pulmonary function or decreased sputum viscosity. Hence, its clinical usefulness is questionable. Guaifenesin is administered orally. The usual dose of guaifenesin as an expectorant in adults and children 12 years of age and older is 200–400 mg orally every 4 hours, not to exceed 2.4 g daily. The usual dosage of guaifenesin as an expectorant for children 6 years to younger than 12 years of age is 100–200 mg every 4 hours, not to exceed 1.2 g daily. Children 2 years to younger than 6 years may receive 50–100 mg every 4 hours, not to exceed 600 mg daily. Dosage in children younger than 2 years of age is undetermined. Doses of guaifenesin larger than those required for expectorant action may produce emesis, but GI upset at ordinary doses is rare. Common antitussive and antitussive combinations are listed in Tables 57.6 to 57.8; sore throat preparations are found in Table 57.9.

Table 57.25.
Dosage and Side Effects of Decongestants and Antihistamines

Drug	Equivalent Adult Dose (mg)	Pediatric Dose (mg/kg/24 hours)	CNS
Common Decongestants:			Stimulation
Ephedrine	50	3	+ + +
Phenylephrine (Neo-Synephrine)	10–25	4	—
Phenylpropanolamine	50	3	+
Pseudoephedrine (Sudafed)	60	1–2	+ +
Common Antihistamines:			Sedation
Ethanolamines			
Bromodiphenhydramine	25	2.5	+ + +
Carbinoxamine (Clistin)	4	0.4	+
Diphenhydramine (Benadryl)	50	5.0	+ + +
Doxylamine	12–25	2.0	+ + +
Clemastine (Tavist)	1[a]	—	+ +
Ethylenediamines			
Methaphrilene	50–100	5.0	+
Pyrilamine (NiSaval)	50	2.5	+ +
Tripelennamine (PBZ)	50	5.0	+ +
Alkylamines			
Brompheniramine (Dimetane)	4	0.5	+
Chlorpheniramine (Chlor-Trimeton)	4	0.35	+
Dexchlorpheniramine (Polaramine)	2	0.25	+
Triprolidine (Actidil)	2.5[b]	0.2	+
Phenothiazines			
Promethazine (Phenergan)	25[b]	1.5	+ + +
Piperidines			
Cyproheptadine (Periactin)	4	0.25	+
azatidine (Optimine)[a]	1–2	—	+ +
Miscellaneous			
Terfenadine (Seldane)[a]	60[a]	30–60 6–12 yrs 3–6 yrs 15	±
astemizole (Hismanal)[c]	10	—	±

All taken TID–QUID except as noted.
[a]Taken BID.
[b]Taken BID–TID.
[c]Taken QD.

Table 57.26.
Pediatric Antitussive Combinations

Product	Decongestant	Antihistamine	Antitussive	Other	Manufacturer
Hycomine Pediatric Syrup	12.5 mg phenylpropanolamine HCl		12.5 mg hydrocodone bitartrate		DuPont
Tricodene Pediatric Liquid	12.5 mg phenylpropanolamine HCl		10 mg dextromethorphan HBr		Pfeiffer
Snaplets-DM Granules	6.25 mg phenylpropanolamine HCl		5 mg dextromethorphan HBr		Baker-Cummins
Contact Jr. Non-Drowsy Cold Liquid	15 mg pseudoephedrine HCl		5 mg dextromethorphan HBr	160 mg acetaminophen	Sk? Beecham
PediaCare, Night Rest Liquid Triaminic Nite Lite Liquid	15 mg pseudoephedrine HCl	1 mg chlorpheniramine maleate	7.5 mg dextromethorphan HBr		McNeil-CPC Sandoz
Children's NyQuil Cold/Cough Liquid	10 mg pseudoephedrine HCl	0.67 mg chlorpheniramine	5 mg dextromethorphan HBr		Richardson-Vicks
Pedia Care Cold/ Cough Liquid	15 mg pseudoephedrine HCl	1 mg chlorpheniramine maleate	5 mg dextromethorphan HBr		McNeil CPC
Aspirin-free St. Joseph Complete Nightime Cold Relief Liquid	15 mg pseudoephedrine HCl	1 mg chlorpheniramine maleate	5 mg dextromethorphan HBr		Schering-Plough
Randec-DM Drops	25 mg pseudoephedrine HCl	2 mg carbinoxamine maleate	4 mg dextromethorphan HBr		McNeil-CPC
Rynatuss Pediatric Suspension	5 mg phenylephrine tannate 5 mg ephedrine tannate	4 mg chlorpheniramine tannate	30 mg carbetapentamine tannate		
PediaCare Cough/Cold Chewable tablets	7.5 mg pseudoephedrine HCl	0.5 mg chlorpheniramine maleate	2.5 mg dextromethorphan HBr		McNeil-CPC
Snaplets-multi Granules	6.25 mg phenylpropanolamine	1 mg chlorpheniramine maleate	5 mg dextromethorphan HBr		Baker-Cummins

Table 57.27.

	Pediatric Antitussive and Expectorant Combinations			
Product	Decongestant	Antitussive	Expectorant	Manufacturer
Entuss-D Jr Liquid	30 mg pseudo-ephedrine HCl	2.5 mg hydrocodone bitartrate	100 mg guaifenesin	Hauck
Naldecon DX Children's Syrup	6.25 phenyl-propanolamine HCl	5 mg dextro-methorphan	100 mg guaifenesin	Apothecon
Dorcol Children's Cough Syrup	15 mg pseudo-ephedrine HCl	5 mg dextro-methorphan	50 mg guaifenesin	Sandoz
Ipsatol Cough Formula for Children	9 mg phenyl-propanolamine HCl	10 mg dextro-methorphan HBr	100 mg guaifenesin	Kenwood
Naldecon DX Pediatric Drops	6.25 phenyl-propanolamine HCl	5 mg dextro-methorphan HBr	50 mg guaifenesin	Apothecon

Table 57.27. *continued*

Pediatric Expectorant Combinations

Product	Decongestant	Antihistamine	Expectorant	Other	Manufacturer
Triaminic Expectorant Liquid (not pediatric)	12.5 mg phenyl-propanolamine		100 mg guaifenesin		Sandoz
Fedahist Expectorant Pediatric Drops	7.5 mg pseudo-ephedrine HCl		40 mg guaifenesin		Schwarz Pharma Kremers Urban
Naldecon Ex Children Syrup	6.25 mg phenyl-propanolamine HCl		100 mg guaifenesin	alcohol: 5%	Apothecon
Naldecon Ex Pediatric Drops	6.25 mg phenyl-propanolamine HCl		50 mg guaifenesin		Apothecon
Snaplets-Ex Granules	6.25 mg phenyl-propanolamine HCl		50 mg guaifenesin		Baker-Cummins
Donatussin Drops	2 mg phenylephrine	1 mg chlor-pheniramine maleate	20 mg guaifenesin		Laser

Pediatric Narcotic Antitussive with Expectorant Combinations

Product	Decongestant	Antihistamine	Antitussive	Expectorant	Manufacturer
Nucofed Pediatric Expectorant Syrup	30 mg pseudo-ephedrine HCl		10 mg codeine phosphate	100 mg guaifenesin	Sk-Beecham
Nucotuss Pediatric Expectorant Liquid	30 mg pseudo-ephrine HCl		10 mg codeine phosphate	100 mg guaifenesin	Barre-National
Pediacof Syrup	2.5 mg phenyl-ephrine HCl	0.75 mg chlorphen-iramine maleate	5 mg codeine phosphate	75 mg potassium iodide	Winthrop
Pedituss Cough Syrup	2.5 mg phenyl-ephrine HCl	0.75 mg chlorphen-iramine maleate	5 mg codeine phosphate	75 mg potassium iodide	Major

Pediatric Non-Narcotic Antitussives with Expectorants

Product	Antitussive	Antihistamine	Expectorant	Other	Manufacturer
Children's Formula Cough Syrup	5 mg dextromethorphan HBr		50 mg guaifenesin		Pharmakon
Meditussin Pediatric Cough	5 mg dextromethorphan HBr		50 mg guaifenesin		Del-Med
Vicks Childrens Cough Syrup	3.5 mg dextromethorphan HBr		50 mg guaifenesin		Richardson-Vicks
Vicks Pediatric Formula 44e	3.3 mg dextromethorphan HBr		33.3 mg guaifenesin		Richardson-Vicks

Table 57.28.
Anti-Tussive Preparations

Product Name	Formulation	Manufacturer
Dextromethorphan: (Pediatric dose): 1 mg/kg/24 hours divided TID-QID		
Mediquell	Chewy Squares: 15 mg	Warner-Lampert
Sucrets Cough Control	Lozenges: 5 mg	Beecham
Hold	Lozenges: 5 mg	Beecham
Benylin DM	Syrup: 10 mg/5 ml	Parke-Davis
St. Joseph Cough	Syrup: 7.5 mg/5 ml	Plough
Congespirin for Children	Syrup: 5 mg/5 ml	Bristol-Meyers
PediaCare Cough	Syrup: 5 mg/5 ml	McNeil
Vicks Formula 44 Pediatric	Syrup: 15 mg/5 ml	Richardson Vicks
Delsym	Liquid, sustained action 30 mg/5 ml	McNeil
Diphenhydramine: (Pediatric dose): 5 mg/kg/day divided q6 hours		
Benylin Cough	Syrup: 12.5 mg/5 ml Alcohol: 5%	Parke-Davis
Benadryl Elixir	Elixir: 12.5 mg/5 ml Alcohol: 14%	Parke-Davis

Table 57.29.
Sore Throat Preparations

Product Name	Active Ingredient	Manufacturer
Sorettes	Lozenges(L): 32 mg benzocaine, 8 mg licorice extract and 0.5 mg menthol	Lannett
Mycinettes	Lozenges(L): 15 mg benzocaine cetylpridinium chloride, terpin hydrate, sodium citrate and sorbitol in a demulcent base	Pfeiffer
Spect-T	Lozenges(L): 10 mg benzocaine	Squibb
Oradex-C	Troches(T): 10 mg benzocaine and 2.5 mg cetylpyridium chloride	Commerce
Trocaine	Lozenges(L): 10 mg benzocaine, 2.5 mg cetylpyridium chloride and 15 mg terpin hydrate	Vortech
Cepacol Anesthetic	Troches(T): 10 mg benzocaine and 0.07% cetylpyridium Cl	Lakeside
Oracin	(L) 6.25 mg benzocaine and 0.1% menthol in a sorbitol base	Vicks
Children's Chloroseptic	(L) 5 mg benzocaine	Vicks
Vicks Throat	(L) 5 mg bencozaine, 1.66 mg cetylpyridium Cl, menthol, camphor, and eucalyptus oil	Vicks
Sucrets Maximum Strength	(L) 3 mg dyclonine	Beecham
Listerine Maximum Strength Throat	(L) 4 mg hexylresorcinol	Warner-Lampert (WL)
Listerine Aniseptic	(L) 2.4 mg hexylresorcinol	WL
Sucrets Sore Throat		Beecham
Cepastat	(L) 1.45% phenol, 0.12% menthol, eucalyptus oil	Lakeside
Chloraseptic	(L) 32.5 mg phenol	Vicks
Halls, Vicks, and Nice	Menthol	Various

REFERENCES

1. Bergstrand H. Phosphodiesterase inhibition and theophylline. *Eur J Respir Dis* 1980; 61(Suppl 109):37–44.
2. Horrobin DF, Manku MS, Franks DJ, et al. Methyl-xanthine phosphodiesterase inhibitors behave as prostaglandin antagonists in a perfused rat mesentenc artery preparation. *Prostaglandins* 1977; 13:33–40.
3. Brisson GR, Malaisse-Lagae F, Malaisse WJ. The stimulus–secretion coupling of glucose induced insulin release. VII. A proposed site of action for adenosine 3's–cyclic monophosphate. *J Clin Invest* 1972; 51:232–241.
4. Miech RP, Niedzwicki JG, Smith TR. Effect of theophylline on the binding of CAMP to soluble protein from trachea/smooth muscle. *Biochem Pharmacol* 1979; 28:3687–3688.
5. Satchell C and Smith R. Adenosine causes contractions in spiral strips and relaxation in transverse strips of guinea-pig trachea: studies on mechanism of action. *Eur J Pharmacol* 1984; 101:243.
6. Lunell E, Svedmyr N, Anderson KE, Persson CGA. Effects of enprofylline, a xanthine lacking adenosine receptor antagonism, in patients with chronic obstructive lung disease. *Eur J Clin Pharmacol* 1982; 22:395–402.
7. Hendeles L, Massanari M, Weinberger M. Update on the pharmacodynamics and pharmacokinetics of theophylline. *Chest* 1985; 885:1035.
8. Aubier M, DeTroyer A, Sampson M, Macklem PT, Roussos C. Diaphragm NEJM Aminophylline improves diaphragmatic contractility. *N Engl J Med* 1981; 305:249–252.
9. Hendles L, Weinberger M, Bighley L. Absolute bioavailability of oral theophylline. *Am J Hosp Pharmacol* 1977; 34:525–527.
10. Jonkman JGH, Berg WC, Schoenmaker R, Greving JE, DeZeeuw RA, Orie NON. Disposition and clinical pharmacokinetics of microcrystalline theophylline. *Eur J Clin Pharmacol* 1980; 17:379–384.
11. Upton RA, Sansom L, Guentert TW, et al. Evaluation of the absorption from 15 commercial theophylline products indicating deficiencies in currently applied bioavailability criteria. *J Pharmacokinet Biopharm* 1980; 8:229–242.
12. Koysooko R, Ellis EF, Levy G. Effect of ethanol on theophylline absorption in humans. *J Pharm Sci* 1975; 64:299–301.
13. Apold J and Bakke OM. Is microcrystalline theophylline really better? [Letter]. *Lancet* 1979; 1:667–668.
14. Sansom LN, Milne RW, Cooper D. Comparative bioavailability of a microcrystalline theophylline tablet and uncoated aminophylline tablets. *Eur J Clin Pharmacol* 1979; 16:417–421.
15. Welling PG, Lyons LL, Craig WA, Trochta GA. Influence of diet and fluid on bioavailability of theophylline. *Clin Pharmacol Ther* 1975; 17:475–480.
16. Arnold LA, Spurbeck GH, Shelver WH, Henderson WM. Effect of an antacid on gastrointestinal absorption of theophylline. *Am J Hosp Pharm* 1979; 36:1059–1062.
17. Rohr WJ, Henderson WM, Shelver WH. In vitro Absorption of theophylline by antacids. *Am J Hosp Pharm* 1981; 38:1779–1780.
18. Karim A, Burns T, Wearley L, et al. Food induced charges in theophylline absorption from controlled release formulations. Part I. Substantial increased and decreased absorption with Uniphyl tablets and TheoDur sprinkle. *Clin Pharmacol Ther* 1985; 38:77–83.
19. Howick J, Kelly HW, Menendez R, Murphy S. Absorption characteristics of a new sustained-release theophylline (SRT) sprinkle for infants and young children [Abstract]. *J Allergy Clin Immunol* 1983; 71:130.
20. Pedersen S and Moller–Peterson J. Erratic absorption of a slow release theophylline sprinkle product. *Pediatrics* 1984; 74:534–538.
21. Pedersen S. Absorption of Theo-Dur sprinkle with food: importance of types of meals and medication times. *J Allergy Clin Immunol* 1986; 78:653–660.
22. Pedersen S. Food and fasting intake of sustained release theophylline preparations. *Br J Clin Pract* 1984; 38(Suppl 35):37–39.
23. Karim A. Effects of food on the bioavailability of theophylline from controlled-release products in adults. *J Allergy Clin Immunol* 1986; 78:695–703.
24. Leeds NH, Gal P, Purohit AA, Walter JB. Effect on food on the bioavailability and pattern of release of a sustained-release theophylline tablet. *J Clin Pharmacol* 1982; 22:196–200.
25. Sips AP, Edelbroek Pm, Kulstads S, deWolff FA, Dijkman JH. Food does not effect bioavailability of theophylline from Theolin Retard. *Eur J Clin Pharmacol* 1984; 26:504–507.
26. Osman MA, Patel RB, Irwin DS, Welling PG. Absorption of theophylline from enteric coated and sustained release formulations in fasted and non–fasted subjects. *Biopharm Drug Dispos* 1983; 4:63–72.
27. Pederson S and Moller–Pederson J. Influence on food on the absorption of theophylline from somophyllin (R). *Clin Allergy* 1985; 15:253–259.
28. Birkett DJ, Coulthard KP, Lines D, Grgurinovich N. Circadian Variation in the absorption of three sustained release theophylline products in asthmatic children and the effect of food on the absorption of somophylline CRT. *Br J Clin Pract* 1984; 38(Suppl 35):17–23.
29. Weinberger M. Clinical and pharmacokinetic concerns of 24–hour dosing with theophylline. *Ann Allergy* 1986; 56:2–8.
30. Hendeles L, Weinberger M, Milavetz G, Hill M, Vaughan L. Food induced dumping from a "once-a-day" theophylline product as a cause of theophylline toxicity. *Chest* 1985; 85:758–765.
31. Weinberger M. Theophylline qid, tid, bid and now qd? A report on 24-hour dosing with slow release theophylline formulations with emphasis on analysis of data used to obtain Food and Drug Administration approval for Theo-24. *Pharmacotherapy* 1984; 4:181–198.
32. Steffensen G and Pedersen S. Food induced changes in theophylline absorption from a once-a-day theophylline product. *Br J Clin Pharmacol* 1986; 22:571–577.
33. Pederson S. Effects of food on the absorption of theophylline in children. *J Allergy Clin Immunol* 1986; 78:704–709.
34. Pederson S, Moeller-Peterson J. Influence of food on the absorption rate and bioavailability of a sustained release theophylline preparation. *Allergy* 1982; 37:531–534.
35. Myhre KI and Walstad RI. The influence of antacid on absorption of two different sustained release formulations of theophylline. *Br J Clin Pharmacol* 1983; 15:683–687.
36. Shargel L, Stevens JA, Fuchs JE, Yu ABC. Effect of antacid on bioavailability of theophylline from

rapid and time-release drug products. *J Pharm Sci* 1981; 70:559–602.

37. Mason WD, Lanman RC, Amick EN, Arnold J, March L. Bioavailability of theophylline following a rectally administered concentrated aminophylline solution. *J Allergy Clin Immunol* 1980; 66:119–121.

38. Bolme P, Edlund PO, Ericksson M, Paalzow L, Winblach B. Pharmacokinetics of theophylline in young children with asthma: Comparison of rectal enema and suppositories. *Eur J Clin Pharmacol* 1979; 16:133–139.

39. Waxler SH and Shack JA. Administration of aminophylline (theophylline ethylenediamine). *JAMA* 1980; 143:736–739.

40. Levy G and Koysooko R. Pharmacokinetic analysis of the effect of theophylline on pulmonary function in asthmatic children. *J Pediatr* 1975; 86:789–793.

41. Simons KJ, Simons FER, Briggs CL, Lo L. Theophylline protein binding in humans. *J Pharm Sci* 1979; 68:252–53.

42. Arwood LL, Dasta JF, Friedman C. Placental transfer of theophylline: Two case reports. *Pediatrics* 1979; 63:844–846.

43. Veh TF and Pildes RS. Transplacental aminophylline toxicity in a neonate [Letter]. *Lancet* 1977; 1:910.

44. Vurchak AM and Jusko WJ. Theophylline secretion in to breast milk. *Pediatrics* 1976; 57:518–520.

45. Stec GP, Greenberger P, Rou TI, et al. Kinetics of theophylline transfer into breast milk. *Clin Pharmacol Ther* 1980; 28:404–408.

46. Aranda JV, Sitar DS, Parsons WD, Loughnan DM, Neims AH. Pharmacokinetic aspects of theophylline in premature newborns. *N Engl J Med* 1976; 295:413–416.

47. Ellis EF, Koysooko R, Levy G. Pharmacokinetics of theophylline in children with asthma. *Pediatrics* 1976; 58:542–547.

48. Neims AH. Pharmacokinetic analysis of the disposition of intravenous theophylline in young children. *J Pediatr* 1976; 88:874–879.

49. Mitenko PA and Ogilvie RI. Pharmacokinetics of intravenous theophylline. *Clin Pharmacol Ther* 1973; 14:509–513.

50. Cornish HH and Christman AA. A study of the metabolism of theobromine, theophylline and caffeine in man. *J Biol Chem* 1975; 228:315–323.

51. Tan-Liu DOS, Williams RL, Riegelman S. Nonlinear theophylline elimination. *Clin Pharmacol Ther* 1982; 31:358–369.

52. Bada HS, Khanna NN, Somani SM, Tin AA. Interconversion of theophylline to caffeine in newborn infants. *J Pediatr* 1979; 94:993–995.

53. Ogilvie RI. Clinical pharmacokinetics of theophylline. *Clin Pharmacokinet* 1978; 3:267–293.

54. Levy G and Koysooko R. Renal clearance of theophylline in man. *J Clin Pharmacol* 1976; 16:329–332.

55. Decourt S, Fodor F, Flouvat B, et al. Pharmacokinetics of theophylline in night workers. *Br J Clin Pharmacol* 1982; 13:567–569.

56. Jonkman JH, VanderBoon W. Nocturnal theophylline plasma concentrations. *Lancet* 1983; 1:1278.

57. Taylor Dr, Duffin D, Kinney CD, et al. Investigation of diurnal changes in the disposition of theophylline. *Br J Clin Pharmacol* 1983; 16:413–416.

58. Hendeles L, Massanari M, Weinberger M. Theophylline. In Evans WE, Schentag JJ, Jasko WJ, eds. *Applied pharmacokinetics.* San Francisco, Applied Therapeutics, 1986, pp 1105–1188.

59. Nassif EG, Weinberger M, Guiang SF. Theophylline disposition in infancy. *J Pediatr* 1981; 98:158–161.

60. Jusko WJ, Schentag JJ, Clark JH, Gardner M, Vurchak AM. Enhanced biotransformation of theophylline in marijuana and tobacco smokers. *Clin Pharmacol Ther* 1978; 24:405–410.

61. Powell JR, Thiercelin JF, Vozeh S, Sansom L, Riegelman S. The influence of cigarette smoking and sex on theophylline disposition. *Am Rev Respir Dis* 1977; 116:17–23.

62. Giacoia B, Jusko WJ, Menke J, Koup JR. Theophylline pharmacokinetics in premature infants with apnea. *J Pediatr* 1976; 89:829–832.

63. Wyatt R, Weinberger M, Hendeles L. Oral theophylline dosage for the management of chronic asthma. *J Pediatr* 1978; 92:125–130.

64. Chang KC, Lauer BA, Bell TD, Chai H. Altered theophylline pharmacokinetics during acute respiratory viral illness. *Lancet* 1978; 1:1132–1133.

65. Mangione A, Imhoff TE, Lee RV, Shum LY, Jusko WJ. Pharmacokinetics of theophylline in hepatic disease. *Chest* 1978; 73:616–622.

66. Piafsky KM, Sitar DS, Rangro RE, Ogilvie RI. Theophylline disposition in patients with hepatic cirrhosis. *N Engl J Med* 1977; 296:1495–1497.

67. Staib AH, Schuppan D, Lissner R, Zilly W, Bomhard GV, Richter E. Pharmacokinetics and metabolism of theophylline in patients with liver disease. *Int J Clin Pharmacol Ther Toxicol* 1980; 18:500–502.

68. Jenne JW, Chick TW, Miller BA, Strickland RD. Apparent theophylline half-life fluctuations during treatment of acute left ventricular failure. *Am J Hosp Pharm* 1977; 34:408–409.

69. Powell JR, Vozeh S, Hopewell P, Costello J, Sheiner LB. Riegelman S. Theophylline disposition in acutely ill hospitalized patients. The effect of smoking, heart-failure, severe airway obstruction, and pneumonia. *Am Rev Respir Dis* 1978; 118:229–238.

70. Vicuna N, McNay JL, Ludden TM, Schwertner H. Impaired theophylline clearance in patients with cor pulmonale. *Br J Clin Pharmacol* 1979; 7:33–37.

71. Isles A, Shpjino M, Tabachnik E. Theophylline disposition in cystic fibrosis. *Am Rev Respir Dis* 1983; 127:417–421.

72. Vozeh S, Otten M, Staub JJ, Follath F. Influence of thyroid function on theophylline kinetics. *Clin Pharmacol Ther* 1984; 36:623–640.

73. Upton RA. Pharmacokinetic interactions between theophylline and other medications (Part I). *Clin Pharmacokinet* 1991; 20:66–80.

74. Upton RA. Pharmacokinetic interactions between theophylline and other medications (Part II). *Clin Pharmacokinet* 1991; 20:135–150.

75. Weinberger MM, Bronsky EA. Interaction of ephedrine and theophylline. *Clin Pharmacol Ther* 1975; 17:585–592.

76. Laaban JP, Iung B, Chauvet JP, Psychoyos I, Proteau J, Rochemaure J. Cardiac arrhythmias during combined use of intravenous aminophylline and terbutaline in status asthmaticus. *Chest* 1988; 94:496–502.

77. Victoria MS, Tayaba RG, Nangia BS. Isoproterenol infusion in the management of respiratory failure in children with status asthmaticus: Experience in a small community hospital and review of the literature. *J Asthma* 1991; 28:103–108.

78. Hendeles L, Wyatt R, Weinberger M, Schottelius O, Fincham R. Decreased oral phenytoin absorption following concurrent theophylline administration. *J Allergy Clin Immunol* 1979; 63:156.

79. Thomsen K and Schou M. Renal lithium excretion in man. *Am J Physiol* 1968; 315:823–827.

80. Albert S. Aminophylline toxicity. *Pediatr Clin North Am* 1987; 34:61–73.
81. Olson KR, Bonaoltz NL, Woo OF. Theophylline overdose: Acute single ingestion versus chronic repeated overdedication. *Am J Emerg Med* 1985; 3:386–394.
82. Weitmen S, Farrington EA, Barry DE, Kamen BA. Drug monitoring and pharmacokinetics. In Levin, Moriss, eds. *Essential guide to pediatric intensive care.* St. Louis, Quality Medical Publishing, 1990, pp 38–45.
83. Rossing TH, Fanta CH, Goldstein OH, Snapper JR, McFadden ER. Emergency therapy of asthma: Comparison of the acute effects of parental and inhaled sympathomimetics and infused aminophylline. *Am Rev Respir Dis* 1980; 122:365–371.
84. Fanta CH, Rossing TH, McFadden ER. Emergency room treatment of asthma. *Am J Med* 1982; 72:416.
85. Rossing TH, Fanta CA, McFadden ER. A controlled trial of the use of single versus combined drug therapy in the treatment of acute episodes of asthma. *Am Rev Respir Dis* 1981; 123:190–194.
86. Svedmyr K and Svedmyr N. Does theophylline potentiate inhaled beta₂ agonists? *Allergy* 1982; 37:101–110.
87. Rieder MJ and Koren G. The pharmacotherapy of acute and chronic asthma. In Nussbaum E, ed. *Pediatric intensive care.* Mount Kisco, NY, Future Publishing, 1989, pp 887–913.
88. Johnson MH, Burkle WS. Evaluation of the Chiou method for determining theophylline dosages. *Clin Pharmacol* 1984; 3:174.
89. Jones RAK, Baillie E. Dosage schedule for intravenous aminophylline in apnea of prematurity, based on pharmacokinetic studies. *Arch Dis Child* 1979; 54:190.
90. Anonymous. Use of theophylline in infants. *FDA Drug Bull* 1985; 15:16–17.
91. Murphy JE, Erkan NV, Fakhreddine S. New FDA guidelines for theophylline dosing in infants. *Clin Pharmacol* 1986; 5:16.
92. Gorodischer R and Karplus M. Pharmacokinetic aspects of caffeine in premature infants with apnea. *Eur J Clin Pharmacol* 1982; 22:47.
93. Orygiel JJ, Birkett DJ. Effect of age on patterns of theophylline metabolism. *Clin Pharmacol Ther* 1980; 28:456.
94. Aranda JV, Borman W, Bergsteisson H, Gunn T. Efficacy of caffeine in treatment of apnea in the low-birth-weight infant. *J Pediatr* 1977; 90:467–472.
95. Rall TW. Central nervous system stimulants: The xanthines. In Gilman AG, Goodman LS, Gilman A, eds. *The pharmacologic basis of therapeutics*, 8th ed. New York, MacMillan, 1985, pp 345–382.
96. Sigrist S, Thomas D, Howell S. The effect of aminophylline on inspiratory muscle contractility. *Am Rev Respir Dis* 1982; 126:46–50.
97. Lopes JM, LeSouef PN, Bryan MH. The effects of theophylline on diaphragmatic fatigue in the newborn. *Pediatr Res* 1982; 16:355A.
98. Shannon DC, Gotay F, Stein IM. Prevention of apnea and bradycardia in low-birthweight infants. *Pediatrics* 1975; 55:589–594.
99. Roberts RJ. *Methylxanthine therapy: Caffeine and theophylline. Drug therapy in infants.* Philadelphia, WB Saunders, 1984:119–137.
100. Andersson KE, Johannesson N, Karlber B. Increase in free fatty acids and natriuresis by xanthines may reflect adenosine antagonism. *Eur J Clin Pharmacol* 1984; 26:33–38.
101. Parsons WJ and Stiles GL. Methylxanthines as adenosine receptor antagonists. *Ann Intern Med* 1985; 103:462.
102. Arnada JV, Cook CE, Gorman W. Pharmacokinetic profile of caffeine in the premature newborn infant with apnea. *J Pediatr* 1979; 94:663–668.
103. Arnada JV and Turmen T. Methylxanthines in apnea of prematurity. *Clin Perinatol* 1979; 6:87–108.
104. Banner W and Czajka PA. Acute caffeine overdose in the neonate. *Am J Dis Child* 1980; 134:495.
105. Aranda JV, Collinge JM, Zinman R, Watters G. Maturation of caffeine elimination in infancy. *Arch Dis Child* 1979; 54:946–949.
106. Kriter KE and Blanchard J. Management of apnea in infants. *Clin Pharmacol* 1989; 8:577–587.
107. Hayakawa F, Hakamaola S, Kunok, Nakashima T, Miyachi Y. Doxapram treatment of idiopathic apnea of prematurity: Desirable dosage and serum concentrations. *J Pediatr* 1986; 109:138–140.
108. Barrington KJ, Finer NN, Torok-Both G, Jamali F, Coutts R. Dose–response relationship of doxapram in the therapy of idiopathic apnea of prematurity. *Pediatrics* 1987; 80:22–27.
109. Beaudry NA, Bradly JM, Gramlich LM. Pharmacokinetics of doxapram in idiopathic apnea of prematurity. *Dev Pharmacol Ther* 1988; 11:65–72.
110. Eyal F, Alpan G, Sagi E, Glick B, Peleg O, Dgani V, Arad I. Aminophylline versus doxapram in idiopathic apnea of prematurity: a double blind controlled study. *Pediatrics* 1985; 75:709–713.
111. Gershanik J, Boecler B, Ensley H, McCloskey S, George W. The gasping syndrome and benzyl alcohol poisoning. *N Engl J Med* 1982; 307:1384–1388.
112. Food and Drug Administration Bulletin, Department of Health and Human Services, May 28, 1982.
113. Lofdahl CG, Svedmyer N. Selectivity of B–adrenergic stimulation and blocking agents. *Eur J Respir Dis* 1984; 65:101–113.
114. Church MK, Featherstone RL, Cushley MJ. Relationship between adenosine, cyclic nucleotides, and xanthines in asthma. *J Allergy Clin Immunol* 1986; 78:670–675.
115. Galant SP: Current status of Beta–adrenergic agonists in bronchial asthma. *Pediatr Clin North Am* 1983; 30:931.
116. Santa Cruz R, Landa J, Hirsch J, Sackner MA. Trachea/mucus velocity in normal man and patients with obstructive lung disease: Effects of terbutaline. *Am Rev Respir Dis* 1974; 109:458–463.
117. Barnes PJ. A new approach to the treatment of asthma. *N Engl J Med* 1989; 321:1517–1527.
118. Seligman M. Bronchodilators. In Chernow B, ed. *The pharmacologic approach to the critically ill patient*, 2nd ed. Baltimore, Williams & Wilkins, 1988, pp 436–450.
119. McFadden ER. Beta–2 receptor agonist: Metabolism and pharmacology. *J Allergy Clin Immunol* 1981; 68:91–97.
120. Newhouse MT, Dolovich MB. Control of asthma by aerosols. *N Engl J Med* 1986; 315:870–874.
121. Kelly HW. New beta–2–adrenergic agonist aerosols. *Clin Pharmacol* 1985; 4:393–403.
122. Sly RM, Anderson JA, Bierman CW. Adverse effects and complications of treatment of beta–adrenergic agonists drugs. *J Allergy Clin Immunol* 1985; 75:443–449.
123. Reed CE. Adrenergic bronchodilators: Pharmacology and toxicology. *J Allergy Clin Immunol* 1985; 76:335–341.
124. Lefkowitz RJ, Caron MG, Stiles GL. Biochemical, physiological, and clinical insights derived from

studies of the adrenergic receptors. *N Engl J Med* 1984; 310:1570–1579.

125. Shim C. Inhalation aids of metered dose inhalers. *Chest* 1987; 91:315–316.

126. Newman SP, Moren F, Pavia D, Little F, Clark SW. Deposition of pressurized suspension aerosols inhaled through extension devices. *Am Rev Respir Dis* 1981; 124:317–320.

127. Pedersen S, Stevensen G. Simplification of inhalation therapy in asthmatic children: A comparison of two regimes. *Allergy* 1986; 41:296–301.

128. Pedersen S, Frost L, Arnfred T. Errors in inhalation technique and efficacy in inhaler use in asthmatic children. *Allergy* 1986; 41:118–124.

129. Pedersen S. Aerosol treatment of bronchoconstriction in children with or without a tube spacer. *N Engl J Med* 1983; 308:1328–1330.

130. Lee H, Evans HE. Evaluation of inhalation ards of metered dose inhalers in asthmatic children. *Chest* 1987; 91:366–369.

131. Kemp JP, Furukawa CT, Bronsky EA. Albuterol treatment for children with asthma: A comparison of inhaled powder and aerosol. *J Allergy Clin Immunol* 1989; 83:697–702.

132. Chambers S, Dunbar J, Taylor B. Inhaled powder compared with aerosol administration of fenoterol in asthmatic children. *Arch Dis Child* 1990; 65:401–403.

133. Rau JL. Delivery of aerosolized drugs to neonatal and pediatric patients. *Respir Care* 1991; 36:514–545.

134. Compton GK. Problems patients have using pressurized aerosol inhalers. *Eur J Respir Dis* 1982; 63(Suppl 119):101–104.

135. Kelling JS, Strohl KD, Smith RL, Altose MD. Physician knowledge in the use of canister nebulizers. *Chest* 1983; 83:612–614.

136. Papa V. Beta–Adrenergic Drugs. *Clin Chest Med* 1986; 7:313–329.

137. Milledge JS, Morris JA. A comparison of slow release salbutamol with slow release aminophylline in nocturnal asthma. *J Int Med Res* 1979; 7:106–110.

138. Heins M, Kurtinl, Ollerich M. Nocturnal asthma: Slow release terbutaline versus slow–release theophylline therapy. *Eur Respir J* 1988; 1:306–310.

139. Sly R, Badie B, Faciano J. Comparison of subcutaneous terbutaline with epinephrine in the treatment of asthma in children. *J Allergy Clin Immunol* 1977; 59:128–135.

140. Victoria MS, Tayaba RG, Nangia BS. Isoproterenol infusion in the management of respiratory failure in children with status asthmaticus: Experience in a small community hospital and review of the literature. *J Asthma* 1991; 28:103–108.

141. Fuglsang G, Pedersen S, Borgstrom L. Dose relationship of intravenously administered terbutaline in children with asthma. *J Pediatr* 1989; 114:315–329.

142. Bohn D, Kalloghlian A, Jenkins J. Intravenous salbutamol in the treatment of status asthmaticus in children. *Crit Care Med* 1984; 12:391–396.

143. Barnes PJ. A new approach to the treatment of asthma. *N Engl J Med* 1989; 321:1517–1527.

144. Kaliner M. Mechanisms of glucocorticosteroid action in bronchial asthma. *J Allergy Clin Immunol* 1985; 76:321–329.

145. Munck A, Mendel DB, Smith LI, Orti E. Corticosteroid receptors and actions. *Am Rev Respir Dis* 1990; 141:S2–S10.

146. Morris HG. Mechanisms of glucocorticoid action in pulmonary disease. *Chest* 1985; 88(Suppl):133S–141S.

147. Cockcroft DW, Murdock KY. Comparison of the effects of inhaled salbutamol, sodium cromoglycate, and beclomethasone dipropionate on allergen induced early asthmatic response, late asthmatic responses, and increased bronchial responsiveness to histamine. *J Allergy Clin Immunol* 1987; 79:734–740.

148. Sertl K, Cark T, Kaliner M, eds. Corticosteroids: Their biologic mechanisms and application to the treatment of asthma. *Am Rev Respir Dis* 1990; 141(Suppl):51–596.

149. Kelly HW, Murphy S. Corticosteroids for acute severe asthma. *DICP* 1991; 25:72–79.

150. Anderson SD. Exercise induced asthma: The state of the art. *Chest* 1985; 87(Suppl):191–195.

151. Mattoli S, Rosanti G, Mormile F, Ciappi G. The immediate and short-term effects of corticosteroids on cholinergic hyper-reactivity and pulmonary function in subjects with well controlled asthma. *J Allergy Clin Immunol* 1985; 76:214–222.

152. Hayes RC, Murad F. Adrenocorticotropic hormone: Adrenocortical steroids and their synthetic analogs; inhibitors of adrenocortical steroid biosynthesis. In Gilman AG, Goodman LS, Rall TW, eds. *The pharmacological basis of therapeutics*, 7th ed. New York, MacMillan, 1985, pp 1459–1489.

153. Rieder MJ, Koren G. The pharmacotherapy of acute and chronic asthma. In Nussbaum E, ed. *Pediatric intensive care*, 2nd ed. Mount Kisco, NY, Future Publishing, 1989, pp 887–913.

154. Chang KC, Miklich DR, Barwise G, et al. Linear growth of chronic asthmatic children: The effects of the disease and various forms of steroid therapy. *Clin Allergy* 1982; 12:369–378.

155. Bhagat RG, Chai H. Development of posterior subcapsular cataracts in asthmatic children. *Pediatrics* 1984; 73:626–630.

156. Bisgaard H, Nielson MD, Anderson B, et al. Adrenal function in children with bronchial asthma treated with beclomethasone dipropionate or budesonide. *J Allergy Clin Immunol* 1988; 81:1088–1095.

157. Prahl P, Jensen T. Decreased adreno-cortical suppression utilizing the Nebuhaler for inhalation of steroid aerosols. *Clin Allergy* 1987; 17:393–398.

158. Littlewood JM, Johnson AW, Edwards PA, et al. Growth retardation in asthmatic children treated with inhaled beclomethasone dipropionate. *Lancet* 1988; 1:115–116.

159. Wolthers OD, Pederson S. Growth of asthmatic children during treatment with budesonide: A double blind trial. *BMJ* 1991; 303:163–165.

160. Pierson WE, Bierman CW, Kelley VC. A double blind trial of corticosteroid therapy in status asthmaticus. *Pediatrics* 1974; 54:282.

161. Haynes RC. Adrenocorticotropic hormone: Adrenocorticosteroids and their synthetic analogs: Inhibitors of adrenocortical steroid biosynthesis. In Gilman AG, Goodman LS, Rall TW, et al., eds. *The pharmacological basis of therapeutics*, 7th ed. New York, MacMillan, 1985, pp 1459–1489.

162. Littenberg B, Gluck GH. A controlled trial of methylprednisolone in the treatment of acute asthma. *N Engl J Med* 1986; 314:150.

163. Harnes JB, Wienberger MM, Nassif E. Early interventions with short courses of prednisone to prevent progression of asthma in ambulatory patients incompletely responsive to bronchodilators. *J Pediatr* 1987; 110:627–633.

164. Wyatt R, Waschek J, Weinberger M. Effects of inhaled beclomethasone dipropionate and alternate day prednisone on pituitary–adrenal function in children with chronic asthma. *N Engl J Med* 1978; 299:1387–1392.

165. Nassif E, Weinberger M, Sherman B. Extrapulmonary effects of maintenance corticosteroid therapy with alternate day prednisone and inhaled beclomethasone in children with chronic asthma. *J Allergy Clin Immunol* 1987; 80:518–529.

166. Tunnessen WV, Feinstein AR. The steroid croup controversy: An analytical review of methodological problems. *J Pediatr* 1980; 96:751–756.

167. Super DM, Cartelli NA, Brooks LJ. A prospective double-blind, randomized study to evaluate the effect of dexamethasone in acute laryngotracheitis. *J Pediatr* 1989; 115:323–329.

168. Busse WW. Actions and effects of corticosteroids in allergic rhinitis. *J Respir Dis* 1991; 12(Suppl 3A):536–538.

169. Holgate ST. Reflections on the mechanism(s) of action of sodium cromoglycate (Intal) and the role of mast cells in asthma. *Respir Med* 1989; 83(Suppl):25–31.

170. Foreman JC, Garland LG. Cromoglycate and other antiallergic drugs: Possible mechanism of action. *Br Med J* 1976; 1:820–821.

171. Bungaard A, Bach-Mortensen N, Schmidt A. The effect of sodium cromoglycate delivered by spinhaler and pressurized aerosol on exercise induced asthma in children. *Clin Allergy* 1982; 12:601–605.

172. Breslin FJ, McFadden ER, Ingram RH. The effects of cromolyn sodium on the airway response to hyperpnea and cold air asthma. *Am Rev Respir Dis* 1980; 112:11–16.

173. Cockcroft DW, Murdock KY. Comparative effects of inhaled salbutamol, sodium cromoglycate, and beclomethasone dipropionate on allergy induced early asthmatic responses, late asthmatic responses, and increased bronchial responsiveness to histamine. *J Allergy Clin Immunol* 1987; 79:734–740.

174. Weinberger MM, Hendeles L, Ahrens R. Clinical pharmacokinetics of drugs used in asthma. *Pediatr Clin North Am* 1981; 28:47–75.

175. Murphy S, Kelly W. Cromolyn sodium: a review of mechanisms and clinical use in asthma. *Drug Intell Clin Pharm* 1987; 21–35.

176. Shapiro GB, Konig P. Cromolyn sodium: A review. *Pharmacotherapy* 1985; 5:156–176.

177. Brown LA, Kaplan RA, Benjamin PA. Immunolglobuln E–medicated anaphylaxis with inhaled cromolyn sodium. *J Allergy Clin Immunol* 1981; 68:416–420.

178. Lesko LJ, Miller AK. Physical-chemical compatibility of cromolyn sodium nebulizer solution–bronchodilator inhalent solution admixtures. *Ann Allergy* 1984; 53:236–238.

179. Thompson. Nedocromil sodium: An overview. *Respir Med* 1989; 83:269–276.

180. Holgate ST. Clinical evaluation of nedocromil sodium in asthma. *Eur J Respir Dis* 1986; 69(Suppl 147):149–159.

181. Ruggleri F, Patalano F. Nedocromil sodium: A review of clinical studies. *Eur Respir J* 1989; 2(Suppl 6):568s–571s.

182. Cugell DW. Clinical pharmacology and toxicology of ipratropium bromide. *Am J Med* 1986; 81(Suppl 5A):18–22.

183. Engelhardt A. Pharmacology and toxicology of atrovent. *Scand J Respir Dis* 1979; 103(Suppl):110–115.

184. Hensley MJ, O'Cain CF, McFadden ER. Distribution of bronchodilation in normal subjects: Beta agonist versus atropine. *J Appl Physiol* 1978; 45:778–782.

185. Santamaria J, Guillemi S, Osborne S. Site of bronchodilation with inhaled ipratropium bromide and fenoterol in normal subjects. *Chest* 1987; 91:86–91.

186. Wanner A. Effect of ipratropium bromide on airway mucociliary function. *Am J Med* 1986; 81(Suppl 5A):23–27.

187. Ziment I, Au JP. Anticholinergic agents. *Clin Chest Med* 1986; 7:355–366.

188. Gal TJ, Suratt PM, Lu JL. Glycopyrrolate and atropine inhalation: Comparative effects on normal airway function. *Am Rev Respir Dis* 1984; 192:871–873.

189. Walker FB, Kaiser DL, Kowal MB, Surratt PM. Prolonged effect of inhaled glycopyrrolate in asthma. *Chest* 1987; 91:49–51.

190. Schroeckenstein DC, Bush RK, Chervinsky P, Busse WW. Twelve–hour bronchodilation in asthma with a single aerosol dose of the anticholinergic compound glycopyrrolate. *J Allergy Clin Immunol* 1988; 82:115–119.

191. Middleton E. Calcium antagonists and asthma. *J Allergy Clin Immunol* 1985; 76:341–346.

192. Rafferty R, Holgate ST. Terfenadine (seldane) is a potent and selective histamine H_1 receptor antagonist in asthmatic airways. *Am Rev Respir Dis* 1987; 135:181–184.

193. Cookson WOCM. Bronchodilator action of anti–histamine terfenadine. *Br J Clin Pharmacol* 1987; 24:120–121.

194. Holgate ST, Emanuel MB, Howarth PH. Astemizole and other H_1–antihistaminic drug treatments of asthma. *J Allergy Clin Immunol* 1985; 76:375–380.

195. Septcor SL, Altman R. Cetirizine, a novel antihistamine. *Am J Rhinol* 1987; 3:147–149.

196. Kemp JP, Meltzer EO, Orgel A. Dose response study of bronchodilator action of azelastine in asthma. *J Allergy Clin Immunol* 1987; 79:893–899.

197. Craps LP. Immunologic and therapeutic aspects of ketotifen. *J Allergy Clin Immunol* 1985; 76:389–393.

198. Loftus BC, Price LF. Long-term placebo-controlled trial of ketotifen in the management of preschool children with asthma. *J Allergy Clin Immunol* 1987; 79:350–355.

199. Jolivet J, Cowan KH, Curt GA. The pharmacology and clinical use of methotrexate. *N Engl J Med* 1983; 309:1094–1106.

200. Mullarkey MF, Webb OR, Pardee NE. Methotrexate in the treatment of steroid dependent asthma. *Ann Allergy* 1985; 56:347–351.

201. Mullarkey MF, Blumenstein BA, Anderade WP, Bailey GA, Olason I, Wetzel CG. Methotrexate in the treatment of corticosteroid dependent asthma: a double blind crossover study. *N Engl J Med* 1988; 318:603–607.

202. Mullarkey MF, Lammert JK, Blumenstein BA. Long-term methotrexate in corticosteroid-dependent asthma. *Ann Intern Med* 1990; 112:577–583.

203. Lammert JK, Mullarkey MF. promises and problems with the use of methotrexate in asthmatic patients. *Immunol Allergy Clin North Am* 1991; 1:65–79.

204. Bernstein DI, Bernstein Il. Use of gold in the severe asthmatic patient. *Immunol Allergy Clin North Am* 1991; 11:81–90.

205. Muranaka M, Mivamoto T, Shida T. Gold salt in the treatment of bronchial asthma—A double blind study. *Ann Allergy* 1978; 40:132–137.

206. Bernstein DI, Bernstein IL, Bodenheimer SS, Pitrusko RG. An open study of auranofin in the treatment of steroid dependent asthma. *J Allergy Clin Immunol* 1988; 81:6–16.

207. Naclerio RM, Proud D, Kagey-Sobotka A. Is histamine responsible for the symptoms of rhinovirus colds? A look at the inflammatory mediators following infection. *Pediatr Infect Dis J* 1988; 7:215–242.

58

Comprehensive Home Care

JEAN H. ZANDER

As increasing numbers of critically ill children survive the acute phase of disease, many are found to be incapable of maintaining independent physiologic function without the supportive technology of monitoring, supplemental oxygen, and/or mechanical ventilation. Care of the O_2-dependent child (1–5), the tracheotomized child (6–8), and the ventilator-assisted child (9–16) is complex and requires great planning and a well organized team. This discussion will focus on general elements of home care planning for children and then review special needs of care for these three groups.

PATIENT SELECTION

Prior to discharge, an infant or child must demonstrate medical stability according to some predetermined criteria (Table 58.1). The child should have appropriate growth and development for gestational age and disease state, have a dietary management plan that provides adequate caloric intake, and have documentation of therapeutic levels of medications.

An assessment of the family's resources and willingness to care for the child should be an ongoing one, made by clinical nurse specialist or social worker. Stein (17) suggests that the "functional burden" of home care be assessed

in order to determine the readiness for home care. The functional burden consists of two components—the child's health condition and the family's resources and ability to cope (Table 58.2). By a careful assessment of these factors and a balance between burden and resources, achieving a successful home care program is more likely.

The family's *willingness* to undertake the complex home care program must be carefully and *directly* explored. The child's discharge to home must always be seen by the family as an *alternative* for them. They must be willing to undergo extensive training, and to live with the commitment of physical and emotional care. This commitment often involves surrendering much personal time and perhaps even a career.

The physical environment of the home should be assessed by a home care nurse or RT who is familiar with the requirements for high-tech home care. Room size and arrangements, adequacy of electrical wiring, and geo-

Table 58.1.
Discharge Criteria

Disease process stable on reasonable careplan
Stable blood gases
Stable O_2 requirements or ventilator settings
Stable growth
Established nutrition and medication schedules

Table 58.2.
Assessment of "Functional Burden"

1. Child's health condition
   - Need for medical/nursing care
   - Fixed deficits
   - Age-inappropriate dependency in APL
   - Potential for disruptions in normal family routine due to care needs
   - Psychologic burden or prognosis

2. Family's resources and ability to cope
   - Resources of primary caretaker: physical, emotional, educational
   - Social supports and help available
   - Competing demands for time and energy

From Stein REK. Homecare: A challenging opportunity. *Child Health Care* 1985; 14:90–95.

graphic location are all important elements to consider.

Community resources must also be assessed and their assistance evaluated early in the planning process. The essential resources are listed in Table 58.3.

HOME NURSING CARE

Most families of technology-dependent children will require the assistance of home care nurses, either by having nurses work shifts in the house or by visiting periodically, depending on their capabilities and the needs of their child. The nursing care will offer some respite for the parents, enabling them to maintain some outside activities and/or employment.

Home care nursing may be secured through a local agency or the family may hire individual nurses by advertising in the local media. An agency provides the advantage of assuming the responsibility for such tasks as scheduling and payroll, which the parents must undertake if they hire nurses independently. However, some parents feel that they must surrender too much control in working with an agency. If an agency is selected, it is essential that the administrator and his or her home care team understand the home care philosophy and goals for the child. The parents, nursing agency, and home care planning team should meet at the start of the discharge process to discuss mutual expectations.

If the parents elect to hire nurses independently, they may find it helpful to contact the hospital employment office, which often will have a file of nurses seeking part-time flexible employment.

No matter which route the family chooses to secure home care nursing assistance, the parents should interview each nurse prior to

Table 58.3.
Community Resources in High-Tech Home Care

Primary care physician

Home care nursing agency

Home care equipment vendor, respiratory therapist

Local hospital and emergency medical services

Utilities (phone, electricity, water, heat, and air-conditioning

School

OT, PT, speech therapy

Infant stimulation program

Psychologic/Psychiatric evaluation and support

selection for their child's care (Table 58.4). This requirement should be understood by the nursing agency. A nurse or social worker at the discharging hospital may assist the family to prepare for this by role-playing employment interviews with them.

Few have had the opportunity to supervise employees in their home, and problems may arise when parents establish *friendship* as the basis for their relationship with the home care nurses. It is best for parents to maintain some *professional* distance with the home care nurses, and they should be instructed in ways this may be done. All caretakers, parents, friends, and nurses alike should participate in thorough technical training prior to discharge. This training should include sessions in ventilator management, respiratory care, growth and development, etc. Each caregiver should then be requested to demonstrate back their skills in operating all equipment and specialized care techniques for the child prior to discharge. The home care program for occupational therapy (OT), physical therapy (PT), and speech therapy should also be reviewed with them.

HOME RESPIRATORY CARE

The home respiratory care equipment vendor should be selected according to parameters delineated by the discharging institution, but it is essential that the family be given a choice of vendors. The company should participate in all pre-discharge meetings and in the assessment of the home physical environment and have *pediatric* respiratory therapists on staff with 24-hour availability and who make house calls for maintenance and trouble shooting. Equipment should be delivered to the home at least 24 hours before discharge.

REIMBURSEMENT ISSUES

Issues associated with third party payment are often the greatest source of frustration and stress to families and staff working with technology-dependent children. In a study to identify factors predictive of family stress associated with home care of the ventilator-assisted child, Wegener and Aday (18) found the only predictive variable to be the availability and comprehensiveness of the child's insurance coverage. As the needs of these children become more widely known,

Table 58.4.
Sample Interview Questions

- What is your current nursing licensure (state, license no.)?
- Where were you educated?
- Where have you worked? Do you have background in pediatrics and/or ICU? (If not: Why are you applying for *this* position without that experience?)
- How are you qualified for *this* position?
- What do you like/dislike about nursing?
- If this is an employment change, why are you changing?
- Describe a crisis you handled well.
- What nursing skills are you most proud of?
- What do you think would be the biggest adjustment for you in coming to care for our child?
- What about yourself would you like to improve or strengthen?
- What type of patients give you the most satisfaction? Most frustration?
- What do you expect as a typical shift in working in our home?
- What activities outside nursing do you think have helped make you a better nurse?
- Do you smoke? Do you like dogs, cats? (if applicable)

From Lund CH, ed. Bronchopulmonary dysplasia: *Strategies for total parent care.* Petaluma, Neonatal Network, 1990.

more third party payors are developing case management programs to plan for the needs of these children. In addition, as the advantages of home care are recognized, more companies are willing to approve some home care coverage outside the bounds of their original coverage contracts.

PSYCHOSOCIAL ISSUES

Family life of chronically ill children and their parents has been well studied (19–21). Studies specific to ventilator-assisted children and their families have reported the advantages the parents have found in caring for their child in the home (10, 18). Among those mentioned are improvements in the child's emotional and medical condition, and "feeling more like a family."

Despite the potential advantages, families do report a significant level of stress with high-risk home care. Families suddenly assume the burden of responsibility for their child's physical care. When they are fortunate enough to receive assistance from private duty nurses, they are faced with another set of challenges, including their need for privacy as a couple, and as a family, and their need to define the boundaries of the nurses' rights and responsibilities. Many families experience social isolation because of their care commitments at home. In addition, parents often have established intense long-term relationships with the ICU staff that they find hard to leave

behind. This may contribute to the family's feelings of isolation and abandonment.

Wegener and Aday identified seven predictors of caregiver and family stress in ventilator-assisted children (Table 58.5) and suggest that these be used to plan pre-discharge interventions.

HOME OXYGEN THERAPY

Home oxygen therapy has been employed for many years in the care of adults with chronic obstructive pulmonary disease (COPD), and recent advances in technology have enabled this therapy to be made available to children (1, 3, 4, 22, 23).

Unlike their adult counterparts, children are often unable to state specifically that they are short of breath; they must be assessed for increased respiratory rate and effort (nasal flaring, head bobbing) diaphoresis, pallor, and poor feeding. Older children may report sleepiness during the day, decreased attention span, deterioration in school performance, or headaches upon arising in the morning, reflecting nocturnal hypoxia.

In order to determine the need for home oxygen therapy, the adequacy of oxygenation must be assessed at rest, with activity, during feedings, and during sleep; this is most commonly done by pulse oximetry. Oxygen is then prescribed for each level of activity, to be adjusted as needed. The goal should be to maintain arterial oxygen saturation at or above

Table 58.5.
Predictors of Caregiver and Family Stress in the Ventilator-Assisted Pediatric Population

Family finances
- Family states that finances are a serious problem for them.
- Family identifies large amount of out-of-pocket expenses during child's initial hospitalization (transportation, lost work time, parking, food, phone, etc.)

Social and physical environment
- Recent hospital discharge of child
- Large number of extended family members in household

Comprehensiveness of discharge plan
- Families without a designated nurse care manager at discharge (families either have no care manager or it is not a nurse)
- Families whose discharge planning included fewer elements of the AAP's Ad Hoc Task on Home Care of Chronically Ill Infants and Children guidelines
- Families whose children had seen a large number of physicians (i.e., an number of specialists or rotation of residents in a tertiary care institution)

From Wegener DH, Aday LV. Home care for ventilator assisted children: Predicting family stress. *Pediatr Nurs* 1989; 15:371–376.

92%. By paying close attention to ensuring good oxygenation, occult hypoxia may be relieved and growth and development promoted (2, 5).

When selecting a home oxygen system a variety of factors must be considered (Table 58.6), including the advantages and disadvantages of various O_2 sources (Table 58.7). Compressed gas may be the source of choice when oxygen is used infrequently. However, as a continuous system the large tanks are inconvenient, bulky, and potentially dangerous. Liquid oxygen is a safer alternative, and the small portable units are easily filled from a large reservoir. Oxygen concentrators provide a lower flow of oxygen. If one of these systems is prescribed, a portable source must also be available to allow mobility within and outside the home.

Tents and hoods, most commonly used within the hospital, are not the prime choice

Table 58.6.
Factors to Consider in Selecting Home O_2 Systems

Intended usage
Weight of system
Ease of refills
Low flow capability
Need for backup
Home environment
Local supply and service
Economics and reimbursement

From Lund CH, ed. *Bronchopulmonary dysplasia: Strategies for total parent care*. Petaluma, Neonatal Network, 1990.

for home use. They prevent parent-child interaction, may become uncomfortably warm in summer weather, and are expensive to use. Masks also interfere with activities of daily living. Huts may be acceptable for home use during sleep but restrict the hand to mouth movements so important for infants.

The nasal cannula is the most popular home O_2 delivery system for the child without a tracheostomy. Small squares of Stomahesive should be applied to the face when the cannula is taped in place; this prevents the inevitable skin irritation associated with long-term cannula use. The tape is changed as necessary; the stomahesive is changed one or two times per week.

As with any home care technology, many parents fear the use of O_2 and question their ability to provide safe care for their child. Parents of infants with bronchopulmonary dysplasia (BPD) may attribute the presence of chronic lung disease to the use of oxygen in the neonatal period, and thus are reluctant to continue O_2 therapy at home. Extreme care must be taken in explaining the rationale for O_2 use and the importance of O_2 to the child's overall recovery, including growth, cardiac health, and brain development. The dangers of premature discontinuation of O_2 must be clearly detailed.

Prior to discharge, a respiratory therapist visits the home and delivers the equipment; parents are taught the use and maintenance of each component. They are cautioned to store O_2 away from extreme heat and cold,

Table 58.7.
Advantages and Disadvantages of Oxygen Sources

Oxygen System	Advantages	Disadvantages
Compressed gas (tanks)	• Long shelf-life • Easily available	• Heavy • Need refills • High pressure (2000 PSI) • Low volume for size when compared to liquid system
Liquid oxygen	• Low pressure (20 PSI) • Portability • Easy home refilling	• Evaporation • Potential for frostbite during refilling • Technical problems such as ice
Oxygen Concentrators/Enrichers	• Simple, easy to use • Mobile	• Heavy • Not portable • Need power source

From Lund CH, ed. *Bronchopulmonary dysplasia: Strategies for total parent care.* Petaluma, Neonatal Network, 1990.

and sources of combustion. Tanks of compressed gas are well secured to prevent accidental damage and explosion.

When growth and development are good, and Sao$_2$ is $\geq 95\%$ while awake, O$_2$ may be discontinued during the waking hours. Sleeping O$_2$ saturation is later evaluated to determine the need for O$_2$ at night and during naps.

HOME TRACHEOSTOMY CARE

As with the other home technologies discussed here, long-term tracheostomy and care in the home has become more common because of technologic advances, improved survival rates for very ill neonates and children, and the increased recognition of the effects of chronic upper airway obstruction in neurologically impaired children.

Prior to discharge from the hospital, the parents and other home caretakers must demonstrate a variety of skills required for care of their child. These skills are listed in Table 58.8 and are described in detail below.

1. Parents are able to state the reason for their child's tracheostomy.

Because of the variety of indications for long-term pediatric tracheostomy, parents must have a clear understanding of the reason for *their* child's tracheostomy. This explanation can also be set forth in context of their child's long-term prognosis and health care needs.

2. Parent must explain basic anatomy of trachea and relationship of tracheostomy tube to vocal cords and esophagus.

Parents must have a basic understanding of the relationship between the trachea and the lungs. If parents are shown the placement of

the tracheostomy tube in relationship to the vocal cords, they will have a greater understanding of why of their child cannot vocalize.

3. Parents state elements of respiratory assessment and signs of illness.

Parents must be able to correctly count respiratory rate and apical heart rate. The signs of increased respiratory distress and/or illness are listed in Table 58.9.

Most respiratory infections in tracheotomized children are viral in nature, manifested as an increase in the amount and tenacity of tracheal secretions. Green, foul-smelling mucus is often attributed to bacterial infection and treated empirically with antibiotics. Tracheal aspirate cultures reflect chronic colonization and do not indicate true infection, but may assist in the choice of antibiotics in the event of acute, severe illness.

4. Parent states actions to be taken in the event of tube obstruction, accidental decannulation, and/ or bleeding.

Tube obstruction is the most common cause of severe respiratory distress in the child with a tracheostomy and must be treated as an emergency.

Equipment for an emergency tracheostomy change (suction machine and catheter; clean extra tracheostomy tube and one size smaller, with string, ready for insertion; and scissors) must *always* be available, even when the family is traveling. The child must *never* be left alone with a caregiver who is unable to perform an emergency tracheostomy change.

The parent must be able to assess correctly for the possibility of obstruction by recognizing the presence of dyspnea, diaphoresis, cyanosis, restlessness, and decreased or absent

Table 58.8.
Home Care Skills for a Child with a Tracheostomy

Prior to discharge, the parents must demonstrate the following skills:

1. Explain basic anatomy of trachea and relationship to adjoining structures.
2. State reason for tracheostomy.
3. State elements of respiratory assessment and signs of illness.
4. State actions to be taken in the event of tube obstruction, accidental decannulation, and/or bleeding.
5. Demonstrate CPR.
6. Name type of tracheostomy tube, parts of tube, and purpose of each part. Demonstrate proper use of trach tube cuff if applicable.
7. State importance of humidification, method of delivery, and care of equipment.
8. Assess need for suctioning, demonstrate suction technique using catheter and bulb syringe, state indications and technique for normal saline lavage, demonstrate methods for cleaning inner cannula and suction equipment.
9. Demonstrate correct technique for changing trach tube.
10. State principles and techniques of skin care and general safety, including feeding.
11. State importance of verbal stimulation and know communication/speech therapy home plan for child.
12. State plans regarding decannulation timetable.

From Lund CH, ed. *Bronchopulmonary dysplasia: Strategies for total parent care.* Petaluma, Neonatal Network, 1990.

Table 58.9.
Signs of Increased Respiratory Distress or Illness

- Fever
- Change in amount, color, consistency, odor of secretions
- Hemoptysis
- Change in respiratory rate, rhythms (including retractions, nasal flaring)
- Diaphoresis
- Color change (pallor, cyanosis—cyanosis is a *late, inconsistent* sign)
- Restlessness

Adapted from the Home Care Teaching Program, James Whitcomb Riley Hospital for Children.

breath sounds. If obstruction is suspected the caregiver quickly calls for help, if readily available. An attempt is made to suction. If the child's distress is not relieved, the tracheostomy tapes are quickly cut, the old tube is removed, and a new one is immediately inserted. The adult manually ventilates the child while assessing breath sounds. Depending on the status at the conclusion of the procedure, the parent secures the tube or begins other emergency measures, such as CPR.

Blood-tinged secretions are not uncommon because of drying and irritation of the airway—increased humidification may be indicated. Frank bleeding may indicate tracheal lesion of an adjoining vessel such as the innominate artery, and a physician must be notified immediately.

5. Parents are able to name type of tracheostomy tube, the parts of the tube, and the purpose of each part. They demonstrate proper inflation and deflation of cuff, if applicable.

The most common types of tubes currently in use in children are those constructed of polyvinyl chloride (PVC); these tubes soften at body temperature, conforming to the contours of the airway and producing less airway trauma. They are labeled as "disposable" tubes but with meticulous technique are often cleansed and reused as long as tube integrity persists. They are available in a variety of pediatric and neonatal sizes, the larger size with a low pressure cuff and/or cannula.

Metal tubes, such as the Jackson and Hollinger types, are less frequently used in children. Parents must be advised that tube parts are *not* interchangeable between sets. In addition, the metal tube does not accommodate the 15-mm adapter on a standard resuscitation bag and a specialized adapter must be available *at all times* in the event assisted ventilation is required.

Cuffed tracheostomy tubes, although used infrequently, may be necessary to prevent aspiration and/or ventilation leak. When needed, a pre-stretched, low-pressure cuff will provide an effective seal with minimal pressure on the trachea. The caregivers should be instructed to deflate the cuff two or three times each day for approximately 30 minutes in order to prevent mucosal trauma.

An inner cannula is used with metal tracheostomies, larger size tubes, and fenestrated tubes (see below). This inner cannula fits into the larger, outer cannula and can be removed for cleaning and suctioning.

A fenestrated tracheostomy tube has an opening in the superior aspect of the outer cannula to allow air flow through the upper airway. When the tracheostomy lumen is capped, this upwardly directed flow permits vocalization. However, a long inner cannula that occludes the fenestration must be used when the child is manually/mechanically ventilated or suctioned. If the inner cannula is not used and assisted ventilation is supplied via the trach tube, air will escape through the upper airway, resulting in inadequate lung inflation. Thus, parents must be warned of the need for an inner cannula, especially in an emergency.

The use of a fenestrated tracheostomy tube may also allow for the development of granulation tissue within the fenestration itself. The long inner cannula should be in place whenever vocalization is not likely (i.e., at night).

6. Understand importance of humidification, method of oxygen delivery, and care of equipment.

The administration of humidity protects the trachea from drying, irritation, and some foreign particles. One commonly available device, the Humidivent ("artificial nose"), is easily portable and is disposed of when soiled. Units that supply humidification directly to the tracheostomy are used in conjunction with tracheostomy collars. The units must be cleaned meticulously according to a well-defined procedure to avoid bacterial contamination. Ultrasonic units must be avoided as the very small water particles may trigger bronchospasm in patients with hyper-reactive airways.

7. Parents assess need for suctioning, demonstrate suctioning technique using suction catheter, method of cleaning inner cannula, and suction machine.

Indications of the need for suctioning include increased respiratory rate and/or effort, diaphoresis, restlessness, persistent cough, and cyanosis. Parents are cautioned to avoid *too* frequent suctioning as this may result in tracheal irritation, copious secretions, and the need for even *more* suctioning. As a general rule, parents should suction by using a cathe-ter when secretions cannot be cleared by cough or with a small bulb syringe.

Rather than the sterile technique used in the hospital, clean suctioning technique is used in the home. The array of microbacterial flora to which the patient is exposed differs from hospital to home; with careful technique gloves are not necessary and suction catheters may be reused for several days. This practice simplifies the procedure for the family and results in significant cost savings.

Equipment for suctioning must be available *at all times.* Normal saline lavage may be used when secretions are tenacious. The inner cannula should be cleaned BID-TID with hydrogen peroxide and a pipe cleaner, then thoroughly rinsed in normal saline. When reinserted it must be *locked* in place.

8. Parents demonstrate correct technique for changing tracheostomy tube.

Two trained adults must be present for a tracheostomy tube change. Supplies are assembled and the steps are followed as specified in Tables 58.10 and 58.11. The frequency of tube changes is determined by the policies of the discharging institution.

9. Parents state principles and techniques of skin care and general safety, including feeding.

Generally, the trach tube is secured by the use of twill tape, tied in a triple knot, encircling the neck. Skin irritation may result in sensitive individuals if the tapes are tied too snugly. The short, fat necks of infants are particularly vulnerable to breakdown from snug ties or irritation due to diaphoresis. Commercial velcro ties are easy to use and cause less skin irritation but may be easily unfastened by a curious, active child. Twill tape ties may be threaded through latex rubber tubing or sponge hair rollers to provide another alterna-

Table 58.10.
Supplies for Changing a Trach Tube[a]

- Clean tube with trach stings in place
- Tube that is one size smaller with trach strings in place
- Scissors
- Obturator
- Water-soluble lubricant
- Suction equipment
- Small roll for shoulders

[a]These supplies are to be kept with child at all times as part of his "travel kit." Adapted from the Home Care Teaching Program, James Whitcomb Riley Hospital for Children.

Table 58.11.
Changing the Tracheostomy Tube

- Assemble supplies
- Place obturator in new tube; check cuff integrity; check tube integrity
- Suction child's trach tube
- Position neck in slight extension, using small roll under shoulders
- Deflate cuff (if present) in old tube
- Cut strings
- Remove tube in upward and outward arc
- Insert new tube in inward, downward arc
- *Immediately* remove obturator
- Reposition head in neutral position by removing shoulder roll
- Tie strings in triple knot with one finger space between neck and strip
- Inflate cuff
- Lock inner cannula in place

tive. Sponge rollers are preferable to the latex method in that the sponges absorb moisture, thereby affording more protection to the neck. Stomahesive, manufactured for protection of peri-stomal areas, may be applied to the neck beneath the ties to provide a "cushion" for the skin.

Meticulous care should be directed toward keeping the skin of the neck clean and dry. The area should be inspected and cleansed several times each day; areas caked with dried secretions are cleansed with half-strength hydrogen peroxide. Powders and the routine use of ointments should be avoided. If the skin or stoma becomes irritated or "weepy," hydrocortisone cream should be tried followed by topical antibacterials or antifungals.

The child with a tracheostomy tube may be bathed in a tub with water 1–2 inches in depth. The child must *never* be left unattended.

Clothing and bedding should be selected so not to occlude the tracheostomy tube and should not be "fuzzy." A scarf or bandanna can be draped loosely around the neck to protect the tracheostomy when the child is outdoors on a dusty, windy, or cold day. Parents must be warned to avoid dust, smoke, lint, pet hair, powders, and other environmental contaminants. All standing water presents a hazard to the child with a tracheostomy, so parents must be aware of the potential dangers of pools, toilets, and buckets. Siblings must

be carefully supervised to prevent them from inserting foreign objects into the tube.

Infants and children who have small tracheostomy tubes in place (less than Shiley size 2) are discharged with a cardiac/apnea monitor to be used during sleep or when unattended. If the small tube becomes obstructed by secretions, apnea will not be detected because the monitor will interpret the child's efforts against an obstructed airway as respirations. However, as the distress persists and bradycardia occurs, the bradycardia alarm will be activated.

Parents should be taught to time feedings to be given after uncomfortable procedures such as suctioning or tube changes. The child should be positioned so as to avoid aspiration. Small foods that are easily aspirated, such as raisins and nuts, should be avoided. The parents should observe for the occurrence of any foods or liquids suctioned from the tracheostomy tube.

10. Parents state importance of verbal stimulation and know communication speech therapy home plan for child.

The increased number of children with tracheostomy tubes and the increase in the duration of cannulation has resulted in a growing population at risk for delayed speech (24, 25). Early verbal stimulation is essential for the child with a tracheostomy; speech/communication therapy should be instituted at age 6–9 months. Simple sign language can be successfully taught to toddlers unable to move adequate air past the vocal cords to achieve verbalization. Passey-Muir one-way valves or fenestrated tracheostomy tubes increase air flow past the vocal cords and are helpful to the older child. Because these devices may increase the work of breathing, they may not be tolerated in a child who cannot accommodate increased respiratory work, such as one with neuromuscular disease. Parents may, understandably, be concerned about a baby's inability to cry and that they will not hear them at night. Small bells sewn on an infant's socks will alert the parent to an awake, restless, kicking infant, especially when used in conjunction with commercially available nursery monitors. In addition, even an older infant quickly learns to summon his parents by disconnecting the chest leads for his cardiac/apnea monitor, thereby triggering an alarm!

11. Parent demonstrates CPR.

Basic life support—"airway, breathing, and circulation"—are adapted for the child with a tracheostomy. Ventilation can be supplied by mouth to tracheostomy breathing or by resuscitation bag to tracheostomy tube. If there is *any* doubt as to the position of the tracheostomy tube (see above), it should be changed. Children who have a patent airway above the trach can be ventilated via mouth-to-mouth resuscitation if the tracheostomy tube cannot be changed; care must be taken to occlude the stoma. In an emergency, medical personnel can intubate the child orally or an endotracheal tube can be passed through the stoma to secure an airway.

12. Parents state plans regarding decannulation timetable.

In order for tracheostomy decannulation to be attempted, the underlying condition that necessitated the tracheostomy must be gone or improved. Additionally, the child must have good control of both oral and respiratory secretions.

The airway is inspected for patency and the presence of granulation tissue by the use of fiberoptic bronchoscopy. If the airway is judged to be adequate, tracheostomy size may be gradually decreased to allow gradual increase in the use of the upper airway, especially vocal cords. The child is observed in the hospital for 24–48 hours after decannulation to ensure that there are no subsequent problems, such as airway obstruction or hypoxia.

Performing a sleep study with a down-sized tracheostomy tube in place can be useful in detecting obstructive sleep apnea that is not otherwise recognized. This and the fact that some children will hypoventilate when asked to breath through the upper airway makes sleep studying of selected patients a useful tool to use prior to decannulation.

HOME VENTILATION

Chronic alveolar hypoventilation resulting in hypoxia and hypercapnia is the primary indication for home mechanical ventilation (HMV). Chronic respiratory failure may be the result of parenchymal disease (e.g., BPD), abnormalities of central respiratory control, mechanical impairment, or neuromuscular disease (26). The evaluation of such patients is discussed elsewhere.

Negative Pressure Ventilation

Ventilation may be provided by negative pressure machines, particularly in the child who requires assistance only at night (15). Negative pressure devices, such as the iron lung, chest cuirass, and poncho wrap, were initially a subject of research during the late nineteenth century (27). Their use became widespread during the polio epidemics of the mid-twentieth century. The chest is enclosed in a sealed device (tank or wrap) and the head remains exposed. As sub-atmospheric pressure is applied to the chest, inspiration takes place. Expiration takes place passively as the pressure within the tank is allowed to return to atmosphere.

Tank ventilators are durable and require little maintenance. They are easy to operate and offer the possibility of hand-operation by crank in the event of a power failure. In addition, an artificial airway is not usually required, thereby eliminating the danger of airway disconnection and reduces the risk of infection via water reservoir. However, upper airway obstruction has been reported when using tank respirators.

Disadvantages to the tank include its size and weight. Many families find that their homes are not able to accommodate the machine because of inadequate room size or the need for additional floor support. Ventilation is provided only by the control mode, and in many machines the I/E ratio is locked in at 1:1.

Tank shock may develop when an iron lung is used. As negative pressure is applied within the tank, it effects the abdomen, specifically resulting in venous pooling in the splanchnic bed. Hypotension may then result secondary to decreased venous return and decreased cardiac output. Tank shock may be avoided by applying 3–5 cm of expiratory pressure to prevent splanchnic pooling.

A cuirass or wrap has several advantages over the tank. Movement is less restricted and nursing care is easier because the entire body is not encased. Some wraps also have the advantage of providing an "assist" mode of ventilation. However, the cuirass may not generate adequate pressure to supply a full tidal volume to the patient, resulting in hypoventilation.

If a negative pressure ventilator is selected, an effective neck seal is essential. Plastic iris diaphragm collars are commonly available, or collars may be custom sewn from chamois cloth to accommodate individual children's machines.

Despite the fact that a tracheostomy tube is not required for negative pressure ventilation, many children will have a tracheostomy tube in place to decrease ventilatory work during the day. In addition, the tracheostomy tube supplies a ready suction port in the child with a weak cough. In children old enough to accommodate one, a fenestrated tracheostomy tube is particularly useful. When placed in the iron lung, the short, red-tipped cannula is used to plug the trach. This is an important safety feature, for if the open tracheostomy were to slip down the tank's collar, a seal would no longer be maintained and ventilation would not take place. In a child with a trach tube, extreme care must be taken in positioning, to ensure that the child does not slip into the tank.

Customized padding is helpful in positioning the scoliosis patient and achieving a comfortable, effective seal. Sandbags beneath the child's buttocks prevent movement during the ventilatory cycle.

Positive Pressure Ventilation

Positive pressure devices are more complex to operate and more expensive but offer finer adjustments of volumes and pressures. These machines enhance visibility and mobility for the child, essential elements when *continuous* mechanical ventilation is required and when close attention is paid to developmental needs. Some models are small enough to be mounted on the back of a modified wheelchair.

Among the major disadvantages to positive pressure ventilation are the need for a tracheostomy tube and the need for external humidification. In addition, compressed air and O_2 must be selected to accommodate the specific ventilator.

HOME CARE PLANNING

In addition to the ventilator and its accessories, the child who is vent-dependent may require a feeding pump, wheelchair, ramp, hospital bed, or car seat. At the onset of the discharge planning process, the parents and all members of the multidisciplinary team involved in the child's care should meet (9, 16) (Table 58.12) to compile a list of necessary equipment and services that will be needed in the home. A teaching plan is developed to include all nursing care skills and to delineate when the parents must demonstrate skills, including feeding, tracheostomy care, and medications. While the equipment is being obtained from home care vendors, and reimbursement is secured from the third party payer, the parents begin their training in these skills. During this interval, home care nurses are hired and, prior to discharge, complete a ventilator training course with the parents. This course should include classroom instruction in the operation of all equipment and several days (for each adult) in providing bedside care to the child using classroom skills.

DISCHARGE AND OUTPATIENT VISITS

Prior to discharge, all caregivers must satisfactorily complete the training program. The discharging physician, having been in regular contact with the local primary care physician, ensures that a current discharge summary is sent to the local physician and a copy is given to the parents. Parents transport the child home in the family car, rather than an ambulance, and a home care nurse awaits their arrival.

Outpatient visits to the multidisciplinary "home vent" clinic are scheduled for every 1–2 months. The program of care is assessed and revised every month. Particular attention is paid to family stress and adjustment, and to problems of chronic illness such as skin irritation and breakdown, problems with elimination, and nutrition.

WEANING FROM THE VENTILATOR

The underlying illness may make it impossible for some children to be weaned from the ventilator. For the remainder, the criteria for readiness to wean may not be well defined. A decrease in respiratory rate, a decrease in arterial P_{CO_2}, regular weight gain, and freedom from acute illness may be signals that the child requires less mechanical assistance. While one is monitoring with an end-tidal CO_2 monitor and pulse oximeter, the ventilator rate during awake hours can be decreased by one breath per minute every 2 weeks. Once

Table 58.12.
Multidisciplinary Planning Checklist for Home Ventilator Program

Date/Initials

_____   1.   Pulmonologist meets with family for initial discussion/consideration of home ventilator program.

           2.   Team members notified and established as follows:
- _____ primary physician
- _____ nurse specialist
- _____ respiratory therapist (continuing care specialist)
- _____ social worker
- _____ primary nurse
- _____ occupational therapist
- _____ physical therapist
- _____ nutritionist
- _____ speech therapist
- _____
- _____
- _____

_____   3.   Nurse specialist and primary nurse meet with family to provide overview of program and planning process.

_____   4.   Multidisciplinary planning meeting scheduled by nurse specialist and held. Decisions made regarding ventilator, oxygen, hospital bed, wheelchair, nursing, monitor, trach, etc.

_____   5.   Primary nurse develops home care plan.

_____   6.   Primary nurse determines skills to be taught, obtains documentation sheets.

_____   7.   Nature of third-party payment determined by social worker.

_____   8.   Initial contact with third-party payer made by nurse specialist.

_____   9.   List of respiratory home care equipment compiled by respiratory therapist and reviewed by nurse speialist and primary physician.

_____   10. Bid letters submitted to appropriate vendors by respiratory therapist.

_____   11. Bids received and reviewed with family, vendor selected and notified, bid forwarded to nurse specialist.

_____   12. Nurse specialist arranges meeting with vendor and family.

_____   13. Family, assisted by primary nurse, clinical nurse specialist, and respiratory therapist, devises schedule for equipment maintenance at home.

_____   14. Family makes decision about home nursing care, with consultation from nurse specialist and primary nurse.

_____   15. Proposal submitted to third-party payer by nurse specialist.

_____   16. Proposal accepted.

_____   17. Nurse specialist and primary nurse plan home care teaching program for all caregivers.

_____   18. Primary nurse, clinical nurse specialist, and parents meet with home care nursing agency.

_____   19. Training schedule circulated to family and team members. Primary nurse assigns preceptors for all caregivers. Agenda for first day of training:
- _____ Nursing care plan presented
- _____ Introduction to family dynamics, program philosophy
- _____ Introduction to team members
- _____ Training schedule

_____   20. Respiratory care equipment manuals provided to family.

_____   21. Prior to discharge, all caretakers must demonstrate proficiency in the following skills (on each of three separate dates):
- _____ Cardiopulmonary resuscitation
- _____ All respiratory equipment
- _____ Trach care
- _____ Gastrotomy tube care or other feeding procedures
- _____ Respiratory assessment and intervention
- _____ Administration of all medications
- _____ Other specialized instruction

_____   22. Primary nurse ensures that family has home care plan for occupational therapy, physical therapy, dietary, and speech therapy.

_____   23. Nurse specialist coordinates and schedules first follow-up visit.

_____   24. Primary nurse arranges meeting with nurse specialist, vendor, nursing agency, family, primary nurse, and respiratory therapist.

From Lund CH, ed. *Bronchopulmonary dysplasia: Strategies for total parent care.* Petaluma, Neonatal Network, 1990.

weaned from awake support, similar steps are used to decrease the sleep time rate. Careful attention must also be paid to heart rate, respiratory rate, respiratory effort, color, appetite, and general mood. Weaning from O_2 is the final step, accomplished as described earlier.

REFERENCES

1. Abman SH, Accurso FJ, Koops BL. Experience with home oxygen in the management of infants with BPD. *Clin Pediatr* 1984; 23:471–476.
2. Markestad T, Firtzhardinge PM. Growth and development in children recovering from BPD. *J Pediatr* 1981; 98:597–602.
3. Penry JK. Cost effectiveness of home management of BPD. *Pediatrics* 1982; 70:330–331.
4. Pinny MA, Cotton EK. Home management of BPD. *Pediatrics* 1970; 58:856–59.
5. Weinstein MR, Oh W. Oxygen consumption in infants with BPD. *J Pediatr* 1981; 99:958–961.
6. Aradene CE. Homecare for young children with long term tracheostomies. *Matern Child Nurs* J 1980; 121–125.
7. Foster S, Hoskins D. Home care of the child with a tracheostomy tube. *Pediatr Clin North Am* 1981; 28:855.
8. Lichenstein MA. Pediatric home tracheostomy care: A parents guide. *Pediatr Nurs* 1986; 12:41.
9. Zander JH. Home ventilation for the infant with BPD. In Lund CH, ed. *Bronchopulmonary dysplasia: Strategies for total parent care.* Petaluma, Neonatal Network, 1990, pp 189–205.
10. Burr BH, Guyer B, Todres ID, Abrahams B, Chiodo T. Home care for children on respirators. *N Engl J Med* 1983; 309:1319.
11. Goldberg AI, Faure EAM, Vaughn CJ, Snarski R, Seleny FL. Homecare for life-supported persons: An approach to program development. *J Pediatr 1984; 104:785–795.*
12. *Frates RC, Splaingard ML, Smith EO, Harrison GM. Outcome of home mechanical ventilation in children. J Pediatr 1985; 106:850–856.*
13. Schreiner MS, Donar ME, Kettrick RG. Pediatric home mechanical ventilation. *Pediatr Clin North Am* 1987; 34:47–60.
14. Splaingard ML, Frates RC, Harrison GM, Carter RE, Jefferson LS. Home positive-pressure ventilation. Twenty years experience. *Chest* 1983; 84:376–382.
15. Splaingard ML, Frates Rc, Jefferson LS, Rosen CL, Harrison GM. Home negative pressure ventilation: Report of 20 years experience in patients with neuromuscular disease. *Arch Phys Med Rehabil* 1985; 6:239–242.
16. Eigen H, Zander JE. Home mechanical ventilation of pediatric patients. *Am Rev Respir Dis* 1990; 141:258–259.
17. Stein REK. Homecare: A challenging opportunity. *Child Health Care* 1985; 14:90–95.
18. Wegener DH, Aday LU. Home care for ventilator assisted children: Predicting family stress. *Pediatr Nurs* 1989; 15:371–376.
19. Patterson JM. Chronic illness in children and the impact on families. In Chilmann S, Cox FM, Minnally EW, eds. *Chronic illness and disability.* Newbury Park, Sage Publications, 1988; 69–107.
20. Satterwhite BB. Impact of chronic illness on child and family: An overview of 5 surveys with implications for management. *Int J Rehabil Res* 1978; 1:7–17.
21. Mattsson A. Long term physical illness in children: A challenge to psychosocial adaptation. *Pediatrics* 1972;50:801–811.
22. Sauve RS, McMillan DD, Mitchell I, Creighton D, Hindle NW, Young L. Home oxygen therapy: Outcome of infants discharged from NICU on continuous therapy. *Clin Pediatr* 1989; 28:113–118.
23. Hudak BB, Allen MC, Hudak ML, Loughlin GM. Home oxygen therapy for chronic lung disease in extremely low birth weight infants. *Am J Dis Child* 1989; 143:357–360.
24. Hill BD, Singer LT. Speech and language development in infant tracheostomy. *J Speech Hear Disord* 1990; 55:1–20.
25. Singer LT, Kercsmar C, Legris G, Orlowski JP, Hill BP, Doerschuk C. Developmental sequelae of long-term infant tracheostomy. *Dev Med Child Neurol* 1989; 31:224–230.
26. Garay RM, Turino GM, Godring RM. Sustained reversal of chronic hypercapnia in patients with alveolar hypoventilation syndromes. *Am J Med* 1981; 70:269–274.
27. Wollam CHM. The development of apparatus for intermittent negative measure respiration. *Anaesthesia* 1976; 31:537–547.

59

Pulmonary Rehabilitation

MARK SPLAINGARD

A basic rehabilitation principle is that there is no direct correlation between a specific disease and the spectrum of disability associated with it. Ventilator-dependent children now attend school, and adolescents with asthma win Olympic medals. The degree of disability (or lost function) of these children depends not only on their residual physiologic capacity but their personal and community's capability for psychologic and sociologic adaption.

Pulmonary rehabilitation is defined by the American Thoracic Society as the

> art of medical practice wherein an individually tailored, multidisciplinary program is formulated which through accurate diagnosis, therapy, emotional support, and education stabilizes or reverses both the physio- and psychopathology of pulmonary disease and attempts to return the patient to the highest possible functional capacity allowed by the pulmonary handicap and overall life situation.(1)

True pulmonary rehabilitation, then, is not simply breathing exercises or strengthening techniques but a comprehensive attempt to maximize the functional abilities of a child with pulmonary disease, allowing participation at the highest possible societal level.

PRINCIPLES

Basic objectives of a pulmonary rehabilitative program include the following:

1. Patient selection—which children would benefit from interventions
2. Patient evaluation:
   a. Medical evaluation may include chest radiograph, pulmonary function testing, arterial blood gases, pulse oximetry, exercise testing, and therapeutic drug evaluations

   b. Psychosocial evaluation, including an assessment of the child's developmental ability, family and community strengths and limitations, environmental barriers, and misconceptions about the disease.
3. Determination of appropriate functional goals for the child and family
4. Development of a specific rehabilitation program for each child
5. Periodic evaluation of patient/family progress
6. Long-term follow-up with anticipatory guidance addressing expected developmental, medical, and social issues

The components of a pediatric pulmonary rehabilitation program are shown in Table 59.1.

BRONCHIAL ASTHMA

Bronchial asthma is the most common pediatric pulmonary disorder referred for pulmonary rehabilitation. An optimal asthma rehabilitation program includes the following:

1. Comprehensive pharmacologic therapy
2. Preventive/environmental controls to avoid acute exacerbations (avoid smoking and other pollutants)

Table 59.1.
Components of a Pediatric Pulmonary Rehabilitation Program

Patient and family education
Respiratory therapy
   Equipment use and maintenance
   Correct techniques for metered dose inhalers
   Oxygen administration
   Chest physiotherapy
Physical therapy
   Exercise training and conditioning
   Ventilatory muscle training
   Breathing exercise
Psychosocial counseling of child and family

3. Child and family education of the pathophysiology, symptoms, and treatments of asthma
4. Objective measures for patients/family to assess the severity of asthma and monitor therapy results
5. Specific exercise prescriptions to prevent the physical deconditioning common in asthmatics

Appropriate rehabilitation goals for children with asthma include improving physical fitness, developing gross motor skills, helping the child cope with the psychologic consequences of the disease, and educating the child/caretakers regarding preventative steps to minimize dyspnea.

Children with asthma are frequently and inappropriately exempted from physical education and may avoid leisure sports because of the fear of precipitating asthma attacks. Parents may be overprotective of their "vulnerable child." Physical exercise for asthmatic children has only recently gained wide acceptance in pediatrics. There are two main reasons that acceptance has been slow to develop:

1. The incidence of exercise-induced bronchospasm (EIB) is 40–95% in children with asthma (2–5), making physicians reluctant to allow child with asthma to participate in strenuous exercise program
2. Pediatric training does not routinely provide knowledge about specific exercise routines and techniques for asthmatics; conventional swimming techniques, for example, may fail in asthmatic children due to dyspnea (6); program modifications such as initially teaching the backstroke or sidestroke may alleviate dyspnea and allow initial success

Numerous studies have shown that a regular exercise training program can substantially improve the physical conditioning of the child with asthma (Table 59.2). Exercise programs focusing on either general improvement in physical fitness or strengthening of specific respiratory muscles have been developed for asthmatics. The benefits of exercise therapy in children with asthma can be evaluated in five areas (14):

1. Health history from parent (and child if possible)
2. Clinical examination
3. Physiologic measurements
4. Medication requirements
5. Restrictions in daily activities

Improvements may also be seen in duration and number of hospitalizations and school absences.

Exercise-Induced Bronchospasm (EIB) and Exercise in Asthmatics

There is no good correlation between the degree of EIB and a child's baseline spirometry (15). Physical exercise of 1–2 minutes duration increases forced expiratory volumes and peak flows in both normal and children with asthma, whereas exercise of longer duration (6–8 minutes) may cause post-exercise bronchoconstriction in many children with asthma (16).

The incidence of EIB is significantly influenced by the type of exercise. Free running induces more EIB than an equivalent amount of work performed by cycling (17). Swimming has a lower incidence of EIB than any comparable aerobic activity. The severity of EIB after running is unchanged by swimming training (11).

Refractoriness to episodes of EIB can occur after mild warm-up exercises (jogging, stretching, or calisthenics for a few minutes) that do not induce asthma. Participation in these activities before engaging in more strenuous activities can reduce or prevent EIB in some children. This refractory period, lasting up to 1 hour, occurs in up to 40% of asthmatics and can be a useful adjunct to exercise (18, 19). In addition, many children with asthma learn to "run through" their initial chest "tightness," which may diminish or disappear. An exercise prescription to reduce EIB in children with asthma is shown in Table 59.3.

General Exercise Program and Asthma

Although beneficial effects of exercise for asthmatic children have been shown using a variety of different programs, including jogging (13), running (2, 12), cycling (10), canoeing (20), and swimming (6, 8), no study has documented significant improvement in pulmonary function. There may be a decrease in the number of asthmatic attacks and the need for medications, however (11). Aerobic training may decrease the amount of ventilation required for a specific work load, increasing the threshold of activity at which EIB occurs. An increase in total work performance with a concomitant improvement in psychologic well

Table 59.2.
Effect of Exercise Training in Asthma

Author	Number of Subjects	Ages	Mean FEV$_1$%	Steroids	Prophylactic Medication	Type of Training	Duration	Effect
Svenonius et al., 1983 (7)	40	8–17	95–96%	None	Yes	30 minute interval and 30-minute swim 2 ×/week	12–16 weeks	11–21% improvement in physical working capacity
Ramazanoglu et al., 1985 (2)	23	6–15	83% ± 9%	3 inhaled	No	3 hrs regular PE/ week, 1.5 hours/ week running and respiratory muscle training	15 weeks	SGAW improved by 8.5%; VO$_2$/kg improved 22%
Szentagothai et al., 1987 (8)	121	5–14	NS	6 oral	Yes	Swimming 2 hours/ week, gymnastics 1 hour/week, running 1/hour week	1 year	Number of children with > 60 days/ year symptoms decreased from 45.5% to 9.1%
Oseid & Haaland, 1978 (9)	10	11–16	NS	NS	Yes	Muscle strengthening 12 weeks & endurance training 2–3×/week	12 weeks	16% increase in VO$_2$; 34% increase in total dynamic muscle strength score
Ludwick et al., 1986 (10)	32	8–17	6 < 80%	65%	Yes	12 minutes bicycling 2–4×/week	2–17 weeks	84% of children with scores < 2SD below achieved normal workload
Fitch el al., 1976 (11)	46	9–16	NS	NS	NS	Swimming 5 hours/ week	20 weeks	Improvement in VO$_2$
Orenstein et al., 1985 (12)	20	6–16	$\frac{FEV_1}{FVC} = 83$	None	Yes	Running 30 minutes/ day, 3 days/week	16 weeks	14% increase in VO$_2$
Nickerson et al., 1983 (13)	15	7–14	69%	2 oral 10 inhaled	NS	Jogged 2 miles 4 days/week	6 weeks	10% increase in distance covered in 12-minute run

NS = Not stated in Report

Table 59.3.
General Guidelines for Asthmatics to Prevent EIB

Maintain good compliance with regular medications

Beta-adrenergic agonist and/or cromolyn sodium 15 minutes before exercise

Two-minute "warm up" of moderate exercise before vigorus exercise

If symptoms develop with exercise, an attempt to "run through" symptoms may result in clinical improvement

When exercising in cold weather, use a cold weather mask or large scarf over nose and mouth; if problems still occur, try indoor exercise of swimming as alternative

being is frequently reported (20). The psychologic benefits of exercise programs should not be overlooked since they result in improvements in the child's self-confidence and motivation for increased physical activity. Parents are reportedly less fearful about their child's health after participation in an exercise program.

In assessing significant conditioning, the duration of training appears to be the most important factor; supervised instruction in technique is important initially. Prophylactic inhaled bronchodilators may allow a beneficial training effect (21).

Ventilatory Muscle Training

Voluntarily contracting the abdominal muscles elevates the diaphragm and increases diaphragmatic vertical excursion and expansion of the lower thorax. This "belly breathing" (Fig. 59.1) can improve ventilation in asthmatics. Few children with asthma consciously use their abdominal muscles during expiration, even when dyspneic (22, 23). Although belly breathing may be useful for short-term relief of dyspnea from asthma, it is difficult to incorporate consistently and rarely of long-term usefulness in children with asthma. No controlled study has ever verified a long-term benefit of ventilatory muscle exercises in children with asthma.

Specific exercises have been designed to prevent or overcome the rounded shoulder, kyphotic appearance of many children with moderate and severe asthma. Exercises that increase thoracic cage mobility, improve shoulder girdle flexibility, and strengthen trunk extensor muscles are useful in improving

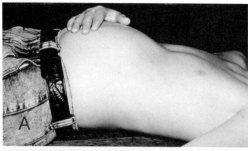

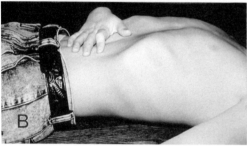

Figure 59.1. Abdominal breathing technique. *A*, Inspiration. *B*, Expiration.

posture (24, 25). Muscle relaxation and stretching techniques for the anterior chest wall also are useful in older children.

Whether focusing on specific muscle groups or generalized conditioning, it is essential that the program be tailored to the child's ability and developmental level. Generally programs that are fun and incorporate the training into leisure activities such as aerobics, dance, and karate will have a greater degree of acceptance and lead to better long-term compliance by a child.

CYSTIC FIBROSIS

An excellent example of incorporation of the principles of comprehensive rehabilitation is found in the care of pediatric patients with cystic fibrosis (CF) in CF centers. The success of these programs is demonstrated by the findings of a recent study comparing psychosocial functioning in adults with CF to age-matched peers in which the activities of the patients with CF were found to be appropriate and "on par" with those of healthy adults (26). The focus on global "wellness" of patients with CF and not simply their nutritional status or pulmonary function tests is basic. Recent work has attempted to quantify the quality of well-being (QWB) in patients with CF by

measuring factors such as mobility, physical activity, and social activity (27).

Exercise Training in Cystic Fibrosis

The limitation of ventilatory capacity plays a major role in limiting maximal exercise capacity in CF. Although maximal exercise capacity may be normal in some patients, strenuous exertion may induce dangerous arterial desaturation in advanced CF, worsening pulmonary hypertension and triggering ventricular arrhythmias. A Taussig score of less than 60, forced vital capacity (FVC) < 60% predicted, and forced expiratory volume in 1 second (FEV_1) < 36% and a FEV_1/FVC < 50% are all associated with significant risk for profound oxygen desaturation and progressive hypercapnia with strenuous exercise (28, 29). A supervised exercise test with ear oximetry saturation monitoring is recommended in patients meeting these criteria before undertaking a physical training program. The exercise program should be structured to prevent arterial desaturation of more than 5% and to maintain absolute oxygen saturation greater than 80% (28).

Maximum work capacity in CF depends on lung function, nutritional status, and presence of resting hypoxia. Cardiac function is not a limiting factor (30). Patients with CF who have even moderately advanced lung disease have shown improvements in work capacity, without significant changes in pulmonary function, after participating in exercise programs incorporating jogging (31), upper body strengthening (32), or swimming (33). Consistent gains are almost universally reported (34, 35) along with a significant improvement in sputum clearance while participating in regular aerobic exercise (36). The mechanism responsible for improvement (improvements in motor skills, coordination, patient motivation, or peripheral tissue changes) is unknown.

Exercise limitation in moderately severe CF appears mainly related to air flow obstruction. Exercise capacity is worse in females than males irrespective of resting pulmonary functions (37). Interestingly, inspiratory muscle training, performed by breathing through a series of inspiratory resistors for 15 minutes twice a day for 1 month, does not improve exercise endurance (38).

Reduced joint mobility and trunk flexibility is common in moderately affected CF patients and should be assessed before instituting and during exercise programs (39). Malnutrition, common in CF, may lead to loss of skeletal muscle mass with a reduction in respiratory muscle strength. Since respiratory muscle strength does increases with improved nutrition, optimal caloric intake should accompany any exercise training program (40). Salt depletion may occur in CF patients exercising in hot weather, and measures should be taken to prevent and recognize this complication.

The bronchoconstriction induced by exercise that occurs in patients with CF is less predictable and generally less responsive to therapy than in asthma, and occurs less frequently (41). Exercise-induced bronchoconstriction occurs, but much less frequently ($< 10\%$) than in children with asthma (41). Although true bronchoconstriction is not a major contribution, dynamic airway collapse may result in air trapping and decrease small airway flows, which will limit exercise capacity (42, 43).

Oxygen Therapy

There are no clearly established guidelines for the use of supplemental oxygen in patients with CF. Patient acceptance is often poor, and documenting long-term benefit is difficult. If a patient demonstrates reduced exercise tolerance and hypoxia during a formal study, supplemental oxygen should be prescribed (44). Although long-term nocturnal use of oxygen does not decrease mortality, delay progression of the disease, or reduce the frequency of hospitalizations (45), oxygen supplementation of patients with resting arterial $Po_2 < 65$ mm Hg and $FEF_{25-75} < 25\%$ predicted allowed a significantly greater number of patients to remain at work or school longer. Oxygen supplementation may improve exercise tolerance in some patients with CF (45). Although this suggests some potential "quality of life" benefit from oxygen therapy, further study is needed.

Chest Physiotherapy

Several studies of chest physiotherapy have documented short-and long-term benefits (46, 47). Physiotherapy techniques vary but generally consist of postural drainage of all bronchopulmonary segments with manual or mechanical percussion and vibration, deep breathing, and coughing. New approaches in chest physiotherapy CF include autogenic drainage (48), a positive expiratory pressure (PEP) mask (49), and high-frequency chest compression (50). These are discussed in detail in Chapter 62.

SPINAL CORD INJURY

Although many muscle groups are involved in ventilation (Table 59.4) intact, innervated diaphragms generally provide 70% of quiet resting ventilation in the newborn and 50% of resting ventilatory function in the alert adult. In patients with spinal cord lesions above the fourth cervical level (C4), the diaphragm (innervated by the phrenic nerve from cervical nerves 3, 4, and 5) does not function adequately. Children who are quadriplegic from lesions at C4 or higher usually experience respiratory failure and require prolonged mechanical ventilatory support.

In these children, pulmonary rehabilitation is directed at achieving as much time free of assisted ventilation as possible. Children older than 10 years can generally be taught either glossopharyngeal breathing ("frog breathing") (51) or can use their neck flexors ("neck breathing") (52) to provide adequate ventilation for a few hours a day without ventilatory support. Failure to master these maneuvers limits tolerance to only a few minutes without ventilatory support.

An alternative approach involves inspiratory muscle training (Table 59.5) In patients with C4-C8 quadriplegia muscle training results in improvements in ventilatory muscle

Table 59.4.
Respiratory Muscles

Inspiratory Muscles	Expiratory Muscles
Primary	*Primary*
Diaphragm	Internal oblique
External intercostal	External oblique
	Rectus abdominis
	Transversus abdominis
Accessory	*Accessory*
Sternocleidomastoid	Internal intercostal
Trapezius	
Scalenus	
Pectoralis minor	
Posterior neck muscles	
Platysma	

Table 59.5.
Muscle Training Techniques in Patients with Spinal Cord Injury

- Sub-fatiguing breathing through inspiratory resistance
- Forced expirations and inspirations through resistance
- Pectoralis major muscle strengthening exercises
- Abdominal binder
- Incentive spirometry
- Graded inspiratory resistance exercises
- Passive forced insufflation with IPPB to improve compliance

strength and endurance and has been useful in weaning children with high quadriplegia from mechanical ventilation (53). Techniques include training by sub-fatiguing breathing (work insufficient to produce EMG evidence of muscle fatigue) through inspiratory resistances at a resting ventilatory rate for 15 minutes twice daily (54). Performing forced expirations and inspirations through resistances in combination with regular IPBB has also shown to improve forced vital capacity. A strengthening program specifically for the pectoralis muscles has also been used (55).

Other approaches to strengthening ventilatory muscles that may be useful in the pulmonary rehabilitation of a child who is quadriplegic include use of an abdominal binder to splint the abdomen while allowing rib cage excursion. A program of inspiratory training, either in the form of incentive spirometry or graded inspiratory resistance exercises, strengthens the diaphragm and accessory muscles. Passive forced lung insufflation with IPPB to prevent decreased chest wall compliance is performed while muscle training is undertaken. Depending on the level of the spinal injury, expiratory muscle strengthening may also be useful in improving cough (Table 59.5). The improvements achieved with these techniques diminish quickly if training is discontinued. Hence, a training program should be used indefinitely in patients with a spinal chord injury that affects the respiratory muscles.

Electrophrenic respiration (EPR) by diaphragmatic stimulation has been used successfully in children with high cord injury (56). Patients using EPR require intact phrenic nerves. These can be documented by phrenic nerve conduction studies prior to implantation of pacers. Tracheostomy is usually required since simulation of the diaphragm without upper airway muscle activation during sleep may lead to collapse and upper airway obstruction with resulting hypoventilation.

In children with quadriplegia requiring long-term mechanical ventilation, intensive caregiver training incorporating all aspects of a comprehensive pulmonary rehabilitation program with spinal cord management is required before hospital discharge (57, 58). Psychologic evaluation and continued plans for long-term psychologic support of the ventilator-dependent spinal cord injured child and his or her family should begin as soon as possible after injury. Fostering independence in the child with a spinal cord injury and his family is critical to successful management.

HEREDITARY NEUROMUSCULAR DISEASES

Symptoms of decreased ventilatory reserve in children with neuromuscular disease may be masked because of their general decrease in physical activity. Respiratory deterioration may present in different ways, depending on the disease. Disturbance of respiration during sleep or easy fatiguability may be the earliest signs of respiratory muscle weakness in patients with less severe skeletal muscle weakness. Impairment of ventilation is determined largely by respiratory muscles involved (diaphragm, intercostals, and abdominals) and their degree of weakness (Fig. 59.2). Since the diaphragm is the principle muscle of inspiration and almost wholly responsible for quiet tidal breathing, diseases affecting it early in their course may cause significant respiratory impairment. In nemaline myopathy, for example, a child may be ambulatory yet the diaphragm may be so severely weakened that respiratory failure occurs. In contrast, in Duchenne muscular dystrophy, diaphragmatic function is spared until relatively late in the course of the disease, when the patient may already have been confined to a wheelchair for some time.

If the vital capacity is less than three times resting tidal volume in the child with neuromuscular disease, cough is significantly impaired and clearance of bronchial secretions becomes inadequate. If bulbar muscles are affected, protective pharyngeal and laryngeal

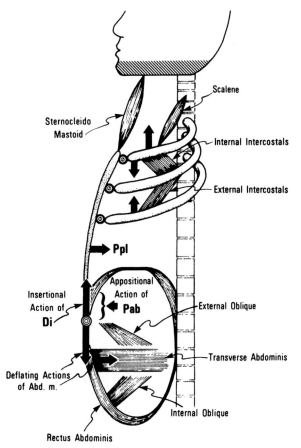

Figure 59.2. Diagrammatic representations of actions of inspiratory and expiratory muscles. (From Roussos C. Function and fatigue of respiratory muscles. *Chest* 1985:88(Suppl):125S.)

reflexes are diminished, and aspiration of oral secretions and upper airway obstruction may occur. Heart failure due to cardiomyopathy (Duchenne muscular dystrophy) or from chronic hypoxia and cor pulmonale may further compromise respiratory function.

Treatment is aimed at improving ventilation, oxygenation, and endurance. The major pulmonary rehabilitation goal in children with hereditary neuromuscular diseases is to extend the patient's life expectancy while improving stamina, function, and patient comfort. Chest physiotherapy is usually unnecessary early in the course of neuromuscular disease since these children generally do not have significant increased airway secretions. It may become useful when atelectasis or pneumonia is present. Assessment of swallowing function is important since dysfunctional swallowing is common and increases the risk of recurrent

aspiration. Breathing exercises appear to benefit some patients (59). Glossopharyngeal breathing is a useful technique for patients without bulbar paralysis to increase ventilation and maintain independence. If a tracheostomy becomes necessary for suctioning, a Passey-Muir valve is useful for allowing speech in these children.

There is controversy among physicians regarding providing long-term ventilation in patients with neuromuscular disease (60). The patient and his or her family should be involved in any decision regarding long-term ventilatory support (61). Factors such as patient age, severity of global central nervous system (CNS) injury, and natural course of the hereditary neuromuscular disease and family resources should be considered in the decision making process. Tracheostomy with positive pressure ventilation (61, 62) or negative pressure ventilator (63) has been a traditional mode of therapy. Noninvasive nasal or mask positive pressure ventilation has been advocated to provide elective respiratory support for adults with neuromuscular disease (64). Care of these children at home with minimal disruption of family life, a comfortable extension of life expectancy, and participation in the activities of the community is the ultimate goal.

REFERENCES

1. Hodgkin J, Farrell M, Gibson S, et al. Pulmonary rehabilitation. Official ATS statement. *Am Rev Respir Dis* 1981; 124:663–666.
2. Ramazanoglu Y, Kraemer R. Cardiorespiratory response to physical conditioning in children with bronchial asthma. *Pediatr Pulmonol* 1985; 1:272–277.
3. Sly RM, Harper RT, Rosselot I. The effect of physical conditioning upon asthmatic children. *Ann Allergy* 1972; 30:86–94.
4. Fitch KD. Sport, physical activity and the asthmatic. In Oseid S, Edwards AM, eds. *The asthmatic child in play and sport.* London, Pitman, 1983, pp 246–258.
5. Kawalori I, Pierson WE, Conquest LL, Bierman CW. Incidence of exercise-induced asthma in children. *J Allergy Clin Immunol* 1976; 58:447–455.
6. Fitch KD. Swimming, medicine, and asthma. In Erikson B, ed. *Furberg beds. Swimming medicine IV.* Baltimore, University Park Press, 1977, pp 16–31.
7. Svenonius E, Kautto R, Arborelius M. Improvement after training of children with exercise induced asthma. *Acta Paediatr Scand* 1983; 72:23–30.
8. Szentagothai K, Gyene I, Szocska M, Osvath P. Physical exercise program for children with bronchial asthma. *Pediatr Pulmonol* 1987; 3:166–172.
9. Oseid S, Hasland K. Exercise studies on asthmatic children before and after regular physical training. *Swim Med* 1978; 4:32–41. International Series on Sports Sciences.
10. Ludwick S, Jones J, Jones T, Fukuhara V, Strunk R. Normalization of cardiopulmonary endurance in severely asthmatic children after bicycle ergometry therapy. *J Pediatr* 1986; 109:446–451.
11. Fitch KD, Morton AR, Blanksby B. Effects of swimming training on children with asthma. *Arch Dis Child* 1976; 51:190–194.
12. Orenstein D, Reed M, Grogan F, Crawford L. Exercise conditioning in children with asthma. *J Pediatr* 1985; 106:556–560.
13. Nickerson B, Bautista D, Namey M, Richards W, Keens T. Distance running improves fitness in asthmatic children without pulmonary complication or changes in exercise-induced bronchospasm. *Pediatrics* 1983; 71:147–152.
14. Chai H, Purcell K, Brady K, Falliers CV. Therapeutic and investigational evaluation of asthmatic children. *J Allergy* 1968; 41:23–36.
15. Silverman M, Anderson SD. Standardization of exercise tests in asthmatic children. *Arch Dis Child* 1972; 47:882–889.
16. Cropp GJ. Grading, time course, and incidence of exercise-induced airway obstruction and hyperinfla-

tion in asthmatic children. *Pediatrics* 1975; 56(Suppl):868–879.
17. Anderson SD, Connolly NM, Godfrey S. Comparison of bronchoconstriction induced by cycling and running. *Thorax* 1971; 26:396–401.
18. Anderson SD, Schoeffel R. Respiratory heat and water loss during exercise in patients with asthma: Effects of repeated exercise challenge. *Eur J Respir Dis* 1982; 63:472–480.
19. Ben-Dov I, Bar-Yishay E, Godfrey S. Refractory period after exercise induced asthma unexplained by respiratory heat loss. *Am Rev Respir Dis* 1982; 125:530–534.
20. Keens TG. Exercise training programs for pediatric patients with chronic lung disease. *Pediatr Clin North Am* 1979; 26:517–524.
21. Latimer K, O'Byrne P, Morris MM, Roberts R, Hargrave F. Bronchoconstriction stimulated by airway cooling: Better protection with combined inhalation of terbutaline sulfate and cromolyn sodium than with either alone. *Am Rev Respir Dis* 1983; 128:440–443.
22. Strick L. Breathing and physical fitness exercises for asthmatic children. *Pediatr Clin North Am* 1969; 16:31–42.
23. Livingstone J. The value of breathing exercises in asthma. *Lancet* 1935; 2:705–708.
24. Kisner C, Colby L. *Therapeutic exercise: Foundations and techniques.* Philadelphia, FA Davis, 1985, pp 536–550.
25. Frounfelter D. *Chest physical therapy and pulmonary rehabilitation.* Chicago, Year Book, 1978, pp 153–176.
26. Sheperd S, Hovell M, Harwood I, et al. A comparative study of the psychosocial assets of adults with CF and their healthy peers. *Chest* 1990; 97:1310–1316.
27. Orenstein D, Nixon P, Ross E, Kaplan R. The quality of well being in CF. *Chest* 1989; 95:344–347.
28. Cropp GJ, Pullano TP, Cerny FJ, Nathanson I. Exercise tolerance and cardiorespiratory adjustment at peak work capacity in CF. *Am Rev Respir Dis* 1982; 126:211–216.
29. Henke K, Orenstein D. Oxygen saturation during exercise in CF. *Am Rev Respir Dis* 1984; 129:708–711.
30. Marcotte J, Grisdale R, Levison H, Coates A, Canny G. Multiple factors limit exercise capacity in CF. *Pediatr Pulmonol* 1986; 2:274–281.
31. Orenstein D, Franklin B, Doershuk C, et al. Exercise conditioning and cardiopulmonary fitness in CF. *Chest* 1981; 80:392–398.
32. Keens T, Kasten I, Wannmoler E, Levison H, Crozier D, Bryan A. Ventilatory muscle endurance training in normal subjects and patients with CF. *Am Rev Respir Dis* 1977; 116:853–866.
33. Edlund L, French R, Herbst J, Ruttenberg H, Ruhling R, Adams T. Effect of a swimming program on children with CF. *Am J Dis Child* 1986; 140:80–83.
34. O'Neill P, Dodds M, Phillips B, Poole J, Well A. Regular exercise and reduction of breathlessness in patients with CF. *Br J Dis Chest* 1987; 81:62–69.
35. Braggion C, Cornacchia M, Miano A, Schena F, Verlato G, Mastella G. Exercise tolerance and effects of training in young patients with CF and mild airway obstruction. *Pediatr Pulmonol* 1989; 7:145–152.
36. Bonforte R. *Guide to diagnosis and management of CF.* Atlanta, CF Foundation, 1977.

37. Orenstein D, Nixon P. Exercise performance and breathing patterns in CF: Male-female differences and influence of resting pulmonary function. *Pediatr Pulmonol* 1991; 10:101–105.

38. Asher M, Pardy R, Coates A, Thomas E, Macklem P. The effects of inspiratory muscle training in patients with CF. *Am Rev Respir Dis* 1982; 126:855–859.

39. Rose J, Gamble J, Schultz A, Lewiston W. Backpain and spinal deformity in CF. *Am J Dis Child* 1987; 141:1313–1316.

40. Mansell AL, Anderson J, Mullart C, et al. Short-term pulmonary effects of total parenteral nutrition in children with CF. *J Pediatr* 1984; 104:700–705.

41. MacFarlane P, Heaf D. Changes in airflow obstruction and oxygen saturation in response to exercise and bronchodilators in CF. *Pediatr Pulmonol* 1990; 8:4–11.

42. Loughlin GM, Cota KA, Taussig LM. The relationship between flow transients and bronchial lability in CF. *Chest* 1981; 79:206–210.

43. Zach M, Oberwaldner B, Forche G, Polgar G. Bronchodilators increase airway instability in CF. *Am Rev Respir Dis* 1985; 31:537–543.

44. Zinman R, Corey M, Coates A, et al. Nocturnal home oxygen in the treatment of hypoxemic CF patients. *J Pediatr* 1989; 114:368–377.

45. Coates A, Boyce P, Muller D, Mearns M, Godfrey S. The role of nutritional status, airway obstruction, hypoxia, and abnormalities in serum lipid composition in limiting exercise tolerance in children with CF. *Acta Paediatr Scand* 1980; 69:353–358.

46. Desmond K, Schwenk WF, Thomas E, Beaudry P, Coates A. Immediate and long-term effects of chest physiotherapy in patients with CF. *J Pediatr* 1983; 103:538–542.

47. Reisman J, Rivington-Law B, Corey M, et al. Role of conventional physiotherapy in CF. *J Pediatr* 1988; 113:632–636.

48. Chevalier J. Autogenic drainage. In Lawson D, ed. *Cystic Fibrosis: Horizons.* Chichester, John Wiley, 1984, pp 235–240.

49. Lapen A. Chest physical therapy in CF: A review. *Cardiopul Phys Ther* 1990; 1:11–13.

50. Warwick W, Hansen L. Vest bronchial drainage therapy 2 year follow up. *Pediatr Pulmonol* 1990; 5:251.

51. Collier C, Dail CW, Affeldt J. Mechanics of glossopharyngeal breathing. *J Appl Physiol* 1956; 8:580–584.

52. Gilgoff I, Barras D, Jones M, Adkins RPT. Neck breathing: A form of voluntary respiration for the spine-injured ventilator–dependent quadriplegic child. *Pediatrics* 1988; 82:741–745.

53. Lerman R, Weiss M. Progressive resistive exercise in weaning high quadriplegics for the ventilator. *Paraplegia* 1987; 25:130–135.

54. Gross D, Ladd H, Riley E, Macklem P, Grossino A. The effect of training on strength and endurance of the diaphragm in quadriplegia. *Am J Med* 1980; 68:27–35.

55. Detroyer A, Estenne M, Heilporn A. Mechanism of active expiration in tetraplegic subjects. *N Eng J Med* 1986; 314:740–744.

56. Weese-Mayer D, Morrow A, Brouillette R, Ilbawi M, Hunt C. Diaphragm pacing in infants and children: A life table analysis of implanted components. *Am Rev Respir Dis* 1989; 139:974–979.

57. Splaingard M, Frates R, Harrison GM, Carter RE, Jefferson LS. Home positive pressure ventilation: Twenty years experience. *Chest* 1983; 84:376–382.

58. Schreiner M, Donar M, Kettrick R. Pediatrics home mechanical ventilation. *Pediatr Clin North Am* 1987; 34:47–60.

59. DeMarco A, Lelling J, Sujouic M, Jacobs I, Shields R, Altose M. Respiratory muscle training in muscular dystrophy. *Clin Res* 1982; 36:169–174.

60. Colbert A, Schock N. Respirator use in progressive neuromuscular disease. *Arch Phys Med Rehabil* 1985; 66:760–762.

61. Baydur A, Gilgoff I, Prentice W, Carlson M, Fischer A. Decline in respiratory function and experience with long–term assisted ventilation in advanced Duchenne's muscular dystrophy. *Chest* 1990; 97:884–889.

62. Bach J, Alba A, Pilkington L, Lee M. Long–term rehabilitation in advanced stages of childhood onset, rapidly progressive muscular dystrophy. *Arch Phys Med Rehabil* 1981; 62:328–331.

63. Splaingard M, Frates R, Jefferson L, Rosen C, Harrison G. Home negative pressure ventilation: Report of 20 year of experience in patients with neuromuscular disease. *Arch Phys Med Rehabil* 1985; 66:239–242.

64. Bach JR, O'Brien J, Krotenberg R, Alba A. Management of end stage respiratory failure in Duchenne muscular dystrophy. *Muscle Nerve* 1987; 10:177–182.

60

Preoperative and Postoperative Care

GLENNA B. WINNIE

Children are at greater risk than adults of developing pulmonary complications during and after anesthesia because of structural differences and smaller size. This chapter briefly delineates the effects of anesthesia on pulmonary mechanics, mucociliary clearance, and alveolar macrophage function; discusses preoperative evaluation of children with pre-existing pulmonary disease; and outlines a plan for postoperative management.

EFFECTS OF ANESTHESIA ON PULMONARY FUNCTION

The induction of general anesthesia causes changes in chest wall function as well as alterations in diaphragmatic configuration and movement. Since the chest wall and lungs function as a unit, changes in the shape or motion of the chest wall affect the lungs, and the nonproportional changes in chest wall shape that occur with anesthesia alter regional lung volumes, distribution of inspired gases, and pleural pressure. There is decreased functional residual capacity and diminished pulmonary compliance (1). Intercostal muscle function may be suppressed more than diaphragmatic function, causing decreased rib cage expansion and consequently paradoxical ventilation (2–4). In addition, loss of diaphragmatic tonic activity during anesthesia causes a cephalad shift of the end expiratory position of the diaphragm. Although application of positive end expiratory pressure moves the diaphragm more caudally, it does not return the diaphragm to the awake functional residual capacity position. Similarly, large mechanical breaths do not duplicate the pattern of displacement observed during spontaneous ventilation (5). The alterations in ventilation associated with these changes in chest wall and diaphragmatic mechanics are not accompanied by appropriate changes in perfusion, resulting in the development of ventilation-perfusion mismatch. Atelectasis and impairment of hypoxic pulmonary vasoconstriction further contribute to ventilation-perfusion mismatch (6).

Atelectasis is a common perioperative complication and is the result of failure of normal mechanisms to maintain the stability of air containing lung units (7). Computed tomography has revealed that induction of anesthesia is followed by rapid development of atelectasis in dependent lung regions, and intrapulmonary shunting due to diffuse closure of terminal lung units (8, 9). These areas of atelectasis may persist more than 24 hours after anesthesia. Decreased expiratory reserve volume, lack of sighing, and retained secretions further contribute to atelectasis during anesthesia. Because oxygen is resorbed more quickly than nitrogen distal to the site of airway occlusion, patients receiving supplemental oxygen are at greater risk for atelectasis. Postoperative changes in ventilatory pattern also contribute to the development of atelectasis. Sighing may be decreased by chest wall splinting caused by pain, narcotic analgesics, and residual anesthetic agents. This can lead to a reduction in functional residual capacity and atelectasis, and decreased pulmonary compliance. Postoperatively, expiratory reserve volume is also decreased, which may bring the end-tidal point lower than the closing volume, increasing the risk of atelectasis.

Postoperative changes in ventilation are determined in part by the site of the operative incision. More frequent pulmonary complications occur after thoracic than abdominal surgery, and fewer complications occur after operations on an extremity. After abdominal surgery, total lung capacity and its subdivisions are decreased, with larger changes occurring after upper abdominal surgery as compared to lower (10). There is a reduction of tidal volume on the first postoperative day, with a compensatory increase in respiratory rate and no change in minute ventilation (11). Vital capacity is reduced by approximately 45% 1–2 days after surgery and does not return to preoperative levels for 1–2 weeks. Residual volume and functional residual capacity also are decreased postoperatively and are at their lowest levels on the 4th postoperative day (11, 12).

EFFECTS OF ANESTHESIA ON PULMONARY DEFENSE MECHANISMS

Anesthesia alters nonspecific pulmonary defense mechanisms, including cough, mucociliary clearance, and phagocytosis by alveolar macrophages. Intubation completely bypasses normal upper airway mechanical barriers, and mucociliary clearance is depressed by general anesthesia. It may remain so for more than 48 hours postoperatively, particularly in patients who have had abdominal operations or who are exposed to prolonged anesthesia (13). Endotracheal tubes damage the epithelium of the larynx and trachea, and the accompanying suctioning can denude the respiratory epithelium, cause edema, and bring about the formation of inflammatory exudates (14). Exposure of tracheal epithelium to dry air is associated with ultrastructural changes in the ciliated epithelial cells, with sloughing of these cells and the presence of submucosal inflammation (15, 16). Inspiration of high concentrations of oxygen decreases tracheal mucous velocity (17), and halothane, tetracaine, atropine, and opiates impair mucociliary clearance. The bactericidal activity of the alveolar macrophage, which protects the host against inhalation of particulate matter and infectious agents, is depressed by halothane, methoxyflurane, and cyclopropane (18, 19). Local anesthetics, including lidocaine and tetracaine, also impair alveolar macrophage function. Hypoxia, which may occur in the intraoperative or postoperative period, impairs macrophage phagocytosis and killing (20). These alterations in pulmonary defense mechanisms contribute to the risk of retained secretions, atelectasis, hyp-

oxia, and pneumonia during the postoperative period.

FACTORS THAT PLACE CHILDREN AT INCREASED RISK OF PERIOPERATIVE PULMONARY COMPLICATIONS

Children are at greater risk of perioperative pulmonary complications than adults, and younger children are at greater risk than older children. There are multiple reasons for this. Decreased collateral ventilation due to fewer pores of Kohn, increased peripheral airways resistance, high chest wall compliance, and high closing volume place the child at higher risk for atelectasis. Relative muscle weakness combined with an inability to recruit intercostal muscles, a more easily fatigued diaphragmatic muscle, and immaturity of ventilatory control add to the risk of complications, including apnea and respiratory failure. Peripheral airways resistance is relatively high in children less than 5 years of age because the total cross-sectional area of the peripheral airways relative to the proximal airways is proportionally less than in older children and adults. Cartilaginous support of the airways is deficient in infancy and childhood, allowing greater dynamic compression of the bronchi and trachea. A given degree of airway narrowing causes a greater increase in airway resistance in the smaller airways of children than in the larger airways of adults. Moreover, a given length of endotracheal tube extending beyond the mouth causes a proportionally greater increase in airway resistance in a child than it does in an adult.

Infants have highly compliant chest walls, resulting in lower functional residual capacity and increased risk of atelectasis. Because of the highly compliant chest wall, the normal newborn infant's closing volume occurs above functional residual capacity and may be above the end-tidal resting point. Therefore, some airways are closed during a portion of tidal breathing, placing the normal infant at risk of atelectasis. During the first year of life, the normal infant maintains functional residual capacity above residual volume by maintaining respiratory muscle tone throughout much of expiration, and by using partial closure of the vocal cords to increase intraluminal pressure (21). Changes in chest wall mechanics induced by anesthesia may increase the closing volume further to above the end inspiratory level, causing closure of dependent airways throughout tidal breathing. The highly compliant chest wall of infants also creates a mechanical disadvantage. Although intercostal muscles are recruited to help stabilize the chest wall, it may be distorted by contraction of the diaphragm and creation of negative intra-thoracic pressure during inspiration. This wastes some of the force of diaphragmatic contraction and increases the work of breathing. Chest wall compliance diminishes through childhood, and total respiratory system compliance and lung elastic recoil approach adult levels by approximately age 15, although there is large intersubject variation (22).

The higher airway resistance, more compliant chest wall, and higher closing volume in children can adversely affect the postoperative course of pediatric patients. Postoperative edema, bronchospasm, and secretions further increase airway resistance, as does an endotracheal tube. However, when an infant must compensate for this increased work of breathing, there may be failure to recruit intercostal muscles (23) and development of diaphragmatic fatigue with consequent respiratory failure. After 10–20 minutes of breathing with increased airways resistance, normal newborns may fail to maintain minute ventilation and tidal volume (24). Thus, increased airway resistance for only a short time may be associated postoperatively with atelectasis, hypoxia, and respiratory failure in the young child.

PREOPERATIVE EVALUATION OF PEDIATRIC PATIENTS

A careful preoperative assessment is essential for all children, and should include history, physical examination, and pertinent laboratory studies. A history of respiratory tract symptoms is obtained, especially focusing on evidence of reactive airways disease. A history of respiratory tract infections, asthma, bronchopulmonary dysplasia, stridor or airway abnormalities, congenital heart disease, or neuromuscular disease is sought. Pulmonary complications of previous surgery are noted. If the patient has reactive airways disease, the severity of the disease and adequacy of control are determined. Symptom pattern, history of hospitalization for pulmonary disease, medication history including steroid use, and allergies are ascertained. Physical examination

includes assessment for chest hyper-inflation, prolonged expiratory time, retractions, adventitious sounds, adequacy and symmetry of aeration, and digital clubbing. In addition, adequacy of gag reflex, cough, and general muscle strength are determined. The patient's physical and intellectual capability for cooperating with postoperative pulmonary therapy are evaluated. When appropriate, the patient should be psychologically prepared for the operation.

The preoperative laboratory evaluation should be tailored to the patient. Complete blood count and oximetry are performed on all patients. Patients with any history of lung disease should have pulmonary function tests if capable of performing them. However, normal preoperative spirometry does not assure an uncomplicated postoperative course. A chest radiograph is obtained if there are abnormalities on physical examination, pulmonary function tests, or oximetry, or if the last chest radiograph performed on the patient was abnormal. It has not been determined if a chest radiograph is of value in a child who is asymptomatic. Spirometry before and after a bronchodilator aerosol is performed on patients with a history suggestive of reactive airways disease. Arterial blood gas determination or oximetry, and measurement of maximal inspiratory and expiratory mouth pressures, are performed on children with neuromuscular disease. Electrolytes are measured in patients with cystic fibrosis or bronchopulmonary dysplasia, and in those on diuretics. Total protein and albumin, liver function studies, and clotting studies are also obtained in patients with cystic fibrosis.

Patients at high risk for pulmonary complications should have a thorough evaluation within 24 hours before surgery. A child with an abnormal pulmonary examination, hypoxia on room air, suboptimal control of bronchospasm, electrolyte abnormalities, or cor pulmonale is admitted at least 1 day prior to surgery in order to maximize pulmonary status before anesthesia. If the patient is able to participate in his or her care, the planned operation and postoperative management are described. The necessity for postoperative chest physiotherapy and cough is explained, and when appropriate the child is taught incentive spirometry and the other respiratory care techniques that will be used postoperatively.

INTRAOPERATIVE MANAGEMENT

Patients with significant lung disease should have an intravenous line in place at the time of induction of anesthesia. Warm humidified gases used throughout the procedure help prevent hypothermia and postoperative complications in infants and children (38). Ventilation should be controlled during surgery so that chest expansion equals or exceeds chest expansion at rest. In cystic fibrosis patients not provided with ventilatory assistance during anesthesia, tidal volume decreases, and atelectasis or hypoventilation may develop (35). Such individuals often have low pulmonary compliance, and it may be difficult to maintain adequate ventilation. In all patients, breath sounds should be monitored continuously and the adequacy of gas exchange assessed by arterial or venous blood gases, or end-tidal CO_2 monitoring and oximetry. Increased pulmonary resistance during anesthesia is most commonly caused by bronchospasm, but mucus plugging and pneumothorax must be considered as possible etiologies. In patients with reactive airways disease, airway stimulation under light anesthesia may precipitate bronchospasm; this can be treated by deepening anesthesia and increasing the inspired oxygen concentration. In addition, treatment with intravenous aminophylline, inhalation of a beta-2 agonist, or use of intravenous steroids may be indicated. Intravenous isoproterenol or subcutaneous terbutaline may be useful but may precipitate arrhythmias; ketamine and lidocaine have been used with success. During anesthesia frequent suctioning of the lower respiratory tract may be required to remove excessive secretions, especially in patients with cystic fibrosis; a specimen should be sent for stain and culture.

POSTOPERATIVE MANAGEMENT

The most common postoperative pulmonary complications are hypoxemia, atelectasis, and pneumonia. Airway obstruction, bronchospasm, apnea, and respiratory failure may also occur. Careful management can decrease the incidence of these complications. Although hypoxia may be caused by ventilation-perfusion mismatch and atelectasis, fluid overload and respiratory depression secondary to analgesia may contribute. It is especially important to maintain adequate oxygenation with supplemental humidified oxygen in children to prevent muscle fatigue and periods of respiratory instability. During weaning from the ventilator, the endotracheal tube should not remain in place without either intermittent mandatory ventilation or pressure support, and a T-tube should not be used, since the increased airway resistance may precipitate atelectasis and respiratory failure, for reasons explained earlier. Prevention and vigorous treatment of bronchospasm is also important.

Postoperative pain should be controlled in all patients, as it may compromise respiratory status through chest wall splinting, decreased cough, and exacerbation of bronchospasm. Pain may also contribute to cardiovascular instability, particularly in infants. Opiates must be used carefully, as they may thicken secretions and depress respirations. Continuous intravenous infusion of medication may decrease the amount of medication required and improve pain control after major surgery. Other techniques that are useful in selected patients include infusion of medication through an indwelling epidural catheter, and patient-controlled administration of drugs.

Chest physiotherapy is an important means of prevention and treatment of postoperative pulmonary complications (39). There are several modalities of chest physiotherapy that may be applied, and the form most appropriate for each patient should be selected. Chest percussion and postural drainage is used in young children because they are unable to participate in most other forms of therapy. Incentive spirometry is effective in the older cooperative patient, and is preferred because it is less labor-intensive; preoperative instruction increases the chance of successful performance postoperatively. Coughing exercises may also be used. Intermittent positive pressure breathing can decrease pulmonary complications. However, since it is associated with more frequent bloating and abdominal distension than other forms of chest physiotherapy (39), it is usually restricted to use in those patients who are unable to inspire fully, particularly patients with neuromuscular weakness. Periodic face mask administration of positive expiratory pressure (PEP) or continuous positive airway pressure (CPAP) are more efficacious than incentive spirometry in decreasing postoperative $(A-a)O_2$ gradient, maintaining lung volumes, and preventing atelectasis after upper abdominal surgery (40). Nasal CPAP may also effectively treat atelectasis when chest physiotherapy and IPPB have failed (41). Complications of chest physiotherapy include (a) pain, which may contribute to cardiovascular instability, (b) decreased PaO_2, particularly in patients who mobilize thick secretions with therapy, and (c) bronchospasm, particularly if the child with asthma is placed in a head-down position. Despite these possible complications, chest physiotherapy is an important treatment modality.

The following outline is suggested for the postoperative pulmonary care of the pediatric patient:

1. Maintain adequate ventilation. Extubate when appropriate from a low ventilator rate or pressure support; do not use a T tube to wean a pediatric patient. Significant upper airway obstruction secondary to edema may be treated acutely with epinephrine aerosol.

2. Maintain adequate oxygenation. Monitor oxygen saturation continuously by pulse oximetry until the patient is fully awake, then as appropriate for the individual. Fully humidified oxygen should be administered until the child is awake, and then as needed.

3. Control pain.

4. Prevent bronchospasm, and treat it aggressively when it occurs. Administer bronchodilator aerosols every 4 hours for the first 24 hours to children with known reactive airways disease, and then four times daily for the next 48 hours. Theophylline and steroids should be given if the child received them preoperatively, or if aerosolized bronchodilators are inadequate. This regimen may be intensified when required.

5. Prevent atelectasis and promote clearance of secretions. Chest physiotherapy should be done at least every 4 hours for the first 24 hours and four times daily for the next 48 hours in children who are at increased risk of complications, and in those who have had chest or abdominal surgery or prolonged anesthesia. Incentive spirometry can be used on the same schedule if the patient is awake, cooperative, and has normal secretions. Suctioning should be done as needed. Cough, deep breathing, and early ambulation are encouraged.

6. Treat complications aggressively. If atelectasis develops, intensification of chest physiotherapy is indicated. CPAP or PEP may be added. Maximize control of bronchospasm. Mucolytic aerosols or bronchoscopy with lavage are indicated only in selected cases. Secretions should be obtained for Gram stain and culture, and infection treated vigorously.

CHILDREN AT HIGH RISK FOR PERIOPERATIVE COMPLICATIONS

All children are at risk for peri-operative complications. However, pre-existing respiratory tract disease further increases the likelihood of postoperative pulmonary problems.

Respiratory Tract Infection

Children with acute upper or lower respiratory tract infections are at increased risk for postoperative pulmonary complications. Therefore elective surgery should be deferred during a respiratory tract infection and for at least 2 weeks thereafter (25).

Asthma

The risk of intraoperative and postoperative complications is increased in children with asthma. The most frequent problem is bronchospasm, but laryngospasm, hypoxia, excessive secretions, atelectasis, and intraoperative arrhythmias may also occur. A therapeutic theophylline level should be achieved preoperatively in patients with asthma who require theophylline. Intravenous steroids beginning either before surgery or close to the time of induction are administered for prophylaxis against bronchospasm and to prevent perioperative adrenal insufficiency in patients receiving oral or inhaled steroids. Hydrocortisone hemisuccinate (5 mg/kg) or an equivalent drug is given every 6–8 hours for at least 24 hours. It is unclear whether children who have received steroids in the previous year should receive such treatment, although there is evidence that high-dose steroids given for 5 days to adults can cause adrenal suppression, which may persist for up to 1 year (26).

Prematurity

The most frequent perioperative pulmonary complication in premature infants is apnea, which may occur up to 12 hours postoperatively. Other complications include atelectasis, aspiration, pneumonia, stridor, excessive secretions, coughing, and cyanosis (27). In addition, postoperative bradycardia and periodic breathing may occur in the formerly premature infant. Nonessential surgery should be delayed for pre-term infants until they are beyond 44 weeks conceptional age. If surgery cannot be delayed, even the asymptomatic pre-term infant should be monitored for apnea and bradycardia for at least 18 hours postoperatively, and the hospital should be equipped to provide appropriate mechanical ventilation of the premature infant if necessary (28). Infants with an endotracheal tube in place postoperatively should always receive support with at least a low ventilator rate. Premature infants who are extubated from a low ventilator rate are successfully extubated, whereas 50% of those who are placed on positive airway pressure by endotracheal tube without intermittent ventilator breaths for 6 hours fail extubation (29).

Bronchopulmonary Dysplasia

Histopathologic changes in bronchopulmonary dysplasia include squamous metaplasia of the bronchiolar epithelium, derangement of alveolar architecture, areas of atelectasis alternating with emphysema, bronchiolar and bronchial smooth muscle hypertrophy, and medial hypertrophy of small pulmonary arteries (30). There exist ventilation and perfusion abnormalities, increased work of breathing, an abnormally reactive pulmonary vascular bed, and sometimes cor pulmonale (31). Mucociliary clearance is impaired, and often obstructive airways disease complicated by large airways collapse and reactive airways disease is present (32). Because of these abnormalities, the child with bronchopulmonary dysplasia is at high risk for perioperative pulmonary complications. Preoperatively, the child's general pulmonary and cardiovascular status should be thoroughly evaluated, including adequacy of oxygenation and ventilation, control of airways reactivity, and fluid and electrolyte status. It may be necessary to hospitalize the child for 1–2 days prior to surgery for evaluation. Elective surgery should be delayed in the presence of uncontrolled bronchospasm, any respiratory tract infection, or cardiovascular instability. Children with bronchopulmonary

dysplasia require meticulous postoperative care.

Neuromuscular Disease

Patients with neuromuscular disease are at high risk for postoperative pulmonary complications. There may be a history of frequent lower respiratory tract infections. Swallowing is often poorly coordinated, and cough weak. Difficulty in clearing secretions and chronic aspiration may also be present. There may be respiratory muscle weakness. Patients who have chronic respiratory muscle weakness, which is often not evident on general examination, may have abnormalities in pulmonary mechanics, including reduced lung volumes, microatelectasis, scoliosis, decreased chest wall compliance, ventilation-perfusion mismatch, and decreased pulmonary compliance (33). Central hypoventilation or hypoventilation caused by muscle weakness may be present. In addition, patients with neuromuscular disease may develop anaesthetic complications unrelated to their pulmonary status, including malignant hyperthermia, cardiac arrhythmias, excessive potassium release, and myoglobinuria (34).

Preoperative measurement of vital capacity and negative inspiratory force will help predict the degree of postoperative difficulty to be expected; however, we have successfully performed scoliosis repair on patients with vital capacity as low as 22% of predicted. Intermittent positive pressure breathing (IPPB) can be particularly helpful postoperatively, since these individuals may lack the strength to inhale maximally. This technique and incentive spirometry should be taught preoperatively. A temporary tracheostomy may be necessary to wean an extremely weak patient from ventilatory support.

Developmental Delay

Children with severe development delay or marked spasticity present a challenge in perioperative pulmonary care. Poor or absent gag reflex, weak cough, chronic aspiration of saliva, and inability to protect the airway increase the risk of postoperative atelectasis, pneumonia, and ventilator dependence. Gastroesophageal reflux is frequently present, sometimes triggering bronchospasm and often associated with aspiration of gastric contents. Such children may have abnormal breathing patterns, which must be documented before surgery so that postoperative expectations are appropriate. These children are often unable to cooperate with their postoperative care.

Cystic Fibrosis

Patients with cystic fibrosis are at increased risk of perioperative pulmonary complications (35, 36). There may be difficulty with ventilation during surgery, or intraoperative bronchospasm. Patients are prone to develop atelectasis, respiratory or circulatory depression, cyanosis, bradycardia, or airway obstruction. Other possible complications include pneumothorax, atelectasis, respiratory failure, and respiratory arrest. As expected, greater deterioration in pulmonary function is observed in patients with cystic fibrosis after general anesthesia than is seen in normal individuals (37). Therefore, it is advisable to admit even stable patients with this disease at least 24 hours before surgery in order to begin intravenous antibiotics and intensive chest physiotherapy. Individuals with significant lung disease may require even longer preoperative therapy to maximize pulmonary function and assure adequate bronchodilation before surgery. Because of the increased risk of atelectasis, pneumonia, and respiratory compromise due to excessive secretions in the perioperative period, local or regional anesthesia should be used whenever practical.

REFERENCES

1. Westbrook PR, Stubbs SE, Sessler AD, et al. Effects of anesthesia and muscle paralysis on respiratory mechanics in normal man. *J Appl Physiol* 1973; 34:81–86.
2. Jones JG, Faithfull D, Jordan C, et al. Rib cage movement during halothane anaesthesia in man. *Br J Anaesth* 1979; 51:399–406.
3. Rehder K, Sessler AD, Rodarte JR. Regional intrapulmonary gas distribution in awake and anesthetized-paralyzed man. J Appl Physiol 1977;42:391–402.
4. Tusiewicz K, Bryan AC, Froese AB. Contributions of changing rib cage–diaphragm interactions to the ventilatory depression of halothane anesthesia. *Anesthesiology* 1977; 47:327–337.
5. Froese AB, Bryan AC. Effects of anesthesia and paralysis on diaphragmatic mechanics in man. *Anesthesiology* 1974; 41:242–255.
6. Mathers J, Benumof JL, Wahrenbrock EA. General anesthetics and regional hypoxic pulmonary vasoconstriction. *Anesthesiology* 1977; 46:111–114.
7. Tisi G. Preoperative evaluation of pulmonary function: validity, indications and benefits. *Am Rev Respir Dis* 1979; 119:293–310.
8. Brismar B, Hedenstierna G, Lundquist H, et al. Pulmonary densities during anesthesia with muscular relaxation: A proposal of atelectasis. *Anesthesiology* 1985; 62:422–428.
9. Hedenstierna G, Strandberg A, Tokics L, et al. Correlation of gas exchange impairment to development of atelectasis during anaesthesia and muscle paralysis. *Acta Anaesthesiol Scand* 1986; 30:183–191.
10. Anscombe AR, Buxton R. Effect of abdominal operations on total lung capacity and its subdivisions. *Br Med J* 1958; 2:84–87.
11. Beecher HK. The measured effect of laparotomy on the respiration. *J Clin Invest* 1933; 12:639–650.
12. Beecher HK. Effect of laparotomy on lung volume: Demonstration of a new type of pulmonary collapse. *J Clin Invest* 1933; 12:651–658.
13. Gamsu G, Singer MM, Vincent HH, et al. Postoperative impairment of mucous transport in the lung. *Am Rev Respir Dis* 1976; 114:673–679.
14. Amikam B, Landa J, West J, Sackner MA. Bronchofiberscopic observations of the tracheobronchial tree during intubation. *Am Rev Respir Dis* 1972; 105:747–755.
15. Burton JDK. Effect of dry anesthetic gases on the respiratory mucous membrane. *Lancet* 1962; 1:235–238.
16. Hirsch JA, Tokayer JL, Robinson MJ, Sackner MA. Effects of dry air and subsequent humidification on tracheal mucous velocity in dogs. *J Appl Physiol* 1975; 39:242–246.
17. Sackner MA, Landa J, Hirsch MS, Zapata A. Pulmonary effects of oxygen breathing: A 6-hour study in normal men. *Ann Intern Med* 1975; 82:40–43.
18. Goldstein E, Munson ES, Eagle C, et al. The effects of anesthetic agents on murine pulmonary bactericidal activity. *Anesthesiology* 1971; 34:344–352.
19. Manawadu BR, LaForce FM. Impairment of pulmonary antibacterial defense mechanisms by halothane anesthesia. *Chest* 1979; 75:242–243.
20. Harris GD, Johanson WG, Pierce AK. Bacterial lung clearance in hypoxic mice. *Am Rev Respir Dis* 1975; 111:910.
21. Mortola JP, Milic–Emili J, Noworaj A, et al. Muscle pressure and flow during expiration in infants. *Am Rev Respir Dis* 1984; 129:49–53.
22. Sharp JT, Druz WS, Balagot RC, et al. Total respiratory compliance in infants and children. *J Appl Physiol* 1970; 29:775–779.
23. Lopes JM, Muller NL, Bryan MH, Bryan AC. Synergistic behavior of inspiratory muscles after diaphragmatic fatigue in the newborn. *J Appl Physiol* 1981; 51:547–551.
24. LaFramboise WA, Standaert TA, Guthrie RD, Woodrum DE. Developmental changes in the ventilatory response of the newborn to added airway resistance. *Am Rev Respir Dis* 1987; 136:1075–1083.
25. McGill WA, Coveler LA, Epstein BS. Subacute upper respiratory infection in small children. *Anesth Analg* 1979; 58:331–333.
26. Fung DL, Schatz M. Surgery in allergic patients, in Bierman CW, Pearlman DS, ed. *Allergic diseases from infancy to adulthood*, ed 2. Philadelphia, WB Saunders, 1988, pp 748–759.

27. Steward DJ. Preterm infants are more prone to complications following minor surgery than are term infants. *Anesthesiology* 1982; 56:304–306.

28. Gregory FA, Steward DJ. Life-threatening perioperative apnea in the ex-"premie." *Anesthesiology* 1983; 59:495–498.

29. Kim EH, Boutwell WC. Successful direct extubation of very low birth weight infants from low intermittent mandatory ventilation rate. *Pediatrics* 1987; 80:409–414.

30. Northway WH, Rosan RC, Porter DY. Pulmonary disease following respirator therapy of hyaline-membrane disease: bronchopulmonary dysplasia. *N Eng J Med* 1967; 276:357–368.

31. Abman SH, Wolfe RR, Accurso FJ, et al. Pulmonary vascular response to oxygen in infants with severe bronchopulmonary dysplasia. *Pediatrics* 1985; 75:80–83.

32. McCubbin M, Frey EE, Wagener JS, et al. Large airway collapse in bronchopulmonary dysplasia. *J Pediatr* 1989; 114:304–307.

33. Smith PE, Calverley PM, Edwards RH, et al. Practical problems in the respiratory care of patients with muscular dystrophy. *N Engl J Med* 1987; 316:1197–1205.

34. Kafer ER. Respiratory and cardiovascular functions in scoliosis and the principles of anesthetic management. *Anesthesiology* 1980; 52:339–351.

35. Doershuk CF, Reyes AL, Regan AG, Matthews LW. Anesthesia and surgery in cystic fibrosis. *Anesth Analg* 1972; 51:413–421.

36. Lamberty JM, Rubin BK. The management of anaesthesia for patients with cystic fibrosis. *Anaesthesia* 1985; 40:448–459.

37. Richardson VF, Robertson CF, Mowat AP, et al. Deterioration in lung function after general anaesthesia in patients with cystic fibrosis. *Acta Paediatr Scand* 1984; 73:75–79.

38. Rashad KF, Benson DW. Role of humidity in prevention of hypothermia in infants and children. *Anesth Analg* 1967; 46:712–718.

39. Celli BR, Rodriguez KS, Snider GL. A controlled trial of intermittent positive pressure breathing, incentive spirometry, and deep breathing exercises in preventing pulmonary complications after abdominal surgery. *Am Rev Respir Dis* 1984; 130:12–15.

40. Ricksten SE, Bengtsson A, Soderberg C, et al. Effects of periodic positive airway pressure by mask on postoperative pulmonary function. *Chest* 1986; 89:774–781.

41. Duncan SR, Negrin RS, Mihm FG, et al. Nasal continuous positive airway pressure in atelectasis. *Chest* 1987; 92:621–624.

61

Nutritional Management in Pediatric Pulmonary Disease

DIANE L. BARSKY and VIRGINIA A. STALLINGS

NUTRITIONAL ASSESSMENT

The purpose of nutritional assessment of the child with pulmonary disease is to determine who is malnourished and who is at risk for becoming malnourished so that preventative measures can be implemented. Since almost all children with chronic pulmonary disease have some nutritional component to their care, this discussion is directed toward the chronically ill child. Comprehensive reviews of nutritional assessment are available for further detail (1–3).

Nutritional assessment includes documentation of anthropometric and biochemical data, dietary intake, and clinical status. Assessment of anthropometric data in children includes the documentation and interpretation of changes in body weight and linear growth. It is essential that a member of the health care team be trained to obtain accurate weight, supine length, standing height, and head circumference, and to interpret these data in a clinically meaningful way. Weight and height (or length) should be obtained at each evaluation. If there is concern about growth, measurements should be obtained by trained personnel at more frequent intervals than routine clinic visits. If the patient is found not to be gaining normal increments in weight and/or stature (4, 5) or if the patient is losing weight, then a complete nutritional assessment should be part of the evaluation for failure to thrive. A complete nutritional assessment includes evaluation of additional anthropometric measurements (midarm circumference, tricep, and subscapular skinfold measurements)

and pubertal status, as well as usual dietary intake and nutrition practices, serum biochemical data, and evaluation for drug-nutrient interactions (6).

The cornerstone of optimal nutritional care for infants, children, and adolescents with chronic pulmonary disease is the promotion of normal growth and development as well as the early detection of malnutrition, which may adversely affect the course and outcome of the primary disease process (7) and affect immune status and wound healing. Finally, for families with chronically ill children and for the patients themselves, having a positive body image and experiencing normal pubertal development contributes greatly to a sense of well-being and to quality of life. The elements of complete nutritional assessment, evaluation, and plan are based on the standard pediatric evaluation:

1. Medical history that includes a nutrition history, a "typical" day's food intake, past nutrition history, use of nutritional supplements, use of vitamin or mineral supplements, unusual food practices by the child or family, problems of emesis or elimination
2. Physical examination that includes present and past weight, height or length, head circumference, midarm circumference, skinfold measurements
3. Laboratory evaluation
4. Evaluation of anthropometric and nutritional data using appropriate reference data
5. Plan that includes further evaluation, treatment, and follow-up care

Each component offers information needed by the physician to make an accurate assessment and to plan therapy. For non-hospitalized children a detailed nutrition history should be obtained by a registered dietitian, and may include an evaluation of a 3- to 5-day measured food intake record, especially if the child has been losing weight or gaining weight at a slower than desired rate. This information can be analyzed for energy, protein, and "at risk" nutrients such as, iron, calcium, and vitamins A and C. The nutrients that are at risk for being deficient vary with disease and therapy. For hospitalized children, inpatient calorie counts or a recall of a typical day's intake also may be useful in evaluating usual dietary intake, but offer less reliable information than a measured food record. The nutrition history should include information about unusual food practices by the child or family, vitamin or mineral supplements, and problems associated with emesis or elimination (i.e., diarrhea or constipation). Frequently used medications also may be reviewed for possible drug-nutrient interactions (Table 61.1) (6).

The nutritionally focused physical examination should include the standard anthropometric measurements (weight, height or length, and head circumference [birth–3

years]) with correction made for prematurity, if necessary. Correction for prematurity generally is made until the child has reached a corrected age of approximately 3 years. When available, previous weights, lengths or heights, and growth patterns provide important information. Additional anthropometric measurements such as midarm circumference, tricep, and subscapular skinfold measurements may be included in the nutritional evaluation. The midarm circumference, the derived midarm muscle circumference, and muscle area are indicators of muscle stores (fat-free compartment) and are related to dietary intake of both energy and protein. The tricep and subscapular skinfolds and derived fat area are measures of energy stored as subcutaneous fat and of the adequacy of energy in the diet. Skinfold measurements should be obtained only by trained examiners, otherwise the anthropometric data obtained may be inaccurate and even misleading. Anthropometric measures require high-quality, calibrated equipment (scale, lengthboard, stadiometer, calipers, non-cloth tape measure) and careful attention to the exact protocol for each measurement (8). Precise and accurate measurements are essential for obtaining reliable, longitudinal data. The physical examination also should include careful assessment of pubertal development by the Tanner method (9) beginning at approximately 10 years of age.

No group of laboratory tests reliably categorizes children into poorly or adequately nourished groups, particularly in reference to the adequacy of energy and protein in the diet. Measures of protein status (e.g., serum albumin) indicate both protein and energy status but often are influenced by other aspects of disease. Albumin, with a long half-life (15–20 days) and a large pool size, indicates protein-energy status over the previous weeks to months. In instances of chronic protein energy malnutrition, however, an adaptive process occurs in which albumin concentrations may be preserved at marginal or low ranges of normal (2.9–3.2 g/dl) in some children with obvious tissue wasting, and therefore may not be a sensitive indicator of the patient's nutritional status. Other protein energy measurements include transferrin (half-life 8 days), thyroxine-binding prealbumin (half-life 2–3 days), and retinol binding protein (half-life 12 hours); all have character-

Table 61.1.
Drug-Nutrient Interactions

Drug	Nutrient Affected
Anticonvulsants	
Dilantin	Folate, vitamins B_{12}, B_6, D Vitamin C, calcium
Phenobarbital	Folate, vitamins B_{12}, B_6, K Vitamin C, calcium
Anti-Inflammatory Agents	
Aspirin	Vitamin C, iron
Corticosteroids	Protein, fat, zinc, sodium, potassium, calcium, glucose
Antimicrobials	
Isoniazid	Vitamin B_6, niacin
Trimethoprime	Folate
Penicillin	Potassium
Cholestyramine	Vitamins A, D, E, K, calcium, fat
Cathartics	
Mineral oil	Vitamins A, D, E, K, carotene, calcium
Other	
Digitalis	Potassium, magnesium, calcium
Furosemide	Zinc, calcium, sodium, potassium
Antacids	Phosphate, calcium, vitamin A, iron

istics that limit their usefulness in routine assessment. Vitamin assays may be indicated in specific conditions, such as fat-soluble vitamin levels for children with cystic fibrosis (CF) and malabsorptive losses of fat. Determination of iron stores is indicated, particularly for children with chronic hypoxia, as hemoglobin plays a vital role in oxygen transport. Iron status may be assessed with a series of tests, alone or in combination: complete blood count, serum iron, total iron-binding capacity, transferrin, serum ferritin, and free-erythrocyte protoporphyrin. Serum ferritin appears to be the most useful single test in assessing iron stores. Plasma zinc levels should be monitored in children with marginal intake and growth failure, chronic diarrhea, or malabsorption.

Finally, the use of indirect calorimetry for determining energy expenditure, and thus, the energy needs of an individual patient, is becoming a part of clinical care. This method is based on the principle of cellular oxidative energy metabolism and the ability, under strict testing conditions, to measure oxygen consumption and carbon dioxide production from all metabolic processes. The resting energy expenditure (kcal/day) is calculated from these measurements. The respiratory quotient (RQ) can also be determined; RQ is the ratio of carbon dioxide produced to the oxygen, and reflects the pattern of substrate utilization. The RQ of fat is 0.7, protein 0.8, carbohydrate 1.0, and a "mixed" diet 0.85. An optimal range is considered to be 0.8–0.9. If the RQ is less than 0.7, this may be indicative of underfeeding, lipolysis, or oxidation of ketones. If the RQ is greater than 1.0, this may be indicative of overfeeding, lipogenesis, or excess production of carbon dioxide. Development of standardized, practical testing methods for children and developing reference data for healthy children will facilitate the use of energy expenditure measurements in clinical care.

Once the nutrition history, physical examination, and laboratory assessment are complete, the clinician must interpret these findings and formulate a care plan using reference information from appropriate sources and multiple data points for each child. For weight, length or height, and head circumference, the most accepted standard curves are from the National Center for Health Statistics (10). The calculation at each outpatient visit of the weight for height, by the method of Waterlow (11) or by the method of ideal body weight for actual height (i.e., if height is at the 25th percentile, the actual weight is compared to the 25th percentile weight for age), is very useful in assessing changes in weight in relation to the changes in height. During the annual nutritional evaluation, the arm circumference and skinfold measurements may be compared to the standards published by Frischano (12) for healthy children. Growth velocity (change over time) may be compared to the standard curves developed by Tanner (13) or by the incremental growth charts (14). Height and weight velocity may also be calculated.

The other component of nutritional assessment is to determine the adequacy of the diet and to set individualized dietary goals for the patient. Our discussion will be limited to energy requirements, since poor energy intake is the most common cause of malnutrition in patients with respiratory disease. The finding of isolated deficiencies of protein, vitamins, or minerals in these patients is rare, and often predictable (e.g., fat-soluble vitamin deficiencies in children with CF).

Intake recommendations for energy, protein, and many vitamins and minerals of the population of healthy people in the United States are presented as the Recommended Dietary Allowances (RDA) (15). Table 61.2 lists the median recommended intake for age and gender in subjects with light physical activity, and thus may include large ranges to account for individual variation. The RDA is not a precise tool with which to assess an individual patient's energy intake, or to predict the patient's energy needs. Yet, even with these limitations, dietary intake may be compared to the RDA and thus provide useful screening information. The energy intake data of healthy children also is useful in evaluating the average energy intake of children (16). These data are reported in smaller, more defined age ranges (compared to the RDA's ranges) as well as by percentile of energy intake.

Another method, more suited for determining the individual patient's energy expenditure, and thus estimation of energy needs, has been proposed by the World Health Organization (17). The energy required for basic body functions (basal metabolic rate [BMR])

Table 61.2.
Recommended Dietary Allowance for Energy

	Age (years)	REE (kcal/day)	Multiple of REE	Energy Allowance[a]		
				kal/kg/day	k/cal/day	Range
Infants	0.5–0.5	320	2.03	108	kgx108	(520–780)
	0.5–1.0	500				
Children	1–3	740	1.76	102	1300	(1040–1560)
	4–6	950	1.89	90	1800	(1440–2160)
	7–10	1130	1.77	70	2000	(1600–2400)
Males	11–14	1440	1.70	55	2500	(2000–3000)
	15–18	1760	1.67	45	3000	(2400–3600)
Females	11–14	1310	1.67	47	2200	(1760–2640)
	15–18	1370	1.60	40	2200	(1760–2640)

[a]The calculation of kcal/kg/day in children $\geq$ 3 years of age is based on the average of a wide range of acceptable intakes. Appropriate rates of growth may occur at energy intake levels above and below this estimate.
Adapted from Beal VA. Nutritional intake. In McCammon RW, ed. *Human growth and development.* Springfield IL, Charles C. Thomas, 1970, pp 63–100.

is estimated based on gender, age, and actual weight; the total daily energy needs (kcal/day) is calculated by multiplying the BMR by a factor reflecting the physical activity and, with some illnesses, the change in energy requirements related to the disease process (Table 61.3). For most disease processes (other than multiple trauma, untreated sepsis, and burn injury), the factors are modest, ranging from 1.1 to 1.3. Since children with a significant acute episode or an active chronic illness often decrease voluntary physical activity, the final adjustment for the BMR reflecting both physical activity and disease process may be in the range of 1.3–1.5, less than that for a normally

Table 61.3.
WHO Equations for Predicting Basal Metabolic Rate from Body Weight

Age range (years)	Kcal/day
Males	
0–3	60.9 W − 54[a]
3–10	22.7 W + 495
10–18	17.5 W + 495
18–30	15.3 W + 679
30–60	11.6 W + 879
> 60	13.5 W + 487
Females	
0–3	61.0 W − 51
3–10	22.5 W + 499
10–18	12.2 W + 746
18–30	14.7 W + 496
30–60	8.7 W + 829
> 60	10.5 W + 596

[a]W = body weight in kg.
Adapted from Hamill PVV, Drizd TA, Johnson CL, Reed RB, Roche AF, Moore WM. Physical Growth National Center for Health Statistics percentiles. *Am J Clin Nutr* 1979; 32:607–629.

active child. In children with normal pulmonary function, respiration constitutes only 2–3% of resting energy expenditure. However, with chronic lung disease, the workload of breathing increases as accessory respiratory muscles are used and respiratory rate increases. These responses require additional calories, but the increase is small in relationship to the total daily requirement, except in the late stages of chronic pulmonary disease.

If the child is found not to be nourished adequately and growing well, nutritional intervention should be initiated. Increased consumption of calorically dense foods is recommended initially with the use of enteral support using various supplemental formulas and enteral tubes as the second choice. Parenteral nutrition serves as the last option. There are constant advances in specialty nutritional formulas for children and adults, including higher fat, lower carbohydrate products for patients with chronic lung disease, and products designed for children. In addition, there are continued changes and improvements in the various enteral feeding tubes and buttons. Children who cannot ingest or digest adequate amounts of food or formula to support normal growth are potential candidates for tube feeding or parenteral nutrition.

CYSTIC FIBROSIS

Patients with cystic fibrosis (CF) present with a variety of nutrition-related symptoms, usually secondary to pancreatic insufficiency. Although 85% of patients with CF suffer from some degree of pancreatic insufficiency, presenting symptoms can range from mild malabsorption to significant steatorrhea with severe growth failure (18). The etiology of malnutrition in patients with CF may be multifactorial. The primary reason is maldigestion secondary to pancreatic insufficiency. Negative energy balance also may occur because of inadequate caloric intake, increased energy requirements, or both. The increased energy requirements may be caused by recurrent infections, increased workload of breathing from chronic pulmonary disease, and maldigestion related to pancreatic insufficiency and impaired bile salt metabolism (19).

As persons with CF now are living longer, the associated malnutrition and growth failure is becoming more apparent. Studies indicate that protein energy malnutrition diminishes long-term survival. Corey and associates (7) compared survival, growth, and pulmonary function in two groups of patients with CF, one followed in Boston and the other in Toronto. Although both groups had similar age-specific pulmonary functions, the median age of survival in the Toronto group was 30 years, but only 21 years in the Boston patients with CF. The main difference between the two groups was approach to diet: the Toronto group received a high-calorie, unrestricted fat diet with a higher number of enzyme capsules per meal, whereas the Boston group consumed a lower-fat, high-calorie diet. The Toronto patients with CF were found to have improved growth and better nutritional status than the Boston patients, which was felt to contribute to longer survival.

Persons with CF often consume less than their daily energy requirement. Luder et al. (20) studied a high-energy (greater than 120% RDA), unrestricted fat diet following 37 patients (ages 2–27 years) over 4 years after initial nutrition education intervention. Mean energy intake increased from 94% of the RDA to greater than 120%, and fat consumption rose from 32% to 39% of total caloric intake. Nutritional anthropometrics indicated weight gain, height maintenance, and normal onset of puberty. Lung function stabilized after having deteriorated during the 2 years prior to intervention.

Acute illness often interferes with the food intake of patients with CF. Chronic pulmonary infections, acute respiratory exacerbations, or both cause anorexia and nausea.

Decreased appetite and weight loss often are the first signs of an acute pulmonary infection. Esophagitis, dysphagia, chest pain, and symptoms associated with gastroesophageal reflux may interfere with food intake. Other complications of CF, pancreatitis, biliary dyskinesia, cirrhosis, and cholangitis may also result in anorexia, recurrent abdominal pain, and nausea (21).

In addition to having a reduced energy intake, the majority of patients with CF maldigest nutrients because of pancreatic insufficiency. Fat malabsorption also is caused by inadequate pancreatic bicarbonate secretion, resulting in a loss of buffer to gastric acid entering the duodenum. In this acidic environment, bile acids precipitate, rendering them unavailable for micelle formation and fat absorption. Pancreatic enzymes also become inactive when exposed to an acidic environment. Recent improvements including enteric-coated pancreatic enzyme microspheres greatly reduce inactivation of pancreatic enzymes. Fat malabsorption also results in fat-soluble vitamin deficiencies. Insufficient pancreatic chymotrypsin and trypsin secretion results in protein maldigestion, as defined by stool nitrogen losses, which are at least twice normal. Although patients with CF lack adequate amounts of pancreatic amylase, most carbohydrate is well tolerated since alpha amylase in saliva and glucoamylase present in the intestinal brush border efficiently hydrolyze starch and glucose polymers (22).

Some patients with CF also demonstrate higher metabolic rates than expected for age. Vaisman et al. (23) measured the resting energy expenditures (REEs) in 71 patients with CF with clinically significant lung disease (pulmonary function tests < 80% of predicted). REE values in all the patients with CF were significantly elevated, which was attributed by the authors to a greater workload of breathing. However, the study sampled a heterogenous population and did not separate the group according to severity of pulmonary disease, nutritional status, or pubertal development. Therefore, as pulmonary status deteriorated, REE rose. Shepherd et al. (24) determined total energy expenditure (TEE) in nine infants with CF without apparent lung disease compared to 16 control infants who did not have CF and were apparently healthy, using the doubly labeled water technique. Patients with CF had a 24% higher TEE than age-matched controls and a 27% higher TEE than weight-matched controls. A basic cellular defect was hypothesized as the cause of elevated energy expenditure. These conclusions are limited by the small sample size, lack of objective measurements of pulmonary function, nutritional status, and body composition, all of which affect TEE.

Chronic pulmonary disease raises the metabolic rates of some patients with CF, resulting in increased energy demands. If these demands are not met, malnutrition develops, which reduces respiratory muscle strength, diminishes diaphragm muscle mass, impairs immune defenses, and compromises normal growth and pubertal development (25).

Patients with CF are at risk for protein energy malnutrition. Aggressive nutrition intervention should be initiated when a patient reaches 85–90% of ideal weight for height (26). A comprehensive nutritional evaluation should be completed on each patient with CF annually, with weight and height (or length) measurements taken at each clinic visit. The yearly nutrition assessment for a child with CF is presented in Table 61.4. If the patient appears to be experiencing maldigestion with resultant malabsorption, a 72-hour fecal fat malabsorption study would be indicated. Steatorrhea is defined as a coefficient of fat absorption less than 93% (90% in infants). Recent studies have demonstrated that larger doses of pancreatic enzymes are safe and effective in decreasing steatorrhea and correcting maldigestion in patients with CF (27, 28). Laboratory data should include

Table 61.4.
Annual Comprehensive Nutritional Assessment in CF

- Detailed 3- to 5-day diet history including recent dietary pattern changes
- Plot current and past height and weight
- Evaluate rate of growth
- Pancreatic enzyme supplementation (type, number, compliance)
- Stool pattern—number, frequency, consistency
- Other symptoms of malabsorption/maldigestion (flatus, abdominal pain, oily discharge, rectal prolapse)
- Vitamin and mineral supplements (types and quantities)
- Medications (types and doses)

a fasting serum glucose, albumin, zinc, prothrombin time, vitamin E, electrolytes, and liver function tests.

Nutritional management of the child with CF includes a diet adequate in energy and all essential nutrients, adequate pancreatic enzyme replacement, appropriate vitamin supplementation, and salt replacement (Table 61.5). Malabsorption of the fat-soluble vitamins A, D, E, and K may lead to clinical deficiencies. As shown in Table 61.2, some vitamin supplements must be provided in each age group. Most patients with CF will receive adequate vitamin supplementation from a multiple-vitamin preparation (26). Infants receiving commercial formula require 1 ml of a liquid multivitamin daily, whereas two multivitamins per day (chewable) are recommended for older children receiving a regular diet. Adults require a standard adult multivitamin preparation, one or two tablets per day. If prothrombin time is abnormal, or if serum vitamin A or E levels are found to be low, additional supplementation with water miscible forms of vitamin A, E, or K may be administered.

Salt replacement should be given to infants (12.5–23 mEq sodium per day; 1/8–1/4 teaspoon salt) because formula, breast milk, and commercial baby foods contain insufficient sodium chloride to offset losses via the sweat. Once the child begins to consume table foods, consumption of salty foods and generous use of the salt shaker should be encouraged. Salt tablets are generally considered unnecessary.

With adequate pancreatic enzyme replacement, many infants with CF will tolerate standard formula with iron. Breast milk can successfully support normal growth with adequate pancreatic enzyme supplementation. However, because of the low protein content of human milk and losses of protein from maldigestion, infants who are breast fed should be monitored closely for complications of failure to thrive, hypoproteinemia, and hyponatremic alkalosis. High-quality protein from strained baby meat or formula can be added to the diet of a breast fed infant. Semi-elemental formulas such as Pregestimil (Mead Johnson Laboratories) or Alimentum (Ross Laboratories) may be indicated for patients who are malnourished, who have had intestinal resection due to meconium ileus, or who have persistent fat maldigestion despite enzyme

Table 61.5.
Nutritional Management of Cystic Fibrosis

DIET—Adequate in energy and and all essential nutrients

Infants and Toddlers:

Feeding Formula	Comment
Standard formula with iron	Adequate pancreatic enzyme replacement required
Human milk	Monitor closely for failure to thrive, hypoproteinemia, and hyponatremic alkalosis. Consider supplementing with high quality protein such as infant formula and strained baby food meats.
Semi-elemental formulas	May be indicated for patients who are malnourished, S/P intestinal resection, or who have persistent fat maldigestion despite enzyme replacement
Cow's milk	For children > 1 year, with appropriate adjustments made in enzyme dosages, vitamin supplementation, and salt replacement

Children and Adults: A diet that is high in energy and fat and all essential nutrients is recommended.

PANCREATIC ENZYME REPLACEMENT—Determine and adjust on an individual basis

Infants:
An initial dose of 1000–4000 lipase units of an enteric-coated pancreatic enzyme replacement per 4 oz of formula is reasonable. Dosage may be increased based on the infant's growth velocity and stooling pattern. Application of a zinc containing ointment *prior* to initiation of enzymes may help prevent excoriation of patient's peri-anal area due to the enzymes.

Children and Adults:
Adjust dose of enzymes as necessary to achieve a stool goal of one to two well-formed stools per day, and absence of gastrointestinal symptoms suggestive of maldigestion/malabsorption (e.g., excessive flatus, abdominal pain, oily discharge).

VITAMIN SUPPLEMENTATION—To offset losses from maldigestion/malabsorption

Multivitamins	Vitamin E		Vitamin A	Vitamin K
Infants and Toddlers:				
1 ml standard multivitamin preparation daily for infants receiving fortified infant formula. Increase to 2 ml/day when whole cow's milk is introduced (approximately 1 year of age).	3–6 months 6–12 months 1–4 years 4–10 years > 10 years	25 IU/day 50 IU/day 100 IU/day 100–200 IU/day 200–400 IU/day	Indicated for patients who routinely take standard multivitamin preparations yet fail to maintain adequate serum vitamin A concentrations.	It is prudent to prescribe vitamin K to patients receiving antiobiotics, or if cholestatic liver disease ire present. B–12 months 2.5 mg twice weekly > 1 year—adult 5.0 mg twice weekly
Children (2–8 years):				
One standard multivitamin/day containing 400 IU vitamin D and 5000 IU vitamin A.	May not be indicated if serum vitamin E levels are normal and are tested at least one time per year. Excessive doses of vitamin E (> 1000 IU/day) may exacerbate the coagulopathy associated with vitamin K deficiency.			
Older children and adults:				
Two standard multivitamins/day, 1 plain and 1 with iron				

SALT REPLACEMENT—To offset losses in the sweat

Infants:
12.5–23 mEq sodium/day ($^1/_8$–$^1/_4$ teaspoon salt/day) added to formula.

Older Children and Adults:
Encourage consumption of salty foods and generous use of the salt shaker.

Adapted from Ramsey BW, Farrell PM, Pencharz P, et al. Nutritional assessment and management in cystic fibrosis: A consensus report. *Am J Clin Nutr* 1992; 55:108–116.

replacement. These formulas are more expensive and less palatable than standard infant formulas. Whole cow's milk may be introduced for the child who is over 1 year of age, with appropriate adjustments made in enzyme dosages, vitamin supplementation, and salt replacement. For older patients, a diet high in energy and fat and adequate in all essential nutrients is recommended.

Pancreatic enzyme replacement should be determined and adjusted on an individual basis. As a guideline for initiation of enteric coated enzymes in infants, a dose of 1000–4000 lipase units per 4 oz of formula is reasonable. Dosage can be increased according to the infant's growth velocity and stooling pattern. Some clinicians have recommended initial enzyme doses based on units of lipase per kilogram of body weight per meal (28). For children who require large doses of pancreatic enzyme replacement to achieve effective digestion, more concentrated pancreatic enzyme replacement products are available that decrease the number of capsules needed. Table 61.6 summarizes the concentrations of currently available pancreatic enzyme replacements.

A difficult but important decision in nutritional management is when to increase the level of nutritional support to treat growth failure. An increase in nutrition intervention should be initiated if the patient's weight for height falls below 85% of "ideal" (weight for height greater than or equal to the 50th percentile) (26) or if the patient experiences weight loss since the last visit. For the patient with mild weight loss, counseling by the dietitian to increase the caloric density of meals and snacks using the child's favorite foods and supplements is the first step. If this fails to achieve the desired outcome, more aggressive nutritional intervention becomes necessary. One method is to begin nocturnal continuous drip feedings using a nasogastric tube that is replaced each night or one that is left in place for several weeks. Several studies demonstrated that night-time enteral feeds providing either elemental or polymeric formulas improve growth, nutritional status, and body composition in children and adolescents with mild to moderate pulmonary disease (29). Researchers also reported that enteral supplementation stabilized lung disease while pulmonary function continued to deteriorate in the untreated control groups (30). There is concern of a detrimental effect of additional fluid and carbohydrate on an already compromised cardiorespiratory system. Both Kane

Table 61.6.
Concentrations of Pancreatic Enzyme Replacements

Enzyme	Company	USP Units		
		Lipase	Protease	Amylase
Enteric-coated pancreatic enzyme replacements:				
Cotazym-S	Organon	5,000	20,000	20,000
Creon-10	Solvay	10,000	37,500[a]	33,200
Creon-25	Solvay	25,000	62,500[a]	74,700
Pancrease	McNeil	4,000	25,000	20,000
Pancrease MT-4	NcNeil	4,000	12,000	12,000
Pancrease MT-10	NcNeil	10,000	30,000	30,000
Pancrease MT-16	McNeil	16,000	48,000	48,000
Pancrease MT-25	McNeil	25,000	75,000	75,000
Pancrease MT-32	McNeil	32,000	70,000	90,000
Ultrase MT-6	Scandipharm	6,000	19,500	19,500
Ultrase MT-12	Scandipharm	12,000	39,000	39,000
Ultrase MT-18	Scandipharm	18,000	58,500	58,500
Ultrase MT-20	Scandipharm	20,000	65,000	65,000
Ultrase MT-24	Scandipharm	24,000	78,000	78,000
Ultrase MT-30	Scandipharm	30,000	97,500	97,500
Zymase	Organon	12,000	24,000	24,000
Non–enteric-coated pancreatic enzyme replacements:				
Cotazym	Organon	8,000	30,000	30,000
Viokase Powder (1/4 teaspoon)	Robins	16,800	70,000	70,000
Viokase Tablet	Robins	8,000	30,000	30,000

[a]Free and Zymogen-bound Protease

(31) and O'Loughlin (29) supplemented daily oral intake with 12-hour overnight continuous nasogastric feeds. Not only did the patients tolerate the extra volume and substrate without developing pulmonary edema, their long-term prognosis improved. These researchers demonstrated nutritional rehabilitation improved linear growth, stimulated weight gain, and decreased episodes of pneumonia without compromising cardiac function. Nasogastric tubes can be effective but patients often have difficulty keeping them in place and may cough them up during coughing spasms. Relaxation techniques may need to be employed for successful passing of the tube. Nasogastric tubes can also be uncomfortable and unsightly but do obviate the need for surgery. Placement of the tube also can be very traumatic for young children and is not recommended. Gastrostomy provides enteral access and a more permanent route for delivery of enteral supplements. Recent advances in the use of percutaneous endoscopic gastrostomy (PEG) has simplified the decision to place a gastrostomy tube in patients with CF. Concerns about the increased risk of gastroesophageal reflux seen with the traditional surgical gastrostomy appear to be less with the PEG. Furthermore, the duration of anesthesia and postoperative recovery period are shorter than with a surgical tube. In fact, in selected older patients a gastrostomy can be performed using endoscopy while the patient is under intravenous sedation. An evaluation of gastric emptying, the presence of reflux, and an assessment of the patient's ability to tolerate intragastric feedings should be performed prior to tube placement. Once the gastrostomy tube is functioning and the patient is gaining weight, the tube can be converted to a gastrostomy button, which is more convenient, less noticeable, and equally effective.

Any of these forms of enteral access may be used for nocturnal drip feedings or daytime bolus feedings to supplement voluntary daily intake; the amounts that can be given will vary depending on the size of the patient. It is generally recommended to increase the volume gradually over a period of days. To avoid the need for pancreatic enzymes, feedings of elemental formula usually are provided. Full-strength elemental formulas are typically 1 kcal/ml. For daytime bolus feedings, more calorically dense non-elemental nutritional supplements (e.g., 1.5–2.0 kcal/ml) may be administered with appropriate pancreatic enzyme replacement.

If enteral feedings do not result in adequate weight gain or are poorly tolerated, central hyperalimentation may be used. Length of therapy may vary depending on the patient's nutritional status. A surgically placed tunneled line is used, and the family is taught how to manage the infusion. Involvement of a home infusion therapy program can be helpful in monitoring these patients.

BRONCHOPULMONARY DYSPLASIA

Growth failure and malnutrition in infants with bronchopulmonary dysplasia (BPD) continues to be a major clinical problem, especially with the very low birth weight (VLBW) infant (i.e., birth weight < 1500 g). These premature babies require intensive respiratory treatment; thus, other adjuvant therapy such as nutritional support may not receive sufficient attention initially. However, malnutrition exerts deleterious effects on the lung's capacity for growth and repair, further compromising the premature infant's ability to develop healthy lungs and perhaps predisposing him or her to BPD. A National Institute of Health workshop on Nutrition and the Respiratory System (32) issued the statement that "sufficient evidence is available to recommend that greater clinical priority be given to nutrition as a vigorous part of total support of premature infants." Table 61.7 summarizes an approach to the nutritional management of these infants.

VLBW infants are born with minimal energy and protein stores since the majority of nutritional reserves are deposited during the third trimester of pregnancy. In the VLBW infant energy stores consist of approximately 2% body weight as fat and less than 0.5% as glycogen, whereas a full-term infant has 15% body weight as fat and 1.2% as glycogen (33). Early and successful nutritional support facilitates the normally rapid linear and brain growth. Initial support usually consists of parenteral nutrition delivered through a peripheral venous catheter. Optimal intravenous intake for the VLBW infant (80–90 kcal/kg/day, 2.5–3.0 g fat/kg/day, and 2.5–3.0 g protein/kg/day) prevents catabolism and promotes acceptable rates of tissue deposition and growth (33). Enteral feedings should be initi-

Table 61.7.
Nutritional Approach to the BPD Infant

1. Calorie goals
    a. Does the infant require O_2 supplementation and/or ventilatory support?
    b. Does the infant demonstrate tachypnea and/or CO_2 retention?
    If yes to either: start 120–140 kcal/kg/day,
        <1800 g: Premature formula PO/NG
        >1800 g: start fullterm formula with caloric density 24 kcal/oz.
    If fluid restricted: to further increase caloric density, add microlipid 1 ml/oz (4.5 cal/ml) or corn oil (9 kcal/ml).
    If risk of malabsorption: i.e., surgical NEC, cholestasis use elemental formula at 24 kcal and/or supplement
        with medium chain triglyceride 1 ml/oz (7.7 kcal/ml).
2. Energy distribution goals, as percentage of total daily caloric intake
    a. Fat: 50–55%
    b. Protein: 15–20%
    c. Carbohydrate: 25–30%
3. Monitor vitamin and mineral status
    a. Follow serum calcium, phosphorus, alkaline phosphatase: Increased risk of rickets due to prematurity
        and urinary calcium loss induced by diuretics
    b. Multivitamin with iron
4. Weight gain goals
    a. 15–30 g/day depending on age and degree of FTT; advance energy intake up to 180 kcal/kg/day until
        appropriate weight gain for age
5. Formula intolerance
    a. Emesis
        1. Evaluate for gastroesophageal reflux
    b. Diarrhea
        1. Rule out infectious etiology
        2. Reduce volume and/or concentration

ated as early as possible to minimize the risk of atrophy of the intestinal villi, parenteral nutrition–related cholestasis, and catheter-related sepsis. Energy intake should be adjusted as necessary to promote a weight gain of at least 20–30 g/day for a preterm infant (34) and 15–30 g/day for a term infant (35).

Even after the initial stresses of the neonatal period, these infants often continue to grow poorly. Factors that may contribute to decreased energy intake and failure to thrive in infant with BPD include fluid restrictions, frequent respiratory exacerbations, increased energy expenditure, neurologic damage that may interfere with sucking and swallowing, and overly aggressive oxygen weaning (36). Several studies measuring energy expenditure with indirect calorimetry reported increased energy expenditure in infants with BPD who were failing to thrive. Weinstein and Oh (37) demonstrated a 25% increase in mean oxygen consumption VO_2 of eight infants with BPD as compared to controls matched for age and weight. In another study investigating the effects of various glucose intake on the RQ, Yanis and Oh (38) measured six infants with

BPD and found a 20% higher resting energy expenditure (REE) compared to healthy infants matched for age and weight. Other groups have also measured greater energy requirements for infants with BPD and postulated a multifactorial etiology: the metabolic cost for "catch up" growth, increased respiratory effort, chronic heart failure, and acid-base imbalances. Abnormal pulmonary mechanics, especially increased small airway resistance and decreased lung compliance, result in greater workload of breathing and may contribute to increased energy needs.

Most infants with BPD require a high energy intake to promote satisfactory growth, but when carbohydrate constitutes the major nutrient, carbon dioxide production may rise, potentially exceeding the ventilatory capacity of the infant, who may not be able to compensate for the hypercarbia and acidosis. Table 61.8 summarizes general categories of formulas and specific medical indications for use. One should first concentrate the formula to 24 kcal/oz, increasing the caloric density while simultaneously maintaining the volume restriction. The total energy intake can be

Table 61.8.
General Categories of Formulas and Specific Medical Indications for Use

Type of Formula	Indications for Use
Standard formulas Enfamil[b] Similac[c] SMA[d]	Normal term, human milk substitute
Low mineral-electrolyte formulas Similac PM 60/40[b] SMA[d]	Renal, cardiac dysfunction

Lactose-free, casein-free formulas and special milk-based formulas with reduced allergenicity
Soy formulas
  Isomil[c]
  Isomil SF[c]
  Prosobee[b]
  Nursoy[b]
Nutramigen[b]
Alimentum[c]
	Primary or secondary lactase deficiency
	Cow's milk protein allergy
	Galactosemia

Nutramigen[b] Alimentum[c]	Cow's milk and soy protein allergy
Formulas with altered fat, protein, and carbohydrate *Fat alterations*	Steatorrhea (cystic fibrosis, biliary artesia, severe protein energy malnutrition)

Lipisorb[b] (30-40 kcal/oz)
  Portagen[b]
  Pregestimil[b]
  Alimentum[c]
	Intestinal resection
	Intractable diarrhea
	Intestinal lymphangiectasia

Protein alterations
  Casein hydrolysates (Nutramigen[b], Alimentum[c])
  Whey hydrolysate (Goodstart HA)
	Cow's milk and soy protein allergy

Elemental feedings (30 kcal/oz)[h]
  Criticare HN[b]
  Peptamen[e]
  Tolerex[f]
  Vital High Nitrogen[c]
	Extensive bowel resection
	Intractable diarrhea
	Overnigth drip feedings in older children or adults with cystic fibrosis

Premature feedings (24 kcal/oz)
  Milk from a premature baby's own mother with Prematurity fortifier added (Enfamil Human Milk)
  Enfamil Premature Formula[b]
  Similac Special Care[c]
  "Preemie" SMA[d]	

Formula designed for pediatric patients (30 kcal/oz) Pediasure[c]	Lactose-free, isotonic enteral formula designed for children 1–6 years of age
Formulas designed for pulmonary patients (45 kcal/oz) NutriVent[g] Pulmocare[c]	Increased fat, decreased carbohydrate enteral designed to reduce CO_2 production

[a]All formulas are 20 kcal/oz unless otherwise indicated.
[b]Mead Johnson Nutrition Division, Evanston, IN.
[c]Ross Laboratories, Columbus, OH.
[d]Wyeth Laboratories, Philadelphia, PA.
[e]Carnation Company, Los Angeles, CA.
[f]Norwich Eaton Pharmaceuticals, Norwich, NY.
[g]Clintec Nutrition Company, Deerfield, IL.
[h]Recommend administering at diluted strength (i.e., two-thirds to three-fourths strength) if administered to toddlers or young children, with appropriate adjustments made in vitamin and mineral supplementation. If elemental feedings are the sole source of nutrition, one must ensure that essential fatty acid requirements are met.
From Ernst JA, Gross SJ. Types and methods of feeding for infants. In Polin RA, Fox WM, eds. *Fetal and neonatal physiology.* Philadelphia, WB Saunders, 1991, pp 257–276.

increased further by supplementing the formula with modular components (e.g., glucose polymers [Polycose, Ross Laboratories] and/ or MCT or vegetable oil). Care must be taken to balance the distribution of calories from protein, carbohydrate, and fat so that steatorrhea from excess fat or osmotic diarrhea from a too-high carbohydrate load is prevented. It is also important to avoid protein inadequacy (ratio of protein per unit of energy) from dilution of the formula with fat and carbohydrate. Calorically dense infant formula recipes with acceptable ranges of carbohydrate, protein, and fat are presented in Table 61.9. Providing fat as the predominant energy source, 50–55% of daily caloric intake, and restricting carbohydrate to 25–30% of total calories, improves caloric intake without overwhelming the lung's capacity to exhale CO_2. Since fat constitutes the most calorically dense substrate at 9 kcal/g with the lowest RQ (0.7), adding additional calories to the formula as fat facilitates meeting the greater energy needs of the infant with BPD by increasing the caloric concentration without excess CO_2 production. Since infants with BPD frequently have difficulty tolerating increased fluid volumes, the approach to increasing calories is based on increasing concentration rather than volume. The caloric density may be increased gradually to 30 kcal/oz, depending on response to the lower caloric density formula. Rarely does one need to exceed 30 kcal/oz in order to achieve acceptable growth.

Other researchers investigated the association of specific nutrient deficiencies and development of BPD. Shenai et al. (39) hypothesized that vitamin A deficiency may lead to BPD. Vitamin A augments epithelial tissue repair through inducing differentiation of basal epithelium into the appropriate mucosal cell type and preventing replication of fibroblasts. The researchers supplemented 40 VLBW infants with either intramuscular vitamin A or a saline placebo and demonstrated reduced lung disease in the supplemented group. Further studies are required to investigate the potential for vitamin A administration to reduce the incidence of chronic pulmonary disease in preterm infants. Vitamin E (alpha tocopherol) has not been shown to prevent or ameliorate BPD. Still, many neonatologists advocate following serum vitamin E levels and correcting any deficiency (< 0.5 mg/dl)

because of vitamin E's important role as an oxygen free-radical scavenger and membrane stabilizer (40). Megadoses of vitamins should be avoided because of possible deleterious affects. It should be noted that many of the studies published on nutrition as it relates to BPD consist of small populations, and further investigation continues to be done in this area.

For the older infant with BPD, long-term nutritional management may include the placement of an enteral tube (e.g., gastrostomy tube) to assist in part, or entirely, with feeding the infant. A decision to incorporate long-term tube feedings into the care plan is frequently resisted by families who are most interested in the life of an infant who has been through so much already. However, a careful explanation of the risks of malnutrition and the benefits of tube feeding in terms of increasing caloric intake will usually convince parents of the necessity of such a seemingly aggressive therapeutic approach. Infants with BPD are often developmentally delayed, with dysfunctional swallowing and/or feeding refusal further interfering with their ability to consume orally the increased quantities of formula required for growth. The issue of feeding refusal should not be minimized in these patients since eliminating the refusal will facilitate the nutritional plan, avoiding (it is hoped) the use of enteral tubes. A feeding team may need to be consulted to work with difficult infant and parent. Caloric delivery should be carefully evaluated and revised as needed since the nutritional goal is to promote a steady rate of weight gain and linear growth while maintaining the patient's weight for length within an appropriate range (i.e., 50th–90th percentile). Since infants fed through enteral tubes cannot control their own energy intake, patient nutritional status should be closely followed to prevent obesity.

ASTHMA

Cohen et al. (41) initially described the association between chronic asthma and short stature in 1940. Both cross-sectional and longitudinal studies confirmed growth delay in asthmatics. A study of longitudinal growth patterns of 531 asthmatic boys over 11 years in a residential school for asthmatics demonstrated growth delay associated with delayed puberty. These boys entered puberty at a later age with relative short stature, which cor-

Table 61.9.
Calorically Dense Infant Formula Recipes

Formula Caloric Density	Measures in Hospital	Household Measures	Distribution of Calories		
			% Pro	% CHO	% Fat
24 kcal/oz Using liquid concentrate	145 ml formula liquid concentrate 95 ml water Yields 240 ml	13 oz formula liquid concentrate (1 can) 9 oz water Yields 22 oz	9–12	40–43	47–50
24 kcal/oz Using formula powder	1 cup (120–140 g)[a] formula powder 690 ml water Yields 780 ml *or*, for a smaller volume: 1 scoop (8.3–9.7 g)[a] formula powder 48 cc's water Yields 55 ml	1 cup formula powder 23 oz water Yields 26 oz *or*, for a smaller volume: 2 scoops formula powder 3 oz water Yields 3$\frac{1}{2}$ oz	9–14	35–52	40–50
27 kcal/oz Made with added fat	240 ml 24 kcal/oz formula 3.2 ml MCT[b] or vegetable oil	13 oz formula liquid concentrate (1 can) 9 oz water 2 teaspoons MCT or vegetable oil *or* 1 cup formula powder 23 oz water 2$\frac{1}{2}$ teaspoons MCT or vegetable oil	7–12	30–46	47–56
27 kcal/oz Made with added carbohydrate	240 ml 24 kcal/oz formula 20 ml Polycose[c] liquid or 7.5 g Polycose powder	13 oz formula liquid concentrate (1 can) 9 oz water 3$\frac{1}{2}$ tablespoons Polycose powder *or* 1 cup formula powder 23 oz water 4 tablespoons Polycose powder	7–11	46–60	33–41
30 kcal/oz Made with added fat and carbohydrate	240 ml 24 kcal/oz formula 3.2 ml MCT or vegetable oil 20 ml Polycose liquid or 7.5 g Polycose powder	13 oz formula liquid concentrate (1 can) 9 oz water 2 teaspoon MCT or vegetable oil 3$\frac{1}{2}$ tablespoons Polycose powder *or* 1 cup formula powder 23 oz water 2$\frac{1}{2}$ teaspoons MCT or vegetable oil 4 tablespoons Polycose powder	6.5–10	41–53	39–46

[a]Gram weight/scoop or cup varies with type of formula
[b]MCT Oil (Medium Chain Triglyceride) (Oil), Mead Johnson Nutritional Division, Evansville, IN
[c]Polycose (Glucose Polymers), Ross Laboratories, Columbus, OH
Adapted from Ernst JA, Gross SJ. Types and methods of feeding for infants. In Polin RA, For WM, eds. *Fetal and neonatal physiology*. Phildelphia, WB Saunders, 1991, pp 257–276.

rected after the delayed pubertal growth spurt was completed (42). Cross-sectional studies identified the risk factors for retarded growth in asthmatics: early age of onset, frequent episodes of wheezing, low arterial oxygen saturation, anorexia, reduced spirometry, and chest deformity (43). A review of the medical records of approximately 3400 asthmatics examined for the Israeli military at age 17 found that these adolescents had demonstrated retarded growth and maturation but did ultimately reach normal height and weight (44). Weight and height were more retarded in the severe asthmatics, although this difference was not significant. Balfour-Lynn demonstrated this in a 13-year prospective study of 66 children with chronic asthma; weight gain tended to be reduced in the more severe asthmatics; however, only one-half of the children demonstrated growth retardation secondary to the decelerated growth velocity of delayed puberty (45). After the onset of puberty, all the children attained predicted adult height. Although some of the studies anecdotally describe anorexia and poor weight gain during acute attacks and in the severe asthmatics, none has measured nutritional status in asthmatics. Other studies investigated the effects of asthma on dietary intake, energy requirements, and subsequently long-term growth.

Some medications used to treat asthma are associated with adverse affects on linear velocity. Growth suppression is a known complication associated with steroid therapy. Wolthers and Pederson (46) performed a random double-blind crossover trial investigating linear growth by measuring lower leg lengths of asthmatics taking either placebo or prednisolone (2.5 mg or 5.0 mg twice each day) for 2 weeks. By allowing patients to serve as their own control, the investigators demonstrated the short-term growth suppressive effect of steroids, especially seen with the higher prednisolone dose. Oberger (47) followed 40 children with asthma severe enough to require long-term glucocorticoid or ACTH therapy, and observed linear stunting continuing into adulthood in patients receiving long-term prednisolone therapy. Withdrawal of the glucocorticoid prior to the pubertal growth spurt was associated with the achievement of normal adult height. Inhaled steroids do not seem to exert the same detrimental affect on growth.

Brown et al. (48) retrospectively reviewed growth data on 82 asthmatic children treated with triamcinolone aerosol for 1 year. These height velocities equaled the predicted rate for healthy children of the same age and gender. Other studies also suggest little or no effect of inhaled corticosteroids on the linear growth velocity of children with asthma. None of these studies addressed the interaction of steroid-induced appetite stimulation, dietary intake, and nutritional status.

Investigators have also studied the affects of theophylline therapy on growth. Initial studies challenged healthy children with theophylline to study short-term pharmacologic action on growth hormone (GH) secretion. Theophylline blunted the growth hormone response to stimulation tests, along with diminishing the basal GH secretion in normal subjects (49). Few long-term studies investigated the effect of theophylline on growth hormone levels in asthmatics. Tokuyama et al. (50) studied the effects of theophylline on the growth hormone dependent peptide, insulin-like growth factor 1 (IGF-1). They did not find a statistical difference in IGF-1 levels between asthmatics with and without theophylline therapy. Further studies will be required to determine the etiology of growth delay in asthmatics. The impact of asthma and therapeutic interventions on the energy requirements, nutrient intake, and overall nutritional status of the patient still need to be elucidated.

CONCLUSIONS

Principles of nutritional assessment apply to the examination of the chronically ill child. Adequate nutrition serves as the vital force in stimulating growth and development. Following the pattern of weight gain, linear velocity, and head circumference growth proves a tool to detect changes in the patient's condition. Especially in children with chronic disease, adequate nutritional support provides a crucial component of the total therapeutic regimen. As this chapter illustrates, the disease state and associated therapy impact on the patient's nutritional requirements and growth velocity. Early identification of these interactions and aggressive nutritional intervention may prevent growth failure and improve overall prognosis.

REFERENCES

1. LeLeiko NS, Stawski C, Benkou K, Luder E, NcNierney M. Nutrition assessment of the pediatric patient. In Grand RJ, Stuphen JL, Dietz WH, eds. Boston, Butterworth, 1987, pp 395–420.
2. Walker WA, Hendricks KM. *Manual of pediatric nutrition.* Philadelphia, WB Saunders, 1985, pp 1–62.
3. Gibson RS. *Principles of nutritional assessment.* New York, Oxford University Press, 1990.
4. Roche AF, Himes JH. Incremental growth charts. *Am J Clin Nutr* 1980; 33:2041–2052.
5. Baumgartner RN, Roche AF, Himes JH. Incremental growth tables: Supplementary to previously published charts. *Am J Clin Nutr* 1986; 43:711–722.
6. Roe DA, Campbell TC, eds. *Drugs and nutrients: The interactive effects.* New York, Marcel Dekker, 1984.
7. Corey M, McLaughlin FJ, Williams M. A comparison of survival growth and pulmonary function inpatients with cystic fibrosis in Boston and Toronto. *J Clin Epidimiol* 1988; 41:583–591.
8. Cameron N. The methods of auxological anthropometry. In Falkner F, Tanner JM, eds. *Human growth. A comprehensive treatise,* vol 3. New York, Plenum Press, 1986, pp 3–46.
9. Falkner F, Tanner JM, eds. *Human growth,* vol 2. New York, Plenum Press, 1978.
10. Hamill PVV, Drizd TA, Johnson CL, Reed RB, Roche AF, Moore WM. Physical growth: National Center for Health Statistics percentiles. *Am J Clin* 1979; 32:607–629.
11. Waterlow JC. Classification and definition of protein calorie malnutrition. *Br Med J* 1972; 566.
12. Frisancho AR. New norms of upper limb fat and muscle area for assessment of nutritional status. *Am J Clin Nutr* 1981; 34:2540–2545.
13. Tanner JM, Davis PSW. Clinical longitudinal standards for height and height velocity for North American children. *Pediatrics* 1985; 107:317–329.
14. Hamill PVV, Drizd TA, Johnson CL, Reed RB, Roche AF, Moore WM. Physical Growth National Center for Health Statistics percentiles. *Am J Clin Nutr* 1979; 32:607–629.
15. National Research Council Food and Nutrition Board. *Recommended dietary allowance,* 10th ed. Washington, DC, National Academy of Sciences, 1989.
16. Beal VA. Nutritional intake. In McCammon RW, ed. *Human growth and development.* Springfield, IL, Charles C Thomas, 1970, pp 63–100.
17. FAO/WHO/UNO Expert Consultation. *Energy and protein requirements.* Geneva, Would Health Organization 1985, pp 71–112.
18. Forstner G, Durie PR. Cystic fibrosis. In Walker VA, Durie PR, Hamilton JR, Walker-Smith J, Watkins J, eds. *Pediatric gastrointestinal disease.* Philadelphia, BC Decker, 1991, pp 1179–1197.
19. Lloyd–Still JD. Cystic fibrosis. In Lebenthal E, ed. *Textbook of gastroenterology and nutrition.* New York, Raven Press, 1989, p 831.
20. Luder E. Kattan, Thornton J, Koehler K, Bonforte R. Efficacy of a nonrestricted fat diet in patients with cystic fibrosis. *Arch Dis Child* 1989; 143:458–464.
21. Forstner G, Durie P. Nutrition in cystic fibrosis. In Grand R, Stuphen S, Dietz W, eds. *Pediatric nutrition.* Boston, Butterworth, 1987, pp 501–512.
22. Roy CC, Darling P, Weber A. A rational approach to meeting macro and micronutrient needs in cystic fibrosis. *J Pediatr Gastro Nutr* 1984; 3(Suppl):S154.
23. Vaisman N, Pencharz P, Corey M, Canny G, Hahn E. Energy expenditure of patients with cystic fibrosis. *J Pediatr* 1987; 111:496–500.
24. Shepherd R, Vasques-Velasquez L, Prentice A, Holt T, Coward W, Lucas A. Increased energy expenditure in patients with cystic fibrosis. *Lancet* 1988; 1:1300–1303.
25. Durie PR, Pencharz PB. A rational approach to the nutritional care of patients with cystic fibrosis. *J Roy Soc Med* 1989; 82:11–20.
26. Ramsey BW, Farrell PM, Pencharz P, et al. Nutritional assessment and management in cystic fibrosis: A consensus report. *Am J Clin Nutr* 1992; 55:108–116.
27. Beker LT, Fink RJ, Chaney H, Kluft J, Schidlow D, Evans E. The efficacy of high-dose pancrease MT in the treatment of steatorrhea. *Pediatr Pulmonol* 1990; 5:26S(290).
28. Brady MS, Rickard K, Yu P, Eigen H. Effectiveness and safety a of small versus large doses of enteric-coated pancreatic enzymes in reducing steatorrhea in children with cystic fibrosis: A prospective randomized study. *Pediatr Pulmonol* 1991; 10:79–85.
29. O'Loughlin E, Forbes D, Parsons H, Scott B, Cooper D, Gall G. Nutritional rehabilitation of malnourished patients with cystic fibrosis. *Am J Clin Nutr* 1986; 43:732–737.
30. Shepherd RW, Holt TL, Thomas BJ et al. Nutritional rehabilitation in cystic fibrosis: Controlled studies of effects on nutritional growth retardation, body protein turnover, and course of pulmonary disease. *J Pediatr* 1986; 109:788–794.
31. Kane RE, Hobbs PJ, Black PG. Comparison of low, medium and high carbohydrate formulas for night-time enteral feedings in cystic fibrosis patients. *JPEN* 1990; 14:47–52.
32. Frank L, Sosenko I. Undernutrition as a major contributing factor to the pathogenesis of bronchopulmonary dysplasia. *Am Rev Respir Dis* 1988; 138:725–729.
33. Georgieff M, Mills M, Lindeke L, Iverson S, Johnson D, Thompson T. Changes in nutritional management and outcome of very-low-birth-weight infants. *Am J Dis Child* 1989; 143:82–85.
34. Ziegler EE, O'Donnell AM, Nelson SE, Famon SJ. Body composition of the reference fetus. *Growth* 1976; 40:329–334.
35. Guo S, Roche AF, Famon SJ, et al. Reference data on gains in weight and length during the first two years of life. *J Pediatr* 1991; 119:355–362.
36. Covelli HD. Respiratory failure precipitated by high carbohydrate loads. *Ann Intern Med* 1981; 95:579–581.
37. Wienstein MR, Oh W. Oxygen consumption in infants with bronchopulmonary dysplasia. *J Pediatr* 1981; 99:958–961.
38. Yanis KA, Oh W. Effects of intravenous glucose loading on oxygen consumption, carbon dioxide production and resting energy expenditure in infants with bronchopulmonary dysplasia. *J Pediatr* 1989; 115:127–130.
39. Shenai JP, Kennedy K, Chytil F, Stahlman M. Clinical trial of vitamin A supplementation in infants sus-

ceptible to bronchopulmonary dysplasia in the tiny infant. *Clin Perinatol* 1986; 13:315–327.

40. Escobedo MB, Gonzalez A. Bronchopulmonary dysplasia in the tiny infant. *Clin Perinatol* 1986; 13:315–327.

41. Cohen M, Welles R, Cohen S. Anthropometry in Children. Progress in allergic children as shown by increments in height, weight and maturity. *Am J Dis Child* 1940; 60:1058–1061.

42. Huaspie R, Suzanne C, Alexander F. A mixed longitudinal study of the growth in height and weight in asthmatic children. *Hum Biol* 1976; 48:271–274.

43. Preece MA, Law CM, Davies PSW. The growth of children with chronic pediatric disease. *Clin Endo Metab* 1986; 15:453–471.

44. Shohat M, Shohat T, Kedem R, Mimouni M, Danon YL. Childhood asthma and growth outcome. *Arch Dis Child* 1987; 62:63–65.

45. Balfour–Lynn L. Growth and childhood asthma. *Arch Dis Child* 1986; 61:1049–1055.

46. Wolthers OD, Pedersen S. Short term linear growth in asthmatic children during treatment with prednisone. *Br Med J* 1990; 301:145–147.

47. Oberger E, Engstrom I, Karlberg J. Long term treatment with glucocorticoids/ACTH in asthmatic children. *Acta Paediatr Scand* 1990; 79:77–83.

48. Brown DCP, Savacool Am, Letizia CM. A retrospective review of the effects of one year of triamcinolone acetonide aerosol treatment on the growth patterns of asthmatic children. *Ann Allergy* 1989; 63:47–51.

49. Losa M, Huss R, Konig A, et al Theophylline blunts the GH response to growth hormone releasing hormone in normal subjects. *Acta Endocrinol* 1986; 112:473–490.

50. Tokuyama K, Nagashima K, Yagi H, et al. Effect of theophylline on insulin-like growth factor 1 in children with asthma. *J Pediatr* 1987; 111:612–614.

51. Ernst JA, Gross SJ. Types and methods of feeding for infants. In Polin RA, Fox WM, eds. *Fetal and neonatal physiology.* Philadelphia, WB Saunders, 1991, pp 257–276.

62

Chest Physical Therapy: New Techniques

MAGGIE McILWAINE

Increasingly, physical therapy is being prescribed by the physician as an important component in the overall management of respiratory conditions. Yet only within the past decade has adequate research been conducted to allow proper assessment and identification of the efficacy of techniques in the treatment of pediatric respiratory conditions.

The purpose of this chapter is to identify for the physician those pediatric patients and respiratory conditions that benefit significantly from physical therapy intervention. It also discusses the relative benefits of a variety of physical therapy techniques currently being applied in the treatment of specific respiratory conditions. The goals of chest physical therapy are to prevent respiratory complications and improve pulmonary function through the following measures: (a) maintaining normal movement of the thorax, (b) strengthening and re-educating the muscles of respiration, (c) mobilizing secretions, and (d) maintaining or improving exercise tolerance. It is hoped that by understanding these goals, the physician can identify problems that may be alleviated through the use of physical therapy. The first part of this chapter describes the various physical therapy techniques used in the treatment of pediatric patients with respiratory dysfunction. The second part of this chapter discusses the application of these techniques to specific respiratory conditions.

PHYSICAL THERAPY TECHNIQUES

The six most common physical therapy techniques used to treat pediatric patients are (a) positioning, (b) bronchial drainage, (c) huffing, coughing, suctioning, (d) breathing exercises (e) postural and thoracic mobility exercises, and (f) physical exercise.

Positioning

Proper positioning of the patient can assist in mobilizing secretions, thereby improving ventilation and oxygenation. Postural changes affect regional ventilation differently in children and adults. When adults are positioned on their sides, ventilation and perfusion are increased to the dependent lung. However, the opposite occurs in infants and young children. Studies of infants between the ages of 2 days and 2 years have shown that ventilation is preferentially distributed to the uppermost lung regardless of any lung disease (1, 2). Thus by placing a young child with unilateral lung disease in side-lying position with the unaffected lung uppermost, oxygen saturation will be improved. However, when the affected lung needs to be placed uppermost, as in children requiring postural drainage to clear secretions, care must be taken to avoid oxygen desaturation. Further research is needed to determine the age at which the adult pattern first emerges.

Other methods of positioning may also improve oxygen saturation. Studies of neonates with respiratory distress syndrome (RDS) (3) have found that by simply turning the patient from supine to prone position, arterial oxygenation is usually increased. Positioning as an aid to clearing secretions will be discussed under bronchial drainage techniques.

Bronchial Drainage Techniques

POSTURAL DRAINAGE WITH PERCUSSION (CONVENTIONAL CPT)

Conventional CPT consists of placing the patient in various gravity-assisted positions to drain secretions from the affected segments of the lung. While the patient is in these positions, other auxiliary techniques are applied. The chest wall is percussed over the lung segment being drained, followed by vibration of the chest wall on expiration. In some patients, vibration alone may be the choice of treatment. In the patient who is able to cooperate, percussion and vibration are followed by deep breathing, huffing, and coughing (4) (Fig. 62.1). Modification of these techniques will vary depending on the age and condition of the patient.

In studies conducted to assess the benefits of postural drainage with percussion, it has been noted that airway obstruction can be reduced and pulmonary function improved in patients with excessive bronchial secretions (5–7). In addition, in a 3-year study (8) with cystic fibrosis (CF) patients, pulmonary function declined at a faster rate when postural drainage was discontinued in favor of breathing exercises only.

In patients with chronic obstructive lung disease, a home program of postural drainage and percussion may have to be instituted. However, experience has shown that there is a high degree of noncompliance in these patients arising from the need for the assis-

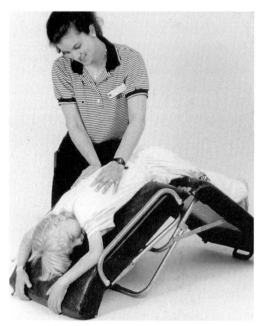

Figure 62.1. Patient receiving postural drainage, percussion and vibration, using a postural drainage board.

tance of a second person, the level of discomfort experienced in being placed in various positions, and the time it takes to perform the treatment (9). In the 1980s, in an attempt to increase the level of compliance and enhance the removal of secretions, four new techniques emerged, namely: (a) active cycle of breathing, (b) autogenic drainage, (c) low-pressure positive expiratory pressure (PEP), and (d) oscillating PEP-flutter. The use of these alternative techniques has mostly been confined to Europe, but gradually they are gaining acceptance on the North American continent, particularly for patients in whom conventional CPT has proven ineffectual.

ACTIVE CYCLE OF BREATHING (ACB)

ACB, formerly referred to as the "forced expiration technique," combines an active cycle of breathing exercises with postural drainage. It may also include a degree of auto percussion. In the active cycle of breathing, the patient is required to inhale to mid lung volume followed by a forced expiration down to low lung volume, repeated once or twice and interspersed with periods of controlled diaphramatic breathing. When secretions are mobilized they are cleared with a huff from high lung volume.

The theory of ACB is based on the equal pressure point principle—that is, huffing puts pressure on the airways, causing them to compress. As the patient huffs from a mid to low lung volume this causes a wave of compression to move downstream, thus pushing secretions upstream toward the larger airways (10). Pryor and Webber in an extensive study of the technique at the Brompton hospital in England found it to be as effective as conventional CPT in mobilizing secretions (10, 11). Because of the significant level of patient cooperation required for ACB to be effective, it should be introduced only in the older child or adolescent. Although it can be performed independently, the accompanying postural drainage and auto percussion may be undesirable for some patients in spite of their ability to cooperate to the degree required.

AUTOGENIC DRAINAGE (AD)

Autogenic drainage, which means self-drainage, utilizes the expiratory airflow to move secretions. First introduced by Chevaillier to treat asthmatic patients in Belgium, AD is performed in a sitting position (Fig. 62.2). Its objective is to reach the highest possible airflow in the different generations of bronchi through the use of controlled breathing (12, 13). There are three phases to this exercise: (a) low lung volume breathing to "loosen" the peripheral mucus, (b) low to mid lung volume breathing to "collect" the mucus in the middle airways, and (c) mid to high lung volume breathing to "evacuate" the mucus from the central airways (Fig. 62.3). Through proprioceptive, sensory, and auditory signals, the patient quickly learns the level of bronchi at which the secretions are localized. Once secretions are expectorated the sequence is repeated until as much mucus as possible is cleared. At the end of each inspiration a pause of 2–3 seconds ensures equal filling of all lung segments.

The theory behind the AD technique is best explained using flow-volume curves. The flow-volume curves demonstrate that higher flows of longer duration can be achieved while performing the AD technique. As a result, the mucus moves centrally at a more rapid rate and for a longer duration during expiration (13). Published short- and long-term studies comparing AD to other drainage techniques have found AD to be highly effective in clearing secretions in patients with asthma and CF (14–17). These studies have also shown that AD mobilized significantly more sputum than conventional CPT or ACB. In particular, AD has been shown to be very useful in mobilizing secretions when conventional CPT has been ineffective. Such patients tend to be those with reactive airway disease or who have easily compressible large airways (PEP is also very effective with the latter patient—see the discussion below under "PEP").

Like ACB, AD demands a high degree of patient concentration and self-discipline. It is therefore not recommended for the younger child. Since it is performed in the sitting position and does not require any equipment, it can be done anywhere. However, a physical therapist trained in the principles of AD is required to teach the technique effectively.

POSITIVE EXPIRATORY PRESSURE (PEP)

The PEP mask was first used as a method to re-expand collapsed portions of the lung in postoperative patients (18). However, it also proved to have secretion removal effects. The PEP mask utilizes a one-way valve with a resistor attached to the expiratory valve, producing a positive pressure within the lungs of 10–20 cm of water. The patient is positioned sitting in a chair, with arms resting on a table, as he breathes in and out through the mask 10–15 times. This is followed by forced expiration maneuvers consisting of huffing interspersed with relaxed diaphragmatic breathing with the mask removed. The entire cycle is repeated five or six times or until as much sputum is cleared as possible (Fig. 62.4). The underlying theory of PEP is that by using the collateral ventilation channels (pores of Kohn and canals of Lambert) to allow the air to move behind the obstruction, the secretions are forced centrally towards the larger airways (19).

Patients with reactive airway disease or who otherwise require a bronchodilator prior to physical therapy can be given the nebulized bronchodilator through the PEP mask. In patients with severe bronchospasm, this method of delivery has been shown to be the most effective means of administration (20,

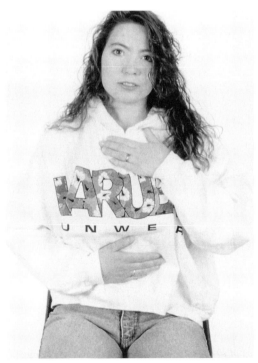

Figure 62.2. Patient performing autogenic drainage, using hands for proprioceptive feedback.

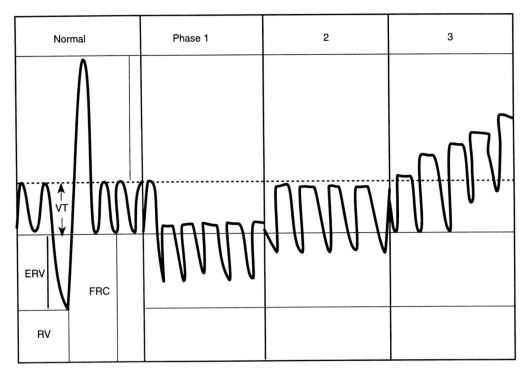

Figure 62.3. Phases of autogenic drainage shown on a spirogram of a normal person. *Phase 1:* loosen, or unstick, phase. *2:* collect. *3:* evacute. (Vt = tidal volume, ERV = expiratory reserve volume, RV = reserve volume, FRC = functional residual capacity, IRV = inspiratory reserve volume).

21) because of better dispersment in the peripheral airways.

Both short- and long-term studies comparing PEP to conventional CPT (15, 22, 23) report no significant difference in pulmonary function or sputum production between either technique. However, PEP has the advantage of being the easiest method to teach and perform. It requires no assistance and can be performed in any environment. It may even be used with young children once they have learned to huff effectively. For patients with gastroesophageal reflux, in whom postural drainage in the Trendelenburg position may increase the tendency to aspirate, PEP may be used as an alternative form of therapy. It is also well accepted by the patient with advanced disease who does not tolerate conventional CPT due to oxygen desaturation during postural drainage positions or for whom percussion is too painful.

OSCILLATING PEP-FLUTTER

The Flutter VRP1 is a pocket device that generates a controlled oscillating positive pressure and interrupts expiratory flow when one breathes out through it. The device is made of a mouthpiece, a plastic cone, a steel ball, and a perforated protective cover.

Although several studies have been conducted to assess the effect of the Flutter VRP1, to date *none have yielded postitive results.* Several other studies are currently underway, but until there is postitive literature to support the use of the Flutter device, *the Flutter should not be used as an alternative form of physiotherapy.* It may be helpful in some cases, but should only then be used as an adjunct to other forms of therapy.

Huffing, Coughing, Suctioning

The patient should be able to cough and clear secretions that have been mobilized to the upper respiratory tract using any of the above bronchial drainage techniques. Problems arise, however, when patients are unable to cough, which results in partial obstruction caused by pooling of secretions in the larger airways (25). (For causes of ineffective cough see Table 62.1.) Huffing, assisted cough,

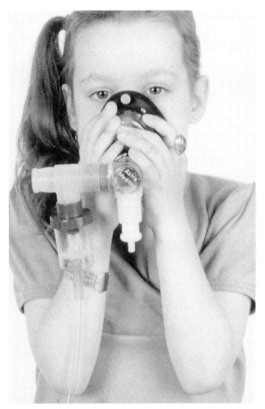

Figure 62.4. Patient using a positive expiratory pressure mask with a nebulizer containing a bronchodilator connected to the inspiratory valve and a resistor connected to the expiratory valve.

Table 62.1.
Causes of Ineffective Coughing

Causes	Conditions
Weak abdominal and respiratory muscles	Neuromuscular disease Spinal cord injury Cerebral palsy Prolonged mechanical ventilation
Brain dysfunction	Unconscious patient Head injury Cerebral palsy
Pain	Postoperative patients Trauma
Bronchospasm	Chronic obstructive airway disease
Premature airway closure	Asthma

tracheal stimulation, or suctioning can assist the patient to expectorate secretions when there is an impaired cough. Huffing is more effectual in patients with high closing volumes. For these patients, controlled huffing stabilizes the airways while moving secretions (10).

Tracheal stimulation (26) is effective with the young child who does not understand the concept of coughing. It does, however, require a physical therapist trained in the technique. Suctioning is a traumatic, invasive technique that may induce atelectasis, bronchospasm, bradycardia, or hypoxia (27), and should be used only as a last resort. In the unconscious patient or the young child with copious secretions in the upper airways, however, it may be the only effective method of clearing the secretions.

Breathing Exercises

Breathing exercises as a technique of physical therapy have been used since World War I with the objectives of the promotion of a normal relaxed pattern of breathing, re-expansion of aveoli, improvement in both ventilation and oxygenation, and mobilization of the thoracic cage. There are several types of breathing exercises, which are discussed below.

DIAPHRAGMATIC BREATHING

With the patient in a relaxed half-lying position and the abdominal wall relaxed, the exercise emphasizes gentle diaphragmatic breathing with a minimum of effort and the avoidance of accessory muscle action. Expiration should be passive (4). Although the effectiveness of this exercise continues to be controversial, it has proven effective in improving lower lung zone ventilation in well trained patients (28). Most noticable is its effect in reducing the rate of postoperative pulmonary complications (29). However, it has failed to alter the distribution of ventilation in chronically obstructed patients (30).

INCENTIVE INSPIROMETERS

The incentive inspirometer is a breathing apparatus that provides the patient with visual feedback of the volume of air inspired during maximal inspiration. It is used as an adjunct to breathing exercises. The patient is encouraged to practice deep inspiration with the inspirometer, pausing for 3 seconds at the end of inspiration to allow for even filling of all segments of the lung. Inspirometers have been most successfully used in the treatment of postoperative atelectasis (31).

SEGMENTAL BREATHING

Segmental breathing exercises presume that inspired air can be directed at a predetermined area. Studies have failed to show any change in the distribution of ventilation using this method (32). Effectiveness is therefore very doubtful.

Postural and Thoracic Mobility Exercises

Thoracic mobility and postural re-education exercises are important components of physical therapy in patients with chronic obstructive lung disease. These patients often present with round shoulders, kyphotic posture, and barrel-shaped chest produced by chronic hyper-inflation due to air trapping and an abnormal breathing pattern. If this condition is left untreated, vertebral wedging with resulting back pain may occur (33). It is important to reduce the degree of air trapping by other means prior to the commencement of these exercises.

Physical Exercise

In the normal child, physical exercise has been associated with improved cardiovascular and metabolic function as well as a more positive self-esteem and improved mental condition (34). Children with chronic lung disease tend to remain sedentary, resulting in decreased cardiovascular fitness and endurance (35). Research now shows that these patients may safely engage in some form of physical exercise and, although pulmonary function tests may not be improved, respiratory muscle function and exercise capacity are generally enhanced, particularly with running and swimming (36, 37). In patients with severe respiratory disease the limiting factor tends to be ventilation rather than heart rate. Although most of these patients can tolerate even maximal exercise without significant oxygen desaturation, patients with a forced expiratory volume in 1 second (FEV_1) of less than 50% of FVC should have an exercise test performed with

oximetry before undertaking a physical exercise program (38). Any physical exercise prescription for children with pulmonary disease should include stretching, strengthening, and aerobic components.

APPLICATIONS IN DISEASE

The second part of this chapter discusses the application of the physical therapy techniques described above, in the management of specific pediatric respiratory conditions (see Table 62.2 for an overview).

Aspiration

Common causes of aspiration into the lungs include meconium aspiration, aspiration of foreign body, tracheoesophageal fistula, gastroesophageal reflux, and near-drowning. The appropriate treatment depends on the cause of the aspiration. For example, aspiration of a foreign body first necessitates its immediate removal. A tracheoesophageal fistula requires immediate surgical repair when possible. However, the medical management of these patients can be assisted by using a combination of bronchial drainage, breathing exercise, and positioning (Fig. 62.5, 62.6).

Foreign Body Aspiration

Physical therapy should never be used as a method of removing a foreign body from the lungs, since it can lead to cardiopulmonary arrest (39). Bronchoscopy is the recommended treatment. Physical therapy techniques beginning with bronchial drainage being applied to the affected area can and should be started as soon as the foreign body is removed and continued until the pneumonic process has resolved. Deep breathing exercises and the use of inspirometers will aid re-expansion of those collapsed portions of the lung distal to the aspirated foreign body. Occasionally, when aspiration of a foreign body has gone unrecognized, lung damage with bronchiectasis may occur (40), in which case bronchial drainage should be continued for an indefinite period.

Gastroesophageal Reflux (GER)

GER is common in patients with cystic fibrosis, bronchopulmonary dysplasia, or cerebral palsy, and in patients with other abnormal neurologic deficits. The main concern with

Table 62.2.
Use of Physical Therapy Techniques in the Treatment of Pediatric Respiratory Conditions.

Conditions	Physical Therapy Techniques			
	Positioning	Bronchial Drainage	Breathing Exercises	Posture Exercise
ASPIRATION				
Pneumonia	Yes	Yes	Yes	No
Foreign Body	Post Removal	Post Removal	Yes	No
TE Fistula	Depends on type	Modified	Too Young	No
ASTHMA				
Early stage	Maybe	No	No	No
Chronic stage	Yes	Only if secretions present	Yes	Yes
BRONCHIECTASIS	Yes	Yes	Yes	Yes
BRONCHOPULMONARY DYSPLASIA	Yes	Only if secretions present	Too Young	Maybe when older
CYSTIC FIBROSIS	Yes	Yes	Yes	Yes
RESPIRATORY TRACT INFECTIONS				
Bronchiolitis				
Early stage	Yes	No	Too young	No
Later	Yes	Only if secretions present		No
Pneumonia	Yes	Only if secretions present	Maybe	Yes

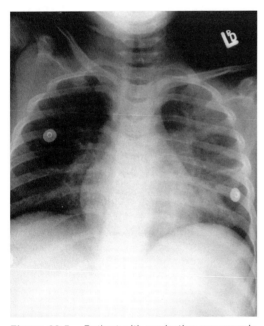

Figure 62.5. Patient with aspiration pneumonia affecting the left lingula.

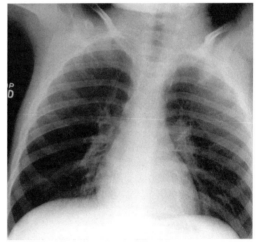

Figure 62.6. Same patient as in Figure 62.5, 3 weeks later. Treatment consisted of antibiotics and physical therapy.

GER is that the gastric contents of the stomach may be aspirated into the lungs, causing aspiration pneumonitis.

Because of continued reflux in patients with GER, the physical therapy treatment program may need to be adjusted in the following ways.

When the lower lung is affected, bronchial drainage may necessitate a modified side-lying position, and should be performed no earlier than 1 hour after a meal and preferably beforehand. In the older child, PEP may be used as an alternative technique. Conservative medical management may require the child to remain in an upright prone position of 30° after feeding, thereby lessening the tendency to reflux (41). For infants, the prone position also encourages extensor muscle activity and strengthening, which is of benefit in motor development. This is particularly important in treating the neurologically impaired infant or any patient experiencing prolonged periods of hospitalization, and for whom developmental delay is a significant problem. The physical therapy program should also include developmental stimulation.

Asthma

Physical therapy treatment of asthma depends on the condition of the patient at the time of referral. In an acute attack, medical treatment with drug therapy is of primary importance. However, physical therapy can assist in reducing the severity of the attack (42) through the use of relaxation and controlled diaphragmatic breathing, resulting in more efficient breathing control.

ACUTE ATTACK

During the bronchodilator therapy, physical therapy should be directed toward reassurance and relaxation only. Any other physical therapy intervention is contraindicated until the medications have taken effect. Thereafter, the patient can be encouraged in gentle breathing exercises with emphasis on exhalation, in a side-lying position. In this position the accessory muscles are stabilized and the patient more effectively uses his or her diaphragm during inspiration. Other relaxation positions may be used as the patient regains some control of his or her breathing pattern (43) (see Fig. 62.7). Removal of secretions, if present, is important in order to avoid severe lung obstruction as well as secondary consolidation and atelectasis. Postural drainage and percussion are contraindicated in the acute stage as they are likely to induce more bronchospasm (44). The method of choice is either gentle vibrations in a half side-lying position or autogenic drainage used in a sitting position (13).

CHRONIC STAGE

In the chronic stage, the goal of physical therapy is to prevent or at least minimize asthmatic attacks by educating both parent and child in methods to abort and control attacks. This can be achieved, in part, by teaching them about the disease in general and about effective and efficient breathing control in a relaxed position. Correcting posture and maintaining thoracic mobility are also important components, along with teaching confident participation in physical exercise (45). Methods to abort an attack include stopping all activity, assuming a relaxed position, and taking prescribed medications, while using controlled diaphragmatic breathing. This breathing technique should not only be used during an acute attack, but should be incorporated into all activities of the patient's life. Because it takes time to become confident in these techniques, it is recommended that the patient enroll in one of the many Family Asthma Programs that exist throughout North America (46).

EXERCISE

The child with exercise-induced asthma can be taught safe participation in exercise by adhering to certain rules. The primary rule is that inhaler medication should always be taken prior to exercise. Next, exercise should begin with a small number of warm-up periods so that the exercise-induced wheeze becomes refractory (47). The physical therapist should follow up to check for correct procedure.

The type of exercise selected and the duration are important considerations because of their varying effect on induced bronchospasm. The greatest degree of bronchospasm occurs with running, less with cycling and walking, and the least with swimming (48). Short periods of low-intensity exercise lasting 2–3 minutes are less likely to cause bronchospasm than continuous exercise of 6–8 minutes' duration (47). The result is that a variety of exercises such as walking, swimming, circuit training, and team games can be incoporated into a conditioning program to improve the physical fitness of asthmatic children and increase their self-confidence.

Bronchopulmonary Dysplasia (BPD)

BPD is a respiratory disease with a multifactorial etiology. It affects infants who require intensive respiratory support, including those infants who receive high concentrations of oxygen and mechanical support as a neonate (49, 50). Patients with BPD are susceptible to developing lower respiratory tract infections, atelectasis, recurrent reflux, aspiration, and

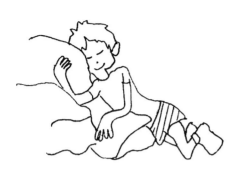

A Side-lying with knees bent, either flat or with head inclined up.

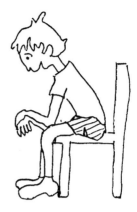

B Sitting on a small stool or chair, forearms resting on knees.

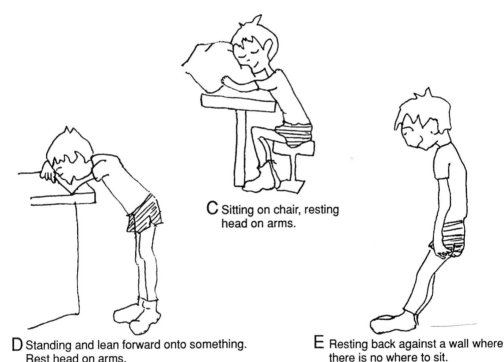

C Sitting on chair, resting head on arms.

D Standing and lean forward onto something. Rest head on arms.

E Resting back against a wall where there is no where to sit.

Figure 62.7. Relaxation positions that may be used for relaxed breathing. *A,* Side-lying with knees bent, either flat or with head inclined up. *B,* Sitting on a small stool or chair, forearms resting on knees. *C,* Sitting on chair resting head on arms. *D,* Stand and lean forward onto something. Rest head on arms. *E,* Resting back against a wall where there is nowhere to sit.

inadequate mucus clearance. Physical therapy is important in preventing atelectasis and in aiding mucus clearance in a manner similar to the previously discussed conditions.

Several studies have proven that physical therapy in BPD immediately following extubation is effective in preventing atelectasis (51, 52). Although there are no studies proving the efficacy of physical therapy as a prophylactic measure in BPD patients after discharge from the hospital, physical therapy should be taught to parents of infants with BPD who have problems in clearing secretions (26). The literature describes a variety of methods used in physical therapy for BPD and respiratory distress syndrome (RDS). They include different combinations of postural drainage, percussion, and vibrations (51–54). Factors determining the appropriate postural drainage positions for a patient include chest radiograph, auscultation findings, and a review of the patient's past course, identifying the most susceptible areas of the lung to disease.

Cystic Fibrosis (CF)

Medical management of the pulmonary disease in CF is directed toward mobilization of secretions and control of pulmonary infection through the use of physical therapy and antibiotics. The importance of physical therapy in the treatment of CF is well documented (55). It utilizes a variety of techniques such as bronchial drainage, breathing exercises, thoracic mobility exercises, and general conditioning exercises, all adapted to meet the needs of the patient with CF.

BRONCHIAL DRAINAGE TECHNIQUES

The technique of combining postural drainage, percussion, vibration, deep breathing, and coughing (collectively referred to as "conventional CPT") was first introduced to the management of CF in the 1950s. It is still the technique of choice and was recently termed the "gold standard" (8). Although ACB, AD, and PEP all have advantages over conventional CPT, and may prove more effective for certain patients, they all require patient participation and therefore cannot be introduced until the patient is 5 or 6 years old. In any event, all patients should be taught the technique of huffing at the earliest possible age, as a method of mobilizing secretions from the large airways. It is important that the physical therapy technique prescribed for any CF patient be tailored by type and frequency to be compatible with the individual's needs. This will enhance compliance (9). Therefore, when assessing the patient, psychologic and social needs should be considered as well as the severity of disease. Nevertheless, it is important to remember that bronchial drainage is prophylactic in keeping the chest clear and also familiarizes the patient with this part of the treatment. For these reasons bronchial drainage should be instituted as soon as the diagnosis is made, at which time both parents

should be instructed in the techniques by an experienced physical therapist. Thereafter, the physical therapy program may be adjusted to the patient's needs. In some instances, twice-daily bronchial drainage would be preferable. Because of the family environment, however, once-daily bronchial drainage may be all that is possible.

Patients with moderate to severe lung disease, who produce sputum regularly, should have bronchial drainage two or three times per day. Patients with mild lung disease may only require bronchial drainage once per day. There are also a few CF patients who, at 10–12 years of age, still have a normal chest radiograph and pulmonary function, and are nonproductive. For these patients, exercise alone may be all that is required as long as they are educated in drainage techniques and understand that if there is any change in lung function, bronchial drainage needs to be re-instituted.

EXERCISE

Although physical exercise is increasingly being advocated as part of the CF regimen, it should not be considered a substitute for bronchial drainage, but merely an adjunct. Only one study has shown exercise on its own to be as effective as bronchial drainage in clearing sputum in patients with mild disease (56). However, in this study the patients had to participate in an extremely intensive program of physical exercise that included 2 hours swimming, a 2-hour hike, and a 10-km jog per day, as well as other activities.

Respiratory Tract Infections

Whether physical therapy is of benefit to patients with respiratory tract infections such as bronchiolitis or pneumonia has been much debated. Today, with health care dollars at a premium, careful consideration should be given to the selection of the theraputic program (i.e., the most beneficial program for the patient) before being prescribed by the physician. This is of particular importance in the use of physical therapy for the treatment of respiratory tract infections. Recent studies have reported that physical therapy may be deleterious to some patients and cause bronchospasm or hypoxia (57, 58).

BRONCHIOLITIS

Existing literature neither supports nor refutes the use of physical therapy in the treatment of bronchilitis. Nevertheless, there are certain guidelines for the physician to follow in determining the likely benefit of physical therapy in the treatment of a patient with bronchiolitis. If scant secretions are present, physical therapy is not indicated, but in cases exhibiting copious secretions that may cause airway obstruction, the pros and cons of physical therapy must be carefully considered. Physical therapy will aid the removal of secretions but may cause bronchospasm or increase hypoxia. Physical therapy should *never* be commenced in the early stages of the disease, when wheeze predominates. During the resolution stage, when secretions are present, a trial of physical therapy, utilizing an oximeter, may prove worthwhile. While monitoring the patient's respiratory status, one can employ a variety of techniques including postural drainage, vibrations in alternate side-lying, and passive autogenic drainage (Fig. 62.8). The patient should be continually assessed to determine which technique results in

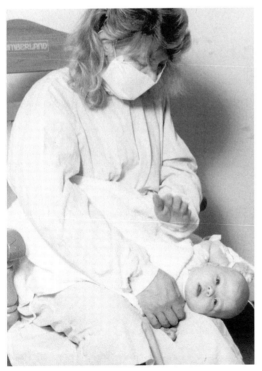

Figure 62.8.   Baby with bronchiolitis receiving postural drainage with percussion on the therapist's lap.

improved respiratory function and patient tolerance.

PNEUMONIA

Physical therapy in the acute stage of uncomplicated lobar pneumonia is ineffective and often is painful. A study by Graham and Bradley (59) concluded that physical therapy did not hasten the resolution of pneumonia in patients who have no other underlying disorder such as bronchiectasis, cystic fibrosis, or aspiration. This finding is now widely accepted in the management of uncomplicated pneumonia (60). Physical therapy may be of benefit when resolution begins and secretions are present. The techniques to be used include bronchial drainage techniques, percussion, vibration, and/or localized breathing exercises. Mechanical vibrations have actually been found to increase arterial oxygenation in acutely ill patients with atelectasis or pneumonia (61).

Because of the different pathology of bronchopneumonia, which is more widespread than lobar pneumonia and characterized by atelectasis and collapse due to increased sputum production, these patients are more successfully managed by physical therapy (62).

Bronchiectasis

Bronchiectasis is a chronic lung condition that usually occurs secondary to an infection, aspiration, BPD, pneumonia, a tumor, or genetic diseases such as cystic fibrosis, agammaglobulinemia, and disorders of the cilia. It is characterized by a persistent cough and copious sputum production. Since bronchial drainage has been shown to be effective when excessive secretions are present (6, 7) a vigorous daily program of physical therapy should be instituted similar to that used for CF. Combined with antibiotics, bronchial drainage is usually effectual in keeping the disease under control. If postural drainage is used, it need only be targeted to the areas that are bronchiectatic. Since ventilation may be severely reduced, or absent in bronchiectasis, care must be taken to avoid hypoxia while performing physical therapy.

Patients with bronchietasis have a limited maximum expiratory flow rate (63), which may result in an ineffective cough. Therefore, once secretions are loosened and mobilized centrally, patients may require instruction on how to expectorate effectively. The best means of achieving this is huffing since it provides stabilization to the airways, enhancing secretion clearance (10). Patients with bronchiectasis should also undergo an exercise evaluation and posture assessment, which should be followed by a program that incorporates these two components of physical therapy.

CONCLUSIONS

As documented in this chapter, research has revealed that physical therapy has proven successful in the management of certain respiratory conditions such as aspiration, CF, and bronchiectasis. However, research has also shown, in other conditions, that it is only effective when certain prerequisites have been met (i.e., in bronchopulmonary dysplasia, bronchiolitis, and pneumonia, secretions need to be present; in asthma and bronchiolitis, the bronchospasm needs to be medically managed prior to the introduction of physical therapy). Finally, there are some patients and certain respiratory conditions for which physical therapy may be of no benefit; in fact, the patient may be adversely effected by its introduction (e.g., in a patient with an acute asthmatic attack, postural drainage will induce bronchospasm). For these reasons, the physician should give careful consideration to the benefits of physical therapy before prescribing it for a patient. Even within those respiratory conditions for which physical therapy has proven beneficial, some techniques have proven more effective than others. This is partly due to the effect that the patient's personality and maturity has on the level of compliance. In some instances, various physical therapy techniques need to be combined to achieve the optimal effect. It is also important that the perscribed techniques are administered by a physical therapist skilled in those techniques.

When properly used, with the appropriate techniques applied to the right condition, physical therapy can be an effective component in the overall management of the patient with respiratory dysfunction.

ACKNOWLEDGMENTS

I would like to thank the entire physiotherapy staff at the British Columbia Children's Hospital for their inspiration and help in writing this chapter. I would particularly like to mention Jennifer Lenard-Granikovas for her contribution to the section on bronchopulmonary dysplasia and Mary Cross, former Director of Physiotherapy, for her support and valued advice. I am also appreciative of the valued academic advice and many ideas provided to me by Dr. Michael Sears, Pauline Bingham, Dr. Mary Bennet, Dr. Domlin Peacock, and Mark Gray. Most important has been the tireless proofreading and support of my husband, Fred Morris.

REFERENCES

1. Heaf DP, et al. Postural effects of gas exchange in infants. *N Engl J Med* 1983; 308:1505.
2. Davies H, et al. Regional ventilation in infancy—Reversal of adult pattern. *N Engl J Med* 1985; 313:1626.
3. Martin RJ, Herrell N, et al. Effect of supine and prone positions on arterial oxygen tension in the preterm infant. *Pediatrics* 1979; 64:528–531.
4. Gaskell DV, Webber BA. *The Brompton Hospital guide to chest physiotherapy*, 4th ed. London, Blackwell Scientific, 1980.
5. Cochrane M, Webber BA, Clarke SW. Effects of sputum on pulmonary function. *Br Med J* 1977; 2:1181–1183.
6. Lorin MI, Denning CR. Evaluation of postural drainage by measurement of sputum volume and consistency. *Am J Phys Med* 1971; 50:215.
7. Murray JF. The ketchup bottle method. *N Engl J Med* 1979; 300:1155.
8. Reisman JJ, Rivington-Law B, Corey M, et al. Role of conventional physiotherapy in cystic fibrosis. *J Pediatr* 1988; 113:632–636.
9. Muszynski-Kwan AT, Perlman R, Rivington-Law BA. Compliance with and effectiveness of chest physiotherapy in cystic fibrosis. *Physiother Can* 1988; 40:28–32.
10. Pryor JA, Webber BA. An evaluation of the forced expiratory technique as an adjunct to postural drainage. *Physiotherapy* 1979; 65:304.
11. Webber BA, Hofmeyr JL, Morgan MDL, Hodson ME. Effects of postural drainage incoporating the forced expiration technique on pulmonary function in cystic fibrosis. *Br J Dis Chest* 1986; 80:353–359.
12. Chevaillier J. Autogenic drainage. In Lawson D, ed. *Cystic fibrosis horizons.* Chichester, John Wiley, 1985, p 235.
13. Schoni MH. Autogenic drainage: A modern approach to physiotherapy in cystic fibrosis. *J R Soc Med* 1989; 82(Suppl 16).
14. Dab I, Alexander F. Evaluation of the effectiveness of a particular bronchial drainage procedure called autogenic drainage. *Cystic Fibrosis* 1977; 185–187.
15. McIlwaine PM, Davidson AGF, Wong LTK, et al. Comparison of positve expiratory pressure and autogenic drainage with conventional percussion and drainage therapy in the treatment of CF. *Abstr Pediatr Pulmonol* 1988; 132(Suppl 2):137.

16. Davidson AGF, McIlwaine PM, Wong LTK, et al. Long-term comparative trial of conventional percussion and drainage techniques. *Abstr Pediatr Pulmonol* 1992; 298(Suppl 8):235.

17. Miller S, Hall D, Clayton CB, Nelson R. Chest physiotherapy in cystic fibrosis. A comparative study of autogenic drainage and active cycle of breathing. [In press.]

18. Paul WL, Downs JB. Postoperative atelectasis, I.P.P.B., incentive inspirometry and positive end-expiratory pressure. *Arch Surg* 1981; 116:861–863.

19. Malkem PT. Airway obstruction and collateral ventilation. *Physiol Rev* 1971; S1:368–436.

20. Anderson JG, Klausen NO. A new mode of administration of nebulized bronchodilator in severe bronchospasm. *Eur J Respir Dis* 1982; Suppl 119:63.

21. Christensen EF, Norregaard O, Dahl R. Treatment of bronchial asthma with terbutaline inhaled by conespacer combined with positive expiratory pressure mask. *Chest* 1991; 100:317–321.

22. Falk M, Kelstrup M, Anderson JB. Improving the ketchup bottle method with postive expiratory pressure. A controlled study in patients with cystic fibrosis. *Eur J Respir Dis* 1982; 53:58.

23. Mortensen J, Falk M, Groth S, Jensen C. The effects of postural drainage and positive expiratory pressure physiotherapy on tracheobronchial clearance. *Chest* 1991; 100:1350–1357.

24. Althaus P. The bronchial hygiene assisted by the Flutter VRP1. *Eur Respir J* 2(Suppl 8):693.

25. Irwin RS, et al. Cough: A comprehensive review. *Arch Intern Med* 1977; 137:1186–1191.

26. Tecklin JS, Irwin S. *Cardiopulmonary physical therapy*, 2nd ed. St. Louis, CV Mosby, 1990.

27. Jacquette G. To reduce hazards of trachael suctioning. *Am J Nurs* 1971; 71:2362–2364.

28. Shearer MC, et al. Lung ventilation during diaghramatic breathing. *Phys Ther* 1972; 52:139.

29. Vraciu JK, Vraciu RA. Effectiveness of breathing exercises in preventing pulmonary complications following open-heart surgery. *Phys Ther* 1977; 57:1367.

30. Sachner MA, et al. Distribution of ventilation during diaghramatic breathing in obstructive lung disease. *Am Rev Respir Dis* 1974; 109:331.

31. Craven JL, Evans GA, Davenport PJ, Williams RHP. The evaluation of the incentive inspirometer in the management of postoperative pulmonary complications. *Br J Surg* 1974; 61:793.

32. Martin CJ, Ripley H, Reynolds J, et al. Chest physiotherapy and the distribution of ventilation. *Chest* 1976; 69:2.

33. Denton JR, Tietjen R, Gaerlan RF. Thoracic kyphosis in cystic fibrosis. *Clin Orthop Relat Res* 1981; 155:71–74.

34. Eide R. The relationship between body image, self image and physical activity. *Scand J Soc Med* 1982; Suppl 29:109.

35. Strunk RC, Rubin D, Kelly L, et al. Determination of fitness in children with asthma: Use of standardised tests for functional endurance, body fat composition, flexibility, and abdominal strength. *Am J Dis Child* 1988; 142:940–944.

36. Orenstein DM, et al. Exercise conditioning in children with asthma. *J Pediatr* 1985; 106:556–560.

37. Cerny FJ, Pullano TP, Cropp GJA. Cardiorespiratory adaptations to exercise in cystic fibrosis. *Am Rev Respir Dis* 1982; 126:217.

38. Henke KG, Orenstein DM. Oxygen saturation during exercise in cystic fibrosis. *Am Rev Respir Dis* 1984; 129:708–711.

39. Kosloske AM. Tracheobronchial foreign bodies in children: Back to the bronchoscope and a ballon. *Pediatrics* 1980; 66:21.

40. Cohen SR, Herbert WI, Lewis GB Jr, Geller KA. Foreign bodies in the airway. Five year retrospective study with special reference to management. *Ann Otol Rhinol Laryngol* 1980; 89:437–442.

41. Orenstein SR, Whittington PE. Positioning for prevention of infant gastroesophageal reflux. *J Pediatr* 1983; 103:534.

42. Bolton JH, Gandevia B, Ross M. The rationale of breathing exercises in asthma with results of a controlled clinical trial. *Med J Aust* 1956; 2:675–680.

43. *Cash's textbook of chest, heart and vascular disorders for physiotherapists*. London, Faber & Faber, 1977.

44. Kang B, et al. Evaluation of postural drainage with percussion in chronic obstructive lung disease. *J Allergy Clin Immunol* 1974; 53:109.

45. Magee MS. Physical therapy for the child with asthma. *Pediatr Phys Ther* 1991; 3:23–28.

46. *Asthma care training for kids*. Washington, DC, Asthma and Allergy Foundation of America, 1984.

47. Schnall RP, Landau LI. The protective effects of short sprints in exercise induced asthma. *Thorax* 1980; 35:828.

48. Fitch D, Norton AR. Specificity of exercise in exercise induced asthma. *Br Med J* 1971; 4:577.

49. Dinwiddie R. *The diagnosis and management of paediatric respiratory disease*. London, Churchill Livingstone, 1990.

50. Bancalari E, Abdenour GE, Feller R, Gannon J. Bronchopulmonary dysplasia: Clinical presentation. *J Pediatr* 1979; 95:819–823.

51. Vivian-Beresford A, King C, Macauley H. Neonatal post-extubation complications: The preventitive role of physiotherapy. *Physiother Can* 1987; 39:184–190.

52. Finer NN, Moriarley RR, Boyd J, et al. Atelectasis: A retrospective review and a prospective controlled study. *J Pediatr* 1979; 94:110–115.

53. Finer NN, Boyd J. Chest physiotherapy in the neonate: A controlled study. *Pediatrics* 1978; 61:282–285.

54. Crane LD. Comparison of chest physical therapy techniques in infants with hyaline membrane disease [Abstract]. *Pediatr Res* 1978; 12:559.

55. Holsclaw DS. Recognition and management of cystic fibrosis. *Pediatr Ann* 1978; 7:19–27.

56. Zach M, Oberwaldner B, Hausler F. Cystic fibrosis: Physical exercise versus chest physiotherapy. *Arch Dis Child* 1982; 57:587.

57. Cambell AH. The effect of chest physiotherapy on FEV1 in chronic bronchitis. *Med J Aust* 1975; 1:33.

58. Connors AF. Chest physical therapy: The immediate effect on oxygenation in acutely ill patients. *Chest* 1980; 78:559.

59. Graham WGB, Bradley D, Efficacy of chest physiotherapy and intermittent positive pressure breathing in the resolution of pneumonia. *N Engl J Med* 1978; 299:624–627.

60. Britton S. Chest physiotherapy in primary pneumonia. *Br Med J* 1985; 290:1703–1704.

61. Holody B, Goldberg HS. The effect of mechanical vibration physiotherapy on arterial oxygenation in acutely ill patients with atelectasis or pneumonia. *Am Rev Respir Dis* 1981; 124:372–375.

62. Sutton PP, et al. Chest physiotherapy. A review. *Eur J Respir Dis* 1982; 63:188–201.

63. Macklem PT. Physiology of cough. *Ann Otol* 1974; 83:761–768.

Index

Page numbers followed by *t* and *f* indicate tables and figures, respectively